Dr. McCalla
Hope this is helpful in your practice.

Melvin-~~Fatlin~~
Bayer

Nasal and Sinus
SURGERY

Nasal and Sinus SURGERY

Steven C. Marks, MD

Associate Professor, Department of Otolaryngology
Wayne State University School of Medicine
Grace Hospital
Detroit, Michigan

William A. Loechel, Artist

W.B. SAUNDERS COMPANY
A HARCOURT HEALTH SCIENCES COMPANY
Philadelphia London New York St. Louis Sydney Toronto

W.B. SAUNDERS COMPANY
A Harcourt Health Sciences Company

The Curtis Center
Independence Square West
Philadelphia, Pennsylvania 19106

Library of Congress Cataloging-in-Publication Data

Marks, Steven C.

Nasal and sinus surgery / Steven C. Marks.

p. ; cm.

ISBN 0-7216-7804-1

1. Nose—Surgery. 2. Paranasal sinuses—Surgery. 3. Rhinoplasty. I. Title. [DNLM: 1. Nose Diseases—surgery. 2. Paranasal Sinuses—surgery. 3. Rhinoplasty—methods. WV 300 M346n 2001]

RF350 .M385 2001
617.5′23059—dc21 00-038803

Acquisitions Editor: Stephanie Smith Donley
Editorial Assistant: Sophie Brookover
Production Manager: Donna L. Morrissey

NASAL AND SINUS SURGERY ISBN 0-7216-7804-1

Printed in the United States of America

Last digit is the print number: 9 8 7 6 5 4 3 2 1

I would like to dedicate this book to my past, current, and future residents, who were the inspiration for this book, and to my wife Diane and children Brian and Andrea, who are the inspiration for my life.

CONTRIBUTORS

Richard L. Arden, MD
Department of Otolaryngology–Head and Neck Surgery
Wayne State University
Detroit, Michigan

Chapter 14: Nasal Reconstruction

Jeffrey Wilseck, DO
Department of Radiology
Wayne State University
Detroit, Michigan

Chapter 3: Radiology of the Nose and Sinuses

ACKNOWLEDGMENTS

This book could not have been written without the help of a number of dedicated individuals. I want to thank Denise Ventura and Dawn Wheeler for their secretarial help; Stephanie Smith Donley from Saunders for her guidance throughout the publishing process; Dr. Robert Mathog, my friend, colleague, and chairman for his encouragement and support; and William Loechel, my friend and illustrator for his incredible talent and ability to put my thoughts into understandable pictures. Thank you all.

PREFACE

Why write a textbook of nasal and sinus surgery? Furthermore, why a single author book, and why me? The decision to write this textbook came from my residents. As they are apt to do, residents frequently ask me for references on how to do various rhinologic procedures. Which textbook should they buy? Where can they read more about a particular technique? I couldn't always answer them. I would say, this technique was learned from this teacher; that technique from another. This skill I adapted from what I read here, and that surgery was from a course at the Academy meeting. But, there has never been a single text that covers all of this information.

I looked for alternatives and could not find a current book that could do what I had in mind. Certainly, comprehensive books in otolaryngology exist, many with well-written sections on rhinologic topics. There are also a number of excellent texts on endoscopic sinus surgery by authors more experienced and famous than I am. But, there are no comprehensive books on surgery in rhinology, as there are in otology, head and neck surgery, pediatric otolaryngology, and facial plastic surgery. So, why not me, if no one else will do it?

During my medical school years when I set out to become an otolaryngologist, the last things I considered were the nose and sinuses. Like many young physicians, I was drawn to the field by the power and intrigue of major head and neck cancer surgery. Later, during my training in otolaryngology, I was fascinated by the realm of the microscope and the otologist. I never considered a career in rhinology. After all, the field of rhinology was going nowhere. The sign on the door of our department said, "Otolaryngology–Head and Neck Surgery" and the certifying board of our specialty is the American Board of Otolaryngology. Serious residents interested in academic careers were interested in cancer or the ear. The nose was to be left to the private practitioner.

All of that changed with the introduction of endoscopic sinus surgery. While I was a medical student and resident at Johns Hopkins University, David Kennedy traveled to Europe to learn about this new surgery and began perfecting the techniques. What he brought back to Baltimore was more than a new trick or technique in surgery; it was a new interest in a long dormant field. The field of rhinology never really went away. However, from the days of innovation at the beginning of the twentieth century with the introduction of the Caldwell-Luc procedure, the frontoethmoidectomy, the maxillectomy, and many other procedures, the luster had certainly fallen off the shine of rhinology. Today that shine is back. The greatest technological advancements in the field, the greatest gains in the quality of care, and the greatest growth in interest in the field of otolaryngology–head and neck surgery are in rhinology.

I began my academic career with an interest in otology and neurootology. I took a position at Wayne State University having already made a commitment to take a year off to study under the great Professor Ugo Fisch in Switzerland. I agreed with my chairman, Robert Mathog, to practice endoscopic sinus surgery and to teach the residents this still relatively new technique for the two years prior to my departure for Europe. Up to that time, the department at Wayne State had not had a trained endoscopic sinus surgeon, and the residents were anxious to learn what I could teach them.

Fortunately, as a beneficiary of a residency experience that is still the model of education for teaching endoscopic sinus surgery, I was prepared for this task. We had access to the best cadaver dissection course, the best equipment, and, of course, Dr. Kennedy. During my residency, I was able to observe his technique on dozens of occasions. Later in my training, Mary Loury joined the faculty and took over much of the responsibility for teaching the residents the hands-on techniques. It is to these two individuals that I owe my expertise in sinus surgery. The lessons they taught me continue in my practice today.

In 1997, I found myself as an academic otolaryngologist with a specialization in nasal and sinus surgery who had unique training and experience. The need for the textbook I had in mind was real, and I decided to begin writing this book in September of that year.

I always intended *Nasal and Sinus Surgery* to be more than a book of endoscopic sinus surgery. I wanted to cover the entire field of rhinology: rhinoplasty, septoplasty, trauma surgery, tumor surgery, traditional sinus surgery, allergy, and medical care—all of which are part of the day-to-day practice in this field. To address all of these aspects of rhinology in a single text, I decided to discuss each technique in the context of the disease to be treated. Therefore, the book is organized into sections: general considerations (basic science), surgery for inflammatory conditions, plastic and reconstructive surgery, tumors, and special procedures.

Each chapter is organized to allow the reader easy access to the topic of immediate interest. Thus, the reader can use the text as a day-to-day reference to help prepare for surgery. When I think about a particular surgery, I consider the diagnosis and decision to perform the surgery, the preoperative care, the technical aspects, the postoperative care, and complications. Because the surgical chapters have been organized in this way, the reader should be able to adopt this philosophy and better coordinate the overall care of the patient.

I hope that the reader of *Nasal and Sinus Surgery* uses this book as a starting point and a general guide. Although I have been quite specific in the details of the procedures, certain goals can be achieved in more than one way. Much of the book is opinion. The reader can be assured, however, that what is written in this book is what I use in practice and in most situations, have used repeatedly through the years with good results. In the absence of their own experience, readers can rely on these procedures and recommendations to provide them with at least one alternative method.

Steven C. Marks

NOTICE

CONTENTS

SECTION ONE

General Considerations

SECTION TWO

Surgery for Inflammatory Conditions

SECTION THREE

Plastic and Reconstructive Surgery

SECTION FOUR

Tumors

SECTION FIVE

Special Procedures

Nasal and Sinus
SURGERY

SECTION ONE

General Considerations

CHAPTER 1

Anatomy of the Nose and Sinuses

The basis for all surgery throughout the body is a thorough understanding of anatomy. For this reason, this textbook begins with a review of the regional anatomy of the nose, sinuses, and adjoining structures. The anatomy of the nose and sinuses is at one time consistent and extremely variable. Certain relationships such as the alignment and orientation of the major bony structures, are highly conserved, whereas other aspects of the anatomy, like the aeration of the ethmoid cells, are individually unique. The anatomy of the nose and sinuses is, in addition to the variability, one of the most complex aspects of human anatomy. The three-dimensional relationships of this area are challenging to understand and require a lifetime of study to master. In the following pages, the anatomy of the nose and sinuses is covered in detail. This chapter is divided into sections: development, soft tissues, orbital soft tissues, mucosa, osteology, vasculature, and innervation. The nomenclature in this chapter is that used by the author, in anatomic textbooks,[1] and in common practice, and is that endorsed by the Anatomic Terminology Group.[2]

DEVELOPMENT

The first nasal structures are initially identifiable in the 4-week-old embryo.[3] At this stage, the facial area of the embryo includes paired lateral nasal placodes derived from ectodermal cells and the midline frontonasal process derived from mesodermal cells. The nasal placodes eventually will develop into the nasal cavities and lining, and the frontonasal process will become the nasal septum. During the ensuing weeks, the nasal placodes invaginate to form the nasal pits. These pits extend back into the oral cavity but remain separated from the oral cavity by the bucconasal membrane. Later in development, the bucconasal membrane will undergo reabsorption to create the posterior choanae. Failure of this membrane to perforate results in choanal atresia.

Anteriorly, the maxillary process fuses with the lateral and medial nasal processes to form the anterior nares.[4] Laterally, the nasolacrimal groove is formed between the maxillary process and the lateral nasal process. Eventually, this invaginates and reabsorbs to form the nasolacrimal duct.

By the seventh gestational week, the lateral nasal wall begins to develop. The maxilloturbinal appears first, followed by the five ethmoturbinals and the nasoturbinal. The maxilloturbinal later forms the inferior turbinate, the ethmoturbinals form the structures of the ethmoid sinus, and the nasoturbinal delineates into structures of the anterior lateral wall, including the agger nasi.[3, 4] Eventually, the first ethmoturbinal forms the uncinate process, the second becomes the ethmoid bulla, the third ethmoturbinal develops into the basal lamella of the middle turbinate, the fourth ethmoturbinal becomes the superior turbinate, and the fifth the supreme turbinate. The ethmoid infundibulum derives from the inferior part of the space between the first and second turbinals, whereas the superior aspect of this space forms the frontal recess. The space between the second and third ethmoturbinals becomes the sinus lateralis; similarly, the space between the third and fourth turbinals becomes the sphenoethmoidal recess.

Between the 9th and 10th weeks of development, the ossification and chondrification of the nasal and sinus structures begin. The maxillary sinus forms from an ingrowth of cells from the lateral wall into the middle meatus. This begins sometime after the 10th week of gestation. The anterior ethmoid cells start to pneumatize around the 14th week, with sphenoid and frontal sinus aeration occurring after birth.

FACIAL SOFT TISSUE

The soft tissues over the nose and sinuses consist of several layers: skin, subcutaneous tissue, facial muscles, and periosteum. The subcutaneous and muscle layers are separated by a discrete layer of fascia that merges with the parotid fascia and forms the superficial musculoaponeurotic system (SMAS). The soft tissues of the orbit are considered in a separate section.

The face has a number of external landmarks that are useful in describing facial structures and proportions. Figure 1–1 depicts a number of these. In the midline are the trichion, glabella, nasion, rhinion, subnasale, filtrum, and mentum. The medial and lateral canthus, malar eminence, and the melolabial crease are located laterally.

The trichion is defined as the most inferior point of the frontal hairline in the midline. This is important in cosmetic procedures of the upper face. The glabella is the region of the face superior to the nasal bones between the eyebrows. The glabella is defined by the bony ridge that connects the supraorbital ridges. The nasion refers to the maximum point of recess between the frontal and nasal bones. Usually, this is at the point where the frontal and nasal bones join. The rhinion is the inferior point of the nasal bones. Often, there is an identifiable protrusion on the nasal dorsum at this point. The subnasale is the point where the columella and the lip meet, and it represents the inferior attachment of the anterior nasal spine. The mentum refers to the greatest point of projection of the chin on a lateral view.

Skin

The skin of the face is marked by extreme variability in thickness, density of sebaceous glands, and density of hair follicles. Skin thickness is greatest on the tip of the nose and the scalp and is thinnest on the eyelids. The density of sebaceous glands also varies widely. The tip of the nose has the highest density of sebaceous glands in the body which, in certain disease states, can become thickened to a pathologic degree. Rosacea is an early inflammatory stage of this condition, which can progress to rhinophyma. Hair distribution on the face is both genetically varied and hormonally controlled. The primary determinant is the hormonal drive. A higher testosterone level leads to increased density of facial hair growth.

Surface contours and skin creases are determined by several factors. The primary creases form perpendicular to the pull of the underlying muscles. Thus, there are transverse creases across the forehead, radial creases around the eyes, and vertical creases around the mouth and in the glabella. This is the basis for the direction of the relaxed skin tension lines (Fig. 1–2). To achieve ideal cosmetic results from an incision on the face, the incision should be in one of the facial creases or along the relaxed skin tension lines. A second factor that affects facial contour is aging. With aging, the skin and fascia lose their elasticity, resulting in sagging of the soft

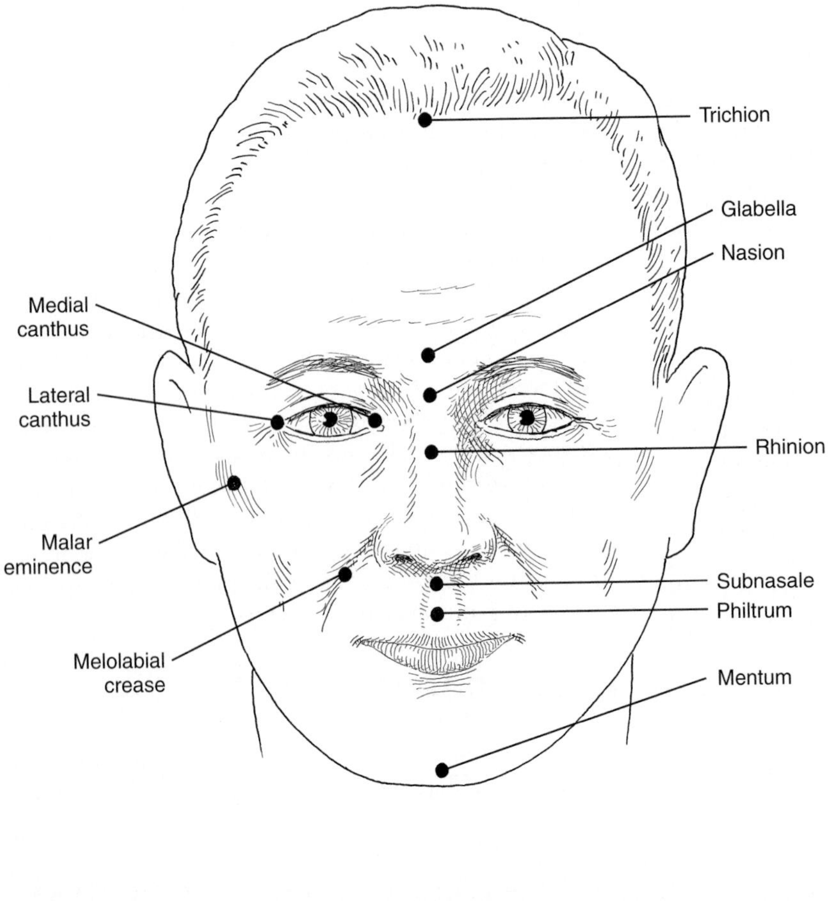

Figure 1–1. Facial landmarks.

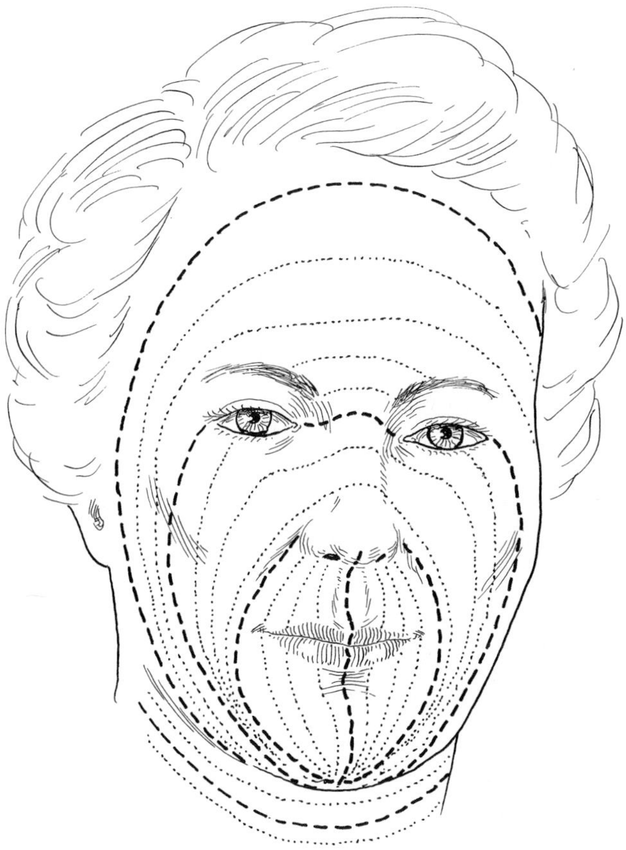

Figure 1–2. Relaxed skin tension lines.

tissues around the face. This tends to accentuate the vertical perioral creases and horizontal forehead creases, and creates so-called bags under the eyes. The third factor is solar damage. Excessive sun exposure leads to actinic changes and development of fine rhytids or wrinkles around the eyes and mouth.

Subcutaneous Tissue

The subcutaneous tissue of the face is composed of a layer of adipose tissue of variable thickness. The thickness of this layer varies depending on the location in the face and from one individual to the next. All patients have this layer to some extent. It can be very thin in thin patients or quite thick in obese people. There are specific areas of accumulation of fat in this layer, also known as fat pads. These are located over the malar eminence, the posterior buccal space, and along the inferior orbital rim.

Muscles

The face is lined by a complex network of fine muscles that provide animation for the face. These are referred to as mimetic muscles. Each is supplied by the facial nerve for motor control. Figure 1–3 demonstrates the orientation of the muscles. The frontalis muscle extends from the eyebrows to above the trichion and, when stimulated, raises the eyebrows. The corrugator supercilii muscle is oriented obliquely under the eyebrow. Contraction of this muscle draws the eyebrow medially and inferiorly, whereas the depressor supercilii muscle pulls the medial eyebrow inferiorly.

The eye is surrounded by the concentrically oriented orbicularis oculi. Contraction closes the eyelids. The orbicularis can be divided into several sections: the palpebralis superiorly, the orbitalis inferiorly, and the lacrimalis medially. During blinking, the palpebralis alone is activated. Activation of the lacrimalis compresses the lacrimal sac, expressing tears into the nasolacrimal duct. Elevation of the eyelid is accomplished by activation of the levator palpebrae muscle, which is innervated by the oculomotor nerve (cranial nerve III).

The nasal muscles consist of the procerus and the nasalis. The procerus is continuous with the frontalis and pulls the skin of the forehead inferiorly and the nasal skin superiorly. The nasalis is divided into a compressor that is oriented transversely above the nasal tip and a dilator that is oriented over the alae. These muscles either compress or dilate the nares.

The mouth and cheek are supplied with a number of muscles. The upper lip is elevated by the levator labii and the levator anguli labii, as well as the zygomaticus majorii and minimii. The lower lip is depressed by the depressor labii and the depressor anguli labii. The lower lip is pushed up and out by the mentalis muscle. The orbicularis oris muscle is the primary muscle that constricts and closes the lips. The buccinator muscle lines the inside of the cheek and tenses the cheek to assist in mastication. The buccinator also pushes the lips out.

The muscles of the face all tend to intertwine and work in concert to develop specific facial motions. These actions result in complex facial expressions, such as the smile, frown, grimace, and others. Anatomists continue to study the complex interaction of these muscles in order to better understand their actions and functions.

Periosteum

The facial skeleton is covered by a thin layer of tough fibrous tissue, the periosteum. This layer provides a smooth surface for the facial muscles to glide against. The periosteum is continuous with the periorbita inside the orbit. The periosteum is perforated by nerves and arteries as they leave the various foramina.

ORBITAL SOFT TISSUES

Eyelids

The upper and lower eyelids are multilayered structures that participate in protection and lubrication of the

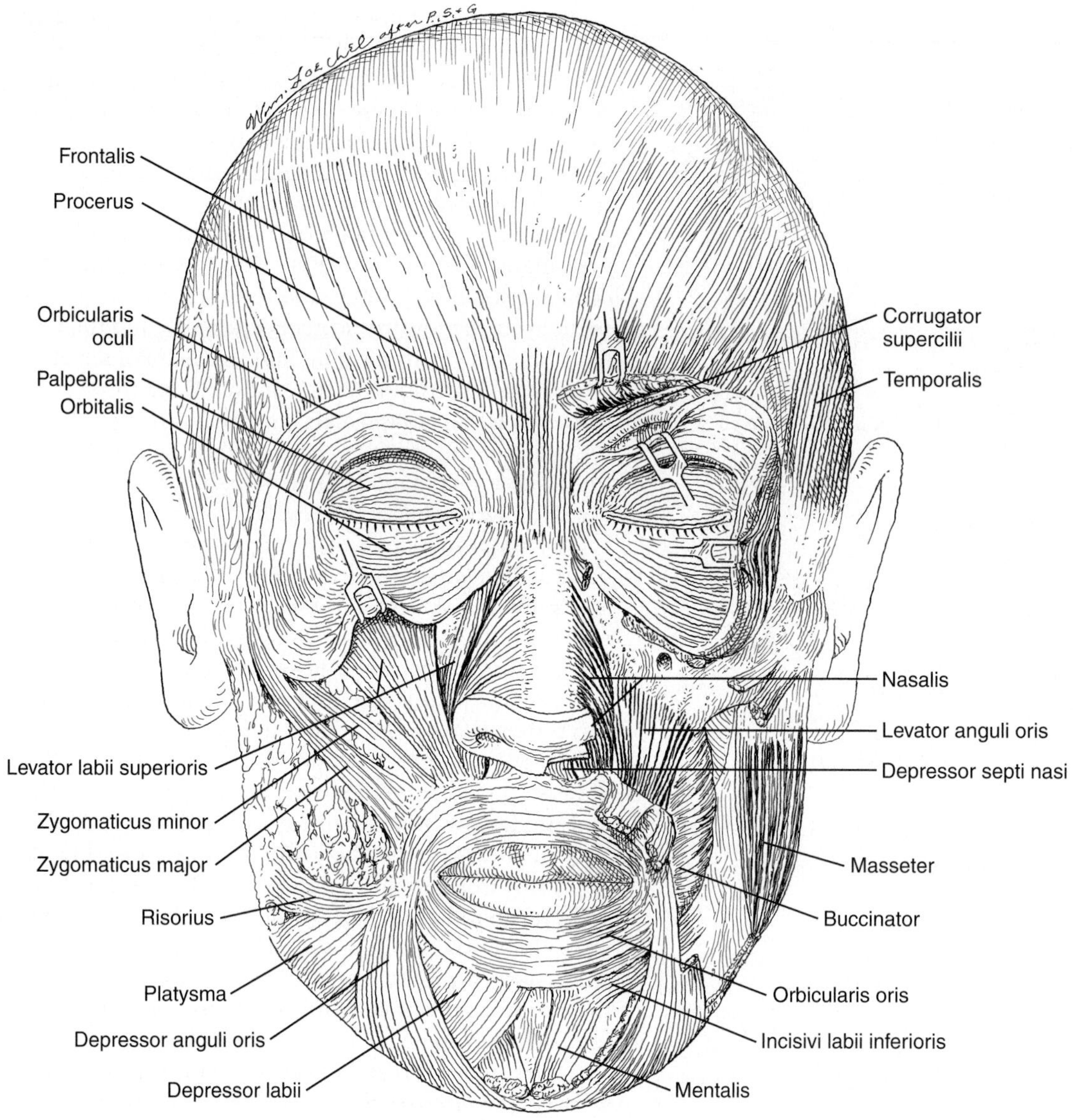

Figure 1–3. Facial mimetic muscles.

cornea. The basic layers are the skin, orbicular muscle, tarsal plate, orbital septum, and orbital fat (Fig. 1–4). The skin is very thin and contains a number of unique features. The upper lid contains the prominent supratarsal crease and the upper lid fold (see Fig. 1–4). The supratarsal crease is formed at the upper edge of the tarsal plate where the levator aponeurosis inserts into the orbital septum and orbicularis muscle. Here, the skin folds owing to the rigidity of the tarsus whenever the upper lid elevates. The upper lid fold is caused by the redundancy of the upper lid skin as the eyelid opens. At the lid margin of both the upper and lower lids are a row of hair follicles producing the eyelashes. This line is called the ciliary line. Just behind the ciliary line is the gray line, which is created by the junction of the squamous epithelium of the lid skin and the columnar epithelium of the conjunctiva. The lower lid contains inconsistent creases due to the variability of the anatomy of the underlying structures with aging. Generally, a fold develops with aging where the fat of the lower orbit bulges outward owing to laxity of the lower lid orbital septum and orbicularis muscle.

The orbicularis oculi is the sphincteric muscle that lines the entire upper and lower eyelid just beneath the skin. Typically, there is a thin layer of subcutaneous tissue under the skin before the muscle is found. This muscle extends from the eyelid margin superiorly and inferiorly to overlap the supraorbital and infraorbital rims.

The orbital septum extends from the orbital rim above and below the eye deep to the orbicularis muscle to merge with the superficial surface of the upper and lower lid tarsal plates. This fibrous layer is continuous with the orbital periosteum and the periosteum of the

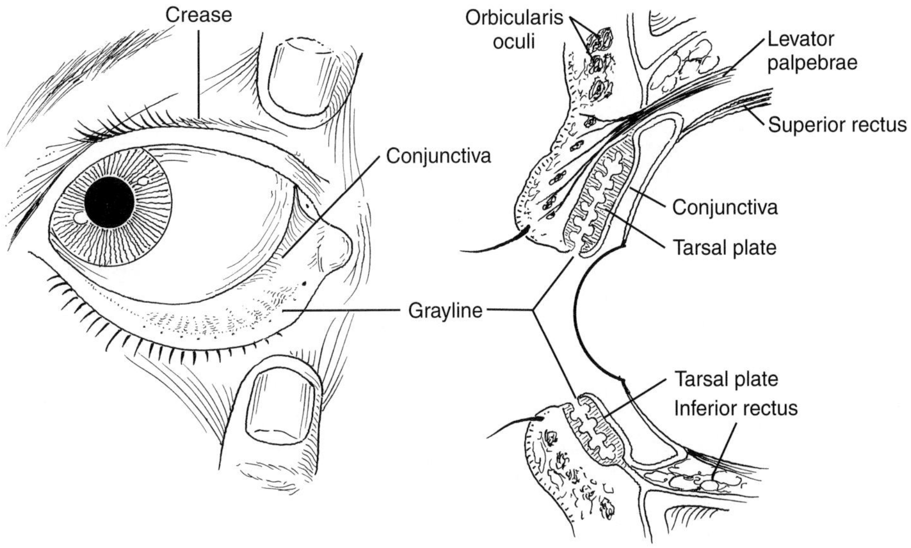

Figure 1–4. Anatomy of the eyelids. The anterior view depicts the supratarsal crease and the gray line. The lateral view shows the cross-sectional layers of the eyelids.

facial bones. It functions to contain the orbital contents. At the free margin of the eyelids, the septum merges with the tarsal plate. The tarsal plate acts as a fibrous skeleton for the eyelids, giving the eyelids a degree of rigidity. The upper lid tarsal plate is normally about 1 cm tall in the midline of the lid, narrowing both medially and laterally. The lower lid tarsus is shorter, typically measuring 5 to 6 mm.

The levator muscle is found deep to the orbital septum in the central area of the upper lid above the tarsus and below the upper orbital fat pad. This is the main muscle for elevating the eyelid. The levator inserts into the orbital septum and merges into the fibers of the orbicularis muscle. The deep aspect of the levator is a separate condensation of the levator known as Müller's muscle. It attaches to the upper edge of the tarsal plate.

Deep to the orbital septum lie the orbital fat pads. Most authorities describe two upper and three lower fat pads. However, many have stated that this is merely an anatomic distinction and that there is really no clinical significance to these divisions. The upper lid has a large central fat pad found lateral and superior to the superior oblique muscle. The upper medial fat pad is smaller and is located medial and inferior to the superior oblique muscle. The lower lid has the medial compartment, which is medial and superior to the inferior oblique muscle, and the central fat pad, which is located inferior and lateral to the inferior oblique muscle. The lower lateral fat pad has no discrete separation from the central fat pad except for a fine fibrous fascial division.

Finally, the eyelids are lined on the inside by the conjunctiva. This stratified columnar epithelium contains numerous glands and provides a lubricated surface to ease the motion of the eye and protect the cornea. It merges with the skin of the eyelids at the gray line. It forms a sulcus for both the upper and lower lids before folding back to attach to the sclera outside the cornea.

Lacrimal System

The lacrimal system consists of two components: the secretory lacrimal gland and the lacrimal collecting system. The lacrimal gland lies in the lacrimal temporal portion of the orbit deep to the orbital septum. It empties through secreting ducts into the lateral aspect of the superior conjunctival sulcus.

The lacrimal collecting system begins with openings or puncta in the margin of the upper and lower eyelids (Fig. 1–5). These are the ends of the lacrimal canaliculi that extend medially through the margin of the eyelids to enter the lacrimal sac. The lacrimal sac lies within the lacrimal fossa in the medial wall of the orbit. The inferior end of the sac opens into the nasolacrimal duct that drains into the apex of the inferior meatus of the nose. The walls of the sac have a relative elasticity that causes the sac to reexpand after compression. With each blink of the eye, the sac is compressed, pumping tears into the nose. After each blink, the eyelids relax, allowing the sac to reexpand and sucking the tears into the collecting ducts.

Oculomotor Muscles

Each eye has six oculomotor muscles that act in coordination to move the eye. These are the superior, inferior, medial and lateral rectus muscles, and the inferior and superior oblique muscles (Fig. 1–6). The rectus muscles attach to the common tendinous ring or annulus of Zinn, which surrounds the optic nerve at the orbital apex within the optic foramen. Each muscle then fans

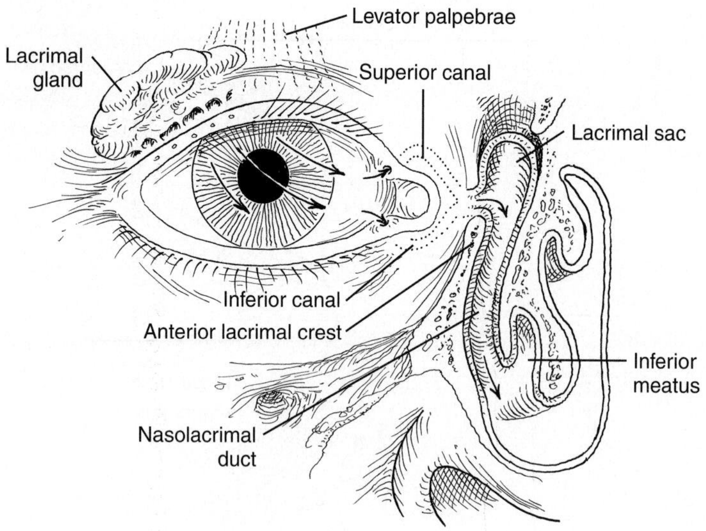

Figure 1–5. Anatomy of the lacrimal system.

out over the surface of the eye to attach according to its name. These muscles form a cone in the retro-ocular orbit through which the optic nerve passes on its way to the optic foramen. The superior oblique muscle extends through a fascial loop attached to the trochlea in the superior medial orbit before attaching horizontally behind the superior rectus muscle. The inferior oblique muscle angles across the inferior portion of the eye outside the inferior rectus to attach to the lateral eye deep to the lateral rectus muscle.

Because of their unique attachments, the six eye muscles have differing actions. The rectus muscles pull the eye in the direction for which they are named. However, the oblique muscles pull the eye differently. The inferior oblique, because it attaches more posteriorly, rolls the eye superiorly and laterally. The superior oblique, which attaches more posteriorly on the superior eye, rolls the eye inferiorly and medially.

MUCOSA

Nose/Sinuses

The nasal and sinus mucosa is a ciliated, pseudostratified, columnar epithelium. It consists of an epithelial

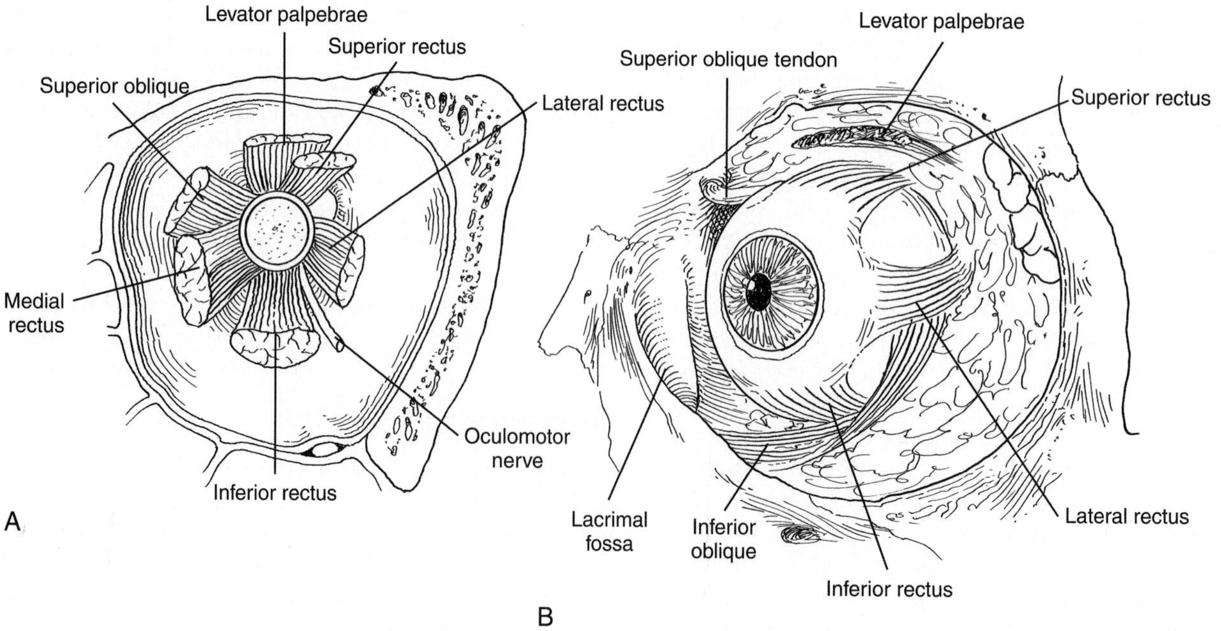

Figure 1–6. Extraocular muscles. *A,* Cross-sectional view. *B,* In situ view.

layer lying on a lamina propria, a submucosal layer, and a periosteal layer. The principle cell type of the epithelium is the ciliated columnar cell. Each of these cells contains a tuft of cilia on the luminal surface. Many of the cells sit on the basement membrane, but some cells either do not have a luminal surface or do not sit on the basement membrane. In addition to the principle ciliated cells, the mucosa contains mucosal glands and goblet cells. The goblet cells produce exocrine secretions that make up the glycoproteins of the mucus; the mucosal glands secrete the serous portion of the mucous blanket.

The submucosal layer lies under the lamina propria. It contains the vessels and nerves of the mucosa in a loose stroma. The submucosal layer varies greatly depending on the area of the sinonasal tract. The thickest natural mucosa is over the inferior turbinates, whereas the thinnest mucosa lies within the cells of the ethmoid sinus. The submucosal layer contains a varying degree of inflammatory cells depending on the location and the individual's recent inflammatory status. The submucosa is separated from the bone by a periosteal or perichondrial layer. This attachment is generally loose, allowing the mucosa to detach easily from the bone.

The mucosa spreads out over the entire lining of the nose and sinuses. The mucus is cleared from the nose and sinuses owing to the action of the cilia. The cilia are specifically oriented and beat in unison to move the mucus in constant patterns. These patterns have been carefully described in animals and humans. The mucus flows through the natural ostia of the sinuses into the nose and then into the nasopharynx. The details of this clearance is covered in Chapter 2.

Olfactory Epithelium

The olfactory epithelium is a specialized, pseudostratified, columnar epithelium resting on a vascular lamina propria without a submucosal layer. The olfactory epithelium is about three times as thick as the adjacent respiratory nasal epithelium. It is located on the surface of the cribriform plate and may extend onto the upper septum and superior turbinate. The total surface area is about 1 cm^2 on each side of the nose. The three main types of cells in the epithelium are the basal cells, the supporting cells, and the bipolar, ciliated, olfactory, receptor cells. A fourth type of cell, the microvilli cell, has been described in humans as well as animals and is a less common type of olfactory receptor cell. Olfactory function will be covered in Chapter 2.

OSTEOLOGY

The osteology of the nose and sinuses refers to the study of the bony and cartilaginous structures of the region. This includes the interrelationships of the bones, the external contours, and the fine details of their structure. The following sections cover these topics in some detail.

Nose

The nose consists of an external skeleton of bone and cartilage and an internal structure consisting of the nasal septum and turbinates.

External Skeleton. The external skeleton of the nose is made up of the paired nasal bones, upper lateral cartilages, lower lateral cartilages, and accessory sesamoid cartilages (Fig. 1–7). The nasal bones are small,

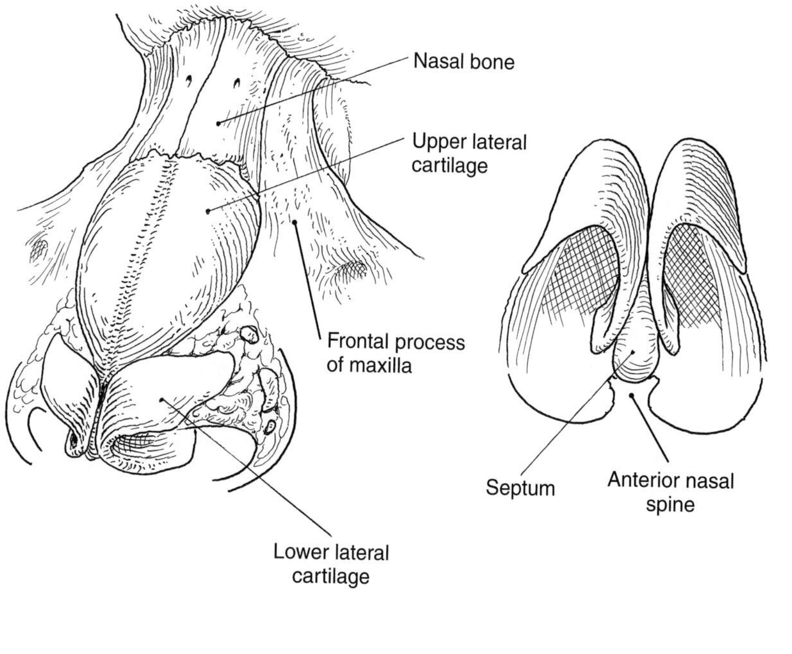

Figure 1–7. External skeleton of the nose, anterior oblique and basal views.

rectangular-shaped structures that join together in the midline. The nasal bones join the frontal bones superiorly and attach to the frontal process of the maxilla laterally. The upper lateral cartilages insert under the inferior edge of the nasal bones and join to the dorsal surface of the quadrangular cartilage of the nasal septum. The inferior edge of the upper lateral cartilages overlap, with the cephalic edge of the lower lateral cartilages in the area inside the nose known as the scroll. The most common variation is for the upper lateral to underlie the lower lateral with an interlocking pattern. In this form, the internal nasal valve correlates to the lower edge of the upper lateral cartilage.

The anatomy of the lower lateral cartilage is complex. Typically, the lower lateral cartilage is described as having a lateral and medial crus. These elements join at the nasal dome. The medial crus flares out inferiorly and provides the skeletal support for the columella. The lateral crus tapers to a point laterally. The caudal edge of the lateral crus fades away from the rim of the nares toward the lateral end of the cartilage (see Fig. 1–7). The dome is the medial aspect of the lateral crus. This transition zone is sometimes referred to as the middle crus, but anatomically, this is a misnomer. The dome of the lateral crus usually has a point, referred to as the tip-defining point, at the maximal dorsal height of the nasal tip. There is a tremendous variety of shapes, sizes, and symmetries of the lower lateral cartilages that give the tip of the nose its unique individual shape.

The sesamoid cartilages are small crescents of cartilage positioned just inside the pyriform aperture. These are sometimes referred to as lesser alar cartilages. These structures help provide some rigidity to the lateral ala to prevent collapse during inspiration. The lower lateral cartilages are suspended from the pyriform aperture by a fibrous matrix that also provides some degree of rigidity to the ala.

Nasal Septum. The nasal septum is the bony and cartilaginous midline structure that provides support for the nasal dorsum and divides the nose into two halves (Fig. 1–8). The septum is made up of the large quadrilateral cartilage anteriorly and the vomer and perpendicular plate of the ethmoid posteriorly. The quadrilateral cartilage extends from the nasal dorsum to the maxillary crest inferiorly. Along the dorsum, the cartilage sits between the upper lateral cartilages and is attached by a tough fibrous connection. The cartilage extends under the inferior edge of the nasal bones for several millimeters. Along the floor of the nose, the septal cartilage sits on the anterior nasal spine and lies within a trough in the maxillary crest. The cartilage is attached to the maxillary crest by a tough fibrous sheath. The cartilage joins the perpendicular plate of the ethmoid for the entire height of the perpendicular plate and sends a process posteriorly between the perpendicular plate and the vomer. This extension is variable in size. In some patients, it may extend almost to the sphenoid, whereas in other individuals, this may be only 1 to 2 cm in length. Posteriorly, the vomer and perpendicular plate merge into the anterior spine of the sphenoid bone.

Lateral Wall. The lateral wall of the nose is a composite structure with contributions from the maxilla, palatine, lacrimal, inferior turbinate, ethmoid, and sphenoid bones (Fig. 1–9). Anterior to the turbinates, the lacrimal bone forms much of the lateral wall. However, most of

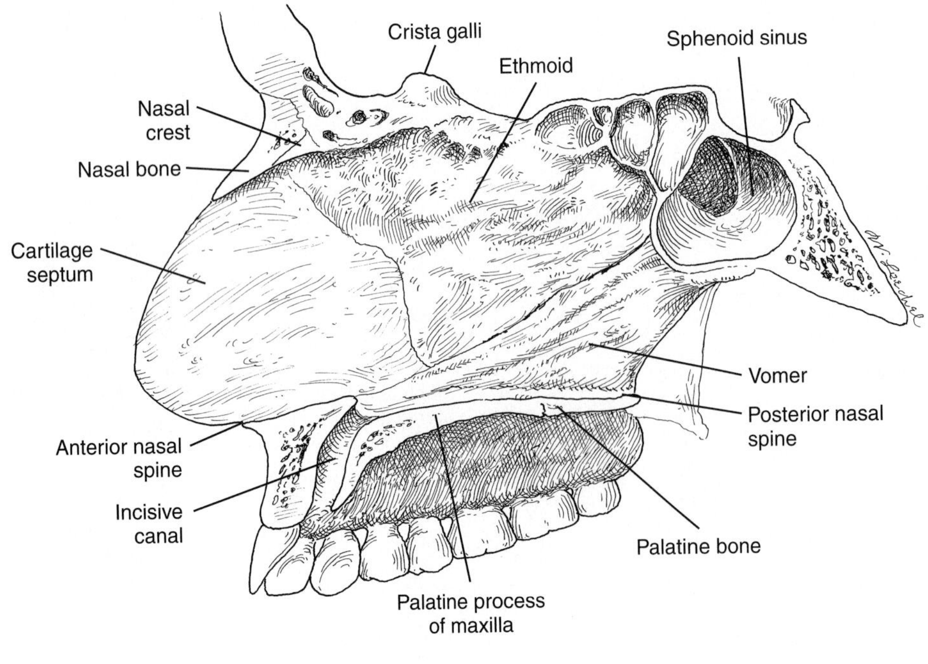

Figure 1–8. Anatomy of the nasal septum. The relationship between the quadrilateral cartilage, vomer, and perpendicular plate of the ethmoid is variable. Often, there is a long tongue of cartilage that extends posteriorly between the two bones.

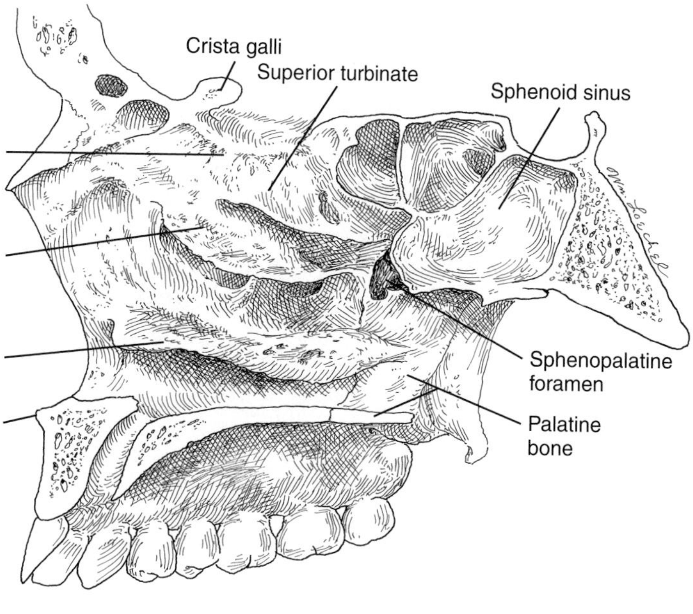

Figure 1–9. Skeletal structures of the lateral wall of the nose. A type 2 sphenopalatine foramen is depicted here passing both above and below the posterior attachment of the middle turbinate. Note the contributions to the lateral wall of seven bones: maxilla, ethmoid, sphenoid, palatine, lacrimal, frontal, and nasal.

the lateral wall is made up of the turbinates. There are usually three turbinates: the inferior, middle, and superior turbinates. The space under each turbinate is referred to as the meatus. The inferior turbinate bone is a separate structure that attaches to the maxilla laterally. It normally has a horizontal projection attached to the lateral wall and a vertical component that extends inferiorly into the nasal airway. In some cases, there is a single, obliquely oriented projection. The lateral wall of the inferior meatus is made up of the palatine bone inferiorly and the maxilla more superiorly. The only structure in the inferior meatus is the opening of the nasolacrimal duct at the apex of the meatus, about 1 to 2 cm posterior to the front of the turbinate.

The middle turbinate is a projection of the ethmoid bone. It attaches anteriorly to the lacrimal bone, superiorly to the ethmoid roof, and posteriorly crosses the ethmoid as the partition between the anterior and posterior ethmoid sinuses. The middle meatus contains the complex anatomy of the ethmoid sinus and the medial wall of the maxillary sinus. This is covered in detail later in the chapter. At the posterior end of the middle turbinate is the sphenopalatine foramen. This is the place of entry into the nose for the sphenopalatine artery and nerve.

The osteology of the sphenopalatine foramen has recently been classified.[5] The most common variation is an oblong ostium that extends from above the posterior attachment of the middle turbinate to just below this point. The other variations described locate the foramen just superior to the posterior attachment of the middle turbinate alone or with a small accessory opening a few millimeters inferior to the primary foramen.

The superior turbinate is a projection of the ethmoid bone and forms the medial wall of the posterior ethmoid sinus. It attaches superiorly to the skull base and posteriorly to the sphenoid bone. The superior meatus contains the posterior ethmoid sinus structures. The posterior end of the superior meatus is sometimes referred to as the sphenoethmoidal recess. Just medial and superior to the posterior and inferior end of the superior turbinate is the ostium of the sphenoid sinus.

In some individuals, there is a small, fourth turbinate that is called the supreme turbinate. This is absent in most noses. When present, it is a process of the ethmoid bone and attaches to the skull base posterior to the superior turbinate.

Cribriform Plate. At the roof of the nose is the cribriform plate (Fig. 1–10). It extends from the sphenoid bone to the frontal bone on either side of the midline for approximately 1 cm. Attached to the inferior side is the perpendicular plate of the ethmoid, which makes up the upper part of the bony septum. On the superior surface in the midline is the crista galli, a ridge of bone that separates the right and left olfactory bulbs. The cribriform plate is perforated by 10 to 12 small holes per side that transmit the olfactory nerves. On the superior surface, the dura surrounds the olfactory nerves and extends into the perforations of the cribriform plate. The undersurface is lined by the special sensory olfactory epithelium, which is continuous with the surrounding mucosa of the septum and turbinates. The cribriform plate itself is only 1 to 2 mm thick. However, the bony attachments of the roof of the ethmoid sinus to the lateral edge of the cribriform plate can be only microns thick and even completely dehiscent in places in certain individuals. The transition zone is one of the areas at high risk for penetration through the skull base during nasal and ethmoid sinus surgery.

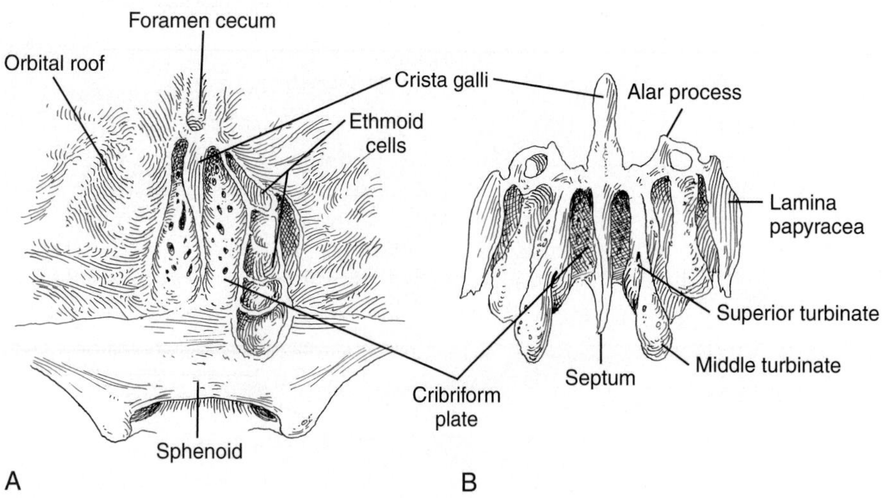

Figure 1–10. Bony anatomy of the ethmoid bone. *A,* superior view. *B,* Anterior view.

Orbit

The bony orbit is made up of contributions from seven different cranial bones (Fig. 1–11). The roof and superior orbital rim are part of the orbital process of the frontal bone. The lateral wall is made up of the zygoma superficially and the greater wing of the sphenoid bone deep to the zygoma. The floor of the orbit is a combination of the zygoma and sphenoid bones laterally, the orbital process of the maxilla medially, and a small projection of the palatine bone posteriorly. The medial wall receives contributions from the frontal process of the maxilla, the lacrimal bone, and the lamina papyracea of the ethmoid bone. The apex of the orbit is formed by the confluence of the lamina papyracea, the frontal bone, and the sphenoid bone.

There are several notable landmarks within the orbit, including several ridges, fissures, and foramina. On the superior rim is the frontal notch, which is located about 1 to 1.5 cm lateral to the nasal bones and which passes the supraorbital nerve. Just inside the superior orbital rim medially is the trochlea where the superior oblique muscle attaches. On the lateral wall, the only structure of note is the sphenozygomatic suture line. The inferior wall or floor is marked by the infraorbital sulcus. This contains the infraorbital nerve and artery. The inferior orbital fissure punctures the floor of the orbit laterally at an oblique angle from lateral toward the apex. This minor fissure transmits the inferior ophthalmic vein.

The medial wall begins superficially with the anterior lacrimal crest. This is the posterior edge of the frontal process of the maxilla. Behind the anterior crest is the lacrimal fossa and then the posterior lacrimal crest. At the inferior extent of the lacrimal fossa is the opening for the nasolacrimal duct. Separating the roof from the medial wall is the frontoethmoidal suture. Usually within or just inferior to this suture are the foramina for the anterior and posterior ethmoid arteries and nerves. The exact distances between these landmarks is a point of interest for the surgeon operating in this region. There is variability, but one rule is to consider the anterior foramen to be 12 mm from the posterior

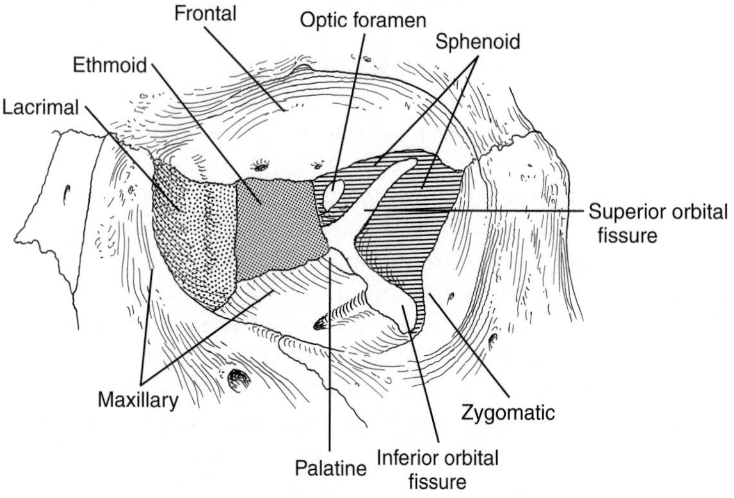

Figure 1–11. Bony anatomy of the orbit. Note the contributions from seven bones: lacrimal, ethmoid, frontal, sphenoid, zygoma, palatine, and maxillary.

lacrimal crest and the posterior foramen to be 12 mm from the anterior foramen. The optic canal is often 6 mm posterior to the posterior foramen.

The orbital apex is highly complex as it includes both the optic foramen and the superior orbital fissure. The optic foramen transmits the optic nerve from the chiasm into the orbit. It is surrounded by the nerve sheath and then the common tendinous insertion of the extraocular muscles. The superior orbital fissure transmits the ophthalmic artery and cranial nerves III, IV, VI, and V1 to the extraocular muscles and orbital structures. Within the fissure, V1 and IV are most superior, III and VI are intermediate, and the ophthalmic artery is most inferior.

Maxilla

The maxilla is the largest and most conspicuous bone of the sinonasal region. It consists of a body and the frontal, orbital, alveolar, and palatal processes (Fig. 1–12). The maxilla forms sutures with the zygoma, frontal bone, lacrimal bone, nasal bone, ethmoid bone, palatal bone, inferior turbinate bone, and vomer. The maxilla contains the largest paranasal sinus and the anterior opening for the nose. It also contains numerous arteries, veins, and nerves, but has only one named foramen, the infraorbital foramen.

The maxilla forms the midface and provides support for the dentition and mastication by its connections to the surrounding skull. The main horizontal buttress of the face is the strong zygomaticomaxillary suture. The vertical buttress is formed by the frontomaxillary suture between the frontal process of the maxilla and the frontal bone. A second vertical buttress is formed by the junction of the maxilla with the vomer, which is supported by the perpendicular plate of the ethmoid and the sphenoid bone.

The anterior surface of the maxilla forms the bulk of the midface. The right and left maxilla fuse in the midline below the nose. Important landmarks include the pyriform aperture and the infraorbital foramen. The maxilla forms the lateral and inferior aspects of the pyriform aperture. In the midline of the inferior aspect of the pyriform aperture is the anterior nasal spine. The roots of the teeth form ridges in the face of the maxilla. The most important of these is the canine ridge. Just lateral to the apex of this ridge is a shallow depression on the face of the maxilla referred to as the canine fossa. This is important in locating the maxillary sinus during surgical procedures.

The alveolar process projects firom the inferior aspect of the body of the maxilla. This houses both the deciduous and permanent upper dentition. The lateral aspect of the alveolar process also forms the floor of the maxillary sinus. This relationship can lead to clinical problems, such as dental-origin infections of the sinus and oral antral fistula when a tooth is pulled that projects into the sinus. The orbital process has been described earlier in reference to the floor of the orbit. It also forms the roof of the maxillary sinus. The palatal

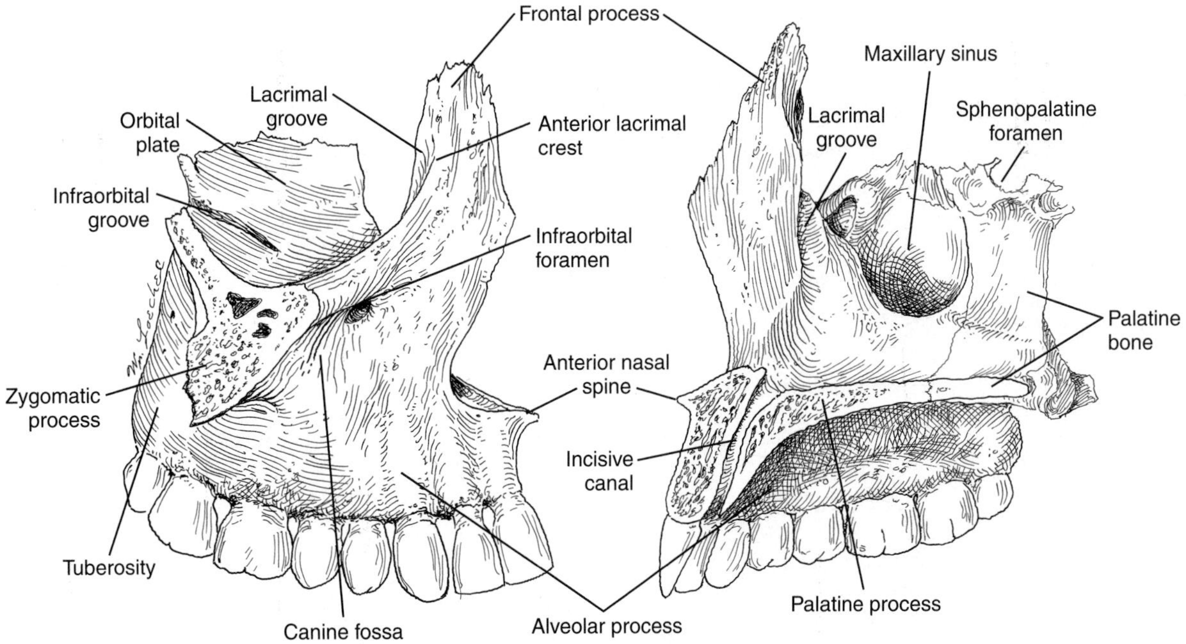

Figure 1–12. Bony anatomy of the maxilla, lateral and medial views. Note the presence of the frontal, zygomatic, alveolar, and palatine processes. The maxilla contains the incisive canal, the infraorbital foramen, and the anterior aspect of the sphenopalatine foramen.

process extends from the alveolar process and body and fuses in the midline to form the anterior part of the hard palate. The incisive foramen that transmits sensory nerves to the palate is found anteriorly in the palatal process of the maxilla. Posteriorly, the palatal process forms a suture with the palatine bone.

The posterior surface of the maxilla forms an attachment to the medial and lateral pterygoid plates of the sphenoid bone. Between the lateral aspect of the posterior wall of the maxilla and the anterior surface of the lateral pterygoid plate is the pterygomaxillary fissure. This important area contains the internal maxillary artery and its terminal branches and cranial nerve V2, as well as the sphenopalatine ganglion. Laterally, this fissure opens into the infratemporal fossa.

The central structure within the maxilla is the maxillary sinus. This is bordered, like a cube, by six walls. The superior wall is the orbital process. The inferior wall is the top of the alveolar process. The anterior, lateral, and posterior walls are from the body of the maxilla. The medial wall is formed by a combination of bone and soft tissue. The bony medial wall contains the ostium of the sinus, the anterior fontanelle, and the posterior fontanelle (Fig. 1–13). The ostium is normally found near the superior aspect of the medial wall about halfway from anterior to posterior. The location is more consistently defined by its relationship to the uncinate process and nasolacrimal duct, where the ostium is found just posterior to the duct and lateral to the uncinate at the anterior apex of the ethmoid infundibulum.

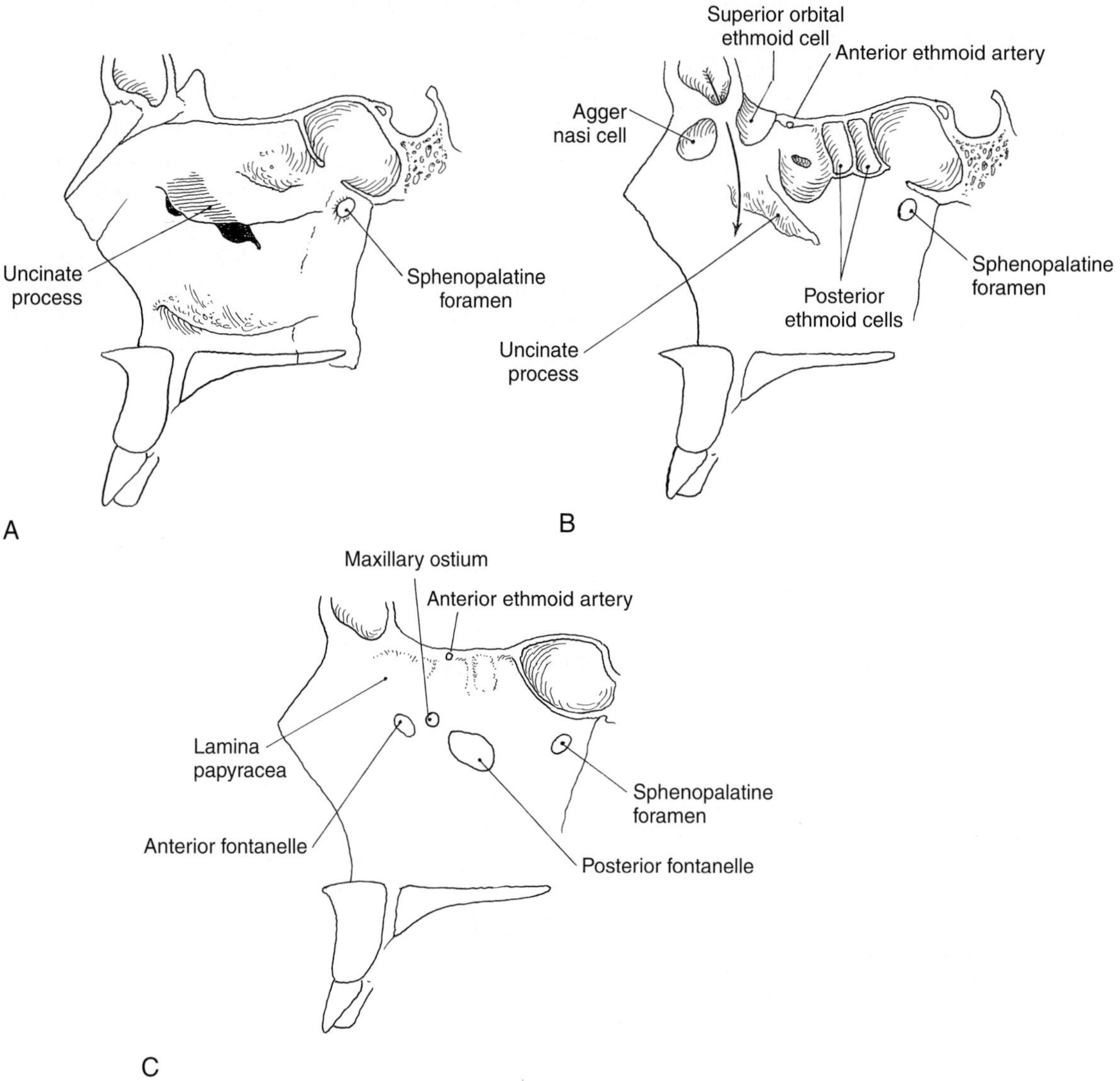

Figure 1–13. Bony anatomy of the sinus ostia. *A,* Sagittal view from the nasal cavity. *B,* Sagittal view through the ethmoid sinus. *C,* Sagittal view at the level of the lamina papyracea.

The ostium is often described as an opening of the maxillary sinus into the ethmoid infundibulum, but more accurately, is a short tunnel.[6] The fontanelles or soft parts of the wall are formed by the mucosa from the nasal and sinus sides of the wall fused together. The anterior fontanelle is small and located anterior to the inferior attachment of the uncinate process. By contrast, the posterior fontanelle is large and found posterior to the ostium and inferior attachment of the uncinate process.[7]

Ethmoid Bone

The ethmoid bone is the central structure of the nose and sinuses. This complex bone contains several components, including the cribriform plate and crista galli, the perpendicular plate of the septum, the lamina papyracea, the middle and superior turbinates, and the ethmoidal labyrinth (see Fig. 1–10). In the midline superiorly, the cribriform plate forms the center of the anterior skull base and roof of the nose. The crista galli is a bony plate that projects superiorly from the midline of the cribriform plate. This provides a platform for the falx cerebri to attach. The cribriform plate is perforated by approximately 10 to 12 openings through which the main branches of the olfactory nerve enter the olfactory epithelium.

The perpendicular plate extends from the midline of the cribriform plate opposite the crista galli. The perpendicular plate extends inferiorly from the entire length of the cribriform plate. The perpendicular plate attaches to the anterior wall of the sphenoid bone posteriorly and the vomer inferiorly. The inferior anterior surface of the perpendicular plate attaches to the quadrilateral cartilage of the septum.

The lamina papyracea is the smooth bony plate that forms the medial wall of the orbit. It is, as its name implies, a paper-thin bone. It separates the orbital contents from the ethmoid sinus. In certain individuals, the lamina papyracea may be exquisitely thin and even dehiscent. A variety of pathologic processes can erode through this thin bone, either by pressure of an expansile lesion, such as a mucocele, or by direct invasion, as in the case of a malignant tumor or an infection.

The middle and superior turbinates project from the medial portion of the ethmoid bone into the nasal cavity. The middle turbinate attaches anteriorly to the lacrimal bone and the anterior aspect of the ethmoid bone, superiorly to the ethmoid roof, and posteriorly to the ethmoid bone just anterior to the sphenopalatine foramen. The superior turbinate is found just posterior and superior to the middle turbinate and attaches similarly to the ethmoid roof and the ethmoid bone anteriorly and posteriorly. Both the middle and superior turbinates can become aerated by the ethmoid sinus. The aerated middle turbinate is referred to as the concha bullosa.

The anatomy of the ethmoid sinus is complex, variable, and the subject of intense study. Rather than viewing the ethmoid sinus as a series of stacked cells, it is more accurate to consider it a series of bony partitions and recesses. Embryologically, the ethmoid sinus is derived from five ethmoturbinals. These turbinals develop into the vertically oriented bony partitions. The five partitions are: the uncinate, the ethmoid bulla, the basal lamella (ground lamella), the superior turbinate, and the supreme turbinate. These partitions can become aerated to a lesser or greater extent, forming well-defined air cells. The agger nasi cell, the ethmoidal bulla, and the concha bullosa are examples. Normally, the uncinate process and the basal lamella do not aerate, but this is not always the case. The bony partitions are separated by a series of recesses: the frontal recess, the infundibulum, the sinus lateralis, and the sphenoethmoidal recess.

Considering these structures from anterior to posterior, the most anterior is the agger nasi. This term refers to the bulge in the lateral wall of the nose where the middle turbinate attaches. The term is literally translated as nasal ledge or shelf. The agger nasi typically aerates with a single cell that is the farthest anterior cell in the ethmoid sinus. It is also the only cell that is normally found anterior to the opening of the frontal recess. Immediately posterior to the agger nasi cell is the opening of the frontal sinus ostium into the frontal recess (see Figs. 1–13 and 1–14). This recess is always found posterior to the agger nasi cell and always anterior to the anterior ethmoid artery as it crosses the skull base from the orbit to the septum. Within this same space is often found a secondary recess separated from the frontal sinus by a bony partition. This is the so-called supraorbital ethmoid cell.[8] These cells can be quite large and may extend far above and behind the orbit. Just anterior to the anterior ethmoid artery is a usually shallow depression in the skull base. This is an important landmark in identifying the ethmoidal artery and the frontal sinus ostium during endoscopic sinus surgery.

The anatomy of this region is complicated by a number of variations that can confuse the surgeon operating to open the frontal sinus. The supraorbital ethmoid cells may be larger than the frontal sinus and extend laterally well beyond the frontal sinus. In addition, there may be intrafrontal ethmoid cells that may narrow or obstruct the frontal opening.[9] These cells have been classified into four types, including a single cell above the agger nasi, multiple tiered cells above the agger nasi, a single large cell pneumatizing into the frontal sinus, and an isolated cell within the frontal sinus. The frontal recess may also aerate into the intersinus septum of the frontal sinus, creating an interfrontal sinus septal cell.[10]

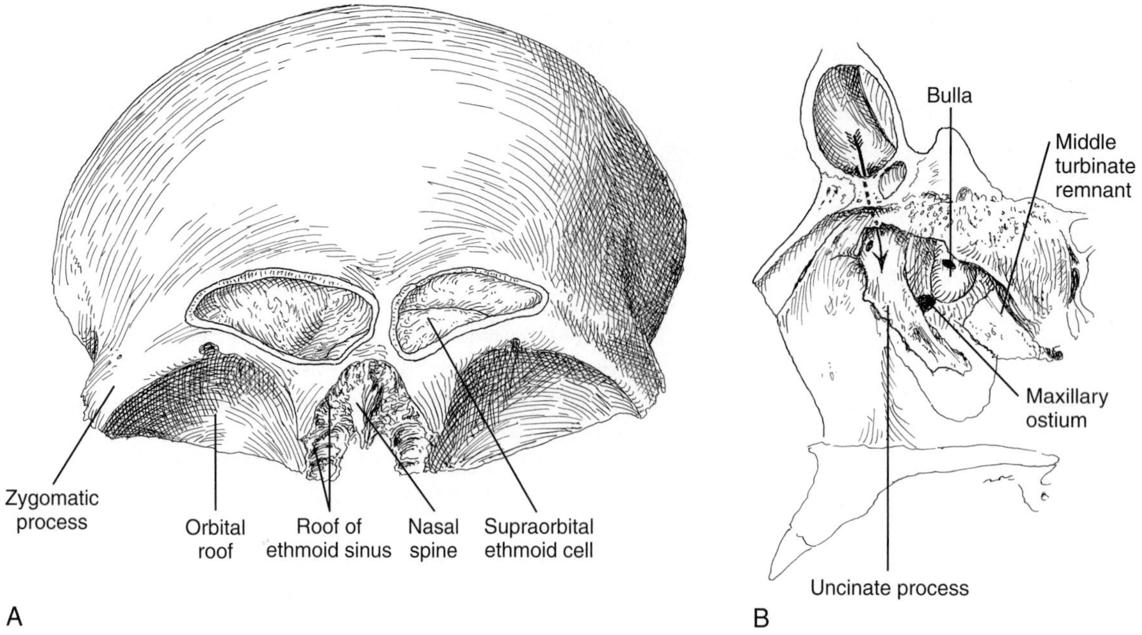

Figure 1–14. Bony anatomy of the frontal bone. *A,* Exploded frontal view. The anterior wall of the frontal sinus has been removed for demonstration purposes. *B,* View of the drainage from the medial side. In this alignment, the sinus drains medial to the uncinate process (one of two possibilities).

The outflow of the frontal sinus has been a subject of some controversy. Early investigators found the frontal sinus to drain predominantly medial and anterior to the uncinate process.[11] However, more recent studies suggest that the frontal sinus drains primarily into the infundibulum in most individuals.[12, 13] These discrepancies may be caused by differences in the populations studied, techniques, and ultimately, anatomic accuracy.

The uncinate process is the next bony partition and is found just inside the middle turbinate (see Figs. 1–13 and 1–14). It is attached to the anterior edge of the lamina papyracea just as the lamina joins the lacrimal bone. The uncinate most often projects posteriorly and medially. The lower end of the uncinate becomes part of the medial wall of the maxillary sinus. The upper end of the uncinate can terminate in one of three ways: it can attach to the skull base, it can attach to the middle turbinate, or it can attach to the lateral wall of the sinus (the lamina papyracea). This last is the most common variation.[14] Just lateral to the uncinate process is the ethmoid infundibulum. This pyramidal space has its apex anteriorly and opens posteriorly. The medial wall of the infundibulum is the uncinate process, the lateral wall is the orbit, and the posterior wall is the ethmoid bulla. A narrow, two-dimensional opening is formed by the posterior edge of the uncinate process and the anterior surface of the bulla. This is referred to as the hiatus semilunaris, or sometimes, the hiatus semilunaris inferior.

At the anterior apex of the infundibulum is the natural ostium of the maxillary sinus. Within the maxillary sinus and adjacent to the natural ostium is often found an extension of the ethmoid sinus called the infraorbital cell or Haller cell.[5] This cell adjoins the floor of the orbit and can block the opening of the maxillary sinus. The openings of the anterior ethmoid sinus cells are always into the posterior aspect of the infundibulum. This small pyramidal space is, therefore, the site where the entire anterior sinus drainage may pass. Blockage of this space can have profound effects by obstructing the other dependent sinuses.

The next bony partition is the ethmoid bulla. This is sometimes referred to as the middle ethmoid cell. However, this is a misnomer as the ethmoid is divided into anterior and posterior sinuses by the basal lamella and there is no anatomic differentiation of a middle ethmoid sinus. The bulla is often the largest ethmoid cell and is the first cell encountered inside the middle turbinate just posterior to the uncinate process. This cell generally extends superiorly to the skull base and anteriorly almost to the anterior ethmoid artery. The bulla drains anteriorly into the infundibulum. The space between the bulla and the middle turbinate is sometimes referred to as the hiatus semilunaris superior.

Immediately posterior to the bulla is the sinus lateralis. This recess is typically narrow inferiorly, widening superiorly at the skull base. In some cases, it may extend over the bulla. In this instance, it is referred to as the suprabullar recess. It is bordered anteriorly by the bulla and posteriorly by the basal lamella. On occasion, the sinus lateralis will invaginate into the posterior ethmoid sinus. The basal lamella, sometimes referred to as the ground lamella or grand lamella, is the lateral extension of the middle turbinate as it attaches to the lamina papyracea. This bony partition divides the anterior and posterior ethmoid sinuses. The basal lamella attaches to the skull base superiorly and the lamina papyracea laterally. The main part of the basal lamella is oriented vertically. Inferiorly, the basal lamella becomes horizontal as it merges into the posterior end of the middle turbinate.

The posterior ethmoid sinus is normally made up of two or three large cells. The anterior wall of the most posterior cell is an important landmark, as it usually indicates the position of the posterior ethmoid artery along the skull base. The posterior wall of this last cell merges with the sphenoid bone. Often, there is a cell that projects posterior or lateral to the anterior extent of the sphenoid sinus. This is the so-called sphenoethmoid or Onodi cell.[16] This is important because the optic nerve may indent the lateral wall of an Onodi cell, crossing this structure rather than the lateral wall of the sphenoid sinus. When Onodi cells are present, there is a high incidence of dehiscence of the bone over the optic nerve. The vertical height of the posterior ethmoid cell is often less than that of the anterior ethmoid, as the skull base slants inferiorly from anterior to posterior. This is important to keep in mind when performing ethmoid sinus surgery. Finally, the skull base of the posterior ethmoid sinus is typically much thicker than that of the anterior ethmoid cells. This provides added safety in identifying the skull base during surgery.

Frontal Bone

The frontal bone is a complex structure that forms the upper part of the face and anterior part of the skull. It consists of a large, flat, squamous portion, called the zygomatic process, and the orbital process (see Fig. 1–14). The frontal bone forms sutures with the parietal bone (coronal suture), the sphenoid bone (posterior orbit, temporal fossa, and floor of the anterior cranial fossa), the zygoma, the ethmoid bone (cribriform plate and orbital surface), the lacrimal bone, the maxilla, and the nasal bone. The frontal bone forms the superior orbital rim, roof of the orbit, the forehead, and the floor of the anterior cranial fossa. Within the supraorbital portion, the frontal bone splits to contain the frontal sinus in between the anterior and posterior tables.

The main squamous portion of the frontal bone extends from the supraorbital rims to the coronal suture at the vertex of the skull. At birth, the frontal bones are separated sagittally by a frontal suture that extends superiorly up to the anterior fontanelle. During early development, the frontal bones fuse together in the midline without forming a well-defined suture. The anterior fontanelle regresses and eventually disappears completely. The only significant foramen in the frontal bone is the supraorbital foramen through which the supraorbital nerve passes before innervating the frontal scalp. This is located 1.5 to 2.5 cm lateral to the nasal bones.

The zygomatic process of the frontal bone connects to the zygoma about one third of the way inferiorly along the lateral orbital rim. This forms one of the principle vertical buttresses of the facial skeleton.

The orbital process forms the roof of the orbit and part of the floor of the anterior cranial fossa posterior to the frontal sinus. Anteriorly, within the frontal sinus, the orbital roof forms the floor of the sinus. This bony plate curves inferiorly to where it joins the sphenoid bone near the apex of the orbit.

The frontal sinus sits in between the anterior and posterior tables of the frontal bone (see Fig. 1–14). The size of the sinus ranges from nil or absent (in 10% of individuals) to 300 mL. The latter measurement is from the author's practice, and was obtained in a patient with microcephaly secondary to shaken baby syndrome. The patient developed massive aeration of the frontal sinus, possibly owing to the lack of development of the frontal lobe of the brain. The average size is 5 to 10 mL per side. The posterior wall of the sinus splits off of the posterior table of the frontal bone at the apex of the sinus. The posterior wall of the sinus extends obliquely inferiorly and posteriorly to where it meets the roof of the orbit. The angle in between the orbit and the posterior wall can be very narrow and deep or shallow and blunt. The natural ostium of the frontal sinus sits in the anteromedial aspect of the floor of the sinus. Usually, there are ethmoid cells that form lateral to the frontal ostium that constitute part of the floor of the sinus. The right and left frontal sinuses are divided by a bony plate that usually sits in the midline. However, this can deviate to either side to place the dividing septum well off the midline. Occasionally, there will be air cells within the frontal sinus that are seemingly unconnected to the ostium of the sinus. These intrafrontal cells can become obstructed and form mucoceles isolated from the natural ostium and ethmoid sinus.

Sphenoid Bone

Perhaps the single most complex bone in the human body is the sphenoid bone. It forms the main component of the central skull base, a portion of the lateral skull, most of the apical portion of the orbit, and the posterior wall of the nasopharynx. The isolated sphenoid bone, when viewed anteriorly, looks like a bird (Fig. 1–15). The sphenoid bone consists of the greater and lesser wings, the medial and lateral pterygoid plates,

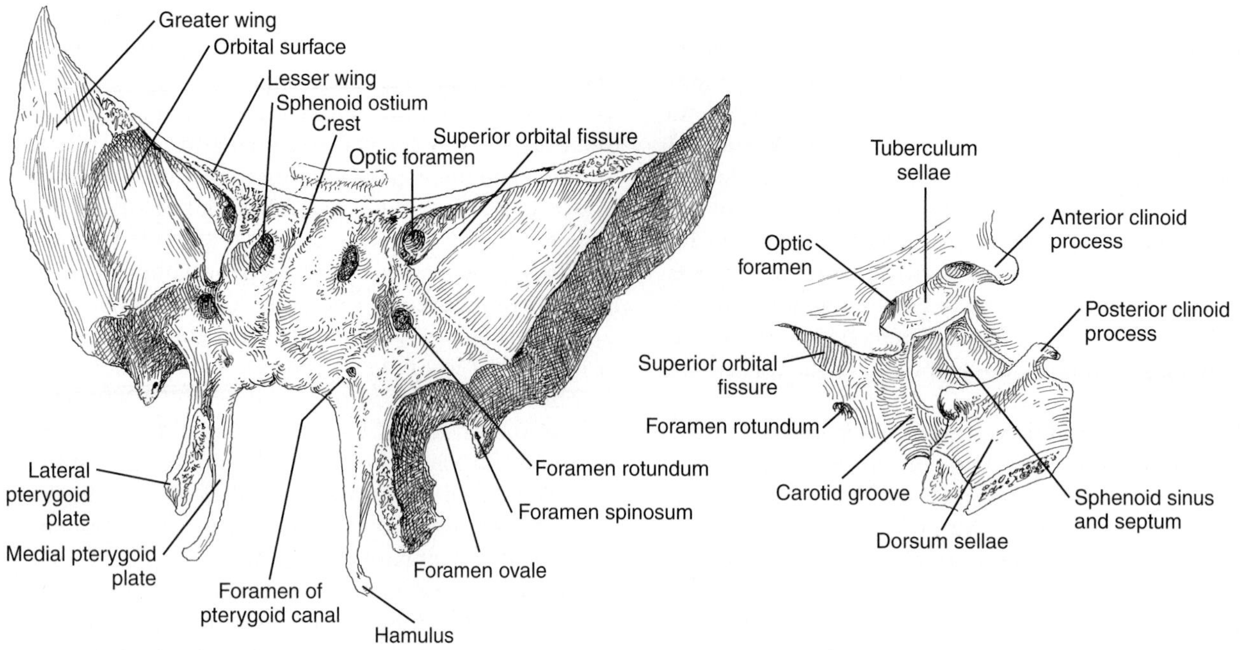

Figure 1–15. Bony anatomy of the sphenoid bone, anterior oblique and superior views. Openings in the sphenoid bone include the ostium of the sinus, the optic canal, the superior orbital fissure, the foramen rotundum, the pterygoid (vidian) canal, foramen ovale, foramen spinosum, and the carotid canal.

the body containing the sphenoid sinus, the structures of the sella, and the upper part of the clivus.

The lesser wings of the sphenoid form the posterior lip of the anterior cranial fossa, a portion of the orbital wall that contains the optic canal, and the anterior clinoid processes (Fig. 1–15). The lesser wing has a broad suture with the frontal bone along the posterior aspect of the anterior cranial fossa. In the midline, the lesser wings join to the cribriform plate of the ethmoid. The small contributions to the posterior, apical portion of the orbit include the optic canal and the superior lip of the superior orbital fissure. The anterior clinoid process extends from the posterior aspect of the lesser wing just lateral to the optic canal. This is an important intracranial landmark for identifying the position of the optic chiasm.

The greater wings constitute the largest portion of the sphenoid bone (see Fig. 1–15). They extend from the body of the sphenoid laterally to form part of the floor of the middle cranial fossa. This portion includes the foramen rotundum, which transmits cranial nerve V2, the foramen ovale, which transmits cranial nerve V3, and the foramen spinosum, which transmits the middle meningeal artery. More anteriorly, the greater wing forms part of the posterior wall of the orbit, including the inferior lip of the superior orbital fissure and the superior lip of the inferior orbital fissure. More posteriorly, the greater wing forms the lateral aspect of the carotid canal. Projecting off the inferior and most posterior aspect of the greater wing is the spine of the sphenoid bone, which is an important landmark during lateral skull base surgery to identify the foramen spinosum. Finally, an extension of the greater wing laterally forms part of the lateral skull anterior to the temporal bone and posterior and inferior to the frontal bone.

The medial and lateral pterygoid plates extend inferiorly from the body of the sphenoid (see Fig. 1–15). These plates attach to the posterior wall of the maxillary sinus on the medial surface to provide horizontal support to the face. These structures also are the origin of the medial and lateral pterygoid muscles that participate in mastication. The medial pterygoid plates also form the lateral walls of the nasopharynx superior to the eustachian tubes. The sphenopalatine foramen is not a true foramen, but an opening between the base of the pterygoid plates and the vertical portion of the palatine bone.

The body of the sphenoid is the central component that contains the sphenoid sinus and forms the floor of the sella turcica (see Fig. 1–15). The sphenoid sinus aerates the sphenoid body and varies in size from 1 to 10 mL. In extreme cases, the sphenoid sinus can aerate into the clivus, into the greater wing, and into the anterior clinoid process. The sinus opens through an ostium in the anterior wall about 4 mm (0 to 9 mm) lateral to the midline and 30 degrees from the floor of the nose.[17] The ostium is usually just posterior to the posterior and inferior edge of the superior turbinate. Typically, the sinus is divided into two equal sides by a midline septum. However, the sides can be markedly asymmetrical, and the septum can slant way off the midline to one side. In some cases, the sphenoid can even have three seemingly equal cells.

The lateral wall of the sphenoid sinus is indented by the carotid artery and the optic nerve (see Fig. 1–26). There is normally a thin layer of bone overlying these structures. In some individuals, this bone may become very thin and even completely dehiscent.[18] The optic nerve crosses from the orbital apex transversely across the lateral wall, coursing anterior to the carotid artery. The carotid artery ascends from the carotid canal and courses vertically to cross posterior and lateral to the optic nerve. Just anterior and inferior to where the carotid and optic nerve cross, there is usually a depression in the lateral wall of the sinus called the optic recess. This useful landmark can help identify the sinus cell as the actual sphenoid sinus and identifies the position of the carotid artery and optic nerve. Inferior to where the carotid artery and optic nerve cross on the lateral wall of the sphenoid sinus is the cavernous sinus. This venous structure is normally protected from the sinus by a thick wall of bone. This makes injury to the cavernous sinus during sphenoid sinus surgery very rare.

The body of the sphenoid bone has a single opening inferior to the sphenoid sinus. This is the pterygoid canal, also referred to as the vidian canal. The vidian nerve passes through the canal as it transmits parasympathetic innervation from the seventh cranial nerve through the greater petrosal nerve to the sphenopalatine ganglion.

The posterior wall of the sphenoid sinus also makes up the floor of the sella turcica, which is also known as the hypophyseal or pituitary fossa (see Fig. 1–15). The anterior lip of the sella is called the tuberculum sella. Posteriorly, the sphenoid bone has a projection that forms the posterior wall of the sella. This is referred to as the dorsum sella. The lateral aspects of the dorsum sella are known as the posterior clinoid processes.

Projecting inferiorly from the body of the sphenoid is the clivus. This is the bony substrate for the posterior wall of the nasopharynx and forms part of the anterior wall of the foramen magnum. The clivus normally has a large marrow space in the bone inferior to the sphenoid sinus. This makes the clivus susceptible to the expansion of mucoceles and invasion by tumors and infectious processes.

VASCULATURE

The blood supply to the nose and sinuses derives from three major arterial sources: the ophthalmic artery from the internal carotid artery, the internal maxillary artery from the external carotid artery, and the facial artery from the external carotid artery. The venous return roughly parallels the arterial supply with a few notable exceptions. The most important is that the ophthalmic and orbital veins drain into the cavernous sinus and eventually into the internal jugular system. In the following sections, the arterial supply of the nose and sinuses is covered in detail.

Internal Carotid Artery

The internal carotid artery (ICA) branches from the common carotid artery at the bifurcation in the upper third of the neck at the level of C-2 to C-3 vertebral bodies. The ICA ascends to the undersurface of the temporal bone where it enters the carotid canal (Fig. 1–16). It then courses through the temporal bone with-

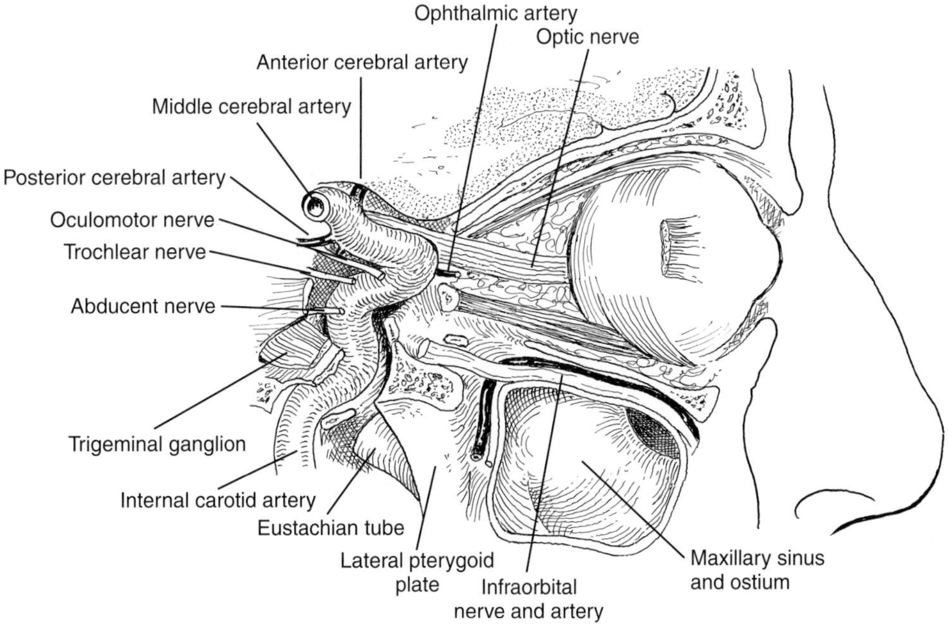

Figure 1–16. Anatomy of the internal carotid artery. The artery enters the temporal bone on the inferior surface and almost immediately takes an anterior bend into the horizontal portion. The artery turns superiorly into the vertical portion and then anteriorly into the cavernous portion. The artery then exits the canal though the sphenoid bone in the middle cranial fossa, where it branches into the main divisions.

out giving off any branches. The ICA has a short vertical portion before it turns anteriorly, at the level of the cochlea, into the horizontal portion. The ICA then turns superiorly again into the cavernous portion of the carotid. At this point, the ICA usually indents the lateral wall of the sphenoid sinus. There is usually an identifiable bulge in the lateral wall that may, in certain individuals, be more or less pronounced. The bone over the ICA in the sphenoid sinus is usually 1 to 2 mm thick, but it can be considerably thinner and, in some cases, may be dehiscent. The ICA passes just posterior to the optic nerve as it exits the cavernous portion and enters the sigmoid portion at the internal foramen of the carotid canal. Just at this point where the ICA bends posteriorly, it gives off its first intracranial branch, the ophthalmic artery (see Figs. 1–16 and 1–17).

Ophthalmic Artery. The ophthalmic artery arises from the ICA just as the latter artery passes through the internal foramen of the carotid canal (Fig. 1–17). This is just at the point where the ICA turns posteriorly and crosses under the optic nerve. The ophthalmic artery immediately courses anteriorly and laterally to enter the orbit through the optic canal lateral to the optic nerve (see Fig. 1–17). The ophthalmic artery immediately begins giving off branches to the various extraocular muscles and the optic nerve sheath. It turns medially and crosses over the optic nerve and then turns anteriorly. The ophthalmic artery gives off the posterior and then anterior ethmoid arteries along the medial wall of the orbit. In its terminal portion, the ophthalmic artery branches into the supratrochlear, supraorbital, and dorsal nasal arteries.

Posterior Ethmoid Artery. The posterior ethmoid artery arises from the ophthalmic artery within the posterior medial orbit. It crosses over the medial rectus and penetrates through an opening in the medial orbital wall into the ethmoid sinus. The posterior ethmoid artery normally is a small vessel, and it may be completely encased within the bone of the roof of the posterior ethmoid sinus. It normally runs through the bone at the anterior wall of the last posterior ethmoid cell. The posterior ethmoid artery can hang down into the sinus and may, in some individuals, be dehiscent. The artery crosses the roof of the ethmoid to descend and break into terminal branches on the posterior part of the nasal septum.

The posterior ethmoid artery supplies the bone and mucosa of the posterior ethmoid sinus and part of the superior and middle turbinates. The artery finally ends on the nasal septum where it contributes a small amount of the total blood flow to the arterial plexus of the posterior part of the septum.

Anterior Ethmoid Artery. The anterior ethmoid artery parallels the course of the posterior ethmoid artery. It arises from the ophthalmic artery in about the middle of the orbit. The anterior ethmoid artery crosses over the medial rectus and penetrates the bone of the medial wall of the orbit. The anterior ethmoid artery crosses the roof of the ethmoid sinus just anterior to the superior

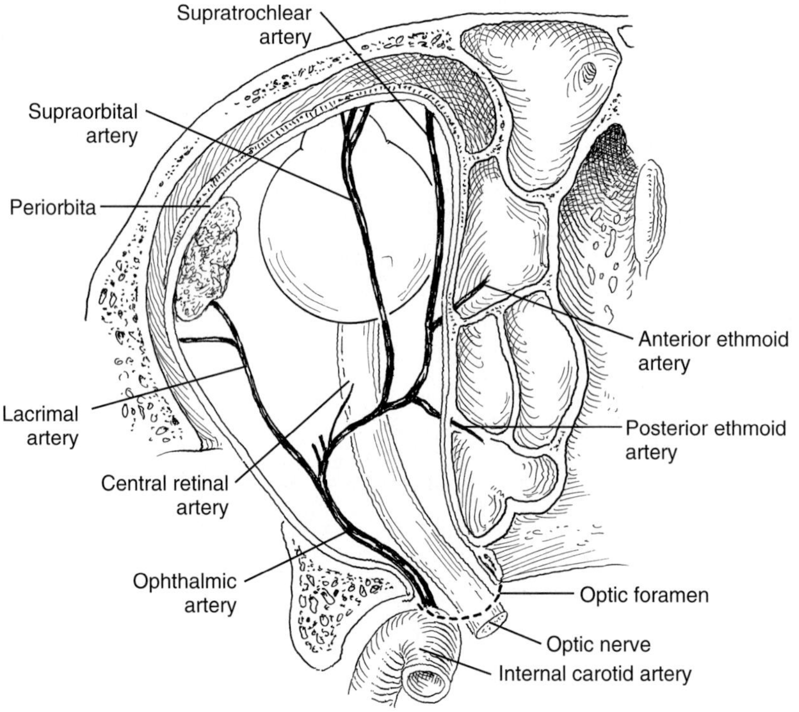

Figure 1–17. The ophthalmic artery.

attachment of the ethmoid bulla. Normally, the anterior ethmoid artery is not encased in bone but is exposed within the sinus. In certain individuals, it may hang well down into the sinus. The artery crosses the roof of the sinus to the anterior part of the nasal septum where it breaks up into terminal branches.

During its course, the anterior ethmoid artery gives off the anterior meningeal artery, which runs along the frontal dura behind the frontal sinus. It also gives off the lateral nasal artery and the external nasal artery. The lateral nasal artery descends from the roof of the ethmoid anterior to the middle turbinate to the nasal vestibule. The external nasal artery runs along the anterior septum to penetrate the undersurface of the nasal bones to help supply the nasal dorsum.

The anterior ethmoid artery supplies much of the blood flow to the anterior ethmoid sinus, as well as to the anterior half of the nasal septum. It supplies minimal blood flow to the anterior aspect of the middle turbinate, but contributes more substantially to the nasal vestibule.

Supraorbital Artery. The ophthalmic artery gives off the supratrochlear, nasal dorsal, and supraorbital arteries. The nasal dorsal artery supplies much of the external soft tissues of the nasal dorsum and medial canthus. The supratrochlear and supraorbital arteries exit the orbit at the supratrochlear and supraorbital foramina. These vessels supply the soft tissues and bone of the forehead up to the vertex of the skull. These vessels run on the undersurface of the frontalis muscle. Numerous small branches cross into the muscle and up to the skin. This allows the frontal skin to act as a myocutaneous axial pattern flap based on these vessels.

External Carotid Artery

The external carotid artery arises at the carotid bifurcation as the primary arterial supply of the extracranial head and neck. The external carotid artery courses superiorly within the neck, giving off branches (Fig. 1–18). It terminates as the superficial temporal artery after giving off the internal maxillary artery just below the external auditory canal. The named branches of the external carotid artery include the ascending pharyngeal, the superior thyroid, the lingual, the facial, the occipital, the posterior auricular, the internal maxillary,

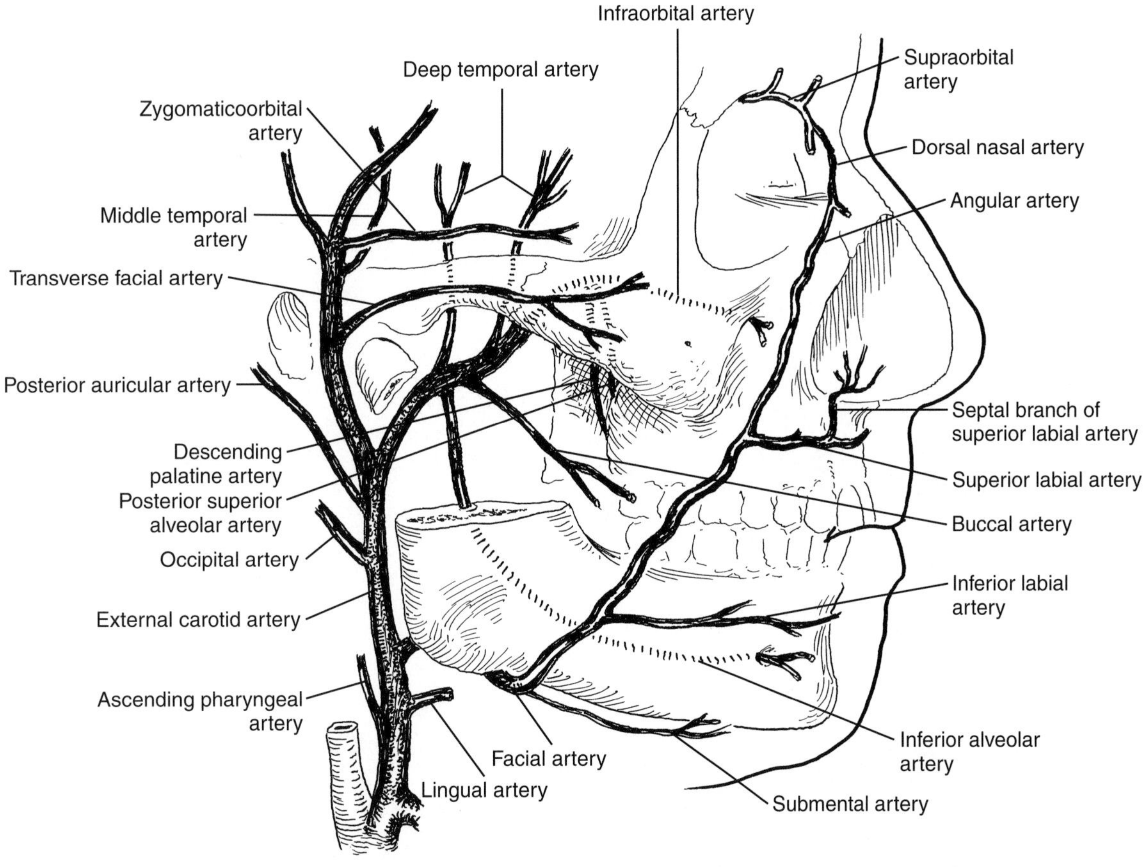

Figure 1–18. External carotid artery. The main branches are the ascending pharyngeal, superior thyroid (not shown), lingual, facial, occipital, postauricular, internal maxillary, and superficial temporal. The facial and internal maxillary arteries supply the majority of the face and sinuses.

and the superficial temporal arteries. The two branches of the external carotid artery that are important for the nose and sinuses are the facial and the internal maxillary arteries.

Facial Artery. The facial artery arises from the medial surface of the external carotid artery at the level of the angle of the mandible. It gives off several branches as it courses anteriorly under the body of the mandible before crossing superiorly over the inferior edge of the mandible. The facial artery gives off the superior labial artery to the upper lip just before it terminates as the angular artery. The superior labial artery runs from lateral to medial within the upper lip. It anastomoses with its counterpart on the opposite side. Close to the midline, it gives off small branches that supply blood flow to the columella and lateral nasal wall. This small but important contribution to nasal blood flow is important in the design of certain reconstructive flaps within the nose. The angular artery courses superiorly in the nasal facial groove. It gives off branches to the nasal sidewall, nasal tip, and nasal dorsum. The terminal branches of the angular artery supply the upper and lower eyelids.

Internal Maxillary. The internal maxillary artery (IMA) is the single most important vascular supply to the nose and sinuses. It arises from the medial surface of the external carotid artery just behind the ramus of the mandible about 1 to 2 cm below the external auditory canal. The IMA courses medially and gives off numerous branches (Fig. 1–19). These are often divided into three divisions. The first division is the portion directly beneath the ramus of the mandible. The deep auricular, anterior tympanic, middle meningeal, and inferior alveolar arteries derive from the first division. The second division lies over the lateral pterygoid muscle. These branches include the deep temporal arteries, the masseteric artery, and the buccal artery. The third division of the IMA lies within the pterygomaxillary fissure with branches that include the posterior superior alveolar artery, the descending palatine artery, the infraorbital artery, and the terminal branch of the IMA, the sphenopalatine artery.

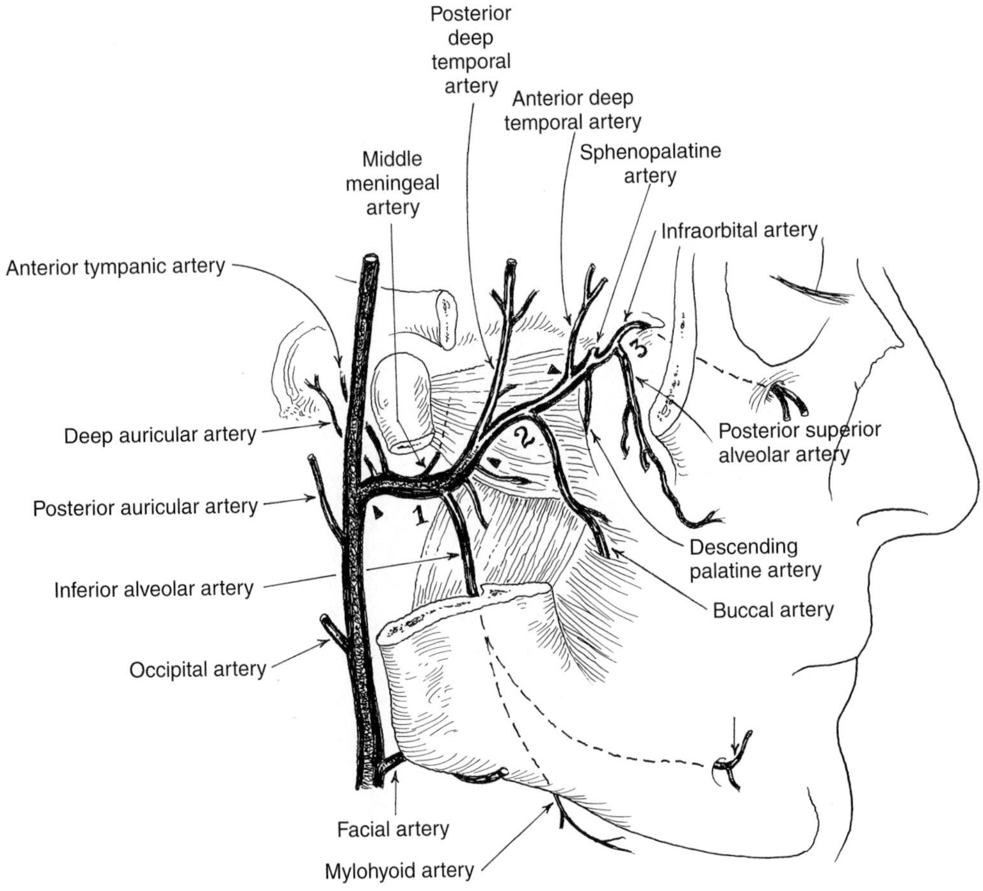

Figure 1–19. Internal maxillary artery. The artery branches widely in three main divisions: (1) medial to the mandible, (2) overlying the pterygoid muscle, and (3) in the pterygomaxillary fissure.

Posterior Superior Alveolar Artery. The posterior superior alveolar artery arises from the IMA just as it enters the pterygomaxillary fissure. The artery breaks into small branches that penetrate the posterior lateral surface of the maxilla just above the third molars. These arteries supply the posterior aspect of the maxilla and the three molar teeth.

Descending Palatine Artery. The descending palatine artery arises from the inferior side of the IMA in the lateral aspect of the pterygomaxillary fissure. It courses vertically and inferiorly along the posterior aspect of the maxilla to the greater palatine foramen. The artery passes through the foramen and becomes the greater palatine artery. The greater palatine artery courses anteriorly through the palate and gives off branches to the soft palate, hard palate, and the premolars and canine teeth.

Infraorbital Artery. The infraorbital artery branches from the IMA from the superior surface. It then extends superiorly, angling over the maxilla to enter the floor of the orbit through the medial aspect of the infraorbital fissure. The infraorbital artery travels through the inferior orbital canal in the roof of the maxillary sinus to the infraorbital foramen in the anterior wall of the maxilla. The intrasinus portion of the artery gives off branches that supply the interior of the maxillary sinus with blood flow. The artery then branches widely to supply the soft tissues of the face.

Sphenopalatine Artery. The terminal branch of the IMA is the sphenopalatine artery. The artery has a short course in the pterygomaxillary fissure before exiting the fissure through the sphenopalatine foramen into the posterior nasal cavity. The foramen is just posterior to the inferior posterior attachment of the middle turbinate. The sphenopalatine artery has branches that go into the middle and inferior turbinates and one branch that enters the maxillary sinus to supply blood flow to the medial wall of the maxillary sinus. Another branch courses posteriorly to cross the anterior wall of the sphenoid sinus. This branch supplies the sphenoid sinus mucosa with blood flow and terminates on the posterior aspect of the nasal septum as the greatest blood supply to the posterior septum (Fig. 1–20). The terminal branch of the sphenopalatine artery is the nasopalatine artery. This artery crosses the floor of the nose at the posterior choanae to contribute to the nasal septum, in addition to sending a branch anteriorly to descend through the incisive canal. This artery supplies blood flow to the anterior hard palate and the incisors. In all, there are usually three main arterioles derived from the sphenopalatine artery that supply the posterior septum.[19] Usually, the superior sphenoid branch splits and supplies two branches, whereas the nasopalatine supplies one inferior branch.

INNERVATION

The nose and sinuses are supplied by a complex network of nerves that serve a variety of functions. These include

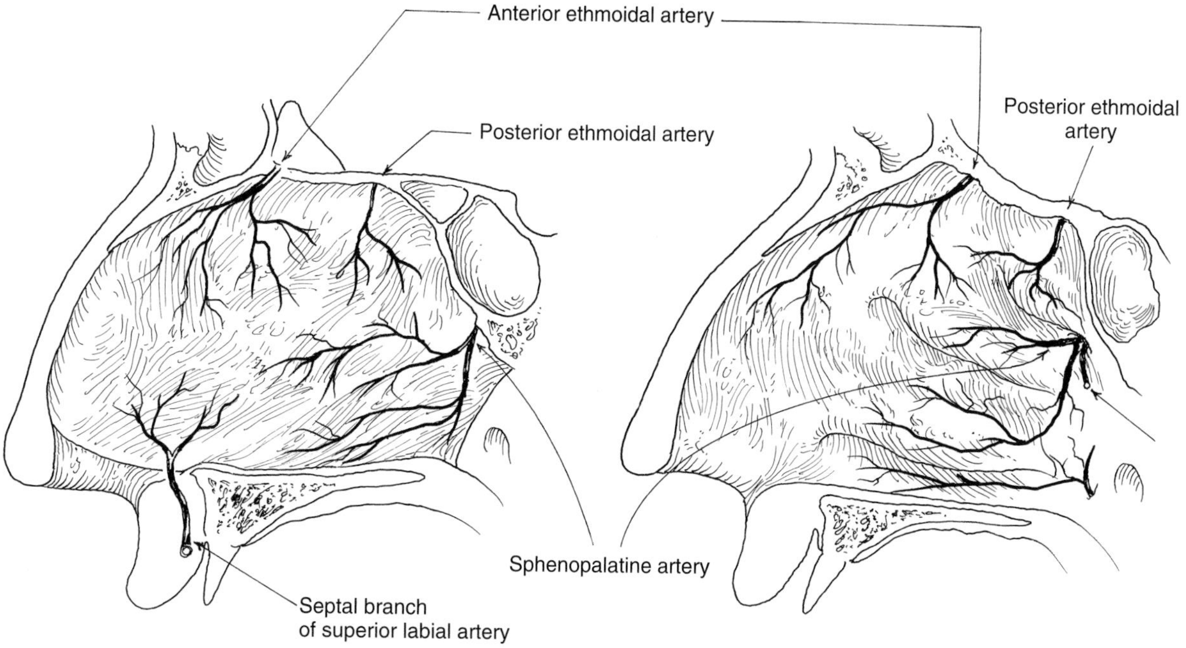

Figure 1–20. Blood supply to the nose. Four major arteries contribute to the septum: the septal branch of the facial artery, the anterior ethmoid, the posterior ethmoid, and the sphenopalatine arteries. The lateral wall of the nose receives blood supply through the anterior and posterior ethmoid arteries and the sphenopalatine.

somatosensory, motor, special sensory, and autonomic innervation. Each of these components of innervation is delivered to the target area through a branch of one of the cranial nerves. The anatomy of innervation of the nose and sinuses is, therefore, the anatomy of the upper cranial nerves. The cranial nerves involved are I, II, V, and VII. In the following sections, the anatomy of the innervation of the nose and sinuses is detailed.

Sensory Innervation

Sensory innervation to the nose and sinuses is carried by the branches of the trigeminal nerve (Fig. 1–21). The trigeminal nerve arises from the ventrolateral surface of the pons. The cell bodies of these sensory neurons are found in the trigeminal ganglion and connect to centrally projecting neurons in the spinal trigeminal and chief sensory nuclei found in the pons. These cells send central projections to the thalamus and then on to the cerebral cortex. The trigeminal nerve exits the pons and runs a short course to a shallow depression in the middle cranial fossa known as Meckel's cave. Within the cave lies the trigeminal ganglion. The trigeminal ganglion then gives off three divisions: the ophthalmic, the maxillary, and the mandibular nerves (V1, V2, V3).

Ophthalmic Nerve. The ophthalmic nerve (V1) courses medially from the trigeminal ganglion to enter the lateral aspect of the cavernous sinus (Fig. 1–22). V1 enters the posterior aspect of the orbit through the superior orbital fissure and lies in the superiormost end of the fissure alongside the trochlear nerve (cranial nerve IV). V1 has several important branches, including the lacrimal nerve, the nasociliary nerve, and the terminal branches: the supratrochlear and supraorbital nerves. The lacrimal nerve arises just inside the superior orbital fissure and courses laterally in the superior orbit to supply the lateral orbit and lacrimal gland with sensory innervation. The nasociliary nerve arises next and turns medially, coursing along the medial wall of the orbit. It gives off both the posterior and anterior ethmoid nerves. The posterior ethmoid nerve enters the ethmoid sinus through the posterior ethmoid foramen along with the posterior ethmoid artery. It supplies the posterior ethmoid sinus, superior turbinate, and a small portion of the posterior nasal septum. The anterior eth-

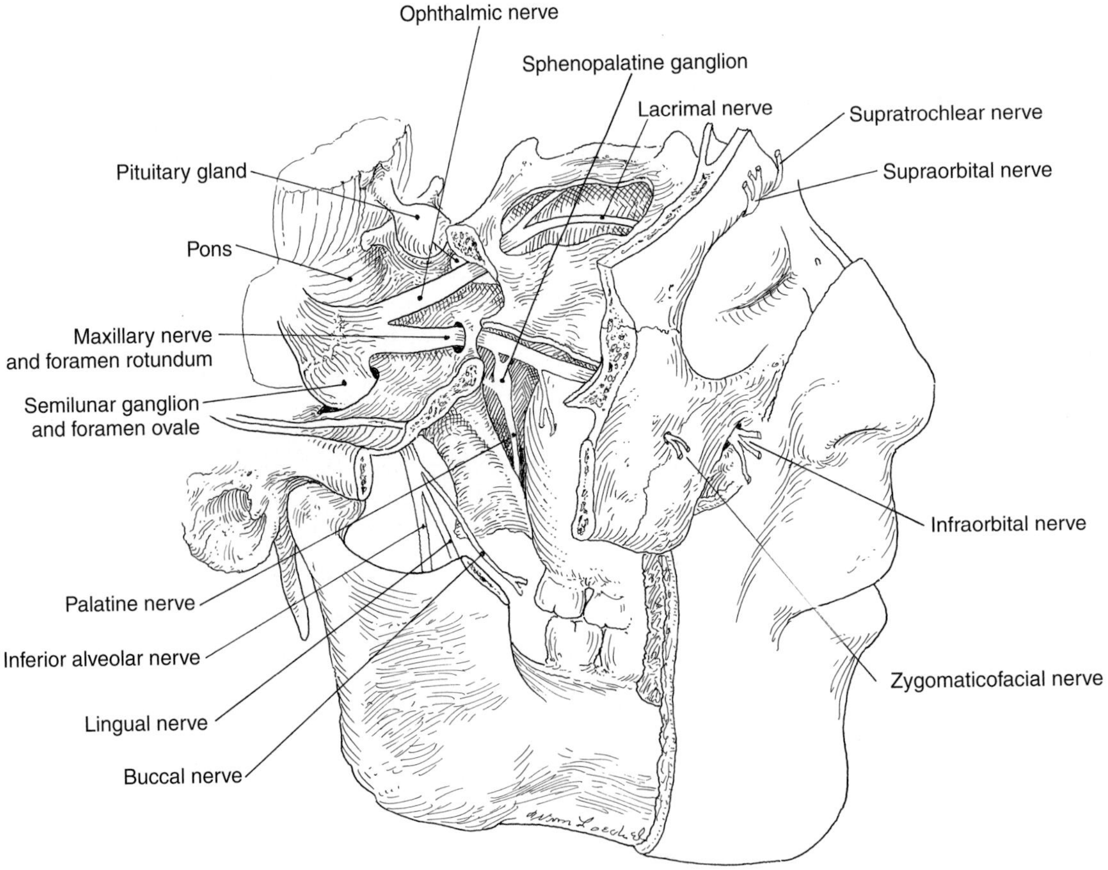

Figure 1–21. The trigeminal nerve. The three main branches are: the ophthalmic (V1), maxillary (V2), and mandibular (V3) nerves.

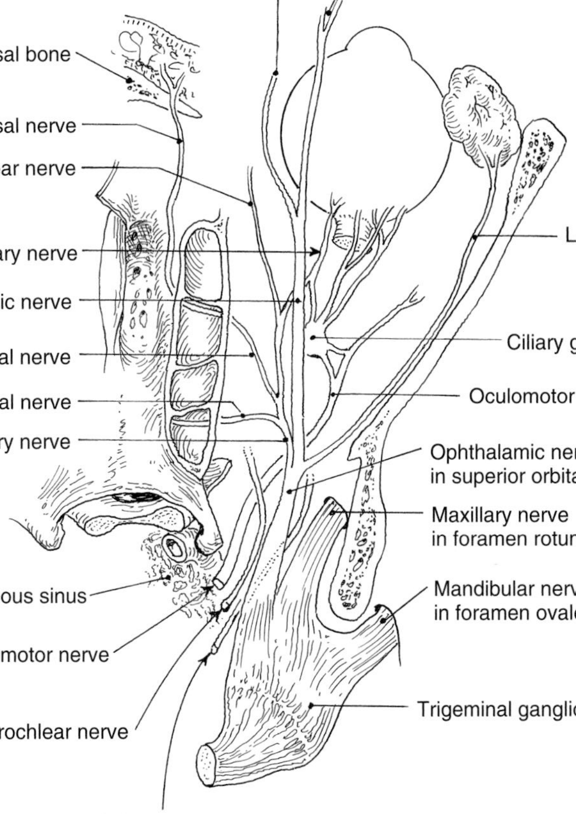

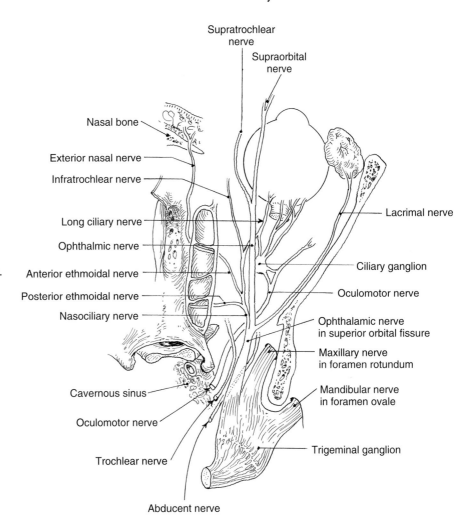

Figure 1–22. The ophthalmic nerve.

moid nerve enters the ethmoid sinus through the anterior ethmoid foramen adjacent to the anterior ethmoid artery. It supplies the anterior ethmoid sinus mucosa, anterior half of the lateral wall of the nose, and the anterior aspect of the nasal septum. A branch of the anterior ethmoid nerve exits the nose between the nasal bone and upper lateral cartilage to innervate the nasal dorsum and tip as the external nasal nerve.

The terminal branch of the ophthalmic nerve courses superiorly within the orbit. Before exiting the orbit, it divides into two main trunks; the smaller, medially directed, supratrochlear nerve and the primary terminal branch, the supraorbital nerve. The supraorbital nerve exits the orbit about 1 to 2 cm lateral to the nasal bones through the supraorbital foramen. This nerve courses on the undersurface of the frontalis muscle with branches extending to innervate the forehead and scalp up to the vertex.

Maxillary Nerve. The second division of the trigeminal nerve (V2) branches from the trigeminal ganglion and courses anteriorly to the foramen rotundum (Fig. 1–23). V2 exits the middle cranial fossa through the foramen rotundum into the posterior apex of the pterygomaxillary fissure. Just within the fissure, branches from the maxillary nerve arise that run a short course to enter the sphenopalatine ganglion. From the ganglion, the descending palatine nerve arises and follows the descending palatine artery inferiorly through the greater and lesser palatine foramina to supply the palate. Branches from the sphenopalatine ganglion course medially through the sphenopalatine foramen into the lateral wall of the nose. Separate branches supply the superior, middle, and inferior turbinates. The nasopalatine nerve courses across the face of the sphenoid to the back of the septum, supplying the posterior and inferior aspects of the septum. The distal end of this nerve runs through the incisive foramen to innervate the anterior hard palate mucosa.

Distally to the sphenopalatine nerve and within the pterygomaxillary fissure, V2 gives off the posterior superior alveolar nerve. This nerve breaks up into two or more branches that enter the back of the maxilla and supply the posterior teeth and gingiva. The maxillary

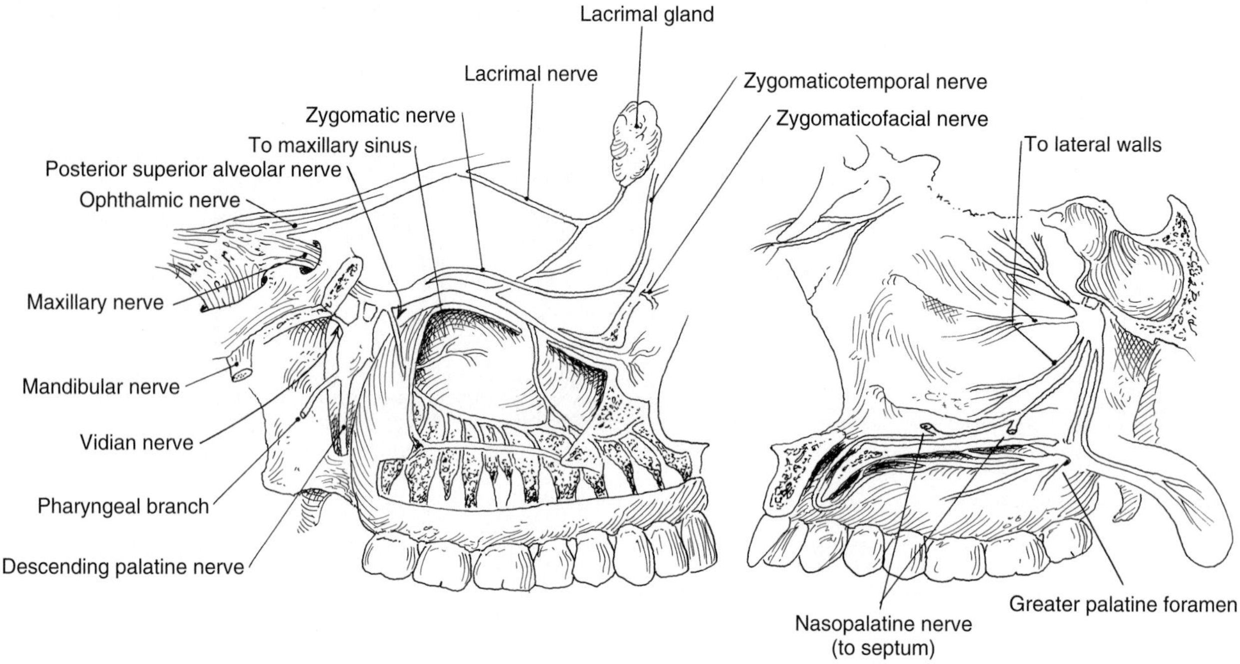

Figure 1–23. The maxillary nerve, lateral and medial view.

nerve then enters the orbit through the inferior orbital fissure. It courses along the floor of the orbit in the inferior orbital groove. In this area, it gives off the anterior superior alveolar nerve that descends within the maxilla to innervate the canine teeth and the central and lateral incisors. In the floor of the orbit, the infraorbital nerve gives off two important branches: the zygomaticofacial and the zygomaticotemporal nerves. The facial branch exits the orbit through a canal in the malar eminence to emerge on the face, supplying the face over the malar eminence (Fig. 1–24). The temporal branch courses to the lacrimal gland, supplying it with parasympathetic innervation. The infraorbital nerve terminates through the infraorbital foramen into the face over the maxilla. It divides into three principle branches that supply the lower eyelid, the nasal sidewall, and the upper lip, as well as the main branch that supplies the cheek.

Mandibular Nerve. The mandibular nerve does not contain any sensory branches to the nose and sinuses. The mandibular nerve does contain motor roots to the muscles of mastication, but does not contain any branches

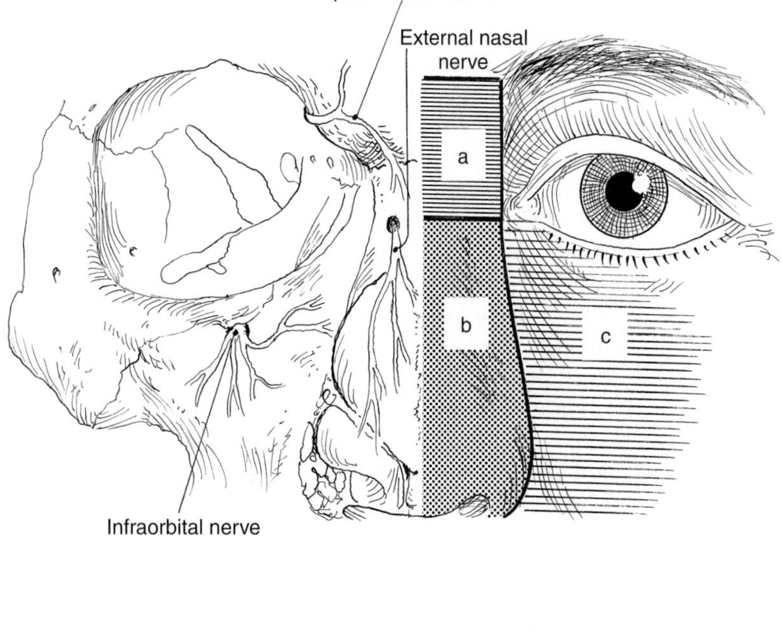

Figure 1–24. Innervation zones of the nose and face: *a,* from the supratrochlear nerve (V1); *b,* from the external nasal nerve (V1); *c,* from the infraorbital nerve (V2).

that are pertinent to the anatomy of the nose and sinuses.

Motor Innervation

The only muscles that are pertinent to this discussion of anatomy are the muscles of the face. These muscles are all innervated by branches of the facial nerve (cranial nerve VII). The facial nerve arises from the motor nucleus of the facial nerve in the ventrolateral pons. The fibers course anteriorly, turn around the abducens nucleus at the internal genu, and then run posteriorly to the surface of the pons, where they exit and form the bulk of the root of the facial nerve. The nerve courses anteriorly with cranial nerve VIII to enter the temporal bone through the porous acousticus on the posterior surface of the bone within the posterior fossa. The nerve courses within the internal auditory canal in the anterior and superior quadrant of the canal.

The facial nerve within the temporal bone is the subject of extensive discussion in otology textbooks and so is not covered here in detail. The important points are that the nerve has three basic segments: the labyrinthine, tympanic, and mastoid segments. At the junction of the labyrinthine and tympanic portions, the nerve makes a sharp posterior turn at the first genu. At this point, at the first genu is the geniculate ganglion. The greater petrosal nerve exits from the geniculate ganglion and runs on the surface of the middle cranial fossa before entering the vidian (pterygoid) canal. At the anterior end of the vidian canal, the nerve enters the pterygomaxillary fissure and joins to the sphenopalatine ganglion.

The facial nerve exits from the temporal bone at the stylomastoid foramen on the undersurface of the temporal bone. The nerve then enters the parotid gland and breaks up, initially into two divisions: the superior and inferior divisions. From this point, the anatomy is variable in the branching pattern. There are numerous patterns possible but several that are most common. With most of the branching patterns, the nerve ends up in five major branches: the frontal, zygomatic, buccal, marginal mandibular, and cervical branches. These nerves innervate all of the facial muscles responsible for mimetic motions.

Special Sensory Innervation

The special senses of interest to the anatomy of the nose and sinuses include olfactory, visual, and gustatory senses. These senses are innervated by cranial nerves I, II, and VII. A portion of the gustatory sense is also transmitted by cranial nerve IX, but this is not relevant to this discussion.

Olfactory Nerve. The olfactory nerve (cranial nerve I) is the shortest of all 12 of the cranial nerves (Fig. 1–25). The nerve arises from the olfactory bulb, which lies on the undersurface of the frontal lobe of the brain as a swelling of the terminal end of the olfactory tract. The bulbs sit over the cribriform plate and send the numerous branches from the bulb through the small perforations in the cribriform plate into the olfactory epithe-

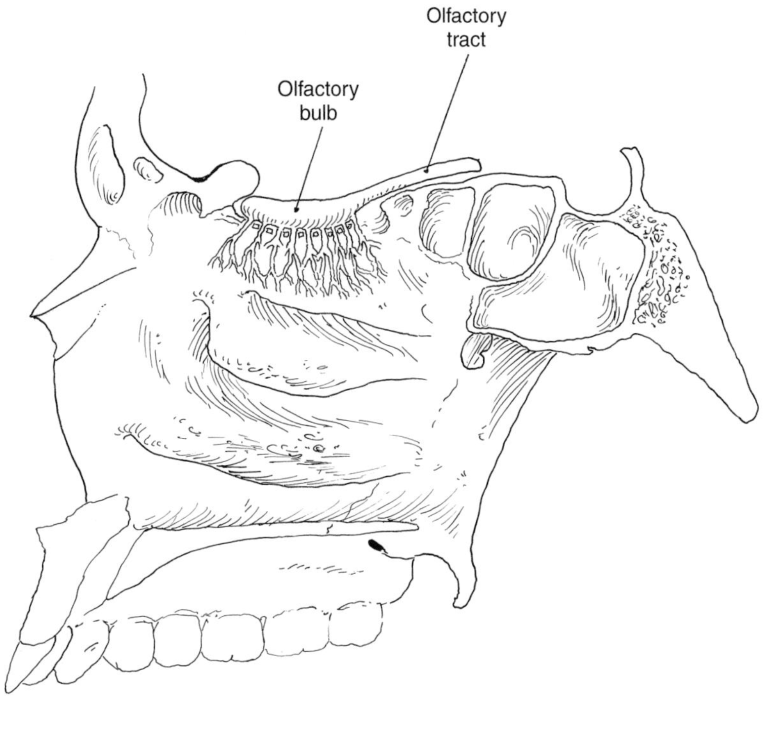

Figure 1–25. Olfactory nerve.

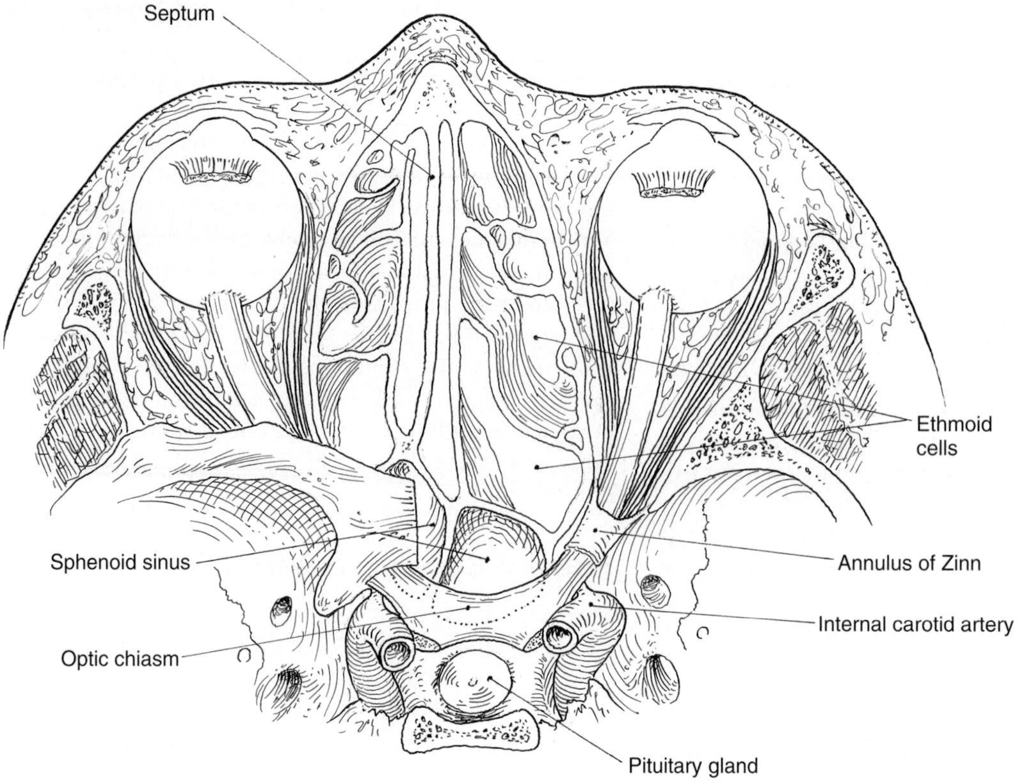

Figure 1–26. Anatomy of the optic nerve. This superior view shows the course of the optic nerve from the chiasm distally.

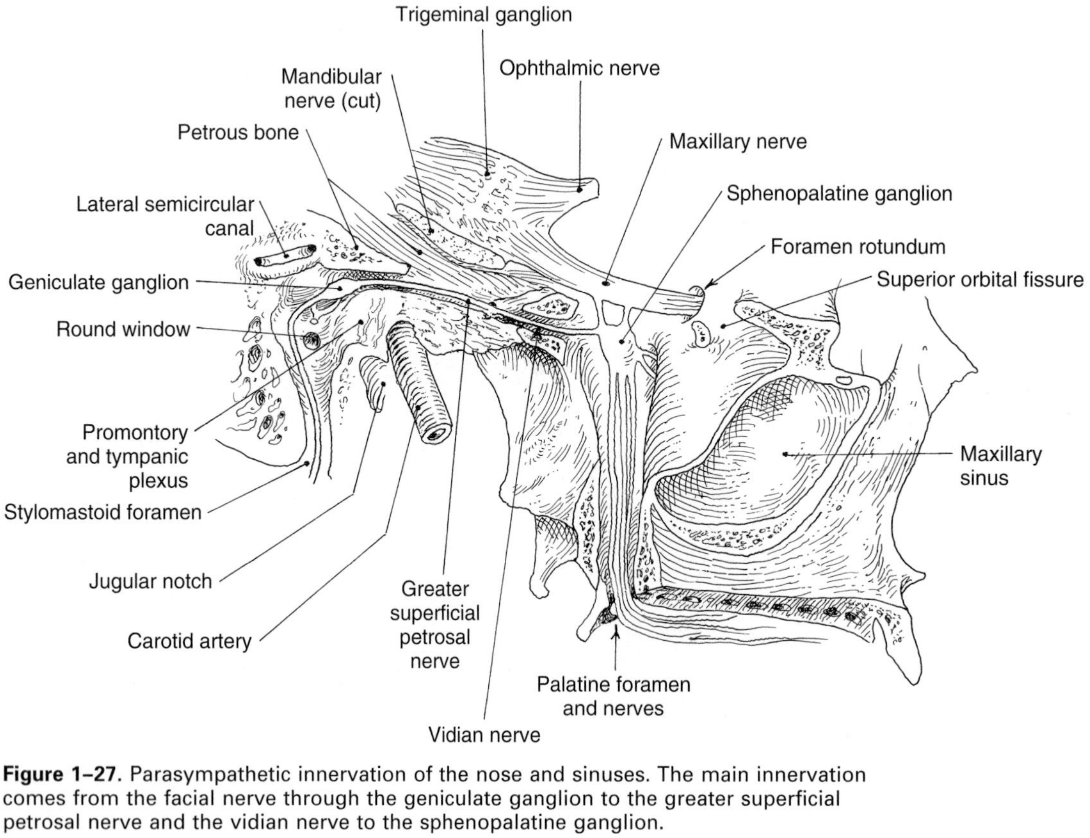

Figure 1–27. Parasympathetic innervation of the nose and sinuses. The main innervation comes from the facial nerve through the geniculate ganglion to the greater superficial petrosal nerve and the vidian nerve to the sphenopalatine ganglion.

lium at the roof of the nose. Each side of the nose has about 20 olfactory nerve bundles that pass through the foramina of the cribriform plate.

Optic Nerve. The optic nerve supplies the eye with special sensory innervation for vision (Fig. 1–26). The nerve originates in the retina as the individual axons of the cones and rods. These fibers coalesce at the optic nerve head and pass posteriorly to form the optic nerve. The nerve courses from the back of the eye toward the optic foramen at the back of the orbit. The length of the optic nerve in the orbit is about half of the depth of the orbit. Toward the apex of the orbit, the ocular muscles form a cone around the optic nerve. The muscles condense into a fibrous sheath called the annulus of Zinn at the orbital apex. The optic foramen is situated toward the medial aspect of the orbit, and the nerve in this area usually lies just lateral to the junction of the sphenoid and posterior ethmoid sinuses.

After it leaves the orbit, the optic nerve courses along the lateral wall of the sphenoid sinus in a superior and medial direction to join with the nerve of the opposite side at the optic chiasm. The chiasm sits anterior to the pituitary gland at the level of the floor of the anterior cranial fossa. From the chiasm, the optic tracts course posteriorly around the midbrain to the lateral geniculate body where the next level of the visual tract ganglion is located. The topographic alignment of the nerves within the optic tracts is a fascinating and well-studied subject. Readers are referred to any ophthalmology text or neuroanatomy text for further details.

Gustatory Nerves. The nerves supplying the special sense of taste arise in the brain in the nucleus of the tractus solitarius. These neurons enter the facial nerve and form two separate tracts. The larger of the tracts is for the anterior two thirds of the tongue. These fibers form the chorda tympani, which branches from the facial nerve in the mastoid segment and crosses under the tympanic membrane. It exits the temporal bone and courses anteriorly to join with the lingual nerve to end in the anterior two thirds of the tongue. The second gustatory tract from the facial nerve exits the temporal bone at the geniculate ganglion to join the greater superficial petrosal nerve. This courses through the vidian canal to join the sphenopalatine ganglion. The

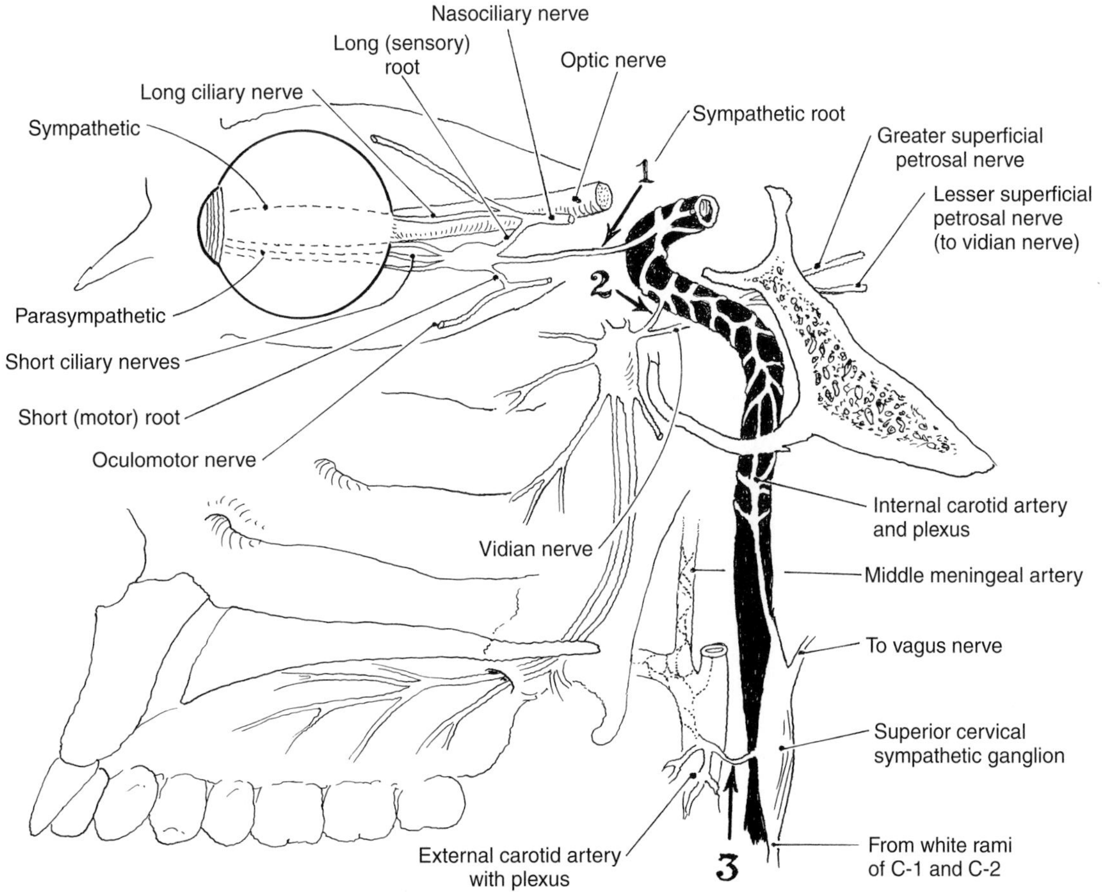

Figure 1–28. Sympathetic innervation. Nerves enter the superior cervical sympathetic ganglion and then course along the internal and external carotid arteries to their destinations.

branches then are directed into the descending palatine nerve through the greater palatine foramen to the special sensory receptors on the surface of the palate.

Autonomic Innervation

The autonomic nervous system consists of sympathetic and parasympathetic components. The areas of the head and neck that are supplied by the autonomic nervous system include the pupil, lacrimal gland, salivary glands, the carotid and jugular baroreceptors, and the sinus and nasal mucosa. This discussion is limited to the salivary glands and the nasal and sinus mucosa.

Parasympathetic Nerves. The parasympathetic innervation for much of the nose and sinuses and adjoining areas arises from the superior and inferior salivatory nuclei. These brain stem nuclei send off neurons that join the nervus intermedius and thence the facial nerve. Some of these fibers branch off the facial nerve into the chorda tympani and then into the lingual nerve. In the floor of the mouth, they branch off to form the submandibular nerve. Other fibers from these ganglia branch off the facial nerve at the geniculate ganglion into the greater superficial petrosal nerve. These fibers end in the sphenopalatine ganglion (Fig. 1–27). One tract carries the lacrimal innervation and runs through the infraorbital nerve to the zygomaticotemporal nerve before innervating the lacrimal gland. A second tract from the sphenopalatine ganglion courses into the sphenopalatine nerve through the sphenopalatine foramen into the posterior aspect of the nose to innervate the nose and sinuses. These fibers terminate on mucous glands and blood vessels within the mucosa. Stimulation leads to increased production of mucus and dilatation of the mucosal blood vessels, resulting in increased congestion.

Sympathetic Nerves. The sympathetic innervation to the nose and sinuses arises in the upper two thoracic segments of the spinal cord. They ascend to the superior cervical sympathetic ganglion. Postganglionic fibers course through the carotid plexus and follow the ICA and external carotid artery to the end destination on small arterioles in the mucosa (Fig. 1–28), where they cause vasoconstriction.

REFERENCES

1. Clemente CD. Anatomy: A Regional Atlas of the Human Body, 2nd ed. Baltimore: Urban & Schwarzenberg, 1981.
2. Stammberger HR, Kennedy DW. Paranasal sinuses: Anatomic terminology and nomenclature. Ann Otol Rhinol Laryngol 167(Oct.):7, 1995.
3. Lee KJ. Essential Otolaryngology Head and Neck Surgery, 4th ed. New York: Elsevier Science Publishing Co., 1987, pp. 280–283.
4. DeArreola GA, Serna NL, Parra RD, Salinas MA. Morphogenesis of the lateral nasal wall from 6 to 36 weeks. Otolaryngol Head Neck Surg 114(1):54, 1996.
5. Wareing MJ, Padgham ND. Osteologic classification of the sphenopalatine foramen. Laryngoscope 108:125, 1998.
6. Kennedy DW, Zinreich SJ, Kuhn F, Shaalan H, Naclerio R. Endoscopic middle meatal antrostomy: Theory, technique, and patency. Laryngoscope 97:1, 1987.
7. Kennedy DW. Functional endoscopic sinus surgery. Arch Otolaryngol 111:643, 1985.
8. Owen RG, Kuhn FA. Supraorbital ethmoid cell. Otolaryngol Head Neck Surg 116(2):254, 1997.
9. Bent JP, Cuilty-Siller C, Kuhn FA. The frontal cell as a cause of frontal sinus obstruction. Am J Rhinol 8(4):185, 1994.
10. Merritt RM, Bent JP, Kuhn FA. The intersinus septal cell: Anatomic, radiologic, and clinical correlation. Am J Rhinol 10(5): 299, 1996.
11. Kasper KA. Nasofrontal connections: A study based on one hundred consecutive dissections. Arch Otolaryngol Head Neck Surg 23:322, 1936.
12. Lang J. Clinical Anatomy of the Nose, Nasal Cavity and Paranasal Sinuses. New York: Thieme Medical Publishers, 1989, pp. 62–68.
13. Lee D, Brody R, Har-El G. Frontal sinus outflow anatomy. Am J Rhinol 11(4):283, 1997.
14. Min YG, Koh TY, Rhee CS, Han MH. Clinical implications of the uncinate process in paranasal sinusitis: Radiologic evaluation. Am J Rhinol 9(3):131, 1995.
15. Stackpole SA, Edelstein DR. The anatomic relevance of the Haller cell in sinusitis. Am J Rhinol 11(3):219, 1997.
16. Weinberger DB, Anand VK, Al-Rawl M, Cheng HJ, Messina AV. Surgical anatomy and variations of the Onodi cell. Am J Rhinol 10(6):365, 1996.
17. Hosemann W, Gross R, Gode U, Kuhnel TH, Rockelein G. The anterior sphenoid wall: Relative anatomy for sphenoidotomy. Am J Rhinol 9(3):137, 1995.
18. Edelstein DR, Liberatore L, Bushkin S, Han JC. Applied anatomy of the posterior sinuses in relation to the optic nerve, trigeminal nerve, and carotid artery. Am J Rhinol 9(6):321, 1995.
19. Fujii M, Goto N, Moriyama H, et al. Demonstration of the nasal septal branches of the sphenopalatine artery by use of a new intravascular injection method. Ann Otol Rhinol Laryngol 105:309, 1996.

CHAPTER 2

Physiology of the Nose and Sinuses

This chapter covers various aspects of the normal function of the nose and sinuses. This is not a topic that one would normally expect to find in a textbook of surgery. However, in order to understand many of the procedures described in this textbook, it is important to understand nasal and sinus physiology. Septoplasty, turbinectomy, endoscopic sinus surgery, and management of epistaxis are all either based on or profoundly affected by sinus and nasal physiology. The areas covered include regulation of airflow, conditioning of inspired air, mucociliary function, mucus composition, immune function, and olfaction.

REGULATION OF AIRFLOW

Regulation of airflow through the nose is a critical factor in the conditioning of inspired air prior to its passage to the remainder of the upper and lower airways. The degree of congestion of the mucosa will determine the surface area of the nasal cavity and resistance to airflow through the nose. The greater the surface area and resistance, the greater the contact between the mucosa and the inspired air. The degree of contact will determine the amount of cleaning, humidification, and warming of the air.

Nasal airway resistance may also play a role in the regulation of minute volume of respiration.[1] The lower the resistance, the shorter the inspiratory phase of respiration, increasing respiratory rate and minute volume. Greater resistance leads to a longer inspiratory phase, which will decrease respiratory rate and decrease minute volume of inspired air. This idealized mechanism is probably of minimal importance in the actual regulation of minute volume. The patient, when dyspneic, can breathe through the mouth with less work of breathing. In this situation, regulation of the expiratory phase will regulate the respiratory rate. However, this study did demonstrate that decreased nasal airflow resulted in a higher end tidal P_{CO_2}, which may protect the individual against sleep apnea.

In the normal nose, maximal airflow is through the middle meatus. Less air flows through the inferior meatus, and airflow through the superior meatus and upper nasal cavity is minimal. Airflow is dependent on the difference in pressure between the nares and the nasopharynx and the nasal resistance. Poiseuille's law states that, for laminar flow of a gas through a tube, the resistance is inversely proportional to the diameter to the fourth power. This means that a decrease in diameter of one half will increase resistance 16-fold. However, normal airflow is turbulent and not laminar. For this reason, the law does not strictly apply, but is generally applicable. This means that the primary determinant of nasal airflow is the minimal cross-sectional area of the nasal cavity.

The minimal cross-sectional area of the nose is determined by the degree of congestion of the nasal mucosa. This varies with the degree of neural tone, the body position, and external and internal factors, such as inflammation, hypertrophy, and secretions. This regulation of nasal airflow is achieved by the nasal mucosa, which acts as a whole organ in its regulation of the congestion and various functions of the nose. To understand the regulation of these functions, it is first necessary to understand the anatomy of the nasal mucosa.

Mucosal Anatomy

The regulation of nasal resistance and nasal airflow is governed by the regulation of blood flow through the nasal mucosa. The mucosa of the nose is a highly complex organ of variable anatomy depending on the location within the nose or sinuses. The sinonasal mucosa contains an epithelial layer, the lamina propria, a submucosal layer, and a thin periosteal layer. The epithelium consists of a ciliated, pseudostratified, columnar epithelium. In some areas, the epithelium may become more of a simple columnar layer, which may be low enough to simulate a cuboidal layer. The epithelium contains a variable number of goblet cells, which produce components of the nasal mucus.[2] The lamina propria is a thin, fibrous layer that forms the basement membrane of the epithelial layer of the mucosa.

The submucosa of the nasal and sinus mucosa contains the vasculature and seromucinous glands, as well as the nerve fibers that innervate the mucosa. The vasculature includes arterioles, capillaries, and venules. The density of these components varies with their location within the nasal anatomy. Consider, for example, the high density of arterioles and capillaries within the anterior septal mucosa, known as Kiesselbach's plexus.

The mucosa of the inferior turbinates is especially unique in that it contains abundant small veins having a relatively thick muscular layer. These veins are referred to as venous sinusoids, cushion veins, or capacitance veins. The high volume capacity of these veins imparts an erectile property to this mucosa. This is the primary mucosa that responds to the regulatory impulses. These veins can either contract to exclude excess blood, leading to decongestion, or they can relax, filling with blood and causing expansion of the erectile tissue. The control of the volume of blood in these vessels is a highly complex, highly regulated system.

Vascular Regulation

Vascular regulation occurs through interaction of sympathetic and parasympathetic innervation.[3] Sensory innervation is also present, but this provides only afferent feedback and does not lead directly to changes in blood flow. The nerves travel along the major vessels, accompanying them through the deep submucosa against the bone. The parasympathetic nerves arise from the brain stem and are carried with the facial nerve to the geniculate ganglion. The parasympathetic nerves course through the vidian nerve to the sphenopalatine ganglion and then into the nose through the sphenopalatine foramen. The sympathetic nerves arise from the upper thoracic spinal column and course to the superior cervical sympathetic ganglion. Fibers run along the carotid artery and branches of the carotid into the nose and sinuses.

The sympathetic nerves are distributed to the arterial vessels and the venous sinusoids of the nasal mucosa.[4] These nerves use norepinephrine as a transmitter, but some evidence exists that the neuropeptide tyrosine can act as a transmitter for some of these neurons.[5] Activation of these sympathetic nerves causes vasoconstriction, which decreases the amount of blood flowing into the capillary bed and the amount of blood in the venous sinusoids. The net effect is to decongest the nasal mucosa, shrinking the mucosa, increasing the size of the nasal airway, and decreasing nasal resistance.

The parasympathetic neurons are mostly distributed to the precapillary arterioles, with sparse distribution to the venous structures.[4] The primary neurotransmitter is acetylcholine. However, there are abundant alternative parasympathetic neurotransmitters, including vasoactive intestinal peptide (VIP) and several neuropeptides.[5] Stimulation of these nerves results in vasodilatation, primarily of the precapillary arterioles. The net effect of this stimulation is to increase the blood in the tissues, swell the nasal tissues, decrease the size of the nasal airway, and increase nasal resistance.

Recently, a new neurotransmitter—nitric oxide (NO)—has been postulated to play a role in the regulation of nasal blood flow and mucous production.[6,7] NO is produced by nitric oxide synthetase (NOS), which is postulated to have three different isoforms, all of which have been found in nasal mucosa. Type I is the neural form found in nerve cells within the nasal mucosa where it is thought to be a neurotransmitter.[8] Type II NOS is an inducible form that responds to inflammation.[9] Type III, the predominant form, is found primarily in ciliated mucosal cells.[10] The function of NO in the regulation of nasal physiology is as yet unknown, although a reasonable guess would be that it participates in vasodilatation. Evidence for this can be found in the ability of NOS inhibitors to block vasodilatation[11] and the decrease in NO levels in exhaled air during heavy exercise that usually is accompanied by vasoconstriction.[12]

Regardless of the neurotransmitters at work, the two limbs (sympathetic and parasympathetic nerves) of the regulation of vascular tone act in concert to create a net effect. Stimuli that induce decongestion activate the sympathetic nerves and inhibit the parasympathetic nerves. Conversely, stimuli that lead to congestion cause increased parasympathetic tone and decreased sympathetic tone. This balance is regulated through a brain stem reflex arc.

Nasal Cycle

The nasal cycle refers to spontaneous, alternating congestion and decongestion on opposite sides of the nose. The nasal cycle was first described by physiologists more than 100 years ago. It is thought to be affected by simultaneous sympathetic and parasympathetic modulation in opposite directions on opposite sides of the nose. The nasal cycle has been theorized to serve several different roles in normal nasal physiology. These include improving mucus clearance from the sinuses and nose, improved filtering and humidification, and acting as a mucosal pump to move plasma through the mucosa.[13] Not all individuals have been found to have a nasal cycle. Studies have shown that the proportion of people with a nasal cycle varies from 20% to 80% depending on the methods used to evaluate and calculate the variation.[14–16]

Many studies have been done to characterize the nasal cycle. One recent study has shown that the maximal decongestion during the nasal cycle is equal to the maximal decongestion that can be achieved through pharmacologic decongestion.[17] Another study has demonstrated that the nasal cycle degenerates with increasing age, becoming less pronounced with increased age.[18] The nasal cycle has also been evaluated in relationship to the menstrual cycle.[19] No effect of changing hormone levels has been observed. However, a separate study found that the nasal cycle tends to oscillate in relation to cardiac output, heart rate, and stroke volume.[20] It has been postulated that the joint regulation is through a hypothalamic ultradian rhythm.

A second normal regulatory adjustment is increased congestion of the dependent side of the nose when supine. This occurs through regulation of the blood flow through the turbinate mucosa. Blood flow studies have shown that blood flow increases when an individual changes position from sitting to supine.[21] In addition, the downward side of the nose has a greater blood flow than the upward side of the nose. A second mechanism for this effect is decreased outflow from the capacitance veins in the downward side of the nose. Both effects lead to increased congestion in the downward side. This increased congestion may be beneficial in preventing airflow through a side of the nose that may be compressed or lying in dirt, or in guarding against potential allergenic antigens.

Nasal Valve

The internal nasal valve is the minimal cross-sectional area of the nose. This normally corresponds to the area of the anterior aspect of the inferior turbinate. This plane usually includes the inferior edge of the upper lateral cartilage. The importance of this area is not only that it imparts the maximum degree of resistance to airflow, but it is also the area where alar collapse can occur. In every individual, there is the possibility of alar collapse. The ala has a natural rigidity that resists collapse. However, sufficiently high negative pressures can lead to collapse. The narrower the nasal valve, the greater the negative pressure that is generated during inspiration. In some individuals, this can lead to the negative pressure exceeding the rigidity of the valve, resulting in collapse.

AIR CONDITIONING

The functions of the nose include not only regulation of airflow, but the conditioning of inspired air to prepare for gas exchange in the lungs. The nose is the primary organ responsible for this air conditioning, which includes warming, humidifying, and cleaning the air. Of course, it is possible to breathe through the mouth, rather than the nose. However, when breathing in this way, the efficiency of the air preparation before arriving in the lungs is much reduced. The effects of lack of conditioning when oral breathing is the predominant method are unknown. Certainly, patients undergoing tracheostomy and laryngectomy, who have even less air preparation than mouth breathers, adapt well and can live indefinitely without the benefits of nasal function. However, it is equally true that the lungs benefit from nasal air conditioning as this process decreases the antigenic load, minimizes exposure to particulate matter, and decreases the drying effect of inspired air. This should, in the long term, increase the health and function of the lungs.

Warming

The nasal mucosa is critical for warming inspired air before it reaches the bronchial mucosa.[22] This warming, effected by transmission of heat across the nasal mucosa, is facilitated by the amount of contact between the mucosa and the air and the nature of the airflow through the nose. For example, compared to a congested nose, a fully decongested nose has less surface area to transfer heat; has greater airflow velocity, thereby decreasing the time of contact; and greater laminar airflow, thereby decreasing the mixing of the air within the nose.

A number of studies have been done in animals and humans to investigate the physiology of the warming function of the nose. In rats, it was discovered that the density of blood vessels in the nasal respiratory mucosa is roughly three times higher than that of the oral mucosa.[23] This implies that the high density of blood vessels may be a primary factor in one's ability to warm inspired air. Presumably, a heat exchange occurs between the inspired air and the blood within these vessels. In humans, it was found that blood flow though the nose increases when body temperature increases.[24] This implies that the nasal mucosa can also dissipate heat as part of the thermoregulatory response to fever. Other investigators have found that the human nasal cavity has a tremendous capacity to warm air, as it was shown not to have reached maximum capacity at even 7 L per minute inspired airflow.[25] Finally, a study on skiers found that the warming of inspired air continues through the respiratory tract into the bronchioles.[22] Despite this, the alveolar air was, in all cases, fully warmed to body temperature. This implies that the lower airways have a great capacity for warming air as a backup to the nasal mucosa, even in the most demanding of circumstances.

Humidification

Humidification of inspired air is perhaps even more important to normal pulmonary function than warming.

Humidification is achieved by the evaporation of moisture from the mucosal surface into the air during inspiration. Once again, airflow regulation is important in this function. The open nasal passage has less surface contact and less turbulent airflow, leading to less humidification. In humidification, an exchange occurs between the mucus and the inspired air. The more liquid the secretions, the more humidification is possible. Using electron microscopy to study rabbit mucosa, it has been found that the vessels in the subepithelial layer contain fenestrations facing only the mucosal side.[26] This is thought to indicate that direct leakage of fluid from the blood contributes to the water content of the mucous blanket and the humidification of the inspired air.

Humidification has been demonstrated to have a significant effect on the gas exchange in the lower airways. In one study comparing nasal to mouth breathing, the end tidal pressure of carbon dioxide (pCO_2) was found to be higher during nasal breathing.[1] This implies that nasal obstruction may lower the expiratory CO_2, thus raising the pCO_2, fostering apneic spells during sleep. A second study found that patients with nasal packing experienced a significant decrease in blood gas pressure of oxygen (pO_2) of 6.9 mm Hg.[27] In other subjects, this decrease was able to be reversed by having the patients breathe humidified air. The total capacity for the nose to humidify air was estimated to require 456 g of water for 24 hours of breathing.[28]

Filtration

The final important function of the nose is filtration of the inspired air to protect the lower airways from particulate matter in the air. By creating turbulent airflow, the nose forces all inspired air to contact a mucosal surface before passing to the lower airways. The filtering aspect of the nose occurs in two stages. The first stage is trapping of large particles in the front of the nose by the nasal vibrissae and nasal valve. This occurs by a straining action of the front of the nose on the air. The second level of filtration occurs as a result of the turbulent flow. Here, particulates impact the mucosa and stick in the mucous blanket.

The ability of the nose to filter the air was evaluated in a recent study.[29] The authors found that the front of the nose is efficient in trapping particles greater than 3 μm in size. The second phase of filtering, the nasal mucus, is effective in trapping particles between 0.5 and 3 μm in diameter. Particles smaller than 0.5 μm seem to be able to pass through the nose into the lower airways without much difficulty. The potential advantage of this process of nasal clearance is underscored by a comparison of transit times in the nose and tracheobronchial tree. Nasal mucus generally is cleared from the front of the nose to the pharynx within minutes. Saccharin clearance times probably underestimate the true clearance of mucus from the nose, but as a rough estimate, the average is usually a few minutes. This is in comparison to the transit time from the lungs, which was recently estimated to range from 2.5 to 24 hours.[30] The significantly shorter clearance time in the nose points out the improved removal of toxins from a functioning nose. This could benefit the species by decreasing the exposure to toxins and pollutants.

NASAL MUCUS

The nasal mucus is integral to the function of the nose. This specialized substance has many functions and roles. In terms of traditional nasal functions, the mucus is the means by which humidification, warming, and filtration occur. Water vaporizes from the mucous blanket into the inspired air. Heat transfer from the nasal mucosa and blood vessels is facilitated by the overlying mucus, which dissipates the heat more rapidly than a dry surface would. Finally, the mucus is responsible for capturing the filtered particles from the air and transporting the filtrate out of the nose and sinuses.

In addition to these well-known functions of the nasal mucus, the mucus also plays a vital role in immune defense of the upper airway. The mucus contains inflammatory cells that participate in regulating and triggering the immune response. Mucus also contains a variety of peptides, inflammatory mediators, and immunologic regulators that modify and control the immune response.

A final function of nasal mucus is to participate in olfaction. The nasal mucus overlying the olfactory epithelium is important in dissolving airborne olfactants into a liquid phase that can initiate the olfactory response.

Composition of Nasal Mucus

Nasal and sinus mucus normally exists in two layers on the surface of the epithelium. The deeper layer is less viscous and thinner than the outer layer. This serves the dual purpose of the mucus well. The inner layer is in direct contact with the cilia and allows the cilia to beat with less resistance. The thicker, more viscous outer layer sits on the inner layer and is better able to trap inhaled particulates and contains a greater density of inflammatory mediators and leukocytes to increase protection against foreign substances and infectious agents.

The number of leukocytes in the nasal mucus has been determined.[31] The number varies depending on the location within the sinonasal tract, level of stimulation, and disease state. A baseline, unstimulated level is typically about 5000 cells/mg of mucus. In the healthy baseline state, the cells are almost exclusively neutrophils. In patients with chronic sinusitis, the cell counts increase to about 25,000 cells/mg of mucus, with eosinophils increasing to about 5%.

The nasal mucus is basically a water-based liquid that contains a large number of dissolved components. The water component is produced by serous glands distributed throughout the mucosa. The predominant dissolved components are glycoproteins. The glycoproteins are produced by the goblet cells. These compounds are what give the mucus its viscosity and elasticity. The higher the concentration of glycoproteins, the greater the viscosity and elasticity of the mucus. Nasal and sinus mucus also contains a large number of other dissolved compounds, including antibodies, immune regulators, and neurotransmitters.

The concentration of glycoproteins and, hence, the viscosity and elasticity of mucus varies depending on the location within the sinonasal tract, the degree of stimulation of the mucosa, and the disease state of the mucosa. Stimulation of the mucosa generally results in increases in the serous component of mucus by direct stimulation of the serous glands. From the baseline, unstimulated state, the nature of the mucus can change dramatically. Consider, for example, the vasomotor response to irritants, which result in secretion of an almost water-like mucus. Allergic rhinitis can also stimulate excessive serous mucus production. Chronic sinusitis, by contrast, usually results in an increase in viscosity caused by an increase in cellular components as well as an increase in goblet cell density and glycoprotein production.[32] This subsequently results in decreased mucociliary clearance.

Production of Mucus

Mucus is a compound substance produced from various sources. The primary sources are the serous glands, which produce much of the serous component, and the goblet cells, which produce most of the glycoproteins. Based on the presence of pores in the luminal side only of the microvasculature, it has been postulated that some proportion of the water component of mucus is directly exuded from the blood. If this were the case, then all components of the serum, including antibodies, albumin, and hormones, would exist in the mucus in proportion to the serum. Finally, the leukocytes exist in the mucus and are produced by an as yet unknown mechanism. The leukocytes may be directly exuded from the blood and may be attracted to the mucous blanket by chemotactic factors in the mucus. Alternatively, there may be specific sources of theses inflammatory cells within the mucosa, comparable to the Peyer's patches found in the small bowel mucosa.

A portion of mucus production is clearly under autonomic neural control. The mucosa contains both sensory and effector nerves that create a feedback loop to enhance control. At the basal state, production of mucus is maintained by a low level of parasympathetic stimulation to the serous glands, as wells as by baseline function of the goblet cells. However, in response to stimulation, the parasympathetic nerves activate the serous glands, resulting in increased production of serous mucus.

A number of potential irritants can lead to parasympathetic stimulation. Direct mechanical or chemical irritation of the mucosa is perceived as a nocioceptive stimulus by the sensory neurons in the mucosa. This leads to a brain stem reflex that increases serous mucus production. On the contrary, there are many pharmacologic agents in use that have an anticholinergic action. These agents (e.g., antihistamines) block the parasympathetic baseline stimulation of the serous glands through inhibition of the acetylcholine-dependent nerve terminals of the parasympathetic nerves in the glands. These agents have as a property a secondary anticholinergic action that results in blockage of the serous gland production of mucus, with thickening and drying of the nasal secretions. The allergic response itself has a direct effect on the production of mucus. This is covered in detail in Chapter 6.

CILIARY FUNCTION

Central to the function of the nose is the activity of the cilia. The cilia on the surface of the epithelium beat constantly to move the mucous blanket on a specific path. This activity is referred to as mucociliary clearance and is essential for normal health of the nose and sinuses. The cilia move the mucus out of the sinuses to prevent stasis of the mucus in the sinuses; in doing so, all the toxic and infectious material trapped in the mucus is moved out of the sinuses and nose. All of the functions of the nose and sinuses depend on adequate ciliary function for normal and healthy operation.

Ciliary Anatomy

The cilia of the respiratory epithelium of the nose and sinuses emerge from the luminal surface of the normal healthy columnar epithelial cell. Each cell has numerous cilia protruding from the surface of the cell and anchored just inside the outer cell membrane. The classic ciliary structure consists of a long axoneme, with a 9 + 2 pattern of microtubule doublets (Fig. 2–1).[33] Just inside the outer membrane of the cilia is a ring of nine pairs of microtubules, which are connected to each adjoining pair by nexin links. In the center of the ring are two pairs of microtubules surrounded by a central sheath. The outer microtubules are connected to the central sheath by radial spokes. Extending from one side of each outer doublet is a dynein arm that contains

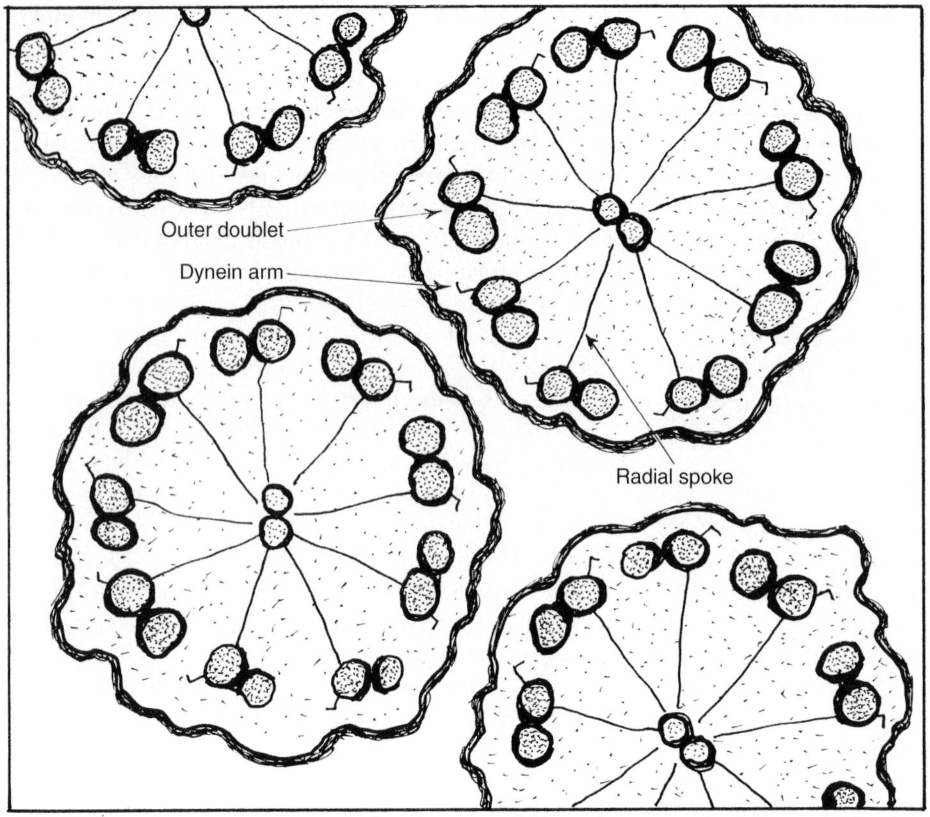

Figure 2–1. Cross-sectional anatomy of human cilia. Nine outer doublets are connected to a single inner doublet by radial spokes. The outer dynein arms contain the energy-utilizing adenosine triphosphatase.

the adenosine triphosphatase activity supplying energy to create ciliary motion.

This classic pattern is necessary for normal ciliary function. Numerous defects in the normal structure have been described that lead to some degree of ciliary dysfunction. These abnormalities can be classified into primary or acquired defects. The most well known of the primary ciliary defects is the lack of outer dynein arms found in Kartagener's syndrome. Other primary ciliary dyskinesias may be caused by abnormalities in the organization of the microtubules or absence of the radial spokes. The abnormalities in acquired ciliary dyskinesias are nonspecific and variable. The most common is the finding of compound cilia. This abnormality occurs when multiple axonemes are surrounded by a common ciliary sheath.

Mucociliary Clearance

Human nasal cilia have been widely studied to determine aspects of function that might impact clinical care. The earliest studies of the modern era were conducted in the 1930s by Proetz, who photo-documented ciliary activity for the first time.[31,35] Later, Hilding described the mucus clearance patterns from the sinuses and nose.[36] These studies have been confirmed repeatedly until now it is a scientific dogma that the mucus clearance patterns of the nose and sinuses are specific and highly conserved. Figures 2–2 and 2–3 demonstrate the patterns described by Hilding in his original work.

In all cases, the mucus moves in the direction of the natural ostia of the sinuses, albeit not necessarily in a straight line. For the frontal sinuses, this is exemplified by the movement of mucus unidirectionally through the ostium from only the lateral side of the ostium. Mucus from the medial side of the ostium must course around the ostium to join the flow of mucus from the lateral side. Both the sphenoid and maxillary sinuses drain in an antigravitational direction. This quirk of development may be related to the direction of aeration of the sinus into the maxilla during development, such that the sinus enlarges into the bone in an inferior direction from the ostium.

It is also well documented that alteration of the anatomy of the sinuses may disrupt the flow of mucus, but ultimately will not tend to alter the direction of the flow toward the original position of the natural ostium. This can be demonstrated by the creation of an inferior nasal antral window, which will ultimately drain only by gravity and will overflow if the natural ostium is not patent. This principle is similarly highlighted by the circuitous motion of mucus after a misplaced surgical antrostomy. In this situation, a surgical antrostomy is placed posterior to the natural ostium of the maxillary sinus but not

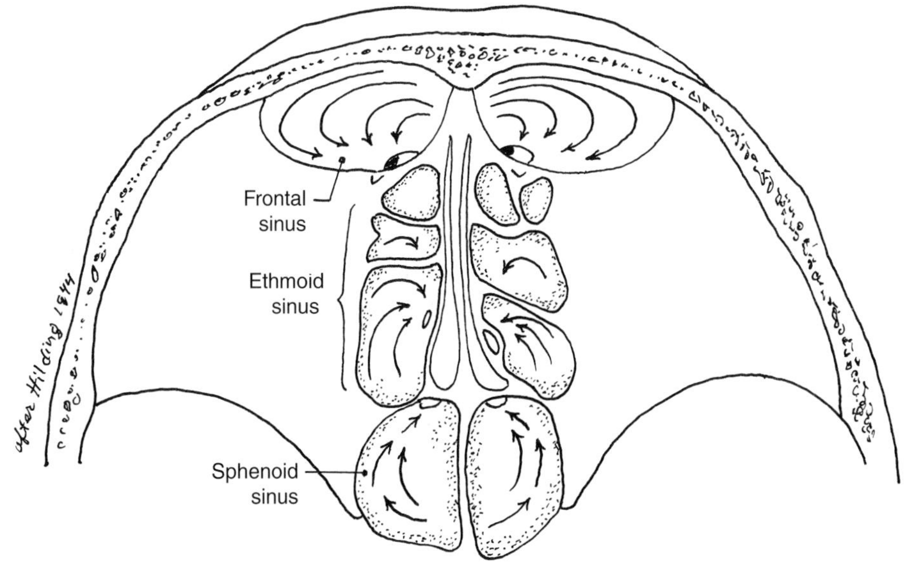

Figure 2–2. Mucociliary clearance patterns of the frontal, ethmoid, and sphenoid sinuses as described by Hilding.[36] Mucus flow is unidirectional and eventually courses toward the natural ostium of the sinus.

connected to the natural ostium. If the natural ostium is patent, the mucus may flow out of the natural ostium and back into the sinus through the surgical ostium, only to circle back to the natural ostium once again.

The pattern of mucus clearance in the nose is always toward the posterior choanae. This is true for all secretions from anywhere within the nose. The mucus from the anterior sinuses exits into the middle meatus and then courses over the inferior turbinate to the nasopharynx anterior to the eustachian tube. The mucus from the posterior sinuses exits into the superior meatus and then courses over the middle turbinate to the nasopharynx posterior to the eustachian tube. Mucus from the floor of the nose courses along the floor directly to the nasopharynx.

Measurement of Ciliary Clearance

There are three separate techniques described for measurement of ciliary activity in vivo. The simplest method is the saccharin test. In this test, a small pellet of artificial sweetener (saccharin) is placed in the front of the nose. As the pellet dissolves, the saccharin is carried back to the nasopharynx and then into the oropharynx, where

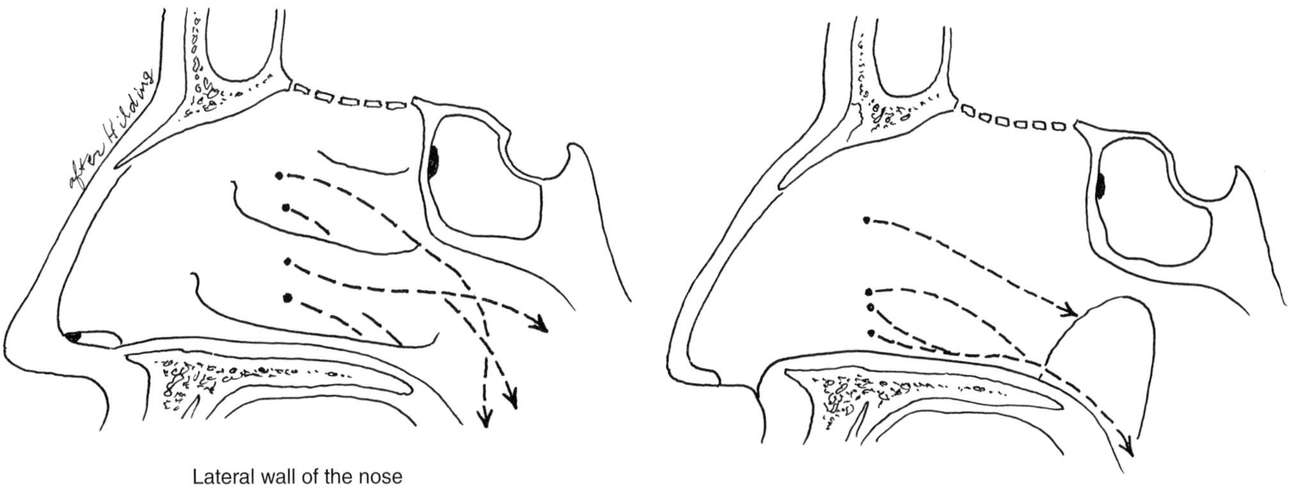

Figure 2–3. Mucociliary clearance patterns of the lateral wall of the nose and septum. This diagram indicates that mucus from the middle meatus courses both anterior and posterior to the eustachian tube, whereas mucus from the superior meatus courses anterior to the eustachian tube. This is contrary to theories accepted today, but is illustrated as shown in the original diagrams by Hilding.[36]

an ultrasweet taste is detected. Normal transport times are less than 20 minutes, with most patients detecting the taste within 10 minutes. A similar test utilizes a small droplet of marker dye, such as methylene blue, which is placed into the front of the nose. The oropharynx is then observed for evidence of the dye color. Again this is usually seen within 20 minutes. This test is more objective than the saccharin test because it does not rely on the perceptions of the patient; however, it is less precise as the oropharynx cannot be observed continuously for up to 20 minutes to detect the dye.

The newest alternative is probably the best of all methods, but it is the most time-consuming and expensive. This procedure relies on the movement of a radioisotope and its detection in the nasopharynx by a radioisotope scanner. This technique allows measurement of mucus movement, which is determined in millimeters of movement per minute. The average movement in a series of normal adults was 9.0 mm/min.[37] Clinically, this test has little utility, but it may be useful as a research tool.

Alteration of Ciliary Function

Ciliary beat frequency (CBF) is a commonly reported measure of ciliary function in animal and human tissue investigation. Although CBF is normally evaluated in vitro using tissue biopsies, in vivo measurement has also been reported.[38] Most studies that evaluate CBF use a photoelectric cell to determine the rate of cilia movement. The normal rate is generally found to be in the range of 750 to 800 ciliary beats/min. This value can change depending on the study, tissue, and species evaluated.

Pharmacologic agents have been well studied. Beta-adrenergic and alpha-adrenergic stimulants have been found to increase the CBF.[39, 40] In one study, terbutaline, a beta-adrenergic agonist, caused a statistically significant increase in CBF. In another study, phenylephrine was reported to increase the CBF in vivo and in vitro in humans. Interestingly, in a separate study, the cholinergic agonist methacholine was found to increase CBF through activation of M1 and M3 muscarinic receptors.[41] Normally, the adrenergic and cholinergic effects on a system are opposite, leading to questions of the true regulation of CBF in human nasal and sinus mucosa.

CBF measurements have been investigated in the presence of infection. In one study, chronic sinusitis was found to have no effect on the CBF of affected patients if patients with no ciliary function were excluded.[42] An opposing study found decreased rates of ciliary function, as well as a reduced ciliated area, in the mucosa of patients with chronic sinusitis.[43] The difference in the studies points out the ongoing controversy in determining the true effect of infection on the ciliary function. The author's clinical experience suggests that there are some individuals who appear to have lost the ability to clear mucous secretions. These patients with severe sinus infection may have lost sufficient ciliary density to lose all function, despite the potential increased CBF in those cilia remaining.

IMMUNE SYSTEM

The immune system of the nose and sinuses is poorly understood. Research is just beginning to address the issues of how the immune system reacts to challenges and how this response is regulated. The components of this system are the cellular and humoral immune systems. The baseline immune system consists of two components. The first is the presence of lymphocytes, mast cells, eosinophils, and basophils scattered throughout the mucosa. These cells are found within the subepithelial layer of all areas of the mucosa of the nose and sinuses. These immune cells generally occur in low densities in uninflamed states. Their number has been determined to be in the range of 15 to 25 cells/high-power field (HPF) using standard histologic analysis of surgical specimens.[44] However, the density can increase dramatically in infection. In certain patients, counts approaching 300 cells/HPF have been observed. This wide variability is attributable to the response of the immune system to the infection present. Presumably, the presence of infection stimulates some of these cells to produce chemotactic factors that recruit additional cells from the blood to migrate through the capillaries into the mucosa. Alternatively, some of the cells may be stem cells that can divide and populate the mucosa. This is less likely to be an important contribution.

The second component of the baseline immune system is found in the conglomeration of lymphocytes into subepithelial nodes or patches. In rabbits, these exist in the floor of the nose, in the nasopharynx, and in certain areas within the sinus and nasal mucosa.[45] In humans, the nasopharyngeal lymphoid tissue is the well-known adenoid pad. Whether there are lymphoid patches in the normal human nose equivalent to those found in the rabbit has yet to be determined.

Both the humoral and cellular immune responses must be initiated through cells residing in the subepithelial layer. Here, the initial response leads to release of inflammatory mediators that result in the cascade of events that is the immune response. Part of this response is the immunoglobulin E (IgE)–mediated immediate hypersensitivity response, or the allergic response. This is detailed in Chapter 6.

OLFACTION

Olfactory Epithelium

The sense of smell is generated from the unique olfactory epithelium. This specialized sensory organ lies in the roof of the nose on either side of the nasal septum overlying the cribriform plate. The total area of the olfactory epithelium is approximately 1 cm^2 on each side. The mucosa has a pseudostratified columnar histologic structure that is two to three times the normal thickness of the surrounding respiratory mucosa. There are four types of cells found in the olfactory epithelium: bipolar olfactory receptor cells, supporting cells, basal cells, and microvillar cells.

The olfactory bipolar receptors are long fusiform cells that perforate the nasal lumen and contain nonmotile cilia. The cells taper to a thin axon that penetrates the lamina propria. Here, the axons are grouped together and bound by Schwann cells into 15 to 20 nerves that perforate the cribriform plate and ascend into the olfactory bulb. Within the olfactory bulb, the nerves separate and synapse with secondary neurons that form the olfactory tracts. The microvillar cells are similar to the bipolar receptor cells, with a tuft of microvilli that protrudes into the mucous blanket and a thin, axonlike projection that enters the lamina propria. Whether these less common cells are functional receptors is not yet fully known.

The supporting cells are situated between the olfactory receptor cells, forming tight junctions with the receptor cells and each other at the mucosal surface. These cells lie on a layer of basal cells that sit on the lamina papyracea. The basal cells can differentiate into either supporting cells or receptor cells to replace lost receptors.

Olfactory Transduction and Coding

Through an explosion in molecular studies of olfaction, the basic steps in odor reception, transduction, and coding are becoming clear. Although there is much yet to be learned, it seems almost certain that odor identification occurs through specific binding of odorants to specific G protein–coupled receptors in the olfactory bipolar cells.[46–48] Odorants are carried to the olfactory epithelium through inspired air that is forced into the nasal roof by turbulent nasal airflow. The odorants dissolve into the mucus over the olfactory epithelium and are carried to the receptor terminals on the bipolar neurons.

On the surface of the bipolar neurons are many different specific binding proteins. These proteins are regulated by a large group of genes controlling olfactory receptor production. There is now increasing evidence that degeneration of olfactory ability in higher-order mammals and primates is related to the accumulation of mutations in these genes, leading to inactivation of this receptor type.[49] The receptors most likely are arranged in specific patterns that allow activation of spatially specific neurons synapsing within specific locations within the olfactory bulb and higher levels of the brain.[50]

The olfactory binding proteins are found coupled to a G-type protein. This implies a second messenger system that is activated upon binding of the specific odorant. Both cyclic adenosine monophosphate (cAMP) and phosphoinositide are probable second messengers that may eventually lead to changes in calcium influx, thereby contributing to depolarization.[51] The exact details of the steps from binding to depolarization are still under study. However, it is likely that continued research in this area will soon elucidate much of this pathway, perhaps even by the time this textbook is published.

Olfactory Recognition

Although molecular biologists have been the ones to dissect the mechanisms involved in signal transduction, psychologists and neurophysiologists have contributed much to our understanding of the way in which the sense of smell works in humans. Whereas prior generations of investigators relied on smell testing and identification, current research utilizes objective measures, such as evoked potential recordings, magnetic resonance imaging, and positron emission tomography (PET).[52–56]

These studies have elucidated many interesting findings. Using evoked potentials in human volunteers, Tateyama et al. found that wave amplitude (i.e., strength of the response) and wave latency (time to response) were increased for higher odorant concentrations.[57] Using perceptual thresholds, Betchen and Doty determined that the left and right sides of the nose do not systematically differ in odorant sensitivity.[58] Several authors have found that olfactory acuity declines with increasing age,[56, 59–61] whereas others have documented the nature and importance of neonatal olfaction.[62, 63] Finally, several studies have begun to investigate the processing of complex sensory input. Small et al. used PET scanning to evaluate the differences between taste, smell, and flavor. They found that flavor processing is not merely a convergence of smell and taste, but a separate processing pattern that involves different brain locations.[64] Sobel and colleagues have reported that the active process of sniffing and the resultant perception of odor utilize different parts of the brain.[65] These findings underscore the complexity of the sense of smell and the tremendous impact it has on our daily lives.

REFERENCES

1. Tanaka Y, Morikawa T, Honda Y. An assessment of nasal functions in control of breathing. J Appl Physiol 65(4):1520, 1988.
2. Tos M. Factors influencing the goblet cell density in paranasal sinuses. Acta Otolaryngol 458:17, 1988.
3. Lund VJ. Nasal physiology: Neurochemical receptors, nasal cycle, and ciliary action. Allergy Asthma Proc 17(4):179, 1996.

4. Riederer A, Fischer A, Knipping S, et al. Basic innervation pattern and distribution of classic autonomic neurotransmitters in human nasal mucosal vasculature. Laryngoscope 106:286, 1996.
5. Baraniuk JN. Neuropeptides. Am J Rhinol 12(1):9, 1998.
6. Ramis I, Lorente J, Rosello-Catafau J, et al. Differential activity of nitric oxide synthase in human nasal mucosa and polyps. Eur Respir J 9:202, 1996.
7. Furukawa K, Harrison DG, Saleh D, et al. Expression of nitric oxide synthase in the human nasal mucosa. Am J Respir Crit Care Med 153:847, 1996.
8. Abel-Jan T, Bogotzki B, Heppt W, Hauser-Kronberger C, Fischer A. Nitric oxide synthase in the innervation of the human nasal mucosa: Correlation with neuropeptides and tyrosine hydroxylase. Laryngoscope 108:128, 1998.
9. Hauser-Kronberger C, Hacker GW, Muss W, et al. Autonomic and peptidergic innervation of human nasal mucosa. Acta Otolaryngol 113:387, 1993.
10. Rosbe KW, Mims JW, Prazma J, et al. Immunohistochemical localization of nitric oxide synthase activity in upper respiratory epithelium. Laryngoscope 106:1075, 1996.
11. Watanabe H, Tsuru H, Kawanoto H, et al. Nitroxidergic vasodilator nerves in the canine nasal mucosa. Life Sci 57:PL109, 1995.
12. Lundberg JO, Rinder J, Weitzberg F, Alving K, Lundberg JM. Heavy physical exercise decreases nitric oxide levels in the nasal airways in humans. Acta Physiol Scand 159(1):51, 1997.
13. Eccles R. A role for the nasal cycle in respiratory defense. Eur Respir J 9(2):371, 1996.
14. Flanagan P, Eccles R. Spontaneous changes of unilateral nasal airflow in man. A re-examination of the 'nasal cycle.' Acta Otolaryngol (Stockh) 117(4)590, 1997.
15. Heetderks DR. Observation on the reaction of normal nasal mucous membrane. Am J Med Sci 174:231, 1927.
16. Stoksted P. The physiologic cycle of the nose under normal and pathologic conditions. Acta Otolaryngol (Stockh) 42:175, 1952.
17. Flanagan P, Eccles R. Physiological versus pharmacological decongestion of the nose in healthy human subjects. Acta Otolaryngol (Stockh) 118(l):110, 1998.
18. Mirza N, Kroger H, Doty RL. Influence of age on the 'nasal cycle.' Laryngoscope 107(l):62, 1997.
19. Paulsson B, Gredmark T, Burian P, Berde M. Nasal mucosal congestion during the menstrual cycle. J Laryngol Otol 111(4): 337, 1997.
20. Shannahoff-Khalsa DS, Kennedy B, Yates FE, Ziegler MG. Ultradian rhythms of autonomic, cardiovascular, and neuroendocrine systems are related in humans. Am J Physiol 270(4 Pt 2):R873, 1996.
21. Bende M. Blood flow with 133Xe in human nasal mucosa in relation to age, sex and body position. Acta Otolaryngol 96: 175, 1983.
22. Latvala JJ, Reijula KE, Clifford PS, Rintamaki HE. Cold-induced responses in the upper respiratory tract. Arctic Med Res 54(1)4, 1995.
23. Yuasa T. Stereographic demonstration of the nasal cavity of the rat with reference to the density of blood vessels. Kaibogaku Zasshi 66(3):191, 1991.
24. White MD, Cabanac M. Nasal mucosal vasodilatation in response to passive hyperthermia in humans. Eur J Appl Physiol 70(3): 207, 1995.
25. Drettner B, Kumlien J. Experimental studies of the human nasal air-conditioning capacity. Acta Otolaryngol 91(5–6):605, 1981.
26. Grevers G. The role of fenestrated vessels for the secretory process in the nasal mucosa: A histological and transmission electron microscopic study in the rabbit. Laryngoscope 103(11 Pt 1): 1255, 1993.
27. Woodson GE, Robbins KT. Nasal obstruction and pulmonary function: The role of humidification. Otolaryngol Head Neck Surg 93(4):505, 1985.
28. Simon H, Drettner B, Falk B. A clinical method of testing the humidifying capacity of the human nose. Laryngol Rhinol Otol 55(12):968, 1976.
29. Schwab JA, Zenkel M. Filtration of particulates in the human nose. Laryngoscope 108(1 Pt 1):120, 1998.
30. Lippmann M, Schlesinger RB. Interspecies comparisons of particle deposition and mucociliary clearance in tracheobronchial airways. J Toxicol Environ Health 13(2–3):441, 1984.
31. Janowski R, Coffinet L, Audouy H, Foliguet B. Leukocyte compartments in the nasal secretion medium. Rhinology 33:203, 1995.
32. Majima Y, Sakakura Y, Hattori M, Hirata K. Rheologic properties of nasal mucus from patients with chronic sinusitis. Am J Rhinol 7(5):217, 1993.
33. McAuley JR, Anand VK. Clinical significance of compound cilia. Otolaryngol Head Neck Surg 118(5):685, 1998.
34. Proetz AW. Motion picture demonstration of ciliary action and other factors in nasal physiology. Trans Am Laryngol Assoc 59: 269, 1932.
35. Proetz AW. Nasal ciliated epithelium, with special reference to infection and treatment. J Laryngol Otol 557, 1934.
36. Hilding AC. The physiology of drainage of nasal mucus. Ann Otolaryngol 53:35, 1944.
37. Karja J, Nuutinen J, Parjalainen P. Radioisotopic method for measurement of nasal mucociliary activity. Arch Otolaryngol 108:99, 1982.
38. Lindberg S, Runer T. Method for in vivo measurement of mucociliary activity in the human nose. Ann Otol Rhinol Laryngol 103: 558, 1994.
39. Phillips PP, McCaffrey TV, Kern EB. The in vivo and in vitro effect of phenylephrine (Neo Synephrine) on nasal ciliary beat frequency and mucociliary transport. Otolaryngol Head Neck Surg 103(4):558, 1990.
40. Ohashi Y, Nakai Y, Zushi K, et al. Enhancement of ciliary action by a β-adrenergic stimulant. Acta Otolaryngol [Suppl] 397:49, 1983.
41. Yang B, McCaffrey T. The roles of muscarinic receptor subtypes in modulation of nasal ciliary action. Rhinology 34:136, 1996.
42. Nuutinen J, Rauch-Toskala E, Saano V, Joki S. Ciliary beating frequency in chronic sinusitis. Arch Otolaryngol Head Neck Surg 119:645, 1993.
43. Saito H, Tsubokawa T. Ciliary activity of nasal polyp and mucosa in chronic sinusitis. Am J Rhinol 5(6):215, 1991.
44. Goldwyn BG, Sakr WA, Marks SC. Histopathological analysis of chronic sinusitis. J Rhinol 9(1):27, 1995.
45. Marks SC. Acute sinusitis in the rabbit: Histologic analysis. Laryngoscope 108:320, 1998.
46. Carver EA, Issel-Tarver L, Rine J, et al. Location of mouse and human genes corresponding to conserved canine olfactory receptor gene subfamilies. Mamm Genome 9(5):349, 1998.
47. Breer H, Wanner I, Strotmann J. Molecular genetics of mammalian olfaction. Behav Genet 26(3):209, 1996.
48. Griff IC, Reed RR. The genetics of olfaction. Curr Opin Genet Dev 5(5)657, 1995.
49. Rouquier S, Friedman C, Delettre L, et al. A gene recently inactivated in human defines a new olfactory receptor family in mammals. Hum Molec Genet 7(9):1337, 1998.
50. Laurent G. Olfactory processing: Maps, time and codes. Curr Opin Neurobiol 7(4):547, 1997.
51. Bruch RC. Phosphoinositide second messengers in olfaction. Comp Biochem Physiol (B) 113(3):451, 1996.
52. Zald DH, Donndelinger MJ, Pardo JV. Elucidating dynamic brain interactions with across-subjects correlation analyses of positron emission tomographic data: The functional connectivity of the amygdala and orbitofrontal cortex during olfactory tasks. J Cereb Blood Flow Metab 18(8):896, 198.
53. Sobel N, Prabhakaran V, Desmend JE, et al. A method for functional magnetic resonance imaging of olfaction. J Neurosci Methods 78(1–2):115, 1997.
54. Levy LM, Henkin RI, Hutter A, et al. Functional MRI of human olfaction. J Comput Assist Tomogr 21(6):849, 1997.
55. Ishimaru T, Shimada T, Sakunoto M, et al. Olfactory evoked potential produced by electrical stimulation of the human olfactory mucosa. Chem Senses 22(1):77, 1997.
56. Evans WJ, Cui L, Starr A. Olfactory event-related potentials in normal human subjects: Effects of age and gender. Electroencephalogr Clin Neurophysiol 95(4):293, 1995.
57. Tateyama T, Hummel T, Roscher S, Post M, Kobal G. Relation of olfactory event-related potentials to changes in stimulus concentration. Electroencephalogr Clin Neurophysiol 108(5):449, 1998.
58. Betchen SA, Doty RI. Bilateral detection thresholds in dextrals and sinistrals reflect the more sensitive side of the nose, which is not lateralized. Chem Senses 23(4):453, 1998.
59. Doty RI. Studies of human olfaction from the University of Pennsylvania Smell and Taste Center. Chem Senses 22(5):565, 1997.

60. Hummel T, Bartz S, Pauli E, Kobal G. Chemosensory event-related potentials change with age. Electroencephalogr Clin Neurophysiol 108(2):208, 1998.
61. Barber CF. Olfactory acuity as a function of age and gender: A comparison of African and American samples. Int J Aging Hum Dev 44(4):317, 1997.
62. Mennella JA, Beauchamp GK. Early flavor experiences: Research update. Nutr Rev 56(7):205, 1998.
63. Marlier L, Schall B, Soussignan R. Neonatal responsiveness to the odor of amniotic and lacteal fluids: A test of perinatal chemosensory continuity. Child Dev 69(3):611, 1998.
64. Small DM, Jones-Gotman M, Zatorre RJ, Petride SM, Evans AC. Flavor processing: More than the sum of its parts. Neuroreport 8(18):3913, 1997.
65. Sobel N, Prabhakaran V. Sniffing and smelling: Separate subsystems in the human olfactory cortex. Nature 392(6673):282, 1998.

CHAPTER 3

Radiology of the Nose and Sinuses

This chapter is co-authored by Jeffrey Wilseck, D.O. His expertise in imaging the nose and sinuses has been relied on, not only in writing this chapter, but also in the author's daily practice of medicine. It is essential for all rhinologists to be able to read and interpret their patients' imaging studies so that they can make sound clinical decisions and so that any surgical procedures are appropriately guided. It is also important for the rhinologist to enlist the aid of an individual radiologist in the hospital or community who can help interpret difficult cases and assist with important clinical judgments. Such a partnership helps both specialists to improve their skills, and ultimately will benefit patients.

This chapter is organized into sections covering the use of imaging to diagnose and guide surgical therapy of the nose and sinuses. In each section, important issues of concern are addressed, along with the role of each imaging modality.

IMAGING MODALITIES

Standard Radiographs (Plain Films)

The conventional paranasal sinus examination remains of value in cases of acute sinusitis and as the initial mode of evaluation for subacute sinusitis. The conventional paranasal sinus examination usually consists of the following radiographic views: Caldwell (posteroanterior), Waters (occipitomental), lateral, and submental vertex (basal) views.

The Caldwell view is used to visualize the frontal and ethmoid sinuses, whereas the Waters view provides the best projection for visualizing the maxillary sinuses. The lateral view is used to evaluate the anterior and posterior walls of the frontal, maxillary, and sphenoid sinuses. The submental view provides an axial view of the maxillary sinuses and their walls, in addition to helping to visualize the ethmoid and sphenoid sinuses. All images should be obtained with the patient in an erect position so that air-fluid levels may be demonstrated.

The plain film examination is limited in the amount of information it can provide. As stated, this study is useful in cases of acute or subacute inflammation. In such situations, radiographic evidence of an air-fluid level or complete opacification of a sinus can help confirm the diagnosis. However, discrepancies may be seen between plain film and computed tomography (CT) imaging studies, especially in cases of chronic inflammation. Such discrepancies may involve an inability to visualize subtle periosteal reaction, misinterpretation of infection versus neoplasm, and an inability to visualize inflammatory or neoplastic spread into the orbit, pterygopalatine fossa, infratemporal fossa, or intracranial cavity.

Computed Tomography (CT) Scans

CT scans provide the best anatomic images for evaluating the paranasal sinuses. Direct coronal imaging optimally displays the complex anatomy of the osteomeatal unit (OMU), the sphenoethmoidal recess, and paranasal sinuses. Direct coronal imaging is especially well suited for the radiologic evaluation of the paranasal sinuses owing to the similar anatomic appearance seen with both imaging and endoscopy. The OMU, a critical area in functional endoscopic sinus surgery, is optimally visualized in the direct coronal plane, as are the bony and soft tissue structures of the sphenoethmoidal recess.

The optimal imaging technique consists of direct coronal images obtained with the patient in the prone position and the head hyperextended (Fig. 3–1). This position allows fluid to move to a dependent position in the sinuses, away from the critical structures of the OMU. Supine coronal images may also be obtained in

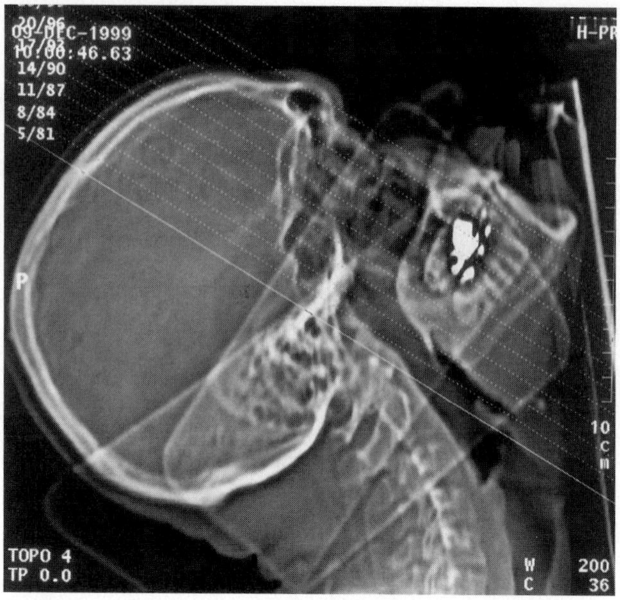

Figure 3–1. CT topogram. The coronal topogram shows the patient in a prone position with the head hyperextended. The imaging plane is perpendicular to the infraorbital meatal angle.

patients who cannot maintain hyperextension of the head, but it must be recognized that fluid may layer into the ethmoid infundibulum, potentially obscuring a polyp or a focus of mucoperiosteal thickening. An alternative approach for patients who cannot tolerate the hyperextended or head-hanging position for direct coronal imaging is spiral imaging (Fig. 3–2). This approach images the sinuses volumetrically at 3-mm slice collimation in the axial plane, with reconstruction every 1.5 mm. Coronal reformations can be processed using volumetric axial data. Although the direct coronal images show better bony detail, reformations are believed to display the OMU adequately.

The optimal angle for scanning in the coronal plane is perpendicular to the canthomeatal line, but the exact angle of scanning is not critical for optimal visualization of the structures of the OMU. This is an important point that allows the imager to vary the coronal angle slightly to help avoid dental amalgam streak artifact. The slice thickness of the coronal scan appears to be the critical factor for optimal visualization in the OMU. The optimal thickness appears to be 3-mm contiguous slices obtained from the nose to the back of the sphenoid sinus. Low-milliampere technique, using 150 to 300 mA, keeps the radiation dose to a minimum. The field of view ranges from 160 to 200 mm. When filming these images, some authors advocate the use of a single intermediate window (2500w/250c - window width/window level). This screening technique, especially the single intermediate window with dedicated soft tissue or bone window settings, has generated considerable debate about the possibility of missing pathologic processes, including intracranial disease related or unrelated to sinus inflammatory disease. The author also obtains a set of images optimized for soft tissue evaluation. The soft

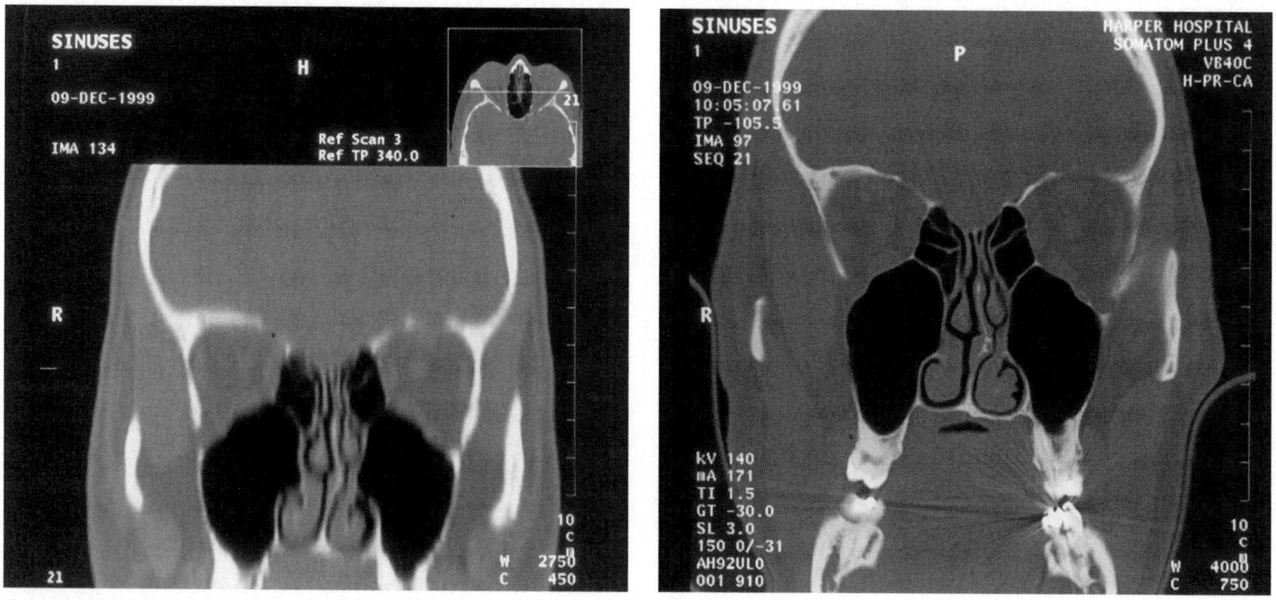

A B

Figure 3–2. *A,* Coronal reformation through the sinuses. The maxillary and ethmoid sinuses are clear. There is a septal deviation to the left. The bony details of the ethmoid septa are poorly defined. *B,* Direct coronal image at the same position. The coronal image shows superior bony definition.

tissue technique allows improved evaluation of mucosal debris, microcalcification, and incidental intracranial pathology. When inflammatory sinus disease is studied pre-endoscopically, intravenous contrast medium is not utilized.

Sinus CT technique is different for patients who are acutely ill or are suspected of having a complication of sinusitis, or when malignant disease of the paranasal sinus or nasal cavity is suspected. In these clinical settings, direct coronal images, as well as direct axial images parallel to the infraorbital meatal line, are obtained from the oral cavity to the superior aspect of the frontal sinus. On the axial images, 3- to 5-mm contiguous slice collimation is utilized, whereas 3-mm slice collimation is used for the coronal study. Both dedicated soft tissue and bone windows should be obtained.

For these indications, intravenous contrast medium is used to improve tissue contrast and specificity. Two general contrast agents are utilized: ionic and nonionic agents. The nonionic preparations, although more costly, are better tolerated by patients and are associated with a decreased incidence of adverse reactions. Intravenous contrast medium enhances normal vascular structures and accumulates in abnormal tissues with increased vascularity. This property is useful when evaluating neoplastic disease and complicated inflammatory processes. Absolute contraindications to intravenous contrast administration include previous adverse reactions and renal insufficiency, particularly in the setting of multiple myeloma or diabetes mellitus.

Magnetic Resonance Imaging (MRI)

MRI studies provide improved soft tissue contrast resolution and tissue characterization when compared with CT. Images can be produced directly in any anatomic plane with the patient remaining in a supine position. Gadolinium-based contrast agent should be used when evaluating complicated sinus disease or malignant lesions to allow improved visualization of intracranial involvement. Cortical bone produces no signal on MRI scans; thus, the thin bony plateaus of the midface are seen only by virtue of their investing mucosa. When compared to CT scans, MRI scans offer better differentiation of benign obstructed secretions from tumor extension. MRI studies also afford better differentiation of postobstructive changes in the paranasal sinuses caused by a primary obstructing mass, delineating the true extent of the mass more clearly than CT images. MRI is also better than CT scanning for visualizing subtle extradural intracranial disease. For these reasons, MRI is the imaging method of choice in the evaluation of soft tissue masses, complicated sinus inflammatory disease, and intracranial or intraorbital extension of sinus pathology.

There are several contraindications to MRI, including the presence of a metallic foreign body, intraorbital metallic fragment, pacemaker, or other electronic device. The MRI compatibility of all implanted metal devices, such as intracranial aneurysm clips, ossicular prosthetics, and the like, must be confirmed prior to placing the patient into the magnetic field.

The author's MRI protocol begins with short TR, short TE (T1-weighted) axial and coronal sequences, and a long TR, long TE (T2-weighted) axial sequence. This is followed by gadolinium contrast enhancement with repeat T1-weighted studies with chemical fat saturation and a T1-weighted coronal sequence. Fat suppression is only used in one plane after contrast administration because of the possible artifact from asymmetric fat suppression. The FOV is 180 and the matrix is 192×256 with a minimum of two acquisitions per sequence. Slice thickness is typically 3 to 4 mm. When evaluating a primary sinonasal malignant lesion, the first- or second-order lymph node groups, such as facial, retropharyngeal, submandibular, or high jugular chain nodes, are included in the imaging field because of the possibility of positive nodal involvement at presentation.

NORMAL SINUS ANATOMY

The goal of most sinus imaging is to provide a surgical road map delineating the anatomy, defining the mucosal pathology, and noting anatomic variants that may predispose the patient to operative complications. With these goals in mind, it is important to understand the complex anatomy of the lateral nasal wall, which is the key to understanding paranasal sinus drainage patterns (Figs. 3–3 through 3–5). The lateral nasal wall contains three projections. These projections are the superior, middle and inferior turbinates. The turbinates divide the superior, middle, and inferior meatus. The superior meatus drains the posterior ethmoid air cells and the sphenoid sinus (via the sphenoethmoidal recess). The middle meatus drains the frontal, maxillary, and anterior ethmoid sinuses. The inferior meatus drains the nasolacrimal duct.

The frontal sinuses are paired, often asymmetric, air cells within the frontal bone. The frontal sinuses drain via the frontal recess, which is a narrowing along the inferior medial aspect of the sinus bordered by the anterior medial portion of the middle meatus. Anterior, lateral, and inferior to the frontal recess is the agger nasi cell. This cell, which is present in nearly all patients, represents the most anterior ethmoid air cell. The agger nasi cell is the anterior floor of the frontal sinus and frontal recess. On coronal CT, it is the air cell immediately anterior to the vertical insertion of the middle turbinate, and it is located medial to the lacrimal fossa.

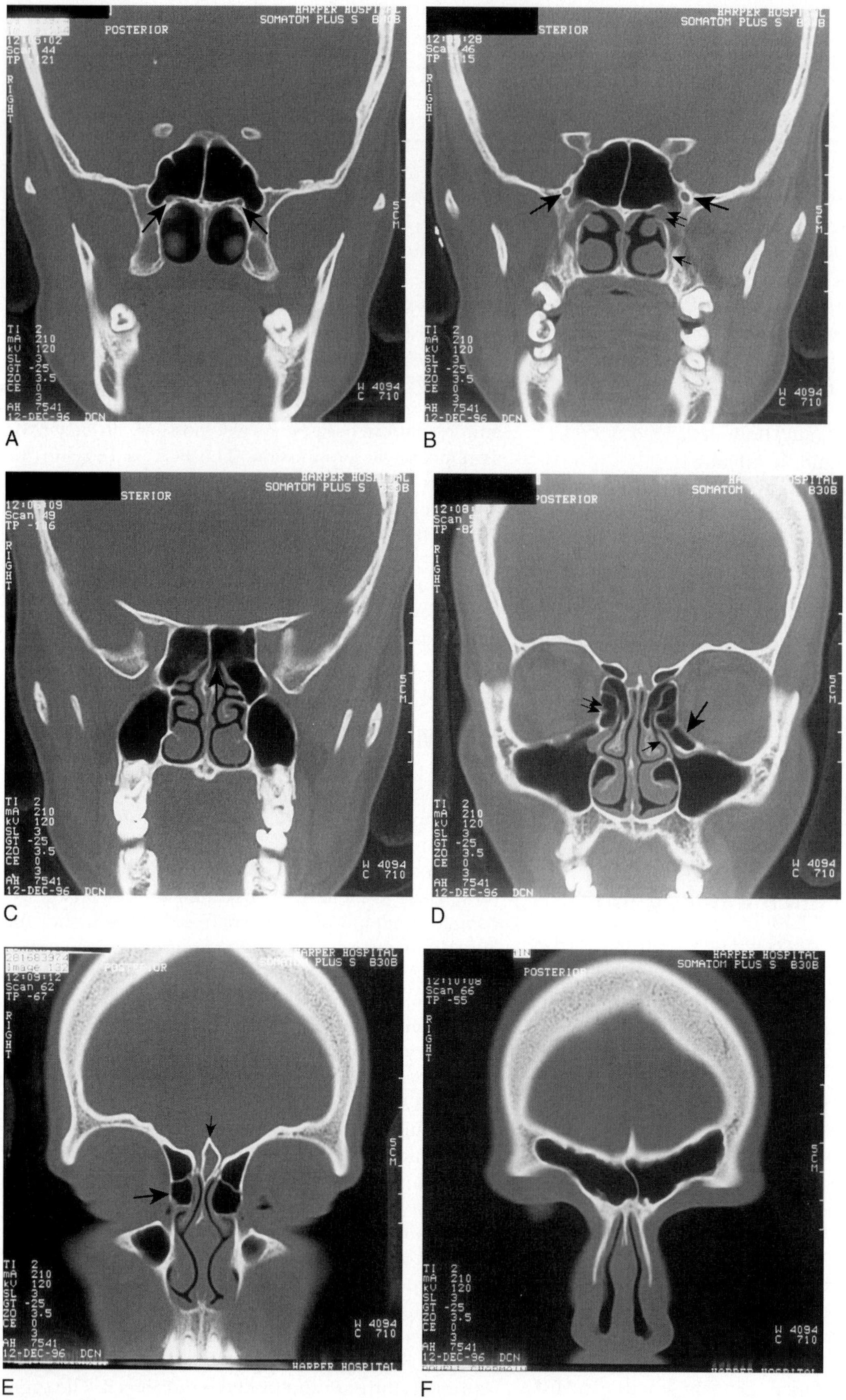

Figure 3–3. Direct coronal scans through the paranasal sinuses from posterior to anterior. *A,* Vidian canals (*arrows*). Note the bony indentation of the canals into the sphenoid sinus. *B,* Foramen rotundum (*large arrows*). The small arrow points to the greater palatine foramen entering the pterygopalatine fossa. The double arrows indicate the sphenopalatine foramen. *C,* The arrow points to the sphenoid ostium. *D,* The small arrow indicates the uncinate process. The Haller cell (*large arrow*) and ethmoid bulla (*double arrows*) are also visible. *E,* Agger nasi cell (*large arrow*). Crista galli (*small arrow*). *F,* Frontal sinus and anterior nasal septum.

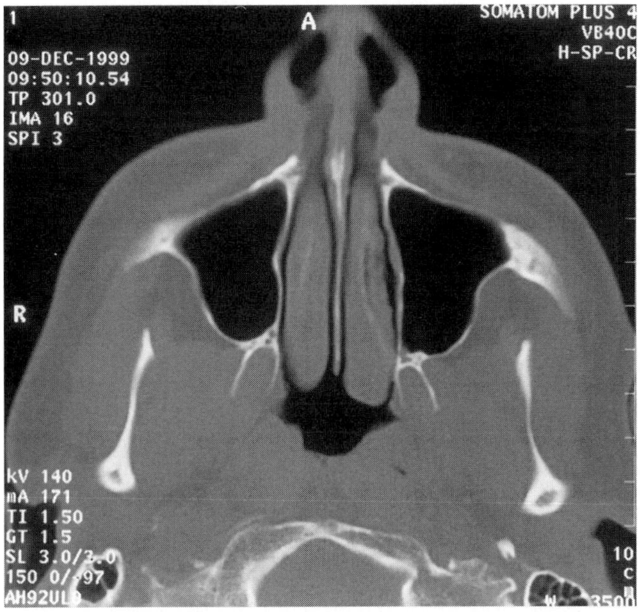

A

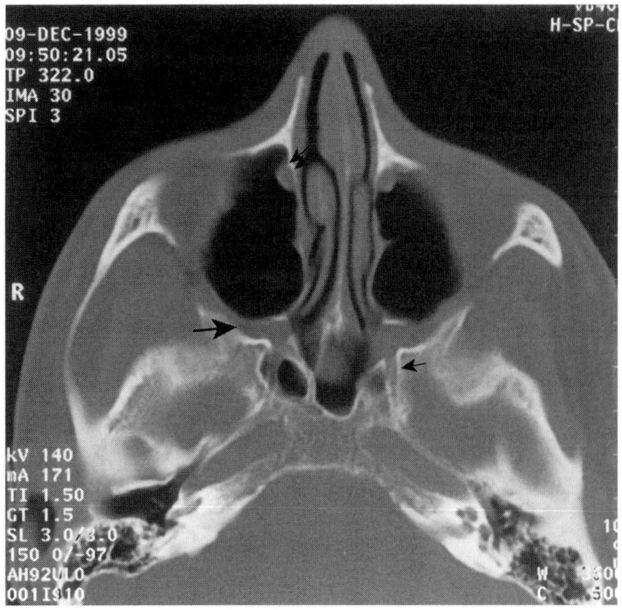

B

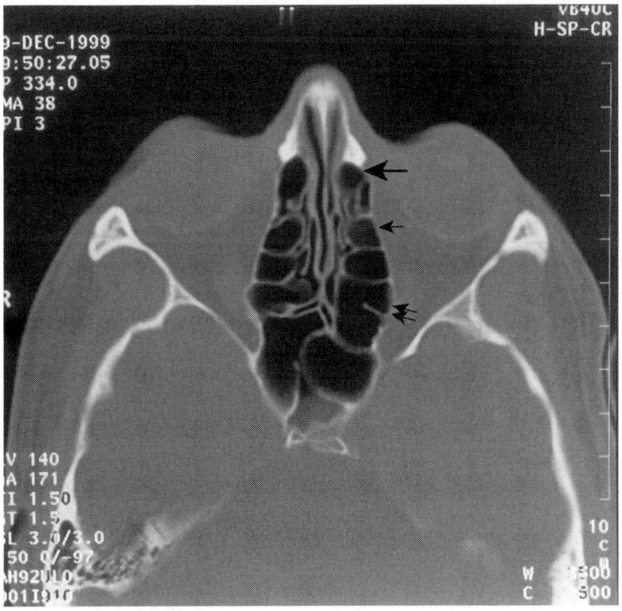

C

Figure 3–4. Axial CT images from inferior to superior. *A,* Maxillary sinuses and inferior turbinates. *B,* Pterygopalatine fossa (*large arrow*). Vidian canal (*small arrow*). Nasolacrimal duct (*double arrows*). *C,* Agger nasi cell (*large arrow*). Anterior ethmoid cells (*small arrow*). Posterior ethmoid cell (*double arrows*).

The agger nasi cell is an important endoscopic landmark.

The maxillary sinuses are paired air cells within the maxilla. The maxillary sinus drains via the maxillary ostium, located at the superior medial aspect of the sinus. This ostia drains into the infundibulum, which is located immediately lateral to the uncinate process, a superior extension of the lateral nasal wall. The lateral superior margin of the infundibulum is bordered by the ethmoid bulla. Anteriorly, the uncinate process fuses with the lacrimal bone. The superior/posterior aspect of the uncinate process is unattached, allowing the infundibulum to communicate with the middle meatus via the hiatus semilunaris (the air space between the ethmoid bulla and the superior free margin of the uncinate process). Accessory ostia are present in the medial maxillary wall in 15% to 40% of individuals.

The structure medial to the middle meatus is the middle turbinate. The middle turbinate attaches anteriorly to the medial wall of the agger nasi cell. Superiorly, the middle turbinate attaches to the lateral aspect of the cribriform plate. As the middle turbinate extends posteriorly, it has a lateral attachment, known as the basal lamella, that fuses with the lamina papyracea. The

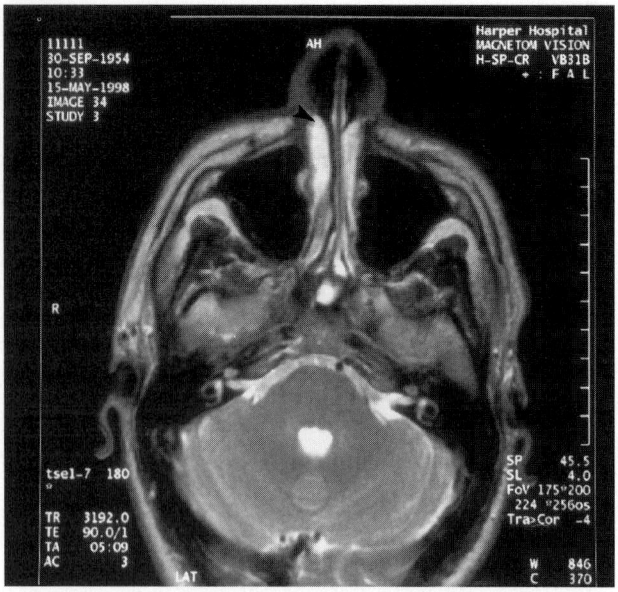

Figure 3–5. Axial T2-weighted MRI scan. The normal hyperintense signal of the nasal turbinates (*arrowhead*) is evident. Note that the osseous sinus walls cannot be directly visualized.

basal lamella demarcates the anterior ethmoid air cells from the posterior ethmoid air cells. The sinus lateralis is the air space located behind an intact ethmoid bulla and anterior to the basal lamella. The posterior ethmoid air cells and the sphenoid sinus drain into the superior meatus behind or near the superior turbinate.

The sphenoid sinuses occupy the medial sphenoid bone. The sinus is typically divided by a septum that lies near the midline anteriorly and may deviate far laterally as it extends posteriorly to divide the sinus asymmetrically. The sphenoid sinuses commonly pneumatize the base of the pterygoid plate, producing lateral recesses in 44% of patients (Fig. 3–6). The sphenoid sinus ostium is located medially in the anterosuperior portion of the anterior wall of the sphenoid sinus. This ostium opens into the sphenoethmoidal recess. This recess is located lateral to the nasal septum and is best visualized on axial images. There are several important neural and vascular anatomic structures that can abut and even indent into the sinus wall, corresponding to the location of the internal carotid artery, the second division of the fifth cranial nerve, the vidian nerve, and optic canal. These structures are at risk from sinus disease or surgical intervention.

The ethmoid sinuses have the most complex and varied drainage pattern because they arise from separate evaginations of the nasal cavity. The ethmoid sinuses are bordered medially by the nasal cavity and laterally by the lamina papyracea (the medial orbital wall). There are 3 to 18 ethmoid air cells in the adult. These cells are grouped into anterior or posterior cells, according to the location of their ostia. The anterior ethmoid air cells' ostia drain into the infundibulum or middle meatus, whereas the posterior ethmoid cells drain into the superior meatus.

ANATOMIC VARIATIONS

Middle Turbinate

Pneumatization of the middle turbinate, termed concha bullosa, is a common variant (Fig. 3–7). If the pneumat-

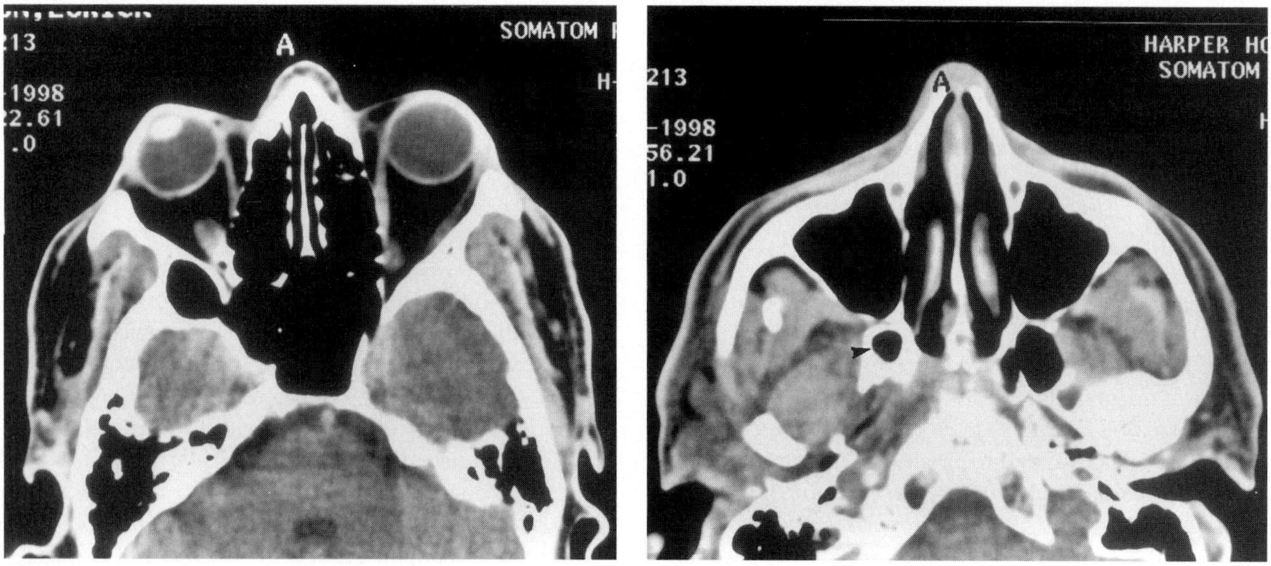

A B

Figure 3–6. Axial soft tissue windowed images. *A,* Lateral pneumatization of the sphenoid sinus. *B,* Pneumatization of the pterygoid plates (*arrowhead*).

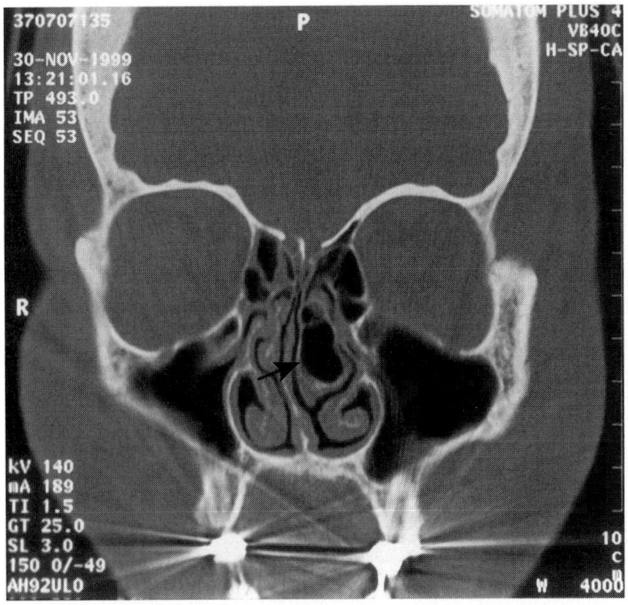

Figure 3–7. Coronal CT scan demonstrating a large concha bullosa (*arrow*) narrowing the middle meatus. Note the deviated septum to the opposite side.

ized concha is large enough, it may obstruct the region of the middle meatus, deviate the nasal septum to the contralateral side, and narrow the contralateral infundibulum. A paradoxical middle turbinate, in which the turbinate curves laterally instead of medially, is a common finding. This can lead to the turbinate encroaching on the middle meatus and infundibulum, causing functional obstruction.

Nasal Septum

Nasal septal deviation and septal spurs are also important variants, as they may prevent endoscopic access to the middle meatus. The CT scan is optimal for visualizing the bony portion of the deviation. However, the cartilaginous septum is poorly demonstrated and is seen primarily because of the enveloping mucosa. The anatomy of septal deviations is extremely variable.

Uncinate Process

Variations of the uncinate process include oblique extension toward the nasal septum and medial extension toward the ethmoid bulla. The free edge of the uncinate process can adhere to the orbital floor or the lamina papyracea. This is known as an atelectatic uncinate process. This variant is typically associated with a hypoplastic maxillary sinus. In rare cases, the uncinate may also pneumatize.

Ethmoid Cells

Haller air cells are found in 10% of the population. Also called infraorbital ethmoid cells, these are ethmoid air cells that extend along the medial orbital floor in the maxillary sinus. When they are large, they may encroach upon the infundibulum. Onodi cells are lateral and posterior extensions of the posterior ethmoid air cells. They may surround the optic nerve as it exits the back of the orbit, making this an important observation for the endoscopist. Pneumatization of the anterior clinoid process can occur (Fig. 3–8). This may result in protrusion of the optic canal into the sphenoid sinus, a condition that has been noted in about 8% of the population. The optic nerve is potentially at risk in these patients.

INFLAMMATORY CONDITIONS

Acute and Chronic Rhinosinusitis

Radiographic evidence of thickening of the sinus mucosa is not a specific indication of acute or chronic inflammatory disease. Typically, mucosal changes secondary to acute sinusitis are seen as smooth or slightly irregular soft tissue thickening within the affected sinus cavity. The presence of an air-fluid level in the absence of recent antral lavage, trauma, or barotrauma is indicative of an acute inflammatory process (Fig. 3–9). These findings must be correlated with the patient's clinical

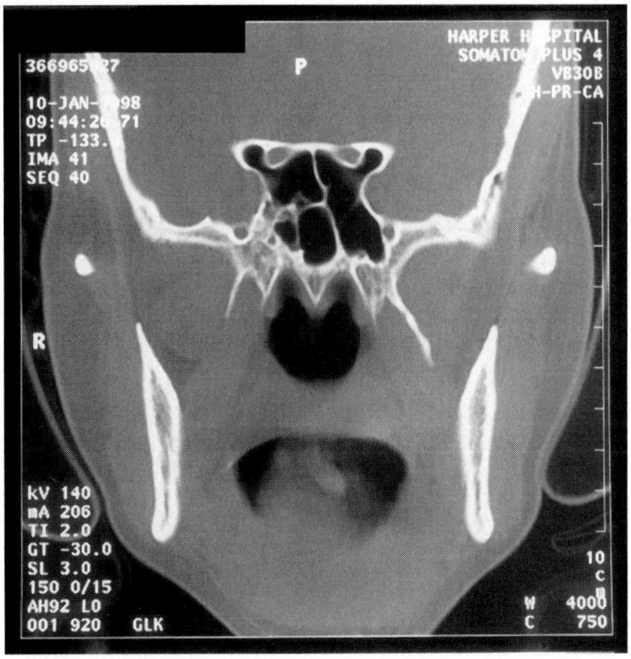

Figure 3–8. Coronal CT scan demonstrating pneumatization of the anterior clinoid process with evagination of the optic canals into the sphenoid sinuses bilaterally.

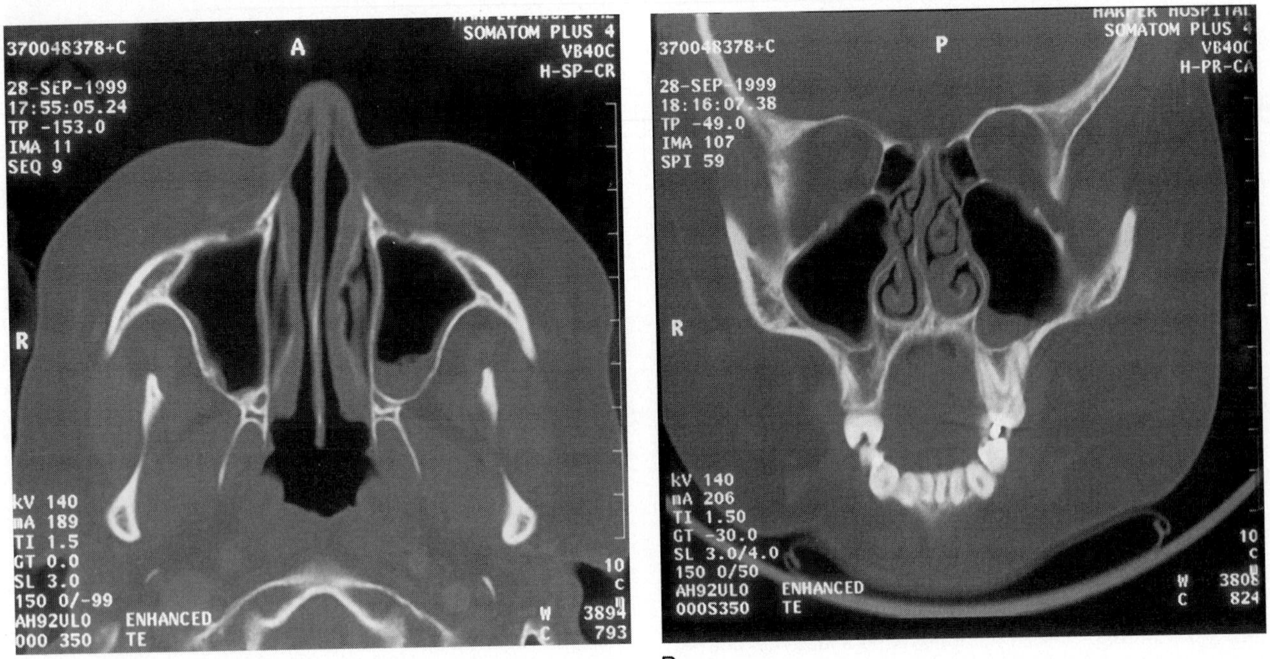

A B

Figure 3–9. Acute bacterial sinusitis. *A*, Axial image. *B*, Coronal image. There is fluid layering within the left maxillary sinus, as well as mucosal thickening of the right maxillary sinus.

presentation and symptoms, so as not to misinterpret the radiographic findings.

Chronic inflammation may result from repeated episodes of acute or subacute disease, or it can result from a progressive, unrelenting illness. The sinus mucosa reflects these insults and usually consists of a combination of hypertrophied polypoid mucosa, fibrotic change, and atrophic changes leading to a more nodular mucosal pattern.

General patterns of sinus inflammatory disease have been described in relationship to the functional drainage patterns of the paranasal sinuses. One pattern is termed the infundibular pattern (Fig. 3–10). If an obstructive process is present at the base of the infundibulum in the region of the maxillary ostium, isolated involvement of the maxillary sinus occurs. Obstructing causes may be secondary to edematous mucosa, polyp, or Haller air cells encroaching on the maxillary sinus ostium. A second major pattern is termed the OMU pattern. The three anatomic structures that may be involved with this pattern include the middle meatus, infundibulum, and nasofrontal recess. Because the middle meatus is the final drainage pathway of the frontal, anterior ethmoid, and maxillary sinuses, all or part of these sinuses may be involved with an abnormality within the OMU. Common abnormalities affecting the OMU include mucosal edema, hypertrophied turbinates, polyps, adhesions, and developmental variants. A third pattern of sinus inflammatory disease is termed the sphenoethmoidal recess pattern. The posterior ethmoid air cells drain into the superior meatus and then into the sphenoethmoidal recess. The sphenoid sinus drains directly into the sphenoethmoidal recess. Abnormalities isolated to the superior meatus and sphenoethmoidal

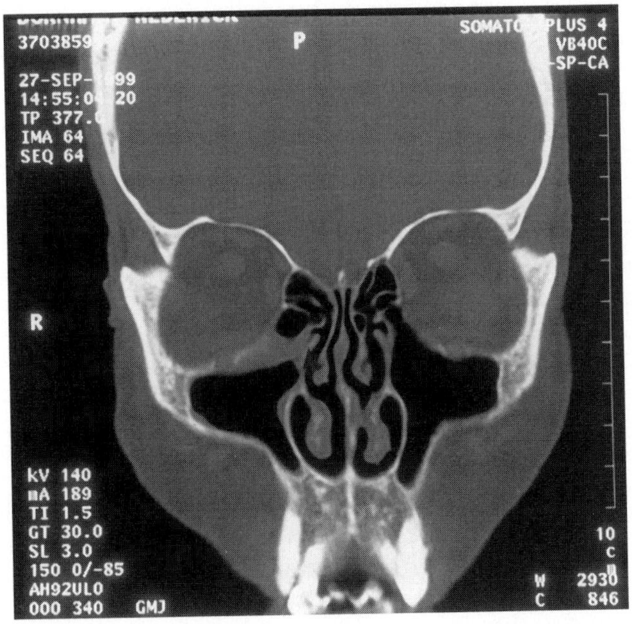

Figure 3–10. Infundibular pattern of chronic sinusitis. The arrow points to infundibular thickening with secondary changes in the maxillary sinus.

recess result in isolated posterior ethmoid and sphenoid sinus disease.

Fungal Sinusitis

The imaging characteristics of fungal sinusitis vary from being nonspecific to being highly suggestive of the diagnosis. There are four clinicopathologic classifications of fungal sinonasal disease: acute invasive (fulminant), chronic invasive, noninvasive colonization (fungus ball), and allergic fungal sinusitis. These four types of infections can be seen with any fungus, but the most common pathogens are Aspergillus species.

Acute fulminant fungal sinusitis may occur in immunosuppressed patients who are typically granulopenic from hematologic malignant disease or in diabetics with ketoacidosis. Clinical symptoms include nasal discharge, sinus pain, and periorbital swelling. Examination of the nasal cavity reveals pale ischemic regions that progress to blackened gangrenous tissue. The fungus spreads via the vasculature and extends to the orbit and intracranial structures. Radiographic findings initially include nonspecific mucosal thickening. The surrounding bone may be thickened and sclerotic, eroded, or remodeled. In advanced cases, frank destruction and orbital or intracranial extension are seen.

Chronic invasive sinusitis can be seen in normal hosts. This entity is most commonly seen in mildly immunosuppressed patients, such as diabetics. The radiographic findings are similar to those in acute fulminant mycotic sinusitis (Fig. 3–11).

Fungal colonization is a benign process that typically occurs within a sinus with altered function, such as that caused by prior surgery, radiotherapy, or opacification. The radiographic findings are typically limited to one sinus and include hyperdense inclusions with significant surrounding mucosal thickening (Fig. 3–12).

Allergic fungal sinusitis is a more diffuse variation of the fungal colonization entity. With this condition, multiple sinuses are involved and intranasal polyps are common. Hyperdense sinus inclusions are usually present. Often, there is bone destruction that follows the pattern of erosion around an expanding process. This occurs more often than focal destruction or an invasive pattern of bone destruction.

Wegener's Granulomatosis

Wegener's granulomatosis is a necrotizing granulomatous vasculitis affecting the upper and lower respiratory tracts and causing a renal glomerulonephritis. This disease may present as a chronic, nonspecific, inflammatory process of the nose and paranasal sinuses. The nasal septum is initially involved and may show soft tissue thickening, which eventually leads to septal erosion and perforation. Sinus involvement is typical of chronic sinusitis.

Mucus Retention Cyst

The most common intrasinus complication of inflammatory disease is a retention cyst. This results from obstruction of the ducts of mucosal serous and/or mucinous glands. The cysts are typically small and are incidental imaging findings. They are estimated to occur in 10% of the population. Radiographic imaging reveals a smooth, convex border, soft tissue lesion, most commonly located in the maxillary sinus. Rarely, these cysts enlarge to fill the sinus cavity. A retention cyst cannot accurately be differentiated from a polyp on cross-sectional imaging.

Mucocele

Mucoceles are expansile cysts of the sinuses that manifest as expansion of an entire sinus or air cell, rather than a cyst within a cell or sinus (Fig. 3–13). Mucoceles are presumed to be caused by obstruction of the ostium of a sinus with accumulation of mucus within the sinus. Radiographically, they appear as a concentric expansion of a cell or sinus. There is usually some evidence of bone erosion around the mucocele. There may be orbital or intracranial expansion. On MRI, the contents of the mucocele may be like water (dark on T1 images, bright on T2 images), or may be inflammatory or mixed. This depends on the contents of the mucocele and the presence of infection (i.e., mucopyocele). Mucoceles cannot reliably be differentiated from cholesterol granuloma on radiographic imaging as both have overlapping presentations.

Antrochoanal Polyp

Occasionally, a polyp can extend through the maxillary sinus ostium into the nasal cavity. This represents an antrochoanal polyp. These lesions are typically unilateral, soft tissue masses filling the maxillary sinus. The region of the infundibulum widens and the soft tissue mass extends into the ipsilateral nasal vault, and eventually into the nasopharynx. This may or may not be accompanied by more diffuse sinus disease.

Sinonasal Polyposis

Sinonasal polyposis (SNP) is an inflammatory condition affecting the mucosa of the nose and paranasal sinuses that has a polypoid endoscopic and radiologic appearance. The polyps in SNP are soft tissue masses, composed of edematous, hyperplastic mucoperiosteum, which have a rounded shape. The polyps also attract intercellular fluid. The cause of SNP is uncertain. Polyps

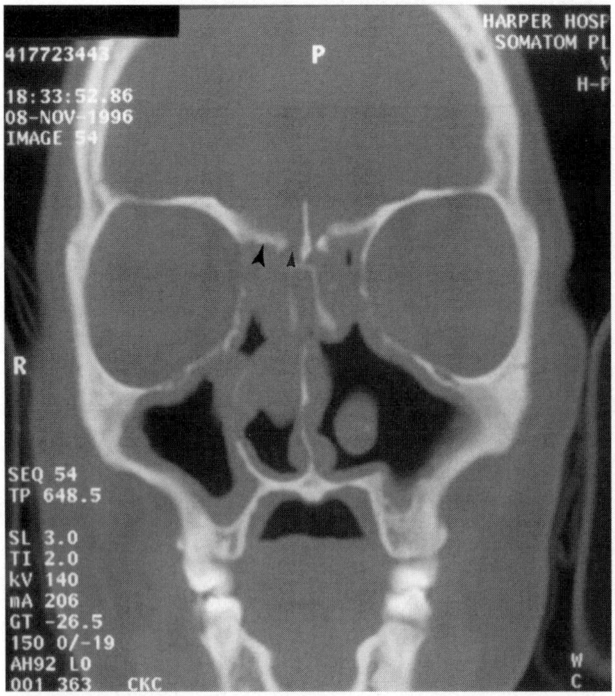

A

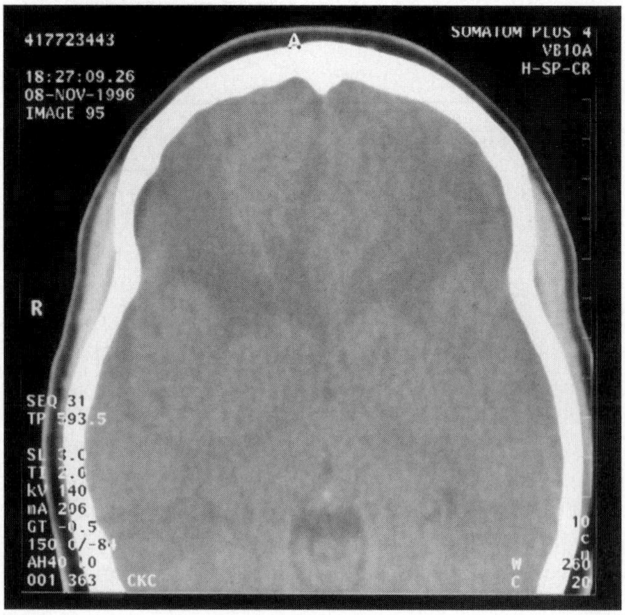

B

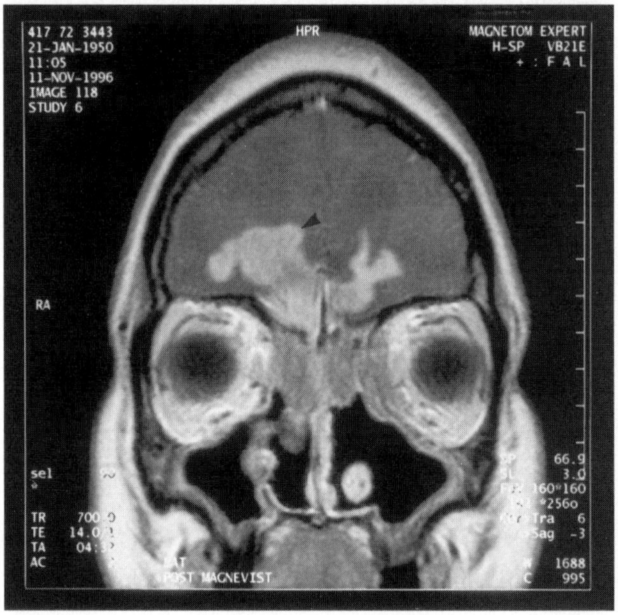

C

Figure 3–11. Chronic invasive fungal sinusitis. *A,* A coronal CT bone window demonstrates a mixed appearance of bony sclerosis (*large arrowhead*) with bony erosion (*small arrowhead*). Note that the adjacent brain parenchyma cannot be seen. *B,* An axial CT soft tissue window reveals the hypodensity that is consistent with parenchymal involvement. *C,* A coronal T1-weighted MRI scan with contrast enhancement reveals the extensive involvement of the brain parenchyma (*arrowhead*) that was not clinically apparent.

are associated with allergic and nonallergic rhinitis, asthma, infection, and aspirin intolerance. SNP is a recognized complication of cystic fibrosis. Symptoms of nasal polyps may precede the diagnosis of cystic fibrosis, leading investigators to suggest that children and young adults with nasal polyps be screened for cystic fibrosis.

There appear to be two major radiographic findings associated with SNP. The first is polypoid soft tissue mass densities with cascading or curvilinear contours. The second is bilateral involvement. Infundibular enlargement is seen in approximately 89% of patients. Minor CT characteristics include ethmoid sinus wall bulging, with or without ethmoid sinus septal osteopenia. The paranasal sinuses may show mixed attenuation with trapping of mucous secretions.

Complications of Sinusitis

Orbital complications from sinusitis may occur in any age range, but are most commonly seen in the pediatric

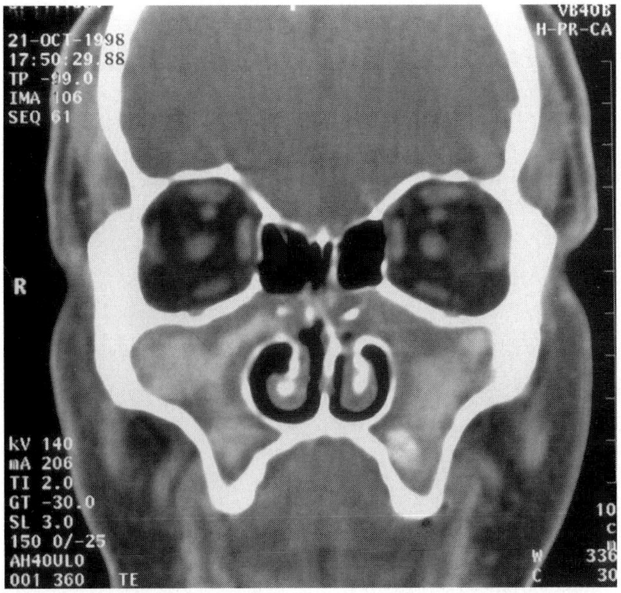

Figure 3–12. Noninvasive fungal colonization. A coronal CT with soft tissue windows shows hyperdense secretions in the maxillary sinus. Note the absence of ethmoid septa middle turbinates and uncinate processes as a result of prior surgery.

population. The most common route of spread is direct extension. Other pathways of infection include trauma, foreign bodies spread from an infectious process of the facial soft tissues, or hematogenous infection. Orbital complications include preseptal cellulitis, postseptal cellulitis, subperiosteal abscess, and orbital abscess. CT scanning is the imaging method of choice because of its superior ability to show bony detail. Intravenous contrast enhancement is helpful.

Imaging findings usually include inflammatory changes of the ethmoid and maxillary sinuses adjacent to the involved orbit. In preseptal cellulitis, there is diffuse swelling of the upper and lower eyelids without abscess formation or involvement of the orbital structures. In these cases, there is no proptosis or swelling of the orbital soft tissues. Orbital cellulitis is recognized by the presence of some degree of change in the orbital soft tissues. In very early cases, this may be indistinguishable from preseptal cellulitis. In more advanced cases, proptosis and edema of the extraocular muscles are seen. The bone of the sinuses is usually intact, and there is diffuse and symmetric involvement of the orbit.

Subperiosteal abscess is best recognized after administration of intravenous contrast medium. In this setting there is displacement of the globe, with a ring-enhancing mass that abuts the laminal papyracea. The degree of soft tissue change within the orbit is variable. Bone erosion abutting the abscess is not always seen, but may be present. Orbital abscess is identified when the abscess cavity is found within the soft tissues of the orbit (Fig. 3–14). There is always significant edema of the extraocular muscles and significant proptosis.

Intracranial complications of sinusitis occur infrequently. These complications include meningitis, epidural abscess, subdural abscess, cerebritis, and cerebral abscess. Intracranial involvement from sinusitis most of-

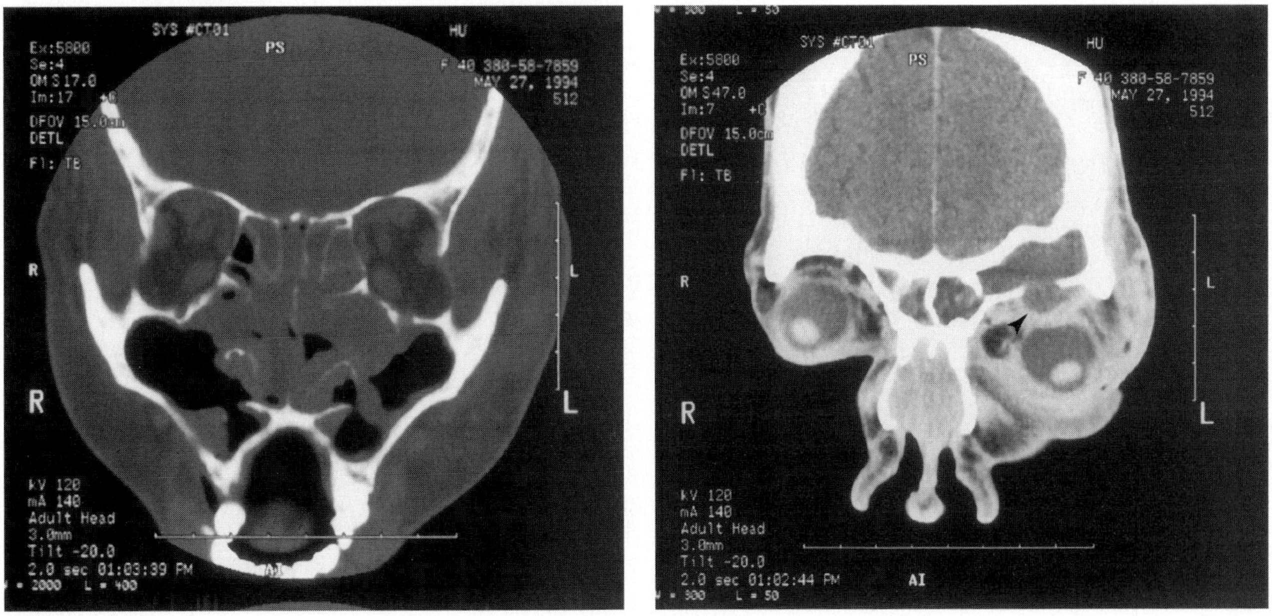

A B

Figure 3–13. Frontal mucocele. *A,* Coronal CT with bone windows. *B,* Coronal CT with soft tissue windows. There are multiple polypoid masses in the sinuses with frontal mucocele (*arrowhead*).

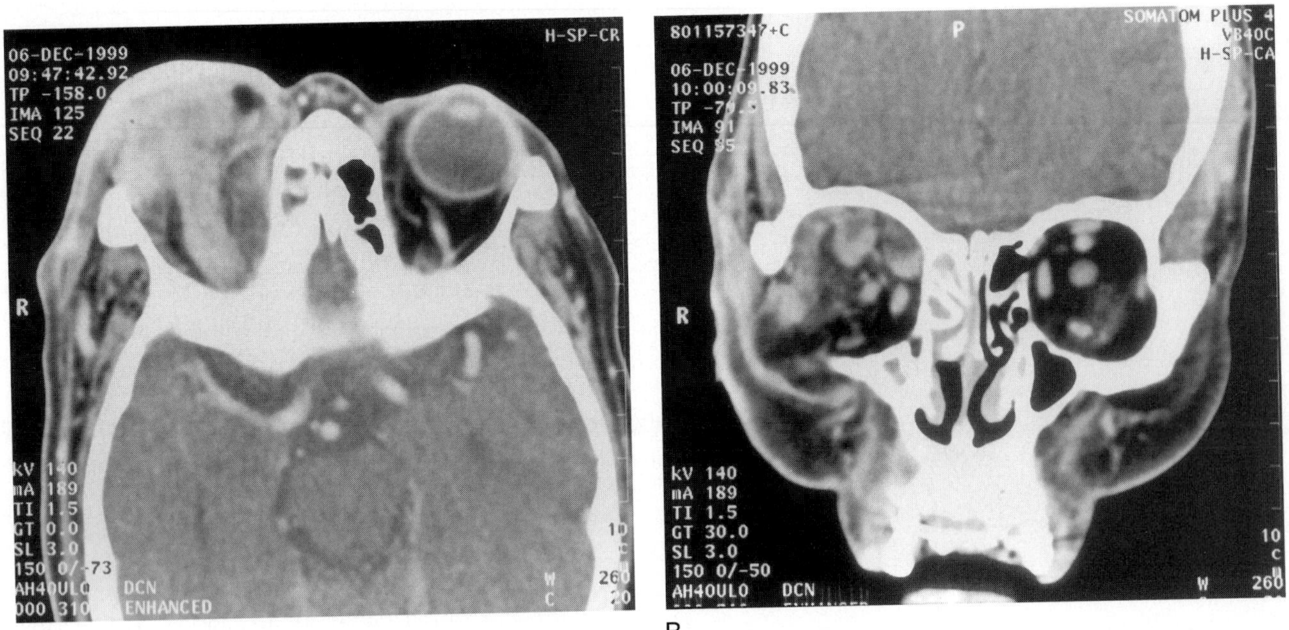

A B

Figure 3–14. Intraorbital abscess secondary to acute sinusitis. *A,* Axial CT with soft tissue window and contrast enhancement. *B,* Coronal CT with contrast enhancement.

ten stems from the frontal sinus. This spread is thought to be secondary to a rich emissary venous network that connects the posterior sinus mucosa with the meninges. CT and MRI scans are complementary in evaluating these complications. Findings are consistent with the specific diagnosis and include a ring-enhancing lesion in the location of the abscess, whether epidural, subdural, or intraparenchymal (Fig. 3–15).

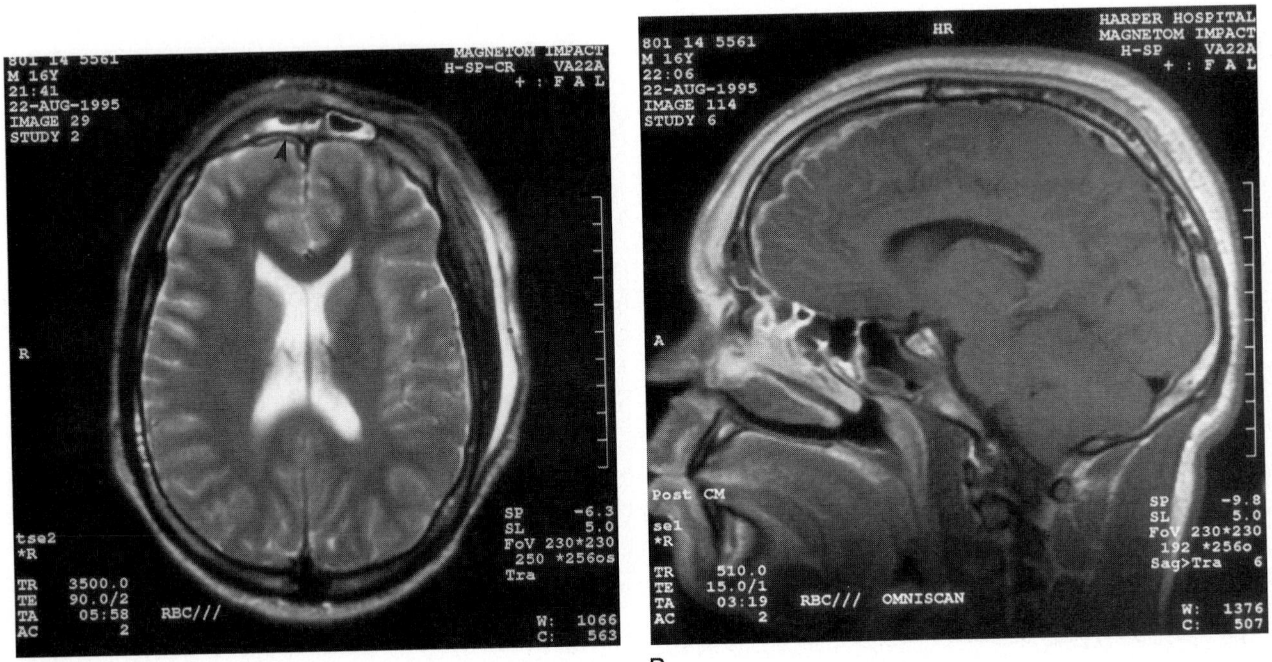

A B

Figure 3–15. Subdural abscess. *A,* T2-weighted axial MRI. Signal with an air-fluid level in the frontal sinuses with subdural empyema (*arrowhead*). Note the loss of diploic fat in the posterior frontal sinus wall, indicating transosseous spread of infection. *B,* T1-weighted, contrast-enhanced, sagittal image.

Osteomyelitis is also a recognized complication of sinusitis. This entity is often encountered in partially treated bacterial or fungal disease. The radiographic findings include focal rarefaction of bone, sequestrum formation, bony sclerosis, and ultimately, bony destruction.

SINONASAL TUMORS

Inverted Papilloma

Inverted papilloma occurs predominantly in men between the ages of 40 and 70 years, but may be found in women and in younger or older men. These lesions arise from the lateral nasal wall near the middle turbinate and extend into the maxillary and ethmoid sinuses. Clinically, inverted papilloma can cause symptoms of nasal obstruction, epistaxis, and anosmia. The reported rate of occurrence for developing squamous cell carcinoma within an inverted papilloma is 10%. The imaging findings range from a small polypoid mass to an expansive nasal mass that remodels the nasal vault and extends into the sinus, causing postobstructive change (Fig. 3–16). The hallmark of this condition is unilateral involvement.

Juvenile Nasopharyngeal Angiofibroma

Juvenile nasopharyngeal angiofibroma is a benign but locally aggressive vascular tumor found exclusively in male individuals between 5 and 25 years of age. Clinically, these lesions present with unilateral nasal obstruction and recurrent, spontaneous epistaxis. This lesion arises adjacent to the sphenopalatine foramen on the lateral nasopharyngeal wall. Local extension can involve the pterygopalatine fossa, infratemporal fossa, sphenoid sinus, posterior nasal fossa, maxillary and ethmoid sinuses, and orbit. Intracranial extension may occur via the foramen rotundum and superior orbital fissure.

CT scanning shows a soft tissue mass lesion remodeling foramina and fissures (Fig. 3–17). The lesion demonstrates immediate and intense contrast enhancement. On MRI, the mass is heterogenous in signal with prominent flow voids. MRI is helpful in differentiating postobstructive change from tumor in the sinuses. Angiography shows a vascular tumor, most commonly fed by the internal maxillary and ascending pharyngeal arteries.

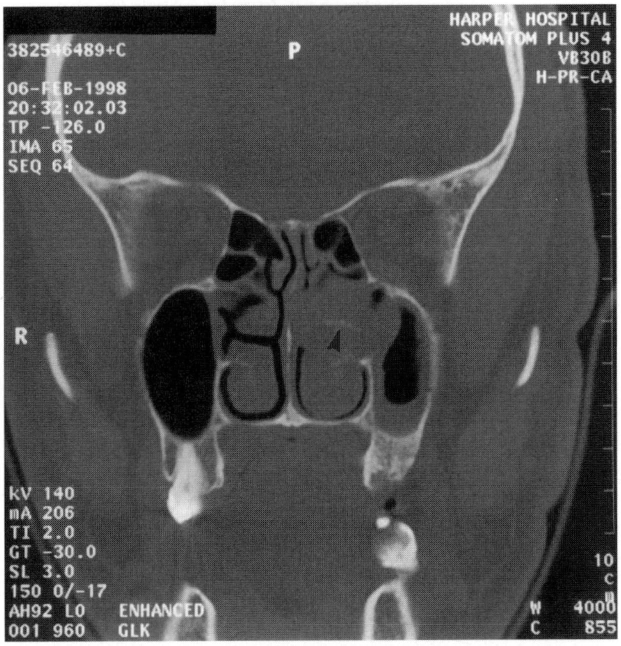

Figure 3–16. Inverted papilloma. A coronal CT with bone window shows a unilateral nasal canal mass with postobstructive changes in the maxillary sinus. Note the osseous fragments in the lesion (*arrowhead*), which represent residual middle turbinate, not ossification within the tumor.

Squamous Cell Carcinoma

Squamous cell carcinoma is the most common malignant lesion of the nose and paranasal sinuses, accounting for approximately 60% of malignant lesions. The maxillary sinus is involved most often, followed by the ethmoid, frontal, and sphenoid sinuses, in that order. The nasal cavity is involved in approximately 25% of squamous cell carcinoma cases. Males are affected more commonly than females, and the condition occurs most commonly in the sixth to seventh decade of life.

The goal of cross-sectional imaging is to visualize the extent of spread beyond the sinus cavity. Contrast enhancement is usually not very helpful because of poor enhancement patterns and the inability to differentiate tumor density from inflammatory reaction, normal soft tissues, and postobstructive changes. CT scanning is helpful in evaluating the osseous structures for erosion or destruction (Fig. 3–18). MRI scans provide excellent delineation of tumor from surrounding soft tissues, inflammatory tissue, and postobstructive sinus secretions. On MRI, these lesions have an intermediate T1-weighted signal and a minimally hyperintense T2-weighted signal intensity. Most neoplasms are homogeneous in signal intensity. These lesions enhance slightly less than normal mucosa.

Esthesioneuroblastoma

Esthesioneuroblastoma is an uncommon tumor of neural crest origin that arises from the olfactory mucosa in the superior nasal fossa. There are two different age peaks for this tumor. The first occurs at 10 to 20 years of age. The second occurs at 50 to 60 years of age. These tumors present unilaterally. The goal of imaging is to map the tumor extent. CT scanning shows an enhancing homogeneous mass that tends to remodel bone. Calcifications can occur in the tumor mass. MRI shows inter-

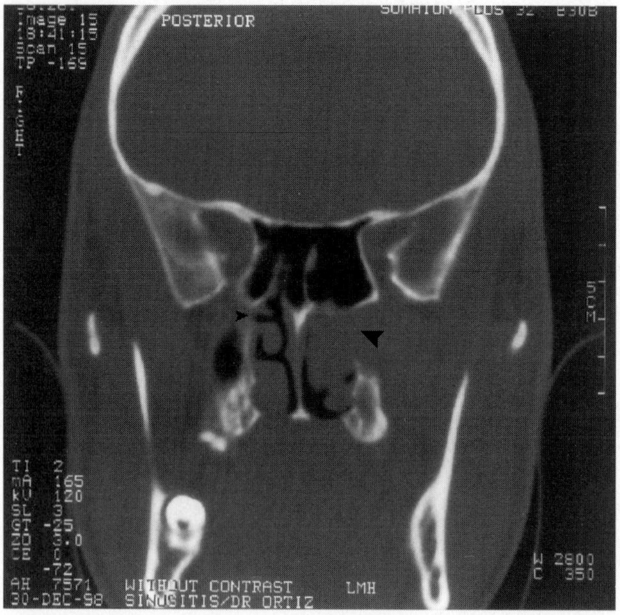

A

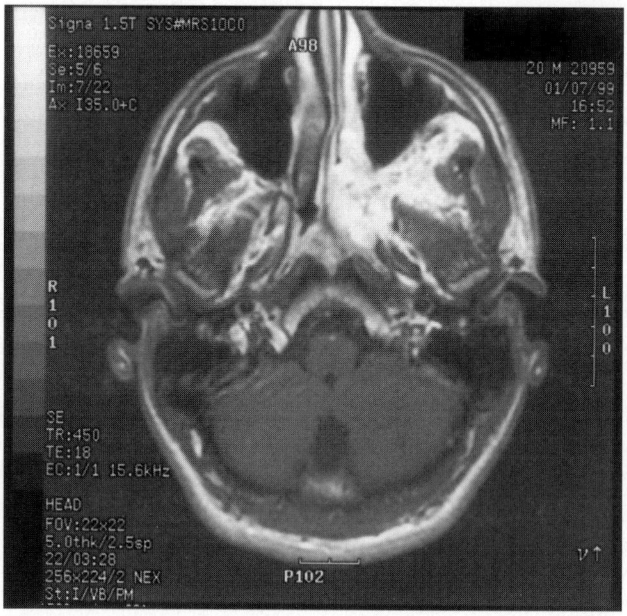

B

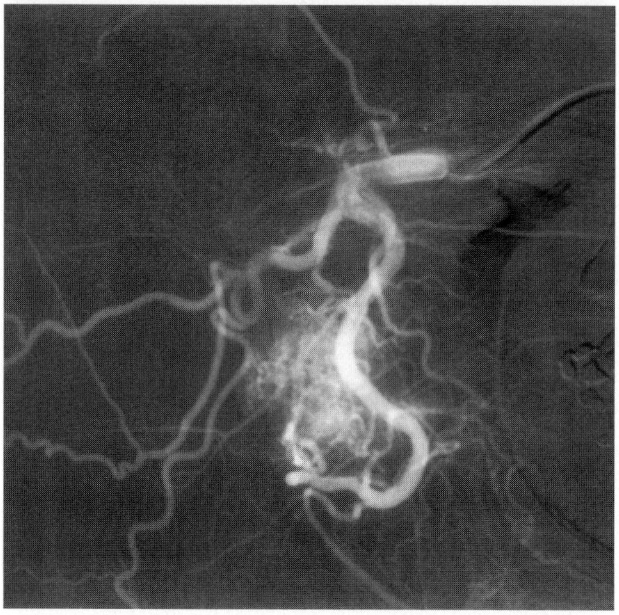

C

Figure 3–17. Juvenile nasopharyngeal angiofibroma. *A,* Coronal CT scan. Note the widening and bony remodeling of the sphenopalatine foramen (*large arrowhead*) compared with the normal right side (*small arrowhead*). *B,* Axial T1-weighted MRI with contrast enhancement. *C,* Lateral selective digital subtraction arteriogram of the left external carotid artery. The MRI reveals the tumor's lateral extension into the masticator space. The black holes in the tumor represent flow voids. The arteriogram confirms the prominent vascularity.

mediate signal intensities on all sequences. These lesions enhance with administration of contrast material. MRI clearly defines intracranial extension and orbital involvement.

Lymphoma

Lymphoma is an uncommon lesion of the nasal fossa and paranasal sinuses. When visualized by imaging, this entity may mimic sinusitis, polyposis, and benign neoplasms. One early finding that may help identify this process is subtle extension outside the bony confines of the sinus with an intact bony wall. Most such lesions involve the nasal fossa and maxillary sinuses.

Plasmacytoma

Extramedullary plasmacytoma is a rare soft tissue malignant lesion composed of plasma cells. Eighty percent of these lesions involve the head and neck. They represent 3% to 4% of all sinonasal cavity tumors. Patients are generally older than 40 years of age at presentation.

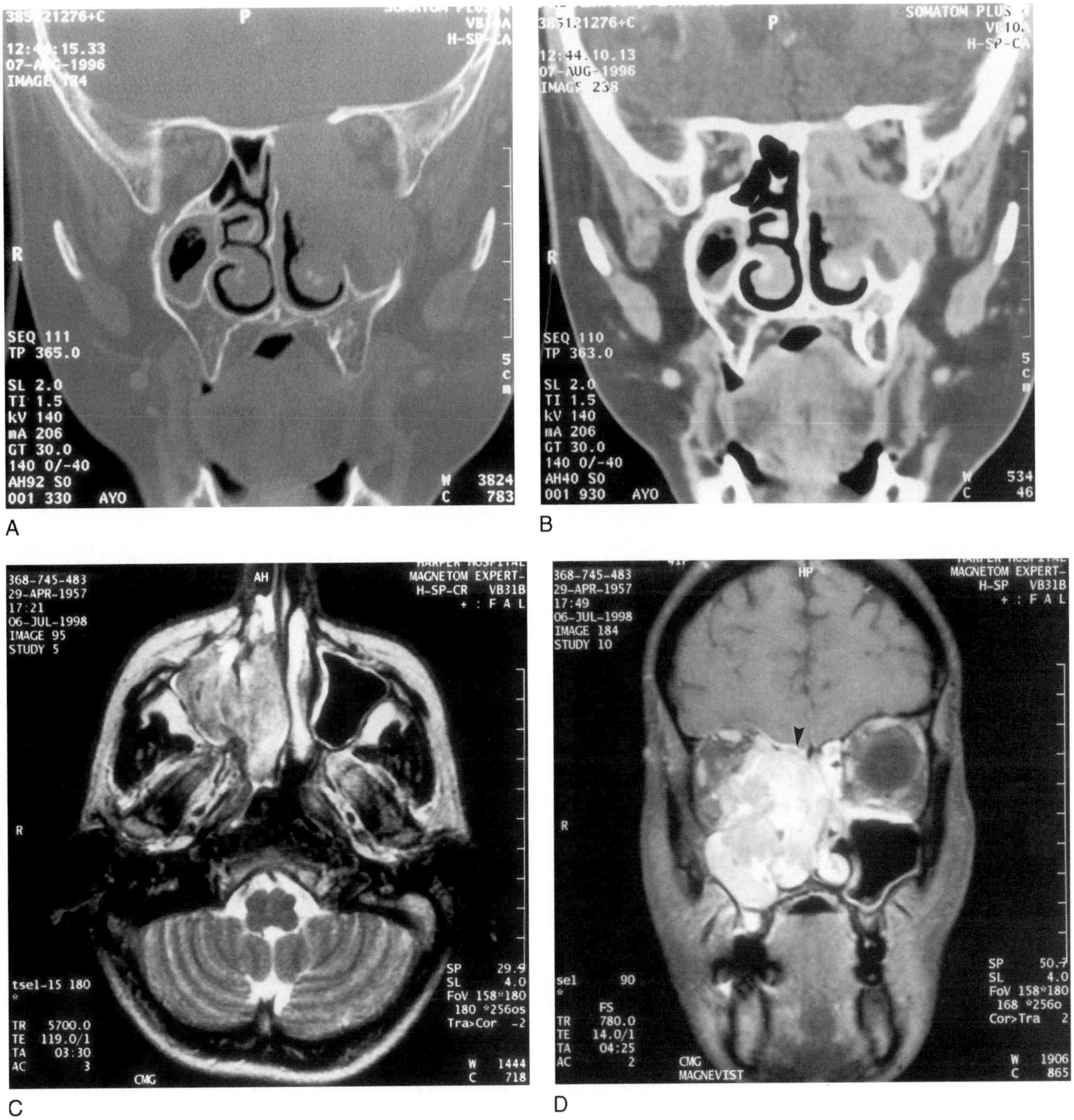

Figure 3–18. Squamous cell carcinoma. *A,* Coronal CT bone window. *B,* Coronal CT postenhancement soft tissue window. The CT image clearly shows the osseous erosion. The soft tissue window shows the neoplasm enhancing similarly to muscle, making it difficult to separate tumor from normal soft tissue structures. C, Axial T2-weighted image. *D,* Coronal T1-weighted image with contrast enhancement in another patient. MRI provides excellent delineation of tumor from normal structures. MRI is also superior to CT in delineating subtle intracranial extension (*arrowhead*).

These lesions are of soft tissue density and tend to remodel bone, but can cause erosion.

Malignant Melanoma

Sinonasal melanomas arise from melanocytes in the nasal mucosa. They occur primarily in the nasal canal and frequently involve the area around the nasal septum. These lesions tend to remodel bone, but erosive changes can be seen. These are vascular lesions that enhance intensely. The MRI signal is typically intermediate on T1- and T2-weighted images, although occasionally a high T1-weighted signal can be seen, caused by hemorrhage and not melanin.

CHAPTER 4

Nasal and Sinus Endoscopy

Nasal and sinus endoscopy has been available to rhinologists since the nineteenth century.[1] Originally, cystoscopes were borrowed from urologists to perform such examinations. Despite the fact that laryngoscopy, bronchoscopy, and esophagoscopy became increasingly popular over the ensuing years, rhinoscopy fell into disfavor. Perhaps the procedure's lack of specific applications or diagnostic utility led to the technique losing popularity. Or, possibly, the lack of a major figure in the field of rhinology willing to champion the use of this technique (as Chavalier Jackson did for bronchoscopy and esophagoscopy) was a critical factor. Regardless of the reason, nasal and sinus endoscopy was a seldom used and rarely discussed technique until the 1970s when Messerklinger, of Graz, Austria, began using the Hopkins rod telescope to evaluate the nose and sinuses.[2]

Since that time, nasal endoscopy has become an indispensable technique in the field of rhinology. Nasal endoscopy is taught in all training programs, fellowships devoted to mastering the techniques of endoscopy and endoscopic surgery are available, and most practicing otolaryngologists rely on nasal and sinus endoscopy on a daily basis in their practices. In this chapter, the indications and technique for and typical findings of endoscopy are discussed.

INDICATIONS

Diagnosis

Endoscopy is routinely performed for the purpose of nasal and sinus diagnosis. Theoretically, endoscopy could be indicated in any patient with either rhinologic or otologic complaints. The evaluation of any symptom complex or any suspected condition affecting the nose and ears could be enhanced by endoscopy. However, in common practice, this is not a practical application of the technology. With the rising cost of medicine and the need to use resources appropriately, if not sparingly, endoscopy for every patient is not a cost-effective policy. This was pointed out in a study examining the incidence of important findings on routine endoscopy of unselected patients presenting with nasal or sinus complaints.[3] In this setting, less than 10% of the patients had additional diagnoses identified or treatment prescribed based on endoscopic examination. Thus, these data support a more restrictive, cost-effective use of endoscopy for specific indications.

Sinusitis. The diagnosis of sinusitis can usually be established from a routine history and anterior rhinoscopy and percussion of the sinuses. However, when the diagnosis remains in doubt after a complete history and routine examination, or if a patient with suspected sinusitis is not responding to medical therapy, endoscopy may be helpful. When the diagnosis is in doubt, it is often acceptable to assume that the diagnosis is sinusitis and treat the patient empirically. However, in certain circumstances, it may be preferable to confirm the diagnosis with endoscopy before prescribing treatment. This is especially true if the patient has had a long history of similar episodes without a definitive diagnosis being established in the past. In the case of the patient who is not responding to medical therapy, endoscopy may be helpful in confirming the diagnosis and in understanding the reasons for the patient's lack of response.

Nasal endoscopy is especially useful in evaluating the patient being considered for sinus surgery. In such cases, an endoscopic examination should be performed and the results compared to those obtained from computed tomography (CT) scans. This examination can help to determine an underlying cause of the sinusitis, as well as to confirm the presence of sinusitis before committing to surgery. An additional benefit of preoperative endoscopy is the ability to evaluate access to the ethmoid sinus. The airway may be found to be narrowed owing to a deviated septum, an abnormal inferior turbinate, or mucosal abnormalities that prevent successful access to the sinuses.

One of the most valuable uses of diagnostic endoscopy is in the assessment of a patient with recurrent infection following endoscopic sinus surgery. Patients may have difficulty distinguishing sinusitis from a routine viral upper respiratory infection after endoscopic sinus surgery. Endoscopy can reliably determine the presence of purulent secretions in the sinuses and the presence of mucosal inflammation or thickening. Similarly, for the patient contemplating revision endoscopic surgery, careful diagnostic endoscopy is critical. In this setting the endoscopic examination is essential in establishing a probable cause for the prior surgical failure. A CT scan alone cannot differentiate between scar tissue and inflamed mucosa or mucous secretions. By contrast, an endoscopic examination can confirm or rule out the presence of synechiae, scar tissue, stenosis, recurrent polyps, and retained secretions. In order to be able to recommend revision surgery with confidence, one must first identify a correctable cause of recurrent or persistent infection. This is only possible with endoscopy.

Rhinitis. The diagnosis of rhinitis usually does not require endoscopy, as in most cases, the diagnosis can routinely be established based on clinical history and anterior rhinoscopy. Endoscopy may be helpful, though, in patients in whom rhinitis and sinusitis are not easily distinguishable. It is in part this difficulty that has led the rhinologic community to adopt rhinosinusitis as the proper nomenclature. However, there is an entire population of patients who suffer from allergic and nonallergic rhinitis but who do not have sinusitis. This differentiation is critical in selecting the best treatment for the patient. In this setting, rhinoscopy is more often performed to rule out sinusitis than to confirm or evaluate rhinitis.

Nasal Polyps. In most cases, the diagnosis of nasal polyps is easily made on the basis of anterior rhinoscopy. The polyp is often visible in the anterior nasal cavity or, in the case of antrochoanal or sphenochoanal polyps, along the floor of the nose in the posterior choanae. Detailed delineation of the extent of polyps and any underlying inflammatory changes in the sinuses is best accomplished with a CT scan rather than endoscopy. However, there are cases when the history is ambiguous and the initial anterior nasal examination yields normal findings. In such instances, endoscopy can reveal small middle or superior meatus polyps that would not otherwise be detected or suspected. In these cases, a knowledge of the presence of these polyps may affect the choice of therapy, as well as the prognosis for the patient. Also, it is possible in some cases to differentiate the origin of a nasal polyp using preoperative or office endoscopy. Identifying a polyp as an antrochoanal polyp may affect the choice of therapy or the surgical approach to the patient.

Epistaxis. The source of epistaxis may be obscure in some patients. This is especially true in patients who report intermittent bleeding or who are not bleeding at the time of examination. In these situations, the source of the bleeding may be difficult to identify. Endoscopy can increase the clinician's ability to determine the bleeding source. Also, in this situation, endoscopy can help rule out tumor as the cause of the epistaxis. A second situation in which the source of bleeding may be difficult to identify is when the bleeding is from the lateral wall of the nose or when posterior epistaxis is noted. When these sites of bleeding are involved, direct visualization of the origin of bleeding is difficult without endoscopy.

Tumor. Diagnosis of a nasal or sinus tumor is rarely aided by endoscopy. The surface characteristics and appearance of the tumor are almost never important in determining appropriate treatment. Rather, the diagnostic evaluation of a tumor usually includes biopsy, CT scan, magnetic resonance imaging, and sometimes, arteriography. Endoscopy may, however, be helpful during the biopsy (see the next section), or in initial detection of a tumor. Rarely, symptoms of obstruction, epistaxis, pain, or sinusitis will prompt a diagnostic endoscopic evaluation, during which a tumor may be incidentally discovered. In this situation, the discovery of an unsuspected tumor is possible only with endoscopy or another imaging technique. The yield in discovering tumors is very low in this setting. However, diagnostic endoscopy should be considered in patients with persistent epistaxis, pain, or obstruction to rule out tumor.

Biopsy

In the modern practice of rhinology, open surgical biopsy is no longer necessary. Prior to endoscopy, it was often necessary to perform a Caldwell-Luc procedure or an external ethmoidectomy to access a tumor for biopsy. Endoscopy has made it possible for tumors in all areas of the nose and sinuses to be accessed, except for the rare lesion high within the frontal sinus that cannot be reached. In most circumstances, the tumor is visible within the nose on endoscopy and a small cup forceps biopsy is easily taken. This can be done in the operating room or in the office setting. Caution should be exercised, however, whenever attempting the biopsy of a nasal mass. The first concern is that any nasal mass could conceivably be an encephalocele or meningocele. Biopsy in this setting could lead to cerebrospinal fluid (CSF) leak or intracranial hemorrhage. For any lesion in which the origin of the tumor is not seen, a CT scan should be performed before biopsy. This will delineate the extent of the tumor before it is violated, and it will also document the origin of the tumor (sinonasal versus intracranial). The second concern in biopsy is the possibility of bleeding. Tumors within the nose may be highly vascular, angiofibromas, or even true hemangiomas. These lesions have a tendency to bleed profusely after biopsy. As long as the endoscopist is prepared for this situation, the bleeding is usually easily controlled and problems can be avoided. For this reason, most tumor biopsies are performed in the operating room where coagulation and packing materials are immediately available.

Surgery

Nasal endoscopy has certainly become well accepted as a visual adjunct for a wide variety of surgical procedures. Table 4–1 lists the indications for surgical endoscopy based on the author's experience. A discussion of the indications for endoscopy during these surgical procedures, as well as when endoscopy is preferred over other techniques, is presented in various chapters throughout this text.

Postoperative Care

Postoperative cleaning of the sinus cavity in the office is an indispensable use of endoscopy. Under endoscopic visualization, it is possible to examine the cavity, both to direct medical therapy as well as to perform manual cleaning of crusts and removal of polyps, cysts, and scar bands. Debridement of the cavity after surgery removes clots and mucus that could lead to stenosis of the ostium, persistent inflammation, or osteitis. In the author's opinion, rigorous postoperative cleaning of the sinus cavity decreases the risk of stenosis and synechiae from greater than 15% to less than 5%.

TABLE 4–1
Indications for Endoscopic Nasal or Sinus Surgery

Chronic sinusitis
Acute sinusitis
Recurrent acute sinusitis
Hypertrophic sinusitis (polyps)
Fungal sinusitis
Mucocele
Inferior turbinectomy
Septoplasty
Rhinoplasty (nasal hump removal)
Nasal tumor resection
Medial maxillectomy
Hypophysectomy
Cerebrospinal fluid leak
Orbital decompression
Optic nerve decompression
Dacryocystorhinostomy
Epistaxis—cautery
Epistaxis—vessel ligation

TECHNIQUE

In this section, the technique for diagnostic nasal endoscopy is described. The details of various surgical procedures are covered in the remaining chapters of the text.

Equipment

The equipment necessary to perform endoscopic examination is minimal. However, optimally, a full office setup should be available, including a motorized examination chair that allows the patient to be placed in a supine position. A standard suction/pressure pump is helpful in applying topical anesthetic and removing any secretions. The array of endoscopes should include a 0-degree, 4-mm scope; a 30-degree, 4-mm scope; a 30-degree, 2.7-mm scope; and a 70-degree, 4-mm scope. Each of these is useful in specific situations. The 0-degree, 4-mm scope is useful in examining the turbinates and the nasopharynx, whereas the 30-degree, 4-mm scope is the workhorse for diagnostic endoscopy because it allows the best view into the middle meatus. The 2.7-mm, 30-degree scope is useful for narrow noses, to navigate around septal deviations, and in children. The 70-degree, 4-mm scope is useful when examining the maxillary sinus and frontal sinus in postoperative patients. A set of instruments including a straight and upturned Blakesley forceps, straight and curved suction catheters, and a giraffe forceps is valuable if postoperative care is to be rendered.

Anesthesia

Diagnostic nasal endoscopy can be performed without any anesthesia. However, in most circumstances, this is uncomfortable for the patient and permits a less complete examination. Thus, decongestion and topical anesthesia are routinely used. By using this combination of treatments, a complete examination can usually be performed easily. The favored combination for outpatient, office-based endoscopic examination is phenylephrine (0.25%) and pontocaine (2%), applied using an atomizer through a pressurized spray bottle. The nose is dilated with a nasal speculum and the decongestant spray is delivered first, followed by the anesthetic. This begins the decongestion and allows the subsequent application of topical anesthesia to penetrate deeper into the nose.

Endoscopic Technique

For most patients, the goal of endoscopic examination will be clear before the procedure. For this reason, a particular scope may be the preferred option. For most diagnostic endoscopic procedures, the 4-mm, 30-degree endoscope provides the widest field, best lighting, and optimal angle of view for observation. Although it is possible to use multiple scopes in a single patient, for practical reasons, it is best to limit the number of scopes used and the number of times the scope is passed to the minimum required for an adequate examination.

On the first pass through the nose, the endoscope is passed over the nasal sill along the floor of the nose to the nasopharynx. This provides an overview and affords the clinician an opportunity to observe any abnormal areas in the nose or nasopharynx. A second pass will take the scope into the middle meatus and superior meatus. Often, it is possible to roll the endoscope under the middle turbinate into the middle meatus. However, in many patients, this is not possible without exerting undue pressure on the turbinate and causing discomfort for the patient. In either case, the area is examined carefully, noting the color and character of the mucosa, the presence of polyps or secretions, and any anatomic abnormalities.

ENDOSCOPIC FINDINGS

Normal Findings

The normal structures of the nose and sinuses that are visible on endoscopy include the turbinates, meati septum, and the nasopharyngeal structures. The mucosa lining the nose and sinuses is pictured in Figures 4–1 through 4–3. The reddish hue is caused by the presence of vessels on a white background. From a distance, the mucosa has a light red or pink color. With magnification, the individual vessels begin to become identifiable, and the background begins to appear white. The normal mucosa is smooth in texture, without irregularities, and is moist, with a slight shine or reflection from the surface.

The turbinates are normally convex medially with a smooth, round, inferior edge. Normal variations of the middle turbinate include concave medial shape (paradoxical turbinate), bifid turbinate, and concha bullosa (aeration of the middle turbinate, Fig. 4–1). This last variation can often be identified by an abnormally widened turbinate or by a step-off between a nonaerated anterior edge and the aerated body of the turbinate, as shown in Figure 4–1.

Beneath and lateral to the middle turbinate are the structures of the middle meatus (Fig. 4–2). These include the uncinate process, ethmoid bulla, and hiatus semilunaris. The uncinate process usually extends posteriorly and medially from its anterior attachment. Variations include medial rotation or lateralization; rarely, the uncinate may be bent anteriorly. The ethmoid bulla is found immediately behind the uncinate process. Aeration is variable. In some patients, there may be an opening into the maxillary sinus through the posterior inferior attachment of the uncinate process. This is known as an accessory ostium. This can be a perforation in the uncinate or the posterior fontanelle.

The nasopharynx is formed by a lateral wall, roof, and posterior wall (Fig. 4–3). The lateral wall consists of the eustachian tube anteriorly and the fossa of Rosenmüller immediately posterior to the eustachian tube. The posterior lip of the eustachian tube is referred to as the torus tubarius. Normally, the lumen of the eustachian tube is collapsed, as shown in Figure 4–3. In waking states, the orifice can open as the palate descends and the tensor tori contract. The fossa of Rosenmüller is usually only a crevice in the lateral wall of the nasopharynx, but it is important as the site of origin of most nasopharyngeal cancers. The posterior wall usually contains adenoidal tissue, or it may have scar bands if the patient has undergone adenoidectomy (see Fig. 4–3).

Pathology of the Nasal Septum

The most common abnormality of the nasal septum is a deviated septum. The variations in septal anatomy of deviated septum are discussed in detail in Chapter 12. Figure 4–4 demonstrates one of the variations, characterized by a sharp septal spur jutting into the inferior turbinate. The inferior turbinate is deformed by an indentation that resembles the size and shape of the spur.

Septal perforations are usually easy to identify with anterior rhinoscopy, but they may be more difficult to identify if they are small or posterior. Figure 4–5 shows an example of a moderately sized anterior perforation. The mucosa around the perforation is healthy, without crust or granulation. The nasal septum is also subject to developing synechiae to the inferior or middle turbinate. Figure 4–6 demonstrates a small adhesion between the septum and the anterior edge of the inferior turbinate.

Inflammatory Conditions

Mucosal inflammation of the nose and sinuses is evident on endoscopic examination based on a number of findings. Acute inflammation is characterized by intense erythema and the presence of mucopurulent or serous secretions. Chronic inflammation is harder to identify, but may be recognized by mucosal edema, mucous secretions, and vessel engorgement. Chronic rhinitis without sinusitis tends to manifest as changes in the inferior turbinate and septal mucosa. Figure 4–7 shows the changes seen in the inferior turbinate. The mucosa is mildly erythematous and marked by numerous deep pits. These pits are the result of hypertrophy of the seromucinous glands and venous sinusoids. Figure 4–8 demonstrates several findings associated with acute and chronic inflammation. A deep furrow is seen in the septum, resulting from a sharp deviation to the opposite side. Thick, mucoid secretions, deep pitting of the inferior turbinate mucosa, and severe erythema of the middle turbinate are also evident. Figure 4–9 shows a high-power view of chronically inflamed mucosa, revealing dilatation of the vessels of the middle turbinate with edema of the mucosa of the uncinate process and the ethmoid bulla.

A variety of secretions may be found in the nose, including CSF, tears, blood, and a full range of mucous secretions. The quality of the mucus, as seen endoscopically, can help establish the underlying condition. Watery, thin mucus suggests rhinitis, whereas purulent, thick, yellow or green secretions suggest sinusitis. Fungal infection is implied by the presence of dark, greasy, inspissated secretions. The origin and location of secretions also may be helpful in assessing the underlying pathology. Infected secretions emanating from the middle meatus usually correlate to sinusitis, whereas secretions found along the floor of the nose or inferior turbinate are typically associated with rhinitis.

Tumors and Masses

Endoscopy is ideal for diagnosing masses and tumors, of which there are many possibilities. Figure 4–10 shows a large polyp in the anterior nares. This polyp is edematous and boggy. There is no inflammation apparent. These findings suggest either allergy or aspirin triad as the cause of the polyp. Figure 4–11 demonstrates a nasal papilloma in the nasal valve area. This mass, which originated in the lateral wall just anterior to the inferior turbinate, was identified as a squamous papilloma on pathologic examination. Inverted papilloma tends to manifest as an inflammatory polyp rather than with the classic appearance of papilloma, as seen in Figure 4–11. Figure 4–12 shows the posterior choanae of the left nasal cavity. Adenoidal hypertrophy, suggested by the presence of stacked lobules or fronds of smooth tissue, is present. The differential diagnosis of this lesion includes nasopharyngeal carcinoma and lymphoma.

A large number of other lesions may be found in the nose or sinuses, including cysts, mucoceles, and malignant lesions. These can often be differentiated based on their endoscopic appearance.

REFERENCES

1. Draf W. Endoscopy of the Paranasal Sinuses. New York: Springer-Verlag, 1983.
2. Messerklinger W. Endoscopy of the Nose. Baltimore: Urban & Schwartzenberg, 1978.
3. Benninger M. Nasal endoscopy: Its role in office diagnosis. Am J Rhinol 11(2):177, 1997.

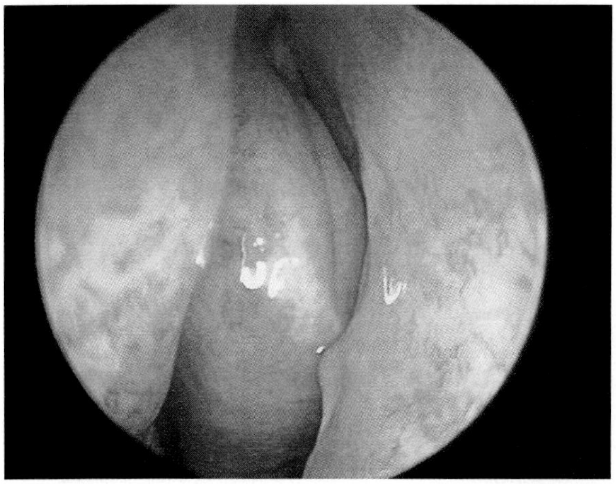

Figure 4–1. Normal-appearing mucosa (*right side*). View of the middle turbinate and nasal septum demonstrating normal mucosa. There is no edema, the color is pink, there are only thin, clear secretions, and the vessels are not engorged. Incidental note is made of a concha bullosa of the middle turbinate.

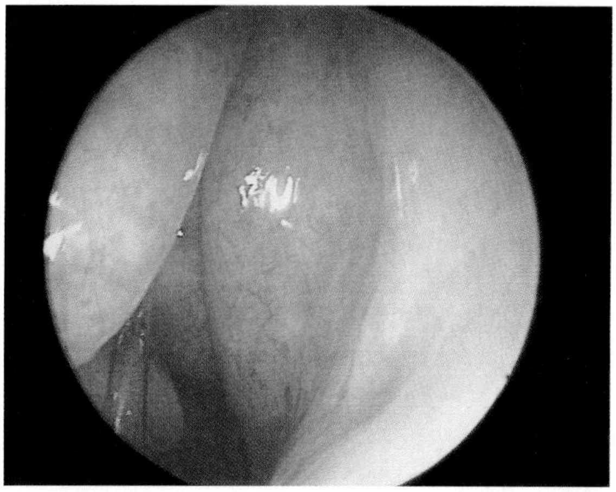

Figure 4–2. Normal middle meatus (*left side*). The uncinate process, middle turbinate, and ethmoid bulla are clearly seen. The mucosa is normal and the secretions are thin and clear.

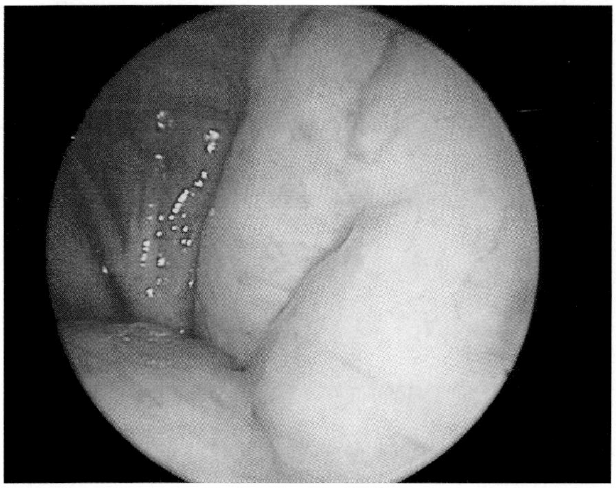

Figure 4–3. Normal nasopharynx (*left side*). The eustachian tube is seen in the center of the field. Scar bands are visible on the posterior wall secondary to previous adenoidectomy.

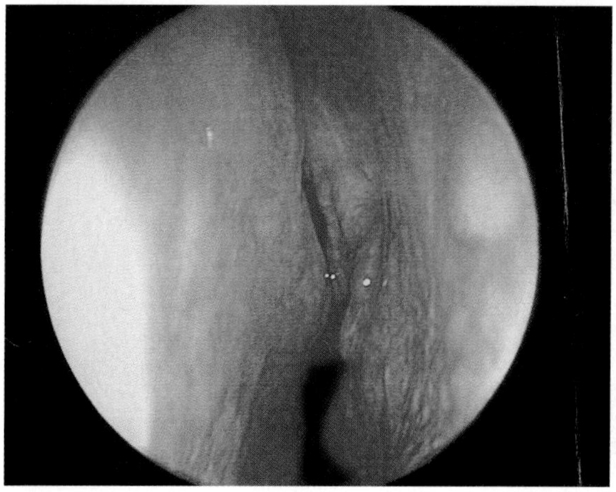

Figure 4–4. Deviated nasal septum (*right side*). The nasal septum is deviated into the nasal cavity; an inferior spur and changes of chronic inflammation are also evident. The inferior turbinate is deformed opposite the spur.

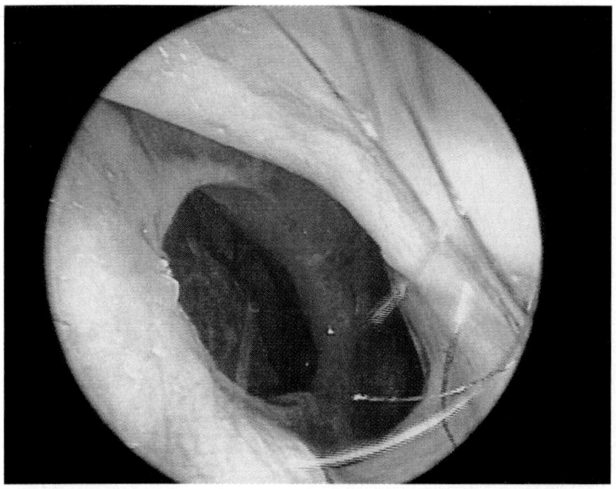

Figure 4–5. Nasal septal perforation (*left side*). A well-delineated, anterior septal perforation is seen. The mucosa on the edge is healthy, without crust, granulation, or secretions.

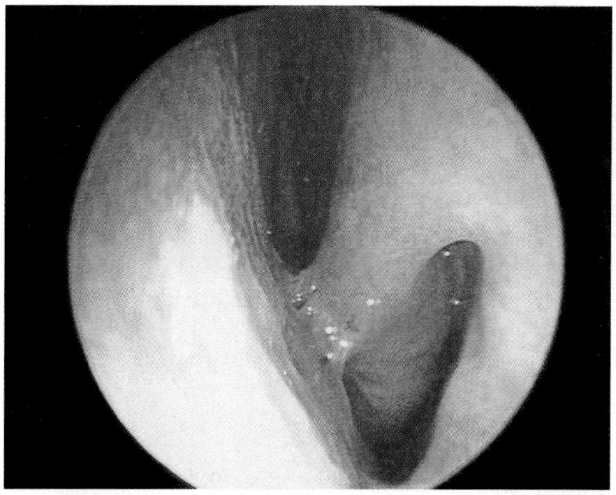

Figure 4–6. Nasal synechiae (*left side*). A scar band secondary to previous nasal surgery is seen to extend from the inferior turbinate to the nasal septum. The mucosa is otherwise healthy.

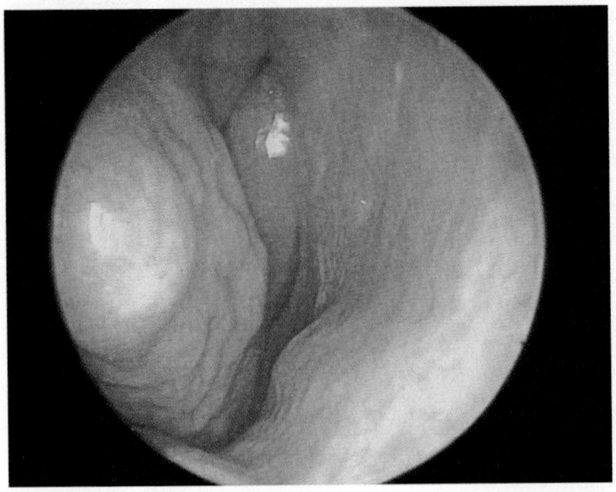

Figure 4–7. Chronic rhinitis (*right side*). The inferior turbinate demonstrates significant changes consistent with chronic rhinitis, including hypertrophy, pitting, and erythema. Secretions were removed prior to obtaining the photograph to better demonstrate the mucosal changes.

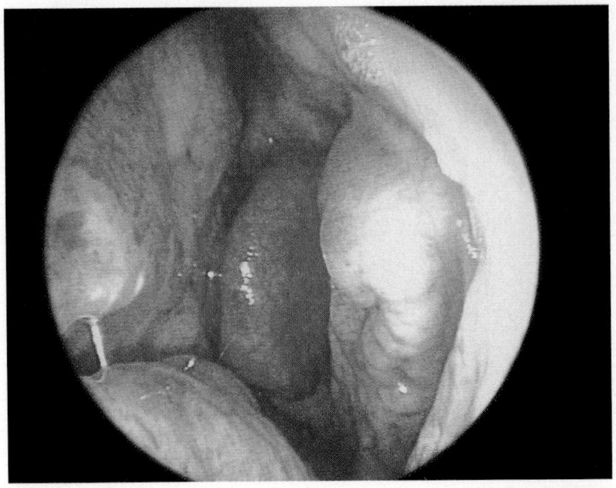

Figure 4–8. Chronic rhinosinusitis (*left side*). The inferior turbinate, middle turbinate, and nasal septum are shown. The septum has a deep furrow corresponding to a sharp septal spur to the opposite side. The inferior turbinate is severely pitted. The mucosa over the entire nasal cavity is erythematous, and thick, mucoid secretions can be seen.

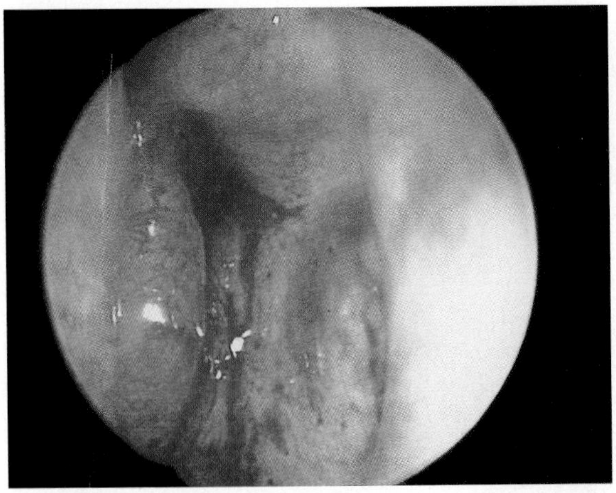

Figure 4–9. Chronic rhinosinusitis (*left side*). A view inside the middle meatus shows the uncinate process in the central region and the middle turbinate on the left side of the image. The mucosa is edematous and erythematous. The hiatus semilunaris is obliterated by edema from the uncinate and ethmoid bulla.

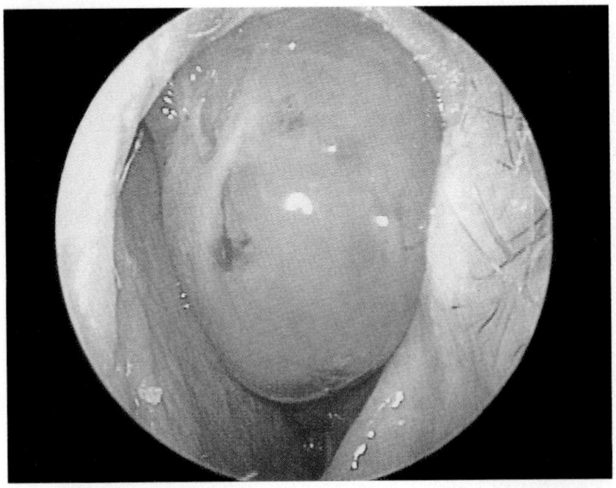

Figure 4–10. Nasal polyp (*right side*). This large, edematous nasal polyp is characterized by watery edema without signs of inflammation. This is consistent with allergy or aspirin triad.

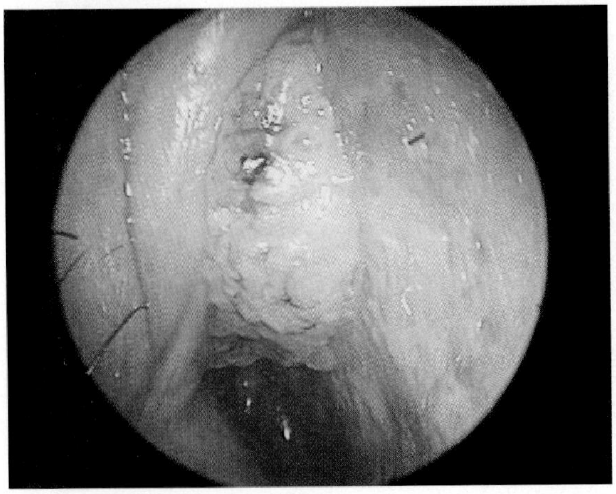

Figure 4–11. Squamous papilloma (*right side*). This shows the typical appearance of nasal papilloma. In this case, the lesion is arising from the lateral nasal wall in the area of the nasal valve.

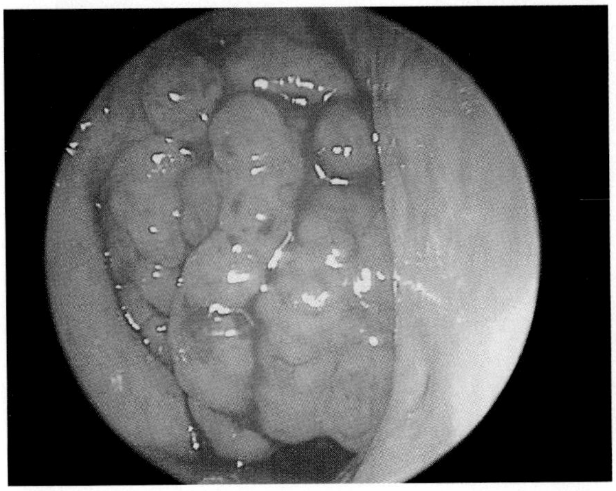

Figure 4–12. Adenoidal hypertrophy (*left side*). Typical appearance of enlarged adenoids in an adult patient. The mucosal folds are smooth, round, and stacked. There are no secretions, and no inflammation is evident. The nasal airway is visible at the bottom of the image.

Through the years, this test has been used in the absence of culture results as the defining measure of the presence of sinusitis. It is, nevertheless, an imperfect measure. The principle weaknesses of this test are the difficulties in interpreting mucosal thickening and the possibility of missing ethmoid and sphenoid mucosal changes. These weaknesses, however, are primarily problems with interpreting chronic sinusitis. When evaluating a patient with acute sinusitis, the findings of an air-fluid level or sinus opacification are highly suggestive of sinusitis and have a high degree of correlation to culture results on sinus puncture.[12, 13]

Nasal endoscopy, a relatively new adjunctive test, has yet to be assigned a definitive role in the diagnosis of acute sinusitis. One study by Benninger et al. demonstrated that endoscopic findings were useful in only 11% of patients undergoing endoscopic examination as part of an initial evaluation for sinus disease, and that, in no case were changes in the diagnosis or treatment made following the endoscopy.[14] However, the American Academy of Otolaryngology, Head and Neck Surgery (AAOHNS), in its consensus statement on the definition of sinusitis, included endoscopic evidence of purulent secretions in the middle meatus as part of the definition of sinusitis. Clearly, in cases in which the diagnosis is in doubt after routine examination, endoscopy can and should be used to help establish the diagnosis. The technical details of performing and interpreting nasal endoscopy are covered in Chapter 4.

Summary. A patient is suspected of having acute rhinosinusitis when there is an illness of immediate onset with symptoms present for less than 4 weeks. If the patient has all three of the hallmark major symptoms and clinical findings consistent with sinusitis, the diagnosis is established without further testing. Alternatively, the diagnosis may be established if two of the major symptoms, two of the minor symptoms, and the physical findings of sinusitis are present. In situations in which the diagnosis is equivocal, testing, including sinus radiographs, nasal endoscopy, or antral aspiration, can be performed to confirm the diagnosis.

The special circumstance of a suspected acute frontal sinusitis warrants performing sinus radiographs. If the x-ray studies demonstrate an opacification or air-fluid level in the frontal sinus, the patient should be diagnosed with acute frontal sinusitis and admitted to the hospital.

Bacteriology

The management of any infectious disease is directed by the microbiologic features of that process. Acute sinusitis is predominantly a bacterial infection with fungi, viruses, and other microbes found far less commonly.[15] The results of studies examining the bacteriology of acute sinusitis vary significantly depending on the population of the patients being studied. Some patients, such as those with hospital-acquired intensive care unit (ICU) infection, human immunodeficiency virus (HIV) infection, cystic fibrosis (CF), and bone marrow transplant, have significantly altered microflora. Also, the method of obtaining the culture is very important. Several studies have compared the results of nasal swab cultures to those derived from direct sinus aspirates,[16–18] and there is generally a poor correlation. This research has helped to establish the direct sinus puncture, either by a canine fossa or inferior meatus approach, as the standard for sinus culture, with endoscopically guided aspiration of the middle meatus a second-best alternative.

However, when evaluating community-acquired acute sinusitis in patients with competent immune systems, the bacteriologic study of direct-puncture samples is quite predictable and very well studied.[19] Table 5–2 lists the more common isolates and their relative incidence. Recently, increasing importance has been placed on the role of antibiotic resistance in acute sinusitis. When present, antibiotic resistance significantly affects the patient's response to routine antimicrobials and the choice of second- and third-line agents for treatment. Whenever possible, the practitioner should become familiar with the susceptibility patterns of the common pathogens in their community.

Medical Management

Most patients with routine community-acquired sinusitis can be treated as outpatients with a combination of oral antibiotics and adjunctive therapies. The results of appropriate therapy are usually prompt relief of the most severe symptoms and gradual resolution of the episode of sinusitis. Inpatient therapy is reserved for

TABLE 5–2
Bacteriology of Acute Sinusitis

Organism	Incidence (%)
Streptococcus pneumonia	41
Hemophilus influenza	35
Anaerobes	7
Streptococcal species	7
Moraxella catarrhalis	4
Staphylococcus aureus	3
Others	4

Reprinted with permission from Gwaltney JM, Scheld WM, Sande MA, Sydnor A. The microbial etiology and antimicrobial therapy of adults with acute community-acquired sinusitis: A 15-year experience at the University of Virginia and review of other selected studies. J Allergy Clin Immunol 90:457, 1992.

three categories of patients: those with complications of sinusitis, patients with altered immunity, and patients with severe sinusitis.

The first category—patients with complications of acute sinusitis—includes patients with orbital or intracranial infection. The need for intravenous antibiotics and close observation or surgery is evident in these patients. In these cases, hospitalization is mandatory.

The second category—patients with altered immunity—includes patients with congenital, severe combined immunodeficiency (SCID), those undergoing chemotherapy or bone marrow transplant, those undergoing organ transplantation with immunosuppression, and HIV-infected patients with low CD4 counts. These patients are at particularly high risk for complications of sinusitis. In addition, these patients have unpredictable bacteriologic examinations with a high risk of opportunistic and resistant infections. For these reasons, a low threshold should be maintained for electing inpatient therapy until the infection can be controlled.

The third category—patients with severe episodes of acute sinusitis—includes patients with acute frontal sinusitis and acute sphenoid sinusitis. Severe acute frontal sinusitis may be identified by severe frontal headache and exquisite tenderness of the frontal sinuses. Usually, an immediate sinus series is taken in this case. If the Caldwell view demonstrates an air-fluid level or opacification of the frontal sinus, the diagnosis is confirmed.

Severe acute sphenoid sinusitis is less obvious and harder to diagnose. These patients may have nonlocalizing headache or vertex, occipital, or temporal headaches. As direct tenderness cannot be elicited, endoscopic evaluation is helpful. Often, plain radiographs will be unrevealing, making a CT scan the only reliable way to confirm the diagnosis.

Once the diagnosis of severe acute frontal or sphenoid sinusitis is made, the patient should be admitted to the hospital for observation and intravenous antibiotics. The primay concern in such cases is the high risk for intracranial complications. Most cases of sinus-related intracranial infection are caused by acute frontal or sphenoid sinusitis. Although most patients would be adequately treated by outpatient therapy, the risk for these patients warrants a short hospitalization to assure the desired outcome. If the patient with this diagnosis does not respond to therapy within 24 to 48 hours (i.e., with marked improvement in headache and tenderness), surgical intervention should be considered.

Antibiotics. The management of acute sinusitis centers around the selection of appropriate antibiotic therapy. To date, only a handful of randomized prospective studies have been performed to address this issue. Despite this, the results of these studies are compelling in that they suggest that amoxicillin alone is the antibiotic of choice for treatment of acute sinusitis.[20–22] Unfortunately, these studies are currently outdated, and their relevance to current practice is questionable. Because of this, expert panels have met to consider the treatment of acute sinusitis and have made alternative recommendations. Table 5–3 shows some of the antibiotic regimens that have been discussed. The author currently favors amoxicillin/clavulinic acid as the first-line oral antibiotic therapy. This is based on the finding that more than 95% of isolates from acute sinusitis are sensitive to this combination antibiotic. Clarithromycin is the customary choice for first-line treatment in penicillin-allergic individuals.

The hospitalized patient with complicated or severe sinusitis will require intravenous antibiotics. The bacteriologic characteristics of these infections are strikingly similar to those of uncomplicated acute sinusitis. However, the severity of the infection warrants more aggressive broad-spectrum coverage. Ampicillin/sulbactam combination or cefuroxime plus clindamycin have been two favored regimens. Alternatively, vancomycin plus an aminoglycoside can be used for penicillin-allergic individuals. When specific culture data are available, these should be used to direct therapy.

The length of treatment remains controversial. Current recommendations range from 10 days to 3 weeks for the initial course of treatment. To date, no study has documented a proven benefit to longer courses of treatment. However, the rationale for prolonged treatment is the high incidence of relapse after short courses of antibiotic therapy. This is thought to be attributable to persistent mucosal edema in the ostial regions of the sinuses, leading to impaired mucociliary clearance. A second factor is the relatively poor penetration of antibiotics into the sinus secretions. This combination of effects leads to recontamination and subsequent reinfection. The prolonged therapeutic course theoretically maintains a sterile environment until the mucosa can heal and normal mucociliary clearance can be restored.

Failure of the initial course of antibiotics is determined by progression of symptoms after 48 hours on the medication, or failure to improve after 5 to 7 days. In either of these circumstances, an empiric trial of a second antibiotic is usually attempted before progressing to a more invasive course of treatment. If the second course of antibiotics proves ineffective after 2 weeks of therapy, investigation of the cause of failure is indicated.

TABLE 5–3
First-Line Antibiotics for Acute Sinusitis

Amoxicillin	Amoxicillin/clavulinic acid
Erythromycin	Cefuroxime
Trimethoprim/ Sulfamethoxazole	Clarithromycin
	Clindamycin

Usually, nasal endoscopy will be performed at this point, and a CT scan of the sinuses will be obtained. Depending on the results of the CT scan, a sinus aspirate may be indicated, or the patient may require admission for a course of intravenous antibiotics. Continued failure of medical therapy will eventually prompt surgical intervention. Alternatively, if the infection progresses despite adequate medical therapy, surgery may be indicated much earlier.

Adjunctive Therapy. Table 5–4 lists some of the available adjunctive therapies. Antihistamines have long been prescribed for patients with acute sinusitis. The rationale is that, by blocking histamine receptors, the inflammatory process will be diminished. This has never been demonstrated in any prospective clinical trial. In fact, the predominant effect of antihistamines is to dehydrate the secretions. Although this may be of some symptomatic benefit in rhinitis, in cases of sinusitis, this is contrary to the goal of promoting mucociliary drainage. Antihistamines are, therefore, not recommended.

Nonsteroidal anti-inflammatory drugs, such as aspirin, acetaminophen, and ibuprofen, have no direct effect on decreasing the duration or severity of a sinus infection. However, they are successful in decreasing headache and are potent antipyretics. In this capacity, they may significantly lessen the symptoms and thus are of value.

Saline irrigations and steam treatments are adjunctive therapies that have gained many supporters despite a lack of scientific data that substantiate a benefit in relieving or hastening the resolution of acute sinusitis. The proposed mechanism of action of irrigations is mechanical removal of secretions with subsequent improvement in mucociliary clearance. Moreover, irrigations are thought to lessen the inflammatory load, resulting in decreased work for the body's natural defenses. Steam purportedly has not only a mucolytic effect, but also a decongestant effect and, possibly, a direct inhibitory effect on the bacteria. Although there is insufficient evidence to suggest these therapies for all cases of acute sinusitis, they appear to be harmless, inexpensive, and readily accessible. Therefore, patients who wish to utilize these therapies should not be discouraged from doing so.

TABLE 5–4
Adjunctive Treatments for Acute Sinusitis

Antihistamines*	Saline irrigations
Oral decongestants	Steam
Topical decongestants	Nasal steroid sprays*
Mucolytics	
Nonsteroidal anti-inflammatory drugs	

* Not recommended by the author, but listed for completeness.

Nasal decongestants come in both topical and oral systemic preparations. The purpose of these medications is to improve mucociliary clearance by shrinking the mucosa and lessening the ostial obstruction. Decongestants also open up the nasal cavity, thus improving nasal breathing, olfaction, and potentially, mucus clearance from the nose. Topical decongestants are generally prescribed for no more than 5 to 7 days. The evidence of an untoward effect of prolonged usage with induction of rhinitis medicamentosum is strong.[23] Because of the potential for patient abuse, the author does not routinely prescribe topical decongestants. Oral decongestants are routinely prescribed. Typically, the decongestant is combined with a mucolytic agent and given for a period of 1 month. The rationale behind the prolonged treatment is to help prevent relapse after the end of the antibiotic course.

Mucolytics (now exclusively in the form of guaifenesin) are thought to improve mucociliary clearance by thinning secretions and allowing the sinuses to clear the mucus more easily. To the author's knowledge, these agents have not been studied in a randomized prospective trial for acute sinusitis. Clinical experience suggests, however, that they are effective and result in decreased symptoms, primarily improving postnasal discharge, throat irritation, and congestion. The dose generally prescribed in combination preparations is only 400 mg twice each day. Maximal mucolytic action is not obtained, though, until three times this amount is taken (1200 mg twice each day).

Nasal steroid sprays are widely prescribed for chronic nasal and sinus diseases. The rationale for their use in acute sinusitis is less clear-cut. These medications decrease nasal inflammation and, therefore, promote mucociliary clearance by decreasing edema around the ostium and directly improving ciliary function. Also, nasal steroid sprays decrease congestion and lessen mucus production. The controversy exists because the onset of action of these drugs is delayed, and peak effect may not be reached until after 10 days of continued use. Most cases of acute sinusitis are nearly resolved by this point. For this reason, nasal steroid sprays are not routinely prescribed for the treatment of isolated acute sinusitis.

Summary. Initial treatment for acute bacterial rhinosinusitis consists of a 2-week course of an appropriate antibiotic and adjunctive therapy for up to 1 month. The author usually prescribes a decongestant/mucolytic combination, nasal saline spray, and nonsteroidal anti-inflammatory medications. Failure to achieve a significant response in the first week will usually prompt a change in the antibiotic and institution of nasal steroid sprays. Continued failure after the second course of antibiotics is an indication for direct culture of the sinus and consideration of a CT scan to investigate the reason for treatment failure.

Sinus Aspiration

Sinus aspiration by direct sinus puncture through either the sublabial canine fossa approach or the transnasal inferior meatus approach is the definitive method for obtaining sinus cultures. The sinus puncture can also be used to allow irrigation of the infected sinus. Although the diagnositc value of this procedure is well established, the evidence to support the therapeutic value of irrigation is not. Theoretically, the irrigation can lessen the inflammatory load of the sinuses and unplug a blocked sinus ostium. Controlled clinical trials, though, are lacking.

Most authors have not recommended this procedure as a part of routine first-line therapy in community-acquired acute rhinosinusitis. The patient who presents with persistent pain and tenderness of the maxillary sinus after at least 1 week of an appropriate antibiotic is a candidate. Alternatively, a second empiric course of antibiotics can be prescribed. Usually, this second-line therapy will involve an antibiotic that will cover beta-lactam–resistant strains and gram-negative bacteria.

The widest use of the direct sinus aspirate is in specialized patient groups, including ICU patients, HIV-infected patients, patients receiving chemotherapy, and those undergoing organ transplantation. All of these groups are routinely treated with suppressive antibiotics and have altered immune function. These factors increase the incidence of atypical or resistant organisms. Management of these patients is greatly facilitated by obtaining accurate culture results to guide therapy.

Aspiration Procedure. The technical aspects of the aspiration procedure are outlined in Figure 5–1. The transnasal route is usually favored owing to the fact that this allows the needle to avoid the infraorbital nerve, the tooth roots, and the sinus laterally. The area of the puncture is anesthetized with a small amount of 1% lidocaine with 1 : 100,000 epinephrine. A 16-gauge angiocatheter or a commerically available trocar is then selected. The needle is firmly grasped and rotated back and forth under constant controlled pressure until it penetrates the bone and enters the sinus. The needle is then withdrawn, leaving the catheter in the sinus. The sinus is aspirated with a syringe attached to the catheter. If the sinus is initially dry, 3 cc to 5 cc of sterile saline are injected into the sinus and then withdrawn.

If irrigation is to be performed following the aspiration, the aspirating syringe is removed and a 20-cc or

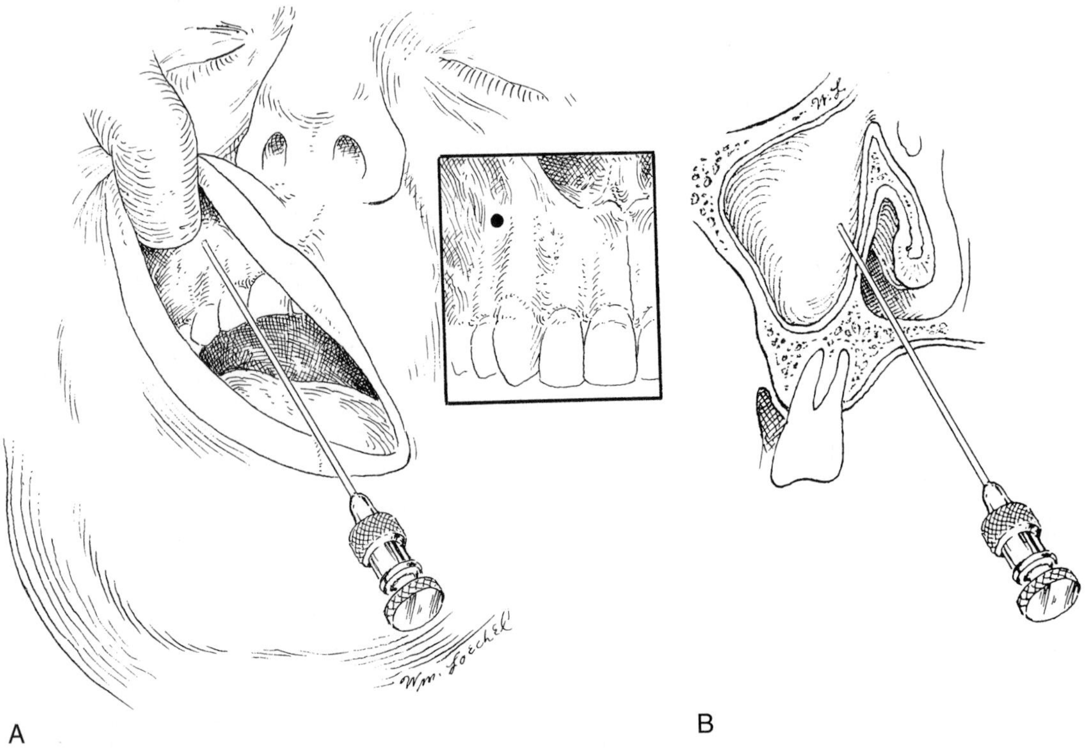

Figure 5–1. *A,* Transoral approach for sinus aspiration. A depression above the root of the canine tooth, referred to as the canine fossa, is punctured in an upward and lateral direction. *B,* Transnasal approach for sinus aspiration. The needle is directed laterally and superiorly through the inferior meatus 1 to 2 cm posterior to the pyriform aperture.

30-cc syringe that has been filled with sterile saline is attached to the catheter. The irrigation must be performed gently and only after confirming that the needle tip is in the sinus by aspirating air or fluid. Firm resistance to the irrigation should be an indication for repositioning the catheter or concluding the procedure.

Aspirates should routinely be sent for aerobic, anaerobic, and fungal cultures. In immunocompromised patients, cultures for tuberculosis and viral incubation should also be obtained. The results of the culture are then used to direct further antibiotic therapy.

CHRONIC SINUSITIS

Definition

Although the diagnosis of acute bacterial rhinosinusitis can be made on the basis of history and physical examination in most cases, the diagnosis of chronic sinusitis is more difficult. Chronic rhinosinusitis is usually defined as an inflammatory process of the sinuses lasting for longer than 12 weeks. In some classification systems, an intermediate category between acute and chronic rhinosinusitis is delineated to include those patients with symptoms lasting between 4 to 12 weeks. This category is known as subacute rhinosinusitis. The basis for differentiating subacute rhinosinusitis is largely practical in that this diagnosis has different treatment implications than chronic rhinosinusitis.

A fourth diagnostic category—recurrent acute rhinosinusitis—is also defined for those patients who develop discrete episodes of acute rhinosinusitis that are separated by periods of normal function and minimal or no symptoms. This condition is usually associated with radiographic studies that demonstrate sinusitis during episodes but are normal between episodes. In order to ensure that the patient does not merely have recurrent viral upper respiratory infection, at least one set of radiographs or CT scans should be obtained during an episode. These studies should clearly document signs consistent with acute rhinosinusitis.

Diagnosis

Clinical Presentation. The signs and symptoms of chronic rhinosinusitis are similar to those of acute rhinosinusitis. The classic symptoms are chronic facial pressure or pressure-type headaches, purulent or mucoid postnasal discharge, and nasal congestion. Commonly associated symptoms include nasal obstruction, anosmia or hyposmia, eustachian tube dysfunction, throat irritation, and cough. Fever, arthralgias, and myalgias are usually absent, although fatigue and malaise are commonly present. Also, most patients with chronic rhinosinusitis have a history of at least one episode of acute rhinosinusitis treated by antibiotics.

The onset of the condition, in some cases, may date back to childhood and include a history of allergies, asthma, or otitis media as a child. Alternatively, the onset may occur in association with an unresolved viral upper respiratory infection or an episode of acute rhinosinusitis that was only partially treated. It is most common to have the onset occur during the third or fourth decade of life; however, pediatric chronic rhinosinusitis and late adult onset chronic rhinosinusitis are also common conditions.

The physical examination findings may vary from entirely normal to massive nasal polyps. Most commonly, the patient has some findings suggestive of the diagnosis. These may include polyps in the nose or middle meatus, purulent or thick mucus draining from the middle meatus into the nasopharynx, and inflammatory changes of the middle turbinate, ethmoid bulla, or uncinate process. Occasionally, an accessory ostium of the maxillary sinus can be seen on endoscopic examination. In some cases, this may be draining mucus or may allow direct inspection of the maxillary sinus. The presence or absence of a deviated septum neither supports nor diminishes the chances of diagnosing chronic sinusitis. It is an important observation, though, and the presence of a severely deviated septum must certainly be considered in the overall management of the patient with chronic rhinosinusitis.

The patient who presents with chronic nasal and sinus symptoms may have one of several possible disease processes (Table 5–5). Classically these syndromes have markedly differing presentations. The patient with chronic rhinosinusitis has pressure headache and thick, postnasal discharge with few findings on anterior rhinoscopy. The patient with allergic rhinitis has sneezing, watery rhinorrhea, seasonal variation, and nasal congestion with boggy, pale or bluish turbinates on examination. The patient with nonallergic rhinitis has watery rhinorrhea, nasal congestion with enlarged turbinates and normal-appearing mucosa, and no seasonal variation. Finally, the patient with an isolated deviated septum has a dry nasal obstruction with obvious septal deformity on examination.

The difficulty in establishing the diagnosis of chronic rhinosinusitis is that the classic syndrome is frequently not present. Patients with allergic rhinitis or isolated deviated septum will often describe headaches or pressure and postnasal discharge, and those with chronic

TABLE 5–5
Differential Diagnosis of Chronic Nasal and Sinus Disease

Chronic sinusitis	Nonallergic rhinitis
Allergic rhinitis	Deviated nasal septum

rhinosinusitis may report seasonal variation. In addition, it is common to have combinations of these classic syndromes present simultaneously. For example, a patient may have allergic rhinitis and a deviated septum in association with chronic rhinosinusitis.

The diagnosis of chronic rhinosinusitis has been facilitated by an algorithm that has been widely adopted. This is published in a number of formats, including the Bulletin of the American Academy of Otolaryngology/Head and Neck Surgery.[24] Table 5–6 shows this algorithm. The important principles are to confirm the history with physical findings and CT scans.

Diagnostic Tests. Adjuvant testing for chronic sinusitis centers around CT scanning of the sinuses. Other studies that may have utility in acute sinusitis, as described earlier, are much less reliable in the setting of chronic sinusitis. Standard sinus radiographs are unreliable because of the lack of detail in the ethmoid sinuses and the difficulty in interpreting mucosal thickening on these studies. The explanation for this is that chronic sinusitis is typically a condition of mucosal thickening. These findings, which are well demonstrated on CT scan, become difficult to discern on plain radiographs, especially in the ethmoid and sphenoid sinuses.

The CT scan using bone windows and direct coronal projections demonstrates the distribution of mucosal abnormalities ideally. In addition, this modality captures the subtle detail of the ethmoid bony labyrinth, enabling diagnosis of the underlying cause of the disease, as well as identification of surgical landmarks, if necessary. A number of studies have now been published that have evaluated the incidence of certain findings in normal and diseased states.[25–29] These factors firmly establish the CT scan as the study of choice for evaluating chronic sinusitis.

TABLE 5–6
Diagnosis of Chronic Rhinosinusitis*

Major Factors	Minor Factors
Facial pain/pressure	Headache
Facial congestion/fullness	Fever
Nasal obstruction/blockage	Halitosis
Nasal discharge/ purulence/discoloration	Fatigue
Postnasal drainage	Dental pain
Hyposmia/anosmia	Cough
Purulence in the nasal cavity on examination	Ear pain/pressure/fullness

* Chronic rhinosinusitis is defined as a condition of greater than 12 weeks' duration that includes two or more major symptoms or at least one major symptom and two or more minor symptoms.

It is essential, though, to correlate the findings on CT to the patient's known history and physical examination. The reason for this is the high incidence of mucosal findings in normal patients without sinusitis. Usually, abnormal findings in normal patients are limited to mucus retention cysts and subtle mucosal changes along the walls of the sinuses. Most patients with chronic sinusitis will demonstrate severe mucosal changes or sinus opacification. The need to correlate the clinical findings with the radiologic examination is underscored by the large number of exceptions to this general rule. Occasionally, a patient will have minimal clinical and radiographic findings that nonetheless lead to recurrent infections and chronic symptoms. Alternatively, some patients will manifest significant but transient changes that may be caused by acute viral infection or allergy. For this reason, it is generally recommended that CT scans be performed only after a course of medical therapy so as to minimize the possibility of obtaining misleading information.

Bacteriology

The bacteriologic characteristics of chronic sinusitis are markedly different from those of acute sinusitis. The technique used to harvest the cultures, as well as the local patterns of disease, will significantly affect the prevalence of different organisms. Table 5–7 shows findings that are typical of reported case series, with the exception that most series report a higher incidence of *Staphylococcus aureus*.[30–32]

The relative incidence of anaerobic bacteria in chronic sinusitis continues to be debated. The incidence ranges from 0 to nearly 100% depending on the series quoted.[33–35] The usual explanations for this wide range are the method used to obtain and transport the cultures and the relative efficacy of the laboratory in isolating anaerobic species. However, it should be noted that patient selection and community variation will also affect the incidence of anaerobes cultured.

It is also common for no growth to result from cultures of patients with chronic sinusitis. The reasons for this are unknown, although possible explanations include noninfectious inflammation, anaerobic infection, and viral infection.

Medical Therapy

Antibiotics. The initial treatment of almost all patients with chronic sinusitis will be medical. The general classes of therapeutic agents are the same as described for acute sinusitis, but the combinations and duration of therapy are markedly different. The first consideration, as with acute sinusitis, is the choice of antibiotic. For initial empiric therapy, the antibiotic must cover the bacteria known to occur in this condition, specifically,

TABLE 5-7
Bacteriology of Chronic Sinusitis

Organism	Incidence (%)
Streptococcus viridans	26
Streptococcus pneumoniae	18
Hemophilus parainfluenza	16
Hemophilus influenza	10
Anaerobes	10
Miscellaneous gram-negative aerobes	19
Staphylococcus aureus	2

Reprinted with permission from Jiang RS, Hsu CY, Leu JF. Bacteriology of ethmoid sinus in chronic sinusitis. Am J Rhinol 11(2):133, 1997.

Staphylococcus, anaerobes, and gram-negative bacilli. For this reason, amoxicillin/clavulinic acid is again the preferred choice. Alternatives include clindamycin, cefuroxime, and clarithromycin. Second-line therapy would include ciprofloxacin, cefprozil, or levofloxacin.

Specific antibiotic therapy may be based on the results of cultures with detailed drug sensitivities. However, obtaining cultures in this setting is difficult. Nasal swabs have been shown to correlate poorly to direct sinus cultures. Puncture of the maxillary sinus may be negative owing to the absence of pooled secretions to aspirate from the sinus. The best method appears to be endoscopically guided middle meatus swabs using a thin, cotton-tipped applicator.[17]

In most cases, the length of therapy will need to be at least 3 weeks. This long interval is required to fully sterilize the sinus cavity during the prolonged resolution of the chronically inflamed mucosa.

Adjunctive Therapy. In most cases, adjunctive therapy will include treatment with nasal steroid sprays. Currently, there are many products available, with no evidence to indicate that any one is better than the others. Initially, the spray is usually administered at the highest dose recommended and continued for at least 1 month. Often, a prolonged treatment course of 3 to 6 months will be prescribed to help prevent recurrence. In patients with hyperplastic sinusitis or severe accompanying allergies, an indefinite course of nasal steroid therapy is prescribed. The safety of this practice has been borne out through clinical practice. The reason for this is the low systemic blood levels detected after use. This results in a very favorable therapeutic ratio of treatment dose to toxic dose and the absence of systemic side effects. The side effects are generally limited to nasal mucosal abrasion or erosion and epistaxis.

A recent report has suggested that topical steroids may lead to open-angle glaucoma.[36] However, this was convincingly demonstrated only with prolonged use of pulmonary aerosols, which generally result in greatly increased blood levels of active drug. A second study of nasal topical steroids only failed to show any increase in risk for ocular complications.[37]

Oral systemic steroids can also be used to treat chronic sinusitis. The dose and duration of therapy need to be adjusted for the specific clinical situation.

Additional therapy consisting of combination decongestant plus guaifenesin is also usually prescribed for the initial therapy of chronic sinusitis. These drugs are prescribed for at least 1 month and often, for 2 to 3 months. Unless the patient has an unusually good response to these agents, they are normally discontinued after the first 2 to 3 months to avoid potential long-term effects of the decongestants on blood pressure.

Treatment Algorithm. Essential to this consideration is the presumptive diagnosis of chronic rhinosinusitis based on the best judgment of the physician at the time of initial evaluation. Treatment begins with a 3-week course of antibiotics combined with 1 month of oral decongestant/mucolytic therapy and topical nasal steroid spray. The patient is reevaluated at the end of 1 month. Following the initial course of therapy, if the patient does not respond adequately, a second and sometimes third full course of therapy is prescribed using a different antibiotic. In addition, if the initial trial is not successful, allergy testing may be considered. If the response is adequate, maintenance therapy is continued for up to 3 to 6 months using the nasal steroid spray before withdrawing treatment. Following two or three full courses of therapy, if the response is not adequate, a CT scan of the sinuses is obtained. If the CT findings correlate to the clinical findings and history, suggesting persistent chronic rhinosinusitis, surgery is offered to the patient. If there is a discrepancy between the CT scan and clinical picture, the patient is reevaluated and alternative diagnoses are assessed, including allergy and atypical facial headache.

MEDICAL MANAGEMENT OF SINONASAL POLYPS

Sinonasal polyps or hyperplastic sinusitis usually require intensive and prolonged medical care to effect symptomatic control. Whether the etiology of the polyps is infection or allergy, simple antihistamines, decongestants, and antibiotics have little or no effect. Two separate patient groups are commonly seen: those with limited middle meatus polyps and those with pansinus sinonasal polyposis.

Patients with more limited disease tend to present on initial diagnosis with nasal obstruction, pressure headache, and postnasal drainage. The examination reveals small to moderately sized polyps limited to the middle meatus and middle turbinate. The CT scan typically shows focal disease with aeration of some of the sinuses. Allergy testing is usually advised, and avoidance therapy or possibly immunotherapy is considered. These patients often respond well to combination medical therapy using nasal steroid spray and antibiotics. After the initial course of therapy, if the patient does respond, then the steroid spray is continued indefinitely. If the patient has an inadequate response, a course of low-dose oral steroids is attempted. Surgery is offered to patients in this category who do not respond to the oral steroids or whose symptoms recur early after withdrawal of the steroids.

Patients with pansinus polyposis almost never respond well to routine medical therapy. In these patients, a specific diagnosis is important for long-term management. Several different underlying diagnoses can be seen. These include allergic fungal sinusitis, severe inhalant allergy, and aspirin triad. Definitive therapy usually includes surgery, perioperative oral steroids, and immunotherapy against specific allergens. All patients undergo a complete CT scan to help delineate the extent of the disease and presence of inspissated secretions. Allergy testing should be done before therapy is initiated. Perioperative oral steroids are normally prescribed. As an isolated therapy apart from surgery, steroids may be successful in medically obliterating the polyps. However, the duration of this effect is typically short-lived; in most cases, complete relapse is seen within months. The dose required to shrink nasal polyps is usually in excess of 0.5 mg/kg/day of prednisone. Typically, a starting dose of 60 mg per day in divided doses is prescribed for 7 days and then tapered over 2 to 3 weeks in 10-mg steps. The side effects of this regimen are usually limited to mild weight gain, acne breakouts, and occasionally, mood disturbance. Other, more serious side effects are possible, however, so the prescribing physician should be well versed in these complications and advise the patient of the risks.

For patients with pansinus polyposis, surgery is almost always necessary. Complete removal of the polyps, together with complete sphenoethmoidectomy (by whatever technique), is usually combined with perioperative oral steroids. The preoperative regimen is often 60 mg/day of prednisone for 10 days prior to surgery. Postoperatively, the dose is tapered from 40 mg/day in 10-mg decrements every 5 days. Long-term maintenance of oral steroids is avoided, but all patients are encouraged to use nasal steroid sprays indefinitely.

The role of immunotherapy in these patients is controversial. If they have significant inhalant allergies, this treatment modality can be tried. Immunotherapy works best as an adjunct to surgery, rather than a replacement for surgery. Similarly, aspirin desensitization for patients with aspirin triad is a treatment modality that may help prevent recurrence of polyps, but is unlikely to result in substantial improvement as a substitute for surgery.

FUNGAL SINUSITIS

Many different species of fungus have been documented to cause human sinus disease. Table 5–8 lists some of the more important. These conditions may present in a number of ways and often mimic acute and chronic sinusitis caused by bacteria, but with dramatically different treatment implications. For this reason, they form a class of sinus infections that can be thought of as a unique category of disease. The following sections describe the more commonly encountered entities.

Fungus Ball

This well-known clinical condition usually presents as a chronic sinus infection involving a single sinus. The maxillary sinus is most commonly involved,[38] followed by the sphenoid[39] and ethmoid.[40] Isolated fungus ball of the frontal sinus is quite rare. This condition occurs due to the implantation of fungus into an otherwise normal sinus. Fungus balls are usually found in immunocompetent individuals without risk factors. Radiologically, this usually manifests as an opacified or partially opacified sinus, often with calcifications or hyperdense areas seen on CT scan. Normally, there is not evidence of bone erosion or expansion. Magnetic resonance imaging (MRI) may show a signal void at the center, but usually there is low signal on T1- and T2-weighted images. Pathologic examination shows a mass of matted fungal hyphae without significant inflammatory exudate. Mucosal biopsies show chronic inflammation but no evidence of invasive fungal infection. Cultures are usually positive for the causative organism.

Treatment of this condition is simple surgical removal. Once the sinus is fully evacuated of the fungal

TABLE 5–8
Human Fungal Sinus Pathogens

Family	Genera	Species
Moniliaceae	Aspergillus	Fumigatus, flavus, niger
Dematiaceae	Bipolaris	Spicifera, senegalensis, hawaiiensis
	Exserohilum	
	Curvularia	Lunata, senegalensis, australiensis
	Alternaria	Alternata
Basidiomycetes	Schizophyllum	Commune
Mucoraceae	Rhizopus, Rhizomucor, Absidia, Mucor, Apophysomyces	

mass and adequate drainage is created through the natural ostium of the sinus, no further antifungal therapy is warranted. Recurrences may arise, possibly related to incomplete evacuation of the fungus or, rarely, reseeding from reexposure.

Allergic Fungal Sinusitis

Allergic fungal sinusitis was first described in 1983 and was named and defined a year later.[41] Essential features of this disease are extramucosal, allergic mucin-containing fungal hyphae; sinonasal polyposis; and allergy to the involved fungus. The histology of the mucin demonstrates abundant, degenerating eosinophils; Charcot-Leyden crystals; and fungal hyphae. Biopsy studies of the involved sinus mucosa reveal severe chronic sinusitis with abundant eosinophils, but no demonstrable fungal invasion. The patient demonstrates hypersensitivity to the appropriate fungal antigen on skin testing, or high circulating levels of specific immunoglobulin E (IgE) on radioallergosorbent testing (RAST).[41–43]

The theoretical pathophysiology of this condition is that the patient has a true allergic hypersensitivity to the inciting fungus. The fungus is inhaled and adheres to the nasal or sinus mucosa, initiating an acute allergic response. The ensuing inflammation traps the fungus in a moist, dark environment that is ideal for growth of the fungus. The cycle of allergic response and growth continues until the full-blown clinical condition is manifested.

The clinical picture on presentation is usually one of a young patient, 15 to 40 years old, with severe chronic sinusitis and nasal polyps. The condition may be unilateral or bilateral, but almost always involves more than one sinus. The CT scans demonstrate severe inflammatory mucosal thickening with opacification and hyperdense areas.[44] Often, there can be bone erosion by pressure necrosis and expansion rather than invasion.

Initial medical treatment is usually unsuccessful, with little or no response to the usual antibiotics and nasal steroid sprays. This is because the inciting fungus is trapped in the sinuses and between inflammatory polyps. Complete surgical extirpation of all fungal elements is a necessary step in the management of this disease.

The best results are usually obtained if oral systemic steroids are combined with surgery. The patient is given a course of steroids immediately before surgery with the standard regimen of 60 mg/day of prednisone for 10 days before surgery. After surgery, the steroids are tapered over a 2- to 3-week period down to 20 mg/day and then kept at that dosage for 3 to 6 months. The purpose of this is to try and effect full healing of the mucosa before withdrawing the steroids. Thereafter, the patient is followed closely and indefinitely at 3-month intervals, with significant relapses being treated with further courses of oral steroids.

An alternative therapy employed by one research group is fungal desensitization using immunotherapy.[42, 45, 46] This group has described creating a serum containing varying amounts of up to nine different known fungal antigens. Repeated injections in increasing doses over a prolonged period apparently have resulted in desensitization to the fungal antigens, based on skin testing and significant clinical response. Definitive demonstration of the superiority of this methodology is pending.

The newest therapy available for allergic fungal sinusitis is long-term treatment with itraconazole. This oral antifungal agent is successful in suppressing the growth of most applicable fungi in the sinuses. This therapy results in prolonged remission from the disease. Unfortunately, upon withdrawal of the itraconazole, the condition rapidly returns. The role of this therapy has yet to be defined.

Chronic Invasive Fungal Sinusitis

Chronic invasive fungal sinusitis is the least common form of fungal sinusitis. Recently, it has been suggested that this disease be separated into two categories: chronic invasive fungal sinusitis and granulomatous fungal sinusitis.[47] However, as both conditions are rare, it may not be practical to distinguish the two entities without additional information that clearly differentiates their clinical courses. The hallmark of this disease is the demonstration of tissue invasion into the sinus mucosa by the fungus in the setting of chronic rhinosinusitis. These patients typically have a prolonged course of chronic rhinosinusitis. CT scans show thickened mucosa with sinus opacification and widespread disease, but not always extramucosal debris and hyperdensities. There may be bone erosion through infiltration rather than expansion.

The invasive nature of the condition may be discovered either by the onset of complications related to intracranial or intraorbital spread or by documentation of tissue invasion on surgical pathologic examination. Tissue histology will demonstrate fungal hyphae in the submucosa. Often, there is a marked granulomatous inflammation with multinucleated giant cells and classic granulomata. A wide variety of fungal pathogens is possible. The most frequent causes are varieties of Aspergillus or one of the dematiaceous fungi. Patients may have a normal immune system or may have altered immune capacity. However, most of these patients will not have a severely impaired immune system. If the immune system is severely depressed, the invasive fungal infection will usually become fulminant.

Treatment of this condition is by surgical removal of all involved sinus mucosa and prolonged antifungal therapy. It is generally not necessary to debride all involved bone or soft tissue if this would require sacrifice of vital structures, such as the skull base, eye, and brain. Antifungal therapy with intravenous amphotericin B is usually advised to a high dose of 2 to 3 g or as tolerated. Alternatively, liposomal amphotericin may be given if the patient develops renal insufficiency or intolerance to the standard amphotericin formulation.

After completing the intravenous course of therapy, a prolonged course of oral antifungal therapy is advisable. Itraconazole is currently the favored agent. This may be continued for up to 12 months or longer if necessary. The endpoint of therapy will be decided by follow-up serial CT or MRI scans until normalization or stabilization is reached. Eventually, a trial of withdrawal of therapy will be needed. The patient should be closely observed during this interval for recurrent disease.

Ultimately, most patients with this disease can be cured if the immune system is normal. In immunocompromised patients, the prognosis is much less certain and mortality has been described.

Fulminant Fungal Sinusitis

Acute or fulminant presentation of fungal sinusitis is a disease seen almost exclusively in immunocompromised patients. This condition is defined by the rapid development of progressive invasive fungal infection. Tissue culture and stains most commonly demonstrate either Mucor or Aspergillus species.[47–49] As these two fungi are associated with different clinical presentations, they are addressed individually.

Mucor. Rhinocerebral mucormycosis presents as a rapidly progressive condition of inflammatory ischemic necrosis. The organism invades blood vessels, causing thrombosis and subsequent ischemic necrosis. The disease occurs in diabetics who are either ketoacidotic or who develop ketoacidosis early in the course of infection, patients undergoing bone marrow transplant, and others with severely altered immune systems. The hallmark clinical findings are dry, black eschar forming over the infected sinus, inferior turbinate, or palate.

The necrotic zone will rapidly spread to involve the entire sinus tract, face, eye, skull base, and brain if left unchecked. This condition is a true surgical emergency and requires immediate and complete debridement of all involved tissues and bone. Subsequently, the underlying immunosuppression must be corrected and high-dose intravenous amphotericin initiated and continued to 3 g or the maximum tolerated dose. In selected cases, surgery can be limited to endoscopic debridement, but frequently, radical surgery with maxillectomy and, possibly, orbital exenteration may need to be performed.[49–51]

Liposomal amphotericin may have distinct advantages in its penetration into ischemic tissues, and case reports suggest cures are even possible with this drug without surgery. However, surgical debridement is still recommended until the exact role and efficacy of this agent are defined.

Aspergillus. This family of fungal agents is known to cause a wide variety of human diseases. In patients undergoing bone marrow transplant and others with immune system dysfunction, a fulminant sinus infection can occur.[52] As opposed to the chronic invasive disease, this entity presents rapidly and progressively without antecedent chronic sinusitis. It may initially present as headache, sinus drainage, and congestion, but it is not diagnosed until complications, sepsis, or tissue invasion noted on biopsy is documented.

It is clearly distinguishable from mucormycosis by the absence of tissue necrosis. This organism does not cause thrombosis and, therefore, does not lead to the formation of black eschar. The predominant tissue reaction is severe inflammation with exceedingly friable and fragile mucosa that is hypervascular and that bleeds excessively when manipulated. In patients with immunosuppression, there is often an accompanying coagulopathy secondary to either low platelet count, coagulation factor deficiency, or both.

This leads to a dilemma in treatment. Antifungal therapy alone will probably be insufficient to resolve the infection, and surgical intervention may be unsafe owing to an unstable patient or severe coagulopathy. Successful treatment will require a combination of antifungal therapy and surgery. Therefore, the patient must be stabilized as quickly as possible, the coagulation system supported with transfusions of red blood cells, platelets, and plasma, and the surgery performed with maximal decongestion and adequate postoperative packing.

The prognosis for this condition is poor. However, if early aggressive intervention can be instituted, the patient may be able to survive.

PREDISPOSING CONDITIONS

Table 5–9 lists some of the conditions that predispose individuals to sinusitis. The management of sinusitis in these patients needs to be individualized to account for the specific combination of factors present. In the

TABLE 5–9
Syndromes Associated with Sinusitis

Cystic fibrosis	Selective immunoglobulin deficiency
HIV infection	Sarcoidosis
Samter's triad	Wegener's granulomatosis
Immotile cilia syndrome	

following sections, a brief discussion of some of the more common syndromes is given.

Cystic Fibrosis

Cystic fibrosis (CF) is an autosomal recessive inherited disorder of the exocrine glands throughout the body. The specific genetic defect is a family of mutations to the gene encoding for the CF transmembrane conductance regulator.[53] This protein helps to control the homeostasis of exocrine secretory cells by regulating the chloride ion transport across the cells' outer membrane.

Affected individuals manifest abnormally thick secretions from target organs, including the pancreas, sweat glands, and respiratory mucosa. The thickened secretions tend to obstruct and become trapped within pancreatic ducts, alveoli, and sinus ostia. The result is a clinical picture of pancreatic failure, recurrent pulmonary infections leading to bronchiectasis, and chronic sinusitis.

Sinusitis is very common in patients with CF, with nearly 100% manifesting some degree of abnormality on CT scan of the sinuses.[54, 55] Sinonasal polyps are also very common in CF, with various studies reporting an incidence ranging from 10% to 67%.[56–60] This frequently presents in early childhood or infancy, but in rare cases, may be diagnosed in young adults without previous history based on their sinusitis. Despite major advances in the medical treatment of CF, the median survival remains only about 30 years. The primary cause of mortality is end-stage pulmonary failure. Currently, both lung transplantation and genetic therapy are under investigation as potential treatments.

The sinus disease must be considered in light of the patient's ultimately poor prognosis, as well as the presence of ongoing chronic pulmonary infection. In addition, the results of surgery in this population are markedly different than in normal patients. Owing to the inability of the sinuses to clear the thickened mucus, even after wide antrostomy, patients uniformly relapse within a few years after surgery.[61] For this reason, the usual indications for surgery have to be adjusted significantly.

Patients with CF and their doctors must be willing to accept some degree of chronic sinus symptoms. Surgery is reserved for those patients who develop symptoms so severe that the patient's lifestyle is significantly altered, preventing them from engaging in normal activities. Most commonly, this manifests as persistent severe headaches, persistent fever, or severe nasal obstruction. Other conditions, such as mucocele and orbital infection, constitute additional indications for surgery.

The medical management of CF-associated sinusitis consists of nasal steroid sprays, high-dose mucolytics, and frequent nasal irrigations. Antibiotics should be reserved for the most severe exacerbations and for perioperative management. The reason for this is that most patients with CF are periodically hospitalized to receive intravenous antibiotics for pulmonary infection. These frequent treatments lead to a high incidence of bacterial resistance to antibiotic. Also, since the antibiotic cannot cure the sinus infection long term, there is a tendency to overtreat the sinusitis with antibiotics. This poses a risk of inducing resistance in the more serious pulmonary infection.

Finally, in managing the patient with CF-related sinusitis, it is important that the otolaryngologist work in close cooperation with the pulmonologist and the remainder of the CF treatment team. Decisions on antibiotic therapy, surgical intervention, and perioperative management need to be made in the context of the overall management plan.

Human Immunodeficiency Virus Infection

Since the advent of the acquired immunodeficiency syndrome (AIDS) epidemic, it has been apparent that these patients have a high incidence of sinonasal disease. Some series estimate that up to 70% of patients with AIDS will have some degree of sinusitis.[62, 63] However, only about one third develop significant symptoms that require specific intervention. Besides the obvious immunodeficiency as a cause of sinusitis, adenoidal hypertrophy and a direct effect on the nasal mucosa are postulated. As part of the HIV infection, many patients develop lymphadenopathy with adenoidal hypertrophy as a manifestation of that process. Also, many patients with HIV will develop a syndrome similar to allergic rhinitis that may be caused by the direct effect of the virus on the nasal mucosa or as part of the immune response to the virus infection.

These patients not only have a high incidence of sinusitis, but as the HIV infection progresses and immune function fails, they develop a high rate of unusual and opportunistic infections in the sinuses.[64] This is a clear indication, especially in highly immunodeficient patients, for direct sinus cultures to be obtained early in the course of therapy. It has been recommended that, if the ambulatory patient with sinusitis does not respond to antibiotics within 1 week, then a sinus puncture should be performed. In hospitalized patients, the puncture should be performed immediately upon diagnosis before antibiotic therapy is started.

In addition to antibiotics, guaifenesin has been shown to offer symptomatic relief in outpatients.[65] In the study cited, patients receiving guaifenesin suffered less severe symptoms than their counterparts who did not receive the drug.

The keys to successful management of patients with HIV are (1) prescribing antibiotics based on culture-proven pathogens and (2) early surgical intervention in antibiotic-resistant cases. As opposed to the patient with a normal immune system, early surgical intervention may be imperative. In one study, 45% of the patients operated on had opportunistic infections, and 100% had organisms that would not respond to the commonly prescribed oral antibiotics.[64]

The early results of surgery in these patients have thus far been rewarding, with most experiencing significant symptomatic improvement. Ultimately, though, these patients will succumb to the disease process. The goal of sinus therapy is to minimize the severity of sinus-related symptoms and maximize quality of life while avoiding major sinus-related morbidity and mortality.

Samter's Triad

Samter's triad, or aspirin triad, is the term used to characterize the association of aspirin intolerance, nasal polyps, and asthma. This condition is thought to be related to an enzyme deficiency in the cyclo-oxygenase pathway of prostaglandin production. This deficiency leads to an overproduction of leukotrienes, which are, in general, proinflammatory mediators. In the presence of aspirin, which inhibits cyclo-oxygenase, the normal precarious balance of the immune system in these patients is disrupted. This creates a systemic reaction similar to anaphylaxis.

The nasal polyps in these patients tend to be refractory to medical management and rapidly recur after surgical removal. The only therapy that can control the growth of the polyps is treatment with oral steroids. Steroids are reserved in this situation for severe exacerbations. As with many other patients with predisposing conditions, these patients should be advised that a certain level of symptoms is to be expected. True symptom-free intervals will be rare, and usually follow treatment with steroids.

Immotile Cilia Syndromes

Immotile cilia syndromes form a family of genetically inherited conditions in which the cilia do not beat normally. This results in impaired mucociliary clearance and recurrent or chronic sinusitis. The most well known of these syndromes is Kartagener's syndrome,[66, 67] which includes the triad of situs inversus, male sterility, and chronic or recurrent sinobronchial infections.

The cornerstone of therapy for these patients is prevention of infection. This can be achieved through the use of decongestants, nasal steroid sprays, and prophylactic antibiotics. In addition, consideration should be given to surgery to create gravity-dependent drainage.

Selective Immunoglobulin Deficiency

In addition to the more severe, life-threatening, combined immunodeficiency states, patients may inherit or develop selective immunoglobulin deficiencies.[68, 69] These conditions are diagnosed by measuring specific quantitative immunoglobulin subtypes. Variations of this problem include IgA, IgG_1, IgG_3, and, most commonly in children, combined IgG_2 and IgG_4 deficiencies. In adults, the IgG_3 selective deficiency is the most commonly observed in the author's practice.

The clinical manifestations of these conditions include, most commonly, relapsing or recurrent acute sinusitis. Often, affected patients are otherwise healthy, but develop frequent episodes of acute infection. The individual episodes seem to respond well to antibiotic therapy, but typically, the infection recurs shortly after withdrawal of antibiotics.

It is unclear whether this syndrome represents a true entity, or alternatively, whether the low immunoglobulin levels may result from the recurrent infections that deplete the circulating immunoglobulin. In either case, patients with this syndrome tend to derive minimal benefit from endoscopic sinus surgery and routine medical management. Prophylactic antibiotics, administered as a once each day suppressive treatment or for 1 week of each month at full dose, have been beneficial. The benefits, though, seem to dissipate once the antibiotics are withdrawn. An alternative therapy consists of immunoglobulin injections. When given at regular intervals, some success has been described with this approach to long-term management.

Sarcoidosis

Sarcoidosis is an idiopathic, systemic, chronic granulomatous disorder that primarily affects the lungs.[70] It is recognized based on its clinical presentation and a pathologic examination demonstrating noncaseating granulomas on biopsy studies of involved tissue. Specific evaluation to rule out other causes of granulomatous inflammation must be completed before the diagnosis can be confirmed.

The nose and sinuses are infrequently involved in this disease, with the incidence ranging from 1% to 6% of patients with sarcoidosis[71–74] However, this low incidence may be attributable to inaccurate diagnosis or failure to appreciate the presence of rhinitis or sinusitis as being related to the underlying disease process.

This idiopathic disease may follow an unpredictable course of relapse and remission, or it may be manifested as progressive chronic disease. Generally, it is not curable, and sinus surgery cannot be expected to be of long-term benefit to the patient. However, it is treatable, and it responds well to systemic steroids, often resulting in complete remission that may last for an extended period.

Patients with sinonasal sarcoidosis may develop classic symptoms of chronic sinusitis and may or may not have a known history of sarcoidosis. The physical findings vary depending on the stage of disease, but the most common finding is the presence of nodularity, dryness, and crusting of the nasal mucosa. This cobblestone pattern is not often seen with other clinical entities. Unfortunately, many cases will be indistinguishable from uncomplicated chronic sinusitis.

A second, more rare form of the disease may be an acute presentation. These patients may develop severe acute sinusitis secondary to the granulomatous process obstructing the sinus drainage. This may lead to orbital and intracranial complications if not treated expeditiously. One form of acute presentation is known as uveoparotid fever or Heerfordt's syndrome. This condition presents with fever, swelling of the parotid glands, and acute uveitis. Failure to recognize this syndrome may result in loss of vision and other complications.

The standard therapy for sarcoid-related acute exacerbations of sinusitis is oral steroids in combination with antibiotics. The steroids are given at a dosage of 0.5 to 1 mg/kg/day of prednisone for 1 to 2 weeks, followed by tapering to a maintenance dose. This regimen almost always results in prompt and complete resolution. Antibiotics are administered as for sinusitis to sterilize any true bacterial component.

Chronic maintenance therapy after withdrawal of systemic steroids consists of nasal steroid sprays in high doses, guaifenesin in high doses, and frequent nasal irrigations. This regimen usually allows the patient to maintain a low to moderate level of symptoms.

Surgeons must resist the temptation to offer surgery for the routine indications. The results are predictably disappointing and may lead to synechiae or ostial stenosis.[75] Rather, surgery is reserved for patients with acute sinusitis that is unresponsive to therapy and for those with complications, such as mucocele or intracranial or orbital infection. Patients with chronic sinusitis who are unable to discontinue systemic steroids may elect surgery. However, careful planning and perioperative high-dose steroids are required to avoid unsatisfactory results.

Wegener's Granulomatosis

Wegener's granulomatosis is an idiopathic systemic disease characterized by the pathologic findings of necrotizing granulomas and perivascular inflammation in the absence of tuberculosis and fungal disease. The disease classically involves the nose and sinuses, lungs, and kidneys. This condition has a generally progressive downhill course if not treated appropriately.

The physical findings in the nose include severe mucosal destruction with ulceration, crusting, and bleeding. Frank necrosis of the nasal structures may occur, leading to septal perforation and saddle nose deformity.

The differential diagnosis includes the syndrome of lethal midline destructive disease. This clinical entity may be histologically consistent with Wegener's granulomatosis or polymorphic reticulosis. The latter is a rare condition that has been known under many names through the years, but now is best thought of as localized lymphoma of the nasal cavity.

Patients with Wegener's granulomatosis have a high incidence of sinus involvement, either through direct infiltration or by ostial obstruction and secondary infection.

Treatment of this disease is largely supportive, with little or no role for surgery. Frequent nasal irrigation is used to debride the crusts, antibiotics are prescribed for complicating sinus infections, and prednisone and cyclophosphamide (Cytoxan) are used to control the disease process. When immunosuppressive agents are initiated, Cytoxan is generally chosen for long-term treatment because it has a better side effect profile than long-term prednisone.

Curiously, the antibiotic combination trimethoprim/sulfamethoxazole was found to be effective in cases of Wegener's granulomatosis. For unknown reasons, this combination agent helps to induce a remission and can be very successful in maintaining a remission.

REFERENCES

1. Dingle JH, Badger GF, Jordan WS Jr. Illness in the home: A study of 25,000 illnesses in a group of Cleveland families. Cleveland: The Press of Western Reserve University; p. 347, 1964.
2. Berg O, Carenfelt C, Rystedt G, Anggard A. Occurrence of asymptomatic sinusitis in common cold and other acute ENT infections. Rhinology 24:223, 1986.
3. Gwaltney JM Jr, Phillips CD, Miller RD, Riker DK. Computed tomographic study of the common cold. N Engl J Med 330(1): 25, 1994.
4. Naclerio RM, deTimeo ML, Baroody FM. Ragweed allergic rhinitis and the paranasal sinuses. Arch Otolaryngol Head Neck Surg 123:193, 1997.
5. Williams JW Jr, Simel DL, Roberts L, Samsa GP. Clinical evaluation for sinusitis. Ann Intern Med 117(9):705, 1992.
6. Williams JW, Simel DL. Does this patient have sinusitis? JAMA 270(10):1242, 1993.
7. Laine K, Maata T, Varonen H, Makela M. Diagnosing acute maxillary sinusitis in primary care: A comparison of ultrasound, clinical examination and radiography. Rhinology 36:2, 1998.
8. Lund VJ, Gwaltney J, Baquero F, et al. Infectious rhinosinusitis in adults: Classification, etiology and management. Ear Nose Throat J 76(12):5, 1997.
9. Shinogi J, Majima Y, Takeuchi K, Harada T, Sakakura Y. Quantitative cytology of nasal secretions with perennial allergic rhinitis in children: Comparison of noninfected and infected conditions. Laryngoscope 108:703, 1998.
10. Shapiro GG, Furukawa CT, Pierson WE, Gilbertson E, Bierman CW. Blinded comparison of maxillary sinus radiography and ultrasound for diagnosis of sinusitis. J Allergy Clin Immunol 77:59, 1986.
11. Landman MD. Ultrasound screening for sinus disease. Otolaryngol Head Neck Surg 94:157, 1986.
12. McNeil RA. Comparison of the findings on transillumination, x-ray, and lavage of the maxillary sinus. J Laryngol 77:1009, 1963.
13. Axelsson A, Grebelius N, Chidekel N, Jense C. The correlation between the radiological examination and the irrigation findings in maxillary sinusitis. Acta Otolaryngol 69:302, 1970.
14. Benninger MS. Nasal endoscopy: Its role in office diagnosis. Rhinology 11:177, 1997.

15. Gwaltney JM Jr. Acute community-acquired sinusitis. Clin Infect Dis 23:1209, 1996.
16. Rontal M, Bernstein JM, Rontal E, Anon J. Bacteriologic findings from the nose, ethmoid, and bloodstream during endoscopic surgery for chronic rhinosinusitis: Implications for antibiotic therapy. Am J Rhinol 13(2):91, 1999.
17. Nadel DM, Lanza DC, Kennedy DW. Endoscopically guided cultures in chronic sinusitis. Am J Rhinol 12(4):1233, 1998.
18. Gold SM, Tami TA. Role of middle meatus aspiration culture in the diagnosis of chronic sinusitis. Laryngoscope 107:1586, 1997.
19. Gwaltney JM Jr, Scheld WM, Sande MA, Sydnor A. The microbial etiology and antimicrobial therapy of adults with acute community-acquired sinusitis: A fifteen-year experience at the University of Virginia and review of other selected studies. J Allergy Clin Immunol 90:457, 1992.
20. Matthews BL. Effectiveness and safety of cefoxime and amoxicillin in adults with acute bacterial sinusitis. Special report: Managing sinusitis. Postgrad Med May:41, 1998.
21. Rimmer D. Efficacy of cefoxime and amoxicillin in adults with acute sinusitis. Special report: Managing sinusitis. Postgrad Med May:50, 1998.
22. Brodie DP, Knight S, Cunningham K. Comparative study of defuroxime axetil and amoxicillin in the treatment of acute sinusitis in general practice. J Intern Med Res 17(6):547, 1989.
23. Yoo JK, Seikaly H, Calhoun KH. Extended use of topical nasal decongestants. Laryngoscope 107:40, 1997.
24. American Academy of Otolaryngology/Head and Neck Surgery-Bulletin 18(10):30, 1999.
25. Basak S, Karaman CA, Akdilli A, et al. Evaluation of some important anatomical variations and dangerous areas of the paranasal sinuses by CT for safer endonasal surgery. Rhinology 36:162, 1998.
26. Bolger WE, Clifford AB, Parsons DS. Paranasal sinus bony anatomic variations and mucosal abnormalities: CT analysis for endoscopic sinus surgery. Laryngoscope 101:56, 1991.
27. Lloyd GAS, Lund VJ, Scadding GK. CT of the paranasal sinuses and functional endoscopic surgery: A critical analysis of 100 symptomatic patients. J Laryngol Otol 105:181, 1991.
28. Calhoun KH, Waggenspack GA, Simpson CB, Hokanson JA, Bailey BJ. CT evaluation of the paranasal sinuses in symptomatic and asymptomatic populations. Otolaryngol Head Neck Surg 104:480, 1991.
29. Meyers RM, Valvassori G. Interpretation of anatomic variations of computed tomography scans of the sinuses: A surgeon's perspective. Laryngoscope 108:422, 1998.
30. Winther B, Vickery CL, Gross CW, Hendley JO. Microbiology of the maxillary sinus in adults with chronic sinus disease. Am J Rhinol 10(6):347, 1996.
31. Jiang RS, Hsu CY, Leu JF. Bacteriology of ethmoid sinus in chronic sinusitis. Am J Rhinol 11(2):133, 1997.
32. Hsu J, Lanza DC, Kennedy DW. Antimicrobial resistance in bacterial chronic sinusitis. Am J Rhinol 12(4):243, 1998.
33. Brook I. Bacteriology of chronic maxillary sinusitis in adults. Ann Otol Rhinol Laryngol 89:426, 1989.
34. Kennedy DW, Zinreich SJ, Rosenbaum AE, Johns ME. Functional endoscopic sinus surgery. Theory and diagnostic evaluation. Arch Otolaryngol Head Neck Surg 111:576, 1985.
35. Frederick J, Braude AL. Anaerobic infection of the paranasal sinuses. N Engl J Med 290:135, 1974.
36. Garbe E, LeLorier J, Bolvin JF, Suissa S. Inhaled and nasal glucocorticoids and the risks of ocular hypertension of open-angle glaucoma. JAMA 277(9):722, 1997.
37. Ozturk F, Yuceturk AV, Kurt E, Unlu HH, Ilker SS. Evaluation of intraocular pressure and cataract formation following the long-term use of nasal corticosteroids. Ear Nose Throat J 77(10):846, 1998.
38. Ferreiro JA, Carlson BA, Cody DT. Paranasal sinus fungus balls. Head Neck 19:481, 1997.
39. Klossek JM, Peloquin L, Fourcroy PJ, Ferrie JC, Fontonel JP. Aspergillomas of the sphenoid sinus: A series of 10 cases treated by endoscopic sinus surgery. Rhinology 34:179, 1996.
40. Rumans TM, Jones M, Ramirez SG. Fungal sinusitis presenting as an ethmoid mucocele. Am J Rhinol 9(5):247, 1995.
41. Katzenstein A, Sale S, Greenberger P. Pathologic findings in allergic aspergillus sinusitis. J Allergy Clin Immunol 72:89, 1983.
42. Mabry RL, Manning SC, Mabry CS. Immunotherapy in the treatment of allergic fungal sinusitis. Otolaryngol Head Neck Surg 116:31, 1997.
43. Manning SC, Mabry RL, Schaefer SD, Close LG. Evidence of IgE-mediated hypersensitivity in allergic fungal sinusitis. Laryngoscope 103:717, 1993.
44. Manning SC, Merkel M, Kriesel K, Vuitch F, Marple B. Computed tomography and magnetic resonance diagnosis of allergic fungal sinusitis. Laryngoscope 107:170, 1997.
45. Folker RJ, Marple BF, Mabry RL, Mabry CS. Treatment of allergic fungal sinusitis: A comparison trial of postoperative immunotherapy with specific fungal antigens. Laryngoscope 108:1623, 1998.
46. Mabry RL, Marple BF, Folker RJ, Mabry CS. Immunotherapy for allergic fungal sinusitis: Three years' experience. Otolaryngol Head Neck Surg 119:648, 1998.
47. DeShaxo RD, O'Brien M, Chapin K, et al. A new classification and diagnostic criteria for invasive fungal sinusitis. Arch Otolaryngol Head Neck Surg 123:1181, 1997.
48. Bendet E, Talmi YP, Kronenberg J. Rhino-orbito-cerebral mucormycosis. Otolaryngol Head Neck Surg 114:830, 1996.
49. Peterson KL, Wang M, Canalis RF, Abemayor E. Rhinocerebral mucormycosis: Evolution of the disease and treatment options. Laryngoscope 107:855, 1997.
50. Gillespie MB, O'Malley BW, Francis HW. An approach to fulminant invasive fungal rhinosinusitis in the immunocompromised host. Arch Otolaryngol Head Neck Surg 124:520, 1998.
51. Jiang RS, Hsu CY. Endoscopic sinus surgery for rhinocerebral mucormycosis. Am J Rhinol 13(2):105, 1999.
52. Saah D, Elidan J, Braverman I, et al. Clinical photographs—Rhinocerebral aspergillosis. Otolaryngol Head Neck Surg 119: 554, 1998.
53. Kerem B, Rommens JM, Buchanan JA, et al. Identification of the cystic fibrosis gene: Genetic analysis. Science 245:1073, 1989.
54. Nishioka GJ, Cook PR, McKinsey JP, Rodriguez FJ. Paranasal sinus computed tomography scan findings in patients with cystic fibrosis. Otolaryngol Head Neck Surg 114(3):394, 1996.
55. Halvorson DJ. Cystic fibrosis: An update for the otolaryngologist. Otolaryngol Head Neck Surg 120:502, 1999.
56. Neely JG, Harrison GM, Jerger JF, et al. The otolaryngologic aspects of cystic fibrosis. Trans Am Acad Ophthalmol Otolaryngol 76:313, 1972.
57. Cepero R, Smith RH, Catlin FI, et al. Cystic fibrosis—An otolaryngologic perspective. Otolaryngol Head Neck Surg 97:356, 1987.
58. Leiberman A, Cole P, Corey M, et al. Otolaryngological and rhinomanometric findings in cystic fibrosis. Am J Rhinol 5:61, 1991.
59. Magid SL, Smith CC, Dolowitz DA. Nasal mucosa in pancreatic cystic fibrosis. Arch Otolaryngol Head Neck Surg 86:106, 1967.
60. Rulon JT, Logan GB. Nasal polyps and cystic fibrosis of the pancreas. Arch Otolaryngol Head Neck Surg 78:192, 1963.
61. Marks SC, Kissner DG. Management of sinusitis in adult cystic fibrosis. Am J Rhinol 11(1):11, 1997.
62. Lamprect J, Wiedbrauk C. Sinusitis und andere typische Erkrankungum im HNO-Bereich im Rahmen des Erworbenen Immundefekt-Syndrome (AIDS). HNO 36:489, 1988.
63. Zurlo JJ, Feuerstein IM, Lebovics R, et al. Sinusitis in HIV-1 infection. Am J Med 93:157, 1992.
64. Upadhyay S, Marks SC, Arden RL, Crane LR, Cohn AM: Bacteriology of sinusitis in human immunodeficiency virus-positive patients: Implications for management. Laryngoscope 105:1058, 1995.
65. Wawrose SF, Tami TA, Amoils CP. The role of guaifenesin in the treatment of sinonasal disease in patients infected with the human immunodeficiency virus (HIV). Laryngoscope 102(11):1225, 1992.
66. Kartagener M. Zur pathologie der bronchiekriasien: Bronkiektasien bei situs viscerum invertus. Beitr Klin Tuberkul Spez 83:489, 1933.
67. Teknos TN, Metson R, Chasse T, Balercia G, Dickersin GR. New developments in the diagnosis of Kartagener's syndrome. Otolaryngol Head Neck Surg 116:68, 1997.
68. Sethi DS, Winkelstein JA, Lederman HL, Loury MC. Immunologic defects in patients with chronic recurrent sinusitis: Diagnosis and management. Otolaryngol Head Neck Surg 112:242, 1995.

69. Eigenmann PA, Ambinder RF, Lederman HM. Chronic sinusitis with acquired immunoglobulin A (IgA) deficiency after bone marrow transplantation. Otolaryngol Head Neck Surg 117(6): S226, 1997.
70. Crystal RG. Sarcoidosis. In Isselbacher KJ, Braunwald E, Wilson JD, et al. (ed). Harrison's Principles of Internal Medicine, 13th ed. New York: McGraw Hill; p. 1679, 1995.
71. Wilson R, Lund V, Sweatmen M, Mackay IS, Mitchell DN. Upper respiratory tract involvement in sarcoidosis and its management. Eur Respir J 1:269, 1988.
72. James DG, Barter S, Jash D, MacKinnon DM, Carstairs LS. Sarcoidosis of the upper respiratory tract (SURT). J Laryngol Otol 96:711, 1982.
73. McCaffrey TV, McDonald TJ. Sarcoidosis of the nose and paranasal sinuses. Laryngoscope 93:1281, 1983.
74. Neville E, Mills RG, Jash KD, et al. Sarcoidosis of the upper respiratory tract and its association with lupus pernio. Thorax 31:660, 1976.
75. Marks SC, Goodman RS. Surgical management of nasal and sinus sarcoidosis. Otolaryngol Head Neck Surg 118:856, 1998.

CHAPTER 6

Allergy Diagnosis and Management

Initially, one might wonder what a detailed chapter on the diagnosis and management of allergy is doing in a surgical textbook of rhinology. However, it is the author's belief that a thorough understanding and appropriate management of allergy is critical to the surgical practice of much of rhinology. Certainly, in terms of decision making prior to turbinate surgery, septoplasty, and most sinus surgery for inflammatory diseases, accounting for allergies is critical. The decision to proceed with these operations in nearly all cases includes an assessment of allergy and the impact that allergy treatment has on the underlying condition and the need for surgery. Additionally, in order for patients undergoing any of these surgeries to enjoy the optimal result from the operation, allergy must be managed appropriately. A septoplasty or turbinate reduction for obstruction in an allergic patient will quickly fail secondary to swelling of the mucosa and obstructing secretions if the allergy is not controlled.

Therefore, as allergy is an essential part of the evaluation and management of rhinologic surgery patients, this textbook includes a discussion of allergy. Many of the recommendations contained in this chapter are based on the opinions of the author. There are many alternative approaches that may be equally valid, or even superior. However, this chapter contains recommendations, as practiced by the author, that have been found to be useful in at least this one experience.

PHYSIOLOGY OF ALLERGY

Immune System and Immunoglobulin E

Allergy begins with an understanding of immunology. The immune system is a complex and carefully regulated combination of cellular and molecular components that protects the body from foreign substances and infectious agents. The cells include lymphocytes, macrophages, eosinophils, basophils, mast cells, and neutrophils (polymorphonuclear leukocytes [PMNs]). Each of these cellular components has a wide variety of functions and can produce and liberate a wide variety of inflammatory mediators. The principle cellular components that relate to the production of immunoglobulin E (IgE) and all antibodies are the lymphocytes and macrophages. Lymphocytes are divided into B-type and T-type cells. The T cells are derived from the thymus and are regulatory and effector cells. The B cells are the precursors to the plasma cells that produce the antibodies or immunoglobulins. Macrophages are important in antigen preparation and presentation for the activation of the immune system. The molecular components of the immune system are many inflammatory mediators and the immunoglobulins. Immunoglobulins are complex molecules that are the products of the immune cells that give the immune system specificity.

The immune system produces five separate classes of immunoglobulins that are different in both structure and function. Each immunoglobulin molecule or antibody will specifically bind to one particular molecule that is the target or antigen. Otherwise, the different classes of immunoglobulins vary considerably in terms of where they are found and what functional role they play. All immunoglobulins, though, share a common basic structure (Fig. 6–1). These molecules are glycoproteins that consist of two heavy protein chains and two light protein chains. The heavy chains are attached to each other by disulfide bonds in the so-called hinge region. The light chains attach to the heavy chains with one light chain for each heavy chain. Each heavy chain consists of three conserved or constant subunits and one variable subunit found on the end of the molecule. Each light chain consists of only one constant and one

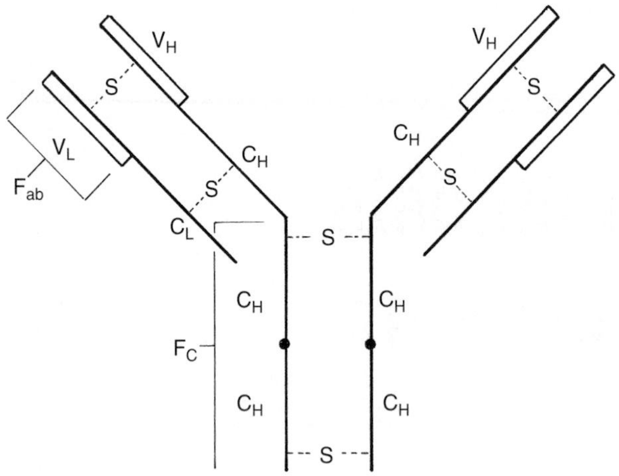

Figure 6–1. Structure of IgG antibody. Note the presence of two heavy and two light chains, each with variable and conserved regions.

variable subunit. The basic structure can be divided into the Fc portion, which conveys the specificity of the immunoglobulin to one of the five classes, and the Fab portion, which conveys the antigen specificity to the immunoglobulin. The variable portions of the light and heavy chains are clustered at one end of the Fab portion and confer the antigen specificity of the antibody.

The IgE class of antibodies is the one that stimulates the Gell and Coombs type 1 inflammatory response (immediate hypersensitivity) and is specified by the presence of the E-type heavy chain. IgE is found circulating in the blood in small amounts and consists of only 0.004% of circulating immunoglobulins.[1] IgE is primarily found in the peripheral tissues attached by the Fc portion to mast cells and basophils. IgE is produced, as are all antibodies, by B lymphocytes or their evolved antibody-producing derivatives, the plasma cells. The IgE antibodies are then bound to basophils or mast cells. Highly allergic patients may be found to have a larger number of copies of a particular IgE antibody on one cell compared to nonallergic individuals. The allergic patient may also have a larger number of mast cells in the target tissue. These apparent differences are what functionally determine which individuals will be allergic. In the presence of high saturation of the cell surface with IgE and a larger number of cells with the IgE antibody, the cell is more likely to encounter the antigen and more likely to react. The more cells that react and the greater the reaction, the greater the clinical response to the antigen exposure.

The number of copies of IgE per cell and the number of mast cells are likely controlled by genetic factors. Allergy itself can be familial, with the incidence of allergy in patients with two nonallergic parents being about 13%, the incidence with one allergic parent 30%, and the incidence with two allergic parents up to 50%.[2] Certain antibodies with known antigen specificities have been linked to specific human leukocyte antigen (HLA) types. This further implies the genetic control of specific allergies.

Individuals become sensitized to an antigen when a specific exposure occurs that results in processing of the antigen and production of IgE specific to that antigen. This processing is a highly complex function that includes the interaction of macrophages, T lymphocytes, and B lymphocytes. The antigen is initially encountered by a macrophage that processes the antigen and presents it to a T helper cell (CD4+). The antigen is then presented to the B cell. The T helper cell also liberates mediators, including interleukin 4 and 13, which stimulate the B cell to synthesize IgE specific to the presented antigen.[2] The specific IgE that is produced then populates the local mast cells and basophils, preparing the area to respond to repeat exposure. On repeat exposure, the acute allergic reaction is initiated by the contact of the antigen with the specific IgE antibody attached to mast cells or basophils. Cross-linking of two or more IgE molecules on the surface of the cell leads to cell changes that initiate the allergic cascade. In addition to this active process, there may be an active downregulation of IgE production by T suppressor cells (CD8+). The T suppressor cells may produce an inflammatory mediator that signals the neighboring immune cells to decrease or completely stop production of specific IgE or IgE in general. Production of allergy may occur when the suppression is released, allowing the plasma cells to synthesize IgE.

The ultimate advantage to the individual or species of having an allergic response is unclear. One could speculate that acute allergic response with stimulation of sneezing, congestion, and rhinorrhea in the nose may help to protect the lower airways by actively expelling the antigen from the nose, thus preventing the allergen from penetrating the lower airways. Pollen, dust, mold, and other substances may cause direct injury to the lungs, thus damaging a vital function. By protecting the lower airway with an allergic reaction, the individual is conferred a survival advantage. The presence of anaphylaxis, skin reactions, and allergic asthma may be an unfortunate side effect of this mechanism, as it is difficult to imagine the survival advantage to these reactions.

Allergy Cascade

The initial event in an allergic reaction is the binding of an antigen to specific basophil- or mast cell–bound IgE antibodies. It is possible that as few as 100 molecules of an antigen may be sufficient to initiate the allergic cascade.[1] Binding of two or more IgE antibodies to an antigen molecule results in cross-linking of the immunoglobulins. This probably results in a deformation in the cell membrane that opens a calcium channel in the cell membrane. The rapid influx of calcium into the cell causes activation of specific cellular proesterase into esterase. This maturation leads to the production of cellular energy supplies. This energy is utilized to activate microfilaments that move granules containing inflammatory mediators into position alongside the microtubules within the cell. The final cellular event is the release of the granules into the extracellular matrix.[1–3]

It is known that cyclic guanine monophosphate (cGMP) promotes this intracellular process.[1] Cyclic GMP is produced by guanylate cyclase, which appears to be under control of the parasymathetic nervous system and is activated by acetylcholine. Conversely, cyclic adenosine monophosphate (cAMP) inhibits the intracellular reaction following antibody cross-linking. Cyclic AMP is known to be produced by adenylate cyclase. This enzyme is stimulated by the sympathetic nervous system and epinephrine. This explains one of the mechanisms by which epinephrine inhibits the allergic reaction. cAMP is metabolized by an enzyme named phosphodiesterase. This activity results in the decrease of available cAMP and an increase in the cellular processes leading to degranulation of the inflammatory mediators. Additionally, phosphodiesterase is known to be inhibited by theophylline. This agent then results in deactivation of the phosphodiesterase with a subsequent increase in cAMP. This, in turn, results in a decrease in the cellular processes involved in degranulation and thus a decrease in the severity of the allergic reaction.

The release of the inflammatory mediator granules in this way results from the cross-linking of IgE antibodies on the surface of the mast cells. A large number of inflammatory mediators are released following degranulation. The most well studied and well known of these is histamine. This small compound is a bioactive amine that stimulates smooth muscle contraction in the bronchioles and small blood vessels. Histamine increases capillary permeability and results in increased nasal and bronchial secretions, itching, and sneezing.

A large number of inflammatory mediators are also released following mast cell degranulation. Some of these compounds are listed in Table 6–1. These mediators can be divided into vasoactive amines, enzymes, and chemotactic factors. The net effect of the vasoactive amines is to increase vascular permeability and smooth muscle contraction. In nasal and sinus tissues, this results in increased vascular permeability. The outcome is an increase in congestion and rhinorrhea. The enzymes released participate in the activation of metabolic pathways, in addition to inflicting tissue damage and assisting in repair. The chemotactic factors recruit primarily eosinophils into the tissues of the nose, but also lead to recruitment of macrophages, basophils, lymphocytes, and neutrophils. The effect of the predomination of eosinophils is to downregulate the inflammatory response by digesting the immune complexes and inactivating the proinflammatory mediators.

TABLE 6–1
Mediators of Acute Phase Allergic Reaction

Vasoactive Mediators
Histamine
Leukotrienes C4, D, and E
Platelet-activating factor
Serotonin (in rodents)
Prostaglandins
Bradykinin
Solubilizing Enzymes
Heparin
Chymase
Arylsulfatases
Beta-glucuronidase
Beta-hexosaminidases
Lysosomal enzymes
Kinin-generating proteases (lead to production of bradykinin)
Chemotactic Mediators
Eosinophilic chemotactic factor
Neutrophilic chemotactic factor
Leukotriene B
Prostaglandin D_2

In the early or acute phase of the allergic response, the action of the vasoactive amines predominate. This accounts for the classic acute symptoms of an acute allergic reaction, including sneezing, congestion, and rhinorrhea. As the reaction progresses, the late phase or delayed phase is entered. In this stage of the reaction, the inflammatory cells, especially the eosinophils, predominate. These cells lead to a cellular infiltration into the tissues, resulting in further congestion, swelling, and thickened secretions. This phase typically takes place 3 to 12 hours after the initiation of the allergic reaction. The late-phase reaction is mediated by the production of a number of mediators, including tumor necrosis factor–alpha (TNF-alpha) and granulocyte macrophage colony-stimulating factor (GM-CSF).[4] Assuming no further exposure to the allergen, the cellular influx will have cleaned up the acute reaction by the end of 6 hours, at which time the tissues will begin to return to the baseline state. However, in the presence of repeated or continuous exposure, as in a true clinical situation, the symptoms of the late phase persist, with periods of exacerbation of acute-phase symptomatology.

CLINICAL SYNDROMES

Allergic Rhinitis

Allergic rhinitis is the most common allergic disorder and among the most common chronic diseases in the

United States. Evidence shows that allergic rhinitis is increasing in incidence internationally, but the highest rate of increase is in the industrialized Western nations. The reasons for this are unclear, but one might speculate that there is a relationship to pollution, diet, or the rise of modern medicine. Prior to modern medicine, patients with severe allergies, especially anaphylactic reactions and asthma, had a definite survival disadvantage. However, with the intervention of modern medicine, these conditions do not confer any tendency to restrict survival or reproduction.

History. Recognition of allergic rhinitis among the various possible explanations for nasal and sinus disease begins with a thorough history. In almost all cases, taking a careful history will lead to a conclusive diagnosis of the presence or absence of clinically significant allergy. The hallmark symptoms of the acute-phase nasal reaction are sneezing, nasal congestion, and watery rhinorrhea. The sneezing is typically frequent, and bouts of multiple consecutive sneezes are common. The nasal congestion may vary from mild to severe with alternating cyclic congestion common. This occurs when one side of the nose is patent and the other is congested and blocked, with the blocked side alternating from side to side periodically. The watery nasal mucus is usually profuse. This leads to the frequently observed "nasal salute." This term refers to the use of the palm of the hand to wipe the base of the nose and help the individual sniff the mucus back into the nose. In children with severe allergies, this action may become habitual. Secondary symptoms may include itchy, watery eyes and headaches. The eyes may be directly involved by conjunctival inflammation or the nasolacrimal duct may be blocked by nasal congestion, leading to excessive tearing. Headache is normally related to pressure within the nose and sinuses secondary to severe congestion. Although true sinus headaches secondary to pressure or infection within the sinuses may occur in allergic patients, this would be expected as part of the late phase or as complications of persistent allergic rhinitis.

The acute-phase reaction is indicative of true allergy, and especially after exposure to a specific agent, these symptoms are highly suggestive of allergy. The symptoms of the late-phase reaction, however, are less specific for allergy. The most common late-phase symptoms are congestion, nasal blockage, and postnasal drip. Many patients experience secondary symptoms of eustachian tube dysfunction, throat irritation, and pressure headaches. In addition, it is common for patients to develop either otitis media or sinusitis secondary to allergy. The difficulty in diagnosis of allergic rhinitis is further compounded by the fact that many patients experience the late-phase symptoms without the acute-phase symptoms or specific recollection of a causative exposure.

Many patients with allergic rhinitis will experience seasonal variation in their symptomatology. This is especially true of patients with allergies to pollens. The classic syndrome of hay fever is related to ragweed pollen allergy and presents with a combination of acute- and late-phase symptoms in the late summer and fall of each year when the ragweed pollen counts are elevated. Other seasonal variations may suggest specific allergies. Examples include tree pollen allergy in the spring, grass pollen allergy in the late spring and summer, and dust and mold allergies in the winter. This last association is related to the use of furnaces and recycled air, which increases the dust and mold counts in indoor air compared to the summer, when open windows and air conditioning decrease recycled air. Some specific allergies may be year-round, such as food allergies or allergies to pets, such as cats, dogs, and horses. In these cases, it is usually possible to elicit a history of acute-phase reaction when heavy contact with the inciting agent occurs.

The past medical history is also important. The presence of previous severe reactions, rashes, eczema, asthma, angioedema, drug reactions, or anaphylaxis will indicate a high likelihood of allergic rhinitis. Most patients will also have some history of taking and benefiting from over-the-counter medications or some other treatment. While this information must be carefully considered, it may provide important clues to the presence of allergy. A family history of allergy is also important. Although the presence of allergy in a family member or the absence of allergy in any family member is not direct evidence of allergy in the particular patient, this can help indicate the likelihood of allergy.

Finally, when obtaining the history of a patient with probable allergy, it is important to investigate the potential sources of allergens in the patient's environment. In this part of the discussion with the patient, the home, work, and/or school environment should be investigated. The type of air handling systems present, the quality of the air, presence of pets, the floor coverings, and condition of the bathrooms and basements will indicate the severity of the exposure in the living situation of the patient. This is important when initiating therapy.

Examination. Examination of the patient with allergic rhinitis should include a complete head and neck evaluation and other aspects of physical examination as indicated. This may include auscultation of the lungs, examination of rashes, and an ophthalmologic examination. With regard to the head and neck examination, the specific findings referable to allergic rhinitis will be in the nose. One common finding, especially in children, is the allergic crease. This is a skin crease in the nasal supratip area created by the frequent, repeated, upward wiping of the nose, known as the "nasal salute." Intranasal examination classically shows congested pale or "blue" inferior turbinates. The turbinate mucosa does not turn a bright blue, but may take on a slight bluish tint. The mucosa, in any case, appears boggy and wet with the anterior nose often blocked by the swollen mucosa of the turbinates. Watery mucus is normally seen in the inferior meatus and around the front end of the inferior turbinate. In most cases of allergic rhinitis, the inferior turbinates shrink dramatically upon treatment with a topical decongestant. This is evidence of the fact that the turbinate is truly congested and not edematous or hypertrophied. After decongestion is achieved, abundant mucoid secretions are usually seen in the middle vault and posterior aspects of the nose. The mucus in these areas is usually much thicker and more turbid than that seen in the front of the nose before decongestion. This is because the deeper mucus is trapped and thus thickens up as it sits in the nose. Polyps may be seen in patients with allergic rhinitis. The polyps may be single, unilateral, or diffuse. The most common pattern in allergic patients is to have severe pansinus polyposis with severe nasal polyposis (see the next section).

On otologic examination, it is common to find evidence of eustachian tube dysfunction or effusion. The effusion is typically serious in nature and may be the direct result of allergic reaction in the middle ear mucosa, rather than secondary to nasal disease with eustachian tube dysfunction. The eye examination may reveal the so-called allergic shiner. This term refers to the edema of the lower eyelids, which may take on a discoloration to suggest recent orbital trauma. This may be secondary to frequent rubbing of the eyes due to itching or from edema of the conjunctiva from allergic conjunctivitis. The pharyngeal wall may appear erythematous and may reveal hypertrophy of lymphoid aggregates, as well as postnasal drip. The chest examination may reveal wheezing consistent with asthma or rhonchi associated with bronchitis.

Sinonasal Polyposis

A small percentage of allergic patients develop a severe form of chronic inflammation manifested by diffuse sinonasal polyposis. This syndrome is distinguished by the presence of bilateral obstructing nasal polyps, pansinus opacification with polypoid mucosa and retained secretions, and severe atopic disease. Not all patients with polyps have this condition. There are patients with polyps, even diffuse polyposis, who are completely nonallergic. In many of these patients, infection is the etiology of their polyps. Others may have Samter's triad (polyps, asthma, and aspirin sensitivity). These syndromes are discussed in greater detail in Chapter 5, as is the general topic of polyps. The discussion here is limited to patients with polyps related to allergy.

These patients are, in general, among the most allergic of all patients. They tend to have numerous, high-grade allergies when tested, have a history of allergies dating back to childhood, and often have other atopic diseases, such as asthma, food allergies, and allergies to drugs and insect bites. These patients may be severely symptomatic of nasal and sinus disease with obstructed breathing, postnasal and anterior rhinorrhea, headaches, and anosmia. Alternatively, some of these patients may have no symptoms other than anosmia and nasal blockage.

Examination of the nose usually reveals large obstructing polyps on both sides of the nose. There may or may not be secretions in the nose. If total obstruction is present, usually there is some pooling of mucus. In advanced cases, the nasal dorsum may actually begin to widen from the pressure of the expanding polyps. These patients may have epiphora if the polyps completely block tear drainage. The polyps are typically very pale and almost translucent, appearing virtually as bags of water. Only when the polyps are very long-standing do they take on a more opaque, fibrous appearance. In the presence of acute complicating sinusitis, the polyps may become inflamed and appear erythematous and friable.

In such cases, computed tomography (CT) scans usually show all sinuses to be opacified. There may also be bone demineralization, making definition of the bony landmarks difficult to interpret. Evidence of expansion within the sinuses may be noted, particularly in the infundibulum, but also in the ethmoid sinus, causing lateral bowing of the lamina papyracea. Normally, the lamina papyracea has a slight medial bow as the orbital walls all normally curve away from the globe. If the polyps are long-standing, the ethmoid will begin to expand, causing the lamina papyracea to bow toward the globe. In severe cases, there may be erosion of the skull base or lamina papyracea. As the polyps grow, there is a slight pressure exerted that can eventually lead to pressure necrosis and erosion of the bony wall.

One particular subcategory of allergic sinonasal polyposis is allergic fungal sinusitis. In these patients, a fungal organism gets trapped in the nose or sinuses either through digital introduction or inhalation. If the patient is allergic to the particular fungus, a severe allergic reaction is initiated. The fungus tends to become trapped within the sinus and, under certain circumstances, will grow instead of being eliminated by the patient's immune response. The result is that the fungus multiplies and induces an even greater allergic reaction. Eventually, the process gets out of control and a severe inflammatory polyposis develops.

These patients may be identified by several specific criteria. The clinical setting is one of severe sinonasal polyposis, usually with severe symptoms. Sampling of the inspissated secretions reveals fungal hyphae in the presence of an allergic-type mucin with degenerating eosinophils and Charcot-Leyden crystals. Culture of the specimen generally reveals a single fungal organism. To confirm the diagnosis, antigen testing may be used to identify specific allergy to the fungus isolated in the culture. In most cases, testing reveals severe allergy with numerous fungal and nonfungal allergens at high levels of allergy. CT scans in patients with allergic fungal sinusitis usually demonstrate fungal concretions in the sinuses, recognized by the presence of increased density or apparent calcification within the lumen of the sinus.

ALLERGY TESTING

One of the most important aspects of allergy management is allergy testing. Testing provides objective evidence of the presence of allergy, a basis for avoidance therapy, and the essential data necessary to formulate immunotherapy. There are a number of methods of allergy testing, including nasal cytology, skin testing, in vitro blood testing, and provocative or challenge testing. The skin testing methods include scratch testing, prick testing, intradermal testing, and skin endpoint titration (SET). Today, the most popular are prick testing and SET. Allergy testing by in vitro analysis using radioallergosorbent testing (RAST) or enzyme-linked immunosorbent assay (ELISA) has recently gained popularity. Challenge testing is rarely used today except in the case of food allergy because it is difficult and potentially dangerous. In the following sections, each of these methods is discussed and the potential role indicated.

Nasal Cytology

Examination of nasal mucus for cellular characteristics is a valuable tool in the diagnosis of allergic rhinitis. In the presence of allergy, the nasal secretions have an abundance of eosinophils and a relative absence of PMNs and bacteria. In acute inflammatory conditions, such as viral rhinitis and sinusitis, the nasal secretions have the opposite constituency, specifically, an absence of eosinophils and abundant PMNs and bacteria. This has been documented repeatedly over the past 70 years since the observations of Hansel.[5] Cytology testing requires certain equipment, including glass slides, fixatives, stains, and a microscope. Proper interpretation requires some experience but is readily learned. The limitation of the test is that it merely suggests allergy. It does not prove the diagnosis, identify the inciting allergens, or imply a particular treatment.

Skin Testing

All skin testing methods are based on the premise that introduction of an antigenic load into the dermis will lead to an immediate type 1 Gell and Coombs reaction, producing a discernible skin reaction. All of these tests require the same prerequisite conditions. The first is that the patient has a clean, dry skin surface devoid of inflammatory changes or markings that would interfere with interpretation of the result. Normally, the upper lateral arm or the back are used for these tests, as these areas provide wide, flat surfaces of uniform skin.

It is also important that the patient be amenable to testing. That is, the patient must have an intact immune system that is capable of reacting to a positive control and must be free of skin disease, such as dermatographia, so that there is no reaction to a negative control. In certain conditions, such as pregnancy, acute upper respiratory infection, and unstable cardiovascular disease, skin testing is contraindicated. Prior to testing, patients should be instructed to avoid certain medications that may interfere with the allergy testing. The most important of these are the antihistamines. Antihistamines successfully block the skin reaction, leading to no reaction or a diminished reaction. Depending on which antihistamine has been taken, a waiting period of up to 4 to 6 weeks may be necessary before skin testing is attempted. The shortest-acting antihistamines are diphenhydramine and chlorpheniramine. These agents impair the skin response for 3 to 5 days. By contrast, terfenadine and fexofenadine will inhibit the skin reaction for up to 2 or 3 weeks, whereas loratidine and astemizole may inhibit the skin testing for up to 4 to 6 weeks. Other medications, such as beta-blockers, may interfere with the skin testing, but it may not be possible to discontinue these essential medications for allergy testing. In such cases, completing the skin testing will be possible as long as the positive control reacts appropriately.

All methods of skin testing are associated with some degree of risk of a systemic reaction, even an anaphylactic reaction. The risk for each of the different methods is the subject of some controversy, but no method is completely without risk. For this reason, all patients should be informed of this possibility and should sign a consent for testing. Most importantly, the office site used for allergy skin testing should be prepared for a life-threatening reaction with all equipment and medications necessary for resuscitation readily available. In addition, a responsible physician trained in resuscitation should be present at the location, and all personnel in the office should be trained in cardiopulmonary resuscitation (CPR).

Scratch Testing. The scratch method of skin testing involves using a needle dipped in a specific antigen to place a small scratch on the skin. The scratches are usually placed on the back. After a short interval, the area is reexamined for erythema and induration. This method is highly subjective and lacks sensitivity. It is also limited in the number of antigens that can be tested. Further limitations include the inability to predict the exact amount of exposure that the patient will get to the antigen applied. In general, however, this method of testing has been found to be relatively safe, with few patients experiencing systemic reactions. However, with the ready availability of other, more precise testing methods, scratch testing is considered to be an inferior method and is not recommended.

Prick Testing. Prick testing has been a standard method for evaluating allergies for more than 70 years.[6] This test can be performed either by placing a drop of antigen solution on the skin and pricking the skin through the drop, or by placing the drop of antigen solution on the needle and then pricking the skin. In either case, a small but predictable amount of extract is introduced into the dermis. After several minutes, the degree of wheal and flair reaction is measured and compared to both positive and negative controls. A semiquantitative scale can be developed by the size of the skin reaction.

For many years, multitest applicators have been available that allow testing of a large number of antigens in a short time period. The most recent studies have shown these tests to have relatively good negative predictive value, but poor positive predictive value.[7] This means the absence of reaction on multitest screening correlates well to the absence of allergy. However, positive results must be confirmed with further testing. This implies that the sensitivity of the prick screening test is good in that most allergic patients will have a positive result on multitest screening; however, the specificity of the test is poor, meaning that the positive result may not be meaningful. This is contrary to the widely held belief that the weakness of the prick testing method is that it fails to detect borderline cases of allergy. The prick method theoretically delivers a lower dose of antigen to the dermis than is possible with intradermal testing, which results in a failure to detect the low-level allergy.

The advantages of the prick technique are that it allows relatively safe testing of a large number of antigens at a low cost in a short period of time. This is the characteristic of a good screening test. The disadvantages of the test are its relative degree of inaccuracy and the difficulty in translating the test results into a starting dose for allergy immunotherapy. As a screening test, though, this method has a high degree of reliability in determining whether or not an individual is allergic. Patients with a completely negative result on multitest screening are highly unlikely to have clinically significant allergy.

Intradermal Testing. Single-dose intradermal testing involves the injection of a test dose of antigen directly into the dermis using a needle and syringe. After a period of time, usually 10 minutes, the size of the wheal is measured and compared to a negative control. A semiquantitative measure of allergy is obtained by determining the size of the reaction compared to the control. The amount injected is typically 0.1 mL. The concentration of antigen used varies, depending on the setting in which the test is applied. When used as a screening test, the intradermal test uses a dilute solution of 1 : 1000 or less. When used as a confirmatory test, the dose is dependent on the degree of reaction observed during screening.

Currently, this method is not often used as a screening test because of the difficulty in determining an appropriate test dose. High-level dosing risks systemic reactions, whereas low-level dosing risks poor sensitivity. However, the method is commonly used as a confirmatory test after prick testing. In this setting, the single-dose intradermal test can serve as either a positive or negative confirmatory test. If the patient has a completely negative reaction to an antigen that the allergist believes the patient may be allergic to, the concentrate of the antigen may be injected to determine that no reaction to the highest dose occurs. Conversely, if the patient has a reaction on prick test that the allergist wishes to confirm with an intradermal test before starting immunotherapy, a more dilute solution based on the size of the reaction to prick testing can be used.

Skin Endpoint Titration. For most otolaryngologists, skin endpoint titration (SET) is the method of choice for allergy testing. This method involves intradermal injection of a test dose in sequentially increasing concentration until evidence of progressive wheal reaction is determined. For each antigen that is tested, a series of injections is used; in each case, 0.1 mL of the dilution is injected to create a 4-mm wheal.

Using the method developed by Rinkle,[8] serial fivefold dilutions of antigen are prepared from the original concentrate and the dilutions are labeled 1 to 10. The No. 1 vial, therefore, contains a 1 : 5 dilution, the No. 2 vial contains 1 : 25, the No. 3 vial contains 1 : 125, and so on up to the 10th vial. One of the more dilute vials is chosen to start the test, usually the No. 6 vial. A 4-mm wheal is created using the No. 6 vial, and 10 minutes later, the size of the wheal is measured. The negative control will usually spread out to 5 mm in this time period. A positive reaction is considered to be a 7-mm wheal or larger. The endpoint is determined as the lowest concentration that elicits a 7-mm wheal. It is customary to confirm the positive reaction by injecting a test dose one vial greater in concentration than the endpoint. The endpoint is confirmed by the presence of a 9-mm wheal using the endpoint +1 vial. This is referred to as the progressive wheal response.

This methodology is somewhat time-consuming, taking up to 60 to 70 minutes to test approximately 12 to 18 antigens in a single session. This is more costly and time-consuming than the multitest prick testing method. However, one can confidently determine the presence or absence of a specific allergy with a high degree of accuracy and reliability with SET testing. SET testing is usually considered to be the gold standard for allergy testing, as it allows one to safely test up to the concentrated antigen to elicit a reaction, and produces a quantitative measure of the degree of allergy by the endpoint determination.

The weakness of the SET method is that it is purported to be a poor screening method, as only a limited number of antigens can be tested; it is also generally more costly to perform than the prick method. However, with careful antigen selection (using the 12 most common antigens in the region of the testing facility), the presence or absence of allergy can be determined with greater than 95% certainty.[9] In other words, because the SET method can determine absolutely whether an individual is allergic to a specific antigen, fewer antigens are necessary to screen effectively. For most of the geographic regions studied, a high percentage of individuals will be allergic to one of the 12 most common allergies in the community, if that individual is actually allergic.

The strategy of most otolaryngologists who use the SET method is to screen with one or two antigens from each of the different classes of antigens in the community during an initial screening test. If the patient is determined to require immunotherapy, a second testing session is used to expand the test for each of the different classes to which the patient is allergic. For example, during an initial screening, a patient may be found to be allergic to mold, grass, and weed pollen, but not allergic to dust, animal, or tree pollen. A second session is then designed to expand the positive areas by including most of the molds, grasses, and weeds found in the geographical region. In this way, the patient is likely to be covered for all of the important antigens.

The final advantage of the SET method is the easy translation from testing to immunotherapy. By determining the endpoint—i.e., the minimum dose that elicits a true reaction—a safe starting dose can conveniently be identified. This dose can then be safely increased in small, measured increments until the maximum tolerated dose is reached.

In Vitro Testing

In vitro testing refers to the use of blood samples to measure circulating IgE antibodies. The total IgE level can be evaluated. In the past, this has been used to help determine whether an individual is likely to be atopic or allergic in general. However, it has been found that the total IgE level corresponds poorly to the presence or absence of clinically significant allergy and provides no information in terms of specific allergies. For this reason, it is not used by many allergists today.

The measurement of circulating, antigen-specific IgE can be performed by a number of different techniques. These methods are all quantitative and extremely specific. That is, the serum concentration of a specific IgE antibody for a specific antigen is measured and the presence of this circulating IgE implies, with a high degree of certainty, that the patient will be allergic to that specific antigen.[10, 11] The sensitivity of these tests is somewhat variable in that there may be locally expressed mast cell–bound IgE that does not circulate in the blood in measurable quantities. This can lead to false-negative test results, which lower the sensitivity of the in vitro methods.[10] However, for most clinically significant allergies, the circulating antibody level is closely correlated to the tissue-bound IgE levels and the degree of local reaction experienced with specific antigens.

The original and most commonly used in vitro test is the RAST. The RAST involves combining the patient's serum with specific allergens bound to a disk. After the serum is washed away, radiolabeled anti-IgE is incubated with the disk. The radiolabeled anti-IgE binds to the specific antigen-bound IgE on the disk. The disk is then measured in a gamma radiation counter to determine the level of radiolabled complexes. In this way, the exact number of molecules of a specific IgE in a measured volume of serum can be determined. The concentration of the antibody is then converted to a simple 0 to 4 or 0 to 6 scale to bring meaning to the value. Most laboratories consider the finding of a RAST level of 0 or 1 to be negative, with a RAST level of 2, 3, or 4 to be clinically significant.

There are now a number of alternatives to the original RAST assay, including modified RAST, ELISA, CAP, and FAST (fluorescent allergosorbent test). Each of these assays effectively measures the quantity of circulating IgE for a specific antigen. Most of these assays have been found to duplicate the specificity of the original RAST, but may have improved sensitivity. In every case, however, the gold standard for determining the presence of allergy will always be skin testing, with the SET method the most accurate and sensitive of all.

The role of in vitro testing remains controversial. In vitro methods have the disadvantages of delayed results, expense, and the possibility of introducing human error in transporting and performing the tests at a remote site. In addition, the in vitro tests are limited by the lower sensitivity of the test and the selection of antigens for testing. Although it is possible to request as many different antigens as desired from the laboratory, this requires additional blood samples and may become very costly. Most users of in vitro methods employ these techniques as a screening tool. Either a 6-, 9-, or 12-antigen screening panel can be devised. These panels will effectively determine the presence or absence of allergy in most patients. The larger the screen, the higher the sensitivity and predictive value of the screen.

In vitro methods can also be used to formulate immunotherapy. The quantitative in vitro techniques translate very accurately to the SET point determined by SET testing. In most cases, the SET endpoint will equal the RAST level + 1. That is, a SET endpoint of 4 usually will translate into a RAST level of 3. This information can then be used to formulate immunotherapy.

Challenge Testing

Challenge testing, a rarely used method of allergy testing, involves exposing the patient to a suspected allergen to determine whether a reaction occurs. Skin testing is the controlled offshoot of this principle. In challenge testing, however, a patient is exposed to the allergen in the target organ of concern. This may be the nasal mucosa, lungs, or gastrointestinal tract. The only form of this method that is currently used is to determine food allergies in the absence of a clear history of reaction. With this technique, the patient is placed on an elimination diet of unseasoned cooked meat, eggs, and water for 3 or 4 days to cleanse the system. These foods are chosen for the elimination portion since they rarely induce allergy. Food groups are added one food at a time for a period of 2 or 3 days per food and the patient is observed for a reaction. In this way, over a 1- to 2-month period, almost all foods in a patient's diet can be individually assessed. This method is time-consuming, inaccurate, and potentially dangerous if the patient has a severe allergy to one of the foods introduced. In modern practice, in vitro testing or skin testing is available to determine the presence of allergies to foods, as well as to inhalant allergens.

Antigen Selection

When considering either in vitro or skin testing, the allergist must choose the appropriate antigens for testing. Careful history taking can provide important clues to the appropriate selection of antigens. All antigens can be divided into one of eight groups. There are six inhalant groups, foods, and insects. The inhalant antigen groups include trees, grass, and weed pollen, mold, dust, and animals. For most otolaryngologists, the inhalant antigens are the most important. For the inhalant antigens, there are a wide variety of commercially available extracts that can be used. The number of extracts that are kept by the individual allergist for clinical use will depend on the nature of the practice. The allergist who uses the multitest prick method will be able to routinely test more than 100 antigens per patient if desired, whereas the allergist who uses the SET method will be able to routinely test only 12 to 18 antigens per screening session, and will be able to keep only 30 to 50 antigens in the office.

The author recommends that individual practitioners research the particular antigens common to their region. Within each of the allergen groups, specific antigens can then be selected that represent the most important ones for that region. This may vary widely from the desert to the tropics to the Midwest to the far north. Table 6–2 lists the antigens in each of the inhalant groups that the author uses for routine allergy screening in the Detroit, Michigan area. The author uses the SET method exclusively in practice; for this reason, fewer antigens are tested on a routine basis. The methodology in most circumstances is to use the 12-antigen screening panel for initial diagnosis. Later, if the patient becomes a candidate for immunotherapy, the groups that were positive on the screening are expanded to the full panel to make sure that all important antigens are included.

The decision of whether or not to test for foods and insect venoms will depend on the philosophy of the physician. Many otolaryngologists shy away from these antigen groups because they have relatively little correlation with otolaryngologic diseases. Conversely, some otolaryngologists believe strongly that food allergies are important to otolaryngologic diseases.

The author remains in doubt. In cases in which certain foods cause individuals to have rashes, asthma attacks, or anaphylactic reactions, the presence of food allergy is easy to understand. However, the concept of a food allergy that affects only the nose, sinuses, or ears is difficult to understand. Foods are absorbed through the intestines, which are loaded with immunoactive submucosal lymph tissue called Peyer's patches. After digestion, the food circulates through the blood, which contains circulating basophils and IgE, and is distributed to the entire body, including the skin and the lungs, which contain IgE bound to mast cells. The question is, in the absence of gastrointestinal symptoms, a rash, asthma, or anaphylaxis, how can an otolaryngologic reaction occur? For this to be true, one would have to postulate that locally bound IgE would not be found in the blood or any other part of the body. Because a complete understanding of the allergic response on a molecular and cellular level is still lacking, this remains

TABLE 6–2
Screening Panel for SET Testing

Dust	**Pollens**
Dermatophagoides farinae	Maple tree
Dermatophagoides pteronyssinus	Cottonwood tree
Mold	Johnson grass
Alternaria	Timothy grass
Aspergillus	Ragweed
Animals	Lamb's quarter weed
Cat	
Dog	

possible. However, concrete demonstration of this phenomenon is also lacking, so skepticism is in order.

ALLERGY THERAPY

The treatment of allergies, specifically allergic rhinitis, usually follows a three-tiered approach. The first tier of therapy is avoidance. Allergies only create symptoms when the patient is exposed to an offending antigen. By avoiding the antigen or eliminating the antigen to the greatest extent possible, antigen exposure is minimized and the symptoms are usually minimized as well. The second tier of allergy therapy is the use of pharmacologic agents. Today, more than ever before, there are a wide variety of medications that have been proven effective against allergies and allergy symptoms. However, this increasing number of medications makes the management of allergic rhinitis more complex. The third tier of allergy management is the use of immunotherapy. Perhaps in modern rhinology, a fourth tier—surgical management—could be added. This therapy, usually reserved for those in whom other treatments have failed, involves procedures performed on the inferior and, rarely, middle turbinates. These options are discussed in Chapter 7. In the following sections, each of the three tiers of allergy therapy is reviewed in detail to provide a framework for thoughtful allergy management.

Antigen Avoidance

Successful avoidance therapy begins with a knowledge of the specific allergies of the patient. Although many of these measures can be utilized without specific knowledge of allergies, most patients have a hard time justifying the expense and trouble without some assurance that their efforts are likely to be rewarded. The specifics of avoidance therapy are discussed based on the antigen class.

Dust Mites. The most common allergy, and one of the most important in terms of avoidance, is dust mite allergy. Dust mites are the microscopic organisms that live in common household dust and constitute the most common antigen found in dust. The mites specifically live off the exfoliated skin cells from people. Skin naturally flakes off at a constant and predictable rate throughout our lives. This exfoliated skin tends to accumulate in areas where dust can deposit, the most important of which are pillows and mattresses. Dust also can accumulate in carpeting, on curtains, and on flat surfaces throughout the house.

The most important measures in dust avoidance involve the bedroom area. People spend more time in their beds than any other single place during life. Not only are we in bed for long periods, but the dust itself is also in close proximity to the nasal mucosa as the head rests on the pillow or against the mattress. The pillow and mattress can accumulate staggering amounts of exfoliated skin and, hence, a heavy concentration of dust mites. To avoid this exposure, the mattress and pillow can be covered with a plastic cover. To improve comfort while sleeping, it is recommended that the mattress be covered directly by the plastic and a mattress pad and sheets be placed over the plastic. The pad and sheets should be washed in hot water once or twice each week to remove the skin and kill the dust mites. It is important that the pad and sheets be washed in hot water to kill the mites; otherwise, they may persist despite the effort. The pillow can be encased in a plastic cover, but then two pillow cases can be used over the plastic to improve comfort. In addition, a new foam pillow should be purchased at least once or twice each year. Feather pillows should be avoided as they tend to accumulate more dust.

Several other measures are helpful in minimizing dust exposure in the home. The first is to avoid deep pile or shag carpet. Low-Pile rugs and carpets or hardwood floors are preferred, as these floor coverings do not tend to trap dust. In addition, daily vacuuming and dusting of all flat surfaces will minimize the dust load in the house. Special dust-inhibiting shampoos for carpeting are also widely available. Preferably, someone other than the allergic individual should perform these household duties, although this may not be practical. Even if allergic patients must do their own dusting and vacuuming, this is preferable to allowing the dust to accumulate. It is also important to make sure that a clean and efficient filter is placed on the furnace every year and that the furnace is cleaned before turning it on each fall. This will help to minimize the circulating dust. The final measure to avoid dust is to have an air cleaner. This is discussed at greater length later in the chapter.

Mold. Mold avoidance is also very important and usually successful. However, molds and fungi are everywhere. They exist on our skin, in our mouths, on our food, in our homes, and in the soil. Molds may be airborne as well. The air mold counts vary during the season and depend largely on the geographic region. In the Midwest the mold counts in the air are at the lowest in the winter, tend to rise in the spring, and peak in the late summer before declining again. The same guidelines that apply to pollen avoidance, described in a later section, also apply to avoidance of airborne mold.

In terms of indoor mold, there are a number of effective measures. Mold tends to grow on wet surfaces and in warm areas. The chief places are in the bathroom, kitchen, and basement. In the bathroom, the floor and shower tiles should be disinfected on a regular basis.

Whenever the molding or tiles begin to show darkening or discoloration, this can be assumed to be mold. Commercially available cleaners, available at any supermarket, can adequately remove or kill this mold. In the kitchen, the most troublesome areas are under the sink and in the refrigerator. The area under the sink is often neglected but should be cleaned regularly to prevent mold. The rubber seal around the inside of the refrigerator door often grows mold, as do the drawers and shelves. Also, old food, especially fruit, tends to grow mold very readily. Cleaning the refrigerator and disposing of old food are important measures in preventing such exposure. Perhaps the most difficult area of the home for controlling mold is the basement. Many basements have damp corners that are rarely cleaned. Merely avoiding going into the basement is inadequate, however, because the basement air is usually sucked into the furnace and circulated throughout the house during winter. Therefore, keeping the basement dry and mold free should be a priority for all patients with mold allergy.

One area of special concern for mold allergy patients is the garden and yard. Gardening is a popular pastime. However, some of the most important allergens in allergic sinonasal diseases are common soil fungi. For this reason, gardening and yardwork should be strictly avoided by individuals with these allergies.

Animal Dander. Animal dander is actually somewhat of a misnomer because today, the actual antigen in animal dander is thought to be a salivary protein, not the hair or skin of the animal. Cats and dogs regularly clean themselves by licking their fur. This action deposits the offending salivary protein on the fur. This dries out, at which point it can become aerosolized. This mechanism explains why long-haired animals are worse than short-haired ones, and why cats are worse than dogs. Because the long hair is cleaned more often, it retains more of the antigen. In addition, cats are much more rigorous about their cleaning and so have a much higher antigen load on their fur. Animal allergies are particularly important because the contact with the antigen is so close and because the animals shed a great deal of hair onto the carpet and furniture. This can lead to a heavy antigenic exposure.

Most patients will not get rid of a pet, no matter how serious their allergy. This is a reality that allergists must face. It is always appropriate for the allergist to suggest removing the animal from the home, but as stated, this is almost never done. There are, however, alternatives. The most important is to keep the animal out of the bedroom, thereby minimizing the antigen load in that one room. A second priority is to avoid rubbing one's face into the animal's fur, as this results in marked exposure. If possible, hands should be washed after petting the animal. Frequent vacuuming of the floor and furniture also helps to decrease the fur content. Finally, shampoos are now available through most pet supply stores that help minimize the antigenic load of the fur. Bathing the animal weekly with one of these products can be beneficial.

Pollens. Pollens are among the most antigenic of potential allergens. Extremely low exposures can lead to significant reactions. This makes avoidance important. Pollens are a problem during the spring, summer, and fall up until the first frost. As the seasons change, or in year-round warm climates, the antigens change as the various plants come into bloom and release their pollen. For patients who have allergies to only one group of pollens—either trees, grasses, or weeds—the period of time of exposure can be relatively short and avoidance measures may be all that is necessary to control the allergy. Conversely, if multiple groups are involved, it may be harder to successfully avoid exposure.

Because the antigens are carried in the air, it is virtually impossible to avoid exposure completely. However, there are days when pollen counts are likely to be high, and on these days, prolonged outdoor exposure can be avoided. The pollen counts tend to be quite high on windy days after a recent rain. The rain tends to stimulate pollen release, the wind increases air carriage, and pollen counts therefore increase. During rain and on dry, windless days, the pollen counts tend to be comparatively low. However, for individuals with severe allergies to pollens, outdoor activities that prolong exposure, such as camping, hiking, and golf, can be avoided.

Air-handling systems are successful in lowering indoor pollen counts. To maximize the benefit, whether in a car or in the home or at work, the windows should be kept closed and the air conditioner should be kept on. If the individual does not have central air conditioning in the home, he or she should be encouraged to get a room air conditioner for the bedroom to avoid keeping a window open in the bedroom. Finally, an air cleaner may be helpful in avoiding pollens in the absence of any air conditioning capability.

Air Cleaners. For patients that have severe allergies and can afford the purchase, a room air cleaner is very helpful. This decreases the dust, mold, and pollen in the air. The most important place to keep it is the bedroom. However, keeping the air cleaner in the bedroom during the night and the most common living area during the day may be even better. The best air cleaners are designated as high-efficiency particulate air filters (HEPAs). These tend to be more expensive, but have the advantage of removing smaller airborne particles, including certain pollens, dust particles, and mold spores. Whenever the individual is buying an air cleaner, it is important to investigate the particle size the filter will protect against. Otherwise, the apparatus may be of little or no use.

Pharmacologic Therapy

Pharmacologic or drug therapy for allergic rhinitis is considered to be the second tier of treatment. In most clinical situations, medications are prescribed at the time of the initial patient visit along with avoidance measures. Avoidance may have long-term benefits and may ultimately relieve the necessity for medical therapy; however, in most cases, its benefits are delayed and do not provide immediate relief for the patient. Therefore, it is customary to begin with medical treatment at the time of initial diagnosis and then decrease the therapy as the situation indicates. In modern medicine, there are a large number of agents available to treat allergies. Generally, they may be classified into six categories. Table 6–3 lists the classes of medications, which are described in the following sections along with the indications for their use and the various agents available.

Antihistamines. Antihistamines are a chemically diverse group of agents that have in common the inhibition of the action of histamine. Their predominant effect is the competitive inhibition of the H1 histamine receptor. Antihistamines were the first class of pharmacologic agents found to have significant benefit in the treatment of patients with allergic rhinitis. The first medication with an acceptable toxicity profile in the class was phenbenzamine (Antergan), which was synthesized in 1942.[12] However, the first agent commonly used for routine treatment of allergic rhinitis was diphenhydramine. Today, this class of agents can be divided into traditional antihistamines, nonsedating antihistamines, and the newest form, topical antihistamines. Table 6–4 shows the most common of these agents used for allergic rhinitis.

Antihistamines are indicated for the symptomatic treatment of allergic rhinitis. Although it was once thought that these agents would inhibit the inflammatory response of allergies and thus block both the early- and late-phase reactions, it is now known that the effect is only on the early- or acute-phase reaction. By blocking histamine at the histamine receptor, these agents inhibit the effects of histamine release, which include sneezing, itching, and rhinorrhea. The late-phase reaction in allergies, as detailed in the earlier sections, is the result of the release of a host of other mediators, including chemotactic factors that draw in inflammatory cells. These factors that are not altered by antihistamines are responsible for the late-phase symptoms of congestion, mucoid rhinorrhea, and postnasal drainage.

In general, antihistamines are used either on an as-needed basis for symptomatic flare-ups or in an ongoing fashion to minimize chronic symptoms. In both cases, the antihistamines can be combined with other classes of agents. In either case, the antihistamines are effective in reducing sneezing, itching, and rhinorrhea in patients with allergic rhinitis. In numerous reports comparing symptoms in a variety of formats, antihistamines have consistently been found superior to placebo.[13–19] Whether one particular antihistamine is superior to the others is more controversial. Published reports can be cited that show conflicting claims. These studies all vary slightly in their methods and outcome measures, making definitive statements difficult.

It has been clearly demonstrated, however, that traditional antihistamine agents tend to cause a degree of unwanted sedation. Of the antihistamines listed in Table 6–4, diphenhydramine causes the most severe sedation. The sedating properties of this agent are so consistent that it is often recommended to help patients sleep. These sedating effects have been linked to problems with driving an automobile, learning in school children, and occupational injuries.[20, 21] The nonsedating antihistamines have been found not to cause any of these difficulties. Although definitive proof of the negative effects of sedation caused by traditional antihistamines is lacking, the suspicion of these effects is strong, and the availability of the nonsedating agents is immediate. For these reasons, when prescribing antihistamines for

TABLE 6–3
Medication Classes

Antihistamines	**Steroids**
Traditional	Topical
Nonsedating	Injected locally
Topical	Systemic
Decongestants	**Cromolyn Compounds**
Oral	**Anticholinergic Agents**
Topical	**Lipoxygenase Pathway Inhibitors**

TABLE 6–4
Antihistamines

Agent	Drug Class
Traditional	
Diphenhydramine	Ethanolamine
Clemastine	Ethanolamine
Chlorpheniramine	Alkylamine
Brompheniramine	Alkylamine
Nonsedating	
Terfenadine	Not classified
Astemizole	Not classified
Loratidine	Piperidine
Cetirizine	Piperazine
Fexofenadine	Not classified
Topical	
Azelastine	Phthalazinone

allergic rhinitis, clinicians are well advised to select one of the nonsedating agents.

The author prefers to use either loratidine, cirtirizine, or fexofenadine owing to the nonsedating properties of these agents. Terfenadine and astemizole have recently fallen into disfavor owing to their prolongation of the Q-T interval in the heart. This effect is amplified to a clinically significant degree in patients who are also taking a macrolide antibiotic or an antifungal agent, both of which increase the serum level of the antihistamine. Within a short period of time, it is possible that both agents will be removed from the market for this reason. Fexofenadine, however, is the active metabolite of terfenadine and does not appear to have this unwanted side effect. For this reason, it is favored over terfenadine.

It is important to remember that, if one antihistamine does not work well for an individual patient, it is worth switching to another antihistamine of a different class. In many cases, the second agent will provide significant relief. The reason for this is unclear, but there may be differences in receptor affinity that are based on slight differences in the receptor, or there may be differences in absorption based on diet or other factors that are not well understood. This variability may be one of the reasons why different studies come to different conclusions with regard to antihistamine efficacy.

The newest additions to the antihistamine class are topical agents. These are now available for patients who either prefer sprays or who cannot or do not benefit from antihistamine pills. The efficacy of the spray form seems to be equal to that of the pills. It remains unclear what effects the topical agent will have on the concomitant use of nasal steroid sprays in terms of efficacy and local side effects on the nasal tissues. One unique circumstance in which the spray may be applicable is in patients who are scheduled for allergy skin testing. The antihistamine pills will block the test, whereas the spray will not. For this reason, sprays can be used up to and including the day of the test in a patient who needs antihistamines for symptomatic relief.

Although antihistamines are typically the first agents prescribed for the treatment of allergic rhinitis, these agents alone are not commonly sufficient. As stated earlier, the antihistamines primarily improve sneezing, itching, and rhinorrhea. Most patients will also suffer from congestion and postnasal drip and may have headache or eustachian tube dysfunction. These symptoms will not be improved by antihistamines. In these cases, additional agents will be necessary. Decongestants are commonly combined with antihistamines in a number of prescription and over-the-counter medications. It is also common to combine antihistamines with nasal steroid sprays.

There are only a few contraindications for using antihistamine drugs. Most of these agents are not yet cleared for use in pregnancy, so they should only be used with the consultation of the patient's obstetrician. A relative contraindication is in the setting of acute or chronic sinusitis. In these situations, the goal of therapy is to promote sinus drainage. Antihistamines, by decreasing mucus production, may increase mucous thickness and retard drainage. Although this is a relatively theoretical argument, many otolaryngologists, including the author, prefer mucolytic agents in the setting of sinus infection. It does not make sense to use both a mucolytic and an antihistamine simultaneously.

Decongestants. Decongestants are sympathomimetic agents that stimulate the alpha-adrenergic receptors of the sympathetic nerves in the nasal mucosa. These drugs result in vasoconstriction of the precapillary arterioles and constriction of the venous sinusoids, decreasing the amount of blood in the tissues. This causes tissue shrinkage or decongestion. Decongestants come in oral medications, either as a single agent or in combination with antihistamines, mucolytics, antitussives, or analgesics. These can be over-the-counter or prescription combinations. Decongestants also come in topical sprays, all of which are over-the-counter medications.

There are only two commonly used oral decongestants: pseudoephedrine and phenylpropanolamine. They are of approximately equal strength and duration of action and can be considered essentially interchangeable, although phenylpropanolamine is, on the basis of effect per milligram, stronger. This is adjusted for by the fact that the tolerated dose before side effects is lower for this drug than for pseudoephedrine. There are three topical decongestants that are most commonly used: phenylephrine, xylometazoline, and oxymetazoline. These agents vary in the time until onset and duration of action, but are essentially equal in their peak decongestant effect.

Oral decongestants are indicated for patients who have symptoms of nasal congestion, nasal obstruction, facial pressure, sinus headaches, and eustachian tube dysfunction. Whenever any of these symptoms are present, the oral decongestants are appropriate to prescribe. The combination medications are used when the congestive symptoms are present in addition to other symptoms not affected by the decongestant. In patients with allergic rhinitis who have rhinorrhea and nasal obstruction or congestion, an antihistamine/decongestant combination is used. These combinations have been demonstrated to be more effective than antihistamines alone in treating allergic rhinitis.[22, 23] The other combinations—decongestants with mucolytics or antitussives and analgesics—are indicated for sinusitis or acute upper respiratory infection.

The limiting factor in the use of oral decongestants is the side effect profile. These agents are associated with numerous problems, including restlessness, jitteriness, insomnia, palpitations, hypertension, and prostate or bladder tension causing urinary retention. The proportion of patients for whom this becomes limiting ranges from 10% to 45% depending on the particular study.[22, 23] In most cases, the side effects are not severe, and patients have the option of working through the side effects or discontinuing the medication. Often, there are easy dosing modifications that make the medications more acceptable. For example, if jitteriness is the problem, a half-dose can be tried, or if the problem is insomnia, the medication can be taken in the morning only.

The topical decongestants are powerful agents in that they produce an almost immediate onset of maximal decongestion. These agents are indicated in the short-term treatment of acute upper respiratory infection, acute sinusitis, or severe exacerbations of allergic rhinitis. In all cases, however, the topical decongestants should be used for only 3 to 5 days per treatment episode. This is because of the well-known complication of these agents, rhinitis medicamentosum. This condition is a severe congestion of the nasal mucosa that results from prolonged treatment with topical decongestants. The mechanism of this effect has been debated. The most commonly accepted explanation is a rebound effect once the medication wears off. The rebound effect occurs when the venous sinusoids and arterioles dilate to a greater-than-baseline degree after the decongestant effect wears off, due to fatigue of the adrenergic receptors. This results in the clinical appearance of extreme congestion. The patient may then feel an increased need to take another dose of the topical decongestant. Eventually, hypertrophy of the mucosa occurs, resulting in a nonreversible increase in baseline congestion. The duration of treatment before rhinitis medicamentous develops varies depending on the agent used and how it is used. The shorter-acting agents have been found to cause the problem in as few as 10 days. The longer-acting agents may be tolerated for longer periods. If the agent is used carefully and only once per day, rhinitis medicamentosum may not develop for up to 30 days.[24]

Steroids. Steroids are the single most powerful agents for reducing the effects of allergy. Steroid medications can be classified as either adrenocorticosteroids or gonadotropic steroids, depending on the organ of origin. The gonadotropic steroids are the sex hormones progesterone, estrogen, testosterone, and the various derivatives. These agents have no activity against allergic rhinitis and so are not discussed here. The adrenocorticosteroids are derived from the adrenal steroid hormones and can further be divided into the mineralocorticoids and the glucocorticoids, depending on their primary effect. The medications used for allergic rhinitis are generally classified as glucocorticoids, but may have some degree of mineralocorticoid effect depending on the particular agent.

The basic glucocorticoid is cortisone. Table 6–5 lists many of the currently available oral and topical derivatives of cortisone. These medications have the ability to completely suppress the symptoms of some patients with allergic rhinitis and have been found to be the most effective of all medications against allergic conditions throughout the body. The effect of topical and systemic glucocorticoids is to diminish primarily the late-phase reaction of allergy.[25] After prolonged treatment, the topical steroids may also suppress the acute-phase reaction.[25]

Topical Nasal Steroids. The topical nasal steroids have become among the most widely prescribed medications in all of rhinology. In recent years, the number of products available for prescription by physicians has increased dramatically (see Table 6–5). Despite the many differences in the medications as marketed, the agents are more similar than they are different. All of these agents work well, and most are usually tolerated well.

All of the topical nasal steroids have the same basic pharmacologic effects. These agents have been shown to block recruitment of inflammatory cells into the mu-

TABLE 6–5
Glucocorticoid Medications

Oral Agents	Relative Potency
Cortisone	1.0
Hydrocortisone	1.25
Prednisone	5.0
Prednisolone	5.0
Methylprednisolone	6.25
Triamcinolone	6.25
Betamethasone	31.25
Dexamethasone	37.5

Topical Agents	Dosing Interval (doses/day)	Therapeutic Ratio*
Beclomethasone	2–4	3†
Flunisolide	2	>2
Triamcinolone	1	>2
Budesonide	1	4
Fluticasone	1	>4
Mometasone	1	>8‡

* Ratio of minimum dose required to suppress hypothalamic-adrenal axis to treatment dose. Calculated from data listed in the Physicians' Desk Reference.
† When given as an oral aerosol.
‡ In single-dose administration, a dose 20 times the recommended therapeutic dose did not cause suppression.

cosa,[26] suppress cytokine production,[27,28] and restore the normal structure of the mucosa.[29] These agents also help to stabilize lysosomal membranes, maintain capillary integrity, and block migration of immune complexes across the basement membranes.[25] The final net effect is to markedly diminish the inflammation in the nasal and sinus mucosa. This effect was demonstrated in one study that involved biopsy examinations of patients before and after 1 year of treatment with mometasone. This study documented a reduction in inflammatory infiltrate, especially eosinophils.[30] The result of this improvement is a suppression of both the acute- and late-phase components of the allergic response. In symptomatic terms, this translates to less itching, sneezing, rhinorrhea, nasal blockage, and congestion.[31–35]

The clinical guidelines for use of nasal steroid sprays in allergic rhinitis are necessarily vague. It is appropriate to use these agents in almost any circumstance because of their low toxicity, excellent safety profile, and high rate of symptomatic relief. The degree of systemic absorption and suppression of the hypothalamic-pituitary-adrenal axis is so low as to be essentially unimportant clinically. There has been some concern that, with very long-term use, these agents may induce cataracts. However, data linking nasal topical steroids to cataracts are distinctly lacking. One study did report that patients taking high doses of oral pulmonary steroid inhalers for long periods had a slight risk of cataracts. However, the same study failed to identify an independent risk associated with the topical nasal steroids. In the author's practice, those patients who have developed presenile cataracts have all been receiving a combination of oral inhalers and intermittent systemic steroids for the treatment of asthma for many years.

The one side effect of topical nasal steroids that is a potential problem with long-term use is mucosal atrophy and erosion. This occurs primarily on the anterior septum and, in rare cases, has reportedly resulted in septal perforation. The clinical experience with these agents is that, in most cases, the irritative effects on the septum can be minimized by careful application of the spray, coating the mucosa with an ointment after each use, and keeping the mucosa moist with nasal saline if necessary. In other cases, a drug holiday of 1 to 2 weeks' duration every 2 to 3 months may be sufficient to allow the mucosa to heal to a point of resuming treatment. There may also be less irritation depending on the formulation of the spray. The aqueous-based sprays tend to be less irritative. Also, once-a-day formulations are less traumatic and may be associated with fewer nasal mucosal problems. These findings favor either the mometasone aqueous, triamcinolone aqueous, or beclomethasone double-strength aqueous formulations.

The author tends to prescribe topical nasal steroid sprays for patients who have failed a trial of avoidance therapy with antihistamines, and for patients with moderate to severe symptoms. The first situation includes patients with mild to moderate symptoms who are seeking primarily seasonal help for exacerbations during peak allergy season. In these patients, nasal steroid sprays are usually very helpful if avoidance and antihistamines do not control the symptoms. These sprays are often used only during peak season and discontinued after the first frost. In patients with moderate to severe symptoms, especially if they demonstrate significant congestion of the turbinates on examination, starting the nasal steroid spray initially may help the patient achieve an earlier response. A trial of discontinuing the spray after the end of the allergy season is reasonable.

In patients with polyps or polypoid mucosa, topical nasal sprays are almost always started on the first visit. In cases of limited polyps, this may be all that is needed to control the symptoms and the polyps. In more severe cases, long-term therapy in conjunction with other modalities, including oral steroids, immunotherapy, and surgery, should be considered.

Topical nasal steroids are very useful after endoscopic sinus surgery. In this situation, the spray is used to help the mucosa heal without inflammation. It is well known that the mucosa in the sinus cavity heals gradually over the first 6 to 12 months after surgery.[36] During this time, there is a tendency for the inflammation from the surgical trauma to cause swelling and polyp formation. The topical nasal steroids help to reduce and control this effect. The usual protocol is to continue the spray for at least 6 months after surgery, and to continue it indefinitely in patients with severe allergies or polyps, or if inflammation in the cavity is observed on follow-up visits.

Finally, topical nasal steroids may become necessary during pregnancy. During pregnancy, many women develop some degree of rhinitis. This is probably caused by the changing hormonal levels related to the pregnancy. In most cases, this can be controlled with standard medications that have been cleared for use in pregnancy, in addition to avoidance. However, in some pregnant patients, especially those with a history of allergic rhinitis that predates the pregnancy, the condition may become severe. In these cases, topical steroids may be prescribed. The topical steroids are officially classified as class C drugs, which means that there is information that suggests that teratogenic effects are possible based on animal studies. For this reason, topical steroids are usually withheld during pregnancy. However, thus far, there are no studies in humans that have documented teratogenic effects or fetal injury in association with the use of topical nasal steroids. If the woman is having severe problems, topical steroids are probably safe to use in the second half of pregnancy. By this time, organogenesis is complete and the risk to the developing fetus is diminished. If the use of topical steroids is contemplated, the woman's obstetrician should be consulted. It is also probably advisable to prescribe mometasone in this population, as it has the highest therapeutic ratio and the lowest systemic absorption, which should minimize the risk.

Injected Steroids. In past years, injected steroids were a popular treatment for seasonal allergic rhinitis. The steroid was injected into the inferior turbinate. This typically led to a period of disease control. Since the introduction of the topical steroids, however, this modality has largely been replaced. The reasons for this are that the same efficacy is usually achieved without a painful injection, and the risk of the injection is avoided. Despite the relative safety of this procedure, there is one risk that is quite severe. A number of patients have suffered blindness as a result of steroid injections into the turbinates, most likely as the result of retrograde embolism of the dose from accidental intravascular injection. In such cases, the full dose or a large part of it is delivered to the microvasculature of the retina or optic nerve, resulting in plugging and subsequent ischemic necrosis. To avoid this risk, suggestions have been made for proper injection technique. Owing to the unnecessary risk, however, intraturbinal steroid injections have largely been abandoned.

Oral Steroids. Oral or systemic steroids are the single most potent treatment for any allergic disease, including allergic rhinitis. Their effect is dose-dependent, and the minimum effective dose will vary depending on the disease treated and the individual patient. All oral steroids are essentially equivalent in effect after adjusting for the strength of the agent by modifying the dose. Table 6–5 shows the relative strength of the commonly used oral steroids. Because of its familiarity, low cost, and availability, prednisone is the most commonly used oral steroid. Prednisone is available in 5-, 10-, and 20-mg tablets that are the most convenient for treating allergic rhinitis.

The dosing of any patient with oral or systemic steroids must take into account the ability of these medications to interfere with the hypothalamic-pituitary-adrenal axis. This system is a feedback loop that regulates the secretion of endogenous glucocorticosteroids. The normal baseline endogenous production of these hormones is in the range of 50 mg of cortisone per day, equalivalent to 10 mg of prednisone per day. Treatment with systemic steroids in excess of this amount will suppress natural endogenous production. This suppressive effect builds up over several days and does not reverse immediately upon withdrawal of the steroids. The suppression also interferes with the body's production of excess glucocorticosteroids in response to stress. In a patient with steroid suppression of adrenal function, acute stress without supplementing steroids or sudden withdrawal of oral steroids will result in acute absence of glucocorticosteroids, a condition referred to as Addison's disease. In Addison's disease, severe metabolic derangements of electrolyte and glucose levels can lead to severe shock and, eventually, to cardiopulmonary arrest.

The amount of steroids that will suppress adrenal function and place the patient at risk for Addison's disease is called the suppressive threshold. If the duration of steroid therapy or the total steroid dose exceeds the suppressive threshold, the steroid dose must be tapered to avoid Addison's disease, or what is referred to as addisonian crisis. The length of time over which the drug is tapered and the speed of the steroid taper must be varied to reflect the duration and total dose of the steroid therapy. For example, a 3-day course of 30 mg/day of prednisone would not be expected to exceed the suppressive threshold of most patients, so no taper is likely to be required. Conversely, after a 3-month course of 20 mg of prednisone per day, almost all patients would have exceeded the suppressive threshold and would require tapering of the dose in small increments every 5 to 7 days.

When treating allergic rhinitis and other allergic nasal and sinus diseases, the starting dose for prednisone therapy is usually in the neighborhood of 1 mg/kg/day, up to 60 mg/day. This is typically very effective for almost all patients. The pattern of dosing and the duration of dosing, though, will vary depending on the severity of the disease being treated. For patients with severe allergic rhinitis without sinusitis or polyps who require a course of steroids to bring their allergic symptoms under control, a short 6-day course is usually prescribed. There are convenient, commercially available, steroid packets that provide this regimen in a prepackaged form that is easy for patients to use.

In patients with severe sinonasal polyposis who are about to undergo surgery, steroids are usually prescribed to help the patient manage the surgery and postoperative recovery with a minimum of problems. In such cases, a course of 60 mg/day for 10 days before the surgery is usually effective. After the operation, a 30-day taper with 5 days at each of six doses (40, 30, 20, 15, 10, and 5 mg/day) is prescribed. The treatment regimen for other conditions requiring oral steroids is usually tailored to the individual patient.

For any patient in whom the duration of oral steroid therapy is to exceed 1 week, a discussion of the risks of steroid use is important. The glucocorticosteroids have many severe risks associated with them. These include Cushing's syndrome, hypertension, peptic ulcers, acne, fatty liver, cataracts, and avascular necrosis of the femoral head. Cushing's syndrome is the complex of findings originally described in the presence of an adrenocorticotropic hormone (ACTH)–secreting pituitary tumor. This includes weight gain, abdominal striae, peripheral edema, and facial edema. There are also classical electrolyte abnormalities associated with this condition. This normally only occurs with prolonged use of suppressive doses of steroids in excess of 2 to 3 months.

Hypertension may be either caused by or exacerbated by steroid use. In both situations, treatment with antihypertensives is warranted if the condition persists and the steroids cannot be withdrawn. In most cases, the hypertension will not be severe enough to warrant changes in therapy or institution of therapy. However, careful observation of the blood pressure is advised. Peptic ulcer disease can also be caused by or exacerbated by oral steroid use. Prevention of this condition usually involves treatment with a type 2 histamine receptor blocker, such as ranitidine or famotidine.

Acne may be caused by cross-reactivity of glucocorticosteroids with testosterone receptors. The acne that occurs usually resolves with cessation of oral steroid therapy, and it rarely leaves acne scars. Acne prophylaxis is usually not indicated, but if desired, doxycycline can be prescribed. Fatty liver is usually seen only in patients who have received long-term steroid treatment. This condition is usually not serious and is reversible once the treatment is terminated. Cataracts have also been associated with chronic steroid use. The minimum dose that causes cataracts is not well understood. This condition usually occurs in patients who have steroid-dependent asthma or systemic lupus erythematosis and who continue moderate-dose steroid therapy for many years. In these cases, the patient clearly requires the treatment and a cataract extraction with lens implant will usually resolve the problem.

Perhaps the most feared complication of steroid use is avascular necrosis of the femoral head. This serious condition is usually brought about by prolonged steroid use; however, there are reports of this occurring in patients after surprisingly short courses and low doses of steroids. The cause is related to vascular damage to the blood vessels in the femoral neck that supply the femoral head with blood. The result is no blood supply to the femoral head, in which case the bone undergoes necrosis. The treatment is surgical replacement with an artificial hip.

Finally, the use of steroids in pregnancy is a common dilemma. Although steroids are sometimes given to the mother to help the baby, routine use of steroids during pregnancy is discouraged. In rare circumstances, oral or systemic steroids may be given to a pregnant patient near the end of gestation. At this point, the baby is probably more tolerant of the treatment. However, this should almost never be necessary in the context of allergic or sinonasal disease alone. If treatment is thought to be necessary, it should only be instituted with the supervision and cooperation of a specialist in high-risk obstetrics.

Cromolyn. Now available over the counter, cromolyn nasal sprays have been proven effective in the treatment of allergic rhinitis.[37] Their proposed mode of action is by blocking mast cell degranulation, although this has not yet been proven definitively.[2] Cromolyn works best as a prophylactic agent when it is used to prevent the acute phase of the allergic response. Unlike antihistamines, cromolyn has some effect on the late phase of the allergic reaction by decreasing degranulation. This results in fewer chemotactic factors in the tissues, which diminishes the degree of inflammation that develops.

Cromolyn compounds are generally considered to have an efficacy that is intermediate to that of antihistamines and topical nasal steroids. For this reason, the role of cromolyn is unclear. For patients who respond to antihistamines and decongestants alone, cromolyn is not indicated. In patients who are unresponsive to antihistamines and decongestants, the nasal steroid sprays are generally most efficacious and most commonly prescribed. Because it is difficult to get patients to use any one nasal spray consistently, it is best to use the most effective spray available. The other disadvantage of using the cromolyn spray over the steroid nasal spray is the frequency of use. Whereas the steroid sprays are effective at only one dose per day, cromolyn requires two to four doses per day.

The one true advantage of cromolyn is its near-total absence of any side effects or complications with use. Of all of the agents prescribed for allergies, cromolyn is perhaps the least toxic, with almost no significant side effects. For this reason, cromolyn may be an appropriate choice in certain individuals who are having problems with the nasal steroid sprays.

Anticholinergic Agents. Anticholinergic agents are theoretically ideal for the treatment of many of the symptoms of allergic rhinitis. Activation of the parasympathetic nerves in the nasal mucosa induces congestion, sneezing, and rhinorrhea. By blocking the parasympathetic cholinergic receptors, anticholinergics can minimize these effects. The most potent action of anticholinergic agents would logically be on rhinorrhea. This is because the mucus glands are enervated predominantly by parasympathetic secretomotor nerves with acetylcholine postsynaptic receptors. The blood vessels that control vascular tone are enervated by both sympathetic and parasympathetic fibers, and the net vascular tone is determined by a balance between these opposing actions. In this system, the sympathetic nerves dominate. Thus, in the clinical setting, increased nasal congestion has more to do with sympathetic blockade than parasympathetic stimulation.

There are a number of anticholinergic agents available. However, most, like atropine, have significant systemic side effects when given orally or intravenously. These side effects, which include tachycardia and hypertension, are common to all systemically applied anticholinergic agents. However, a topical agent (ipratropium), released within the past few years, has been found to have almost no systemic absorption and no systemic effects. This agent is available in 0.03% and 0.06% nasal spray formulations. Clinical research to date has found ipratropium, at the 0.03% dose level, to be effective in the treatment of rhinorrhea in individuals with either allergic or nonallergic rhinitis,[38–40] and, at the 0.06% dose level, to be active against the rhinorrhea of acute viral rhinitis.[41, 42]

The author uses ipratropium nasal spray in selected patients with severe refractory rhinorrhea. Because this agent has minimal or no effect on congestion and sneezing, it is not preferred over the topical nasal steroid sprays for most patients. Occasionally, however, a patient will present for whom severe rhinorrhea is the primary cause for treatment. Also, there are some patients with combinations of symptoms in whom the rhinorrhea will fail to respond to antihistamines and nasal steroid sprays. In these cases, ipratropium nasal spray may provide significant relief. In addition, ipratropium is ideally suited for treating patients with vasomotor rhinitis and uncontrolled, watery rhinorrhea.

Ipratropium nasal spray has very few side effects. The one frequent problem with this agent is nasal irritation, which may progress to bleeding, crusting, and mucosal ulceration. In these cases, the patient should be instructed to apply ointment to the septum after each dose application and to use nasal saline spray, as needed, if the nose feels dry.

Lipoxygenase Pathway Inhibitors. A new class of medications was introduced recently, primarily for the treatment of asthma. These drugs are a diverse group of agents that have in common inhibition of some aspect of the lipoxygenase pathway. Arachidonic acid is a basic root metabolite that can be acted on by one of two enzymes. The first and best known is cyclo-oxygenase. This initiates the arachidonic acid cascade, which culminates in the production of prostaglandins. These agents are mediators of inflammation that, in general, downregulate the inflammatory response. This is not strictly true in that some of the prostaglandins have proinflammatory properties. Cyclo-oxygenase is inhibited by the nonsteroidal anti-inflammatory agents, including acetaminophen and aspirin, with the net effect of inhibiting proinflammatory prostaglandins.

The second enzyme that can act on arachidonic acid is lipoxygenase. The products of this reaction are the leukotrienes, which have a pronounced proinflammatory action. The leukotrienes tend to upregulate the inflammatory response in tissues;[80] inhibitors of this pathway would thus be expected to be anti-inflammatory in action.

Three new medications have been introduced in this family of agents. These medications have been primarily used for asthma. However, there is a theoretical role for lipoxygenase inhibitors in the treatment of all allergic diseases, and particularly Samter's triad, a symptom complex involving asthma, nasal polyps, and aspirin sensitivity. This condition is thought to be related to an enzyme deficiency, possibly in the prostaglandin pathway, that causes shunting of products into the lipoxygenase pathway and, as a result, excess mucosal inflammation. A lipoxygenase inhibitor may balance this deficiency, thereby minimizing the effect of the disorder. To date, the author has not found that patients with Samter's triad experience a significant response to this therapy in terms of shrinking polyps or preventing the return of polyps.

Immunotherapy

The third and last tier of allergy management is immunotherapy. This approach involves the administration of allergy extracts, usually by injection, to effect a desensitization of the patient for the antigen that is being delivered. Allergen immunotherapy was initiated at the turn of the century by Dunbar[12] and Curtis.[43] However, Noon[44] and Freeman[45] have generally been credited with popularizing and standardizing the use of pollen extracts to treat hay fever. Since that time, millions of patients have been treated with allergen immunotherapy using skin injection techniques. Despite the widespread application of this therapy and the proven efficacy of allergen immunotherapy, however, the exact mechanism of how it works remains unknown.

Numerous antibody and immunologic changes have been documented to result from immunotherapy.[46] Most allergists subscribe to the theory that blocking IgG antibodies are important in the response. This is based on a well-documented rise in specific IgG1 antibodies with the onset of immunotherapy and the observation that the higher the IgG level, the greater the blockade of cutaneous reactions to repeated exposure to the antigen.[47, 48] The antigen-specific IgG antibody acts as a blocking antibody by combining with the antigen in the peripheral target tissues. When exposure occurs, instead of the antigen combining with IgE and initiating an allergic response, the IgG combines with the antigen and no subsequent reaction occurs.

In addition to this proposed primary effect, a number of other effects have been demonstrated. This includes increased suppressor activity of T lymphocytes[49, 50] and decreased interleukin-2 production.[51, 52] How these effects are caused and how this relates to the clinical response to allergen immunotherapy is only speculative. Suffice it to say that there remains much to be learned and understood about the mechanisms of allergen immunotherapy.

Indications. Allergy immunotherapy is indicated for any patient with significant symptoms caused by inhalant allergy. For otolaryngologists, this applies to patients with allergic rhinitis, allergic nasal polyposis, and allergic fungal sinusitis. These indications would imply that all patients with these diagnoses should receive immunotherapy. However, in keeping with the three-tier approach to allergy management, only those patients whose symptoms are not controlled by the first two tiers of management will advance to immunotherapy. For allergic rhinitis, this correlates to patients who do not find success with avoidance therapy and for whom pharmacologic therapy is either insufficient or impractical.

Avoidance measures, described in detail earlier in this chapter, are not always possible and not always successful. For example, some patients may not be able to afford to change carpeting, buy expensive air cleaners, or install air conditioners. Others may find it difficult to isolate themselves completely from dust, mold, and pollens, and may be unwilling to get rid of valued family pets. The allergist should always encourage avoidance, but unrealistic expectations and demands in terms of avoidance are not going to be well received and are unlikely to be followed. Pharmacologic therapy is often very successful. However, many patients, especially children, will not be able to be fully compliant with medication regimens. Other patients may experience side effects from medications. Individuals who are steroid-dependent from either topical or systemic treatment may develop long-term complications of steroid use, in which case measures, such as immunotherapy, that are designed to reduce steroid dependency are appropriate.

The efficacy of immunotherapy against a number of specific antigens contributing to allergic rhinitis has been documented by well-controlled clinical trials. These antigens include tree pollen,[53] grass pollen,[54, 55] ragweed pollen,[56] mold,[57, 58] dust and dust mite,[59–61] and animal dander.[62–64] These trials have documented that allergen immunotherapy is effective against a large variety of allergens in many patients. However, there have also been negative results reported in connection with allergen immunotherapy, casting some doubt on the role of this therapy.[65] On balance, though, the current literature supports the use of immunotherapy as a viable alternative in selected patients with allergic rhinitis.

In addition to patients with allergic rhinitis, there are two special groups of individuals who may benefit from allergy immunotherapy. These are patients with allergic sinonasal polyposis and allergic fungal sinusitis. In both of these groups, control of the allergic nature of the condition using immunotherapy may be beneficial regardless of their response to medical therapy. The reason for this is that these patients have an inherently unstable mucosa that tends to form polyps. In these patients, frequent recurrences of polyps requiring surgical debridement or systemic steroids may be related to unpreventable brief exposures to allergens. These recurrences of polyps may be prevented by appropriate immunotherapy,[66] although to date, a prospective randomized trial has not yet been completed to confirm these benefits. The clinical experience of the author does support this practice, however.

Formulating the Serum. The author uses the techniques advocated by the American Academy of Otolaryngologic Allergy (AAOA), which have been taught in certification courses and widely published.[67] The technique can be based on either RAST testing or SET testing. The preferred technique is to use SET testing. The principle is that the first level maintenance dose is equal to 0.5 mL of the endpoint for that specific antigen. The RAST equivalent to this is to use the RAST level −1 method of determining the maintenance dose, that is, a dose of 0.5 mL of the SET vial, which is equal to the RAST level −1 (e.g., RAST level 3 equates to SET vial No. 4). The final maintenance dose is the minimum successful dose that relieves the patient's symptoms. If the first maintenance dose does not completely control the allergy symptoms, the dose may be increased to the maximum tolerated dose.

Normally, it is necessary to treat the patients with more than one allergen extract. In this case, multiple injections may be administered for each treatment, or the injections may be combined in a single treatment vial containing all of the allergens be included in the patient's immunotherapy. It is possible to do this without increasing the total injection volume by using higher concentrations than the SET point. For example, a patient with a SET point of 4 to antigen 1 and a SET point of 5 to antigen 2 can receive an injection containing 0.1 mL of vial No. 3 for antigen 1 and 0.1 mL of vial No. 4 for antigen 2. In cases in which more than 5 allergens are to be included, the SET + 2 vial can be used as the source, with 0.02 mL of the SET + 2 vial. In the above example, this would correspond to 0.02 mL of vial No. 2 for antigen 1 and 0.02 mL of vial No. 3 for antigen 2.

For convenience, most treatment vials are mixed to include 10 treatment doses rather than 1 dose, so that the serum does not have to be freshly mixed each time an injection is given or the patient receives treatment at an outside facility. In the example just presented, the 10-dose treatment vial can be mixed by combining 1.0 mL of vial No. 3 for antigen 1, 1.0 mL, of vial No. 4 for antigen 2, and 3.0 mL of a commercially available diluent. This treatment vial would then contain 10 doses of 0.5 mL which contains the equivalent of 0.5 mL of vial No. 4 for antigen 1 and 0.5 mL of vial No. 5 for antigen 2.

In most cases, the treatment vial will include all of the antigens that the patient reacts to that are clinically significant. These include those antigens that the patient comes in contact with that cause symptoms. Usually, this corresponds to any antigen that reacts at a SET level of 2 or higher (SET level 3, 4, 5, or higher). The patient's exposure level is an important factor in deciding on the inclusion of an antigen in the treatment regimen. For example, a patient who tests positive to dog dander but who does not have a dog and rarely, if ever, plays with dogs does not need to be desensitized to dogs. Similarly, patients who are allergic to a tree pollen that does not grow in their region would not need to be treated. Some experts in immunotherapy do not recommend combining certain extracts—specifically, pollens and molds—in the same vial. This is said to weaken the serum by binding the pollens to the molds. The importance of this is unclear as other experts deny the importance of this issue. As a matter of practical management, it is worthwhile to separate antigens that have a high degree of allergenicity compared to those with low allergenicity. This allows the allergist to more quickly determine the cause of local or systemic reactions if they occur.

Dose Escalation and Maintenance Therapy. Once the immunotherapy is formulated, treatment can be initiated. Usually, for safety reasons, the dose is escalated from a safe lower dose to the full dose. This practice helps to minimize the chances of developing systemic or serious local reactions. The usual method employed is to start, in Week 1, with 0.1 mL of each treatment vial being used. The dose is then escalated by 0.1 mL per week until the first level maintenance dose is reached (a dose equal to 0.5 mL of each treatment vial properly formulated).

Once the first maintenance level is reached, the patient is maintained on this dose until the entire 10-dose treatment vial is used. At this point, it is necessary to determine whether the patient is improving with therapy. If the patient is improving and is satisfied with the benefit of the immunotherapy, this can be considered the minimum successful dose and further escalation is not required. Conversely, if the patient is continuing to have significant symptoms, further dose escalation can be achieved as the second vial is mixed. At this point, the allergist must try to determine the likely source of the problem so that the dose of these antigens can be selectively increased. This can be done by understanding the exposures of the patient during the applicable time period. For example, weed pollen would not be the cause of therapeutic failure during the winter or spring months. The dose is usually increased in half steps rather than full SET levels. For example, antigen 1 may be increased from 0.5 mL equivalent of vial No. 4 to 0.25 mL equivalent of vial No. 3. This would effectively increase the dose by 2.5 times or one-half SET level. This next vial must once again be escalated from a safe dose to the next maintenance level. This is done in 0.1-mL increments starting at the previous dose level.

The final dose is established when the patient's symptoms are controlled or when maximum tolerated dose is reached. The maximum tolerated dose is that which causes a significant local reaction that does not subside over time upon repeated injection. Normally, as desensitization proceeds, the patient will become adapted to the current dose and further escalation becomes possible if desired. If this does not occur, the maximum tolerated dose is established. To be safe, the maximum acceptable local reaction is a 3-cm area of redness or induration that persists for 24 hours.

For most patients, the dosing interval will be one injection per week the first year. After 1 year, the interval can be increased to one injection every 2 weeks. If this increase in interval causes recurrent symptoms, the interval should be returned to one injection per week. If symptoms remain well controlled, the interval can be increased further to one injection per month at the end of the second year. Again, if this is not tolerated, the interval should be returned to the last successful level. One injection per month represents the longest interval that is usually attempted and that is effective.

Safety of Immunotherapy. The safety of allergen immunotherapy has now been well established. However, there does remain a risk of systemic reactions and even death. Adverse reactions to immunotherapy can be classified into three types: (1) transient wheal and flare reactions at the injection site, (2) delayed subcutaneous swelling and itching at the injection site, and (3) systemic reactions. Although the local problems may be irritating and cause discomfort to the patient, these reactions are relatively minor and can be controlled by decreasing the immunotherapy dose, applying ice, or administering antihistamines or topical cortisone cream. By contrast, systemic reactions have the potential to be serious, and may be accompanied by bronchospasm, angioedema, or full-blown anaphylaxis, resulting in cardiopulmonary collapse.

The exact risk of allergy skin testing and allergen immunotherapy is difficult to pinpoint. Almost all studies have found that skin testing is safer than immunotherapy, and that during escalation and maintenance, patients are at approximately equal risk for systemic reactions. Various studies have reported highly divergent rates of reaction ranging from 14% of patients[68] to 0.3% of patients.[69] This great discrepancy can be attributed to several factors, including the definition of a systemic reaction, the methodology used, and the type of patients being treated. The lowest rates of reaction are reported in patients with allergic rhinitis without asthma who have relatively low sensitivity to the antigens,[70] whereas the highest rates of reaction occur in patients with high sensitivity, severe asthma, and pollen allergy. However, overall, the incidence of fatal reactions is exceedingly low, with only 46 reported cases in the literature over nearly a 40-year period.[70] Estimates of mortality risk may, therefore, be as low as 1 in 100,000 to 1 in 1,000,000 patients treated. The risk per injection is even lower than this.

Throughout most of the literature, several suggestions to limit the risks of systemic reactions are consistently presented.

1. Patients with high-level sensitivity or asthma and those receiving beta-blockers should be observed carefully when they receive immunotherapy.

2. The first signs of a systemic reaction are chest tightness, wheezing, urticaria, pruritis, and throat tightness. When any of these signs are present, the patient should be treated for the reaction and observed until stable.

3. Patients who have previously experienced systemic reactions should be treated with lower-dose therapy, and patients who have had multiple systemic reactions should not be treated.

4. Home therapy should be reserved for those patients with low risk for systemic reactions.

REFERENCES

1. Wells JV. Immune mechanisms and tissue damage reactions. In Stites D, Stobo J, Fudenberg HH, Wells JV (eds). Basic and Clinical Immunology, 4th ed. Los Altos, CA: Lange Medical Publications; pp. 136–145, 1982.
2. Naclerio R, Soloman W. Rhinitis and inhalant allergens. JAMA 278(22):1842, 1997.
3. Costa JJ, Weller PF, Galli SJ. The cells of the allergic response. JAMA 278(22):1815, 1997.
4. Belser RB, Fine ED, Boehm KD. Role of tumor necrosis factor and granulocyte-macrophage colony-stimulating factor in the late allergic response in human nasal mucosa. Otolaryngol Head Neck Surg 114(3):418, 1996.
5. Hansel FK. Observations on the cytology of the secretions in allergy of the nose and paranasal sinuses. J Allergy 5:357, 1934.
6. Lewis T, Grant RT. Vascular reactions of the skin to injury. Heart 13:219, 1926.
7. Levine JL, Mabry RL, Mabry CS. Comparison of multi-test device skin testing and modified RAST results. Otolaryngol Head Neck Surg 118(6):797, 1998.
8. Rinkel, HJ. The management of clinical allergy (Parts I, II, III). Arch Otolaryngol 76:491–508, 1962; 77:42–75, 1963; 77:205–235, 1963.
9. Mabry RL. Skin Endpoint Titration. New York: Thieme; p. 19, 1994.
10. Chambers DW, Cook PR, Nishioka GJ, Erhart P. Comparison of mRAST and CAP with skin end point titration for *Alternaria tenuis* and *Dermatophagoides pteronyssinus*. Otolaryngol Head Neck Surg 117(5):471, 1997.
11. Corey JP, Nelson RS, Lai V. Comparison of modified phadezym-RAST, immunoCAP, and serial dilution titration skin testing by receiver operating curve analysis. Otolaryngol Head Neck Surg 112:665, 1995.
12. Passali D, Sperati G. The historical background of allergic rhinopathy therapy. Rhinology 36(3):139, 1998.
13. Thoden WR, Druce HM, Furey SA, et al. Brompheniramine maleate: A double-blind, placebo-controlled comparison with terfenadine for symptoms of allergic rhinitis. Am J Rhinol 12(4):293, 1998.
14. Klein GL, Littlejohn T, Lockhart EA, Furey SA. Brompheniramine, terfenadine, and placebo in allergic rhinitis. Ann Allergy 77:365, 1996.
15. McTavish D, Goa KL, Ferrill M. Terfenadine. An updated review of its pharmacological properties and therapeutic efficacy. Drugs 39:552, 1990.
16. Lockey RF, Widlitz MD, Mitchell DQ, et al. Comparative study of cetirizine and terfenadine versus placebo in the symptomatic management of seasonal allergic rhinitis. Ann Allergy Asthma Immunol 76:448, 1996.
17. Oei HD. Double blind comparison of loratadine, astemizole, and placebo in hay fever with special regard to onset of action. Ann Allergy 61:436, 1996.
18. Meltzer EO, Weiler JM, Waddles MD. Comparative outdoor study of the efficacy, onset, and duration of action and safety of cetirizine, loratadine, and placebo for seasonal allergic rhinitis. J Allergy Clin Immunol 97:617, 1996.
19. Druce HM, Thoden WR, Mure P, et al. Brompheniramine, loratadine, and placebo in allergic rhinitis: A placebo-controlled comparative clinical trial. J Clin Pharmacol 38:382, 1998.
20. Storms WW. Treatment of allergic rhinitis: Effects of allergic rhinitis and antihistamines on performance. Allergy Asthma Proc 18(2):59, 1997.
21. Fireman P. Treatment of allergic rhinitis: Effect on occupation productivity and work force costs. Allergy Asthma Proc 18(2): 63, 1997.
22. Panda NK, Mann SBS. Comparative efficacy and safety of terfenadine with pseudoephedrine and terfenadine alone in allergic rhinitis. Otolaryngol Head Neck Surg 118(2):253, 1998.
23. Backhouse CI, Rosenberg RM, Fidler C. Treatment of seasonal allergic rhinitis. A comparison of a combination tablet of terfenadine and pseudoephedrine with the individual ingredients. Br J Clin Pract 44:274, 1990.
24. Yoo JK, Seikaly H, Calhoun K. Extended use of topical nasal decongestants. Laryngoscope 107:40, 1997.
25. Mabry RL. Pharmacotherapy of allergic rhinitis: Corticosteroids. Otolaryngol Head Neck Surgery 113:1, 1995.
26. Rak S, Jacobson MR, Sudderick RM, et al. Influence of prolonged treatment with topical corticosteroids (fluticasone propionate) on early and late phase nasal responses and cellular infiltration in the nasal mucosa after allergen challenge. Clin Exp Allergy 24:930, 1994.
27. Masuyama K, Jacobson MR, Rak S, et al. Topical glucocorticosteroid (fluticasone propionate) inhibits cells expressing cytokine mRNA for interleukin-4 in the nasal mucosa in allergen-induced rhinitis. Immunology 82:192, 1994.
28. Pipkorn U, Proud D, Lichtenstein LM, et al. Inhibition of mediator release in allergic rhinitis by pretreatment with topical glucocorticosteroids. N Engl J Med 316:1506, 1987.
29. Orgel HA, Meltzer EO, Bierman W, et al. Intranasal fluocortin butyl in patients with perennial rhinitis: A 12-month efficacy and safety study including nasal biopsy. J Allergy Clin Immunol 88:257, 1991.
30. Minshall E, Ghaffar O, Cameron L, O'Brien F, et al. Assessment by nasal biopsy of long-term use of mometasone furoate aqueous nasal spray (Nasonex) in the treatment of perennial rhinitis. Otolaryngol Head Neck Surg 118(5):648, 1998.
31. Siegel SC. Topical corticosteroid therapy in rhinitis. J Allergy Clin Immunol 81:890, 1988.
32. Busse W. New directions and dimensions in the treatment of allergic rhinitis. J Allergy Clin Immunol 82:890, 1988.
33. Scadding GK, Lund VJ, Jacques LA, Richards DH. A placebo-controlled study of fluticasone propionate aqueous nasal spray and beclomethasone dipropionate in perennial rhinitis: Efficacy in allergic and non-allergic perennial rhinitis. Clin Exp Allergy 25:737, 1995.
34. Mygind N. Glucocorticoids and rhinitis. Allergy 48:476, 1993.
35. Rosenthal R, Berger W, Bronsky E, Dockhorn R, et al. Tri-Nasal Triamcinolone Acetonide Nasal Spray 200 and 400, μg qd versus placebo and Nasacort Triamcinolone Acetonide Nasal Aerosol 440 μg qd in patients suffering from seasonal allergic rhinitis during the grass season. Am J Rhinol 12(6):427, 1998.
36. Weber R, Keerl R, Huppmann A, Schick B, Draf W. Investigation of wound healing after paranasal sinus surgery with time lapse video—A pilot study. Am J Rhinol 10(4):235, 1996.
37. Welsh PW, Stricker WE, Chu-Pin C, et al. Efficacy of beclomethasone nasal solution, flunisolide, and cromolyn in relieving symptoms of ragweed allergy. Mayo Clin Proc 62:125, 1987.

38. Finn AF, Aaronson D, Korenblat P, et al. Ipratropium bromide nasal spray 0.03% provides additional relief from rhinorrhea when combined with terfenadine in perennial rhinitis patients: A randomized, double-blind, active-controlled trial. Am J Rhinol 12(6):441, 1998.
39. Bronsky EA, Druce H, Findlay SR, et al. A clinical trial of allergic rhinitis. J Allergy Clin Immunol 95:1117, 1995.
40. Grossman J, Banov C, Boggs P, et al. Use of ipratropium bromide nasal spray in chronic treatment of nonallergic perennial rhinitis, alone and in combination with other perennial rhinitis medications. J Allergy Clin Immunol 95:1123, 1995.
41. Diamond L, Dockhorn RJ, Grossman J, et al. A dose-response study of the efficacy and safety of ipratropium bromide nasal spray in the treatment of the common cold. J Allergy Clin Immunol 95:1139, 1995.
42. Hayden FG, Diamond L, Wood P, et al. Effectiveness and safety of intranasal ipratropium bromide in common colds. Ann Intern Med 125:89, 1996.
43. Curtis HH. The immunizing cure for hay fever. Med News 77:16, 1900.
44. Noon L. Prophylactic inoculation against hay fever. Lancet 1:572, 1911.
45. Freeman J. Further observations on the treatment of hayfever by hypodermic inoculation of pollen vaccine. Lancet 2:814, 1911.
46. Weber RW. Immunotherapy with allergens. JAMA 278(22): 1881, 1997.
47. Djurup R, Osterballe O. IgG subclass antibody response in grass pollen–allergic patients undergoing specific immunotherapy. Allergy 39:433, 1984.
48. Parker WA Jr, Whisman BA, Apaliski SJ, Reid MJ. The relationships between late cutaneous responses and specific antibody responses with outcome of immunotherapy for seasonal allergic rhinitis. J Allergy Clin Immunol 84:667, 1989.
49. Rocklin RE, Sheffer AL, Greineder DK, Melmon KL. Generation of antigen-specific suppressor cells during allergy desensitization. N Engl J Med 302:1213, 1980.
50. Tamir R, Castracane JM, Rocklin RE. Generation of suppressor cells in atopic patients during immunotherapy that modulate IgE synthesis. J Allergy Clin Immunol 79:591, 1987.
51. Hsieh KH. Altered interleukin-2 production and responsiveness after hyposensitization to house dust. J Allergy Clin Immunol 76:188, 1985.
52. Hsieh KH. Decreased production of interleukin-2 receptors after immunotherapy to house dust. J Clin Immunol 8:171, 1988.
53. Pence HL, Mitchell DQ, Greely RL, Udegraff BR, Selfridge HA. Immunotherapy for mountain cedar pollinosis: A double-blind controlled study. J Allergy Clin Immunol 58:39, 1976.
54. Osterballe O. Immunotherapy with grass pollen major allergens. Allergy 87:379, 1982.
55. Frostad AB, Grimmer O, Sandvik L, Moxnes A, Aas K. Clinical effects of hyposensitization using a purified allergen preparation from timothy pollen as compared to crude aqueous extracts from timothy pollen and a four-grass mixture respectively. Clin Allergy 13:337, 1983.
56. Creticos PS, Marsh DG, Proud D, et al. Responses to ragweed-pollen nasal challenge before and after immunotherapy. J Allergy Clin Immunol 84:197, 1989.
57. Malling JH, Dreborg S, Weeke B. Diagnosis and immunotherapy of mold allergy, V: Clinical efficacy and side effects of immunotherapy with *Cladosporium herbarum*. Allergy 41:507, 1986.
58. Horst M, Hejjaoui A, Horst V, Michel FB, Cousquet J. Double-blind, placebo-controlled rush immunotherapy with a standardized Alternaria extract. J Allergy Clin Immunol 85:460, 1990.
59. Aas K. Hyposensitization in house dust allergy asthma: A double-blind controlled study with evaluation of the effect on bronchial sensitivity to house dust. Acta Paediatr Scand 60:264, 1971.
60. Warner JO, Price JF, Soothill JF, Hey EN. Controlled trial of hyposensitization to *Dermatophagoides pteronyssinus* in children with asthma. Lancet 2:912, 1978.
61. Bousquet J, Calvayrac P, Guerin B, et al. Immunotherapy with a standardized *Dermatophagoides pteronyssinus* extract, I: In vivo and in vitro parameters after a short course of treatment. J Allergy Clin Immunol 76:734, 1985.
62. Ohman JL, Findlay SR, Leitermann KM. Immunotherapy in cat-induced asthma. J Allergy Clin Immunol 82:1055, 1984.
63. Van Metre TE Jr, Marsh DDG, Adkinson NF Jr, et al. Immunotherapy for cat asthma. J Allergy Clin Immunol 82:1055, 1988.
64. Hedlin G, Graff-Lonnevig, Heilborn H, et al. Immunotherapy with cat and dog dander extracts, V: Effects of 3 years of treatment. J Allergy Clin Immunol 87:955, 1991.
65. Creticos PS, Reed CE, Norman PS, et al. Ragweed immunotherapy in adult asthma. N Engl J Med 334:501, 1996.
66. Marple BF, Mabry RL. Comprehensive management of allergic fungal sinusitis. Am J Rhinol 12(4):263, 1998.
67. Davis WE, Cook PR, McKinsey JP, et al. Anaphylaxis in immunotherapy. Otolaryngol Head Neck Surg 107:78, 1992.
68. Cook PR, Bryant JL, Davis WE, et al. Systemic reactions to immunotherapy: The AAOA Morbidity and Mortality Survey. Otolaryngol Head Neck Surg 110(6):487, 1994.
69. Reid MJ, Lockey RF, Turkeltaub PC, et al. Survey of fatalities from skin testing and immunotherapy 1985–1989. J Allergy Clin Immunol 92(pt 1):6, 1993.

SECTION TWO

Surgery for Inflammatory Conditions

CHAPTER 7

Turbinate Procedures

INDICATIONS

Turbinate Hypertrophy

Hypertrophy and enlargement of the inferior turbinates are the most common indications for a turbinate reduction procedure. Turbinate enlargement may occur with or without true mucosal hypertrophy. The inferior turbinate bone has a horizontal and vertical projection. Variations in the size of the projections of the inferior turbinate lead to a variety of anatomic configurations. The horizontal part may be minimized and obliquely angled, giving the bone a distinctly vertical profile, or there may be a pronounced horizontal component, projecting the turbinate into the nasal airway and creating a bulbous, wide profile. In the latter instance, the mucosa may be predominantly normal yet may predispose the individual to nasal congestion and obstruction by creating a narrow nasal passageway. In the event of even minimal nasal congestion, severe obstruction may result.

Alternatively, true mucosal hypertrophy can also occur, resulting in the same conditions of obstruction and congestion. Mucosal hypertrophy may be secondary to a number of pathologic processes. One common cause of hypertrophy is a deviated nasal septum. Following acute nasal trauma with septal fracture, the deviated septum leaves one side partially or totally closed and the opposite side overly patent. The inferior turbinate on the patent side will usually undergo mucosal hypertrophy, enlarging the turbinate and increasing the nasal resistance. This may only be a problem in the event that septal reconstruction is performed. In this situation, the straightening of the septum can bring the septum into direct contact with the hypertrophied turbinate, causing obstruction on the preoperatively patent side of the nose.

Rhinitis medica mentosum (RMM) is another possible cause of turbinate hypertrophy. RMM is a form of chronic rhinitis caused by excessive use of topical nasal decongestants. In this condition, the overuse of topical decongestants initiates a pathologic process, resulting in hypertrophy of the turbinate mucosa. This mucosal hypertrophy ultimately leads to increased use of decongestants, initiating a cycle of increased use and tachyphylaxis.

A third but less well-documented cause of noninflammatory hypertrophy of the inferior turbinates is nasal continuous positive airway pressure (CPAP), a form of treatment for obstructive sleep apnea syndrome. In this circumstance, the constant high pressure exerted by the CPAP on the nasal mucosa may trigger compensatory hypertrophy of the mucosa. Although proof of this relationship is lacking, patients treated with CPAP have consistently been found to have enlarged turbinates.

Noninflammatory hypertrophy and enlargement of the inferior turbinates are recognized by the combined clinical symptoms of congestion and obstruction and the absence of inflammatory disease. Physical examination usually reveals a large turbinate without significant mucosal changes that decongests well with application of topical phenylephrine. To confirm the diagnosis, it is necessary to rule out allergic rhinitis, nonallergic rhinitis, and sinusitis.

In patients with a confirmed diagnosis of enlargement or hypertrophy of the turbinates, medical therapy is usually the first line of treatment. Standard treatment would include oral decongestants and nasal steroid sprays.

In most cases, the decision to offer surgery is based on the failure of appropriate medical therapy to control the symptoms. However, if medication is only effective when administered at maximal frequency and doses, the patient may need to decide between surgery or continuous medical treatment with periods of symptomatic nasal obstruction. In such cases, a well-counseled patient who prefers surgical reduction of the inferior turbinate is a reasonable candidate for surgery. Finally, for the patient with deviated septum and contralateral turbinate hypertrophy, some management of the inferior turbinate is justified at the time of septoplasty.

Chronic Rhinitis

Inflammation secondary to allergic and nonallergic rhinitis is the most common disease affecting the inferior turbinates. However, owing to the success of medical therapy, surgical manipulation of the inferior turbinates is not usually the treatment of choice. The diagnosis and medical management of chronic rhinitis are covered in detail in Chapter 6.

The indications for surgical intervention in these diseases are controversial. Essentially, all patients with chronic rhinitis suffering from nasal obstruction or congestion could derive benefit, at least temporarily, from a turbinate procedure. However, long-term results are not easy to predict. This is due to several factors.

One important factor is that chronic rhinitis, whether allergic or nonallergic, has an unpredictable natural history. Patients may have a stable course for many years or a lifetime, may have increasing symptoms over time, decreasing symptoms over time, or a waxing and waning disease course. A change in the severity of the inflammatory hypertrophy of the turbinate mucosa may alter the functional dynamics of the nose and render the turbinate reduction either inadequate or excessive.

A second factor that affects surgical outcome is that patients with chronic rhinitis may have other symptoms that require treatment. This may affect the impact that turbinate reduction has on the primary symptoms that were the indication for the surgery. For example, the patient may undergo turbinate reduction for nasal obstruction, but may continue to have sneezing and rhinorrhea requiring treatment with nasal steroids. The steroids may then overly shrink the turbinates, resulting in inadequate humidification, thickened mucus, and a dry, irritated throat.

Finally, there is the additional factor of the unpredictability of the patients' aging process and its effect on mucociliary function in the nose. Some patients may experience a progressive loss of functional capacity of the nose over time, whereas in others, this functional decline may take place at a much slower rate, or not at all. The effect of the loss of functional capacity incurred by turbinate reduction is, therefore, hard to predict. In some cases, it seems that the functional loss secondary to turbinate reduction is enough to result in significant morbidity many years after the procedure.[1] Symptoms may include mild crusting, thickening of the mucus, and dry throat. However, in some cases, it may result in full-blown atrophic rhinitis with fetid mucus; crusting leading to nasal obstruction; chronic, foul, postnasal discharge; and severe pharyngitis.

Despite these risks, some patients with chronic rhinitis may benefit from turbinate reduction. Simply stated, these patients are the ones that fail maximal attempts at medical therapy. For patients with allergy, maximal therapy would likely include antihistamines, decongestants, nasal steroid spray, and an attempt at immunotherapy. For nonallergic patients, maximal therapy would consist of nasal steroid spray, antihistamines, decongestants, and, probably, a trial of topical anticholinergic spray.

The main symptoms in patients with chronic rhinitis for which turbinate reduction is undertaken are congestion and obstruction. The other symptom is rhinorrhea. Although most studies report success rates approaching 90% for the relief of obstruction and congestion, the success rate for the treatment of rhinorrhea is much lower.[2–4] The reason for this is that the inferior turbinates produce only a portion of the nasal mucus. In fact, the sinuses, septum, and other turbinates produce most of the nasal mucus. Therefore, it is understandable that partial or even total reduction of the inferior turbinate would not have a major impact on this symptom.

PREOPERATIVE CONSIDERATIONS

Anesthesia

The choice of anesthetic technique will vary depending on the precise technique employed and the other procedures to be done in combination with the turbinate procedure. When only the turbinate procedure is to be performed, general anesthesia is rarely necessary. Unless extenuating circumstances exist, a local anesthesia with mild sedation is usually sufficient.

In most cases, 4% cocaine solution is used as a topical agent to decongest the nose and provide some anesthesia of the turbinate mucosa. The solution is applied via cottonoids or cotton pledgets around the turbinate. Alternatives include oxymetazoline or phenylephrine in combination with lidocaine, or a topical decongestant alone. Cocaine flakes are not necessary for isolated turbinate procedures.

Local anesthesia is injected after the topical agent has taken effect. Most commonly, 1% lidocaine with 1:100,000 epinephrine is used. Approximately 3 to 5 cc is injected for each turbinate, divided between the posterior end, the anterior edge, and the medial mucosa.

When the turbinate procedure is performed in combination with other procedures, such as septoplasty or sinus surgery, the selection of anesthesia is based on the requirements of these other procedures.

Choice of Technique

When the decision to perform a turbinate procedure has been made, the choice of which technique to use must be considered. Turbinate procedures can be divided into resection techniques and nonresection techniques. Nonresection techniques include out-fracture,[5, 6] steroid injection,[7] chemical cautery,[8, 9] cryotherapy,[10, 11] electrocautery,[12, 13] and laser treatment.[14–16] Resection techniques include submucous resection,[17] partial turbinectomy,[2, 4, 18] inferior turbinoplasty,[19, 20] and subtotal turbinectomy.[3, 21] Each of these surgical techniques can be performed using traditional instruments or endoscopic techniques. Each of these techniques has its proponents, and each has yielded good results. The nonresection techniques have the advantage of being less invasive, faster to heal, and less likely to result in a dry nose or atrophic rhinitis. The disadvantages are that these techniques provide only small, incremental improvements in nasal airway and, in the long term, are more likely to be associated with recurrent rhinorrhea, congestion, and obstruction secondary to mucosal regrowth and hypertrophy.

The converse is true for the resection techniques. These procedures have the advantage of effecting lasting, major improvements in nasal airway and congestion. However, they are more invasive, take longer to heal, and have the added risk of intraoperative and postoperative hemorrhage. In addition, in some circumstances, nasal dryness and even atrophic rhinitis may result.

Clearly, the more of the turbinate that is removed, the greater the decrease in nasal resistance and the greater the chances of long-term complications related to dryness or atrophic changes. For this reason, total turbinectomy has fallen on disfavor and is not advocated except in circumstances involving tumor resection or severe maxillary sinus infection requiring medial maxillectomy.

The author favors inferior turbinoplasty as the preferred technique for turbinate reduction in patients with hypertrophy and enlargement. The reason for this is that this surgical procedure adequately debulks the turbinate while preserving the entire medial mucosal surface. The inferior turbinoplasty thus simultaneously optimizes the nasal airway and preserves the critical functional mucosa of the medial surface of the turbinate. This procedure has the added benefit of preserving the posterior attachment of the turbinate, which minimizes the risk of hemorrhage and allows more rapid healing than partial or total turbinectomy.

The nonresection techniques have generally proven inadequate for treatment of turbinate hypertrophy and enlargement. If these techniques are performed as intended, they do not remove enough bulk from the turbinate to improve the airway sufficiently. In addition, patients so treated are subject to a high rate of recurrence owing to secondary hypertrophy.

Submucous resection of the inferior turbinate that removes only the turbinate bone is essentially a compromise between resection and nonresection techniques. It, too, is subject to failure owing to inadequate reduction and late recurrence due to secondary hypertrophy.

Out-fracture of the inferior turbinate is a popular method for improving the airway, especially at the time of septoplasty. This technique is very simple, rapid, bloodless, and carries almost no risk of short-term or long-term complications. Unfortunately, it does not have a long-term effect in most patients as the turbinate bone can reform to its original structure, or the mucosa can undergo secondary hypertrophy. Because of this, out-fracture is rarely chosen if true reduction in the turbinate is required.

Partial turbinectomy is a procedure that yields results similar to those achieved with inferior turbinoplasty in terms of airway improvement. The advantage of this technique is that it is very rapid and simple. Its disadvantage is that it involves resection of some of the medial mucosa that is critical to nasal function. Also, it is associated with an increased risk of postoperative bleeding and delayed healing. On balance, this procedure is less favorable than the inferior turbinoplasty for most situations.

The exception to this is the patient with severe septal deformity in which the inferior turbinate is deformed by a large septal spur. The inferior edge below the septal spur may be quite enlarged and require some reduction. In this situation, lateral turbinoplasty can be difficult and may result in laceration of the mucosa at the indentation point. A simple amputation of the inferior edge below the indentation is a reasonable alternative.

Subtotal turbinectomy is rarely, if ever, indicated. Although the degree to which airway resistance is reduced with this procedure is significant, it may lead to complete loss of turbulent flow and a sense of nasal obstruction for the patient. The risk of long-term atrophic changes also makes this technique problematic. Perhaps the only indication for this procedure is in patients who have previously undergone partial turbinectomy that failed due to secondary hypertrophy of the nasal mucosa.

When treating patients with chronic rhinitis, the procedure of choice will depend on the symptoms being treated. If the purpose of the procedure is to treat nasal obstruction and congestion, then inferior turbinoplasty is the procedure of choice for the same reasons as stated earlier. However, if the symptom being treated is refractory mucous discharge or watery rhinorrhea, then one of the nonresection techniques is preferred. In these instances, only the mucous glands need to be treated as a decrease in bulk is not required. Thus, the goals of surgery in such patients are to preserve tissue and to treat only the desired mucosa. In such cases, electrocautery is favored. This instrument is readily available in all operating rooms, is inexpensive to use, and is easy to control. The other techniques, including trichloroacetic acid chemical cautery, laser, and cryotherapy, are all simply different ways to ablate tissue. Each of these work as well as electrocautery, but each has its disadvantages in terms of handling, cost, and availability. However, if a practitioner has easy access to any of these alternative technologies, they may be easily learned and effectively used.

One alternative for the treatment of chronic rhinitis, especially the allergic type, is intraturbinal steroid injection. This procedure has been practiced widely by both otolaryngologists and allergists owing to its simplicity and its applicability to the office setting. The effects of this procedure are usually quite satisfactory, but the benefit is uniformly short-lived; within weeks to months, treated patients return to baseline. This procedure has the added drawback of the risk of blindness.[22, 23] This complication is thought to be caused by the intravascular injection embolizing the ophthalmic vessels, which causes acute effects leading to ischemia and blindness. Because of the short-term effect of the injection and the risk of repeated steroid injections, this procedure is not advocated.

Another alternative for treating rhinorrhea is vidian neurectomy.[24, 25] This operation, once touted as the definitive procedure for the treatment of rhinorrhea associated with vasomotor rhinitis, involves surgical transection of the vidian nerve, which severs the secretomotor innervation of the nasal mucosa. The underlying theory of the procedure was that this would eliminate the efferent arm of the reflex loop that drives nasal secretion in vasomotor rhinitis.

Unfortunately, this procedure failed to live up to its theoretical potential. The procedure was reported to be successful in roughly 50% of cases. The true long-term success rate may even have been lower. The reason postulated for the failure of this procedure is that rhinorrhea can be triggered in a number of ways, not only by efferent nerve impulses. These triggers include all types of local irritation and inflammation and circulating systemic factors.

The greatest drawback to the procedure, however, is the degree of technical difficulty with which it is performed. The operation requires considerable skill on a number of fronts, including avoiding bleeding from the sphenopalatine vessels, preventing injury to the maxillary nerve sensory function, and locating the skull base vidian canal. For these reasons, vidian neurectomy is now rarely offered as a surgical option.

SURGICAL TECHNIQUES

Out-Fracture of the Inferior Turbinate

As out-fracture of the inferior turbinate is generally done in conjunction with other nasal surgery, the mucosa will probably already be decongested. If not, either 4% cocaine solution or a topical decongestant in combination with lidocaine is applied to the turbinate mucosa using cotton pledgets. After adequate decongestion, the turbinate can be anesthetized, if necessary, using 1% lidocaine with 1:100,000 epinephrine. The favored technique for out-fracture is first to displace the turbinate medially, then to lateralize it.

A Freer elevator or a Boise elevator is placed lateral to the turbinate and firmly rotated medially by pushing up and in (Fig. 7–1*A*). The instrument is then reapplied to the medial surface and the turbinate is fully lateralized, making sure that the turbinate bone is fractured along its entire length (Fig. 7–1*B*). Packing is usually not needed, but may be useful in holding the turbinate laterally during initial healing (Fig. 7–1*C*). Little or no postoperative care is required.

Electrocautery of the Inferior Turbinate

Electrocautery can be performed either on the surface of the turbinate or intramucosally. The purpose of surface coagulation is selective ablation of the bulbous mucosa of the turbinate. This is particularly useful in treating mulberry turbinate, which is hypertrophy of the posterior tip of the turbinate. Suction cautery is favored in such cases because the cautery instrument can be bent to improve the angle of approach, has an insulated tip, and evacuates the smoke as it is produced. The latter feature increases visualization and shortens surgery time.

When performing surface cautery, a setting of 20 to 25 mA is used. The cautery is used to vaporize the exact amount of mucosa necessary to achieve the desired effect. After surgery, the patient will usually develop crusting over the cauterized areas. This is treated by manually removing loose crusts and mucus, leaving adherent scabs attached. The patient is encouraged to use saline nasal spray liberally until the scab loosens up, at which time it can be removed. Typically, this takes 3 to 4 weeks, but may take as long as 6 weeks if aggressive mucosal ablation is performed.

Intramucosal cautery is useful when attempting to induce involution of the mucosal glands within the submucosa without damaging the overlying ciliated mucosa. This procedure is indicated for watery rhinorrhea associated with chronic rhinitis. Needle tip cautery is used for this procedure. After adequate anesthesia, the needle is inserted into the submucosa of the turbinate along the inferior edge. The cautery is set for 15 mA and turned on for 30 to 45 seconds. The cautery is then removed and reinserted medially and superiorly a distance of 1 to 2 cm from the initial site. Cautery is repeated in this location and then moved superiorly again and repeated. Three locations along the medial surface are generally used. After this procedure, postoperative care is normally not required.

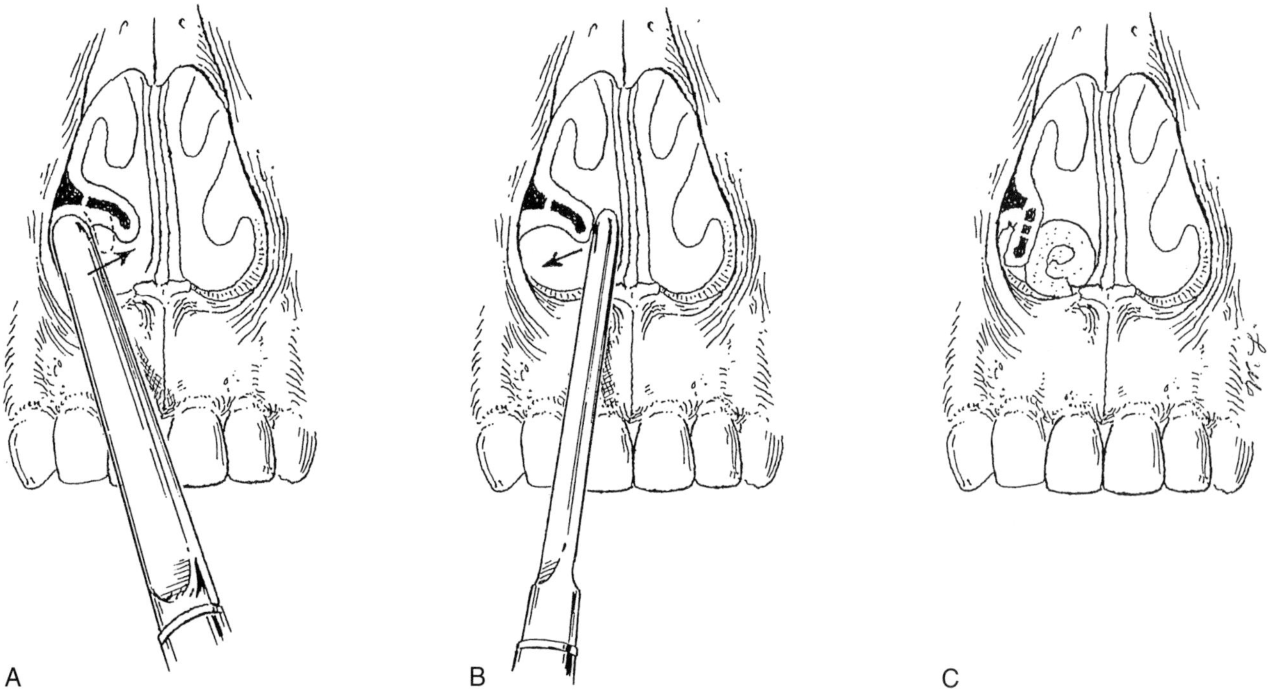

Figure 7–1. Out-fracture of the inferior turbinate. *A,* A Boise elevator is used to first in-fracture the turbinate. A sweeping or rolling motion is used to avoid lateral pressure on the pyriform aperture. *B,* The elevator is replaced medially and the turbinate is pushed laterally. *C,* A rolled Telfa pad is used to stent the turbinate laterally.

Submucous Resection of the Inferior Turbinate

Submucous resection of the inferior turbinate can be performed using a speculum and headlight or nasal endoscopes. After the anesthesia is applied, the incision is made along the inferior edge of the turbinate (Fig. 7–2*A*). The incision is best made with a No. 11 blade. The incision is carried down to bone from as far posterior as can be comfortably reached to anteriorly into the nasal root. The mucosa is then elevated from both the medial and lateral surfaces of the turbinate bone using either a Cottle elevator or an angled turbinate scissors (Fig. 7–2*B*). While retracting the mucosal flaps with the nasal speculum, the turbinate bone is resected. This can be accomplished either by cutting it with the turbinate scissors or using a rongeur to remove the bone piecemeal (Fig. 7–2*C*). The flaps are then cauterized along the raw surface to prevent hemorrhage and laid back together. If necessary, a pack may be placed to stent the flaps during the initial stages of healing (Fig. 7–2*D*). A piece of rolled Telfa is favored for this purpose.

Postoperative care consists of serial removal of crust from the healing incision. This will often only be required on two or three occasions during the postoperative period. As with the cautery procedure described earlier, only loose crusts and mucus should be removed. Adherent scabs should be left in place until they soften and separate naturally. The patient should be encouraged to use normal saline rinses frequently until healing is complete. Topical nasal steroids, decongestants, and antihistamines are withheld until the effect of the procedure is known and the need for these medications is confirmed.

Inferior Turbinoplasty of the Inferior Turbinate

Inferior turbinoplasty of the inferior turbinate can be performed either with the standard headlight and nasal speculum or endoscopically. The anesthesia for this procedure is the same as described earlier. Once adequate anesthesia has been obtained, the standard procedure is performed by making an incision, using a No. 11 scalpel, along the inferior edge of the turbinate up to the anterior attachment. The medial mucosa is next elevated from the turbinate bone using a Cottle elevator (Fig. 7–3*B*). The mucosa of the turbinate is densely adherent to the underlying bone and the surface of the bone is quite irregular, making this elevation somewhat difficult. The elevator should be firmly applied to the bone and the mucosa scraped from the bone. The gentle sweeping motion used to elevate the mucosa from the bone of the posterior septum during septoplasty

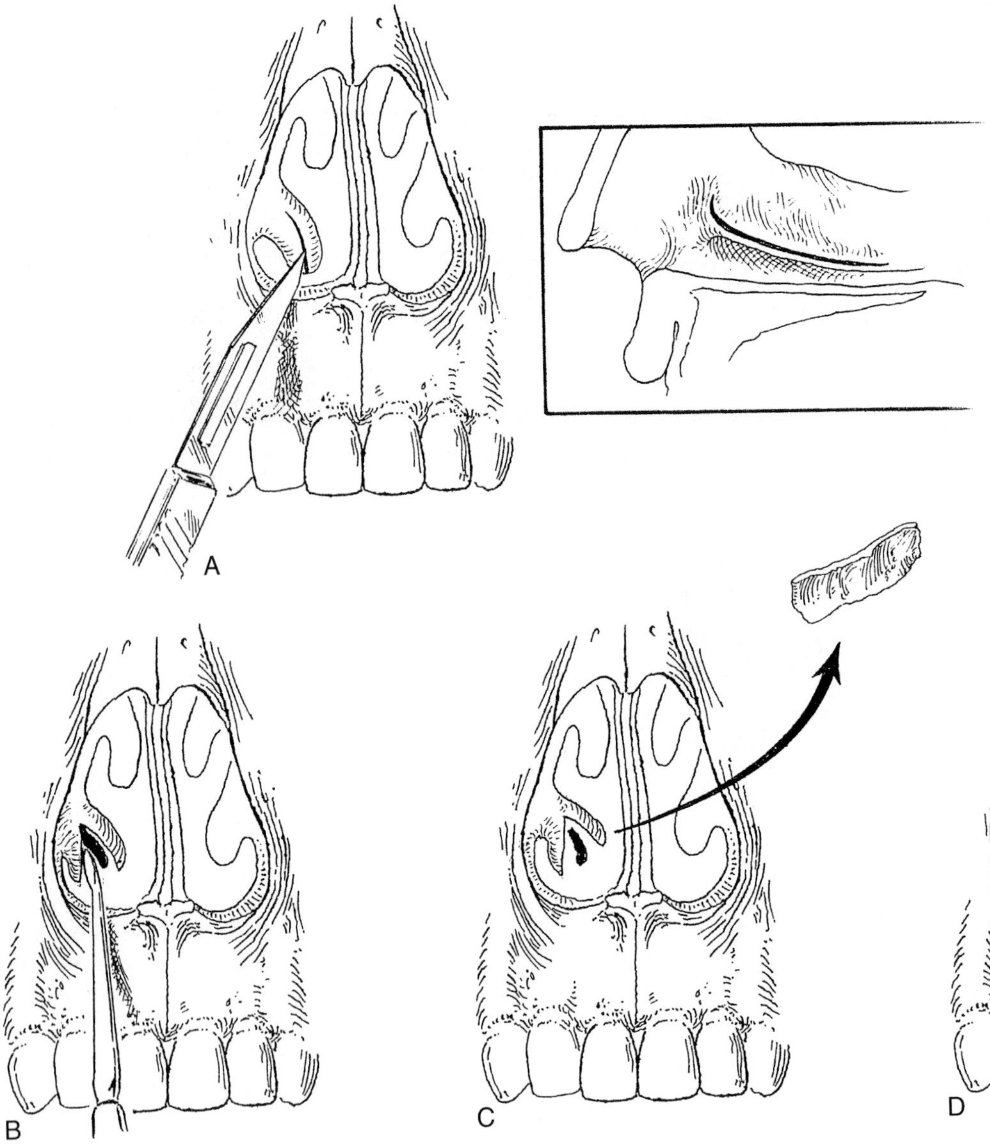

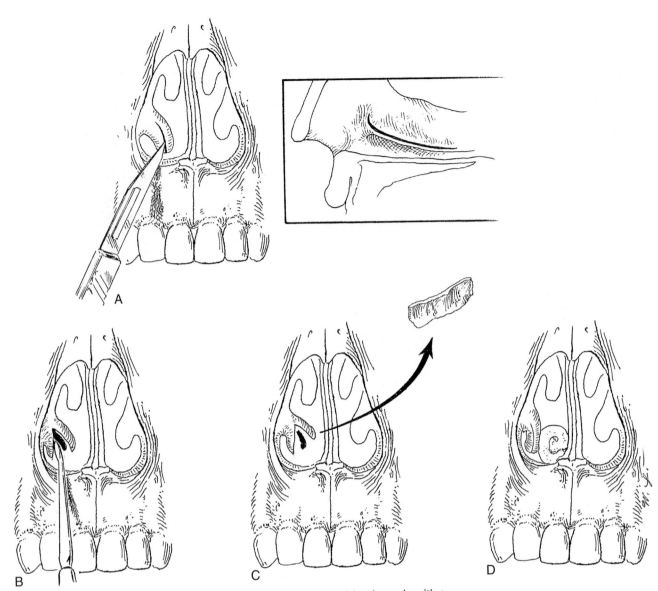

Figure 7–2. Submucous resection of the inferior turbinate. *A,* An incision is made with a No. 11 scalpel blade from as far posteriorly as can be reached into the root of the turbinate. *B,* The medial and lateral mucosal flaps are elevated to expose the turbinate bone. *C,* The bone is excised using scissors or a rongeur. *D,* The flaps are lateralized and held in place by a rolled Telfa pad.

does not work well for this procedure and may result in mucosal tears.

After the mucosa is elevated, there will usually be strands of tissue remaining that connect the mucosa to the bone. These should be lysed with an angled turbinate scissors. The same scissors can be used to extend the flap posteriorly and to release the flap from the posterior aspect of the turbinate.

After the flap is completely elevated, the turbinate scissors are used to excise the bone and lateral mucosa of the anterior two thirds of the turbinate (Fig. 7–3*A,C*). The scissors are first angled superiorly to catch the leading edge of the turbinate bone, then directed posteriorly, parallel to the inferior edge for 1 to 2 cm, and finally inferiorly to come across the inferior edge of the turbinate anterior to the posterior attachment of the turbinate.

After the resection, the free bone edge and deep surface of the flap can be cauterized if necessary. A suction cautery is most useful for this step. Next, the residual turbinate bone is lateralized as much as possible, and the mucosal flap is draped over the bone stump (Fig. 7–3*D*). If cautery has been used and the field is dry, no packing is needed. The final step is to assess the posterior aspect of the turbinate. If this is bulbous and potentially obstructive, suction cautery is used to shrink the mucosa to the desired effect. If there is concern about postoperative hemorrhage, a rolled Telfa pad

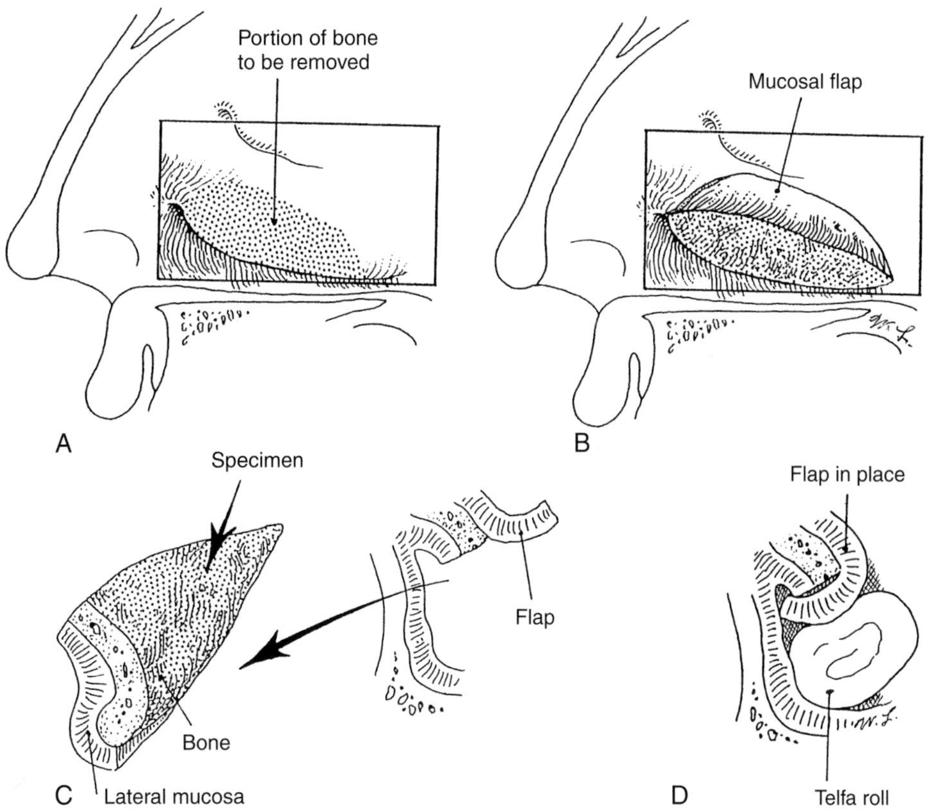

Figure 7–3. Lateral turbinoplasty of the inferior turbinate. *A,* The area of tissue and bone to be removed is shown. *B,* The medial mucosal flap is elevated along the entire medial surface. *C,* The lateral mucosa and bone are removed with care taken to preserve the medial mucosa. *D,* The flap is lateralized by a rolled Telfa pad.

covered with antibiotic ointment is placed under the flap.

Postoperative care is similar to that for submucous resection. If a pack has been placed, it can be removed as early as the morning after surgery. The patient is encouraged to use saline nasal spray liberally until healing is complete. Crusting is manually debrided 1 week and 3 weeks after surgery, but often, that is all that is necessary. Antistaphylococcal antibiotics are given for 1 week if packing is placed, although the evidence to support the need for this is lacking. Typically, no narcotics are needed for this procedure if performed as an isolated operation.

The endoscopic technique is performed in much the same manner as the standard procedure, but with a few modifications. Instead of using a Cottle elevator to raise the medial flap, straight endoscopic scissors are used. These instruments have short blades at the end of a long shaft with a trigger grip. This allows improved visualization and better accuracy when using endoscopic exposure. After the incision, the scissors are used to cut the mucosa from the underlying bone. When the flap is elevated, the same scissors are used to resect the turbinate.

The endoscopic procedure significantly improves visualization during the operation, especially at the posterior end of the turbinate. This facilitates flap elevation and yields improved shaping of the area of resection. The time required to perform the surgery is actually shortened with the use of endoscopic technique, as only one instrument is used and the improved visualization of the back of the nose allows more rapid dissection. The average time of the procedure for each turbinate from incision to resection is about 4 minutes.

Partial and Subtotal Resection of the Inferior Turbinate

Anesthesia is accomplished as for the procedures described earlier. The procedure for both partial and subtotal resection are identical except for the amount of tissue resected. Figure 7–4*A* shows the line of resection for the two variations. When the anesthetic has taken effect, a curved hemostat or Kelly forceps is placed over the turbinate and clamped down over the line of the intended resection (Fig. 7–4*B*). When a partial turbinectomy is performed, the clamp is placed over the anteroinferior two thirds or, according to the amount of resection desired, more or less of the turbinate. For a subtotal resection, the clamp is placed as high on the turbinate as possible, curving down to the inferior edge just anterior to the posterior attachment. The clamp is left there for 2 to 3 minutes and then released. The angled turbinate scissors are then used to cut along the crush line created by the clamp (Fig. 7–4*C*). After the turbinate is resected, suction cautery can be used to

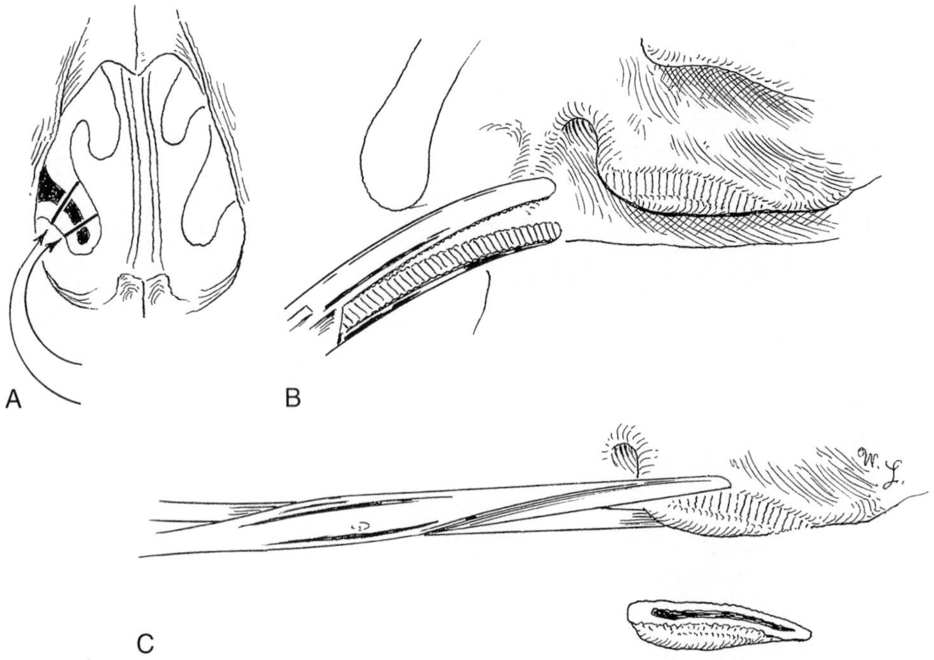

Figure 7–4. Partial and subtotal resection of the inferior turbinate. *A,* The lines of resection are marked for partial and subtotal resection. *B,* A Kelly clamp is used to crush the turbinate along the line of resection. *C,* Angled scissors are used to excise the turbinate.

coagulate the raw edge. This will decrease the incidence of postoperative bleeding and obviate the need for packing the nose.

These operations tend to take longer to heal than the other procedures and, therefore, require more intensive postoperative care. Crusts are removed after 1 week and then every other week until healing is complete. As with the other procedures, frequent nasal saline rinses are encouraged. Postoperative antibiotics are not administered unless packing is used. Postoperative pain medication is not usually needed.

COMPLICATIONS

Hemorrhage

Postoperative hemorrhage is the most common complication of turbinate procedures. The risk of this event, however, is quite low. Although most patients experience some postoperative bleeding, this is usually limited and stops spontaneously within the first few days after surgery. Significant postoperative hemorrhage has been reported after each of the procedures just described. The incidence is generally 1% to 2% or less. The incidence of severe hemorrhage requiring transfusion is low, being less than 1% in all cases. To date, the author has not had to transfuse any patient owing to postoperative bleeding after any form of turbinectomy.

The management of postoperative hemorrhage from the inferior turbinate should be the same as for any patient with epistaxis (see Chapter 22). In brief, the patient should be relaxed and any pain should be well controlled. If, after a period of observation, the bleeding has not stopped, the hemorrhagic source needs to be ascertained. Any existing packing is removed from the nose and, under good headlight illumination, the nose is suctioned free of blood clot and then decongested with a topical solution applied with cotton pledgets. This often is sufficient to stop the bleeding. Bleeding from the turbinate is usually found near the posterior edge of the cut surface where the vessels enter the turbinate. Once the bleeding point is identified, bleeding can be controlled via vasoconstriction, cautery, or packing.

Scarring

Formation of synechiae from the inferior turbinate to the septum or middle turbinate is rare after turbinectomy. However, it may occur if the septal mucosa is abraded adjacent to the raw edge of the turbinate after resection. Blood clot will form between the surfaces, organizing into a fibrous plug. If not removed, this plug will become mucosalized and will mature into a synechia. The incidence of synechiae is hard to ascertain, but if the patient is monitored after surgery as described, this complication can be prevented.

Once a mature synechia is formed, management depends on whether it is symptomatic or not. Usually, these scar bands will need to be removed. It is not generally sufficient merely to incise the synechiae. Most cases require excision from both mucosal surfaces, with some type of postoperative stenting to prevent recurrence. After removal of the stent, careful cleaning should be performed weekly until healed.

Atrophic Rhinitis

The primary function of the nose in respiration is to condition the inhaled air so as to protect the lower airways. This function consists of cleaning, humidifying, and warming the air. According to Kern,[1] the nasal mucosa can be thought of in this role as the organ of nasal function. When any of the nasal mucosa that participates in these functions is removed, the functional capacity of the organ is diminished.

Excessive removal of nasal mucosa results in failure of the nasal organ. This failure is usually manifested by some degree of drying and crusting of the nose. In the extreme, this can result in atrophic rhinitis. This condition is recognized by the persistent production of large nasal crusts. This causes secondary bacterial overgrowth and chronic inflammation of the underlying nasal mucosa. In less severe forms of this condition, the patient may experience only nasal dryness combined with a dry, irritated throat.

These changes may occur many years after the surgical procedure. In a series of more than 200 cases reported by Kern, the mean time of onset was approximately 8 years after the procedure.[1] The reasons for this late onset of complications are speculative, but include the natural loss of nasal function with aging. Another explanation is that the underlying condition necessitating the procedure may lessen over time, resulting in a relative lack of function. Also, there may be ongoing damage to the mucosa from the excess functional stress on the remaining mucosa following the procedure.

Whatever the cause, it seems clear that the more nasal mucosa that is removed, the greater the chance of some degree of atrophic changes. However, the full-blown condition of atrophic rhinitis rarely accompanies any of these procedures, despite the great frequency with which turbinate procedures are performed. It is reasonable to assume that nonresection techniques, such as laser and electrocautery, will almost never result in severe atrophic rhinitis, whereas total turbinectomy has a reported incidence of about 5%.[3, 21] Partial turbinectomy and lateral turbinoplasty, predictably, have an incidence that lies somewhere in between.

When atrophic rhinitis occurs, there is no single method recommended for managing the affected patient. Initially, steps to cleanse the nose and debride the crusts on a daily basis should be tried. Irrigations with normal saline twice each day, saline spray every few hours, and the use of a room humidifier at night are preliminary steps. Antibiotics may be helpful temporarily, but are unlikely to provide lasting relief.

In the worst cases, surgical procedures to close or narrow the nose may be of some benefit. Different surgical options include implants into the lateral nasal wall or floor of the nose.[26, 27] The implant may consist of cartilage, bone, or fat grafts, or silastic implants placed in a submucosal tunnel. Alternatively, the nose may be surgically closed, in part or completely, by creating synechiae from the septum to the lateral nasal wall.[28] Clearly, these procedures are only performed as a last resort.

REFERENCES

1. Kern E. Against turbinectomy. Presentation at the Triologic Society, May 13, 1997; Scottsdale, AZ.
2. Fanous N. Anterior turbinectomy. A new surgical approach to turbinate hypertrophy: A review of 220 cases. Arch Otolaryngol Head Neck Surg 112:850, 1986.
3. Martinez SA, Nissen AJ, Stock CR, et al. Nasal turbinate resection for relief of nasal obstruction. Laryngoscope 93:871, 1983.
4. Spector M. Partial resection of the inferior turbinates. Ear Nose Throat J 61:28, 1982.
5. Marquez F, Cenjor C, Gutierrez R, et al. Multiple submucosal out-fracture of the inferior turbinates: Evaluation of the results by acoustic rhinometry. Am J Rhinol 10:387, 1996.
6. O'Flynn PE, Mifford CA, Mackay IS. Multiple submucosal outfractures of the inferior turbinates. J Laryngol Otol 104:239, 1990.
7. Mabry RL. Intranasal corticosteroid injection: Indications, technique, and complications. Otolaryngol Head Neck Surg 87:207, 1979.
8. Yao K, Shitara T, Takahashi H-o, et al. Chemosurgery with trichloroacetic acid for allergic rhinitis. Am J Rhinol 9, 3:163, 1995.
9. Rinder J, Stjarne P, Lundberg JM. Capsaicin de-sensitization of the human nasal mucosa reduces pain and vascular effects of lactic acid and hypertonic saline. Rhinology 32:173, 1994.
10. Terao A, Meshitsuka K, Suzaki H, et al. Cryosurgery on postganglionic fibers (posterior nasal branches) of the pterygopalatine ganglion for vasomotor rhinitis. Acta Otolaryngol 96:139, 1983.
11. Principato JJ: Chronic vasomotor rhinitis: Cryogenic and other surgical modes of treatment. Laryngoscope 89:619, 1979.
12. Jones AS, Lancer JM. Does submucosal diathermy to the inferior turbinates reduce nasal resistance to airflow in the long term? J Laryngol Otol 101:448, 1987.
13. Jones AS, Lancer JM, Moir AA. The effect of submucosal diathermy to the inferior turbinates or nasal resistance to airflow in allergic and vasomotor rhinitis. Clinical Otolaryngol 10:249, 1985.
14. Kubota I. Nasal function following carbon dioxide laser turbinate surgery for allergy. Am J Rhinol 9(3):155, 1995.
15. Levine HL. The potassium–titanyl phosphate laser treatment of turbinate dysfunction. Otolaryngol Head Neck Surg 104:247, 1991.
16. Fukutake T, Yamashita T, Tomodr K, et al. Laser surgery for allergic rhinitis. Arch Otolaryngol Head Neck Surg 112:1280, 1986.
17. House HP. Submucous resection of the inferior turbinate bone. Laryngoscope 61:637, 1951.
18. Davis WE, Nishioka GJ. Endoscopic partial inferior turbinectomy using a power microcutting instrument. Ear Nose Throat J 75: 49, 1996.
19. Mabry RL. Surgery of the inferior turbinates: How much and when? Otolaryngol Head Neck Surg 92:571, 1984.
20. Mabry RL. "How I do it"—Plastic surgery. Practical suggestions on facial plastic surgery. Inferior turbinoplasty. Laryngoscope 92:459, 1982.
21. Courtiss EH, Goldwyn RM, O'Brien JJ. Resection of obstructing inferior nasal turbinates. Plast Reconstr Surg 62:249, 1978.
22. McCleve D, Goldstein J, Silver S. Corticosteroid injections of the nasal turbinates: Past experience and precautions. Otolaryngology 86:851, 1978.
23. Mabry RL. Intranasal corticosteroid injection: Indications, technique, and complications. Otolaryngol Head Neck Surg 87: 207, 1979.
24. Fernandes CM. Bilateral transnasal vidian neurectomy in the management of chronic rhinitis. J Laryngol Otol 108(7):569, 1994.

25. Kamel R, Zaher S. Endoscopic transnasal vidian neurectomy. Laryngoscope 101(3):316, 1991.
26. Shehata M, Dogheim Y. Surgical treatment of primary chronic atrophic rhinitis (an evaluation of silastic implants). J Laryngol Otol 100:803, 1986.
27. Girgis IH. Surgical treatment of Ozena by dermofat graft. J Laryngol Otol 80:615, 1966.
28. Gadre KC, Bhargava KB, Prudlon RL, et al. Closure of the nostrils (Young's operation) in atrophic rhinitis. J Laryngol Otol 85:711, 1971.

CHAPTER 8

Endoscopic Sinus Surgery

INDICATIONS

Chronic Sinusitis

The most common indication for performing endoscopic sinus surgery (ESS) is chronic sinusitis. The diagnosis and management of chronic sinusitis is covered in detail in Chapter 5. In this chapter, only the indications for surgery are discussed. Some degree of controversy surrounds the appropriate indications for surgery in this group of patients owing to the difficulty in definitively establishing the diagnosis, the high rate of success, and the generally low complication rates for the surgery. Individual surgeons may, in practice, offer surgery to all patients diagnosed with chronic sinusitis under the assumption that surgery will improve their long-term quality of life. However, it is apparent that this surgery, as all others, has an incidence of failure, complications, and bad results that, together with the economic cost of the procedure, make this type of blanket approach both medically inappropriate and ethically unacceptable.

The basic indication for surgery in patients with chronic sinusitis is the failure of medical management to control the symptoms of this disease adequately. In this setting, when the findings on radiologic studies (usually, computed tomgraphy [CT]) and physical examination correlate, the patient is a candidate for surgery.[1–3] If medical therapy can control the patient's symptoms, then the benefit of surgery is difficult to document and, therefore, should be avoided. Likewise, if the CT scan does not correlate to the symptoms and history, then an alternative cause for the patient's condition should be sought.

Even this relatively simple principle is fraught with difficulty, however. To support the contention that, if medical therapy controls the symptoms, then surgery should be avoided, adequate medical therapy needs to be defined. In addition, the cost-versus-benefit ratios for medical therapy and surgery need to be compared, and the possibilities of developing complications with each of the two therapies must be considered.

To date, this type of long-term outcome data is not available. For this reason, the circumstances of each patient need to be individually assessed and the patient must be closely involved in any decision to proceed with surgery.

The initial consideration is what, exactly, constitutes adequate medical therapy. For most patients, this means a minimum of 2 months of continuous therapy that includes at least two antibiotics that, between them, cover the full spectrum of the usual bacterial flora.[4, 5] Typically, a nasal steroid spray and a decongestant/mucolytic combination drug are also prescribed. In most cases, though, prior to arrival in the otolaryngologist's office, the patient has been managed for any number of months or years by internists, pediatricians, family practitioners, or other otolaryngologists. Generally, the patient has already received numerous courses of antibiotics and other adjunctive medications. In this setting, the otolaryngologist must evaluate the quality and appropriateness of this therapy.

The second consideration is the anatomy of the patient's sinuses as defined by radiologic evaluation and its correlation to the history and physical findings.[6, 7] To be a candidate for surgery, the findings on the CT scan should make sense and explain the clinical findings. The amount of mucosal disease is not as critical as the principle that the disease or anatomic abnormality demonstrated by CT scan should correspond to the clinical syndrome with which the patient presents. In general, a CT scan should be obtained after a full course of treatment so as to minimize the mucosal abnormality present and improve the chances of identifying underlying bony abnormalities.

When surgery is elected, the extent of surgery should be based on the extent of disease present in the patient.[2, 8–10] To determine this, both the CT scan and the findings at surgery are considered. The surgery should open up all blocked areas and extend at least one cell layer beyond the finding of disease on CT or at surgery. These concepts may be illustrated by the following clinical examples.

Figure 8–1 demonstrates a patient with minimal radiographic findings that corresponded well to the clinical course. The patient presented with a 2-year history of recurrent right maxillary sinusitis that, despite treatment with antibiotics, was associated with persistent congestion and postnasal drainage. A 3-week trial of intensive medical management, including antibiotics, a decongestant/mucolytic, and nasal steroid spray, resulted in some improvement. A CT scan at this time (Fig. 8–1) demonstrated infundibular thickening with residual minimal maxillary sinus mucosal thickening and an air-fluid level. Owing to the long-standing nature of the problem and the persistent symptoms after therapy, the patient underwent a limited anterior ethmoidectomy with middle meatus antrostomy. In this case, a large Haller cell led to the infundibular disease and was probably the cause of the chronic maxillary sinusitis.

A second patient presented with presistent right frontal headaches, congestion, and postnasal drainage. After a prolonged trial of appropriate medical therapy, a CT scan was obtained (Fig. 8–2). The scan demonstrated anterior ethmoid mucosal thickening with secondary frontal sinus opacification. A large agger nasi cell was the presumed cause of the problem. A complete anterior ethmoidectomy with frontal sinusotomy effectively resolved the problem.

Figure 8–3 is an example of a patient with more diffuse chronic sinusitis. This patient had severe allergies (without polyps), asthma, and symptomatic chronic sinusitis despite maximal medical therapy. This was probably not caused by a single anatomic abnormality, as in the previous two cases, but was likely attributable to a combination of allergy and generally narrow sinus openings. In this case, the persistent symptoms were easily explained by the CT findings. Complete bilateral endoscopic sphenoethmoidectomy with middle meatus antrostomy and intranasal frontal sinusotomy was performed. Together with long-term postoperative medical management, including nasal steroid spray, asthma management, and immunotherapy, the surgery resulted in nearly complete symptomatic relief without episodes of chronic sinusitis.

Hyperplastic Sinusitis (Sinonasal Polyps)

Most patients with sinonasal polyps will eventually come to surgery at some point in their lives. However, the mere presence of a nasal polyp is not an indication to proceed immediately to surgery. Rather, the decision to embark on surgery for sinonasal polyps must be considered carefully, taking into account the same princi-

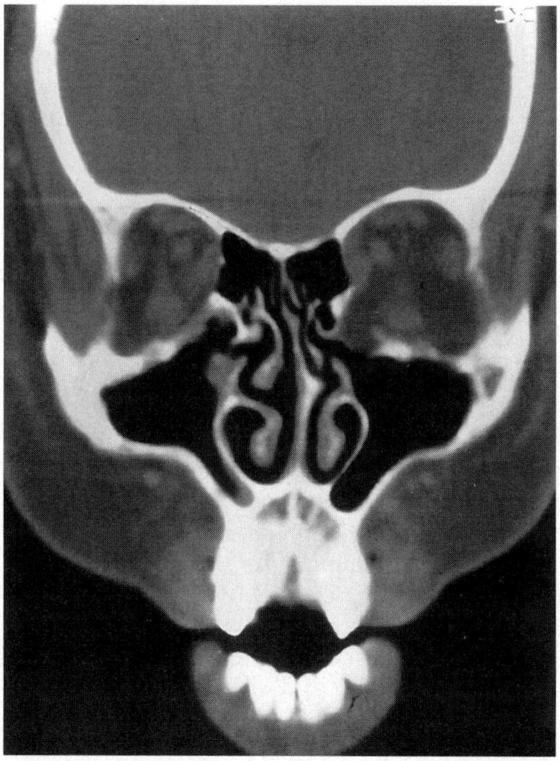

A

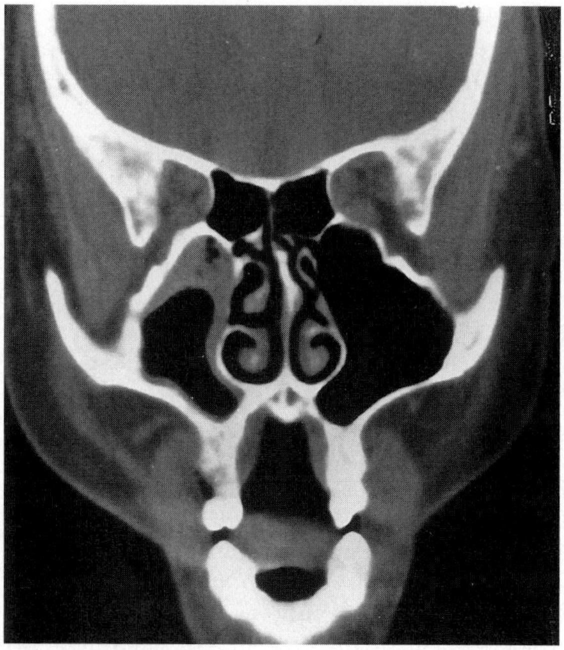

B

Figure 8–1. *A,* CT scan through the infundibulum of the ethmoid sinus. Note the polypoid mass on the lateral surface of the uncinate process. *B,* A CT scan through the mid-maxillary sinus of the same patient as in Figure 8–1*A* demonstrates an air-fluid level.

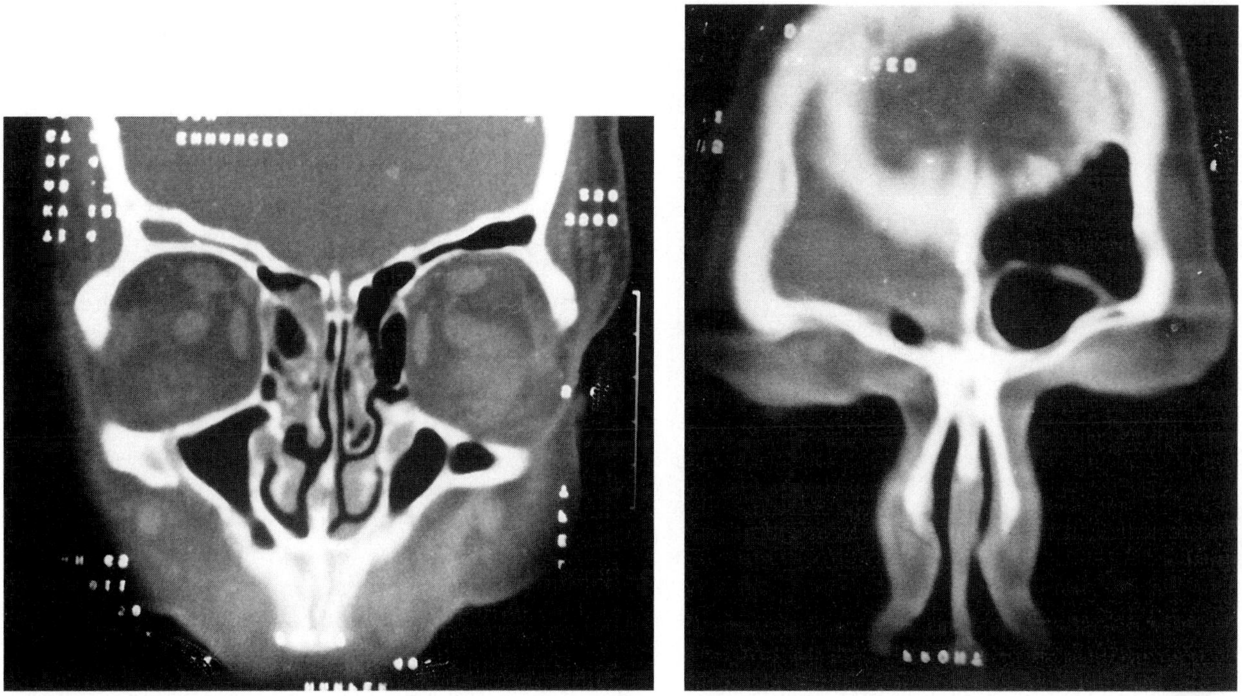

A B

Figure 8–2. *A,* A CT scan through the anterior ethmoid sinus demonstrates a large agger nasi cell with mucosal thickening in the frontal sinus outflow tract. *B,* A CT scan through the frontal sinus of the same patient as in Figure 8–2*A* demonstrates opacification of the frontal sinus.

ples discussed in the section on chronic sinusitis. A patient with small middle meatus polyps may be easily controlled on a single daily dose of nasal steroid spray.[11] Other patients may have medical conditions that complicate the decision to operate. In addition, the patient's symptoms may be surprisingly minimal despite extensive polyps.

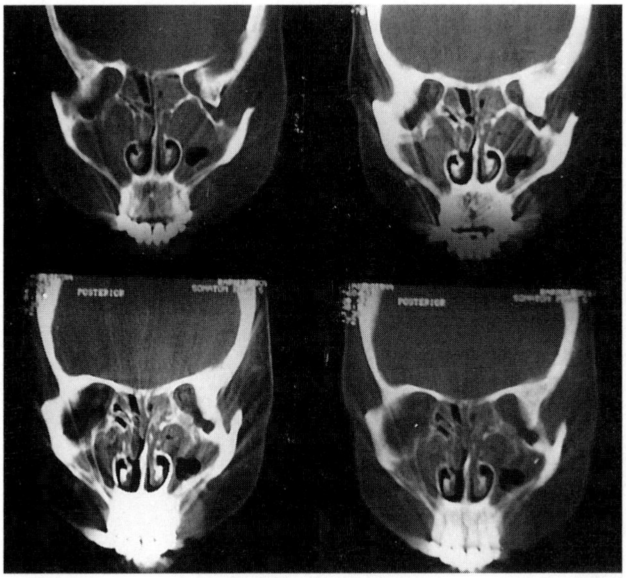

Figure 8–3. CT scan of a patient with severe pansinusitis. Extensive mucosal thickening is present in all sinuses.

Two basic categories of patients are commonly observed: those with pansinus polyposis and those with a limited number of polyps and discontinuous sinus mucosal thickening demonstrated on CT scan.[12] For patients with extensive polyps and pansinus opacification, the decision to offer surgery is relatively straightforward. These patients are typically very symptomatic, presenting with nasal obstruction, anosmia, congestion, and postnasal drainage. Interestingly, many of these patients have a total absence of headache and may have no sense of pressure or fullness despite total nasal obstruction and even expansion of the sinuses from longstanding polyps (Fig. 8–4).

Medical therapy involving the use of topical nasal steroids may have a beneficial effect on polyp size and symptoms, even in cases of massive polyposis, but does not appear to affect the sinuses directly.[13, 14] Conversely, systemic steroids will affect both the nasal and sinus mucosa, improving both.[15, 16] However, the benefits of topical and systemic steroids are short-term in most patients, with recurrence of symptoms typically noted within the first year after withdrawal of therapy.[13, 17] Immunotherapy as a treatment for nasal polyps has not been studied extensively. Experience suggests that most patients will not experience shrinkage of polyps with

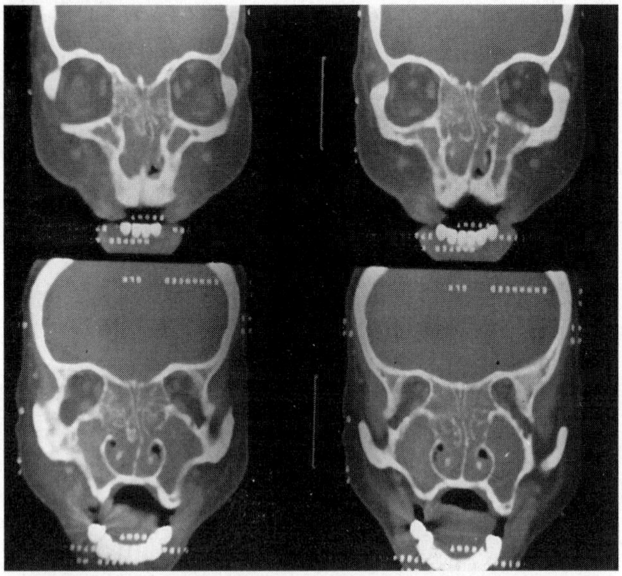

Figure 8–4. CT scan of a patient with extensive sinonasal polyposis. Note the absence of air in all sinuses, with complete nasal obstruction. This patient suffered from anosmia and congestion but did not experience headaches.

immunotherapy, but these agents may have some benefit in the postoperative period.[18]

Untreated extensive polyps do carry a significant long-term risk of complications. If left untreated for decades, the polyps will eventually expand to the point of causing telecanthus, proptosis, and diplopia.[19] Secondary infection may result in either intraorbital or intracranial infection.[20] Secondary mucoceles are also possible.

For these reasons, this group of patients should be treated surgically. The only exceptions would be patients who either cannot tolerate surgery or for whom surgery poses a greater risk than the polyps.

The second category of patients includes those with limited localized polyps. Often, CT scans in these patients demonstrate discontinuous ethmoid disease with localized middle meatus polyps (Fig. 8–5). Although these patients can expect predictably good results from surgery, medical management may result in excellent control of symptoms without substantial risk or cost. The standard approach to these patients is, therefore, a short course of oral steroids followed by a prolonged course of nasal steroid sprays. If this therapy is successful, surgery is unnecessary unless the patient has a subsequent relapse.

When surgery is performed in patients with sinonasal polyps, an aggressive approach is usually warranted. Partial ethmoidectomy with polypectomy will often result in relapse with failure to control the regrowth of the polyps. In this setting, a complete endoscopic sphenoethmoidectomy with wide middle meatus antrostomy and intranasal frontal sinusotomy is the favored approach.

Extramucosal Fungal Sinusitis

Extramucosal fungal sinusitis exists in two distinct clinical forms: allergic fungal sinusitis and fungus ball.[21, 22] Both of these conditions, when diagnosed, are absolute indications for surgery. Allergic fungal sinusitis is essentially nonresponsive to medical management without concomitant surgery.[23, 24] The reason for this is that the fungal elements must be removed to control the allergic response. The patient may have unilateral or bilateral disease. In the case of the former, the extent of surgery should be limited to the side of involvement. Partial

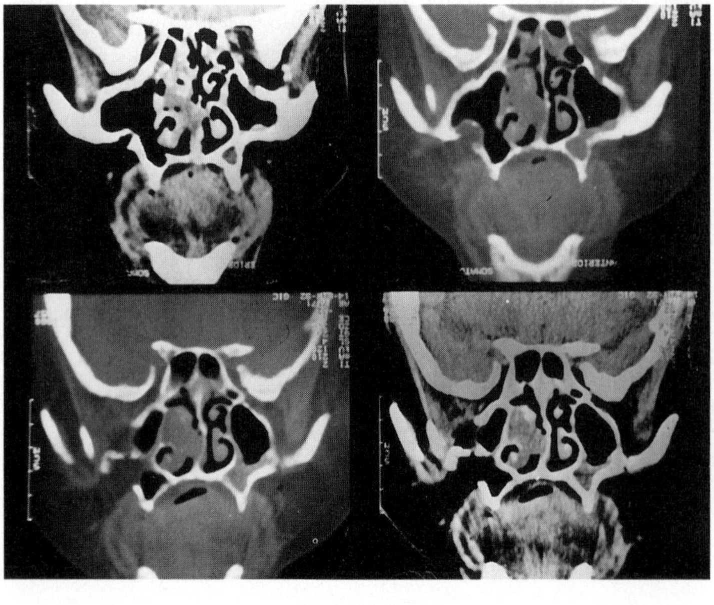

Figure 8–5. CT scan of a patient with middle meatus polyps. The polyps had reportedly been present for more than 50 years without medical treatment over much of that time. The patient had not undergone previous surgery except for an inferior nasal antral window.

surgery in this situation is unlikely to be of lasting benefit. Owing to reexposure to the inciting organism, the pathogenic process is not curable and, despite initial excellent results, eventual relapse is likely.[23] For this reason, complete endoscopic sphenoethmoidectomy, together with wide middle meatus antrostomy and frontal sinusotomy, is warranted in most cases.

Fungus ball is managed quite differently.[22, 25] Only the sinuses that are involved need to be operated on; the goal of surgery is complete removal of all fungal elements. Most commonly, fungus ball is found in the maxillary sinus, so uncinectomy with wide antrostomy is all that is required to remove the inspissated material. However, if the fungus ball is in the sphenoid sinus, then typically, an anterior and posterior ethmoidectomy, with removal of part of the superior turbinate and wide opening of the sphenoid, is performed. This is done to ensure easy access to the sinus after surgery to allow cleaning of the sphenoid and removal of any recurrent debris.

Acute Sinusitis

Most patients with acute sinusitis can be treated effectively with medical therapy, without need for surgical intervention. In select cases, though, surgical drainage is required.[26, 27] Most of those who require surgical intervention have some predisposing factor that is the cause of sinusitis, such as human immunodeficiency virus (HIV), admission to the intensive care unit, or post-transplantation status with immunosuppression.[28, 29] In these patients, the combination of a depressed immune system, exposure to resistant hospital bacteria, and numerous courses of intravenous antibiotics poses a significantly increased risk of medically resistant infection. By contrast, patients with an intact immune system and community-acquired infection only rarely develop a medically resistant infection.

The indications for surgery in both populations are similar. Initially, routine treatment is prescribed for the initial sinus infection. Following this, if the patient remains acutely infected, a second course of empiric antibiotic therapy is usually tried. If this is unsuccessful, direct sinus puncture, with antibiotic therapy based on the culture results, is normally attempted. If this fails, then surgery is often the only recourse. In such cases, endoscopic surgery is often difficult owing to severe mucosal inflammation. Bleeding is often exacerbated and accessibility is limited owing to mucosal swelling. In this setting, the aim of surgery should be limited to achieving drainage of the involved sinuses, as excessive dissection in the frontal recess is likely to result in scarring and subsequent stenosis. In patients with acute frontal sinusitis requiring surgery, consideration should be given to either combining endoscopic surgery with trephination or utilizing external trephination alone for the frontal sinus.

Recurrent Acute Sinusitis

Recurrent acute sinusitis is an uncommon indication for ESS and is difficult to document. This condition is defined by the absence of significant mucosal disease in intervals between episodes of true acute sinusitis. In order to establish the diagnosis, radiologic evidence of acute sinusitis must be documented on at least two separate occasions. CT scans or plain radiographs obtained during infection-free intervals usually reveal no significant mucosal thickening, but often demonstrate anatomic abnormalities that may predispose the patient to episodes of acute infection.

A variety of CT findings have been associated with sinusitis.[30–33] The most common of these are abnormalities of the middle turbinate, including the concha bullosa and paradoxical middle turbinate. Variations of the uncinate process, with either lateralization or pneumatization, may also be found. Unusual or excessive aeration of ethmoid air cells may also significantly limit sinus drainage and predispose the patient to recurrent sinus infection. Examples of this include enlarged Haller cells, agger nasi cells, or hyperaeration of the ethmoidal bulla. Also, a significantly deviated nasal septum may be a cause of narrowing of the infundibulum and subsequent recurrent infection.

Patients with recurrent acute sinusitis without specific anatomic abnormality should be evaluated carefully for medical conditions that could predispose them to recurrent infection. In particular, a careful evaluation of the patient's immune status, with consideration of selective immunoglobulin deficiency and deficits of cellular immunity, is warranted. The possibility of ciliary dyskinesia should also be considered. Other systemic conditions, such as systemic lupus erythematosus and sarcoidosis, may also be associated with normal anatomy and recurrent sinusitis.

Once recurrent acute sinusitis has been documented, management of the disease is based on the underlying cause. For those patients with systemic conditions or immune dysfunction, a course of prophylactic antibiotics is the preferred mode of treatment. The problem with these patients is not anatomic but functional, so an anatomic approach is unlikely to be beneficial. However, for patients with identifiable anatomic abnormalities, surgery is the most sensible approach. In this situation, medical management may help to control the frequency and severity of the infections, but it cannot resolve the problem as surgery can.

When surgery is elected, a limited approach to correct the underlying obstruction is all that is indicated. Usually, the maxillary sinus is the affected sinus. In such cases, surgical intervention requires only uncinectomy and enlargement of the natural ostium of the maxillary sinus. If a deviated septum is part of the problem, then septoplasty should be undertaken. A concha bullosa can be managed by resection of the lateral lamella, whereas a paradoxical turbinate will require partial resection of the middle turbinate to remove the lateralized segment.

Mucocele

Mucoceles are expansile cysts of the sinuses.[34] They are formed by obstruction of the ostium of the sinus, which leads to the sinus filling with mucus. Continued secretion of mucus against a closed ostium eventually leads to increased pressure in the sinus, with bone erosion and expansion into the surrounding tissues.[35, 36] The frontal sinus is most commonly involved, followed, in order of frequency of involvement, by the ethmoid, sphenoid, and maxillary sinus.[37]

Traditionally, the treatment of mucoceles has involved excision of the cyst, with either wide drainage or obliteration of the sinus after excision. [35, 36, 38] However, the introduction of sinus endoscopy has made possible drainage through the natural ostium into the nose, without excision. Numerous articles have described treatment of mucoceles by endoscopic drainage,[37, 39–43] all of which have affirmed that adequate drainage of the mucocele into the nose through the natural ostium can successfully aerate the sinus. To date, though, there has not been sufficient long-term follow-up evaluations to assure that recurrence will not be a problem. Despite this, endoscopic drainage is now widely considered to be the standard of care for the treatment of most mucoceles.

The decision to perform endoscopic surgery is based on several basic principles. The most important principle is that the mucocele must be accessible through the nose. For mucoceles involving the frontal sinus, this means that the mucocele must extend at least to the level of the internal ostium. Rarely, a lateral sinus cell may not be able to be reached through the intranasal route and thus will not be amenable to an endoscopic approach. Other situations may also arise that preclude the endoscopic approach. In the author's practice, these include an osteoma of the frontal sinus blocking the internal os, a post-traumatic mucocele in which the medial orbital wall obstructed the frontal recess, and failed external frontoethmoidectomy with orbital obstruction of the frontal recess.

A second principle affecting the decision to perform endoscopic surgery is that the mucocele must be able to be decompressed completely through the natural ostium. In certain situations, the mucocele may extend outside the sinus, creating nondependent loculations. If this occurs, mere opening of the ostium of the sinus may be insufficient to decompress the mucocele. Consider, for example, the patient with a post-traumatic maxillary sinus mucocele that extends through the lateral wall into the infratemporal fossa and buccal space. Opening the natural ostium in this case would result in a large loculation outside the sinus that might not drain into the nose.

One final principle is that the patient should be one who can reasonably be expected to present for long-term follow-up evaluations. As the long-term viability of this treatment approach to mucoceles has not definitively been established, long-term monitoring is critical. The ideal duration of follow-up evaluation is not known. However, late onset of mucoceles has been reported up to 20 years after frontal sinus obliteration.[44] For this reason, a period of at least 10 years of follow-up evaluation following endoscopic drainage would seem reasonably appropriate.

Headache and Facial Pain

One of the more controversial applications of ESS is for the treatment of headache and facial pain. It has been postulated that, in the absence of sinus inflammation, structural abnormalities that create pressure points within the nose and sinuses may induce a chronic pain syndrome.[45–51] Alternatively, narrowing of a sinus ostium may predispose a patient to intermittent obstruction of the sinus secondary to periodic congestion from the normal nasal cycle. Obstruction of the sinus in this way could, theoretically, cause acute pressure build-up in the sinus, causing baroheadache.

Definitive documentation that these conditions exist is lacking; however, precedence has been established within other organ systems. For example, barotrauma to the ear due to eustachian tube dysfunction during air travel or diving is a well-known phenomenon. Moreover, pressure points within joints secondary to spurs or swollen bursa are known to cause significant pain.

The difficulty with these conditions is accurate diagnosis. In order to determine which patients are appropriate candidates for surgical intervention, the diagnosis must be assured to a reasonable doubt. The patient's history should be highly suggestive, and physical examination and CT scan should clearly identify a probable underlying anatomic cause. Finally, a trial of topical or local anesthesia should have a beneficial effect on the headache.

The typical history is one of unilateral facial pressure or pain that is highly localized over the affected sinus. Symptoms are usually intermittent but sustained, lasting hours per episode. Often, oral or topical decongestants have a beneficial effect. Patients may have been treated repeatedly for sinusitis but invariably have no radiographic evidence of sinusitis.

The examination and CT scan may show numerous different anatomic findings. The most common is a septal spur that projects into the middle or inferior turbinate. Other findings include hyperaeration of ethmoid cells, such as a concha bullosa of the middle turbinate, aeration of the superior turbinate, enlarged ethmoidal bulla, or enlarged agger nasi cell.

The final step in diagnosis is to examine the patient during a typical episode of headache or facial pain. The suspected contact point is then decongested and anesthetized with topical lidocaine or cocaine. The patient should experience prompt relief of symptoms. After this, pressure applied to the contact point should then reproduce the symptoms.

In this setting, an inferred diagnosis of contact point headache can be made. Definitive proof of the association, though, depends on resolution of the syndrome after surgical correction. Despite careful evaluation and screening, it is possible to misdiagnose this condition. Therefore, patients should routinely be treated with a prolonged course of nasal steroid spray and decongestant prior to surgery.

If such a patient ultimately elects to undergo surgery, he or she should always be advised that failure of the surgery to relieve the symptoms is a significant possibility. Even in carefully selected patients, a 10% to 20% failure rate is expected. The procedure itself should be limited to resolving the anatomic problems identified. No single operation is appropriate, but the pressure point or obstructed sinus needs to be corrected.

Revision Endoscopic Sinus Surgery

The decision to perform revision ESS is one of the most difficult in rhinology. The failure of the first procedure must be understood both anatomically and functionally, and clear technical goals for the revision surgery should be outlined before proceeding with the operation. There are two important reasons for hesitancy in performing revision endoscopic sinus surgery: (1) the increased complication rate associated with such procedures and (2) the comparatively lower success rate.

Most experts agree and several studies have shown that revision ESS is associated with a higher complication rate than surgical procedures performed on previously unoperated sinuses.[52–55] The obvious reason is the distortion in anatomy caused by the initial surgery. This may be in the form of loss of landmarks, such as the middle turbinate, the ground lamella, and the uncinate process. Alternatively, this anatomic alteration may involve weakening of the natural barriers to complications, such as dehiscence in the lamina papyracea, septal perforation, or defects in the skull base. In the author's experience, the incidence of cerebrospinal fluid (CSF) leak detected during surgery has been about 1% for revision cases, compared to 0% in unoperated cases. Also, the risk of frontal sinus stenosis is similarly increased.

The success rate of revision surgery has been the subject of some controversy. Some authors have reported success rates with revision ESS that are equivalent to those achieved with the initial operation.[52–54] However, in the author's experience, the success rate of revision ESS has been comparatively lower.[55] This lower success rate was highlighted in an article that documented a statistically lower success rate, as measured by the need for further surgery, that held up in a multivariate analysis.[55] There are several reasons for this lower success rate. First, a proportion of initial failures are the result of inherent disease within the patient. Examples include cystic fibrosis, allergic fungal sinusitis, and aspirin triad. These patients are at high risk for developing recurrent polyposis, despite apparently successful initial surgery, because of their inherent mucosal disease, which cannot be cured by surgery. Revision surgery carries the same risk for failure as the first procedure.

A second reason is that the initial surgery may have failed as a result of difficult anatomy, which may have led to incomplete surgery. The anatomy may be just as challenging during the revision surgery, leading to increased risk of failure due to the same problems encountered during the first procedure. Examples of this problem include narrow access through the anterior nose and narrow access into the frontal recess. In other patients, unusual cell structure, such as high frontal recess cells and intrafrontal sinus cells, may make dissection difficult or impossible.

A third reason that revision ESS may have a higher failure rate than initial surgery is the damage done to mucociliary clearance by the first surgery. Studies of the regeneration of mucosa in animals have demonstrated that the regenerated mucosa is fibrotic, thick, and has decreased ciliary counts and decreased mucociliary clearance.[56–58] Without adequate mucociliary clearance, ESS is doomed to ultimate failure. Examples of this type of complication include previous Caldwell-Luc surgery with aggressive stripping of the sinus mucosa, chronic osteitis of the bone induced by excessive mucosal stripping, and scarring in the sinus outflow areas leading to poor mucociliary clearance. Revision surgery in these cases may be deemed necessary, but may not result in normalization of mucociliary clearance even if anatomically correct drainage is restored.

Finally, the previous surgery may result in obstructing scar formation around the ostia of the sinuses. Presenting the greatest difficulty in the frontal recess, obliterative scarring in this location may be an indication for revision, but will certainly have a lower success rate in restoring mucociliary clearance than if the sinus had never been operated on before.

Owing to these factors, the decision to perform revision surgery must be based on more than the presence of persistent or recurrent mucosal disease. Appropriate management of the patient who fails an initial attempt at surgery is to first maximize medical therapy. This usually involves obtaining directed cultures from the sinus cavity and administering prolonged antibiotic treatment based on the results. Also, allergy management must be maximized, including immunotherapy, if appropriate, and strict avoidance of test-positive antigens. A thorough evaluation for immunodeficiency or contributing systemic disease is also recommended. In addition, in patients with polyps, a 2- to 3-week course of systemic steroids is usually initiated.

If these measures do not result in adequate control, then a high-quality CT scan with thin coronal and axial cuts should be obtained to analyze the residual disease and anatomy. Finally, a careful endoscopic examination should be performed in an attempt to confirm the CT findings and identify possible anatomic causes of surgical failure. The best candidates for revision surgery are those patients who have an identifiable anatomic cause for the recurrent or persistent problem. The most common example of such an anatomic anomaly is a surgical middle meatus antrostomy that does not communicate with the natural ostium of the maxillary sinus. This may set up a recirculation phenomena, leading to persistent infection in the maxillary sinus.[59] The next most common finding is residual disease in the anterior ethmoid and frontal recess. Persistent infection in this location can lead to infection draining down into the lower ethmoids and maxillary sinus, causing reinfection. Other common findings include scarring or synechiae that obstruct the sinus ostia, inspissated secretions that have not been adequately removed, and failure to achieve surgical sphenoidotomy.

When revision surgery is performed, it is essential that a preoperative plan be carefully thought out, including identification of specific goals and an approach to achieve the goals. Preoperative CT scans must be carefully studied prior to the revision and should be available for reference in the operating room. In general, it is best to perform a complete revision in these patients, including a complete sphenoethmoidectomy with intranasal frontal sinusotomy and wide middle meatus antrostomy. In this way, the need for further revision surgery is minimized.

Other

In addition to these well-recognized indications for ESS, there are a number of special procedures and indications for the technique that will be covered in other chapters. These include dacryocystorhinostomy, orbital and optic nerve decompression, repair of CSF leaks, tumor surgery, control of epistaxis, and diagnosis.

PERIOPERATIVE MANAGEMENT

Medical Management

Aside from the treatment considerations involved in the decision to perform ESS, there are also medical management issues to consider in the immediate perioperative period. For one, the patient needs to be assessed as a medical candidate for surgery. This assessment is not unique to this type of surgery, but compared to the usual tonsillectomy or rhinoplasty candidate, the population undergoing ESS tends to be older, with more significant comorbid conditions and a higher incidence of asthma. Attempts should be made to minimize the severity of asthma prior to surgery, given the irritation of anesthesia to the airway, the increase in secretions during the postoperative period, and the possibility of nasal packing, all of which may exacerbate asthma.

Specific to ESS is the need to minimize the amount of sinus inflammation at the time of surgery. The more inflammation present at the time of surgery, the higher the risk of postoperative problems, such as relapse and stenosis.[60] Moreover, the inflamed sinus tends to bleed more, increasing the difficulty of surgery and the inherent risk to the patient from surgery. To control sinus inflammation, it has been suggested that antibiotics be administered for a minimum of 10 days prior to surgery; in patients with polyps, a 10-day course of moderate-dose steroids should be added. Although not documented by a prospective study to date, this practice commonly results in significantly less inflammation at the time of surgery, making the procedure easier and improving the surgical outcome.

Anesthesia

Endoscopic sinus surgery may be performed using either general anesthesia or local anesthesia with intravenous sedation. Many authorities prefer to use local anesthesia with sedation, believing that it is safer for the patient owing to reduced blood loss, which means safer surgery.[2, 61] Despite these claims, these advantages have not been demonstrated in the literature. In fact, multiple studies have reported equivalent rates of complication and success with either form of anesthesia.[9, 62] However, avoiding general anesthesia is a laudable goal in its own right, as local anesthesia with sedation is generally safer, results in less nausea and vomiting, and decreases the length of hospital or surgery center stays.

However, local anesthesia with sedation may add significantly to the surgeon's stress if the patient cannot be kept comfortable. Incomplete surgery may result, as well. In addition, there will usually be some blood in the airway and, in some cases, significant bleeding, which leads to an increased risk of aspiration. In some cases, the length of the procedure may exceed 2 hours; in cases incorporating septoplasty, surgery may take up to 3 hours. Few patients are able to tolerate procedures of this length while awake on the operating table. Finally, in some revision cases, the neuroanatomy may be altered, leading to difficulty in achieving quality nerve block and, thus, inadequate anesthesia.

In the past, general anesthesia was used only in patients undergoing lengthy operations of 2 hours or more, those having revision surgery, and those with an abnormal fear of local sedation. Now, because of the factors just cited, local sedation is used only in those patients undergoing minimal surgery without previous ESS. All others receive general anesthesia.

SURGICAL TECHNIQUE

The technique of ESS described in the following sections is adapted from the techniques of Messerklinger[63] and Stammberger,[8] as taught in the United States first by Kennedy[2] and later by others.[9, 10, 64–66] This technique involves an anterior-to-posterior approach, which has come to be known as functional endoscopic sinus surgery (FESS). This approach to surgery is designed to achieve a functional, intact sinus with the minimal surgical intervention necessary. An alternative technique, known as the Wigand[67] approach, involves a posterior-to-anterior endoscopic dissection, similar to the classic intranasal sphenoethmoidectomy described by Friedman and others.[68–70] The FESS procedure has been the operation that has developed the widest acceptance and greatest use. The advantage of the anterior-to-posterior dissection is that it allows the surgeon to tailor the extent of the surgery to the needs of the patient. This valuable flexibility and versatility are the primary reasons that this technique has gained favor over the Wigand approach.

Instrumentation

Endoscopes have changed little since they were first introduced. All sets should include standard lenses 4 mm in width with 0-, 30-, and 70-degree orientation of the lenses (Fig. 8–6). Some companies have marketed variations on these standard lens angles that are interchangeable with these specifications. Endoscopes are also available in 2.7-mm widths with long and short shafts and additional lens angles, such as 90 and 120 degrees. These extreme angles are difficult to use in actual surgery and, in the author's experience, have not been necessary. The 2.7-mm endoscopes are used predominantly for diagnosis, but may be useful in some pediatric cases, especially in children younger than 5 or 6 years of age.

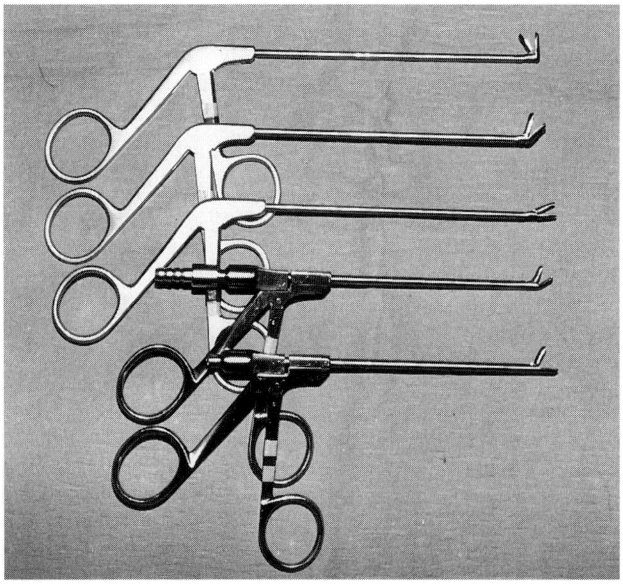

Figure 8–7. Standard Blakesley-type ethmoidectomy forceps. Pictured are 90-, 45-, and 0-degree angle forceps and 45- and 0-degree suction forceps.

The original standard instrumentation for ESS, first introduced in the mid 1980s, has been greatly modified and expanded since that time. The basic set still consists of straight and angled upturned forceps, with and without suction channels (Fig. 8–7). These instruments are

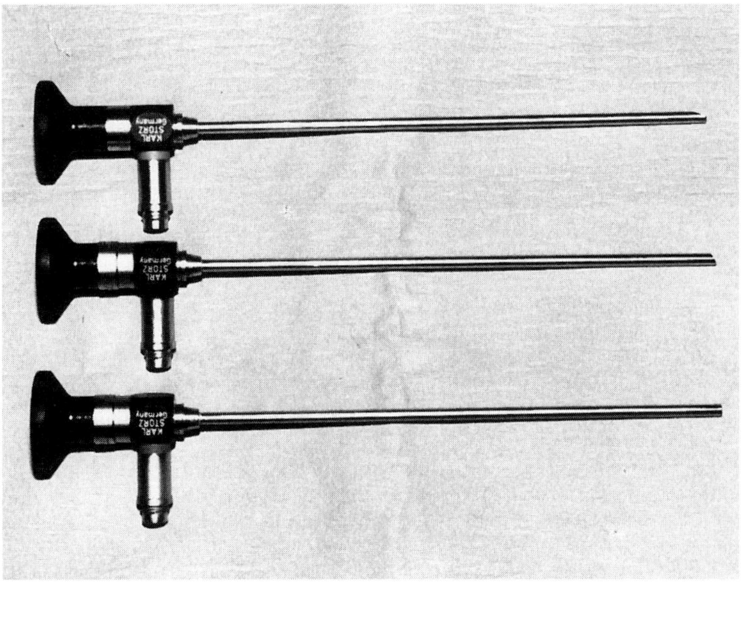

Figure 8–6. Standard 4-mm Hopkins rod telescopes are used in endoscopic sinus surgery. Pictured are 0-, 30-, and 70-degree angle lenses.

the most commonly used. They have a grasping and biting jaw that can bite through bone, but a twisting motion is generally required to bite through tissue. These instruments typically leave a jagged-edge cut and have the tendency to tear and strip mucosa if not used carefully. Variations exist in the size of the biting jaws, the position and orientation of the suction channel, and the exact degree of upturn on the angled forceps, which ranges from 30 to 90 degrees. In addition, these instruments have been modified to offer a through-cutting jaw that acts like a punch, cutting through almost any tissue or bone found in the sinuses without tearing or stripping.

The basic set also contains a back-biting forceps (Fig. 8–8). These instruments have a through-cutting mechanism that prevents tearing and stripping and leaves a smoother cut than the standard grasping/biting jaws. These instruments have been modified since their introduction to have a narrower profile and longer jaw. Other modifications include side-biting and down-biting forceps, and forceps with a rotating head that allows any orientation of the jaws.

The basic set also includes giraffe forceps (Fig. 8–9). These instruments come with a long, thin 70-, 90-, or 120-degree angle shaft, hence the name giraffe forceps. The jaws, which may be either the grasping/biting type or the through-cutting type, are oriented in a horizontal or vertical fashion, and come in 2- and 3-mm jaw sizes.

Other instruments commonly used include the sickle knife, probes, and elevators (Fig. 8–10). The probes are available in several sizes, shapes, and thicknesses depending on whether they are designed for the maxillary or frontal sinus. Curettes are also part of the standard instrument set. These come with a J-shaped cutting jaw mounted on either a straight or long curved shaft. The curved shaft is especially useful for working in the maxillary sinus and frontal recess.

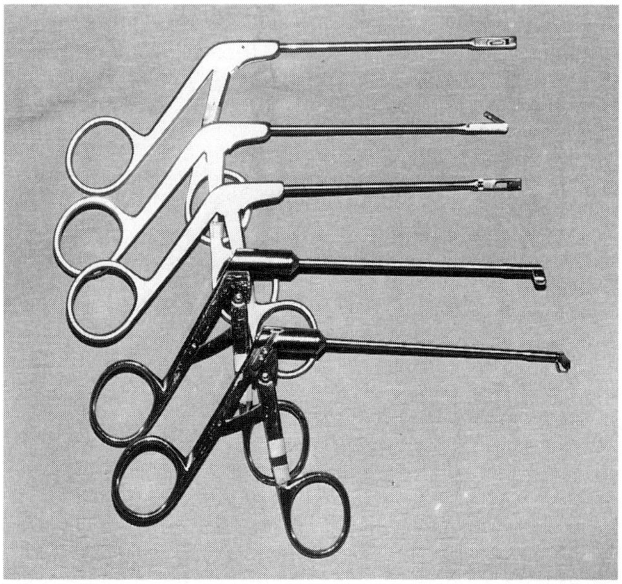

Figure 8–8. Various specialized forceps may be used for endoscopic sinus surgery. Pictured, from the top down, are left back-biting, straight back-biting, right back-biting, left down-biting, and right down-biting forceps.

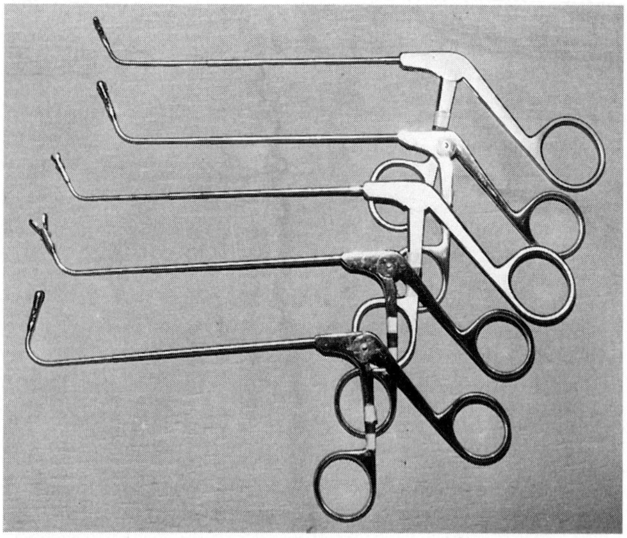

Figure 8–9. Giraffe forceps. Pictured, from the top down, are 70-degree, 2-mm horizontal; 3-mm horizontal; 2-mm vertical; 3-mm vertical; and 120-degree, 3-mm horizontal forceps.

The biggest change in the practice of ESS began in the early 1990s with the introduction of powered instruments.[71–73] Now in their third generation of modifications, these instruments feature an oscillating, cutting blade contained within a metal shaft that supplies continuous irrigation and suction to the tip of the instrument (Fig. 8–11). The original instrument did not cut bone well, but the latest generation cuts through ethmoid bone with little difficulty. Tissue can be excised precisely and suctioned through the shaft into a standard suction line that can be fitted with a tissue trap to retrieve a specimen for pathologic review. These instruments are now available with a variety of attachments, including angled or curved shafts and burrs of various sizes that allow them to be used as drills.

Other adjunctive equipment has also been applied to ESS, including a suction irrigator attachment that is mounted on the endoscope like a pistol grip. Other companies have marketed a foot-controlled irrigation system that rinses the tip of the endoscope to keep it clean of blood and debris.

Since the early days of ESS, video attachments have been modified continuously to improve the visualized endoscopic image. The earliest surgery was performed through the endoscope without video projection. Later, an articulated arm, designed for a single observer, was developed. Still later, the video camera was adapted to the endoscope to allow the image to be monitored continuously on a video screen. Advances in this technology now allow crisp clear images to be viewed in

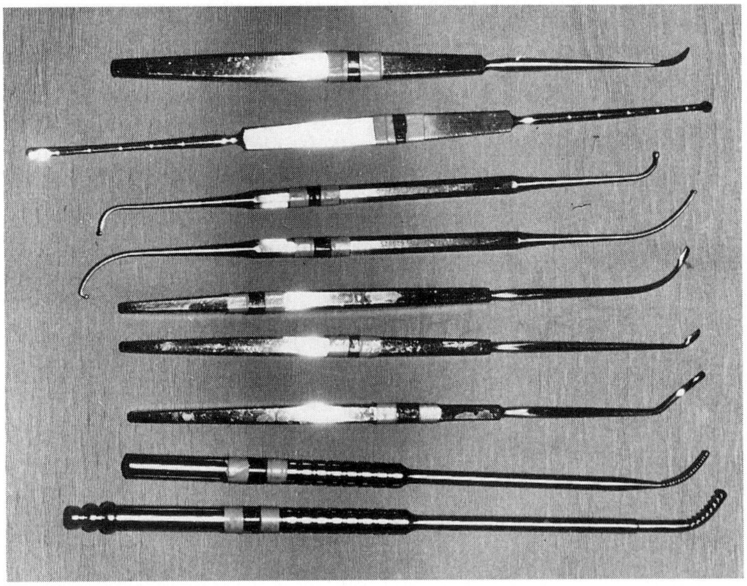

Figure 8–10. Various accessory instruments may also be used in endoscopic sinus surgery. Pictured, from the top down, are the sickle knife; Cottle elevator; maxillary and frontal ostium seekers; curved and straight J-currettes; 45-degree angle ethmoid currette; small, curved, frontal sinus rasp; and large, curved suction rasp.

almost any light or setting. Many surgeons have taken these advances and utilized them to operate from the video image instead of looking into the patient. They believe that the enlarged image improves their operating skill. Other surgeons have steadfastly maintained that use of the endoscope with a beam splitter improves depth perception while still allowing observation and video recording. The direct endoscopic image is also preferred when the operating field is very bloody as the quality of the video image tends to degrade owing to light absorption by the blood. With either technique, the most important consideration is that the surgeon is comfortable and can perform the operation as intended.

The most recent video enhancement is the addition of computer-assisted, image-guided surgery.[74–78] Several systems are available today that allow the surgeon to orient the patient to a magnetic resonance image (MRI) scan or a CT scan with three-dimensional formatting. The surgeon can then, at the touch of a button, orient a probe or endoscope to an exact point in the patient's anatomy. Three basic systems are currently available. The most complex and expensive uses an array of infrared diodes to orient the probe in three dimensions. A remote sensing device localizes the probe in space by recognizing the array on the probe. This can then be oriented to the patient and referenced to a computerized image of the patient's sinuses. This system is accurate to within 1 mm in most cases, but is very costly and time-consuming and not applicable to most sinus surgery.

A second system uses an articulated arm attached to a three-dimensional position finder. The probe or endoscope is attached to the arm and the tip of the

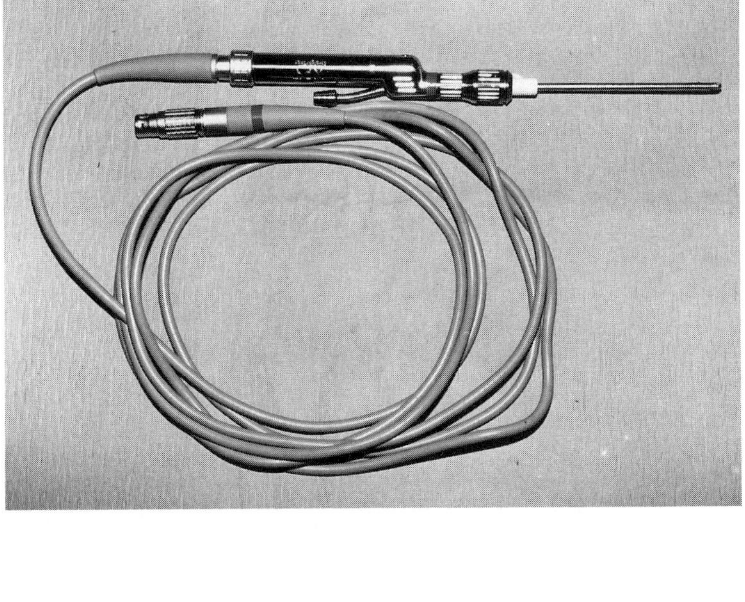

Figure 8–11. Microdebrider with in-line suction and irrigation channels for use in endoscopic sinus surgery. Pictured is the XPS "Straight Shot" (Xomed Corporation, Jacksonville, FL).

probe is oriented to fiducials or external landmarks on the patient's face or skull. Using fiducials improves accuracy, but then requires that the scan be done the same day as the surgery. Using external landmarks makes this technique more applicable but less accurate (usually only to within 2 mm) than the first system described.

The most cost-effective and easiest system utilizes a visor that is mounted on the patient's head, generating a magnetic field. The probe tip is then located within the field by sensors within the visor and the tip of the probe is referenced to a preloaded CT scan. This system has the advantages of not requiring the CT scan to be performed on the day of surgery and not requiring rigid head fixation. Its accuracy is generally within 2 mm, and is often within 1 mm, especially if internal landmarks are used as reference points.

The problem with all these systems is that they are very costly and are not necessary for the routine case. For advanced applications of ESS, however, this type of technology can be very helpful and can significantly improve the safety of the surgery. The burden is now on the manufacturers to produce a cost-effective system.

Standard Ethmoidectomy

The procedure described in this section is complete endoscopic ethmoidectomy, including all cells of the ethmoid sinus, performed with standard instruments. This is in no way meant to infer that complete ethmoidectomy is the standard procedure for all situations. In practice, it is essential to tailor the operation performed to the amount of disease observed on the CT scan and at surgery. A general guideline is to remove one cell layer posterior to the extent of disease. Thus, a patient with maxillary sinus disease alone would need only an infundibulotomy, a patient with infundibular disease would need only an anterior ethmoidectomy, and a patient with disease of the anterior ethmoid would need only an anterior ethmoidectomy with opening of the posterior ethmoid.

Anesthesia

The first step in any endoscopic procedure is to apply topical and local anesthestic. The technique is the same whether local anesthesia/sedation or general anesthesia is administered. The topical anesthestic is applied first. The options include cocaine or oxymetazoline, either alone or in combination with lidocaine. Studies have shown that, in children, oxymetazoline works as well or better than 4% cocaine in achieving decongestion and hemostasis.[79] However, no studies have been done to compare cocaine flakes to any other formulation. Cocaine solution, in concentrations of either 4% or 10% may be applied via pledgets placed throughout the nose. However, this technique provides inconsistent dosing, as absorption and actual drug delivery are unpredictable. By contrast, application of solid cocaine flakes provides a predictable dose of cocaine that can be measured and so is the preferred technique.

Cocaine flakes are applied topically using cotton-tipped metal applicators in three locations (Fig. 8–12).

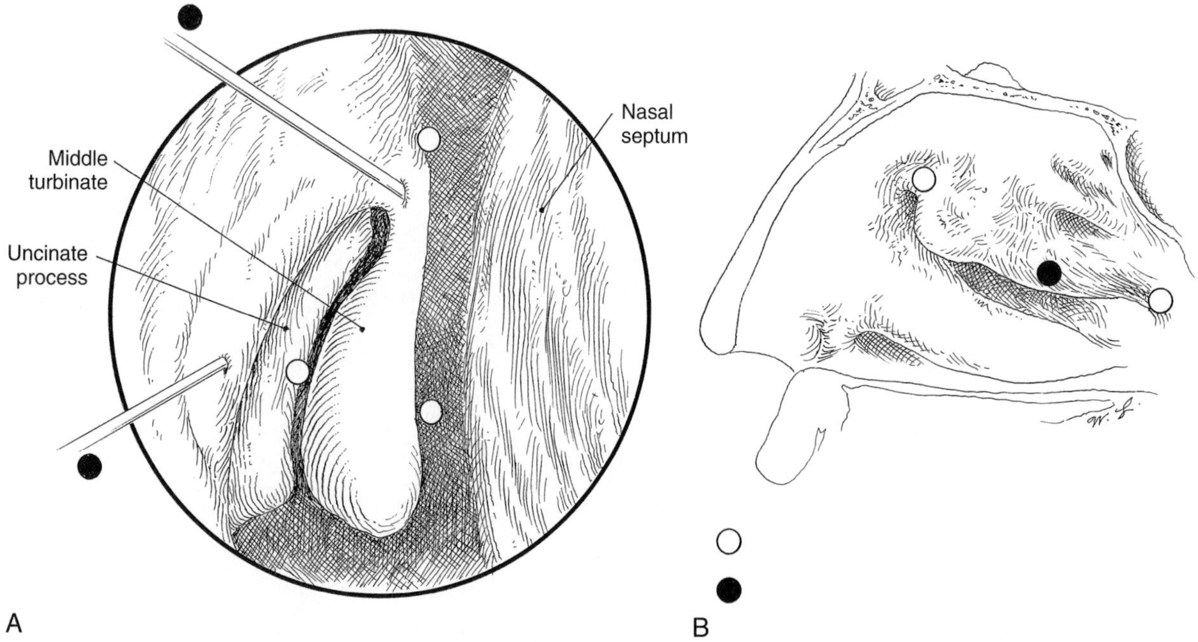

Figure 8–12. Cocaine applicator and needle injection sites used in standard preparation for endoscopic sinus surgery. *A,* Endoscopic view. *B,* Lateral view. The open circles are cocaine sites; black circles are injection sites.

The selected locations are above the anterior end of the middle turbinate to block the anterior ethmoid nerves, inside the middle meatus to decongest the infundibulum, and above the posterior end of the middle turbinate to block the sphenopalatine nerve.

After application of the topical anesthetic, local anesthetic is then injected. The standard formulation is 1% lidocaine with 1 : 100,000 epinephrine, which is injected using a 2-inch, 25-gauge needle. About 2 cc of anesthetic is injected into each of three locations: the anterior attachment of the middle turbinate, a site anterior to the uncinate process, and a site as far posteriorly along the inferior edge of the middle turbinate as possible. If the patient is undergoing sedation anesthesia and posterior ethmoidectomy or sphenoidotomy, a 22-gauge spinal needle or tonsil needle can be used to inject the sphenopalatine ganglion directly, either through the foramen or through the greater palatine foramen.

The topical and local anesthetics are both applied under direct endoscopic visualization, one side at a time, immediately before operating on that side. The local anesthetic is allowed to work for a minimum of 5 minutes before beginning the surgery; however, a 10-minute interval is optimal to achieve the best effect.

The main concern in using cocaine is the risk of cardiac toxicity.[80] Cocaine acts by blocking reuptake of norepinephrine at sympathetic junctions. By itself, it is usually well tolerated at topical doses of up to 200 to 300 mg applied nasally. However, with injection of local anesthetic solution containing epinephrine or with application of concentrated topical epinephrine, a synergistic effect occurs. The epinephrine acts directly on the sympathetic neurons, stimulating the postsynaptic norepinephrine receptors. The combination of reuptake inhibition and direct synaptic stimulation may lead to untoward effects, including tachycardia and hypertension.

This clinical phenomenon is commonly observed with the use of a combination of cocaine flakes and lidocaine with epinephrine injection. Typically, signs are usually limited to transient minor elevations in blood pressure and pulse. In the author's series of cases, only one patient of about 1000 who received this combination sustained a significant alteration that required a change in the treatment plan or medical treatment. In this patient, a 25-year-old woman, bronchospasm and tachycardia persisted for 3 hours and required the administration of supplemental oxygen and bronchodilators in the recovery room. The patient eventually recovered and no further treatment was needed; she was discharged to home that afternoon.

Uncinectomy

The actual surgery begins using the 0-degree endoscope to medialize the middle turbinate. Usually, this is done with a Freer elevator by applying firm pressure against the lateral aspect of the upper part of the turbinate. The procedure begins in earnest with incision of the uncinate process, or infundibulotomy (Fig. 8–13). A sickle knife is preferred, although a Cottle elevator is another option. The incision is made at the anterior attachment of the uncinate process to the lateral nasal wall. A sawing motion is used to extend the incision

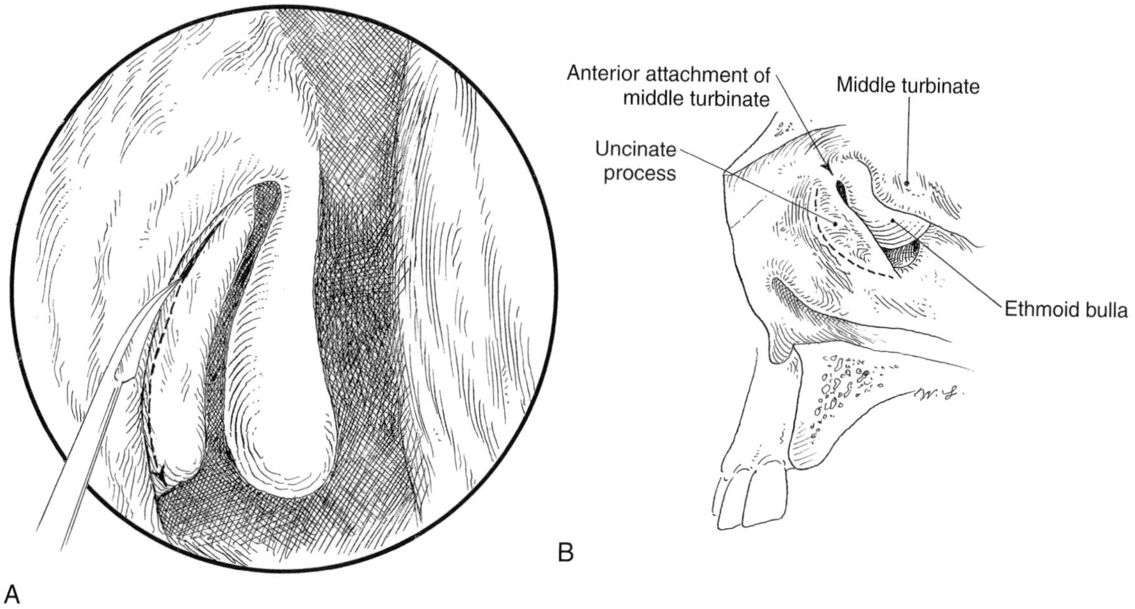

Figure 8–13. Uncinectomy. The dotted line indicates the line of incision. *A,* Endoscopic view. *B,* The anatomy as viewed from an inferior and medial perspective.

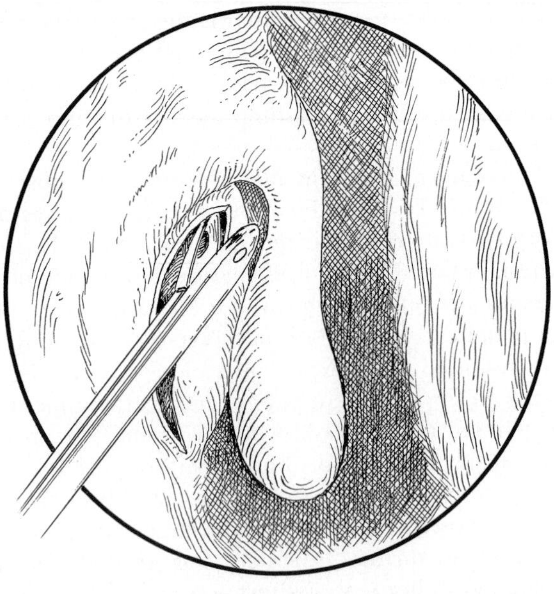

Figure 8–14. Completion of the uncinectomy. An endoscopic view of the removal of the uncinate process after incision using Blakesley forceps.

from the superior attachment inferiorly through the anterior fontanelle. It is important that the knife blade be oriented parallel to the lamina papyracea to avoid orbital penetration. The incised uncinate process is then grasped at the superior attachment and a gentle twisting motion is used to detach the uncinate. The inferior attachment is then grasped and similarly detached using a gentle twisting motion (Fig. 8–14).

Anterior Ethmoidectomy

The bulla ethmoidalis is now easily visualized and approached. A straight Blakesley cup forceps is used to indent and then grasp the medial and inferior edge of the bulla (Fig. 8–15). Throughout the remaining ethmoidectomy, each bite of the forceps is completed by using the same twisting motion to cleanly tear the mucosa and bone. This technique minimizes unwanted tearing and stripping of the tissue as it is removed. The ethmoidectomy proceeds with complete removal of the bulla. With the bulla removed, the lamina papyracea can usually be identified and cleaned of loose tissue fragments.

Posterior Ethmoidectomy

At this point, the ground lamella can generally be visualized (Fig. 8–16). The ground lamella is entered medially and inferiorly, working in the direction of the sphenoid ostium. When the posterior ethmoid is open, the upturned Blakesley forceps is used to work toward the skull base. The forceps are placed behind each partition to verify that the partition is below the skull base. The vertically oriented bony partitions are removed until the skull base or roof of the ethmoid is identified. The skull base is identified both by the relatively smooth contour

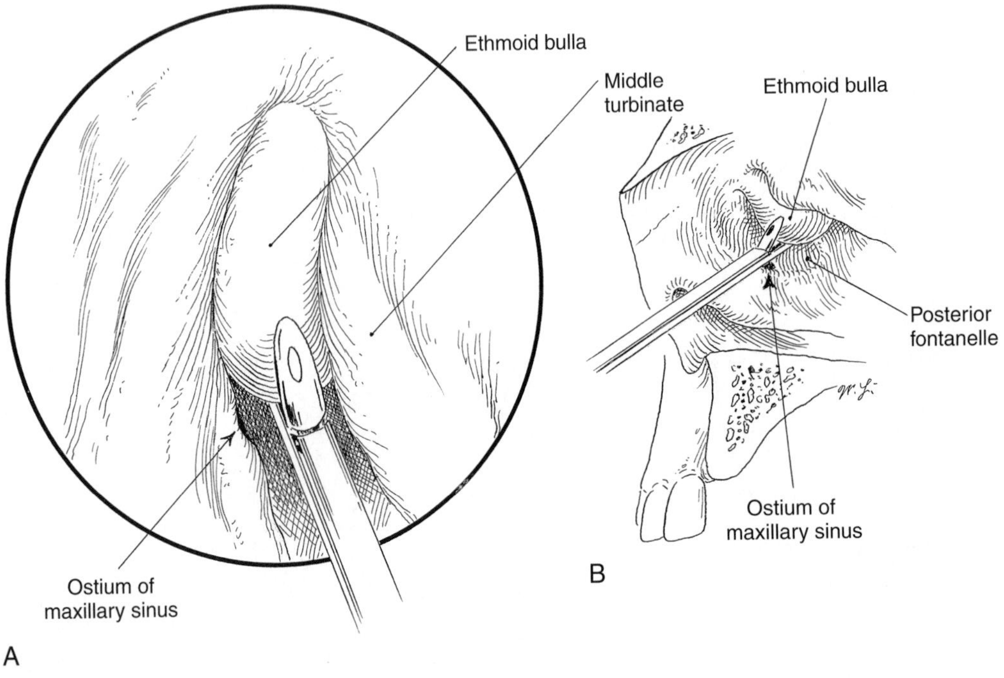

Figure 8–15. Initial step following uncinectomy in standard endoscopic ethmoidectomy. *A,* Blakesley forceps are used to enter the ethmoidal bulla medially and inferiorly. *B,* The anatomy as viewed from an inferior and medial perspective.

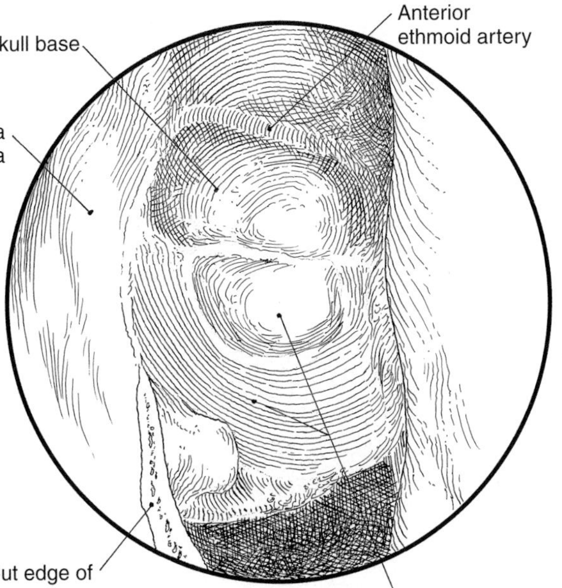

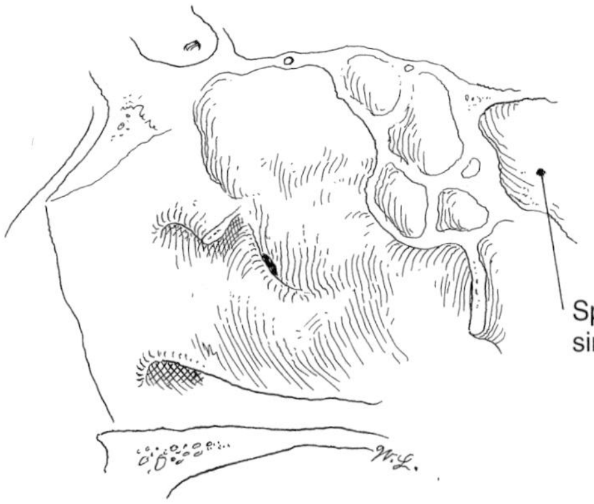

Figure 8–16. Completion of an anterior ethmoidectomy. *A,* Endoscopic view. *B,* Anatomic view from a medial perspective. Note that the middle turbinate has been removed for purposes of illustration in the anatomic view. The ground lamella dividing the ethmoid into anterior and posterior portions is clearly illustrated.

of its surface and the slightly whiter color of the bone. Also the bone of the skull base will typically have a more solid feel to it when palpated with the tip of the angled forceps. The height or depth of the ethmoid should not be used as criterion for judging the skull base location, as precise measurements vary from patient to patient and, while generally accurate, may lead to errors. The best criteria are visual confirmation and the feel of the skull base in the judgment of an experienced operator. This experience is best gained through repeated cadaver dissection and gradual acquisition of experience under the supervision of an experienced mentor.

Unless it is fully hidden within the bone of the skull base, the posterior ethmoid artery can frequently be identified at this point. This landmark identifies the anterior edge of the most posterior ethmoid cell in most patients. With the skull base clearly identified in the posterior ethmoid, this plane can be followed back anteriorly to skeletonize the more anterior skull base. The skull base is then followed anteriorly up to the anterior ethmoid artery. During this process, it is important to remove the bony partitions as close as possible, up to the level of the skull base, without unnecessary removal of the skull base mucosa. Preservation of as much of the skull base mucosa as possible is a basic principle of endoscopic sinus surgery and should be adhered to, to the extent possible. At this point, any residual loose mucosa, bony ridges, and residual cells are removed from the lamina papyracea. Again, the dissection should be completed leaving a smooth surface of the contour of the medial orbital wall, without unnecessary sacrifice of mucosa along this plane (Fig. 8–17).

Middle Turbinate

At this point, the standard ethmoidectomy is completed. In the author's practice, the middle turbinate is routinely preserved, although this approach remains controversial. With the importance of the middle turbinate still unsettled, it is probably best to preserve it unless removal is mandated for some reason. Partial middle turbinectomy is typically required in two specific situations. The first is in the case of a concha bullosa or aeration of the middle turbinate. In this situation, the turbinate is incised along its inferior edge working in a posterior-to-anterior direction using a sickle knife. With the incision completed up to the anterior tip, endoscopic ethmoid scissors are then used to excise the lateral lamella at the superior attachment. The lateral lamella can then be pushed inferiorly to expose the posterior attachment, at which point the ethmoid scissors are used to complete the resection.

The second situation requiring partial middle turbinate resection is in the case of a paradoxical curvature of the middle turbinate. In this instance, the inferior edge of the turbinate curls laterally toward the orbit. To treat this, the turbinate can be fractured medially or resected. When resecting, the curved ethmoid scissors are used to excise only that portion below the lateral

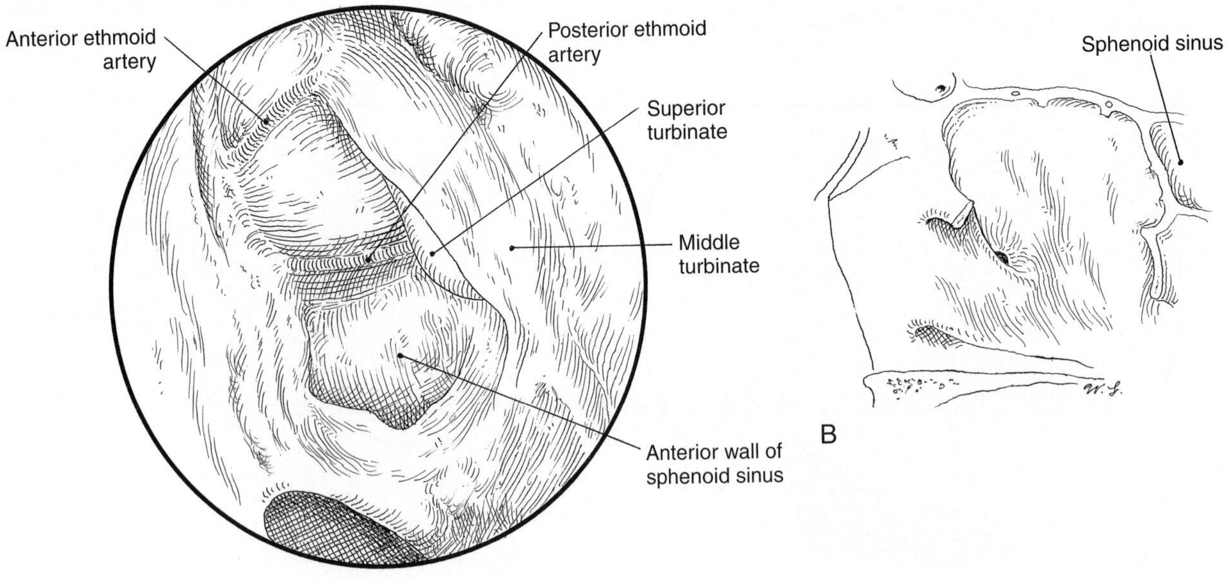

A

B

Figure 8–17. Completion of an anterior and posterior ethmoidectomy. *A,* Endoscopic view. *B,* Anatomic view from a medial perspective. Note that the middle turbinate has been removed in the anatomic view for purposes of illustration only.

projection of the turbinate, thereby preserving the anterior and posterior attachments.

If surgery has resulted in a loose or floppy middle turbinate, rather than resecting the turbinate, it can instead be adhered to the septum by creating opposing abrasions in the mucosa. This technique reliably results in medialization of the turbinate without flail turbinate or lateralization occurring.

Sphenoidectomy

There are two basic approaches to sphenoidectomy and sphenoidotomy: transnasal and transethmoidal. The transnasal procedure is generally used for diagnostic purposes. This approach creates an opening that is adequate for accessing and assessing the sphenoid sinus, but postoperative care is difficult owing to the narrow access, posterior location, and high rate of stenosis. By comparison, the transethmoid approach creates a large opening, allowing easy visualization of the operative site and facilitating debridement, cleaning, and examination in the office. This approach is preferred for treatment of sphenoid sinus disease.

The transethmoid approach to the sphenoid sinus requires preliminary ethmoidectomy. This is done using the standard technique described earlier. The goal is to identify and skeletonize the skull base and lamina papyracea. Once complete ethmoidectomy is accomplished, the sphenoid sinus will be seen to lie medially and inferiorly within the cavity. Typically, with the middle and superior turbinates intact, the natural ostium of the sinus cannot be visualized. However, the sphenoid will usually present as an anteriorly directed contour that projects from the skull base. Two options for entering the sinus exist. If the face of the sphenoid is clearly identified, the sinus can be entered by directly puncturing the anterior wall at the medial and inferior limit of the ethmoid cavity.

The preferred technique, though, is to identify the sphenoid ostium. This is accomplished by resecting the posteroinferior edge of the superior turbinate (Fig. 8–18). The inferior edge of the superior turbinate is identified by placing a probe through the superior meatus. The straight endoscopic scissors are used to excise the desired portion of the turbinate. Once this is completed, the natural ostium of the sphenoid sinus should be able to be identified. The location will be along the septum, just lateral to the anatomic midline and at approximately 30 degrees' elevation from the floor of the nose. If the ostium cannot be seen, it may be located by palpation with the tip of the suction.

After the ostium is identified, the opening is enlarged in a lateral and inferior direction. The initial opening can be made with the straight Blakesley forceps or a J-curette. With the opening enlarged, a rotating sphenoid punch can be inserted into the sinus and the remainder of the anterior wall removed (Fig. 8–19). With the anterior wall completely removed, most pathologic matter

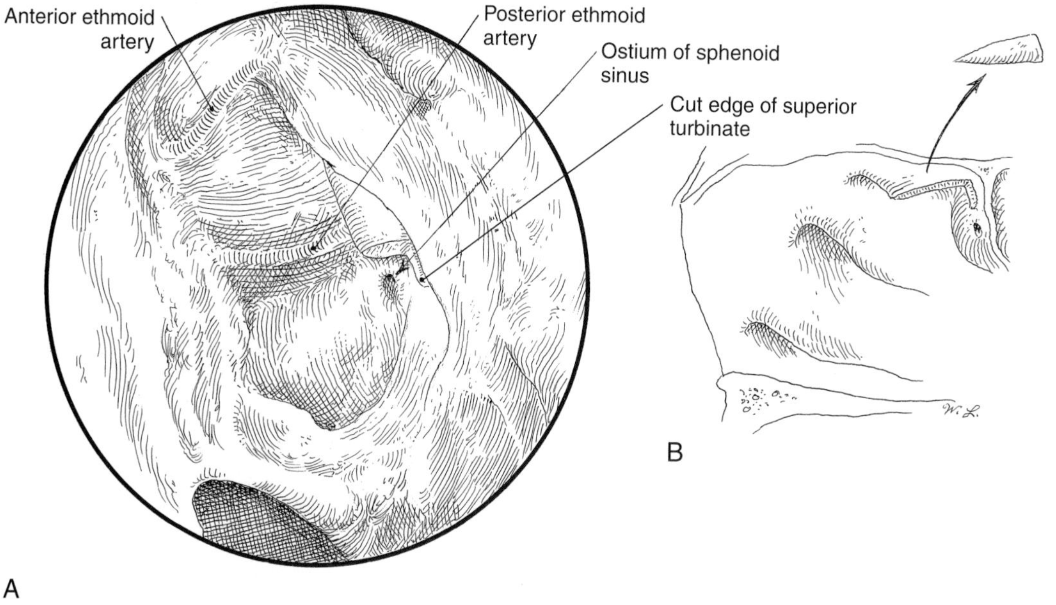

Figure 8–18. Removal of the superior turbinate. *A,* Endoscopic view. *B,* Anatomic view from a medial perspective. After completion of the posterior ethmoidectomy, the inferior and posterior edge of the superior turbinate is excised to expose the sphenoid sinus ostium (indicated by arrow).

within the sinus can be removed. All inspissated secretions or fluid should be debrided completely. Generally, the mucosa within the sinus should be preserved. However, gross polyps or cysts may be excised.

Extreme caution should be used whenever operating in the sphenoid sinus. Both the carotid artery and the optic nerve are located along the lateral and posterior wall, and the bone over these structures can be dehiscent. The sella turcica, which contains the pituitary, is located medial and superior to this structure, and the cavernous sinus is situated laterally. With these critical structures all contained within the walls of the sphenoid sinus, the surgeon must use precise, controlled motions, and visualization must be optimized. However, if the techniques described are carefully followed, complications can be avoided.

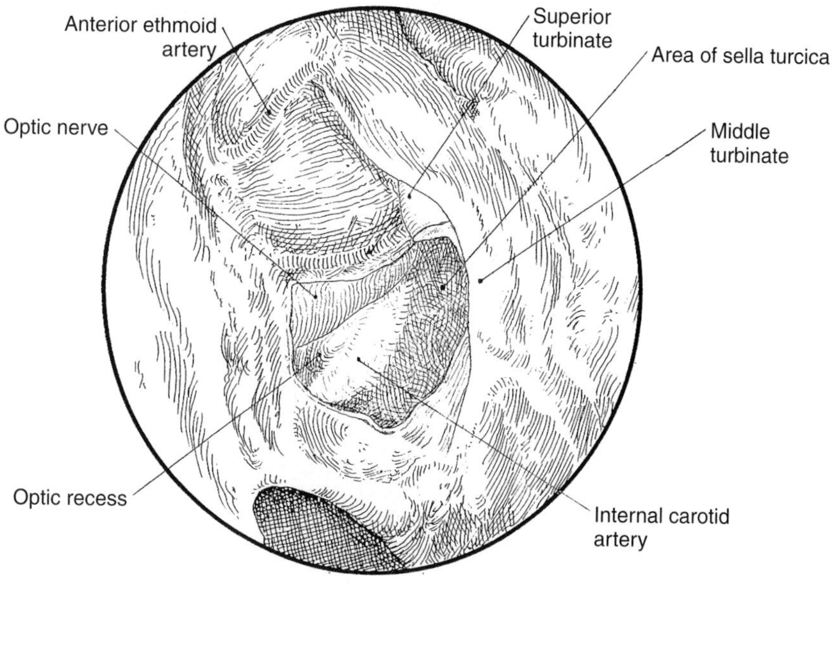

Figure 8–19. Completion of a sphenoidotomy, endoscopic view. The anterior wall of the sphenoid sinus has been removed from the natural ostium laterally, revealing the anatomy of the interior of the sphenoid sinus. The optic recess is a depression in the posterolateral wall of the sinus between the carotid artery and the optic nerve.

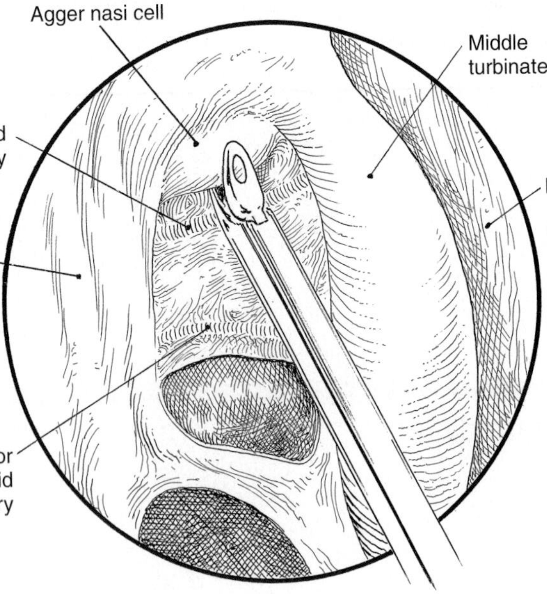

Figure 8–20. Beginning of a frontal sinusotomy. This endoscopic view shows entry into the agger nasi cell of the anterior ethmoid sinus using a 45-degree upturned Blakesley forceps.

Frontal Sinusotomy

Intranasal endoscopic frontal sinusotomy is the most challenging and potentially dangerous procedure performed in routine ESS. Finding the ostium of the frontal sinus can be difficult owing to variations in anatomy. In certain cases, the opening may be very high, anterior, or narrow. In addition, the skull base may be thin or almost dehiscent in this area. Despite these limitations, the dissection of the frontal recess as a means of enlarging the opening into the frontal sinus can be performed safely and reliably.

The keys to performing this procedure successfully are to identify the normal landmarks and to proceed slowly with excellent visualization. Normally, frontal sinusotomy is undertaken after complete ethmoidectomy, with or without sphenoidectomy. If not already done, the anterior ethmoid artery should be identified and the skull base posterior to this point skeletonized. The agger nasi should then be opened using upturned Blakesley forceps (Fig. 8–20). The most common drainage pathway is for the frontal sinus to drain posterior to the posterior wall of the agger nasi cell. In some cases, the frontal sinus drainage may be posterior and medial to the agger nasi cell, but the frontal sinus cannot drain anterior to a true agger nasi cell. Once the agger nasi cell has been opened widely, the posterior wall is then removed using giraffe forceps (Fig. 8–21). This

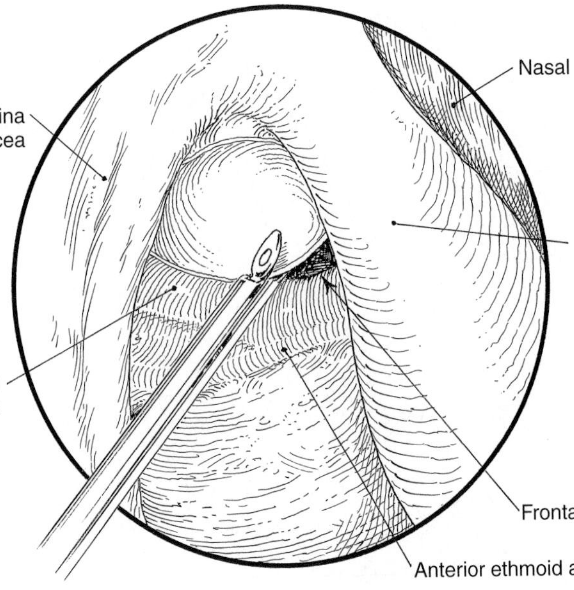

Figure 8–21. Frontal sinusotomy. This endoscopic view shows removal of the posterior wall of the agger nasi cell using a 70-degree, 2-mm, vertical cup, giraffe forceps. The anterior wall and internal contents of the agger nasi cell have already been removed.

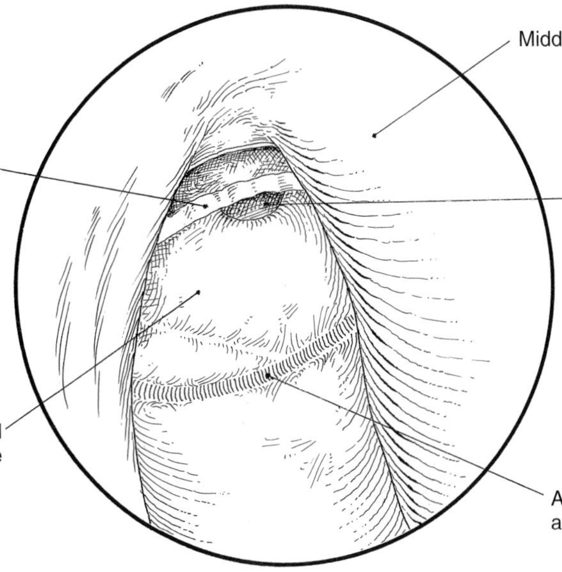

Figure 8–22. Completion of a frontal sinusotomy. This endoscopic view shows the position of the frontal sinus ostium after complete dissection of the frontal recess. The cut edge of the posterior wall of the agger nasi cell or "beak" is indicated.

should be done slowly, one bite at a time, ensuring proper placement of the forceps before each bite.

At this point, if there are residual partitions within the frontal recess, they should be removed, again using the giraffe forceps and proceeding one bite at a time. Normally, this will allow identification of the frontal sinus ostium and adequate opening for most cases (Fig. 8–22). If the opening is not identified by this point, the CT scan should be reviewed to reassess the anatomy. The cavity is then inspected and any loose bone or mucosa is removed. A curved probe, or frontal sinus seeker, can be used to palpate along the skull base, above the anterior ethmoid artery, for the opening.

Usually, if the frontal sinus ostium has not already been identified, the lamina papyracea is carefully skeletonized at this point. By following the orbit superiorly and anteriorly, the opening may be located. However, if there is a supraorbital ethmoid cell, then the frontal will be more medial. In this case, the lateral surface of the middle turbinate is followed superiorly, with removal of the medial wall of the agger nasi cell. If, by this point, the frontal sinus has not been identified, it is advisable to discontinue the procedure and obtain a high-resolution CT scan to help delineate the remaining anatomy. In the author's experience, this has not been necessary, as the frontal sinus opening has eventually been identified in all cases attempted.

Rarely is more than this type of opening into the frontal sinus needed. However, in revision cases undertaken for treatment of stenosis, or in cases in which a very narrow opening is present owing to naturally occurring bony anatomy, more aggressive bone removal is desired. This is always accomplished in an anterior direction extending into the nasal root. Various techniques and equipment are available for removal of bone in this area, including curettes, rasps, and drills. The amount of bone removal can be categorized according to three levels, identified by Draf (Fig. 8–23).[81]

The level III procedure—known as the modified Lothrop procedure or endoscopic Lothrop procedure—has been updated recently by Gross and colleagues.[82, 83] This procedure involves removal of the upper anterior part of the nasal septum. The frontal sinus ostia are identified bilaterally, and the intervening bone is removed across the midline to connect the two ostia. The resulting opening is further enlarged anteriorly to the maximum extent possible.

The endoscopic Lothrop procedure is regarded as a last-chance alternative to osteoplastic frontal sinusectomy with obliteration. The initial results with this procedure are encouraging. However, results are only preliminary, with the long-term outcome being at least a decade away from being well established. Whether this procedure will stand the test of time is uncertain. In the interim, this procedure should be selected with extreme caution.

An interesting variation of the frontal osteotomy, termed the frontal sinus rescue procedure, has been described by Kuhn.[84] This operation is intended to revise a stenosis of the frontal sinus after previous aggressive resection of the middle turbinate. For this procedure, an incision is made along the orbital side of the stenosis. The mucosa is then elevated, working laterally to medially, resulting in a mucosal flap pedicled on the medial surface of the middle turbinate stump. The frontal sinus is then opened widely and the residual turbinate stump is removed right up to the skull base. The mucosal flap is then rotated into the frontal sinus, providing a mucosal lining to the medial wall of the frontal sinus opening.

This new operation is offered as an alternative to the endoscopic Lothrop procedure as a last-chance alterna-

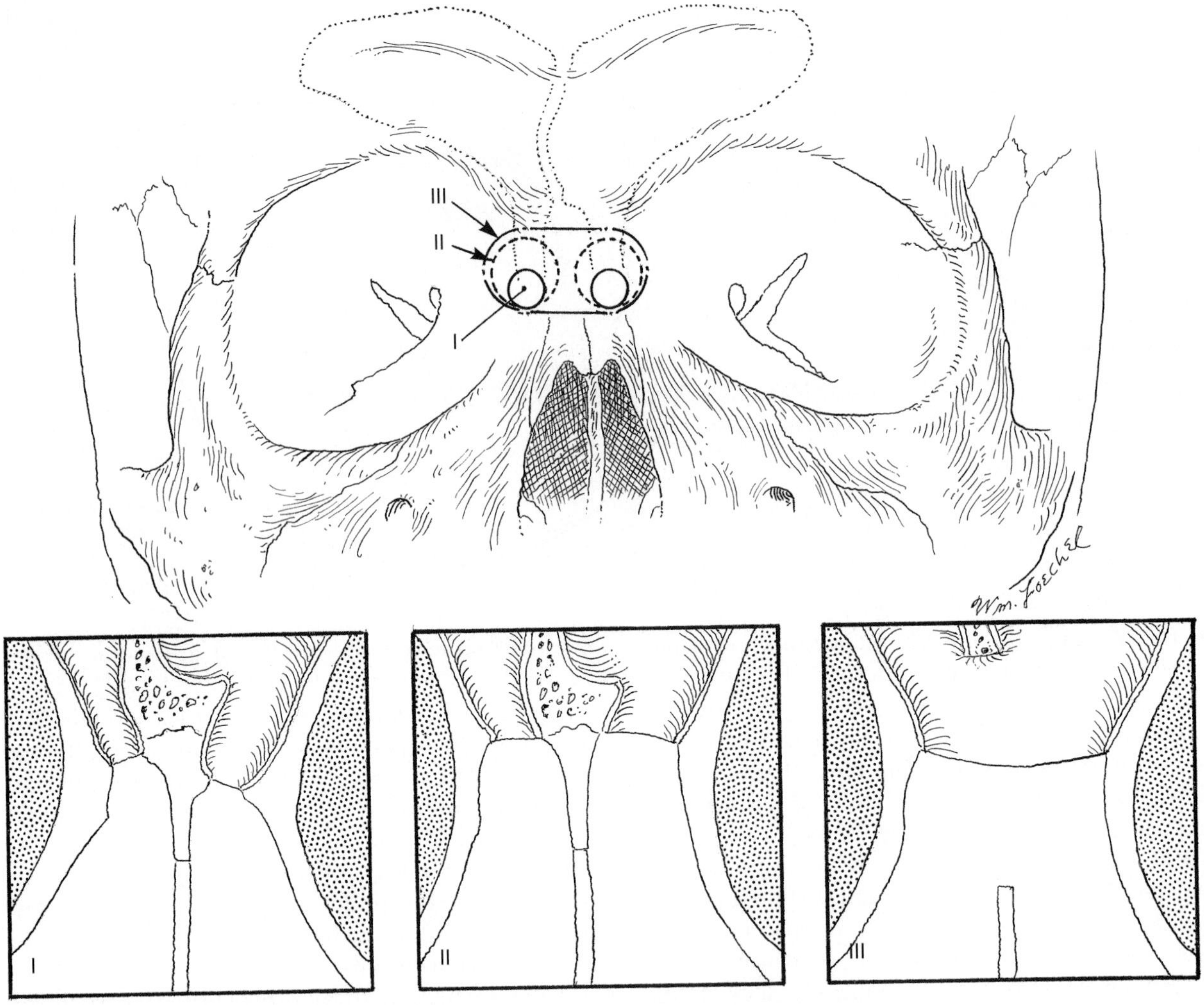

Figure 8–23. Frontal sinusotomy. This illustration demonstrates the different degrees of enlargement of the ostium of the frontal sinus (after Draf).[81] In the illustration at the top, the extent of a type I procedure is represented by the inner solid circles, whereas the type II procedure is indicated by the inner dashed circles and type III by the outer solid circle. The insets at the bottom demonstrate the various stages of anatomic enlargement.

tive to the obliteration option. Results are even more preliminary than those attending the endoscopic Lothrop procedure. However, this operation has the advantage of not requiring resection of the septum or aggressive drilling in the nasal root. The worst thing that could happen in this procedure is that it could fail. As a minimal endoscopic procedure in a desperate situation, this procedure makes sense and, therefore, may be worthwhile despite its unknown success rate.

Antrostomy

The maxillary sinus opening within the middle meatus is a basic part of almost every endoscopic sinus procedure. Even in situations when the maxillary sinuses are not involved, it is best to perform at least a minimal enlargement of the natural ostium of the sinus. If an uncinectomy is performed without enlargement of the maxillary ostium, the patient will be at risk for stenosis, leading to subsequent problems.

In all cases, it is necessary to incorporate the natural ostium into the middle meatus antrostomy. If the surgical antrostomy does not connect to the natural ostium, a recirculation phenomena may occur. In such cases, mucus flows out of the natural ostium, reentering the maxillary sinus through the surgical antrostomy. This recirculation of mucus can lead to chronic inflammation within the sinus.

The key to performing a middle meatus antrostomy is initial identification of the natural ostium. The natural ostium may be obstructed by inflamed mucosa, polyps, or scar tissue, making identification difficult. However, the location of the natural ostium is very consistent, always being anterior and inferior within the middle meatus. If the bulla ethmoidalis is still intact, the ostium will be anterior and inferior to this cell.

The ostium is immediately posterior to the nasolacrimal duct. This relationship is important as it means that enlargement in an anterior direction will open the

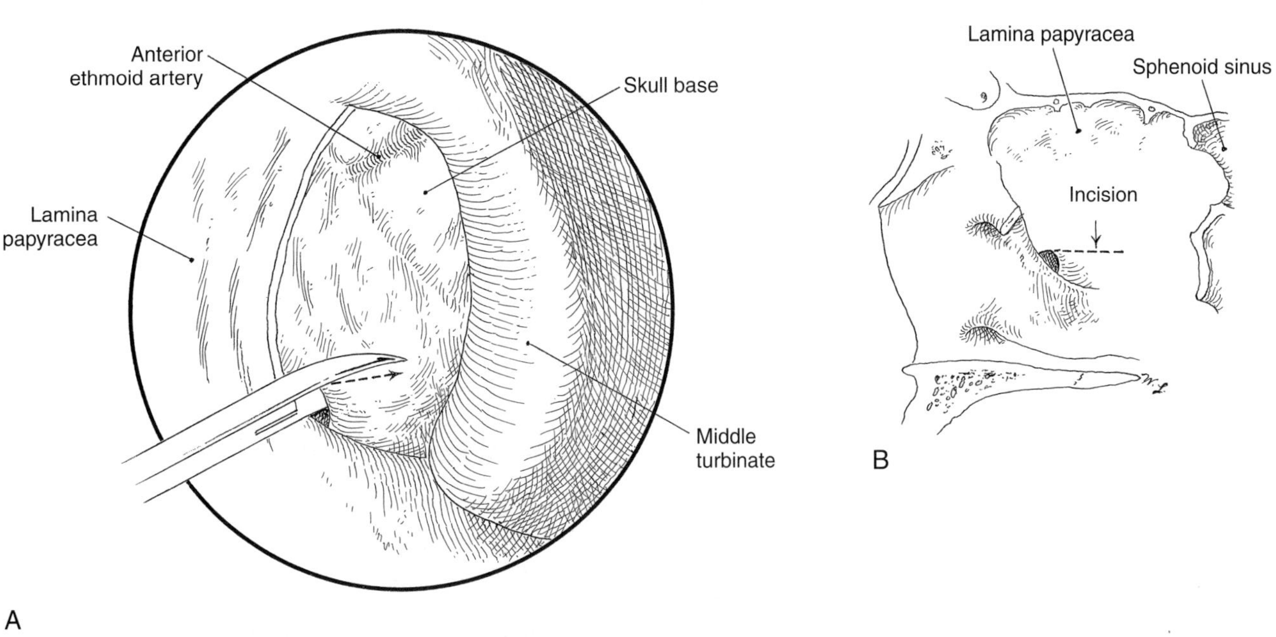

Figure 8–24. Middle meatus antrostomy. *A,* Endoscopic view using a 30-degree endoscope. *B,* Anatomic view from a medial perspective. Note that the middle turbinate has been removed from the anatomic drawing for purposes of illustration only. The initial cut is made, using curved endoscopic scissors, along the floor of the orbit from the maxillary ostium posteriorly through the posterior fontanelle.

nasolacrimal duct into the middle meatus and maxillary sinus. Usually, this does not result in any significant problem. However, it is best avoided because stenosis of the duct can result, causing epiphora or pooling of tears into the sinus with subsequent intermittent drainage of tears.

The first step is complete removal of the uncinate process. If initial excision of the uncinate following incision and removal is incomplete, the residual uncinate can be removed using back-biting forceps. With removal of the uncinate, identification of the natural ostium is best achieved using the 30-degree endoscope. If it is not immediately apparent, the ostium can be located with the ostium seeker. The ostium is then enlarged in the posterior direction. The preferred method for this enlargement is to use the curved endoscopic scissors to incise the posterior fontanelle at the level of the floor of the orbit (Fig. 8–24). Antrostomy is completed by using the back-biting forceps to remove the posterior fontanelle at the level of the inferior turbinate (Fig. 8–25).

In most cases, this opening will be adequate. Through

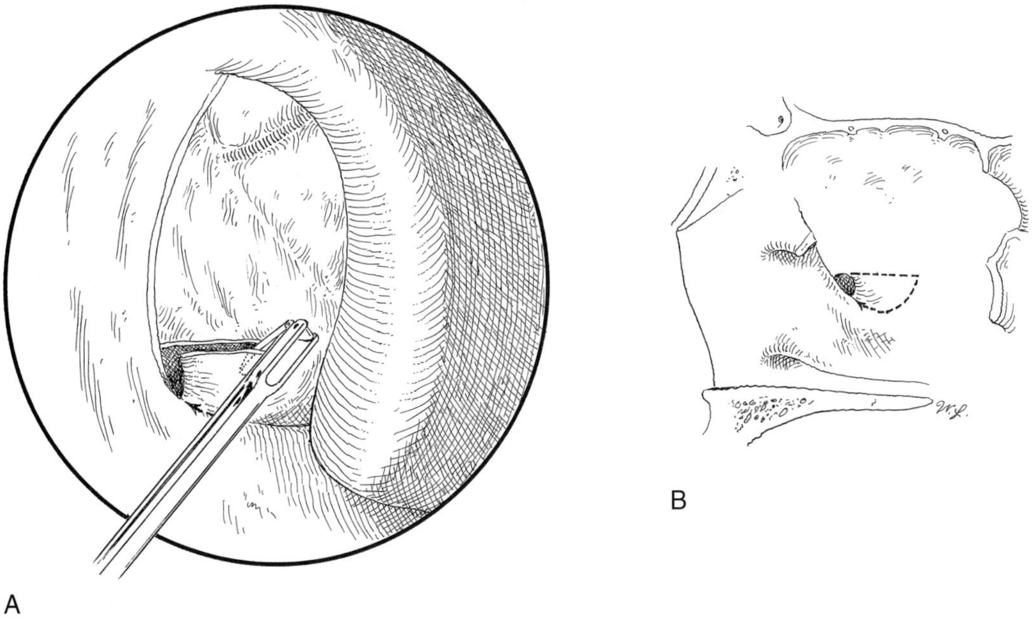

Figure 8–25. Completion of the middle meatus antrostomy. *A,* Endoscopic view using a 30-degree endoscope. *B,* Anatomic view from a medial perspective. Note that the middle turbinate has been removed for the purposes of illustration only. A back-biting forceps is used to excise the posterior fontanelle down to the level of the inferior turbinate and anteriorly to the natural ostium of the maxillary sinus.

this opening, most of the maxillary sinus can be visualized and reached with either curved suction or giraffe forceps. If a larger opening is needed, the inferior turbinate and medial wall of the maxillary sinus can be removed to whatever extent is required. Curved scissors, down-biting forceps, and back-biting forceps are used in combination to perform this step.

Revision Endoscopic Sinus Surgery

Revision surgery is among the most challenging ESS procedure. For most patients undergoing revision surgery, regardless of the type of procedure first performed, it is advisable to convert to a complete sphenoethmoidectomy with frontal sinusotomy and middle meatus antrostomy. One exception to this rule is stenosis of a single sinus, in which case direct reopening of that sinus may be appropriate. Before operating, a repeat high-quality coronal CT scan should be obtained. The results should be available in the operating room and consulted throughout the procedure as necessary. Also before beginning, a goal for the procedure should be documented and a strategy for achieving that goal should be planned carefully.

The basic approach is to start with identification of landmarks. If the middle turbinate is not readily apparent, either from resection or polyps, soft tissue should be removed from around the anterior end of the cavity to identify at least the stump of the anterior edge of the middle turbinate. All work within the ethmoid cavity should remain lateral to this point to avoid injury to the olfactory cleft.

The next landmark to identify is the sphenoid sinus ostium. If the sphenoid has been opened previously, the interior of the sinus can be identified. This is accomplished by direct visualization along the septum at the posterior edge of the cavity, 30 degrees from the floor of the nose. The anterior wall of the sphenoid is then completely removed, along with any tissue to be removed from within the sphenoid.

Identification of the position of the skull base within the sphenoid sinus should then be possible. The skull base is followed anteriorly to the anterior ethmoid artery, with removal of residual ethmoid tissue and bone in the process. The frontal sinusotomy is performed as described previously, as is the antrostomy. It is important to make sure that residual ethmoid cells are removed, especially within the frontal recess, and that the maxillary antrostomy is connected to the natural ostium.

It is difficult to elaborate more on the technical aspects of performing revision surgery as the details of the procedure will vary depending on the previous surgery, the amount of scarring, and the nature of the problem requiring revision. However, several general rules are applicable. Soft tissue removal should be performed before underlying bone is removed. This ensures that the best view of the underlying structure is rendered before it is violated. Small, precise bites should be taken throughout the entire procedure, and landmarks should be identified so as to maintain proper surgical orientation. Excellent visualization and hemostasis should be maintained throughout the procedure. Finally, if in doubt, the procedure should be terminated to minimize risk.

Powered Endoscopic Sinus Surgery

The technique used for powered ESS will depend on the instrument used. The first generation of instruments lacked sufficient power to remove bone easily except in the case of the thinnest, most attenuated bone present in patients with polyps. However, the most recently developed instruments have sufficient power to remove all but the thickest, most osteitic bone. The general technique utilized in all cases involves using the blade in a scraping motion. It is best to start inferiorly, removing tissue in an inferior to superior direction. This is because the cutting surface is on the side, not the tip of the instrument. Therefore, the most controlled excision occurs with the cutting side of the blade visualized from above as it is drawn from posterior to anterior across the inferior edge of the ethmoid or polyp tissue.

The preferred blades are the aggressive 4-mm cutting blade for the straight attachment and a 3.5-mm cutter for the angled-shaft blade. The power is set to 2500 rpm if a variable speed setting is available. The suction line should be equipped with a trap to collect excised tissue for pathologic evaluation.

In polyp cases, the first step is to completely remove the polyps back to the point of origin. With this accomplished, the remaining anatomy can be approached as with nonpolyp cases. If bleeding is significant following initial polyp removal, a temporary pack is placed and the initial polypectomy is performed on the opposite side. The remaining sequence of steps is the same as in the standard procedure, except performed with a powered instrument.

First, the uncinate is excised. The instrument is rolled 90 degrees to orient the cutting surface perpendicular to the uncinate. With the uncinate removed, the bulla and ethmoid are then excised. After the posterior ethmoid is completely removed, the natural ostium of the sphenoid is identified. The tip of the shaft is inserted into the ostium and the anterior wall is taken down in an inferior and lateral direction.

Attention is then directed to the frontal recess. A 30-degree endoscope and angled cutter are used. The agger nasi is entered anteriorly and the cell is exenterated. At this time, it may be necessary to convert to standard instruments if frontal sinusotomy is required. The antrostomy is performed with the angled shaft positioned against the posterior fontanelle to enlarge the natural ostium in a posterior and inferior direction.

POSTOPERATIVE CARE

Postoperative care begins at the conclusion of the surgery with placement of packing material. Many options are available, ranging from no packing to full gauze packing. The author uses a Kennedy sinus pack produced by the Merocel Corporation (Jacksonville, FL). This pack is made of polyvinyl acetal, which is a highly absorbent, inert material. The pack is inserted to stent the middle turbinate medially and to provide pressure, as well as a surface to promote coagulation. In cases of inflammatory polyps with heavy bleeding, two or even three packs can be placed on a single side. The packs are left in place for several days after surgery to help prevent lateralization of the middle turbinate and formation of synechiae from the turbinate to the lateral wall, and to facilitate hemostasis. The packs may be removed 4 to 6 days after surgery, depending on the timing of a follow-up appointment and the degree of bleeding at surgery.

On the night of surgery, the patient is encouraged to remain at rest with the head elevated at least 30 degrees. For the first 10 days after surgery, the patient is limited to nonstressful activities. The recommendation is to avoid active exercise, lifting of more than 10 lb, and sexual activity. After this, the patient is advised to return gradually to normal activity levels. Nose blowing and sneezing are discouraged for the initial postoperative period until the cavity is remucosalized. This helps to avoid the potential complications of pneumocephalus and orbital emphysema. These are risks if very high intranasal pressures are generated, potentially resulting in fracture of unprotected bone. Other than the night of surgery when anesthesia makes emesis a high risk, the diet is not limited.

Medications are prescribed for pain, infection control, and control of inflammation. Pain medication is tailored to the needs of the patient. Most commonly, acetaminophen with codeine is sufficient. Antibiotics are administered for a minimum of 2 weeks after surgery. Empiric selections include amoxicillin/clavulinic acid, clarithromicin, or ciprofloxacin to cover the usual bacteria and *Staphylococcus aureus* that may colonize the packs and lead to toxic shock syndrome.[85] If active infection is found at surgery, then cultures are taken, and as soon as the results are available, the antibiotic regimen is adjusted to cover the cultured bacteria. In cases of severe infection, a prolonged course of antibiotics is indicated; in selected cases, intravenous antibiotics may be administered.

A special consideration is the use of long-term erythromycin after the acute period. Japanese researchers report that erythromycin may have a beneficial effect, in terms of both antibacterial and proimmunity actions, in cases of osteitis.[86] This proimmunity potential is thought to be related to both the inhibition of bacterial binding to epithelial cells and activation of the cellular immune system.[86,87] To date, the benefits of this practice have not been definitively documented. However, this mode of therapy has been a useful adjunct in difficult cases, with some apparent successes observed.

Corticosteroids are used liberally in the postoperative period. All patients with significant polyps before or during surgery are given a 4-week, gradually tapered course of corticosteroid therapy. During this period, the dose is tapered from 40 to 60 mg of prednisone down to 10 mg of prednisone per day in increments of 10 mg. Aside from this standard use, corticosteroids may also be prescribed if significant mucosal edema is detected during the postoperative period.

Once the packs are removed, the patient is started on nasal irrigations, nasal saline spray, and nasal steroid spray. The irrigations begin with normal saline administered with a bulb syringe twice each day and continued until the cavity is healed and crusting subsides. Once the cavity is healed, the formulation of the irrigation can be changed if significant mucosal edema is found. The recommended formula is adapted from Parsons[88] and approximates 3% buffered saline. This may be created at home by adding 3 tsp of salt and 1 tsp of baking soda to 1 qt of boiled water. This hypertonic solution may help resolve mucosal edema by drawing the fluid out of the tissue by osmotic pressure.

The standard postoperative regimen is to have the patient irrigate the nasal passages in the morning and evening. After each irrigation, the patient gently blows the nose to remove loosened crusts and irrigating solution. Nasal steroid spray is then applied. In the interim between the two irrigations, the patient is instructed to use a commercially bottled nasal saline spray every 2 to 3 hours.

An essential part of all ESS is the postoperative cleaning of the sinus cavity. The normal follow-up routine is to clean the sinus cavity at the first postoperative visit following removal of the packs, 2 to 3 weeks after surgery, and again 6 weeks after surgery. Additional follow-up visits may be scheduled depending on the needs of the individual patient, but normally, return visits are scheduled 3, 6, and 12 months after surgery and then every 6 to 12 months after that for an indefinite period of time.

At each cleaning, the sinus cavity is completely debrided of all blood clot, mucus, and inspissated secretions. The regenerating or healing mucosa is preserved with care taken to minimize trauma to the site. Areas of granulation tissue and regenerative mucosal cysts are debrided using suction, and any synechiae are removed sharply. These procedures are uncomfortable for the patient, but with good topical anesthesia and decongestion, combined with gentle, careful technique, almost all patients can be coached through these procedures.

The importance of quality postoperative care cannot be overemphasized. Failure to achieve the desired debridement puts the patient at risk for stenosis, synechiae, and poor outcomes. On the contrary, successful cleaning and debridement will almost always result in normal healing and excellent results.

COMPLICATIONS

Hemorrhage

The most common acute complication after ESS is postoperative hemorrhage. Of a series of 393 operations on 628 sides, significant hemorrhage occurred in five patients, none of whom required transfusion.[89] The most common site of bleeding is from the septal branch of the sphenopalatine artery as it traverses across the face of the sphenoid sinus. Other potential sites include the anterior ethmoid artery, the cut posterior edge of a partially resected middle turbinate, or the inferior turbinate or septum, as a result of associated surgery.

Control of postoperative hemorrhage begins during surgery with preventive measures. Careful technique, adequate decongestion, and local anesthesia will minimize initial bleeding. If arterial bleeding is encountered from the anterior ethmoid or sphenopalatine arteries, suction cautery is recommended to control the hemorrhage. Alternatives, such as temporary packs or cocainization, may result in temporary cessation, but these place the patient at risk for rebleeding in the postoperative period.

In the event of significant bleeding in the postoperative period, attempts should be made to control the bleeding in the office setting. Often, decongestion and locally applied cotton balls will be sufficient to control minor bleeding. If these measures fail, rather than relying on repacking, it is advisable to return the patient to the operating room for direct cautery. The reason for this approach is that repacking almost invariably leads to significant mucosal damage and a high rate of synechiae or stenosis.

The most dreaded vascular complication of ESS is carotid artery laceration. This results in an immediate life-threatening situation. The primary goal is to arrest the massive hemorrhage that accompanies these injuries. This can only be accomplished with rapid application of an occlusive packing. For this reason, strip gauze should always be available in the operating room when performing ESS. If the hemorrhage can be controlled in this manner, the patient is taken immediately to the angiography suite where collateral circulation and the site of injury are assessed. If the crossflow through the circle of Willis is adequate, then embolization is performed. If the patient has inadequate crossflow, then urgent neurosurgical intervention is required. The best alternative is an external-to-internal bypass to the middle cerebral artery with embolization of the internal carotid. Other solutions include leaving the packing in place for several days in the hope of spontaneous resolution or replacing the gauze pack with a dissolvable pack that can be left in place. Clearly, the best approach to this complication is avoidance.

Scarring

Although not strictly an acute complication, scarring (stenosis and synechiae) is the most common cause of failure of ESS provided the initial surgery was adequate. To avoid unwanted scarring, careful preservation of the mucosa within the frontal recess is essential, especially along the skull base above the anterior ethmoid artery. Other steps include sufficient opening of the maxillary and sphenoid ostia, stenting of the middle turbinate, and careful, meticulous, postoperative care.

In the event that scarring does occur, revision is indicated if the scar induces a negative effect. Synechiae should be resected rather than divided. After resection of the scar band, a silastic splint should be placed and kept in place for a minimum of 1 week. Ostial stenosis is more difficult and requires formal revision. Frontal sinus stenosis is the most serious form and the most difficult to revise successfully. If the ostium can be reopened successfully, a decision must be made as to whether to stent the opening after surgery. If circumferential mucosal removal is needed, then stenting with Silastic tubing should be considered. This tubing usually incites formation of granulation tissue and mucosal edema in the frontal recess. The stent should, therefore, be removed periodically and the granulation debrided. Alternatives include the frontal sinus drill-out procedures and the frontal sinus rescue procedure, as described earlier.

Epiphora

Excessive tearing secondary to ESS is an unusual complication that may be caused by injury to the nasolacrimal duct during middle meatus antrostomy. While performing the antrostomy, enlargement in the anterior direction beyond the attachment of the uncinate process can result in disruption of the nasolacrimal duct. In most cases, this causes tear flow to be diverted into the middle meatus or maxillary sinus. Patients with this problem will complain of sudden drainage of clear fluid from the nose upon positional changes from supine to upright or when leaning over.

In rare cases, injury to the nasolacrimal duct will result in stenosis of the duct, which leads to excessive tearing. This is particularly prominent during situations that normally are associated with heavy tearing, as with exposure to cold air or nasal irritants. The incidence of epiphora after ESS has been reported to range from 0 to 1%, depending on the series.[89–94] The true incidence of nasolacrimal duct injury, however, is probably much higher.

Diagnosis and management of epiphora will be covered in detail in a later chapter. If persistent, though, endoscopic dacryocystorhinostomy can usually be performed, with subsequent resolution of the problem.

Orbital Injury

Among the most serious complications of ESS are orbital injuries. Potential orbital injuries can range from orbital fat exposure to retrobulbar hemorrhage leading to ocular emergency and possible vision loss. Injury can occur at any point during ethmoidectomy, but is most common during infundibulotomy or from avulsion of the anterior ethmoid artery at the orbital foramen. In the latter instance, the artery can retract into the orbit, leading to sudden orbital hemorrhage. Direct injury to the optic nerve is much less common, but nevertheless technically possible, particularly during dissection of the posterior ethmoid or sphenoid sinus.

Minimal injury leading to orbital fat exposure requires no specific management. The operation can be completed using careful technique and avoiding suctioning or traction on the exposed fat. If it is unclear, based on visualization, whether orbital fat has been exposed, gentle pressure can be applied to the eye in an attempt to document bulging of the orbital fat into the ethmoid cavity. More serious injury involving periorbital ecchymosis requires more specific evaluation and management.

The initial management of orbital injury should include a complete ophthalmologic examination. Signs of orbital retrobulbar hemorrhage begin with periorbital ecchymosis and then extend to include chemosis, decreased extraocular motion, proptosis, increased intraorbital pressure, and finally, vision loss. If the patient manifests ecchymosis alone, management with cold compresses and close observation is often sufficient. In such cases, the patient should be observed overnight with periodic reexamination.

In the presence of signs of retrobulbar hemorrhage, aggressive and immediate action should be taken. In addition to immediate assessment of intraocular pressure and evaluation for the presence of afferent pupillary defect, ice packs, mannitol, and high-dose steroids should be administered. Any packing within the ethmoid should be removed, and attempts should be made to ascertain the site of orbital penetration. If possible, direct control of the bleeding point is optimal.

In the event of the rapid development of orbital hematoma or signs of vision loss, surgical intervention to expand the orbit and relieve the intraocular pressure is warranted. The best initial step is to perform lateral canthotomy with cantholysis. This can be done under local anesthesia with a scalpel and tenotomy scissors either at the bedside, in the recovery room, or in the operating room. A short incision is made directly in the lateral canthus, followed by division of the lateral canthal tendon. This will result in immediate relief of the orbital pressure. More extensive orbital decompression can be performed if needed. In this setting, inferior and medial decompression can be accomplished through either an endoscopic or sublabial approach. Ultimately, an external ethmoidectomy approach with direct control of the bleeder may be performed.

Intracranial Injury

Intracranial penetration is the most common serious complication associated with ESS. This can occur anywhere along the anterior skull base, but usually occurs either in the frontal recess along the lateral edge of the cribriform plate at the attachment of the middle turbinate or in the cribriform plate itself. In most situations, the injury is recognized immediately by detection of CSF leakage. In the event that CSF leakage is not detected immediately, deeper penetration may occur, with subsequent damage to intracerebral vessels and life-threatening intracranial hemorrhage. Case reports of patients dying on the operating room table subsequent to ESS are usually linked to this type of injury. Management of CSF leakage will be dealt with in a later chapter. The basic principles of management, though, include early identification, direct repair, and postoperative lumbar drainage.

REFERENCES

1. Kennedy DW, Zinreich SJ, Rosenbaum AE, et al. Functional endoscopic sinus surgery. Theory and diagnostic evaluation. Arch Otolaryngol 111:576, 1985.
2. Kennedy DW. Functional endoscopic sinus surgery. Arch Otolaryngol 111:643, 1985.
3. Stammberger H. Endoscopic endonasal surgery—Concepts in treatment of recurring rhinosinusitis. Part I. Anatomic and pathophysiologic considerations. Otolaryngol Head Neck Surg 94:143, 1986.
4. Kennedy DW, Gwaltney JW Jr, Jones JG, et al. Medical management of sinusitis: Educational goals and management guidelines. Ann Otol Rhinol Laryngol 104(10):22, 1995.
5. Kaliner MA. Recurrent sinusitis: Examining medical treatment options. Am J Rhinol 11:123, 1997.
6. Lund VJ, Kennedy DW, Lund VJ, et al. Quantification for staging sinusitis. Ann Otol Rhinol Laryngol 104(10):17, 1995.
7. Casiano RR. Correlation of clinical examination with computer tomography in paranasal sinus disease. Am J Rhinol 11:193, 1997.

8. Stammberger H. Endoscopic endonasal surgery—Concepts in treatment of recurring rhinosinusitis. Part II. Surgical technique. Otolaryngol Head Neck Surg 94:147, 1986.
9. Schaefer SD, Manning S, Close LG. Endoscopic paranasal sinus surgery: Indications and considerations. Laryngoscope 99:1, 1989.
10. Rice DH. Endoscopic sinus surgery: Results at 2-year follow-up. Otolaryngol Head Neck Surg 101:476, 1989.
11. Wiseman LR, Benfield P. Intranasal fluticasone proprionate. A reappraisal of its pharmacology and clinical efficacy in the treatment of rhinitis. Drugs 53:885, 1997.
12. Friedman WH, Katsantonis GP, Bumpous JM. Staging of chronic hyperplastic rhinosinusitis: Treatment strategies. Otolaryngol Head Neck Surg 112:210, 1995.
13. Lildholdt T, Rundcrantz H, Bende M, et al. Glucocorticoid treatment for nasal polyps. The use of topical budesonide powder, intramuscular betamethasone, and surgical treatment. Arch Otolaryngol Head Neck Surg 123:595, 1997.
14. Holmberg K, Juliusson S, Balder B, et al. Fluticasone propionate aqueous nasal spray in the treatment of nasal polyposis. Ann Allergy Asthma Immunol 78:270, 1997.
15. Mygind N, Lildholdt T. Nasal polyps treatment: Medical management. Allergy Asthma Proc 17:275, 1996.
16. Rasp G, Bujia J. Treatment of nasal polyposis with systemic and local corticoids. Acta Otorrinolaring Esp 48(1):37, 1997.
17. van Camp C, Clement PAR. Results of oral steroid treatment in nasal polyposis. Rhinology 32:5, 1994.
18. Nishioka GJ, Cook PR, Davis WE. Immunotherapy in patients undergoing functional endoscopic sinus surgery. Otolaryngol Head Neck Surg 110:406, 1994.
19. McFadden EA, Woodson BT, Massaro BM, et al. Orbital complications of sinusitis in the aspirin triad syndrome. Laryngoscope 106:1103, 1996.
20. Hao SP, Chang C-N, Chen H-C. Transbasal nasal polyposis masquerading as a skull base malignancy. Otolaryngol Head Neck Surg 115:556, 1996.
21. Saeed SR, Brookes GB. Aspergillosis of the paranasal sinuses. Rhinology 33:46, 1995.
22. Ferreiro JA, Carlson BA, Cody DT III. Paranasal sinus fungus balls. Head Neck 19:481, 1997.
23. Kupferberg SB, Bent JP III, Kuhn FA. Prognosis for allergic fungal sinusitis. Otolaryngol Head Neck Surg 117:35, 1997.
24. Quraishi HA, Ramadan HH. Endoscopic treatment of allergic fungal sinusitis. Otolaryngol Head Neck Surg 117:29, 1997.
25. Klossek J-M, Peloquin L, Fourcroy P-J, et al. Aspergillomas of the sphenoid sinus: A series of 10 cases treated by endoscopic sinus surgery. Rhinology 34:179, 1996.
26. Ramadan HH. Endoscopic treatment of acute frontal sinusitis: Indications and limitations. Otolaryngol Head Neck Surg 113: 295, 1995.
27. Turner WJ, Davidson TM. Endoscopic management of acute frontal sinusitis. Ear Nose Throat J 73:594, 1994.
28. Dolan RW, Cohen AF. Acute sinusitis and fever in the HIV-positive patient. Am J Rhinol 9:145, 1995.
29. Kaise T, Sakakura Y, Ukai K. Ability of histamine to increase nasal mucosal permeability to macromolecules in guinea pigs. Ann Otol Rhinol Laryngol 104:969, 1995.
30. April MM, Zinreich SJ, Baroody FM, et al. Coronal CT scan abnormalities in children with chronic sinusitis. Laryngoscope 103:985, 1993.
31. Willner A, Choi SS, Vezina G, et al. Intranasal anatomic variations in pediatric sinusitis. Am J Rhinol 11:355, 1997.
32. Calhoun KH, Waggenspack GA, Simpson CB, et al. CT evaluation of the paranasal sinuses in symptomatic and asymptomatic populations. Otolaryngol Head Neck Surg 104:480, 1991.
33. Bolger WE, Butzin CA, Parsons DS. Paranasal sinus bony anatomic variations and mucosal abnormalities: CT analysis for endoscopic sinus surgery. Laryngoscope 101:56, 1991.
34. Batsaki JG, Sciubba JJ. Pathology. In Blitzer A, Lawson W, Friedman WH (eds). Surgery of the Paranasal Sinuses, 2nd ed. Philadelphia, WB Saunders, 1991, pp. 127–128.
35. Bordley JE, Bosley WR. Mucoceles of the frontal sinus: Causes and treatment. Ann Otol Rhinol Laryngol 82:696, 1973.
36. Evans C. Aetiology and treatment of fronto-ethmoidal mucocele. J Laryngol Otol 95:361, 1981.
37. Marks SC, Latoni JD, Mathog RH. Mucoceles of the maxillary sinus. Otolaryngol Head Neck Surg 117:18, 1997.
38. Nativg K, Larsen TE. Mucocele of the paranasal sinuses. J Laryngol Otol 92:1075, 1978.
39. Kennedy DW, Josephson JS, Zinreich SJ, et al. Endoscopic sinus surgery for mucoceles: A viable alternative. Laryngoscope 99: 885, 1989.
40. Hoffer ME, Kennedy DW. The endoscopic management of sinus mucoceles following orbital decompression. Am J Rhinol 8:61, 1994.
41. Benninger MS, Marks SC. The endoscopic management of sphenoid and ethmoid mucoceles with orbital and intranasal extension. Rhinology 33:157, 1995.
42. Beasley NJP, Jones NS. Paranasal sinus mucoceles: Modern management. Am J Rhinol 9:251, 1995.
43. Terris MH, Davidson TM. Endoscopic management of a large ethmoid mucocele. Ear Nose Throat J 73(8):591, 1994.
44. Hardy JM, Montgomery WW. Osteoplastic frontal sinusectomy: An analysis of 250 operations. Ann Otol 85:523, 1976.
45. Stammberger H, Wolf G. Headaches and sinus disease: The endoscopic approach. Ann Otol Rhinol Laryngol Suppl 134:37, 1988.
46. Greenfield HG. Headache and facial pain associated with nasal and sinus disorders: A diagnostic and therapeutic challenge. Insights Otolaryngol 5:1, 1990.
47. Goldsmith AJ, Zahtz GD, Stegnjajic A, et al. Middle turbinate headache syndrome. Am J Rhinol 7:17, 1993.
48. El-Silimy O. The place of endonasal endoscopy in the relief of middle turbinate sinonasal headache syndrome. Rhinology 33:244, 1995.
49. Chow JM. Rhinologic headaches. Otolaryngol Head Neck Surg 111:211, 1994.
50. Acquardo MA, Montgomery WW. Treatment of chronic paranasal sinus pain with minimal sinus disease. Ann Otol Rhinol Laryngol 105:607, 1996.
51. Clerico DM. Pneumatized superior turbinate as a cause of referred migraine headache. Laryngoscope 106:874, 1996.
52. King JM, Caldarelli DD, Pigato JB. Review of revision functional endoscopic sinus surgery. Laryngoscope 104:404, 1994.
53. Lazar RH, Younis RT, Long TE. Revision functional endonasal sinus surgery. Ear Nose Throat J 71:131, 1992.
54. Kennedy DW. Prognostic factors, outcomes and staging in ethmoid sinus surgery. Laryngoscope 102:1, 1992.
55. Marks SC, Shamsa F. Evaluation of prognostic factors in endoscopic sinus surgery. Am J Rhinol 11:187, 1997.
56. Min Y-G, Kim I-T, Park S-H. Mucociliary activity and ultrastructural abnormalities of regenerated sinus mucosa in rabbits. Laryngoscope 104:1482, 1994.
57. Benninger MS, Schmidt JL, Crissman JD, et al. Mucociliary function following sinus mucosal regeneration. Otolaryngol Head Neck Surg 105:641, 1991.
58. Benninger MS, Sebek BA, Levine HL. Mucosal regeneration of the maxillary sinus after surgery. Otolaryngol Head Neck Surg 101:33, 1989.
59. Coleman JR Jr, Duncavage JA. Extended middle meatal antrostomy: The treatment of circular flow. Laryngoscope 106:1214, 1996.
60. Goldwyn BG, Saker W, Marks SC. Histopathologic analysis of chronic sinusitus. Am J Rhinol 8:37, 1994.
61. Stankiewicz JA. Complications of endoscopic intranasal ethmoidectomy: An update. Laryngoscope 99:686, 1989.
62. Massegur H, Adema JM, Lluansi J, et al. Endoscopic sinus surgery in sinusitis. Rhinology 33:89, 1995.
63. Messerklinger W. Endoscopy of the Nose, 1st ed. Baltimore-Munich: Urban & Schwarzenberg, 1978.
64. Toffel PH, Aroesty DJ, Weinmann RH. Secure endoscopic sinus surgery as an adjunct to functional nasal surgery. Arch Otolaryngol Head Neck Surg 115:822, 1989.
65. Owen RG Jr, Kuhn FA. The maxillary sinus ostium: Demystifying middle meatal antrostomy. Am J Rhinol 9:313, 1995.
66. Schaitkin B, May M, Shapiro A, et al. Endoscopic sinus surgery: 4-Year follow-up on the first 100 patients. Laryngoscope 103:1117, 1993.
67. Wigand ME, Steiner W, Jauman MP. Endonasal sinus surgery with

endoscopic control: From radical operation to rehabilitation of the mucosa. Endoscopy 10:255, 1978.
68. Friedman WH, Katsantonis GP. Intranasal and transantral ethmoidectomy: A 20-year experience. Laryngoscope 100:343, 1990.
69. Lawson W. The intranasal ethmoidectomy: An experience with 1,077 procedures. Laryngoscope 101:367, 1991.
70. Sogg A. Long-term results of ethmoid surgery. Ann Otol Rhinol Laryngol 98:699, 1989.
71. Setliff RC III, Parsons DS. The "Hummer" new instrumentation for functional endoscopic sinus surgery. Am J Rhinol 8(6):275, 1994.
72. Christmas DA, Krouse JH. Powered instrumentation in functional endoscopic sinus surgery. Part I: Surgical technique. Ear Nose Throat J 75:33, 1996.
73. Goode RL. Power microdebrider for functional endoscopic sinus surgery. Otolaryngol Head Neck Surg 114:676, 1996.
74. Roth M, Lanza DC, Zinreich J, et al. Advantages and disadvantages of three-dimensional computed tomography intraoperative localization for functional endoscopic sinus surgery. Laryngoscope 105:1279, 1995.
75. Fried MP, Kleefield J, Jolesz FA, et al. Intraoperative image guidance during endoscopic sinus surgery. Am J Rhinol 10:337, 1996.
76. Gunkel AR, Freysinger W, Martin A, et al. Three-dimensional image-guided endonasal surgery with a microdebrider. Laryngoscope 107:834, 1997.
77. Anon JB, Lipman SP, Opperheim D, et al. Computer-assisted endoscopic sinus surgery. Laryngoscope 104:901, 1994.
78. Carrau RL, Snyderman CH, Curtin HB, et al. Computer-assisted frontal sinusotomy. Otolaryngol Head Neck Surg 111:727, 1994.
79. Tarver CP, Noorily AD, Sakai CS. A comparison of cocaine vs. lidocaine with oxymetazoline for use in nasal procedures. Otolaryngol Head Neck Surg 109:653, 1993.
80. Chiu YC, Brecht K, DasGupta DS. Myocardial infarction with topical cocaine anesthesia for nasal surgery. Arch Otolaryngol Head Neck Surg 112:988, 1986.
81. Draf W. Endonasal micro-endoscopic frontal sinus surgery. The Fulda concept. Operative Tech Otolaryngol Head Neck Surg 2:234, 1991.
82. Gross WE, Gross CW, Becker D, et al. Modified transnasal endoscopic Lothrop procedure as an alternative to frontal sinus obliteration. Otolaryngol Head Neck Surg 113:427, 1995.
83. Becker DG, Moore D, Lindsey WH, et al. Modified transnasal endoscopic Lothrop procedure: Further considerations. Laryngoscope 105:1161, 1995.
84. Kuhn F. Frontal sinus rescue procedure. Presentation at the Cottle International Meeting XVI ISIAN (International Symposium on Infection and Allergy of the Nose); Philadelphia, PA; June, 1997.
85. Younis RT, Lazar RH. Delayed toxic shock syndrome after functional endonasal sinus surgery. Arch Otolaryngol Head Neck Surg 122:83, 1996.
86. Ishida LK, Ikeda K, Tanno N. Erythromycin inhibits adhesion of *Pseudomonas aeruginosa* and *Branhamella catarrhalis* to human nasal epithelial cells. Am J Rhinol 9:53, 1995.
87. Takagita J, Kitanura H, Nishikawer A, et al. Clinical effects of low-dose erythromycin chemotherapy in chronic sinusitis. Pract Otol (Kyote) 84:489, 1991.
88. Talbot AR, Herr TM, Parsons DS. Mucociliary clearance and buffered hypertonic saline solution. Laryngoscope 107:500, 1997.
89. Marks SC. The learning curve in endoscopic sinus surgery. Otolaryngol Head Neck Surg 120:215, 1999.
90. Bolger WE, Parsons DS, Mair EA, et al. Lacrimal drainage system injury in functional endoscopic sinus surgery. Incidence, analysis, and prevention. Arch Otololaryngol 118(11):1179, 1992.
91. Vleming M, Middleweerd RJ, de Vries N. Complications of endoscopic sinus surgery. Arch Otolaryngol 118:617, 1992.
92. Neuman TR, Turner WJ, Davidson TM. Complications of endoscopic surgery. Ear Nose Throat J 73:585, 1994.
93. Kinsella JB, Calhoun KH, Bradfield JJ, et al. Complications of endoscopic sinus surgery in residency training program. Laryngoscope 105:1029, 1995.
94. Gross RD, Sheridan MF, Burgess LP. Endoscopic sinus surgery complications in residency. Laryngoscope 107:1080, 1997.

CHAPTER 9

Sphenoethmoidectomy

Ethmoidectomy and sphenoethmoidectomy can be performed using three basic approaches: intranasal,[1–10] external,[11, 12] and transantral.[13–16] Furthermore, intranasal ethmoidectomy can be performed with a headlight and nasal speculum, microscope, or nasal endoscope for visualization. In the modern practice of rhinology, most surgeons prefer the endoscopic technique. Whichever approach or technique is used, the same principles of anatomy, physiology, and case selection are applied. The particular preference of an individual surgeon for an individual situation will vary. The rhinologist should, however, be well versed in each of these approaches and capable of using them when appropriate. In a previous chapter, the endoscopic approach was presented in detail. In this chapter, the indications and techniques for the other approaches are presented. The microscopic technique is not discussed here as the author has no experience with this approach and there are seemingly no indications for its use for the surgeon who is well versed in the other techniques.

INDICATIONS

Acute Sinusitis

Rarely, cases of acute sinusitis require surgical intervention. The classification of acute sinusitis ranges from mild to moderate to severe.[17] The mild to moderate cases lack frontal sinus tenderness, severe headache, and usually, fever. Affected patients are ordinarily treated with oral antibiotics and do not require surgical intervention until at least several weeks of treatment fail to resolve the infection.[18, 19] By this time, the condition would be classified as subacute or chronic sinusitis. Severe cases of acute sinusitis are marked by fever, severe headache, or significant frontal sinus tenderness. These patients should undergo immediate radiographic evaluation and, if air-fluid levels or opacification of the frontal or sphenoid sinuses are present, the patient should be hospitalized for a course of intravenous antibiotics.[17] Patients who do not improve within 24 to 48 hours may require drainage to avoid complications.

In this clinical setting, the intranasal approach, either by endoscopy or headlight visualization, is complicated by severe congestion, hyperemia, and the tendency for excessive bleeding. Although this will not prevent successful intranasal surgery in most cases, there are situations when the severity of the mucosal reaction makes the intranasal procedure prohibitively difficult. In such cases, an external approach is necessary.

Chronic Sinusitis

The indications for surgery in patients with chronic sinusitis have been discussed in detail in previous chapters. In any of these situations, any one of the three approaches could be utilized. In most cases, the intranasal approach, usually endoscopic, is preferred. The external approach has the disadvantages of leaving an external scar, inferior visualization, and removal of a portion of the orbital wall. Its advantages, however, include early control of the anterior and posterior ethmoidal arteries, which minimizes surgical blood loss, and avoidance of the risk of orbital complications. The transantral approach has the disadvantages of requiring a Caldwell-Luc procedure with sublabial incision and the risk of permanent injury to the teeth or infraorbital nerve, as well as inferior visualization and poor access to the frontal recess and anterior ethmoid sinus. The risks of performing a Caldwell-Luc operation and its associated complications will be discussed in detail in a later chapter. Suffice it to say that the overall risk of permanent injury of some kind has been estimated to be as high as 10% to 15%.[20] The only advantage of the transantral approach is direct access to the maxillary sinus.

On balance, the disadvantages of the external and transantral approaches outweigh their benefits for routine cases. The clinical situations that would dictate the necessity of a nonendoscopic approach are limited, but would include patients in whom transnasal surgery is technically not possible. One case in the author's experience involved a patient with nasal sarcoidosis and enlarged inferior turbinates. The turbinates were infiltrated by granulomas and did not decongest. This patient required a transantral approach because of the inability to pass the endoscope. Another condition that is a relative indication for the external technique is the presence of dehiscence of the lamina papyracea. If this leads to orbital subluxation, use of the external approach may be advisable to allow retraction of the orbital contents, thereby avoiding injury.

Orbital Infection

Sinusitis with associated orbital infection is the strongest indication for the external approach to the ethmoid sinuses. Most reports on the management of orbital infection indicate that preseptal cellulitis can be managed by intravenous antibiotic therapy without surgery.[21, 22] Patients with infection beyond this point, including true orbital cellulitis, subperiosteal abscess, and orbital abscess, require surgery. There have been a few reports of management of orbital cellulitis with antibiotics and observation.[23] However, a proportion of these patients under observation will sustain vision losses that might otherwise have been avoided. For this reason, immediate surgery for orbital cellulitis remains the safest approach. Conversely, subperiosteal abscess and true orbital abscess are absolute indications for surgery, with no serious debate on this issue appearing in the literature.[24–26]

Until recently, surgery for orbital infection always involved external ethmoidectomy. However, reports have now been published suggesting that endoscopic ethmoidectomy, with intentional removal of the lamina papyracea, is adequate for the treatment of orbital cellulitis, and even subperiosteal abscess.[27–30] This is a logical application of the endoscopic technique; however, except in the hands of a very experienced endoscopic sinus surgeon, the safest and most reliable treatment for this surgical emergency remains the standard external ethmoidectomy.

Hyperplastic Sinusitis

Patients with hyperplastic sinusitis or sinonasal polyposis typically require surgery, as previously discussed in Chapter 8. Provided the surgeon is comfortable with the endoscopic technique, these patients are good candidates for this approach. However, a few surgeons, who gained extensive experience treating these patients with the more traditional intranasal sphenoethmoidectomy, continue to prefer the latter method for extensive polyposis.[31, 32] Although there is no convincing data available in the literature to document the superiority of one technique over the other, the combination of powered instrumentation and endoscopes provides far superior visualization and hemostasis to any other technique. It is a basic principle of surgery that the better the exposure and hemostasis, the safer and more successful the surgery. Given these considerations, it is clear that the endoscopic technique will continue to predominate as the preferred technique of most sinus surgeons.

PREOPERATIVE CONSIDERATIONS

Most patients undergoing external ethmoidectomy will undergo general anesthesia. Many of these patients are acutely ill with fever, bacteremia, and, possibly, sepsis. For this reason, a complete medical evaluation is necessary to ensure the safest anesthesia possible. Often, invasive monitoring, such as by arterial line or central venous catheter, is warranted, and a urinary catheter may be placed. With proper preparation and modern anesthesia, the surgery should not pose a significant risk for cardiovascular complications.

Owing to the acute nature of their illness, most of these patients require intravenous antibiotic therapy in the perioperative period. To reduce the incidence of sepsis at the time of surgery, antibiotic therapy should be started at least 1 hour before the operation.

One final consideration is evaluation of the patient's eye. In routine cases without orbital involvement, the risk of orbital complications is minimal. Despite this, it is prudent to perform at least a basic eye examination before the procedure, including an assessment of visual acuity, extraocular movements, and pupillary responses. For patients with orbital infection or known dehiscence of the orbital wall, a complete ophthalmologic examination should be performed by an ophthalmology consultant. This not only serves to document existing deficits, but also allows detection of possible subtle orbital involvement. If orbital exploration is warranted or anticipated, the ophthalmologist should be available to assist during the surgery.

TECHNIQUE

External Ethmoidectomy

Visualization

The typical external approach to the sinuses is performed with a headlight to improve illumination. This permits the operation to be conducted safely under direct vision. However, it is possible to enhance the operative view by utilizing magnification, either with surgical loupes or a microscope. These visual adjuncts are especially useful when operating in the posterior ethmoid and sphenoid sinuses. The distance from the surface in this situation becomes significant and the anatomy smaller, with more critical structures. Although there is no documentation in the literature to support the use of magnification in this setting, it stands to reason that magnification should increase the ease and safety of this part of the operation.

Incision

The incision for external ethmoidectomy is placed approximately halfway between the medial canthus and the nasal dorsum. If a natural fold or crease is present, this can be used to hide the incision. The classic Lynch incision is a curvilinear medial canthal incision designed for external ethmoidectomy (Fig. 9–1). Modifications of this incision have been described to help camouflage the incision or make it less noticeable. Figure 9–2 demonstrates the W-plasty incision used by the author for this purpose. This modification results in a broken-line closure which, after complete healing, results in the incision being less obvious. This also prevents linear contracture, which may result in formation of a ridge or web in the medical canthus. The exposure through the modified incision is identical to the original linear incision and takes only a few extra minutes to design, perform, and later, close.

The skin of the face should be prepared using either PHisoHex or an iodine-containing solution. The field should be draped with the eyes exposed, although they may be protected with either corneal shields or a temporary tarsorrhaphy suture. The incision is drawn on the skin with a marking pen and then infiltrated with local anesthetic, usually 1% lidocaine with 1 : 100,000 epinephrine. Only a small amount (1–2 mL) of local anesthetic should be used to avoid distorting the anatomy. The incision is made with a No. 15 blade through the

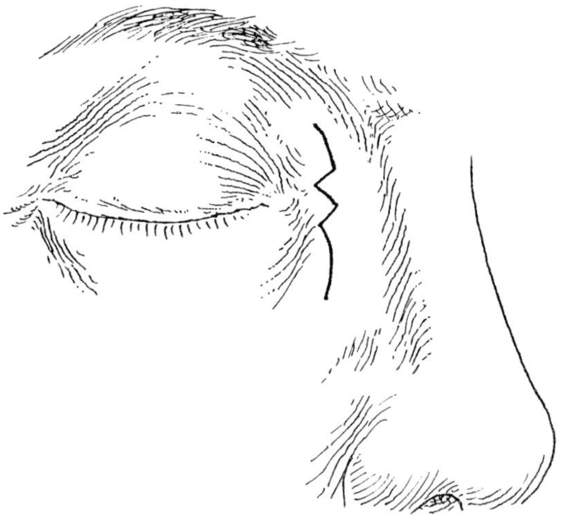

Figure 9–2. W-plasty modification of the Lynch incision.

dermis only. Once the initial incision is made, the skin edges are retracted with a fine, double-hooked retractor. The incision is then spread open with small, sharp, iris scissors. Further retraction can then be effected with a small rake or retractor.

To help minimize bleeding, subcutaneous dissection can then be carried out using needle-tipped electrocautery. The subcutaneous tissue, muscle, and periosteum are divided with cautery down to the bone. A branch of the angular artery crossing this incision in the submuscular layer is usually identified and can either be controlled with a bipolar forceps or clamped, divided, and ligated with suture (Fig. 9–3). The inferior extent of the exposure should carry down to the inferior edge

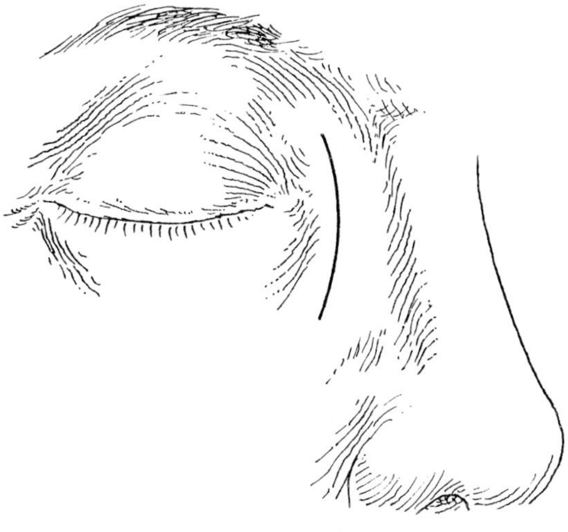

Figure 9–1. The standard Lynch incision for external ethmoidectomy. The incision lies halfway between the nasal dorsum and the medial canthus in the deepest part of the natural hollow of this area.

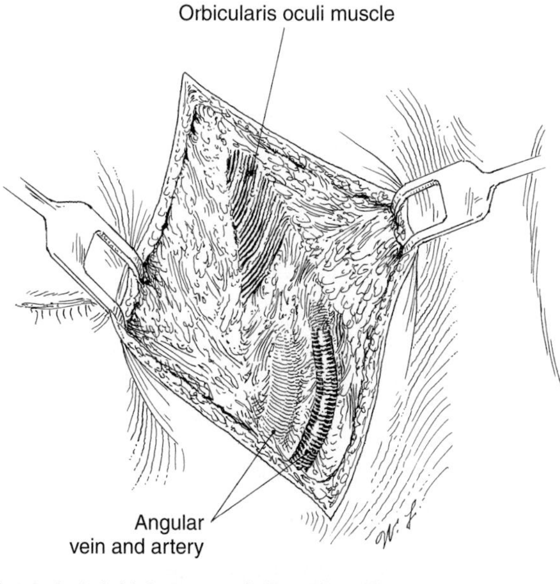

Figure 9–3. Initial stages of dissection. The angular artery and vein are shown inferiorly in the incision. Fibers of the orbicularis muscle are evident superiorly.

of the lacrimal fossa, whereas the superior extent of the incision should be just below the supraorbital foramen. This allows the supraorbital nerve and artery to be preserved.

Exposure

Next, the periosteum should be elevated on the orbital side of the incision. This is accomplished with a Freer elevator and extends inferiorly to the anterior lacrimal crest and superiorly to above the nasal frontal suture line. The orbital contents are then elevated away from the medial orbital wall (Fig. 9–4). Retraction is achieved by using a malleable retractor against the periorbita. The important landmarks include the anterior and posterior lacrimal crests and the frontoethmoidal suture. The superior lacrimal sac should be carefully elevated out of the lacrimal fossa inferiorly to the connection to the nasolacrimal duct. Approximately 15 to 20 mm posterior to the anterior lacrimal crest in the frontoethmoidal suture, the anterior ethmoidal artery will be identified (Fig. 9–5). This artery should be exposed circumferentially by careful periorbital elevation, coagulated with bipolar cautery, and then divided sharply. Alternatively, the artery can be controlled with vascular clips. However, these may fall off during subsequent retraction, leading to troublesome hemorrhage.

The exposure is completed with continued posterior elevation and identification of the posterior ethmoid artery. This is usually situated 5 to 10 mm posterior to the anterior ethmoidal artery in the frontoethmoidal suture (Fig. 9–6). This artery should also be controlled with bipolar forceps.

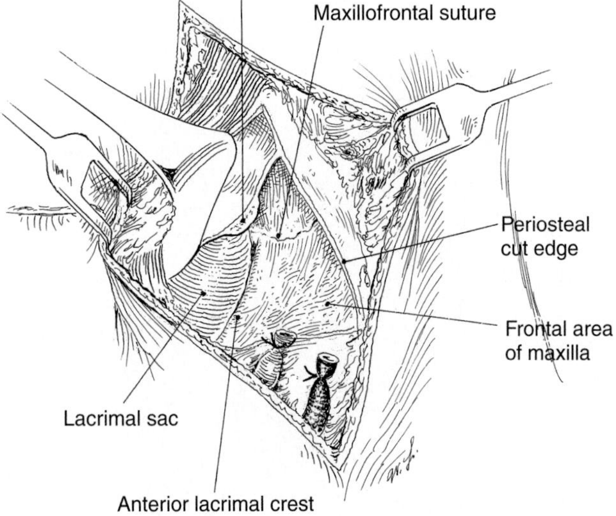

Figure 9–4. Exposure of the medial orbital wall. The lacrimal sac and crest are identified. The frontonasal suture is evident. The medial canthal tendon is identifiable only as a thickening in the cut edge of the periosteum.

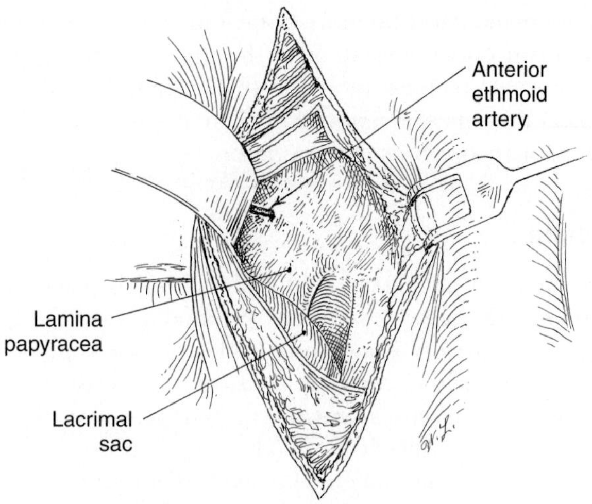

Figure 9–5. Exposure of the anterior ethmoid artery. The lacrimal sac has been elevated out of the lacrimal fossa. The artery is found in the frontoethmoidal suture line.

Ethmoidectomy

The actual resection of the ethmoid sinus is begun by entering the sinus through the lamina papyracea, just inferior to the anterior ethmoid artery, using an upturned forceps (Fig. 9–7). The lamina should be widely removed to the extent needed for adequate visualization of the entire interior of the sinus. This usually requires removal posteriorly to the level of the posterior ethmoidal artery, superiorly to the frontoethmoidal suture, and inferiorly to the maxillary ethmoid junction. Bone removal is easily accomplished using a straight Blakesley forceps or Takahashi forceps (Fig. 9–8).

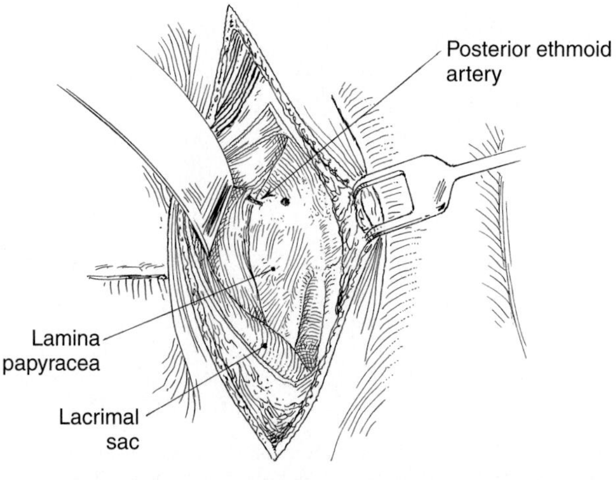

Figure 9–6. Exposure of the posterior ethmoid artery. The anterior ethmoid artery has been cauterized and divided.

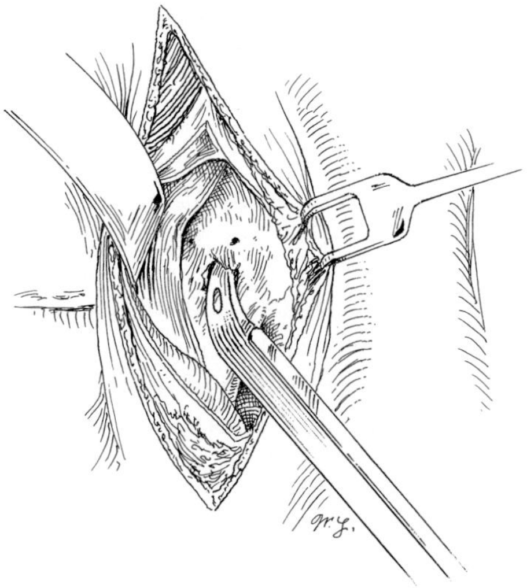

Figure 9–7. Initial entry into the ethmoid sinus. The sinus is entered bluntly in the mid portion of the lamina papyracea.

The next step is to identify the level of the skull base just posterior to the anterior ethmoid artery. This is important to avoid intracranial complications. The operation should then proceed in a superior-to-inferior, anterior-to-posterior direction. Retraction on the orbit should be released every few minutes to minimize orbital trauma. The anterior and posterior ethmoid arteries should be carefully preserved within the sinuses to avoid unwanted hemorrhage from back bleeding. The medial extent of the surgery extends to the middle turbinate. Unless there is reason to remove the middle turbinate, it should be preserved. The posterior extent of the surgery is reached upon identification of the face of the sphenoid sinus. The frontal recess should be approached with caution. The orbital wall anterior to the anterior ethmoid artery should be preserved to prevent orbital collapse into the frontal recess with subsequent stenosis. With this bone preserved, visualization into the frontal recess is difficult. However, by extending the patient's head and viewing the area from a low angle, it is possible to achieve visualization into this recess. An upturned forceps can be used to open the agger nasi and remove some of the cells of the frontal recess. Aggressive dissection through this approach is not encouraged, however, as this would result in a high risk of subsequent stenosis. If more needs to be done to open the frontal sinus at this point, trephination or formal frontoethmoidectomy should be performed.

Sphenoidectomy

After the ethmoidectomy is complete, a sphenoidectomy, if required, is easily accomplished at this point. As stated earlier, use of a microscope or surgical loupes may improve the view and facilitate this step. The sphenoid sinus is easy to identify in this operation by following the orbital wall back to the sinus. Posterior to the posterior ethmoid artery, the orbital apex comes to a point at the optic foramen. The optic nerve then projects posteriorly along the lateral and superior walls of the sphenoid sinus to the optic chiasm. By staying medial and inferior to the optic nerve, the sphenoid may be entered. The landmarks in this area include the posterior ethmoid artery as it crosses the ethmoid roof and the anterior wall of the sphenoid sinus. The slope of the skull base is posterior and inferior in the posterior ethmoid sinus and anterior and inferior on the anterior wall of the sphenoid sinus. This change of slope should allow delineation of the sphenoid sinus. If the anatomy is not clear, the natural ostium of the sphenoid can be identified along the posterior wall of the nose, just lateral to the septum, approximately 30 degrees from the floor of the nose.

Once the sphenoid sinus is identified, the anterior wall may be entered. This can be accomplished either by using a curette or by puncturing it with the suction tip. In either case, only a small opening should be made initially until the exact location in relation to the inside

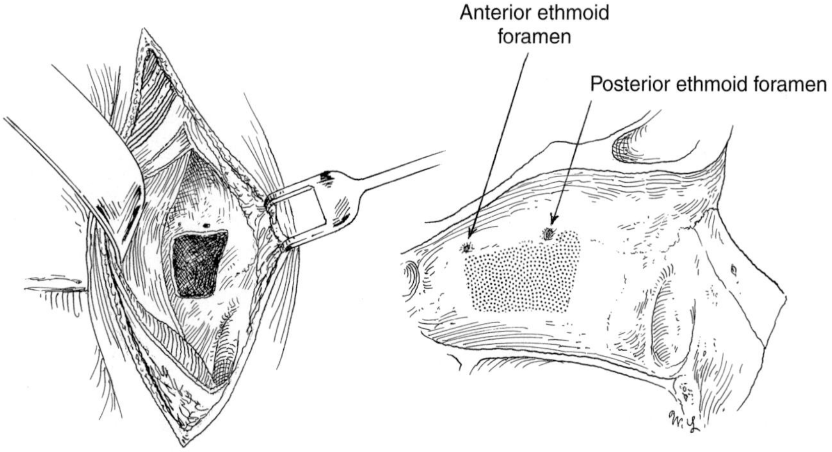

Figure 9–8. Completed resection of the lamina papyracea. The opening is maximized prior to beginning the ethmoidectomy. The lateral view demonstrates the amount of bone that can be removed.

of the sinus can be verified. Once the appropriateness of the opening is established, the remainder of the anterior wall can be removed with a rotating sphenoid punch. The completed sphenoidotomy should connect to the natural ostium, allowing inspection of the entire sinus and additional tissue removal in the sinus, as indicated (Fig. 9–9). Large polyps and cysts or inspissated secretions should be removed, but normal or inflamed mucosa should be preserved.

Closure

After the procedure is completed, the surgeon may proceed with careful cosmetic closure. Before closure, it is necessary to ensure complete hemostasis using the bipolar cautery. Wound irrigation is recommended with normal saline prior to closure. Multiple suture layers are needed. The first layer should reset the position of the medial canthus. The tendon is directly sutured to the periosteum of the nasal bone. The second layer, an interrupted layer of dermal sutures, approximates the incision. Skin closure is achieved with 6-0 nylon in an interrupted fashion.

Transantral Sphenoethmoidectomy

The transantral approach to the ethmoid begins with a sublabial incision and a Caldwell-Luc type procedure. This procedure is covered in detail in Chapter 10. In this section, the technique of ethmoidectomy through the transantral approach is described. Typically, this procedure is done through a generous opening through the anterior wall of the maxillary sinus using retraction of the lip and a headlight to facilitate exposure and illumination, respectively. The author has utilized nasal endoscopes passed transantrally to improve visualization during this procedure and to allow a smaller opening in the anterior wall of the sinus with less retraction. This helps to decrease the risk of complications associated with infraorbital nerve injury and is a logical adaptation for the experienced endoscopic sinus surgeon who has occasion to use this procedure.

Ethmoidectomy

The procedure begins with identification of the natural ostium of the maxillary sinus (Fig. 9–10). The ostium is enlarged in a posterior and inferior direction until the middle turbinate and ethmoidal bulla are identified (Fig. 9–11). The uncinate process can be removed using a back-biting forceps or an upturned Blakesley-type forceps. Next, the ethmoid is entered at the bulla. It is important to identify the medial orbital wall early in the procedure. The angle of approach will be tangential to the lamina papyracea and thus will tend to direct the

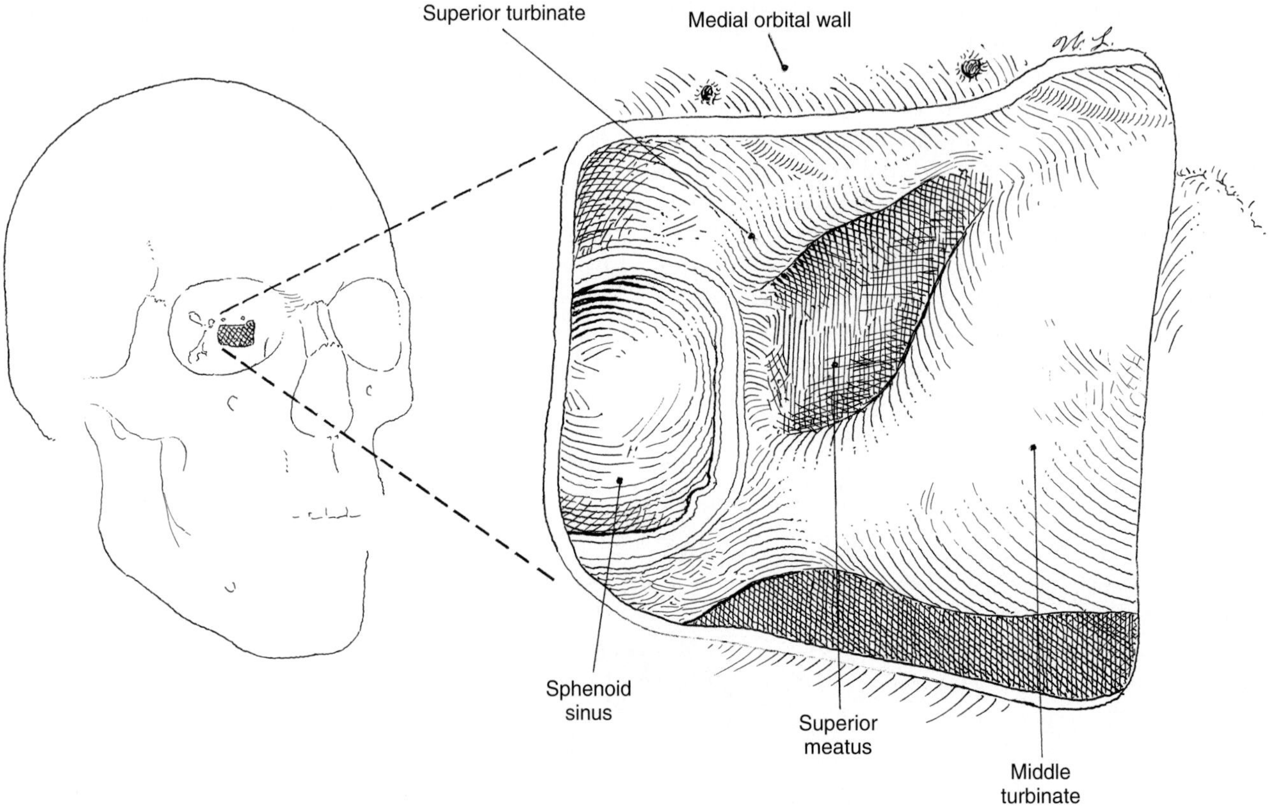

Figure 9–9. Completed sphenoethmoidectomy, magnified view demonstrating the anatomy. The superior meatus and middle meatus are seen, as are the sphenoid sinus and skull base.

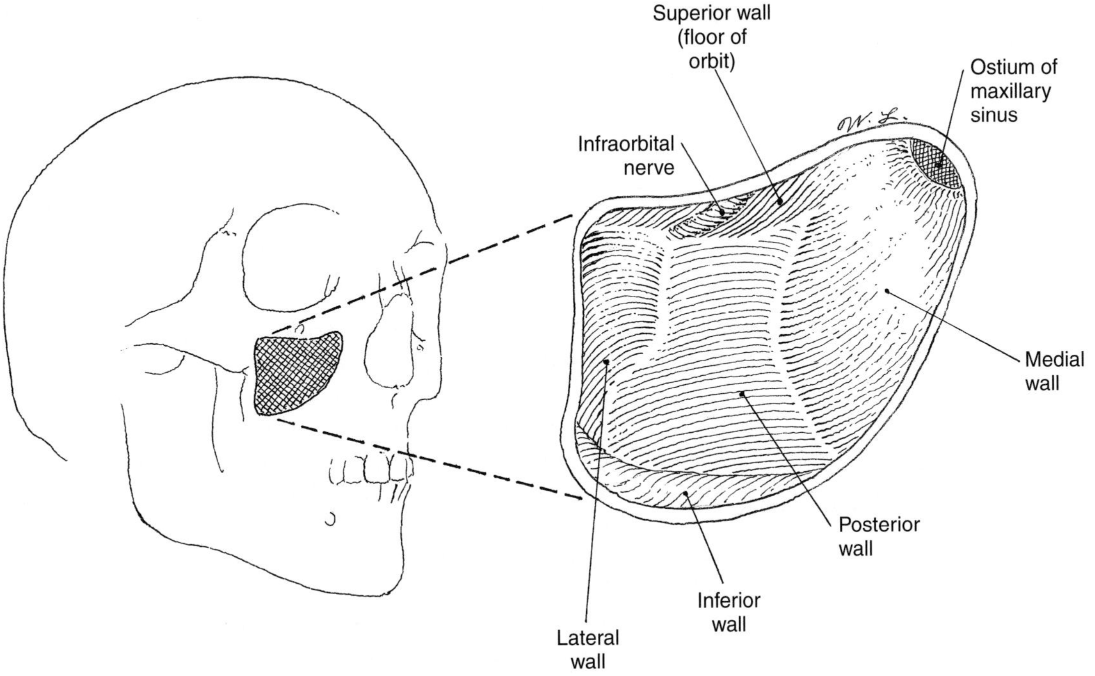

Figure 9–10. Angled view into the maxillary sinus through a standard sublabial approach demonstrates the ostium of the sinus.

surgeon into the middle turbinate and nasal septum. To remain oriented, it is therefore best to work from medial to lateral, skeletonizing the lamina papyracea. The ethmoidectomy proceeds with removal of the ground lamella and the posterior ethmoid cells. The skull base is usually first identified in the posterior ethmoid, but once identified, can be used as a landmark to complete the ethmoidectomy.

The sphenoid ostium can be identified after completion of the posterior ethmoidectomy. To improve visualization, the superior turbinate can be trimmed along its inferior border to expose the natural ostium of the sphenoid sinus. The ostium is located just lateral to the nasal septum at an angle of 30 degrees from the floor of the nose. A rotating sphenoid punch is then used to remove the anterior wall of the sphenoid sinus.

The anterior ethmoid and frontal recess cells cannot be seen through the transantral approach without use of angled nasal endoscopes to augment vision. If these instruments are not in use, the frontal recess can only

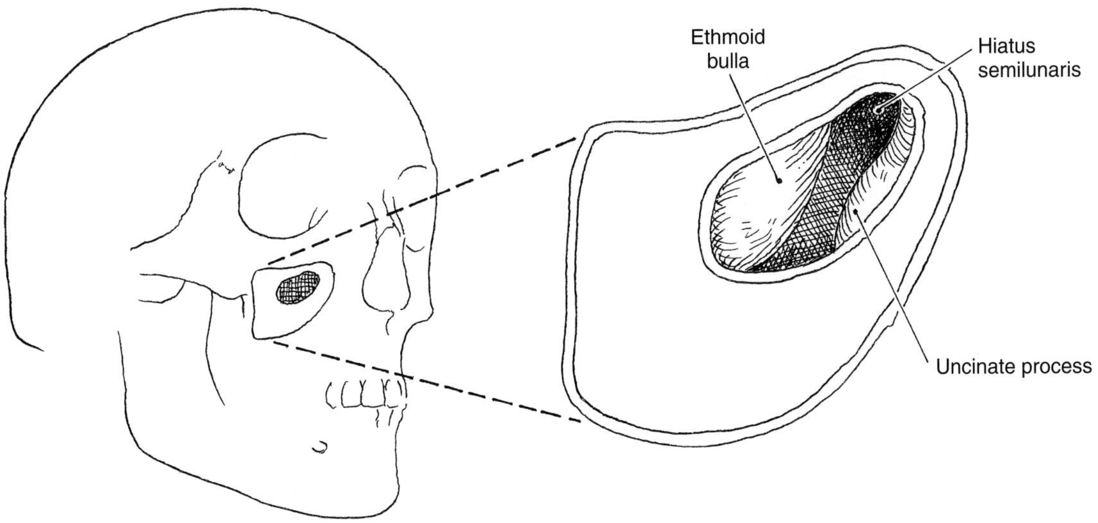

Figure 9–11. Angled view into the ethmoid sinus after the posterior fontanelle has been removed. The uncinate process, ethmoid bulla, and hiatus semilunaris are demonstrated.

be worked on by feel. With the high risk of cerebrospinal fluid (CSF) leak from operating in this area, blind dissection is not recommended. However, by using a 70-degree scope through the sublabial opening, one gains a view that is identical to that afforded by standard intranasal endoscopic surgery.

After surgery, packing is applied as necessary. The ethmoid cavity can be packed separately from the maxillary sinus using an absorbent sponge, or it can be packed with the traditional Vaseline-coated strip gauze that is used to pack the maxillary sinus. The packing is applied by first passing one end of the strip gauze out through the nose, with the remainder packed from medial to lateral.

Intranasal Sphenoethmoidectomy

The operation described here is patterned after that described by Friedman and others.[2, 5, 31] Visualization is achieved using a nasal speculum with a headlight for illumination. Surgical loupes are optional, but by providing magnification, will facilitate identification of the anatomy. Topical and local anesthetics are administered as for endoscopic surgery. Cocaine flakes and 1% lidocaine with 1:100,000 epinephrine are preferred, but other combinations of anesthetic agents are acceptable. The basic surgical method involves a posterior-to-anterior dissection. The first step is removal of any obstructing polyps in order to expose the normal anatomy. This is done with either a polyp snare or Blakesley forceps. Next, angled turbinate scissors are used to excise the middle turbinate (Fig. 9–12) so as to expose the ethmoid and sphenoid rostrum (Fig. 9–13). The natural ostium of the sphenoid sinus is then identified and, using the rotating punch, the anterior wall is completely removed. With this accomplished, the posterior wall of the sphenoid is identified and used as a landmark for the skull base.

The posterior ethmoid is then entered using upturned forceps. The ethmoid cells are removed from a posterior-to-anterior direction up to the skull base. Direct vision is used as much as possible, but the feel of the operation is an essential aspect of this operation. With experience, it is possible to identify the skull base by its feel as much as by its appearance. The skull base has a broad, firm feel if gently palpated with the tip of the upturned forceps. The lamina papyracea should also be identified as early as possible in this procedure so it can be used as a secondary landmark. Without the use of angled endoscopes, it is not possible to see into the frontal recess. However, with the skull base clearly identified and skeletonized to a point as far anterior as possible, it is possible, by feel, to remove much of the anterior ethmoid sinus.

Treatment of the maxillary sinus is not, by definition, part of this procedure. In practice, however, some man-

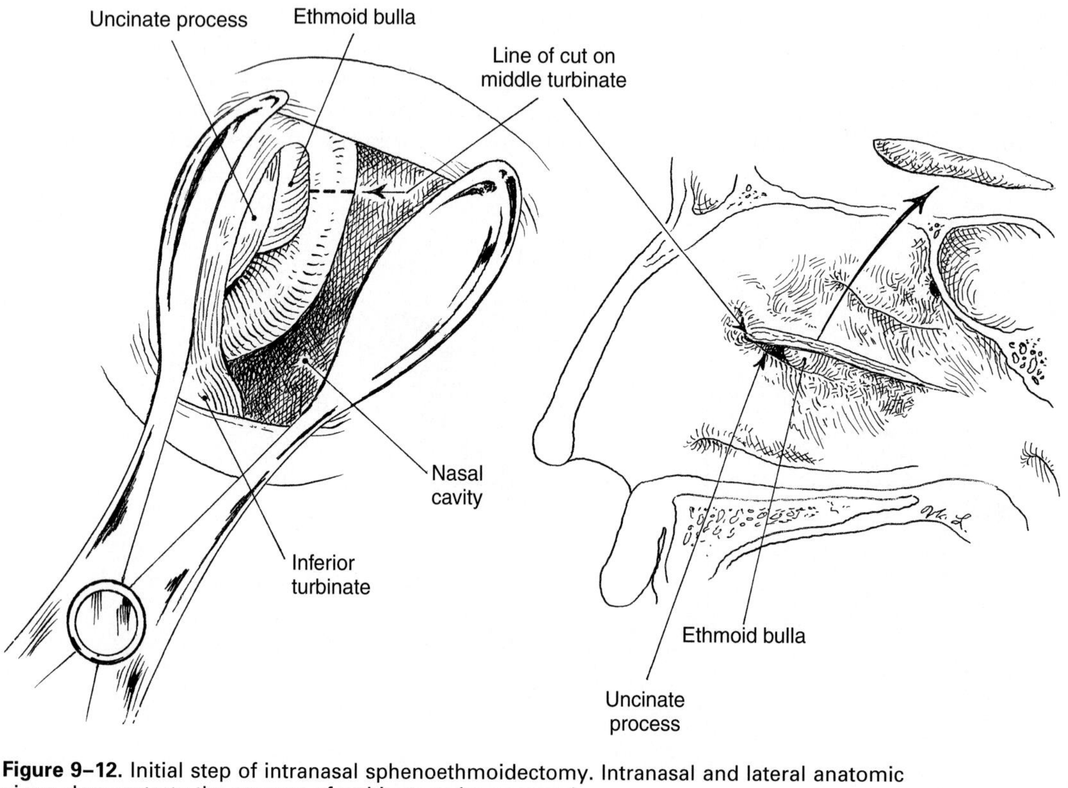

Figure 9–12. Initial step of intranasal sphenoethmoidectomy. Intranasal and lateral anatomic views demonstrate the amount of turbinate to be removed.

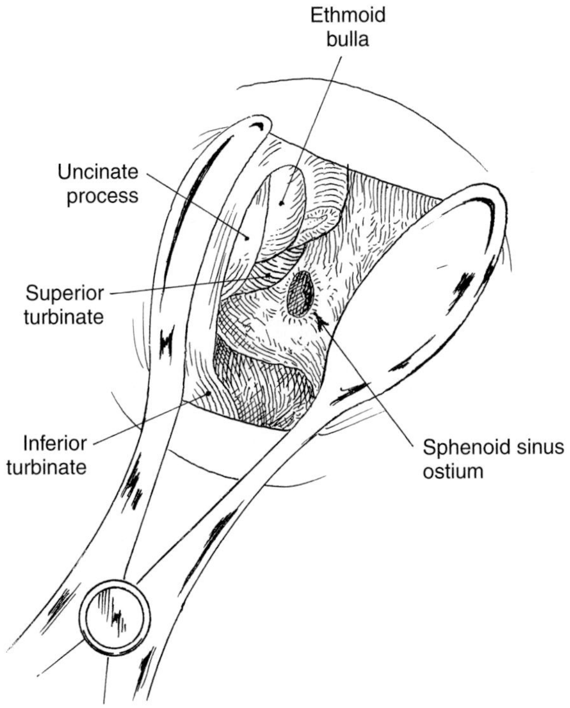

Figure 9–13. Intranasal view after turbinate resection. The ostium of the sphenoid sinus is seen posteriorly at an elevation of 30 degrees from the floor of the nose, immediately lateral to the nasal septum.

agement of the maxillary sinus is indicated. The classic options include a Caldwell-Luc procedure with inferior antrostomy or an inferior antrostomy alone. However, with the recent emphasis on middle meatus antrostomy, this is the primary option for most cases. This is easily performed after the ethmoidectomy is completed. The residual uncinate is removed and the natural ostium is identified using curved olive tip suction. The posterior fontanelle can then be removed to enlarge the sinus ostium.

POSTOPERATIVE CARE

The care of patients after any form of ethmoidectomy is similar. During the first week, the activity level of the patient should be kept at a minimum, although after the first night, bed rest is usually not required. The patient's diet may be advanced over the first day to a regular diet. Nasal packing is maintained for 3 to 5 days according to the schedule for follow-up evaluation. Some bleeding is expected during the first few days, but this normally subsides by the third or fourth day after surgery. Antibiotics are continued for a minimum of 2 weeks, but may be continued longer if the postoperative course warrants an extended course of antibiotics. Oral steroids should be administered in patients with polyps to help prevent early recurrence during the healing period.

At the first postoperative visit, the packing material is removed and the ethmoid cavity is suctioned to remove blood clots and debris. In patients who have undergone external ethmoidectomy, the sutures are also removed. After this, the patient should be started on nasal irrigations. The formulation is either normal saline or hypertonic (3%) saline. Irrigations are continued until the cavities are healed and crusting resolves. As opposed to the postoperative care after endoscopic surgery, which includes periodic debridement in the office until healing is complete, other forms of ethmoidectomy traditionally utilize only debridement by irrigation.

Nasal steroid sprays are recommended for the first 3 to 6 months after surgery to help minimize inflammation during the healing period. In allergic patients and patients with polyps, use of steroid sprays is normally continued indefinitely. There is not convincing evidence that postoperative nasal steroid sprays prevent recurrence. However, in the subgroups of patients with polyps and allergies, the practice is nearly a standard of care.

COMPLICATIONS

The complications of intranasal, transantral, and external ethmoidectomy are similar to those for endoscopic sinus surgery.[4, 33] The most common complications include infection, hemorrhage, scarring, and epiphora. More serious complications include orbital injury, CSF leak, and intracranial bleeding. Headlight-guided intranasal ethmoidectomy has no unique complications, but there has been much debate about whether endoscopic surgery is inherently safer than the headlight procedure. Published reports do not adequately answer this question. Clearly, the endoscopic procedure affords improved visualization which, logically, should make this the safer procedure. However, the increased visualization afforded by endoscopes may prompt the surgeon to perform a more extensive dissection, leading to increased risks for the patient. The individual surgeon's final decision about which technique to use will depend on the training of the surgeon, the knowledge of the patient's anatomy, and the comfort level of the surgeon with each technique. Ultimately, the best technique is the one that the surgeon has the greatest expertise in performing.

Transantral ethmoidectomy carries the added risks associated with the Caldwell-Luc procedure. These risks, which include facial numbness, dental numbness, chronic facial or dental pain, and oroantral fistula, will be addressed in detail in Chapter 10. The risks unique to external ethmoidectomy are related to the incision and may include unsightly scarring secondary to contracture with webbing, hypertrophy of the scar, or poor technique in closure. In any of these situations, scar revision is indicated and is usually easily and successfully performed.

A second problem related to the external approach is telecanthus. During closure of the incision, it is essential that the orbital periosteum be carefully reapproximated to the periosteum of the nose. Failure to do so may result in lateralization of the medial canthus. If necessary, a suture can be placed from the medial canthal tendon through the nose and attached to the opposite medial canthal tendon, as is done during repair of a naso-orbital ethmoid fracture.

Finally, wound infection, hematoma, or wound dehiscence may also occur. The risk of these complications is low, but their occurrence, especially in the case of hematoma or wound infection, warrants emergency intervention to save vision. Prevention is best achieved by administering prophylactic antibiotics and using careful sterile technique. Draining the incision is not generally recommended. However, meticulous hemostasis is mandatory. Bipolar cautery is used effectively for this purpose. If wound infection is detected, reoperation is necessary to drain the infection and decompress the orbit. Orbital hematoma is treated as outlined in Chapters 8 and 21.

REFERENCES

1. Friedman WH, Katsantonis GP. Intranasal and transnasal ethmoidectomy: A 20-year experience. Laryngoscope 100:343, 1990.
2. Eichel BS. The intranasal ethmoidectomy: A 12-year perspective. Otolaryngol Head Neck Surg 90:540, 1982.
3. Morgenstein KM. Intransal sphenoethmoidectomy and antrotomy. Otolaryngol Clin North Am 18(1):69, 1985.
4. Watson DJ, Griffiths MV. The safety and efficacy of intranasal ethmoidectomy. J Laryngol Otol 102(2):802, 1988.
5. Goldman JL. Intranasal sphenoethmoidectomy and antrostomy. In Goldman JL (ed). The Principles and Practice of Rhinology. New York: John Wiley and Sons, 1987.
6. Kennedy DW, Zinreich SJ, Rosenbaum AE, et al. Functional endoscopic sinus surgery. Arch Otolaryngol 111:576, 1985.
7. Kennedy DW. Functional endoscopic sinus surgery. Arch Otolaryngol 111:643, 1985.
8. Stammberger H. Endoscopic endonasal surgery—Concepts in treatment of recurring rhinosinusitis. Part II. Surgical technique. Otolaryngol Head Neck Surg 94:147, 1986.
9. Schaefer SD, Manning S, Close LG. Endoscopic paranasal sinus surgery: Indications and considerations. Laryngoscope 99:1, 1989.
10. Rice DH. Endoscopic sinus surgery: Results at 2-year follow-up. Otolaryngol Head Neck Surg 101:476, 1989.
11. Neal GD. External ethmoidectomy. Otolaryngol Clin North Am 18(1):55, 1985.
12. Wilson WR, Grove AS. A method for combined dacryocystorhinostomy with external ethmoidectomy. Head Neck Surg 4(1):9, 1981.
13. Langenbrunner DJ, Nigri P. Transantral ethoidectomy: An overlooked procedure? Trans Am Acad Ophthalmol Otolaryngol 84(4 Pt 1): ORL-774, 1977.
14. Kimmelman CP, Weisman RA, Osguthorpe JD, et al. The efficacy and safety of transantral ethmoidectomy. Laryngoscope 98(11): 1178, 1988.
15. Friedman WH, Katsantonis GP. Transantral revision of recurrent maxillary and ethmoidal disease following functional intranasal surgery. Otolaryngol Head Neck Surg 106(4):367, 1992.
16. Meloni F, Masala W. Transmaxillary ethmoidectomy: Technic and results. Acta Otorhinolaryngol Ital 8(2):157, 1988.
17. Kennedy DW, Gwaltney JM Jr, Jones JG, et al. Medical management of sinusitis: Educational goals and management guidelines. Ann Otol Rhinol Laryngol 104(10):22, 1995.
18. Kennedy DW (ed). Sinus Disease: Guide to First-line Management. Darien, CT: Health Communications, 1994.
19. Gwaltney JM Jr. State-of-art: Acute community-acquired sinusitis. Clin Infect Dis 23:1209, 1996.
20. Murray JP. Complications after treatment of chronic maxillary sinus disease with Caldwell-Luc procedure. Laryngoscope 93: 282, 1983.
21. Rubinstein JB, Handler SD. Orbital and periorbital cellulitis in children. Head Neck Surg 5(1):15, 1982.
22. Fearon B, Edmonds B, Bird R. Orbital-facial complications of sinusitis in children. Laryngoscope 89(6 Pt 1):947, 1979.
23. Handler LC, Davey JC, Hill JC, et al. The acute orbit: Differentiation of orbital cellulitis from subperiosteal abscess by computerized tomography. Neuroradiology 33(1):15, 1991.
24. Schramm VL, Myers EN, Kennerdell JS. Orbital complications of acute sinusitis: Evaluation, management, and outcome. Otolaryngol 86(2):ORL-221, 1978.
25. Pereira KD, Mitchell RB, Younis RT. Management of medial subperiosteal abscess of the orbit in children—A 5-year experience. Int J Pediatr Otorhinolaryngol 38(3):247, 1997.
26. Arjmand EM, Lusk RP, Muntz HR. Pediatric sinusitis and subperiosteal orbital abscess formation: Diagnosis and treatment. Otolaryngol Head Neck Surg 109(5):886, 1993.
27. El-Silimy O. The place of endonasal endoscopy in the treatment of orbital cellulitis. Rhinology 33:93, 1995.
28. Younis RT, Lazar RH. Endoscopic drainage of subperiosteal abscess in children: A pilot study. Am J Rhinol 10:11, 1996.
29. Froehlich P, Pransky SM, Fontaine P, et al. Minimal endoscopic approach to subperiosteal orbital abscess. Arch Otolaryngol Head Neck Surg 123:280, 1997.
30. Wolf SR, Gode U, Hosemann W. Endonasal endoscopic surgery for rhinogen intraorbital abscess: A report of six cases. Laryngoscope 106:105, 1996.
31. Friedman WH. Surgery for chronic hyperplastic rhinosinusitis. Laryngoscope 85:1999, 1975.
32. Friedman WH, Katsantonis GP. The role of standard technique in modern sinus surgery. Otolaryngol Clin North Am 22:759, 1989.
33. Freedman HM, Kern EB. Complications of intranasal ethmoidectomy: A review of 1,000 consecutive operations. Laryngoscope 89:421, 1979.

CHAPTER 10

Maxillary Sinus Surgery

Inflammatory conditions of the maxillary sinus can be operated on using either an intranasal or sublabial approach. The sublabial approach, or Caldwell-Luc (CL) operation,[1] has been the standard of care for the surgical management of maxillary sinusitis for more than a century. However, beginning in the 1980s, endoscopic sinus surgery (ESS) rapidly gained popularity for the surgical treatment of inflammatory diseases of the maxillary sinus, and today ESS has defined a new standard of care.[2–5] In numerous reports, ESS has clearly been demonstrated as a highly successful treatment for maxillary sinusitis.[6–12] To date, there is only one randomized prospective trial of ESS versus CL.[13] This study, which now includes long-term follow-up results, is imperfect, but the results do tend to support the contention that ESS is as good as the CL procedure without the necessity of an incision or the risk of neural injury.[14] A second retrospective report found ESS to be far superior to the Caldwell-Luc procedure.[15] Despite this fact, there continue to be indications for performing the CL procedure. In this chapter, the CL operation is described in detail, including the author's recommendations for appropriate application of this technique.

CALDWELL-LUC PROCEDURE

Indications

Chronic Sinusitis

The general indications for surgery for chronic sinusitis have been described in detail in previous chapters. For most of the routine cases of chronic sinusitis, ESS with middle meatus antrostomy is recommended, rather than CL. Only in special cases would a CL procedure be indicated,[16–18] as in patients with persistent or recurrent sinusitis. Patients who have undergone technically successful ESS but who still have unremitting infection in the maxillary sinus would also be candidates for this procedure. These patients may have microabscesses in the mucosa, osteitis or osteomyelitis of the maxilla, necrotic tissue within the sinus, or inspissated secretions that are not removable endoscopically. Before performing the CL, several alternatives should be explored. The first is to evaluate the patient for potential revision ESS. The most common causes of failed ESS with persistent maxillary sinusitis are technical.[19–21] If residual infection is present in the frontal recess, the patient should undergo revision surgery before considering a CL procedure. Similarly, if the surgical antrostomy does not connect to the natural ostium of the maxillary sinus, this can lead to recirculation and persistent inflammation. This is easily detected and surgically corrected endoscopically.

When there are no detectable anatomic causes for persistent or recurrent maxillary sinusitis, the patient should be evaluated for systemic causes for failed surgery, such as immunodeficiency, ciliary dyskinesia, or uncontrolled allergy. In the presence of one of these factors, CL will be of limited utility. In addition to this evaluation, patients with persistent maxillary sinusitis should be considered for a prolonged course of intravenous antibiotics directed at culture-specific bacteria. If, after several weeks of culture-specific antibiotic therapy with meticulous office debridement of crusts, secretions, and debris from the maxillary sinus through the middle meatus antrostomy, the patient continues to have chronic infection, then a CL operation should be considered.

Another rare indication for performing a CL procedure in a patient with chronic sinusitis is in the case of inadequate access through the nose to perform the ESS procedure. In this setting, the patient may have stenosis of the anterior nares or hypertrophy of the inferior turbinate, either of which can block passage of the nasal endoscopes. A limited CL procedure may be a reasonable alternative for such patients.

Another possible scenario in which a CL operation would be considered is the patient with fungal sinusitis. If this condition is identified during ESS or prior to surgery and the fungal elements cannot be removed through an enlarged natural ostium, then a CL procedure is indicated to ensure removal of all inspissated fungal elements.[22–24] This procedure might also be considered in cases in which the natural ostium cannot be located endoscopically. In this unlikely scenario, a CL procedure may be performed to locate the natural ostium.

Finally, patients with cystic fibrosis may require a CL operation.[25,26] These patients develop secretions with a unique consistency resembling putty, making suctioning difficult and grasping impossible. In addition, these patients invariably develop severe osteitis and recurrent sinusitis that renders ESS of marginal utility. For many patients with cystic fibrosis, the direct approach yields better results by allowing more thorough cleaning and, perhaps, longer intervals of disease control.

Acute Sinusitis

As discussed in previous chapters, most patients with acute sinusitis can be successfully treated by medical therapy.[27–29] Surgical intervention is only indicated for patients who do not respond to medical therapy, those who develop complications, and those who are hospitalized with persistent fever. This last group of patients includes several common variations, including, most commonly, those cared for in the intensive care unit (ICU). Usually, these patients are intubated, recumbent, and receiving intravenous antibiotics. A consult may be requested to rule out sinusitis, either because of persistent fever or because a computed tomography (CT) or magnetic resonance imaging (MRI) study demonstrates mucosal thickening or opacification. The initial management recommended is to remove any nasal tubes, start the patient on topical decongestants, and obtain sinus cultures by direct sinus aspiration. If subsequent management fails, then surgical intervention is indicated.

Other hospitalized patients with persistent fever that may be attributable to sinusitis include transplant patients and those with human immunodeficiency virus (HIV) infection. Management of these patients is very similar to that of the ICU patient.

When surgery is performed for acute sinusitis, the goal of surgery is to achieve adequate drainage. This can be accomplished by a number of techniques. The traditional standard approach is to drain the maxillary sinus through a simple inferior nasal antral window.[30] In most circumstances, this will result in drainage and resolution of the acute infection. The alternatives include middle meatus antrostomy performed by ESS or a CL procedure. In most cases, ESS is preferred as this is a more physiologic procedure in that it results in augmented natural drainage. There is also the possibility that ESS would resolve the underlying cause of the infection. A CL procedure is not usually performed in this setting. However, a CL operation was performed in one patient with acute sinusitis and a dental abscess of the upper canine tooth resulting in facial abscess, orbital cellulitis, and maxillary sinusitis. Initial ESS revealed the sinus to be filled with gray, watery fluid with necrosis of the mucosa. The CL procedure was performed not only to ensure complete removal of the necrotic mucosa but also to remove the underlying devitalized bone and decompress the orbit.

Mucoceles

The maxillary sinus is the least common site for paranasal sinus mucoceles.[31] Like the other sinuses, mucoceles of the maxillary sinus can be treated by either simple drainage through the natural ostium or by open approaches. The decision of which technique to employ will depend on the specific nature of the mucocele being treated. Mucoceles that fill the sinus and are accessible through a middle meatus antrostomy may be well treated by ESS. Conversely, certain mucoceles may not fill the sinus and may be at a distance from the natural ostium. The classic example of this is the cyst that sometimes develops following a CL procedure. Widely reported throughout Japan[32] but rarely reported in the United States, this condition is thought to be related to mucosa getting trapped in the anterior wall during closure and subsequently growing into a cyst or mucocele.

Another indication for performing the CL procedure to remove a mucocele is extension outside the sinus through the anterior or lateral wall. In these cases, which are usually post-traumatic, drainage through the natural ostium may not completely decompress the entire mucocele if part of the cyst is in a dependent position outside the sinus.

Mucous Retention Cysts

Mucous retention cysts are typically in and of themselves not an indication for surgery. Isolated maxillary retention cysts are extremely common and very slow growing. Most of the time, these cysts will have imperceptible growth from year to year. The need to treat a maxillary retention cyst surgically is dictated by the presence of signs of growth, bone erosion, or enlargement to the point of obstructing the sinus drainage.

When surgery is required, simple drainage will result in only temporary treatment. Subtotal or even total removal may be possible through the natural ostium by ESS.[33] In this case, even if a small remnant of cyst wall is left behind, the cyst may not recur or may recur as a small, slow-growing cyst. If enlargement is sufficient to result in bone erosion, then the logical approach would be a CL procedure.[34] In such cases, a limited opening just large enough to effect complete excision can be created.

Technique

Preoperative Considerations

Candidates for a Caldwell-Luc or nasal antral window procedure typically undergo some type of preoperative radiographic imaging. Prior to the introduction of ESS and CT scanning for sinus surgery, most patients would undergo plain x-ray studies, especially the Waters view. Now, given the easy availability of CT scans, this imaging modality should be considered mandatory prior to any sinus surgery, including a CL or nasal antral window procedure. The goals of CT evaluation include delineation of the distribution of mucosal disease within the sinuses, as well as anatomic definition. Of specific interest to the CL operation is the development and aeration of the maxillary sinus. This information can facilitate initial entry into the sinus and can help avoid injury to the orbit, teeth, and infraorbital nerve.

A second consideration is the use of antibiotics. Because of pre-existing infection, most patients will be receiving antibiotic therapy prior to surgery. In those patients who are not being treated with antibiotics prior to the day of surgery, intravenous antibiotics should be administered 1 hour before surgery. Although the need for prophylactic antibiotics in sinus surgery has not been definitively established, Caldwell-Luc surgery is classified as contaminated surgery and so is among a class of procedures for which perioperative antibiotics are thought to be beneficial.

Most patients undergoing a CL procedure will have general anesthesia, although this is not mandatory. General anesthesia for this procedure has the advantage of allowing the procedure to be performed comfortably and rapidly with no restriction on retraction. The endotracheal tube should be secured to the lower lip just inside the corner of the mouth. If a bilateral CL is to be performed, the tube is secured in the midline.

Preparation

To begin the CL procedure, the patient is positioned on the operating room table with the head angled to the right for a right-handed surgeon and to the left for a left-handed surgeon. The table is turned to allow the assistants to stand on the opposite side. The surgeon should wear a headlight to improve visualization inside the sinus during the procedure. Usually, no skin preparation is necessary to sterilize the skin. Because the incision is made through a contaminated mucous membrane, skin preparation would not be expected to be beneficial.

Topical and injected local anesthetics are both routinely used. The nose is decongested using pledgets and a solution, usually 4% cocaine solution. Oxymetazoline may also be used and has been shown to have similar efficacy. The sublabial mucosa over the incision is injected with 3 to 5 mL of local anesthetic per side to assist in hemostasis. Lidocaine (1%) with epinephrine (1 : 100,000) is the favored compound and is well tolerated in almost every situation. A 25- or 27-gauge needle with a control syringe facilitates accurate and judicious placement of the local anesthetic. Topical and local agents should be administered 5 to 10 minutes before incision to achieve adequate effect.

Incision

Two army-navy retractors are used to expose the undersurface of the lip. The incision is made 5 mm above the gingival labial sulcus (Fig. 10–1). This incisional site is

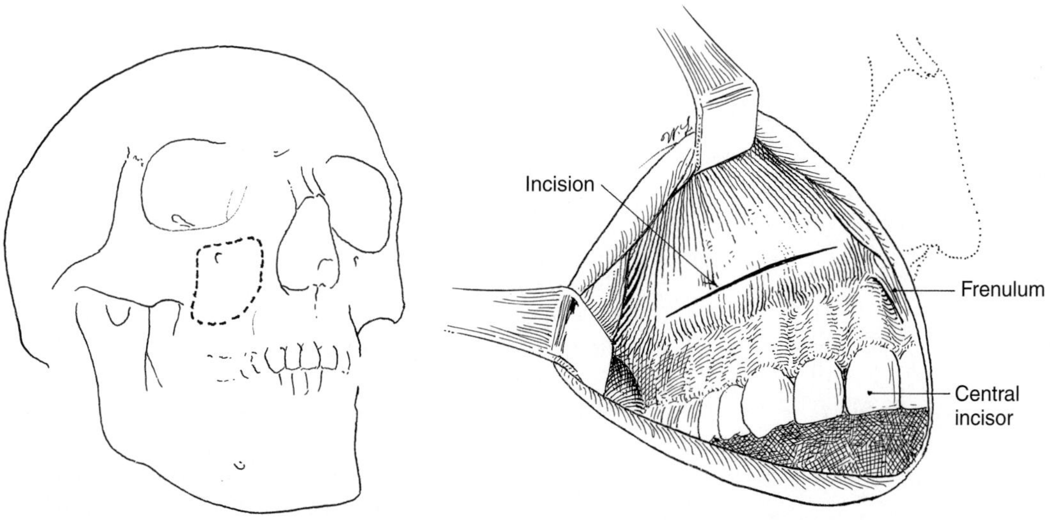

Figure 10–1. Incision for Caldwell-Luc procedure. The incision, which is placed 5 mm above the gingival labial sulcus, extends medially from the lateral incisor to the end of the alveolar ridge laterally.

selected in order to facilitate closure of the wound. By preserving this cuff of mucosa, closure is facilitated by having two mobile surfaces to reapproximate. The gingiva normally has little or no elasticity and does not support a suture, as stitches placed through the gingiva tend to tear and pull out. Also, the creation of an adequate cuff helps to avoid restriction of the lip. The initial incision is made with a No. 15 scalpel. Some surgeons use electrocautery to make this incision, but the advantage of improved hemostasis is more than offset by the excessive damage to the surrounding mucosa. However, once the initial incision is made, the subcutaneous tissues down through the periosteum can be divided with cautery. When cutting through the submucosal tissues, it is important to make sure that the dissection is kept as low as possible to avoid injury to branches of the inferior orbital nerve. The entire length of the incision should extend medially from a site close to the midline to the end of the alveolar ridge laterally. If only a small opening is being made into the sinus, the incision can be limited, but there is no reason to restrict the length of the incision and impair exposure.

Exposure

With the incision through the periosteum completed, the next step is to elevate the periosteum from the maxilla. A Freer elevator or a suitable substitute is used. Small vascular perforators will be avulsed in the process, but these cause little or no bleeding and usually stop bleeding spontaneously. The final exposure should extend from the pyriform aperture medially to the end of the alveolar ridge and superiorly to the infraorbital nerve (Fig. 10–2). During elevation, it is important to proceed slowly in the superior direction until the infraorbital nerve is identified. The nerve is located approximately in the mid-pupillary line about 1 cm below the infraorbital rim. Exposure can be achieved superior to this point if necessary, but this will increase the risk of stretch injury from retraction.

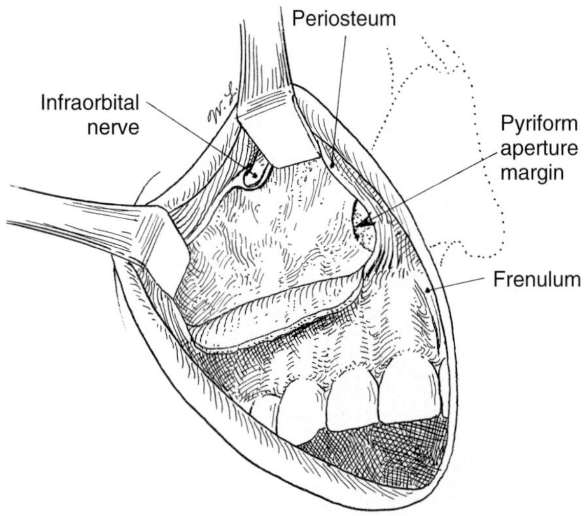

Figure 10–2. Sublabial exposure before osteotomy for Caldwell-Luc procedure. The infraorbital nerve is identified superiorly and preserved.

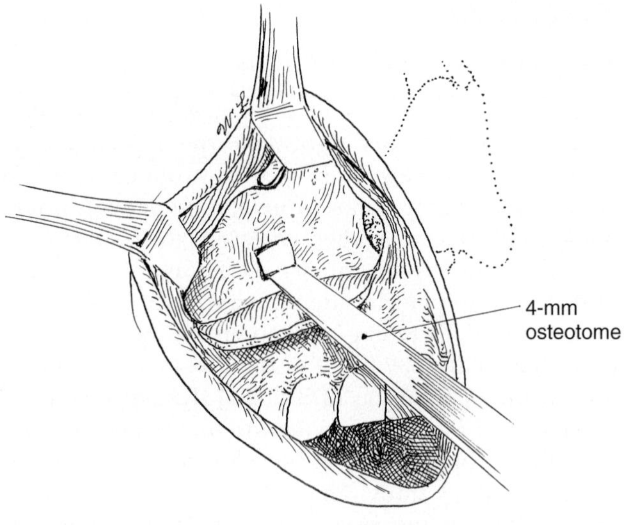

Figure 10–3. Initial osteotomy for Caldwell-Luc procedure. A small window of bone is created through the canine fossa using a 4-mm osteotome.

Entry into the maxillary sinus is initiated through the canine fossa (Fig. 10–3). The preferred technique is to use a small, 4-mm osteotome. Rather than just tear into the sinus at this location, a 5-mm square is outlined in this area with the osteotome and then pushed into the sinus. The bone from this window can subsequently be removed after the window is enlarged. A Kerison rongeur is then used to enlarge the opening into the sinus to the size required for the surgery. The ultimate size of the anterior antrostomy will depend on the procedure being performed. If the goal is to remove inspissated secretions or limited mucosal disease, then only a small opening is needed. However, in the case of a mucocele, extensive mucosal disease, orbital decompression, tumor surgery, or transantral ethmoidectomy, maximal exposure is required. In such cases, the entire anterior wall can be removed, leaving the infraorbital nerve encased by a peninsula of bone (Fig. 10–4).

Osteoplastic Flap

The osteoplastic flap of the anterior wall of the maxillary sinus is an alternative to the traditional Caldwell-Luc procedure.[35–38] This technique was proposed as a method for minimizing trauma to the infraorbital nerve and better preserving the sinus after surgery. Many patients develop contracture and even obliteration of the sinus following CL surgery as a result of collapse of the anterior wall and ingrowth of fibrous tissue secondary to the large anterior wall defect. In this operation, the bone of the anterior wall is preserved and elevated as a flap still attached to the overlying periosteum.

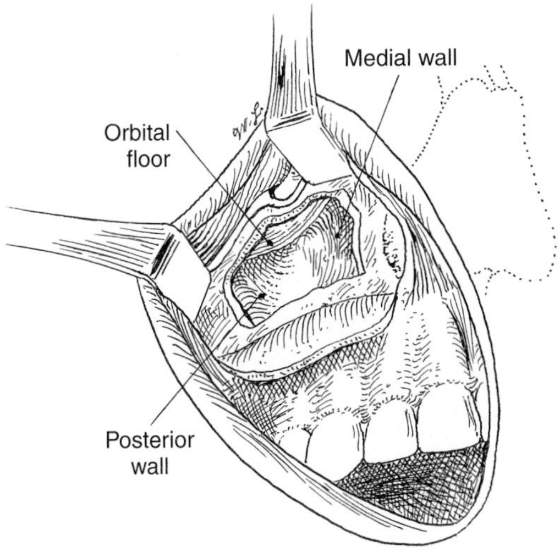

Figure 10–4. Completed anterior antrostomy for Caldwell-Luc procedure. The entire inside of the sinus is visible.

The initial steps are the same as those outlined earlier for the traditional technique through an incision in the periosteum. However, instead of the entire facial soft tissue being elevated from the face of the maxilla, submucosal elevation is performed superficial to the periosteum. Periosteal incisions are created medially along the pyriform aperture and laterally along the maxillary buttress with the central area left attached. Once this is accomplished, either an osteotome or a microsaw is used to create an osteotomy around the anterior surface of the maxilla, through the inferior incision and the medial and lateral periosteal incisions (Fig. 10–5).

With the bone cuts made, the inferior edge of the bone flap is slowly and gently elevated using elevators or osteotomes at several points on the undersurface of the flap. This will create a fracture superiorly, just below the level of the infraorbital nerve. Care must be taken to avoid extending the fracture too far inferiorly, but as long as the fracture is carefully controlled, even if it occurs through the infraorbital foramen, the nerve should be preserved and remain uninjured. The flap is then retracted superiorly using either malleable retractors or a suitable substitute. The remainder of the procedure is carried out as indicated below.

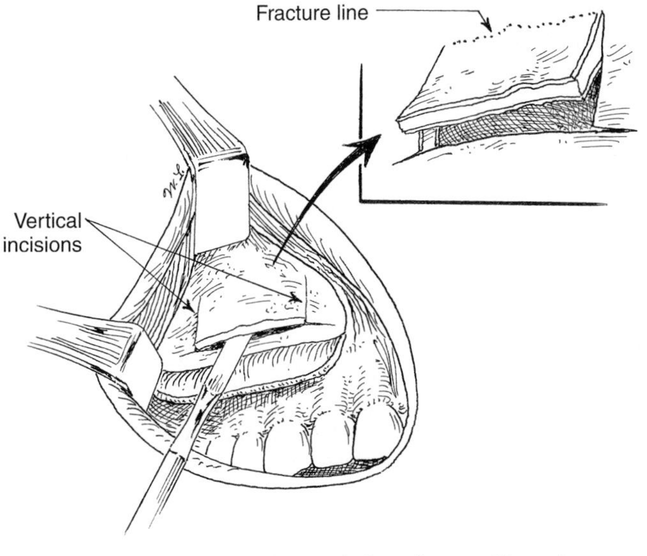

Figure 10–5. Osteoplastic flap technique for maxillary sinus surgery. The initial soft tissue elevation is superficial to the periosteum. Inferior, medial, and lateral osteotomies are created and the bone flap is gently elevated, creating a superior bone fracture at or just below the infraorbital nerve.

Removal of Pathologic Material

The principle of mucosal resection during the Caldwell-Luc procedure is to preserve as much normal mucosa as possible. The minimal procedure allows removal of inspissated secretions only, as may be appropriate in cases of cystic fibrosis or fungal sinusitis. In such cases, a small anterior antrostomy is all that is needed. Large mucous retention cysts can be removed with preservation of all mucosa but the attachment zone of the cyst. The same principle can be applied to cholesterol granulomas and localized polyps. Diffuse, inflammatory swelling and polyps filling the sinus should be approached through an antrostomy that is large enough to allow easy access to the entire sinus. In this situation, rather than complete stripping of the mucosa, it is recommended that intramucosal debridement be performed. In this procedure, the periosteum is preserved but the overlying submucosa and epithelial layer are removed using a curette (Fig. 10–6). This technique has the

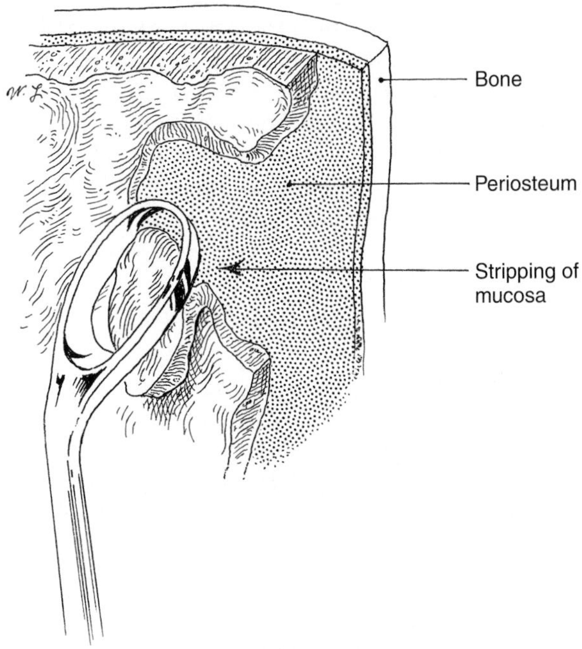

Figure 10–6. Intramucosal dissection. A sharp curette is required for this dissection in which the periosteum is preserved and the overlying mucosa and submucosa are resected. This is possible only with edematous and inflamed mucosa.

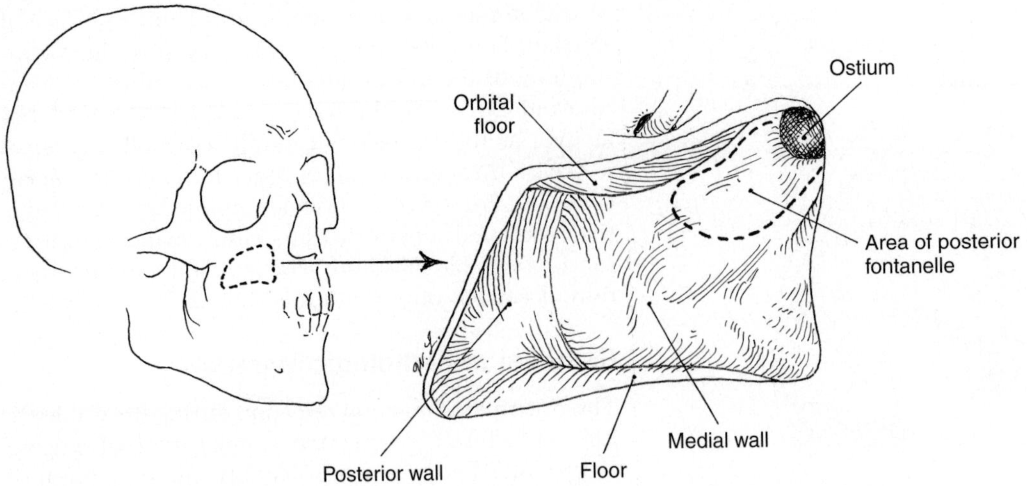

Figure 10–7. Medial wall of the maxillary sinus as viewed from the sublabial approach. The natural ostium lies anterior and superior along the wall. The posterior fontanelle or membranous portion of the medial wall is outlined.

advantage of removal of the inflammatory process without exposure of the underlying bone, thereby minimizing the risk of osteitis and subsequent bone thickening.

Antrostomy

Following the removal of diseased mucosa, an antrostomy must be created for drainage. The traditional site for antrostomy has been the inferior meatus; however, currently, the middle meatus antrostomy is considered to be a more physiologic site, making this the preferred option. In either case, antrostomy through the sublabial approach is a simple procedure. The goal is to create an opening large enough to allow adequate drainage and easy packing removal. The middle meatus antrostomy begins at the natural ostium. The initial step is to incise and remove the posterior fontanelle (Fig. 10–7). This is done in a piecemeal fashion using either a Kerison forceps or scissors to incise the fontanelle along the floor of the orbit and along the top of the inferior turbinate. The fontanelle is left pedicled on the posterior wall of the sinus. This is then cut and the tissue removed. With this accomplished, it is important to remove the uncinate process to make sure that the antrostomy does not close from scarring. The uncinate is removed through the antrostomy using upturned Blakesley forceps (Fig. 10–8). Alternatively, this can be accomplished endoscopically or transnasally using a speculum and headlight.

The more traditional technique is to perform an inferior antrostomy. Done through the sublabial approach, the first step is to identify the entry point (Fig. 10–9). The ideal spot is a few millimeters above the floor of the sinus halfway from anterior to posterior. Any sharp instrument, such as a fine hemostat, J-curette, or rat-tailed rasp, can be used to puncture the wall into the

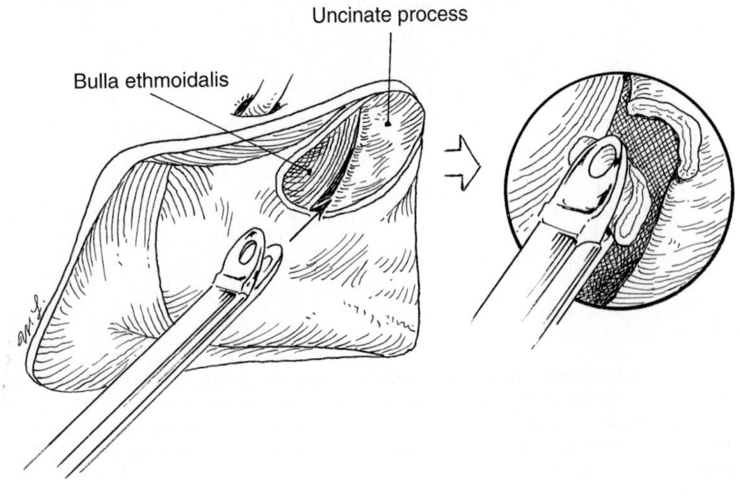

Figure 10–8. Sublabial view through the completed middle meatus antrostomy. The uncinate process and bulla ethmoidalis are exposed.

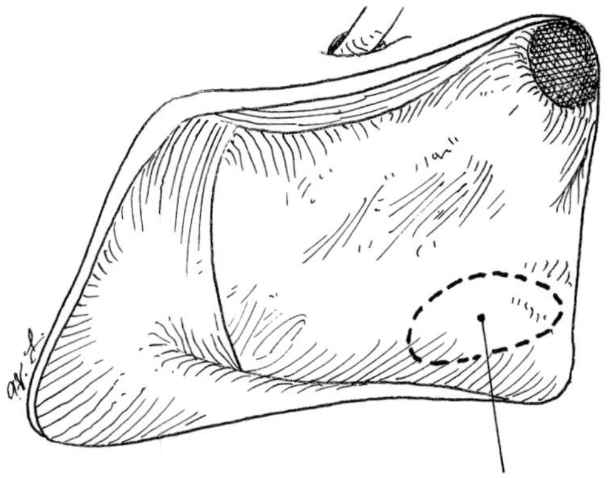

Figure 10–9. Position of an inferior meatus antrostomy as seen from the sublabial view. The dotted area represents the location of the antrostomy on the medial wall of the maxillary sinus.

nose. The opening is then enlarged circumferentially using both Kerison rongeurs and Blakesley forceps.

The same procedure can be performed transnasally. After the nose is decongested and the inferior meatus is injected with local anesthesia, the puncture site is identified. The inferior turbinate can be in-fractured and displaced by the nasal speculum to better expose the surgical area. The ideal site is approximately 1 to 2 cm posterior to the anterior attachment of the inferior turbinate and 5 mm above the floor of the nose (Fig. 10–10). The puncture is made with the same instrument used in the sublabial procedure. The entry is enlarged using Kerison rongeurs in the anterior direction and either Blakesley or Takahashi forceps in the posterior direction.

The last step is to smooth out the edges of the antrostomy. This can be done using any number of techniques and instruments, including a rasp, curette, or rongeurs. The purpose of this is to make sure that loose bone chips and sharp edges are not left behind, as these will cause discomfort upon removal of the packing and increase the risk of stenosis of the antrostomy.

Closure

Prior to closure, some method of hemostasis is required. Cautery can be used to stop bleeding from the mucosal edges, and bone bleeding can be stopped with bone wax. If this is done effectively, the sinus can be filled with antibiotic ointment and the incision closed. The advantage of this technique is that no packing is required. Packing removal is usually painful and bacterial colonization of the pack can occur, delaying healing or causing postoperative infection.

Traditional management involves packing with strip gauze (Fig. 10–11). The packing material is usually coated with either Vaseline or antibiotic ointment to decrease discomfort at removal. Use of an antibiotic ointment may help to decrease bacterial growth on the packing material. One end of the pack is placed through the antrostomy into the nose and brought out of the nose anteriorly. It is worthwhile to slide the packing back and forth across the anterior lip of the antrostomy to make sure that it will not catch on any residual sharp edges. The packing is then layered in anterior-to-posterior strips from medial to lateral until the sinus is filled. The goals are to avoid knotting the packing

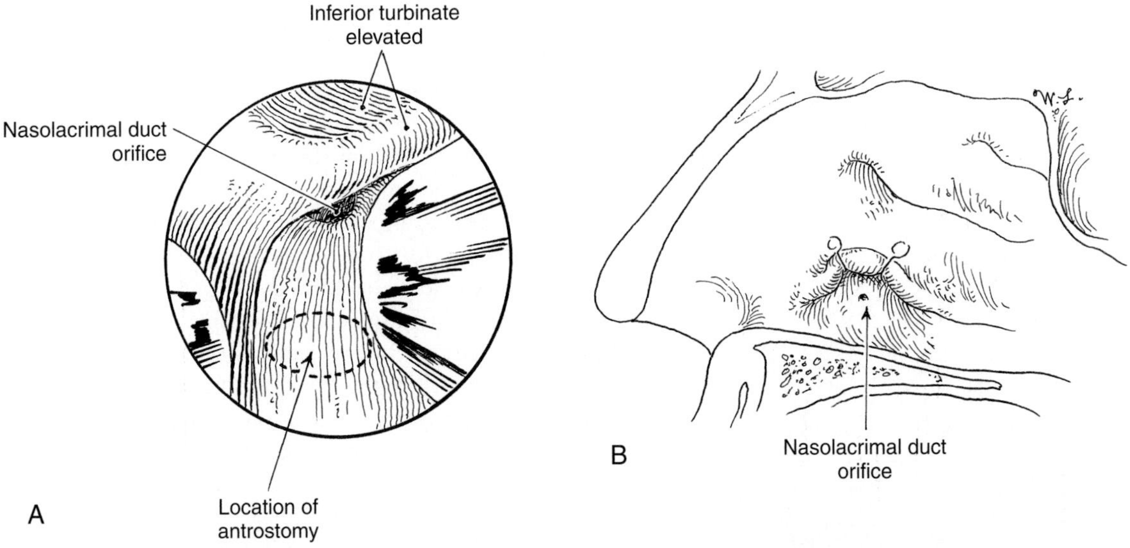

Figure 10–10. Intranasal view of the inferior meatus antrostomy. *A,* Surgical view with the inferior turbinate displaced superiorly by a nasal speculum. At the apex of the inferior meatus, the orifice of the nasolacrimal duct can be seen. *B,* Anatomic view of the location of the orifice of the nasolacrimal duct. The antrostomy is placed inferior to this structure.

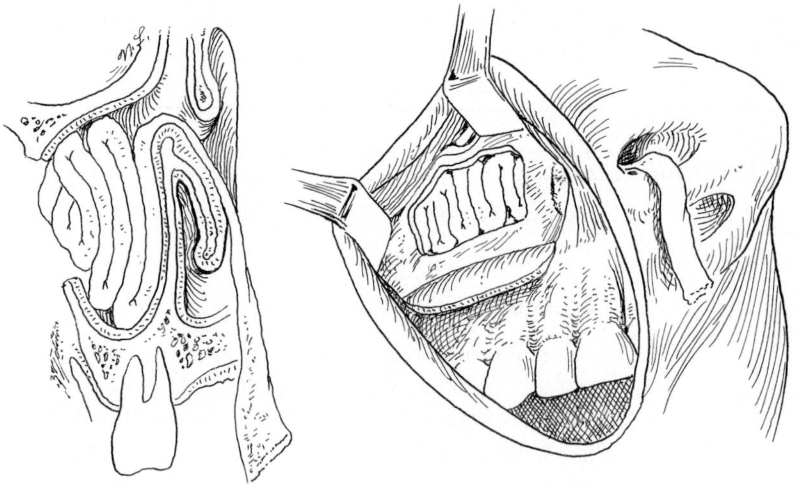

Figure 10–11. Anatomic and surgical views of completed packing. The packing material is layered into the sinus and brought out of the nose through, in this case, a middle meatus antrostomy.

and to ensure that adequate packing is placed to achieve the desired hemostasis.

The incision may then be closed by a variety of techniques (Fig. 10–12). Interrupted or running sutures can be placed using absorbable or permanent suture material. Most surgeons use an interrupted 3-0 chromic suture. However, this loses strength quickly and has been associated with a high risk of dehiscence. For this reason, 3-0 Vicryl sutures on a tapered needle are preferred. It is not necessary to remove this type of suture, but it does tend to persist for up to 4 to 6 weeks before degrading and falling out.

Postoperative Care

Following surgery, the patient may be hospitalized, kept overnight, or discharged. The decision will rest on the duration of surgery, underlying medical problems, and the postoperative recovery of the patient. Most patients will be able to be discharged the day of surgery after only a short period of observation. Immediate postoperative considerations include applying ice to the face, administering adequate pain medication, and monitoring for bleeding.

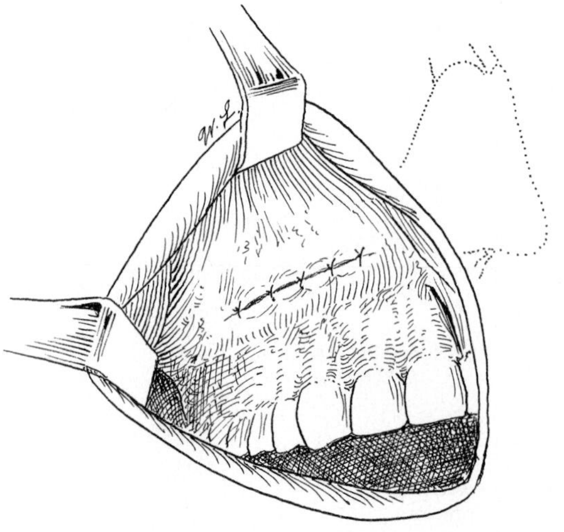

Figure 10–12. Final closure after a Caldwell-Luc procedure.

After discharge, patients should continue to apply ice to the face for 24 hours. Activity should be restricted to bed rest the first night and then nonstrenuous activities for 1 to 2 weeks after that. Diet is generally as tolerated. Oral rinses are prescribed to keep the incision clean beginning the second day after surgery. Medications include only analgesics and antibiotics. Usually, acetaminophen with codeine is all that is necessary for pain relief. However, as with all surgery, the degree of pain perception will vary markedly from individual to individual and the prescription should, in all cases, be adequate for the individual patient. Antibiotics should cover the routine bacteria of chronic sinusitis and any organisms cultured from the sinuses at the time of surgery. Antibiotic therapy should be continued for a minimum of 2 weeks after surgery, with additional treatment as indicated by the clinical course.

Patients are seen back in the office for removal of packing. The packing may be removed as early as 48 hours after surgery but typically is removed 3 to 5 days postoperatively. When removing the packing, the patient should be advised that some bleeding may occur. If bleeding occurs during packing removal, removal should be discontinued until the bleeding stops. After the packing is completely removed, the patient is instructed to do periodic nasal irrigations using normal saline. The patient is then seen back in the office every 2 weeks for cleaning of the antrostomy until crusting subsides and healing is complete.

Complications

The complications associated with the Caldwell-Luc procedure are numerous and frequent.[15, 32, 39–44] The most common complications relate to injuries to the infraorbital nerve or its branches. Such injury has been reported to occur in 9% to 46% of patients undergoing this operation.[40, 41, 44] Damage to the nerve may be attributable either to a stretch injury secondary to retraction or to inadvertent transection. In addition, the branches of the superior alveolar nerve innervating the maxillary teeth can be damaged during creation of the anterior antrostomy if the bone removal extends too far inferiorly.

These injuries most commonly result in anesthesia of the upper lip, face, or teeth. Some affected patients may manifest a chronic pain syndrome related to neuralgia from stretch injury, nerve entrapment by scar tissue, or aberrant nerve regeneration. Management of neuropathic pain is outside the scope of this textbook, but may involve many options ranging from anti-inflammatory medications to tricyclic antidepressants and from nerve decompression to trigeminal neurolysis. The appropriate management of these patients should be decided in consultation with a qualified pain management specialist. The essential job of the otolaryngologist in this setting is to make a correct diagnosis, properly differentiating this injury from recurrent sinusitis. A full spectrum of diagnostic strategies, including CT scan, endoscopy, and serial examination and trial of medication, should be used.

Other complications include facial swelling, fever, bleeding, and infection. Some degree of facial swelling is expected after all Caldwell-Luc operations.[44] In some cases, however, the amount of swelling can be severe, leading to orbital swelling and even eye closure. This severe swelling implies facial hematoma, and should be managed with ice and facial pressure. If continued facial swelling jeopardizes the eye, then reexploration of the wound is indicated to locate the source of hemorrhage and directly control the bleeding.

Normally, postoperative bleeding from the nose, wound, or into the throat is minimal to nonexistent. In cases in which heavy or persistent bleeding is present, however, initial management includes controlling the patient's pain, elevating the head of the bed, and applying ice to the face. If bleeding is persistent despite these measures, nasal packing is added. If this does not control the bleeding, reexploration is warranted to identify the site of hemorrhage and to control it directly by either packing or cautery.

The most dangerous complication of Caldwell-Luc surgery is injury to the eye. This can occur as a result of direct injury during tissue removal or compression from postoperative hemorrhage. The incidence of this type of injury is exceedingly rare. Management of the injury should be performed in consultation with an ophthalmologist and, if related to intraorbital hemorrhage, according to protocols for management of this problem.

MAXILLARY SINUS OBLITERATION AND COLLAPSE

Among the operations for treatment of chronic maxillary sinusitis, sinus obliteration and collapse is seldom used. These operations are similar in terms of both indications and techniques, with the only difference being that one operation involves filling the sinus with an autogenous fat graft and the other involves filling the sinus with local fat from the buccal space and pterygomaxillary fissure. To date, the author has performed this procedure in only five patients, with success being achieved in four of the five.

Indications

Maxillary sinus obliteration and collapse is recommended only as an absolute last resort in patients with refractory chronic sinusitis. The initial surgical treatment of choice for these patients is either the standard endoscopic approach or a Caldwell-Luc operation. However, there are rare instances in which patients do not respond to these more traditional or conservative measures, three examples of which are cited here. In none of these cases was there hope that infection could be resolved with further antibiotic therapy or traditional surgery.

One such patient was a 35-year-old woman with a chronic arthritic condition requiring chronic methotrexate therapy. This resulted in immunosuppression and chronic sinusitis. Over a 3-year period she underwent two endoscopic and two Caldwell-Luc procedures without improvement. She had bilateral pansinusitis which, curiously, spared the right maxillary sinus only. The patient had undergone a total of almost 6 months of intravenous antibiotic therapy without relief. A combination osteoplastic frontal obliteration and left maxillary obliteration was performed. Since surgery, the patient has been without serious infection and off antibiotics for two years.

A second patient was an adult with cystic fibrosis. He had had his first sinus surgery—an endoscopic procedure—at the age of 16. When he was 18 years old, he underwent repeat endoscopic sinus surgery. By the age of 21, recurrent infection was diagnosed, for which he underwent a third endoscopic sinus surgery. Over the ensuing 5 years, he required four more procedures, including a frontal sinus obliteration and Caldwell-Luc procedure on three occasions. At 27 years of age, he underwent a maxillary sinus collapse procedure. Since that time, he has required only routine nasal cleaning, and no further surgery has been needed in the ensuing 18 months.

A third patient was born with combined variable immunodeficiency syndrome. Throughout her life, she has had recurrent sinus, ear, throat, pulmonary, and urinary tract infections. At age 32, she underwent bilateral endoscopic sinus surgery, after which CT scanning revealed a well-healed ethmoid cavity and clear frontal, ethmoid, and sphenoid sinuses. However, bilateral maxillary sinusitis persisted despite a wide-open middle meatus antrostomy and clear ethmoid sinuses. She received intravenous antibiotic therapy for almost a full year with control of the infection. However, every time intravenous antibiotics were discontinued she immediately experienced a relapse and developed pain, drainage, and severe cough. She underwent bilateral maxillary sinus obliteration with autogenous fat grafts and with local mucosal rotation flaps from the roof of the sinus to close the antrostomy. She achieved primary healing and, three months after surgery, is doing well without intravenous antibiotics.

The decision to obliterate with a fat graft versus collapse with local fat is made based on the patient's anatomy. The patient with cystic fibrosis just described had very small, atrophic sinuses measuring about 5 cc or less. By removing the anterior, lateral, and posterior walls of the maxillary sinuses and gently pulling on the fat, the sinus cavity could be completely filled. Postoperative endoscopic examinations reveal that the area of the mucosa smoothly flows from the lamina papyracea onto the inferior turbinate. The other two patients had normal-sized sinuses and, therefore, required autogenous fat grafts for obliteration of the cavities.

Technique

These maxillary sinus operations are performed under general anesthesia after sterile prepping of the face and abdomen. The initial approach follows that of a standard Caldwell-Luc procedure. On initial entry into the sinus, it is important to obtain a direct sample of the sinus contents for culture to ensure that postoperative antibiotic therapy is organism-specific. Once the entire anterior wall has been removed with preservation of the infraorbital foramen, the mucosa is removed. If a large antrostomy is present, then the mucosa from the roof of the sinus (floor of the orbit) is elevated carefully from lateral to medial and rotated down to the upper border of the inferior turbinate. The flap can later be sewn to the inferior turbinate if this is possible.

The initial mucosal removal is done with a Freer elevator and Takahashi forceps. After the mucosa is completely removed, a drill is used to remove bone. The entire inner surface of the sinus is carefully polished with a diamond burr to remove any microscopic mucosal remnants. Special attention is given to several areas, including the area over the infraorbital nerve. If this nerve is dehiscent, microdissection of mucosa from the nerve may be necessary. The area over the tooth roots in the floor of the sinus may contain thin bone, so care should be taken to avoid injury to the innervation and actual tooth roots. The area of the medial wall may be without bone, and the mucosa may be firmly atttached to the nasal mucosa on the undersurface of the mucosa. In this case, cautery can be used to destroy the mucosal remnants without resecting the nasal mucosa.

Special attention is given to the bone on the inside of the sinus in areas where osteitic changes are observed on CT scan or at surgery. All potentially diseased bone is completely resected using cutting or diamond burrs or a Kerison rongeur. This careful extirpation is necessary to avoid reinfection of the graft by the infected bone.

If sinus collapse is indicated, the bone of the lateral and posterior walls is completely removed. This is accomplished without disturbing the zygomatic buttress of the maxilla or the bone of the floor of the orbit. The orbital bone can be thinned, but should be preserved at least as a thin layer. After the bone is removed, the periosteum on the outer surface of the sinus is incised and the underlying fat of the buccal and pterygomaxillary spaces is teased into the sinus cavity.

If sinus obliteration is being performed, the bone is drilled down to remove any osteitic components, but an outer shell is preserved. A fat graft is then harvested from a distant site (usually the abdomen) and placed into the sinus. The graft should be large enough to fill the entire cavity and should bulge slightly into the nose. The mucosal flap from the floor of the orbit will be placed over the surface of the fat graft, but probably will not cover it completely. If the flap is sutured to the inferior turbinate, the graft should gently bulge the flap inward toward the nose.

Postoperative Care

After surgery, postoperative care resembles that for patients undergoing the Caldwell-Luc procedure except that prolonged use of antibiotics is indicated. Culture and sensitivity testing should be used to guide the choice of antibiotic and the route of administration. Oral antibiotics are used if the pathogens are susceptible to oral agents. However, if the organisms that are cultured are resistant to oral antibiotics, a course of intravenous antibiotics therapy will be necessary. Antibiotic therapy should be continued for at least several weeks, and in most cases, a 6-week or longer course of antibiotics is prescribed.

Endoscopic follow-up evaluations to assess the sites of the previous antrostomies are performed at regular intervals until complete healing is achieved, usually within 3 to 6 weeks. The endoscopist should be careful not to debride the site of the antrostomy aggressively, and should remove only loose crusts and secretions. Densely adherent crusts are probably attached to the fat graft and so should be allowed to separate naturally.

Complications

In addition to the routine risks of the Caldwell-Luc procedure, sinus obliteration and collapse procedures are also associated with other risks. The most common complication is injury to the infraorbital nerve. Considering the multiple surgeries most of these patients have undergone prior to this operation, the stretching of the nerve to maximize exposure during the operation, and the drilling over the nerve to remove mucosa, some degree of injury should be expected. The long-term chances of recovery cannot be assessed at this time owing to the lack of patient data; however, normal recovery has been reported.

A second complication is impaired nasolacrimal drainage. If the nasolacrimal duct is anatomically intact at the start of the operation, the duct is likely to incur little or no damage. However, if previous endoscopic sinus surgery has resulted in inadvertent opening of the duct into the middle meatus, closure of the sinus may direct the flow of tears into the maxillary sinus cavity. In the author's experience, this occurred in one patient and caused the loss of the fat graft and failure of the operation.

REFERENCES

1. Caldwell GW. The accessory sinus of the nose, and an improved method of treatment for suppuration of the maxillary antrum. NY Med J 58:526, 1893.
2. Kennedy DW. Functional endoscopic sinus surgery. Technique. Arch Otolaryngol 111:643, 1985.
3. Kennedy DW, Zinreich SJ, Rosenbaum AE, et al. Functional endoscopic sinus surgery. Theory and diagnostic evaluation. Arch Otolaryngol 111:576, 1985.
4. Stammberger H. Endoscopic endonasal surgery—Concepts in treatment of recurring rhinosinusitis. Part I. Anatomic and pathophysiologic considerations. Otolaryngol Head Neck Surg 94:143, 1986.
5. Schaefer SD, Manning S, Close LG. Endoscopic paranasal sinus surgery: Indications and considerations. Laryngoscope 99:1, 1989.
6. Kennedy DW, Zinreich SJ, Kuhn F, et al. Endoscopic middle meatal antrostomy: Theory, technique, and patency. Laryngoscope 97:1, 1987.
7. Kamel RH. Endoscopic transnasal surgery in chronic maxillary sinusitis. J Laryngol Otol 103:492, 1989.
8. Schaitkin B, May M, Shapiro A, et al. Endoscopic sinus surgery: 4-Year follow-up on the first 100 patients. Laryngoscope 103:1117, 1993.
9. Liu C-M, Yeh T-H, Hsu M-M. Clinical evaluation of maxillary diffuse polypoid sinusitis after functional endoscopic sinus surgery. Am J Rhinology 8:7, 1994.
10. Rice DH. Endoscopic sinus surgery: Results at 2-year follow up. Otolaryngol Head Neck Surg 101:476, 1989.
11. Levine HL. Functional endoscopic sinus surgery: Evaluation, surgery, and follow-up of 250 patients. Laryngoscope 100:79, 1990.
12. Downie DB, Walster W. Endoscopic sinus surgery: A comparison of preoperative and postoperative status. Am J Rhinol 9:257, 1995.
13. Penttila MA, Rautiainen ME, Pukander JS, et al. Endoscopic versus Caldwell-Luc approach in chronic maxillary sinusitis: Comparison of symptoms at one-year follow-up. Rhinology 32(4):161, 1994.
14. Pentilla M, Rautianen M, Pukander J, Kataja M. Functional vs radical maxillary surgery. Failures after functional endoscopic sinus surgery. Acta Otolaryngo [Suppl] 529:173, 1997.
15. Unlu HH, Caylan R, Nalca Y, et al. An endoscopic and tomographic evaluation of patients with sinusitis after endoscopic sinus surgery and Caldwell-Luc operation: A comparative study. J Otolaryngol 23(3):197, 1994.
16. Blitzer A, Lawson W. The Caldwell-Luc procedure in 1991. Otolaryngol Head Neck Surg 105(5):717, 1991.
17. Yanagisawa E, Yanagisawa K. The Caldwell-Luc procedure—Is it still indicated in this endoscopic sinus surgery era? Ear Nose Throat J 76:294, 1997.
18. Politi M, Rossetti G, Consolo U, et al. Odontogenic sinusitis. An evaluation and the radiologic checkup protocol after a Caldwell-Luc intervention. Minerva Stomatol 39(2):119, 1990.
19. King JM, Caldarelli DD, Pigato JB. Review of revision functional endoscopic sinus surgery. Laryngoscope 104:404, 1994.
20. Ng M, Rice DH. Revision sinus surgery. Ear Nose Throat J 73(1):44, 1994.
21. Parsons DS, Stivers FE, Talbot AR. The missed ostium sequence and the surgical approach to revision functional endoscopic sinus surgery. Otolaryngol Clin North Am 29(1):169, 1996.
22. Ferreiro JA, Carlson BA, Cody DT III. Paranasal sinus fungus balls. Head Neck 19:481, 1997.
23. Saeed SR, Brookes GB. Aspergillosis of the paranasal sinuses. Rhinology 33:46, 1995.
24. Min Y-G, Kim HS, Lee K-S, et al. Aspergillus sinusitis: Clinical aspects and treatment outcome. Otolaryngol Head Neck Surg 115:49, 1996.
25. Crockett DM, McGill TJ, Friedman EM, et al. Nasal and paranasal sinus surgery in children with cystic fibrosis. Ann Otol Rhinol Laryngol 96:367, 1987.
26. Marks SC, Kissner DG. Management of sinusitis in adult cystic fibrosis. Am J Rhinol 11:11, 1997.
27. International Rhinosinusitis Advisory Board: Infectious rhinosinusitis in adults: Classification, etiology and management. Ear Nose Throat J 76(12):5, 1997.
28. Kennedy DW, Gwaltney JM Jr, Jones JG, et al. Medical management of sinusitis: Educational goals and management guidelines. Ann Otol Rhinol Laryngol 104:22, 1995.
29. Kaliner MA. Recurrent sinusitis: Examining medical treatment options. Am J Rhinol 11:123, 1997.
30. Legler U. Surgical drainage of the maxillary sinus through the inferior meatus. Rhinology 19(1):25, 1981.
31. Marks SC, Latoni JD, Mathog RH. Mucoceles of the maxillary sinus. Otolaryngol Head Neck Surg 117:18, 1997.
32. Iinuma T, Tanaka T, Kase Y, et al. On the postoperative mucocele of the maxillary sinus and its simulating cases. A clinical treatise. J Oto-Rhino-Laryngol Soc Japan 95(5):665, 1992.
33. Hadar T, Feinmesser R, Lisnyansky I, et al. Endoscopic treatment of maxillary sinus cysts. Harefuah 127(10):378, 1994.
34. Rolffs J, Schmelzle R, Schwenzer N, et al. Surgical therapy of odontogenic maxillary sinusitis. Report on 397 cases. Dtsch Zahnarztl Z 34(1):30, 1979.
35. Feldmann H: Osteoplastic operation of maxillary sinus. Laryngologie, Rhinologie, Otologie 57(5):373, 1978.
36. Akuamoa-Boateng E, Niederdellmann H, Fabinger A: Reconstruction of the facial fenestration in the Caldwell-Luc maxillary sinus operation. Rhinology 17(4):237, 1979.
37. Akuamoa-Boateng E, Fabinger A: Results of the reconstructive Caldwell-Luc method of surgery on the maxillary sinus. Dtsch Zahnarztl Z 35(1):134, 1980.
38. Sanderson BA. Physiologic maxillary antrostomy—update. Laryngoscope 93(2):180, 1983.

39. Murray JP. Complications after treatment of chronic maxillary sinus disease with Caldwell-Luc procedure. Laryngoscope 93(3): 282, 1983.
40. Low WK. Complications of the Caldwell-Luc operation and how to avoid them. Aust NZ J Surg 65(8):582, 1995.
41. Ferekidis E, Tzounakos P, Kandiloros D, et al. Modifications of the Caldwell-Luc procedure for the prevention of post-operative sensitivity disorders. J Laryngol Otol 110(3):228, 1996.
42. Walsted A, Raaschou HO, Bonding P. Surgical treatment of chronic maxillary sinusitis. Report of a new surgical technique and an evaluation of results of traditional surgery. Ugeskr Laeger 151(43):2802, 1989.
43. Stefansson P, Andreasson L, Jannert M. Caldwell-Luc operation: Long-term results and sequelaes. Acta Otolaryngol [Suppl] 449: 97, 1988.
44. DeFreitas J, Lucente FE. The Caldwell-Luc procedure: Institutional review of 670 cases: 1975–1985. Laryngoscope 98(12): 1297, 1988.

CHAPTER 11

Frontal Sinus Surgery

Inflammatory conditions of the frontal sinus are among the most serious conditions encountered in the practice of otolaryngology. The imminent possibility of intracranial complications dictates that all such patients be treated promptly and aggressively. Sinus surgery, which is usually elective and performed after extensive medical therapy trials, may become urgent or even emergent if the frontal sinus is involved. In practice, most patients with frontal sinus disease will eventually undergo some form of surgery.

Since the advent of frontal sinus surgery, many procedures have come and gone, failing to stand the test of time. Several reviews and previous publications have described these procedures in detail.[1-5] However, in the modern practice of rhinology, the surgical options have been reduced to the endoscopic procedures described in Chapter 8 and three open procedures: trephination, external frontal ethmoidectomy, and the osteoplastic flap. Each of these procedures has its advocates, specific indications, and well-described techniques. In this chapter, these three open procedures are discussed in detail, with emphasis on indications, surgical techniques, and perioperative management based on the author's experience.

FRONTAL SINUS TREPHINATION

Indications

Acute Frontal Sinusitis

As described in previous chapters, acute sinusitis is typically managed with antibiotics, decongestants, and mucolytics. However, in patients who require drainage, frontal sinus trephination has traditionally been the procedure of choice.[6-12] Many surgeons who are skilled in endoscopic sinus surgery are now advocating endoscopic drainage in lieu of trephination.[13, 14] Theoretically, this avoids a facial incision while promoting drainage and helping to prevent recurrent infections. However, the increased inflammation that is present during acute sinusitis makes the surgery more difficult owing to increased mucosal bleeding. Also, the acutely inflamed mucosa may predispose the patient to scarring and subsequent stenosis of the frontal sinus drainage. Because of these concerns, the relative scarcity of cases reported in the literature, and the minimal follow-up data available, endoscopic management of acute frontal sinusitis should be an option only for the most experienced endoscopic sinus surgeons.

Management of acute frontal sinusitis begins with accurate diagnosis. The most important symptom at the time of initial presentation is frontal headache or pain over the forehead. In a patient with symptoms of acute sinusitis, such as congestion, postnasal drainage, fever, otalgia, or throat irritation, the presence of moderate to severe frontal headache should immediately raise the possibility of acute frontal sinusitis. An examination may demonstrate the typical signs of acute sinusitis with purulent middle meatus secretions, erythema, and congestion. In mild cases, frontal tenderness may be absent; however, in moderate to severe cases, frontal sinus tenderness is usually present.

Plain radiographs of the sinuses may be helpful in further confirming the diagnosis. The best view for evaluating the frontal sinus is the straight anteroposterior view or Caldwell view. The most suggestive findings are either an air-fluid level or opacification of the frontal sinus. Other, less specific findings include mucosal thickening or a diffuse cloudiness. These latter findings are unreliable, however, and should not generally be accepted as evidence of acute frontal sinusitis.

When the diagnosis of acute frontal sinusitis is established, patients should be classified according to the severity of the condition (i.e., mild, moderate, or severe). Those with mild to moderate disease tend to have less frontal pain and headache, as well as negative findings on evaluation with plain radiographs. By contrast, the more severe cases are marked by severe frontal pain, significant tenderness, and findings of air-fluid levels or opacification demonstrated by a Caldwell view of the sinuses. Treatment of mild to moderate cases is the same as for routine sinus infections, and includes oral antibiotics and close monitoring. Patients with severe acute frontal sinusitis require more aggressive care.

Patients with severe acute frontal sinusitis should be hospitalized immediately and started on intravenous antibiotics. Emergent computed tomography (CT) scanning of the sinuses is routinely performed to confirm the diagnosis and delineate the extent of infection and the anatomic details of the sinuses. The choice of antibiotics will depend on various factors specific to the individual patient, including allergies to antibiotics and previous exposure to antibiotics. In straightforward cases, the antibiotic regimen of first choice is either ampicillin/sulbactam, cefuroxime plus clindamycin, or a third-generation cephalosporin with either clindamycin or vancomycin. If other combinations are necessary, then consultation with an infectious disease specialist is warranted. In addition to antibiotics, topical decongestants, nasal saline spray, and mucolytics should be prescribed.

The CT scan should be reviewed carefully for signs of impending complications. If bone erosion or expansion, or any sign of orbital or intracranial complication, is present, then surgery should be undertaken immediately. Trephination of the involved sinuses, whether unilateral or bilateral, should be scheduled as soon as the patient can be stabilized and surgery can be arranged. If no such complications are present, then expectant observation is appropriate. A prompt response with defervescence, decreased pain, and decreased tenderness should be manifested within the first day. In cases in which the response is not immediate, the decision to continue medical therapy alone must be reevaluated every 6 to 12 hours.

A decision to proceed to trephination should be made if the patient fails to improve after 48 hours. In addition, if, during the course of therapy, the symptoms worsen or complications arise, surgery should be performed immediately. Finally, if the acute episode subsides but does not resolve to the point of allowing discharge after 5 to 7 days of intravenous antibiotic therapy, this should be considered a relative indication to proceed to the trephination operation.

Chronic Sinusitis

In the modern practice of rhinology, trephination is not normally performed for chronic sinusitis. However, in some circumstances, trephination may be helpful as an adjunct to endoscopic or other intranasal surgery.[15–17] Trephination has two basic applications in chronic sinusitis. The first is when the frontal sinus contains inspissated secretions that cannot be removed through the natural ostium via an endoscopic approach. Trephination in this case is used to allow direct removal of the inspissated material.

The second situation arises when the internal ostium cannot be located during endoscopic intranasal frontal sinusotomy. In this rare instance, a trephination may be performed that allows the introduction of an instrument or probe into the sinus and through the ostium into the frontal recess. With direct visualization intranasally using an angled endoscope, it should then be possible to locate the internal ostium, allowing safe opening.

Mucocele

Mucoceles may occasionally arise in an inaccessible location, making endoscopic drainage impossible. In such cases, one reasonable option is to utilize either trephination alone or a combined endoscopic/trephination approach. This option is chosen when a mucocele or frontal sinus cyst occurs within a recess or loculation of the frontal sinus. The mucocele may be either lateral or superior within the sinus. Alternatively, an intrafrontal sinus cell may be the site of a mucocele. These cells have been categorized by Kuhn and colleagues.[18] The exact classification is probably not as important as the concept of intrafrontal cells not being accessible through the natural ostium.

If a mucocele of the frontal sinus is to be treated by trephination, the goal of the surgery may be either to resect the mucocele completely or to drain it into the sinus lumen or nasal cavity. In either case, the patient should be monitored closely for several years with repeat CT scans to confirm that the mucocele has not recurred.

Preoperative Considerations

Anesthesia

Frontal sinus trephination can be performed using general anesthesia or local anesthesia with intravenous sedation. For most patients, general anesthesia is preferred to avoid the discomfort associated with drilling on the frontal bone. Also, many of these cases are performed in conjunction with other sinus procedures, such as external ethmoidectomy or a Caldwell-Luc procedure, which typically are done under general anesthesia. Regardless of the form of anesthesia used, it is worthwhile to inject local anesthesia with epinephrine prior to the incision to improve hemostasis. Unless other procedures are being done concurrently, intranasal anesthesia is not necessary.

Preparation

Frontal sinus trephination is considered clean contaminated surgery, but since an external incision is made, the skin should be prepared in a sterile fashion. The technique used varies from region to region, but generally matches the standard of care for facial surgery set by area hospitals.

Antibiotics should be prescribed prior to the start of surgery. Most such patients will have been receiving intravenous antibiotics for several days before surgery, but if the patient is coming directly to the operating room from an outpatient setting, intravenous antibiotics should be started at least 1 hour before the operation.

The patient should be positioned supine with the head of the bed rotated to the right for a right-handed surgeon. The head is tilted toward the right and the neck is slightly extended. A shoulder roll is not necessary.

Technique

Incision

The type of incision made will depend on whether trephination or trephination in combination with an external ethmoidectomy is to be done. The trephination incision is a relatively short, curved incision that can be placed in the inferomedial aspect of the eyebrow (Fig. 11–1). The alternative is the standard Lynch incision with or without a W-plasty (as shown in Figs. 9–1 and 9–2).

After the local anesthetic is injected, an incision is made with a No. 15 scalpel through the skin and dermis. The subcutaneous tissue should be divided carefully to avoid injury to the supraorbital and supratrochlear nerves. These nerves exit the supraorbital foramen on the inferior aspect of the superior orbital rim 1 to 2 cm lateral to the nasion (Fig. 11–2). The supraorbital nerve is the most important and largest and should, in all cases, be preserved. The exact location of the supraorbital foramen can usually be palpated to establish the position. The dissection can be kept inferior and medial to this point to avoid injury. The subcutaneous tissue can be divided with cautery or dissected with scissors or a hemostat.

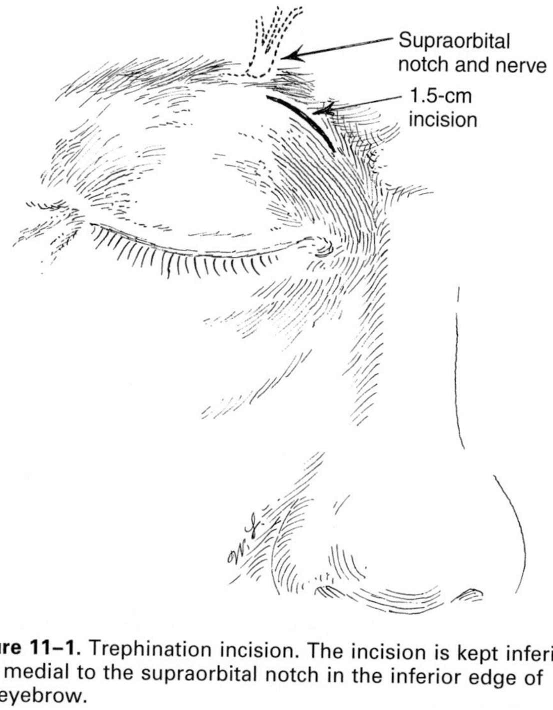

Figure 11–1. Trephination incision. The incision is kept inferior and medial to the supraorbital notch in the inferior edge of the eyebrow.

The periosteum is located and an incision is made approximately 2 cm along the medial orbital rim and nasal root. The periosteum is then elevated to expose the bone of the medial aspect of the superior orbital rim. This can be done with either a Freer or Joseph elevator. Again, it is important to be aware of the location of the supraorbital nerve during this step. The periosteum should be elevated sufficiently to allow a circle of bone measuring up to 1.5 cm in diameter to be exposed (Fig. 11–3).

Drilling

The actual trephination is performed using a drill. Many options are available, but the preferred instrument is an otologic drill with a small cutting burr. The site of trephination is on the underside of the orbital rim at the junction of the medial and superior orbital rims. For drainage alone, the opening need only be 5 mm, but its size may need to increase to up to 1.5 cm if mucocele resection is desired.

The drilling is performed slowly under constant irrigation using a circular motion. The depth of the defect as the drilling progresses should be maintained in an even fashion to avoid a deep hole. As the sinus is approached, the mucosa will create a blue shadow under the bone. When the mucosa is covered only by an eggshell of bone, the contents of the sinus can be aspirated with a needle and syringe. This serves two purposes: to obtain uncontaminated sinus contents for culture and to make sure that the opening is in the sinus and not intracranial. In the unlikely event that the trephination is misplaced, the aspirate will yield clear fluid, indicative of cerebrospinal fluid.

The initial entry into the sinus is made with a curette or drill. With the sinus open, the trephination is enlarged with a drill to a size appropriate for the pathology present. The final appearance of the trephination is illustrated in Figure 11–4. After the opening is completed, a sample of the sinus contents is obtained for culture (if not previously done) and the sinus is thoroughly irrigated.

Closure

Prior to skin closure, drainage catheters are usually placed (Fig. 11–5). An 8-French red rubber catheter is ideal for this purpose, but any suitable catheter is

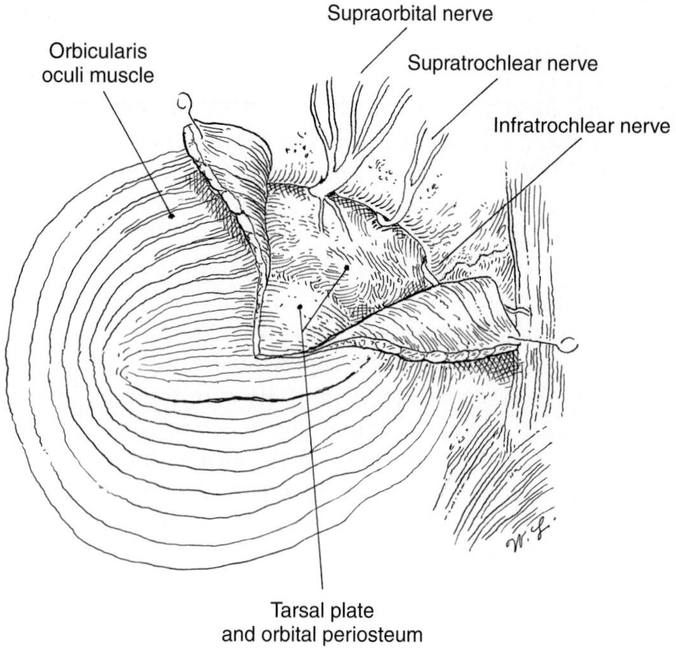

Figure 11–2. Anatomy of the supraorbital and supratrochlear nerves. In this case, there was not a complete annulus of bone around the nerve at the inferior edge of the orbital rim. This represents one of several possible variations.

acceptable. When using 8-French catheters, two short segments of equal length are usually cut and tied together at either end using a silk or nylon suture. The purpose of this is to allow inflow and outflow of irrigation fluid during flushing of the catheters. This prevents pressure build-up inside the sinus during irrigation if the frontal ostium is stenotic owing to edema or narrowing in the frontal recess.

In previously unoperated patients with acute sinusitis, the catheter tip can be positioned in the frontal sinus itself. After surgery, the catheter is irrigated several times per day until the irrigation fluid flows freely into the nose. The catheters can then be removed and the incision closed secondarily.

If the frontal sinus is obstructed, a catheter should be threaded into the frontal recess through the internal ostium of the sinus. This provides ongoing frontal sinus drainage as well as stenting of the frontal sinus outflow tract. After several days, this catheter can either be removed or cut off at the level of the trephination and retained as a stent for several more weeks. To enhance drainage function, side holes should be cut into the catheter prior to placement. When ready to be removed, the catheter is first located intranasally and then extracted through the nose.

Partial skin closure is performed at the time of surgery to close the incision around the catheter. A suture

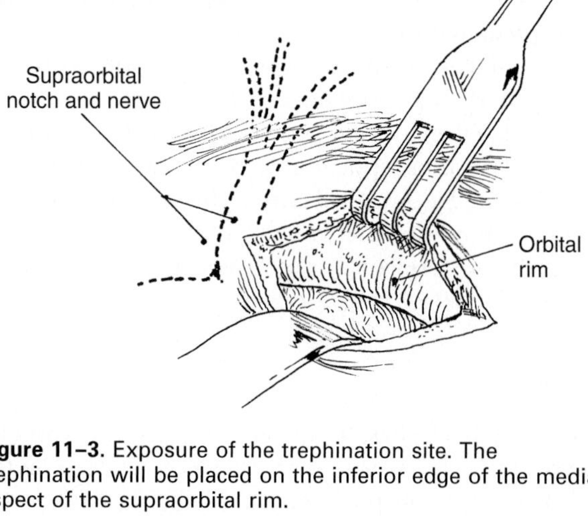

Figure 11–3. Exposure of the trephination site. The trephination will be placed on the inferior edge of the medial aspect of the supraorbital rim.

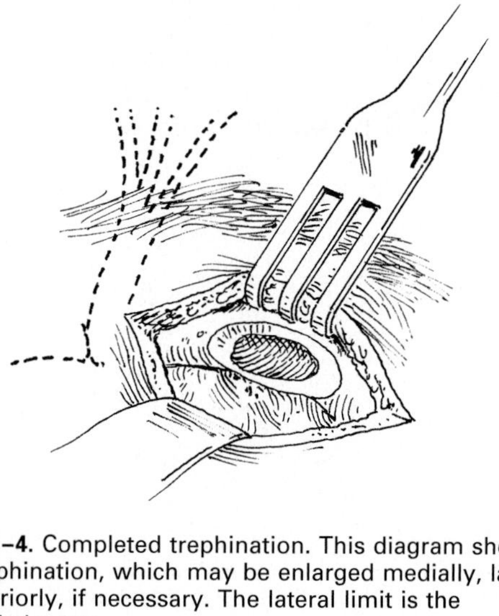

Figure 11–4. Completed trephination. This diagram shows a small trephination, which may be enlarged medially, laterally, and superiorly, if necessary. The lateral limit is the supraorbital nerve.

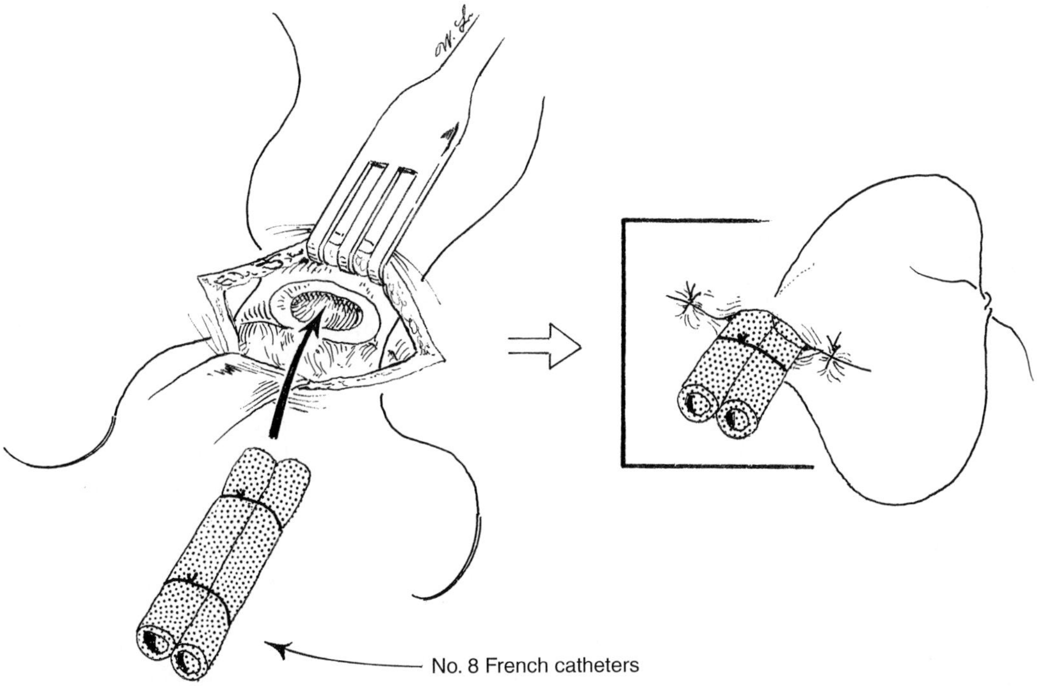

Figure 11–5. Wound closure. This demonstrates the use of double irrigation catheters and a preplaced suture for delayed closure.

can also be looped around the catheter and left loose, to be tied down after the catheter is removed. The incision is usually dressed with antibiotic ointment and a small gauze sponge is placed around the catheters.

Postoperative Care

The management of the frontal irrigation catheter will determine the duration of the postoperative course. The general guideline is to continue irrigations two or three times per day until the irrigation fluid flows freely into the nose. The fluid is usually normal saline, but antibiotic solutions are thought to have some efficacy.

The patient is hospitalized for several days after the surgery. The criteria for discharge include removal of the drains, resolution of the frontal tenderness and headache, and absence of fever with stable vital signs. The length of stay is variable depending on the individual circumstances of the patient.

Intravenous antibiotics are continued throughout the hospitalization and may be continued for an extended period after discharge if necessary. The initial choice of antibiotic is empiric and is based on previous antibiotic exposure and known results from previous cultures. Usually, multiple antibiotics are used to cover a broad spectrum of possible pathogens. When specific culture results are available, the antibiotic regimen is adjusted to reflect the bacteria isolated from the patient. Other medications used may include topical decongestants, oral decongestants, nasal steroid sprays, nasal saline mist, and systemic steroids as indicated.

A follow-up CT scan should be obtained after the surgery. If no other factors intervene, the CT may be delayed until 3 months after the operation. Waiting this long gives the sinus time to settle down from the acute episode, and if aeration is successful, a normal appearance will be able to be documented.

Complications

The complications associated with this procedure are minimal and not serious. The most likely problems are related to failure of the surgery to resolve the infection in the frontal sinus. It is difficult to get an accurate estimation of the risk of failure of this procedure. In the short term, failure of the surgery to resolve the acute sinusitis is unusual. The chances of a subsequent relapse of frontal sinusitis are greater. The chances of relapse after trephination are related to patency of the nasofrontal connection. Investigators from Finland have used rhinomamometry to evaluate the patency of this connection and have found that patency is associated with long-term success, whereas obstruction is associated with relapse.[19, 20]

More serious complications, including hematoma, orbital injury, and intracranial injury, are unlikely and have not been reported in the literature. However, all of these problems are possible if mistakes are made during surgery. The key to management of these injuries is early recognition and prompt appropriate response. The steps of management for each of these complications is covered in other chapters.

The last complication is related to the incision and scarring. If no drain or irrigation catheter is used, then primary closure is performed and the cosmetic result is predictably acceptable. If an irrigation catheter is left in place for several days after surgery, then the scar tends to be wide and can become hypertrophic. The best way to avoid this is by placing a suture at the drain site at the time of surgery and then tying it down at the time of drain removal. If the scar is unsatisfactory, then delayed revision 6 to 12 months after the initial surgery is advised.

FRONTOETHMOIDECTOMY

In years past, the frontoethmoidectomy operation was the most popular method of surgically treating chronic frontal sinusitis.[21–26] However, a combination of factors has led to the decline of this procedure's applicability. These factors include a relatively low success rate, facial scarring, and the introduction of the osteoplastic flap procedures and endoscopic sinus surgery. Indeed, the author chooses not to perform this operation, favoring instead an endoscopic approach for most patients and an osteoplastic flap operation for endoscopic failures. The frontoethmoidectomy, though, does continue to have advocates, mostly among surgeons not well versed in endoscopic techniques. Thus, for the sake of completeness, this procedure is covered in detail, including its indications for use, based on those established by its advocates.

Indications

Chronic Sinusitis

For proponents of the external frontoethmoidectomy, this operation is the primary operation of choice for the management of chronic frontal sinusitis.[26, 27] The indications for operation in this setting are very strict. Only patients who fail prolonged attempts at maximal medical therapy, as well attempts at appropriate lesser procedures, are candidates. Appropriate lesser procedures would include septoplasty and intranasal ethmoidectomy. Most patients scheduled for external frontoethmoidectomy have polyps, hyperplastic sinusitis, or an anatomic obstruction of the frontal sinus drainage as a result of either scar tissue or impingement by abnormal ethmoid cell anatomy. The goal of the operation in this setting is to eliminate the mucosal pathology within the frontal sinus outflow so as to reestablish normal mucociliary clearance.

In the hands of other surgeons, this operation has a lesser role. As a secondary procedure only, the external frontoethmoidectomy is proposed as an alternative to the osteoplastic flap with obliteration for patients in whom endoscopic frontal sinusotomy has failed. This option may be chosen for patients who cannot tolerate the larger osteoplastic operation or who, for some reason, refuse that alternative.

Regardless of the indication, the operation has had mixed success, which has contributed to the hesitancy of many to perform this operation. Success rates have varied depending on the technique used. In cases in which the standard Lynch procedure has been performed, reports indicate a 20% to 30% failure rate associated with stenosis, recurrent infection, and the need for further surgery.[21, 24] When mucosal flaps have been used to reconstruct the nasal frontal connection with ciliated epithelium, an improved success rate of up to 90% has been reported.[26, 27] Others have advocated the use of Silastic sheeting or metallic tubes to stent the new duct as healing occurs.[28–32] Unfortunately, these alternatives have not been widely practiced and few reports in the literature are available to substantiate the benefits of these approaches.

Mucocele

Other than chronic sinusitis, mucocele is the only other usual indication for external frontoethmoidectomy. All patients with frontal sinus mucoceles require some type of surgical treatment. The continued controversy is over which operation to perform. Hypothetically, external frontoethmoidectomy not only achieves adequate drainage or removal of the mucocele, it allows normal mucociliary clearance and the integrity of the sinus to be preserved and obviates the need for the more invasive osteoplastic procedure.

However, as in the case of patients with chronic frontal sinusitis, the choice of external frontoethmoidectomy is a controversial one. Currently, the most popular technique is the endoscopic frontal sinusotomy. Others prefer the osteoplastic approach. Advocates of the external frontoethmoidectomy point out its high degree of reliability in achieving adequate drainage, its acceptable long-term success rate, and its relatively minor nature compared with the osteoplastic flap operation. In the author's practice, however, this procedure would only be selected after failure of the endoscopic approach in a patient unable or unwilling to undergo the osteoplastic operation. To date, such a situation has not presented itself.

Preoperative Considerations

Anesthesia

The original reports of external frontoethmoidectomy all described procedures performed under local anesthesia.[21, 23] In the modern era, though, most surgeons prefer general anesthesia for this surgery. The advantages of general anesthesia are numerous, including control of the airway, complete avoidance of intraoperative pain, and a stabile, compliant patient. Among the reported disadvantages of general anesthesia is increased bleeding secondary to vasodilation. However, this effect is balanced against the possibility of increased bleeding secondary to pain-induced hypertension during local anesthesia with sedation. Moreover, the increased nausea once associated with general anesthesia can easily be avoided with the wide variety of anesthetic agents now available. The sole true advantage of local anesthesia with sedation is the slight decrease in cardiovascular morbidity associated with this technique in patients at high risk for complications.

Regardless of the choice of sedation or general anesthesia, local anesthesia should be administered in all patients. This would include the intranasal application of decongestant and mucosal injection with local anesthesia with epinephrine. The sites of injection are spaced in a manner similar to that used for intranasal ethmoidectomy (see Fig. 8–12). Prior to the start of surgery, the incision should be injected with the same epinephrine-containing solution. The author's preference is to use 1% lidocaine with 1 : 100,000 epinephrine, but other combinations probably induce an equivalent effect.

Preparation

Despite the fact that the sinus to be operated upon is infected and that the surgery is classified as clean contaminated, the face should be prepared thoroughly with either an iodine-containing solution or a suitable alternative and then draped in a sterile fashion. Intravenous antibiotics should be initiated before the initial incision is made. Antibiotic coverage should be geared toward the usual sinus bacteriology, any specific culture data established in the preoperative period, and normal skin flora, including staphylococcus.

Technique

Incision

The incision for this procedure is a variation of that illustrated in Chapter 9 for standard external ethmoidectomy. The difference is that, in this procedure, the incision must extend superiorly far enough to allow adequate access to the frontal sinus (Fig. 11–6). In essence, the incision is a combination of the incision for external ethmoidectomy and that for trephination. After the incision site is outlined and infiltrated with the local injection, an incision is made with a No. 15 blade. The subcutaneous tissues are divided with ligation of the angular artery and vein inferiorly. Superiorly, the supraorbital nerve must be carefully avoided. The subcutaneous tissues can be divided with electrocautery or dissected using Metzenbaum scissors. Cutting directly down to the bone with the scalpel is not recommended as this leads to unnecessary bleeding.

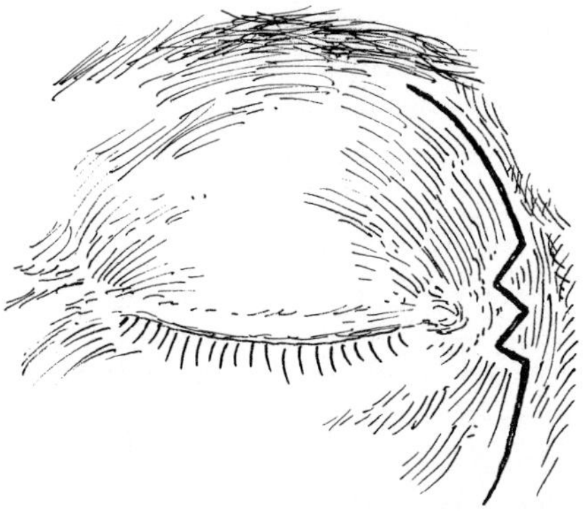

Figure 11–6. The W-plasty incision for external frontoethmoidectomy. The W can be elongated, if necessary.

Exposure

After the periosteum is incised, subperiosteal dissection is carried out to expose the surgical field completely, including the lacrimal fossa, lamina papyracea, and the medial supraorbital rim. When elevation is complete, the exposure will duplicate that described in Chapter 9 for external ethmoidectomy in combination with that shown in Figure 11–3 for the trephination procedure. The dissection should be performed carefully with a Freer elevator using a malleable retractor to hold the orbit away from the lamina papyracea. Throughout this step, hemostasis is maintained with bayonet-style, bipolar electrocautery.

During elevation of the orbit, both the anterior and posterior ethmoidal arteries will be encountered at the level of the frontal ethmoidal suture line. The anterior artery is usually 15 to 20 mm from the posterior lacrimal crest, whereas the posterior artery is usually 5 to 10 mm posterior to the anterior artery. Control of these arteries may be accomplished with either clips or bipolar cautery. Clips are easy and straightforward; however, they carry the risk of falling off during the procedure, with resultant uncontrolled bleeding.

Resection

Ethmoidectomy should be performed next. The details of this procedure have already been presented in Chapter 9. The important steps are briefly reiterated here. The first step is to carefully remove the lamina papyracea from the posterior ethmoid artery posteriorly to the posterior lacrimal crest anteriorly, and from the frontoethmoidal suture line superiorly to the maxillary junction inferiorly. The cells of the ethmoid are then removed as completely as possible. It is important to fully skeletonize the skull base anteriorly to the limits of visualization.

After the ethmoidectomy is completed, the frontal sinus is trephinated, as previously described in this chapter. The opening into the frontal sinus is extended laterally and medially to enlarge the opening into the frontal sinus (Fig. 11–7). At this point, the pathologic area within the frontal sinus is removed. The same concepts as delineated for maxillary sinus surgery apply to this procedure as well, including maximal mucosal preservation and intramucosal resection with periosteal preservation.

The critical part of the surgery comes next and entails opening the nasofrontal connection. If possible, this is done with an intact bridge of bone by reaching up into the frontal recess with an up-biting forceps and reaching down from above. Every attempt should be made to preserve the mucosa overlying the skull base within the frontal recess. As in endoscopic sinus surgery, circumferential removal of the mucosa in this area will almost always result in stenosis. On the other hand, it is essential to achieve an adequate opening from the frontal sinus into the ethmoid sinus.

If an adequate connection cannot be achieved with an intact bridge of bone, the bone can be drilled away. This is accomplished by working from the opening in the frontal sinus superiorly. As bone removal proceeds, the path of the frontal sinus is followed inferiorly until the opening in the frontal sinus is joined with the opening in the lamina papyracea (Fig. 11–8). With the bridge removed, the entire frontal outflow tract can be visualized fully and all cells can be exenterated completely. The disadvantage of the complete frontoethmoidectomy is that the lateral wall of the frontal recess that usually separates the sinus from the orbit is removed. Because of this, there is a high risk of collapse of the frontal recess, resulting in stenosis.

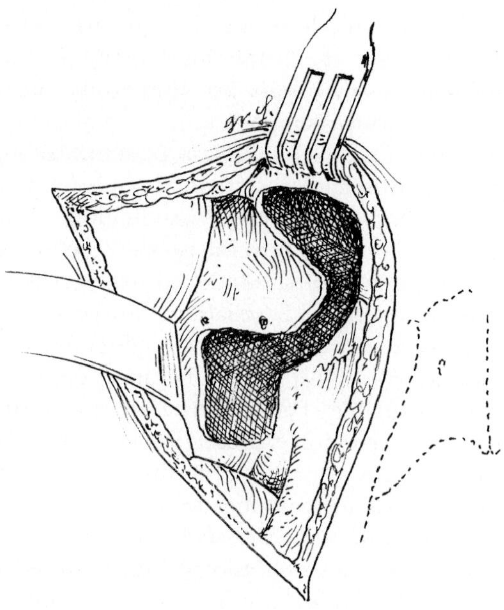

Figure 11–8. Completed frontoethmoidectomy. The trephination has been connected to the ethmoidectomy defect by removal of intervening bone.

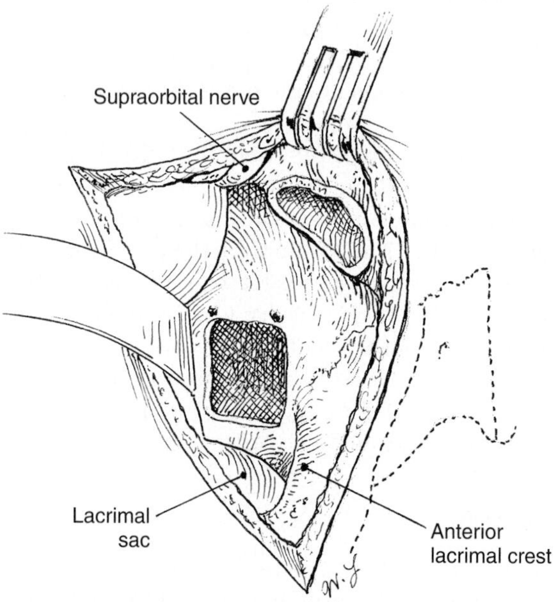

Figure 11–7. Completed exposure: appearance of the surgical field after elevation of the orbit, ethmoidectomy, and trephination. The positions of the anterior and posterior ethmoid artery stumps are shown at the superior edge of the ethmoidectomy defect.

Reconstruction

The reconstruction phase of surgery varies for the two situations of intact bridge and complete frontoethmoidectomy. When the lateral wall of the frontal recess is preserved, the risk of collapse is removed; however, the risk of stenosis persists, especially if circumferential mucosal damage occurs. The standard approach in this situation is to place a stent through the frontal ostium into the nose. Most descriptions of this procedure suggest the use of Silastic or rubber tubing that can be sutured to the lateral nasal wall to stent the duct.[25, 26, 28, 32] The tubing is left in place for a period of 1 to 6 weeks, depending on the condition of the mucosa at the end of the procedure and the patient's tolerance of the stent. To promote drainage, multiple side holes can be cut into the stent's frontal and nasal portions, leaving the central portion in the frontal recess smooth. As an alternative to tubing, rolled Silastic or rubber sheeting may be placed as a stent. Neel et al. have reported on the outcome of the frontoethmoidectomy procedure using either tubing or sheeting as the stent. They found that the rolled sheeting resulted in a relatively higher rate of patency.[26, 28]

As an alternative to the stent, several different types of mucosal flaps have been described. The flap described by Sewell[33] and later named the Sewell-Boyden flap has been the most frequently used, and has been associated with a long-term patency rate as high as 90%.[25, 27] The flap is developed from the lateral nasal wall anterior to the turbinates, using full-thickness mucosa (Fig. 11–9). The design may vary somewhat depending on the distance from the flap to the mucosal edge in the frontal sinus. The flap is initially elevated through the external incision and window into the frontal recess. When the mucosa has been elevated, the shape of the flap is outlined inside the nose using a scalpel to cut down on the elevator passed externally. With the flap completely elevated, it is then rotated into position, pulling the distal end of the flap back on itself laterally and superiorly into the frontal sinus through the external incision (Fig. 11–10). The flap will line the medial and posterior surface of the frontal recess, with the mucosa facing the lumen of the frontal sinus. With the flap in position, the usual frontal stent is placed and secured to the lateral nasal wall.

Closure

Routine wound closure is performed. The first sutures are placed through the medial canthal tendon and secured to the periosteum over the anterior lacrimal crest. Usually, two interrupted 3-0 Vicryl sutures are used to set the position of the orbit and the medial canthus. A Penrose drain is placed into the ethmoid defect to avoid orbital hematoma if postoperative bleeding is a concern,

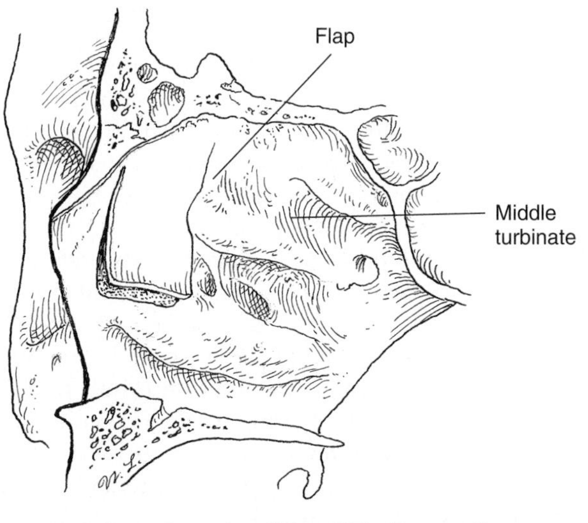

Figure 11–9. Lateral nasal wall flap. This diagram illustrates the outline of the classic lateral nasal wall flap according to Sewell.

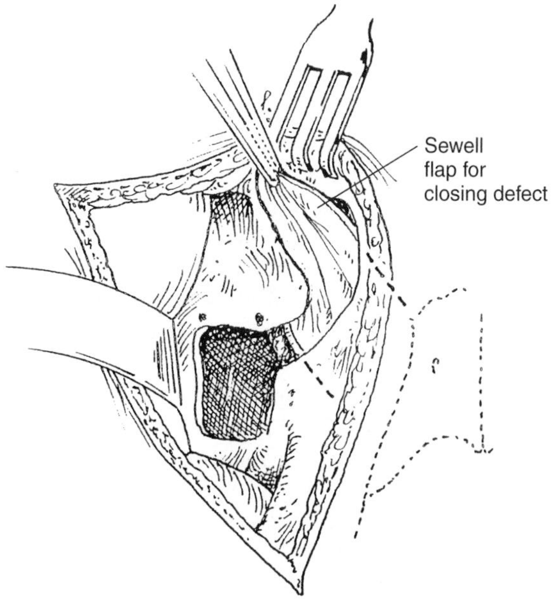

Figure 11–10. Positioning the flap. The Sewell flap has been pulled back on itself into the frontal recess to line the frontoethmoid connection.

and nasal packing is routinely placed to control bleeding from the ethmoid sinus. Skin closure is performed in two layers using subcutaneous 3-0 or 4-0 Vicryl and then interrupted 6-0 nylon suture for the final closure.

Postoperative Care

For most patients, an overnight hospital stay is advisable. Whether or not a drain is placed, the possibility of orbital hemorrhage mandates a period of observation. Provided there is no problem, the patient can be discharged the morning after surgery. If a drain is placed, output will need to be monitored to determine the appropriate time for drain removal.

The most critical question of postoperative care will be how long to leave the nasal frontal stent in place. If excellent mucosal preservation is achieved at surgery with an intact bridge of bone over the frontal recess, then the stent can be removed as early as 5 to 7 days after surgery. If significant mucosal damage occurs or a complete frontoethmoidectomy is done, then a much longer period of stenting will be necessary, in some cases, up to 6 weeks or more. The final circumstance is when a flap is used to line the lateral wall of the frontal outflow tract. When this is done, stenting is usually continued for a period of 1 to 2 weeks. These recommendations are somewhat arbitrary, but are based on the principle that the higher the risk of stenosis, the greater the need for stenting.

The duration of postoperative antibiotics will correspond to the duration of stenting. As with most sinus surgery, at least 2 weeks of antibiotics should be prescribed. The course of treatment should continue as long as the stent is in place. Cultures should routinely be taken during surgery and the results used to direct the choice of postoperative antibiotics.

To help prevent the build-up of crust and blood clot in the ethmoid cavity, postoperative irrigations should be instituted when the packs are removed within the first few days after surgery. Typically, normal saline is used for irrigation and is instilled with either a rubber bulb syringe or a suitable alternative. These irrigations should continue until healing is complete and the stent is removed.

One final consideration is the need for follow-up radiographic studies. With a failure rate ranging from 10% to 40%, long-term evaluation is necessary. Traditionally, plain x-ray studies have been used for this purpose, but CT scans are unquestionably more reliable and so are preferred. The first evaluation should be scheduled 3 months after surgery. If the sinus is opacified at this point, the chances of subsequent aeration are not favorable, and some type of revision surgery should be considered. Conversely, if the sinus is aerated at the time of the 3-month evaluation, then follow-up studies should be planned for 1 year after the operation. Provided the results remain satisfactory, follow-up studies are scheduled annually for a minimum of 5 years.

Complications

External frontoethmoidectomy is an operation with a high risk of complications, the most common of which are a poor cosmetic result from the facial incision and a high risk of recurrent infection. If the incision is strictly curvilinear, without any notching or interruption, the tendency is for a ridge or web to form secondary to contracture. By placing a W-plasty in the incision, this risk is minimized but not completeley eliminated. The risk of recurrent infection or mucocele has been found to range widely. On average, about 30% of patients require subsequent surgery for nasal frontal drainage.[34–36] Other authors have reported up to a 90% long-term patency rate.[25, 27] The predominant cause of failure in all series is stenosis of the frontal outflow from scar tissue and medial orbital collapse.[23, 26]

Excluding these two problems, the complications are the same as those associated with ethmoidectomy in general. These are delineated in detail in Chapters 8 and 9.

OSTEOPLASTIC FLAP

Since the popularization of this operation in the United States by Montgomery and colleagues,[37–41] the osteoplastic flap with frontal sinusectomy and obliteration has enjoyed a premier role in the management of frontal sinus disease. Through the years, there have been many variations of this procedure described, including varying options for incisions, flap creation, sinusectomy, ostial obstruction, obliteration, and closure. In this chapter, the technique employed by the author will be presented. This particular approach is not necessarily better than many other surgical techniques described in the literature. However, in the author's experience, which is based on up to 6 years of follow-up study, this technique has proven to be both reliable and safe. To date, there have been no cases of early or late failure caused by infection, mucocele, or reaeration. Indeed, the only complications reported include one antibiotic-related seizure caused by impipenem on the second postoperative day, and one patient with chronic headaches that were thought to be related to migraines. Although the technique described here is neither simple nor easy to perform, the additional steps taken add to the safety and security of the procedure, as evidenced by the outcome data.

Indications

Acute Sinusitis

Uncomplicated acute sinusitis is never appropriately treated by an osteoplastic flap procedure. However, there are several clinical circumstances in which this operation is indicated. The first is acute frontal sinusitis with intracranial or orbital complication. When intracranial complication of frontal sinusitis is suspected, the diagnosis can be established by a combination of CT scan and lumbar puncture. Immediate management of this situation calls for intravenous antibiotics, neurosurgical consultation, and trephination at the first indication that the patient is stable enough to be transported safely to the operating room. Once the episode of life-threatening infection resolves, definitive surgical management of the frontal sinus must ensue. Some authorities advocate either endoscopic surgery or external frontoethmoidectomy in this situation. However, serious consideration should be given the osteoplastic flap with sinusectomy and obliteration, as this operation most reliably eliminates the risk of further episodes of life-threatening infection. Despite the invasiveness of the operation, no other procedure affords such a high level of control. In the author's series, two patients presented with postneurosurgical intracranial complications. One of these patients had a frontal lobe abscess of the brain secondary to a frontal sinus infection that was drained via a frontal craniotomy. The craniotomy crossed the upper outer corner of the sinus, which caused pneumocephalus to develop whenever the patient blew his nose or sneezed.

A second situation that may require osteoplastic flap with obliteration is recurrent acute frontal sinusitis. If an anatomic cause for this condition can be identified and addressed by endoscopic surgery, this approach would be preferred. On the other hand, if the CT scan does not reveal a predisposing cause or if endoscopic surgery fails, obliteration should be considered.

Chronic Sinusitis

The most common indication for the osteoplastic flap procedure is chronic sinusitis. Although this procedure is rarely performed as a first option, it is the best option for patients in whom endoscopic surgery or frontoethmoidectomy has failed. The best protocol for surgical management of chronic frontal sinusitis is first to attempt endoscopic sinusotomy. If this fails, the reason for failure should be ascertained. Failures secondary to scar tissue or inadequate opening can often be revised endoscopically with success. Patients with open frontal ostia but recurrent or persistent infection are good candidates for osteoplastic obliteration, as are those in whom revision endoscopic surgery aimed at achieving a patent frontal recess has failed.

There are several other circumstances in which the use of the osteoplastic flap may be indicated. One is an inability to approach the frontal sinus endoscopically because of anatomic limitations. An example is a narrow, high frontal recess not approachable endoscopically. In addition, if the frontal sinus ostium cannot be located during endoscopic surgery, then osteoplastic flap is an option. In each of these situations, a technical failure is the reason adequate frontal sinus drainage is not achieved.

Other clinical situations that warrant consideration of an osteoplastic flap include patients with an inherent mucosal disease (e.g., cystic fibrosis, ciliary dyskinesia, or sarcoidosis) that precludes functional restoration of the frontal sinus. In each of these conditions, regardless of the size of the opening into the frontal sinus, normal mucociliary clearance cannot be achieved. In cystic fibrosis, this is because of abnormally thick secretions that do not drain. In ciliary dyskinesia, the cilia are immotile and thus are unable to clear secretions. In sarcoidosis, the mucosa becomes infiltrated with granuloma in a process independent of mucociliary clearance. In these diseases and others that create similar problems, the osteoplastic flap is the best option if chronic frontal sinusitis persists despite adequate medical therapy.

Allergic Fungal Sinusitis

Most cases of allergic fungal sinusitis can be managed by an endoscopic sinusotomy with trephination, if necessary, to remove inspissated secretions. Usually, the fungal elements do not actually invade the lumen of the frontal sinus, but the sinus is obstructed by disease in the anterior ethmoid and nasal cavity. Despite even the best initial results with this disease, there is a tendency for recurrence of fungal infection leading to the accumulation of trapped secretions and polyps in the frontal sinus. In some patients, persistent infection in the frontal sinus may lead to chronic drainage into the lower sinuses, thereby inciting relapse in that location. In situations in which this continually recurs, the osteoplastic flap with obliteration may be the only way to achieve long-term control of the disease and avoid complications and excessive steroid use.

This was the case for one of the patients from the author's series. This patient underwent apparently successful endoscopic sinus surgery in 1992. However, 6 months after the surgery, she had her initial relapse. Over the ensuing 5 years, she had repeated relapses every 3 to 4 months, each marked by frontal recess swelling, purulent discharge, and frontal headache. Every time, she responded to oral steroids and antibiotic therapy with complete resolution of the symptoms and no endoscopic evidence of mucosal disease. A CT scan taken during an asymptomatic period in early 1997 demonstrated opacification of the frontal sinus with density changes consistent with fungal inspissation. The patient then elected to undergo frontal sinus obliteration, at which time fungal elements within the background of classic allergic inflammatory exudate were identified. Although she continues to have periodic relapses, the frontal headache and the severity of the relapses, to date, have improved.

Mucocele

As with most other pathologic processes within the sinuses, mucoceles are best treated by endoscopic means. Numerous studies in the literature, beginning with that of Kennedy et al.[42] in 1989, have documented the success and value of this procedure.[43–45] There are patients, though, who are not amenable to endoscopic drainage, including those with loculated mucoceles that do not connect to the frontal recess area or those with anatomic limitations that prevent the surgeon from approaching the frontal sinus endoscopically. Although the author's series has not included any patients with loculated mucoceles, three patients with the second scenario have been treated.

One patient had an osteoma in the frontal recess that obstructed the frontal sinus. The osteoma arose from the skull base and completely blocked the frontal recess, making an endoscopic approach unsafe. A second patient had a previous history of failed complete external frontoethmoidectomy with takedown of the frontal recess lateral wall. In this patient, the orbit prolapsed medially, obstructing access to the frontal sinus from below. The third patient had severe sinonasal sarcoidosis with severe chronic sinusitis and secondary mucocele. Her nasal passage was obstructed by enlarged turbinates. It was technically impossible to pass an endoscope into the middle meatus without causing significant bleeding from the friable mucosa; thus, the endoscopic approach was untenable.

Preoperative Considerations

Anesthesia

All patients undergoing the osteoplastic flap procedure will require a general anesthetic. Using the technique described in this chapter, the time of surgery will range from 4 to 6 hours. Expected blood loss is moderate, ranging from a minimum of 100 to 200 cc to a maximum of up to 500 cc. Although this is not enough to warrant transfusion, the combination of the length of the surgery and the blood loss will necessitate invasive monitoring in most patients. This includes a bladder catheter and, if the patient has any cardiovascular disease, an arterial line and central venous line to monitor blood pressure and central venous pressure.

Whichever incision is used, it should be injected locally with the standard solution to improve hemostasis. Scalp incisions tend to bleed heavily. With preoperative injection, this source of blood loss is minimized.

Preparation

Because the frontal sinus is usually infected, the operation is normally classified as either clean contaminated or contaminated. These cases, therefore, require prophylactic antibiotics. One of the major concerns is the management of hair during the operation. One tactic is simply to shave the anterior scalp up to the vertex of the skull. This is an option for patients undergoing a bicoronal incision who are not overly concerned about their hair. The other main option is to create a line or part through the hair behind the frontal hairline. To avoid getting hair in the wound, the patient is instructed to braid the hair into numerous, parallel, small braids that create a stripe of exposed scalp in between rows of braids, known as cornrows. This is a time-consuming procedure that the patient should be instructed to complete before coming to the hospital. This option is usually chosen by young women with long hair. Older women tend to be more accepting of either a complete frontal shave or a wide stripe of hair shaved behind the hairline, and often use a scarf or wig to conceal the hair loss until the hair grows back.

The head should be positioned in a horseshoe-shaped head holder wrapped with gauze to provide extra padding, and flexed slightly forward to begin the operation. Later the patient's head can be extended to improve exposure into the frontal sinus. All limbs should be carefully secured and the endotracheal tube taped down onto the mandible. The surgical field is widely prepped with betadyne solution from the vertex to the upper lip and laterally down over the ears and the surgical field sterilely draped. Draping preferences vary from surgeon to surgeon. For this procedure, a sterile towel is stapled to the scalp to keep the hair back out of the wound. A second towel is placed under the nose down to the table. A split sheet is placed around the head, and sheets are hung to wall off the anesthesia from surgical areas.

Technique

Incision

There are three basic incisions used for this operation: the brow incision, the mid-forehead incision, and the bicoronal incision (Fig. 11–11). The choice of the incision will depend on the patient and the surgeon's preference. The advantages of the bicoronal incision are that it best preserves sensation to the forehead and is hidden by the patient's hair. The mid-forehead incision is the most apparent incision for most patients, but does preserve some sensation of the forehead. The brow incision is cosmetically well hidden, but routinely sacrifices sensation to the forehead. The bicoronal incision is preferred for most patients. Except for men with bald-

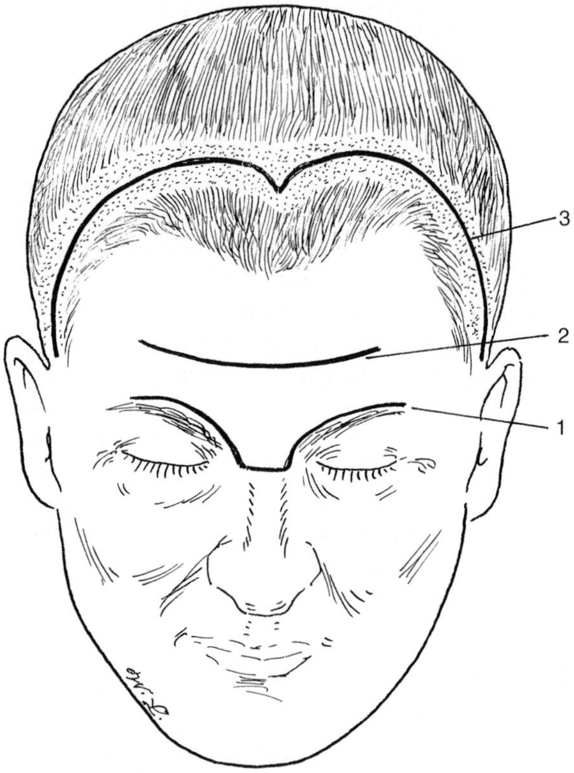

Figure 11–11. Incisions for the osteoplastic flap procedure. *1,* Gull wing brow incision. *2,* Mid-forehead incision. *3,* Bicoronal incision.

ness, this approach combines the best cosmetic result with the best preservation of sensation. One indication for the mid-forehead incision is the presence of anterior or frontal baldness in a man with deep forehead creases. In such cases, the bicoronal incision may be too apparent and cosmetically unappealing. Some men, however, still elect that option, preferring to wear a hat in public. The brow incision, which is rarely used, is indicated in bald men without forehead creases. The different incisions are illustrated in Figure 11–11; only the bicoronal incision will be described in detail.

The bicoronal incision should be placed at least 2 to 3 cm behind the hairline. If the patient is to have the head shaved before the procedure, then the hairline should be marked out prior to cutting any hair to make sure the incision is properly placed. The incision is designed to come to a point in the midline. This helps to orient the flap for closure. The point need not be exaggerated, as even a subtle point will allow accurate realignment. Laterally, the incision is carried down to the level of the preauricular crease, just past the attachment of the auricle. The incision is made with a No. 10 blade, working from the midline toward the surgeon. Initially, the incision should be limited to about 5 cm in length. The layers of the scalp are divided until the subgaleal plane is identified (Fig. 11–12). One useful technique is to cut only through the epidermis and dermis initially. The skin edges are then retracted with skin hooks to elevate the scalp from the periosteum. This makes identification of the subgaleal plane simple and rapid.

With the correct plane identified, an assistant can undermine the incision with a curved hemostat. This makes completion of the incision rapid and safe. Laterally, the incision will stay superficial to the temporalis fascia. Close to the inferior extent of the incision, the superficial temporal artery crosses the line of the incision. Occasionally, the artery can be preserved. In most cases, however, it is best to identify and ligate the artery in routine course.

Hemostasis is important at this stage of the procedure. By incising the flap in stages and preoperatively injecting local anesthetic into the incision, bleeding is minimized. Typically, the incision is performed in four stages, with hemostasis achieved between each step. The fastest and best technique is to coagulate large vessels on the undersurface of the galea and to control skin bleeding with scalp clips. Several roughly equivalent brands are available, and no preference has been noted. (Whatever is used by the neurosurgeons in an individual hospital should suffice.) The clips are placed contiguously on both sides of the incision. When one fourth of the incision is completed, then the next stage is performed.

Flap Elevation

With the incision completed from ear to ear, the elevation of the flap is performed. This can be done with a

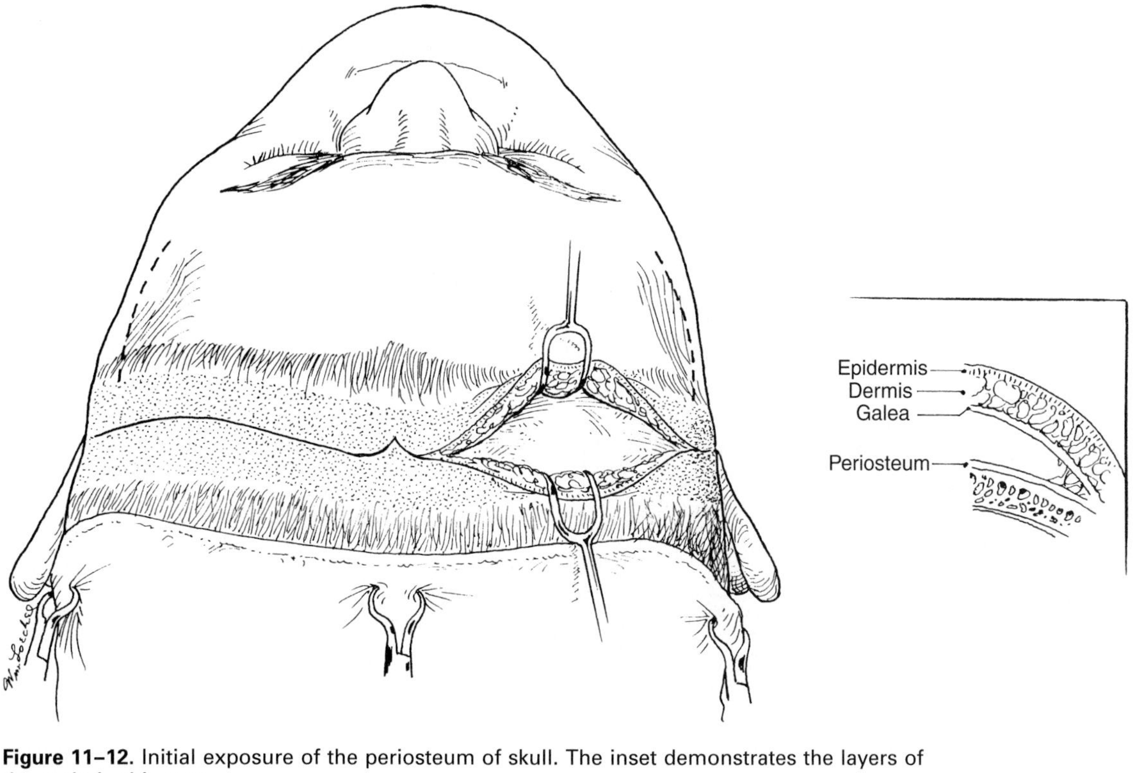

Figure 11–12. Initial exposure of the periosteum of skull. The inset demonstrates the layers of the scalp in this area.

knife, scissors, or electrocautery. Electrocautery is the author's preference because it maintains hemostasis and is very fast. Provided the correct plane is followed, cautery poses no measurably increased risk for wound healing or flap complications. In using cautery for this purpose, several points are worth emphasizing. The first is that cautery is used in coagulation mode and moved slowly but constantly along the dissection plane. As long as the cautery is kept moving, the overlying tissue does not heat up. Allowing the cautery to remain in one place for too long will cause unnecessary thermal damage to the overlying tissues. The second point is to ensure continuously tight traction on the flap during elevation. This stretches the fascial plane and allows minimal thermal energy to be used to lyse the fascial bands (Fig. 11–13). Finally, it is important not to chase bleeding vessels into the flap with the cautery. Instead the vessel should be grasped with forceps and pulled away from the flap, at which point the forceps can then be touched by the cautery to coagulate the vessel. Alternatively, bipolar cautery can be used.

As the flap is elevated, the dissection proceeds first on one side then the other. The surgeon works back and forth from side to side until the elevation reaches the supraorbital rims. When the temporalis is reached, the plane is easily elevated with gentle blunt dissection using a finger. The usual stopping point for the dissection laterally is at the level of the supraorbital rims. This is several centimeters above the zygomatic arch and at a safe level for avoiding the frontal branch of the facial nerve. If, for some reason, the flap needs to be elevated down to the level of the zygomatic arch, as in trauma surgery, then about 2 to 3 cm above the arch, the plane of dissection dives deep to the temporalis fascia. This is necessary to avoid injury to the frontal branch of the facial nerve. For osteoplastic flap procedures, this is generally not needed. At the conclusion of flap elevation, the supraorbital rims can be clearly palpated from the nasion to the temporal fossa (Fig. 11–14).

The next step is elevation of the periosteal flap. A broad-based, large flap is preferred to maximize exposure of the frontal bone. The periosteum is incised with a scalpel from the temporal fossa on one side to the temporal fossa of the other (see Fig. 11–14). This flap should not be incised or elevated with cautery as this would cause shrinkage of the edges of the flap, which would impair closure at the end of the procedure. The periosteal flap is elevated using a Freer or periosteal elevator. Here, the elevation is carried down onto the nasal dorsum in the midline and to the orbital rims on each side. Inferiorly, on the undersurface of the orbital rim, is the supraorbital foramen and nerve (see Fig. 11–14), which should be carefully preserved. To maximize inferior exposure, the supraorbital nerves can be delivered from the foramina. Delivery is easily accomplished with a 2-mm osteotome used to gently remove the orbital bone over the nerve. By mobilizing the nerves from the foramina, the bicoronal flap can be folded inferiorly to expose the entire nasal dorsum. However, this carries no advantage in the osteoplastic flap operation and should, therefore, be avoided.

Osteoplastic Flap

The next part of the operation is to outline and create the osteoplastic flap. To outline the flap accurately, a

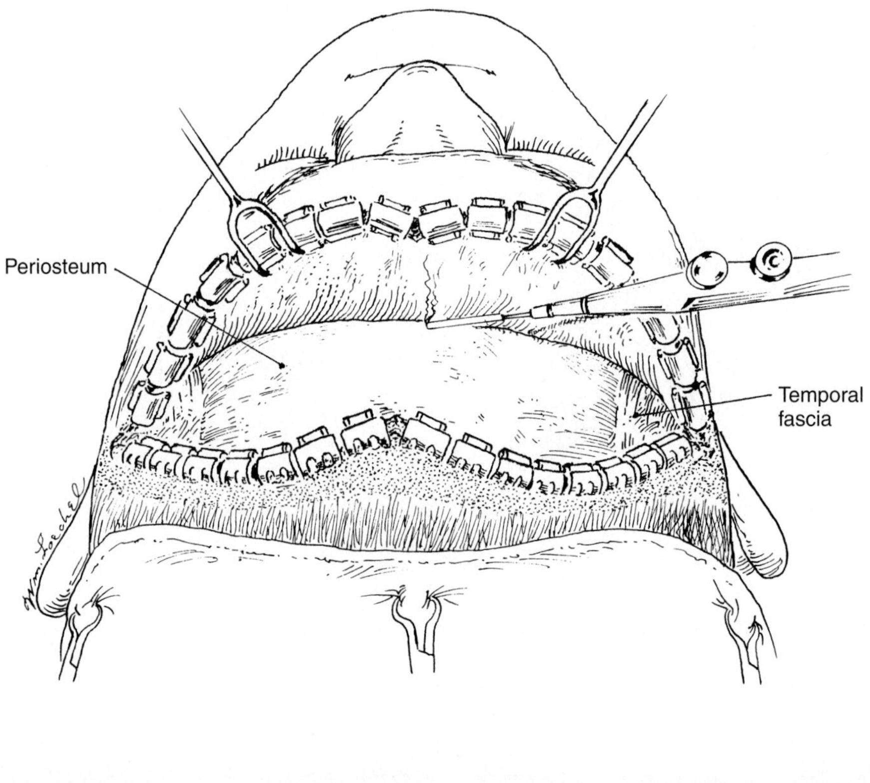

Figure 11–13. Flap elevation. The plane of dissection is maintained between the galea and frontal muscle layer and the periosteum. Laterally, the plane develops on the surface of the temporalis fascia.

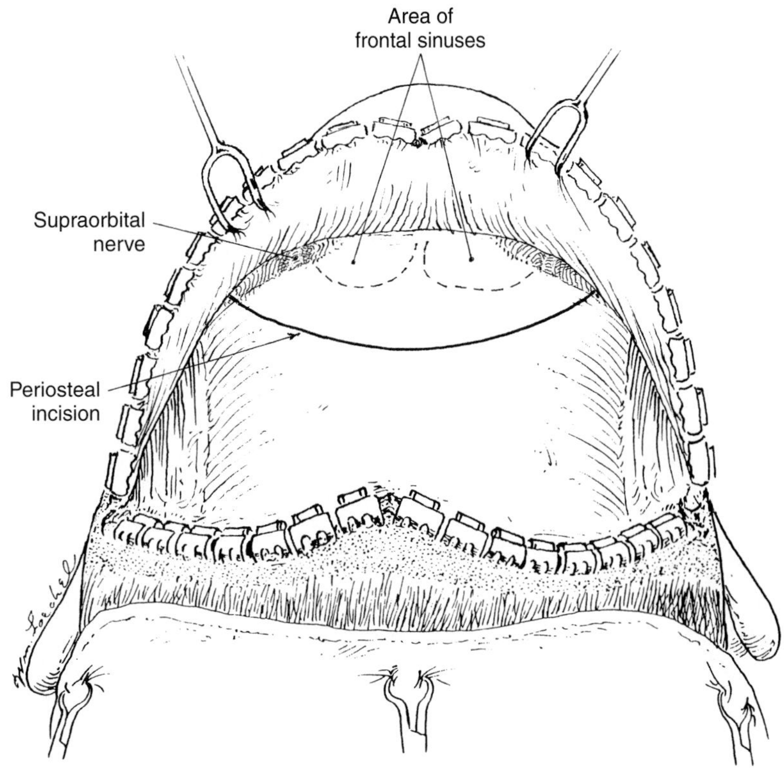

Figure 11–14. Periosteal incision. The flap elevation is complete and the periosteal incision is outlined. The area of the frontal sinus is indicated, as is the location of the left supraorbital nerve.

template of the sinus is required. This is created from a 6-foot Caldwell view of the sinuses. When obtaining the radiograph, a coin is taped to the forehead right above the nasion. This allows comparison of the spot size of the coin on the x-ray film to that of the actual coin. If there is a perfect fit, then the radiograph is a true 1 : 1 representation of the patient's skull. With the appropriate x-ray studies, the template is created by cutting out the shape of the frontal sinus. Before starting, the x-ray film should always be marked with an indelible marker to orient right from left and the midline. One useful technique is to draw the outline of the sinus onto the x-ray film while it is held in a view box. The orbital rims and the nasal bones are left attached to the frontal sinus to help in orienting the template to the patient's skull.

The radiographic template is then held against the frontal bone with the midline mark on the template through the nasal bones used to adjust the right-left orientation, and the junction of the frontal sinus to the supraorbital rim used to judge the superoinferior orientation. With the template carefully held in place, the frontal sinus is traced onto the skull with a marker (Fig. 11–15).

The next step is to create the osteoplastic flap. The bone can be cut with any number of instruments, including osteotome, drills, and saws. The preferred method is to use an oscillating microsagittal saw with a 1-cm wide blade (Fig. 11–16). The blade is held at a very acute angle to the frontal bone, perhaps at 30 degrees, to create a beveled cut into the sinus. The blade is traced along the outlined sinus, maintaining the tangential orientation of the blade at all times (see Fig. 11–16). Rather than work in one limited area, the osteotomy is developed along the entire length of the sinus one side at a time. Using this technique, intracranial entry is avoided. The cut should be carried inferiorly down to and through the supraorbital rim. When the osteotomy is complete, the only attachments will be along the supraorbital rim, across the nasion and the intersinus septum.

A 1-cm curved osteotome is used to cut the intersinus septum. As this is done, the flap will begin to elevate. In order to complete the elevation, the flap is levered up at three points simultaneously (Fig. 11–17). This is done to avoid cracking the flap in the wrong place. As the bone flap is gently elevated, the attachments to the supraorbital rim will fracture, usually just inside the orbit. The flap is then free to rotate inferiorly, where it can be supported by a retractor or fish hook.

Mucosal Resection

In order to obliterate the frontal sinus safely, it is necessary to excise all mucosal tissue completely. Even microscopic fragments of mucosa could potentially lead to late recurrence of a mucocele. The first step, though, after opening the sinus is to culture the contents of the sinus. The mucosa is then elevated from the walls of the sinus using a Freer elevator. A systematic approach

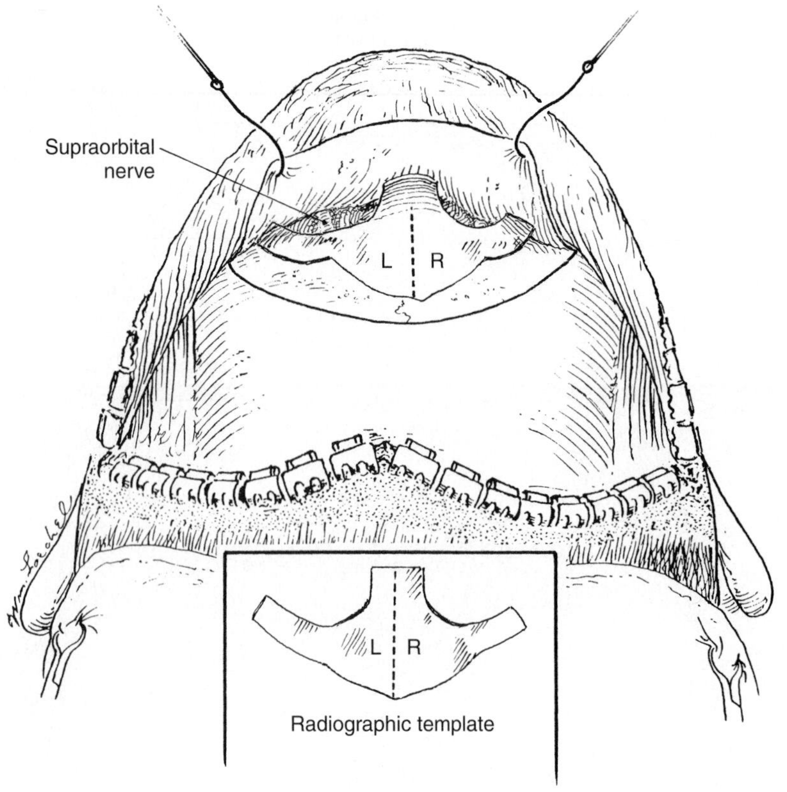

Figure 11–15. Placement of the radiographic template. The template is oriented to the patient by the midline mark and the positions of the junction of the frontal sinus and the supraorbital rim.

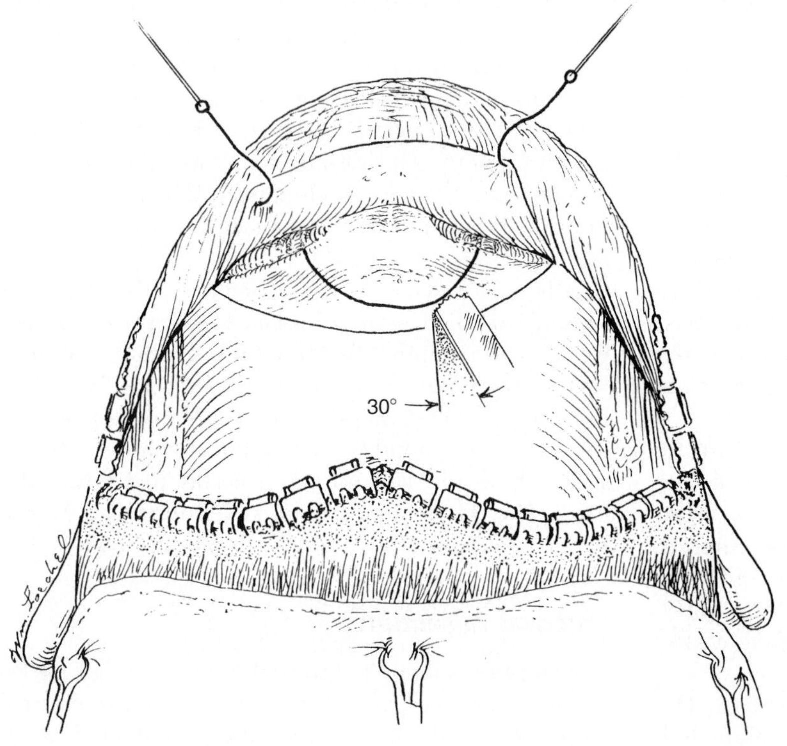

Figure 11–16. Creating the osteoplastic flap. A rounded, thin, saw blade 1 cm in width is held 30 degrees from the plane of the skull.

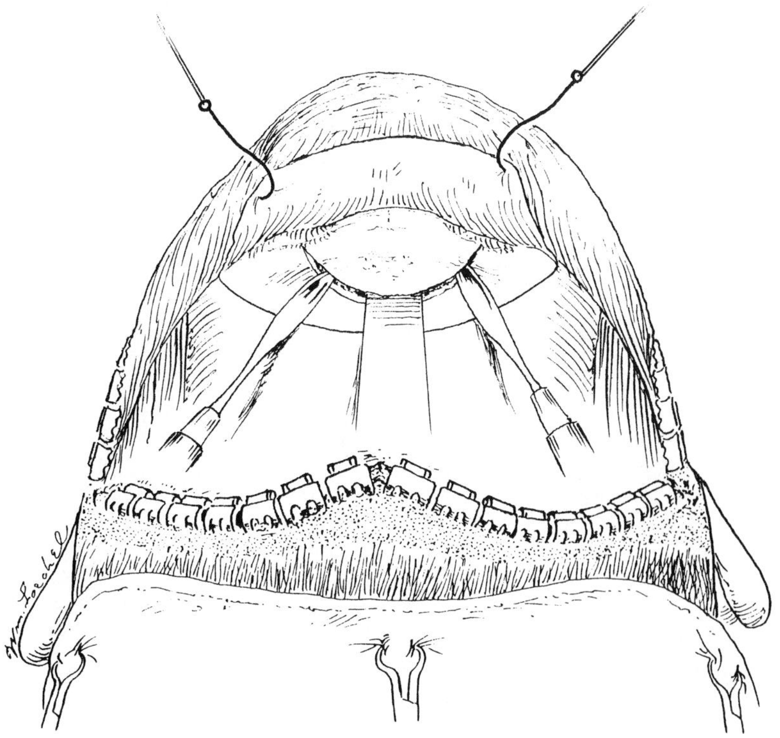

Figure 11–17. Elevation of the osteoplastic flap. The bone flap is supported at three points during this step to help control the line of fracture.

to mucosal removal should be used to make sure that all areas are covered.

One of the main concerns in completely removing the mucosa are mucosal invaginations into the bone of the posterior wall of the sinus around small vascular perforators. These structures are known as the foramina of Luschka and, in order to completely account for the mucosa within them, the bone must be drilled down to a thin shell over the dura. The preferred technique is to use an otologic drill with diamond and cutting burrs.

The first step is to drill down the interior surface of the anterior wall. A large cutting burr can be used for this step. The cutting burr can also be used to take down the intersinus septum and remove any bony overhang at the edges of the sinus (Fig. 11–18). At this point, the orbital and cranial surfaces of the sinus are drilled. A diamond burr is used on these thin and delicate surfaces. In order to be certain that mucosa has been removed without orbital or intracranial penetration, a microscope should be used.

After this step is completed, the frontal recess must be addressed. This area is complicated by the presence of supraorbital ethmoid cells. Sometimes, these cells create a deep, narrow crevice between the orbit and the anterior cranial fossa. To clear these cells, the patient should be placed in the Trendelenberg position, the head extended, and the smallest diamond burr applied under sufficient magnification. Great care must be taken during this step to ensure that injury to the eye and brain does not occur.

It is worthwhile to continue the drilling well down into the ethmoid sinus. Although it is not necessary to drill out the entire ethmoid sinus completely, it is important to maximally enlarge the opening of the frontal sinus into the nose. In addition, the intersinus septum is drilled down to the crista galli posteriorly and the nasal septum anteriorly and inferiorly. This is done to make sure that small intersinus cells are not left unknowingly. The completed resection should leave a clean, smooth surface with the entire bilateral sinus seamlessly connected (Fig. 11–19).

Obliteration

Obliteration of the sinus can be done in many ways and includes harvesting of fat, muscle, and bone. The technique described here was developed as a modification of existing techniques to maximize the chances of a long-term, stable obliteration without reabsorption or reaeration. The obliteration is achieved in four layers: muscle, bone, fascia, and fat. The fascia, muscle, and bone can all be harvested locally within the surgical field, whereas the fat is harvested from an abdominal or thigh incision. The first layer is a plug of muscle that is harvested from the temporalis muscle. The plug should be sized to sit down into the ethmoid sinus at the level of the anterior ethmoidal artery. It is anticipated that this will eventually resorb, but at the time of surgery, it acts as a platform on which to build the permanent layers.

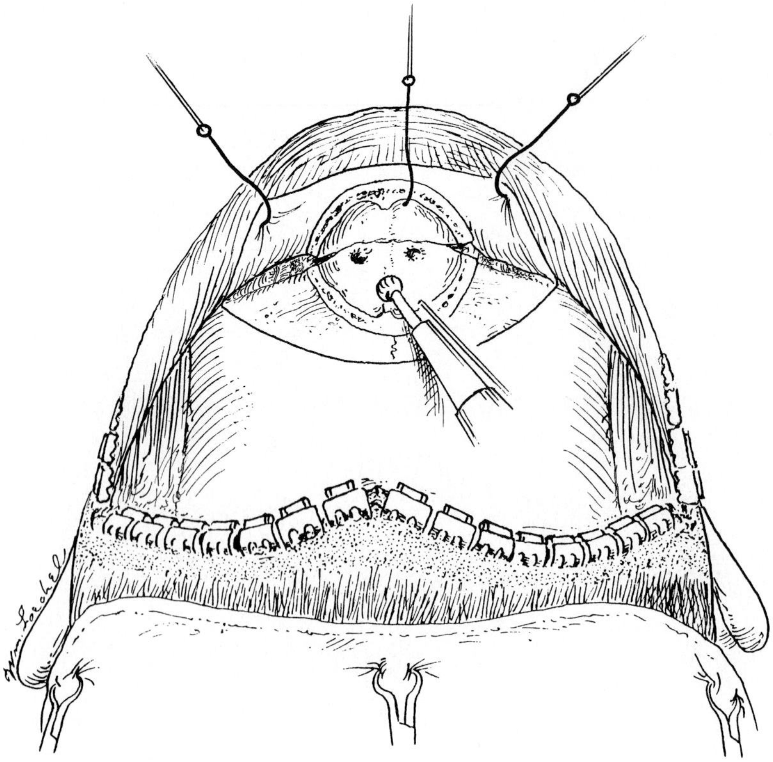

Figure 11–18. Mucosal resection. The inside of the sinus is burred down first using a 2- to 3-mm cutting burr to remove the intersinus septum and to take down any significant bony overhang at the edge of the osteotomy. Final removal of mucosa over the brain and eye is accomplished with diamond burrs.

The second layer is bone. The preferred bone is a split calvarial graft harvested from the calvarium of the parietal bone. This is easily exposed within the surgical field. The graft is harvested using an otologic drill with cutting burrs. The first step is to create a trench around the graft, usually measuring 1.5 × 5 cm. A medium-sized cutting burr is used for this, and the trench is cut only through the outer cortex into the diploic space. The diploic space is easily identified by the change in bone consistency and the occurrence of bleeding when the space is entered. Using a 1-mm cutting burr, the graft is then undermined within the diploic space (Fig. 11–20). When the graft is attached only by a central area, curved osteotomies are used to free the graft. In this instance, it is not critical to elevate the graft in one piece, but it is preferable.

During graft harvest, the bone dust that is created is carefully harvested and saved for later use. The graft is then broken up into small, 2- to 3-mm pieces that are packed into the frontal recess above the muscle plugs on either side. The bone dust is used to fill in the gaps, much like mortar and bricks. The long-term result of this technique is that the bone forms an osseous and fibrous plug that will permanently resist ingrowth of mucosa from below.

A large temporalis fascia graft is harvested from the exposed temporalis muscle. This is laid over the bone across the midline to form a smooth shelf over the frontal recesses. This is done as a security measure in case the bone graft reabsorbs, as the fascia will form a support to hold up the fat graft. Lastly, the fat graft is packed into the sinus over the fascia graft (Fig. 11–21). The fat should fill the sinus completely, with smaller pieces being pushed into the lateral shelves above the eyes, if present. Enough fat should be placed so that when the osteoplastic flap is replaced, it forces the fat to push out from under the edges.

Closure

Closure of the wounds begins with replacement of the osteoplastic flap. This is rotated back into position and adjusted so that the flap fits securely back in its original position. The flap is secured by two 26-gauge wires passed through the flap and the edge of the sinus at 2 and 10 o'clock. Wire is preferred because it is simple, fast, and inexpensive. More high-tech methods are available, but offer no discernible advantages.

The periosteal flap is secured back in place using interrupted 3-0 Vicryl. By carefully reapproximating this layer, the smooth contour of the forehead is assured. This also helps to stabilize the osteoplastic flap. Drains are placed next. Suction drains are preferred, with the usual selection being 10-mm wide, flat, white, Jackson-Pratt drains that have been fully perforated. The drains are placed through the skin posterior to the inferior aspect of the incision. One drain is placed over the

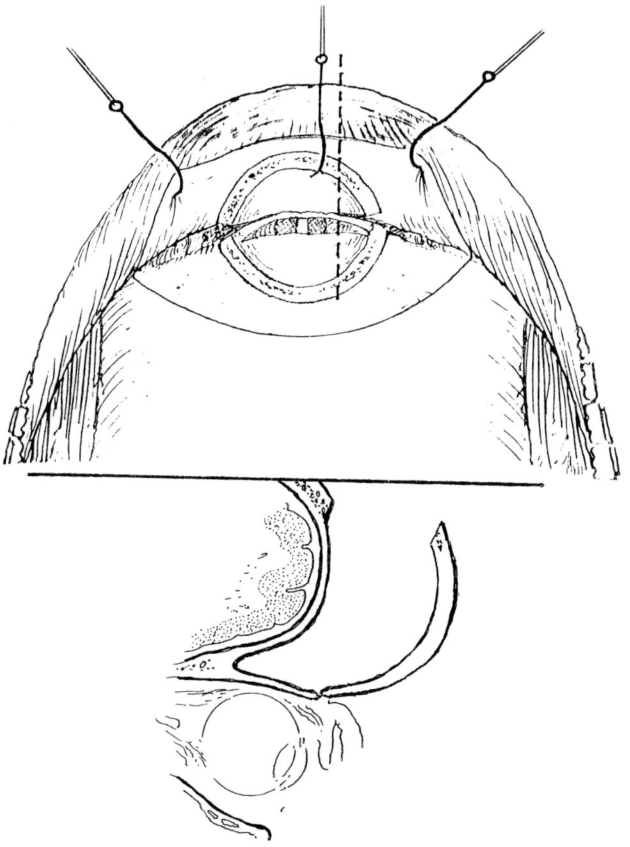

Figure 11–19. Completed drilling. The inside of the sinus is smooth and seamless. The supraorbital ethmoid cells have been drilled away. The intersinus septum is taken down to the nasal septum. The lower portion of the figure is a parasagittal view showing the depth of the supraorbital ethmoid recess.

eyebrows and the other across the top of the skull behind the incision.

At this point, the wound should be irrigated thoroughly with saline solution to remove blood clots and contaminating material from the wound. The scalp clips are then removed. These are removed two or three at a time, with the edges of the scalp wiped off and large vessels coagulated. Excessive coagulation of the skin edge is neither necessary nor desirable. The skin bleeding will always stop when the skin is closed. It is important, though, to make sure that any galeal vessels are thoroughly coagulated, as they can lead to hematoma and wound complications.

The final closure of the skin is achieved in two layers: a deep layer of interrupted 3-0 Vicryl and skin staples. The only important points to remember in closure are that the midline should be reset first and that the deep sutures need to incorporate the galea.

Postoperative Care

Following the surgery, the wound is dressed with antibiotic ointment only. Constricting head bandages are not necessary and only serve to compromise blood flow to the flap. With two suction drains in place and meticulous care taken during closure to ensure hemostasis, no instances of postoperative hemorrhage or hematoma have been observed in the author's series. The drains are immediately connected to an intermediate level of wall suction to ensure that all blood and secretions are collected.

Initial care of the patient may be either in the intensive care unit (ICU) or a surgical nursing unit. The decision to use the ICU will be made based on the patient's medical condition and the course of events in the operating room and recovery room. Length of hospitalization is expected to be 4 days, with some patients requiring 5 or 6 days. The key issue that determines the length of stay is the amount of drainage. Usually, after the first 24 to 48 hours, output has decreased to less than 50 mL per day and the drains are then taken off wall suction and connected directly to closed-bulb suction. This decreases the suction on the drains and minimizes the amount of serous exudate. The drains are removed when the output is less than 20 mL of serous exudate per day. This usually occurs on the third and fourth days. As a routine practice, the drains are never removed on the same day, and the superior drain is removed first.

The patient will experience a progressive amount of facial and orbital swelling during the first 3 days after surgery. Ice packs to the eyes may help minimize this problem. Most patients experience only mild to moderate swelling; however, a few patients have developed severe swelling but none that progressed to eye closure. During this period, the eyes should be checked every 6 to 12 hours to make sure that orbital hematoma is not occurring.

Pain management during the postoperative course is essential. Initially, most patients will require parenteral narcotics. Patient-controlled analgesia (PCA) by an intravenous pump is helpful for the first 2 or 3 days and is welcomed by most patients. By the end of the third day, the patient should be weaned to oral analgesics. Most patients are discharged with a prescription for acetaminophen with codeine elixir or pills.

Postoperative intravenous antibiotics should be continued during hospitalization or at least until the results of intraoperative cultures are obtained. When these are available, they should be used to direct subsequent treatment. Most patients will be able to be discharged on a 2-week course of oral antibiotics. However, if frank bone infection is detected at surgery or if Pseudomonas infection is documented, a prolonged course of intravenous antibiotics is recommended.

Clear liquids are allowed the night of surgery, with a regular diet initiated the morning after surgery if desired. The diet can be advanced as tolerated by the patient. Activity levels after surgery are gradually in-

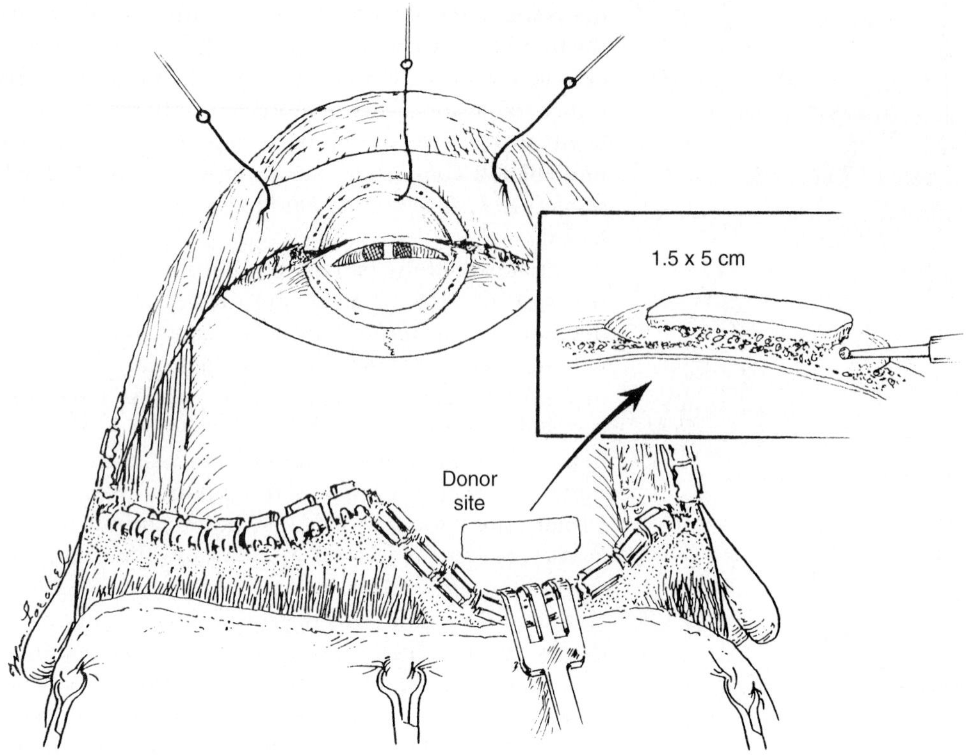

Figure 11–20. Harvesting the calvarial bone graft. The donor site is shown posterior to the incision, but it may be located more anteriorly to avoid excessive elevation of the scalp posteriorly. The inset shows the undercutting of the graft after the outer trench has been created.

creased after the first night, when bed rest is usually prescribed. The patient should be out of bed the day after surgery unless medical complications prevent this. Ambulation is initiated either on the evening of the first postoperative day or the next morning. Most patients take 2 full weeks to resume normal activity and return to work. Contact sports, diving, and sports involving balls are delayed from 6 weeks to 3 months depending on the activity requested.

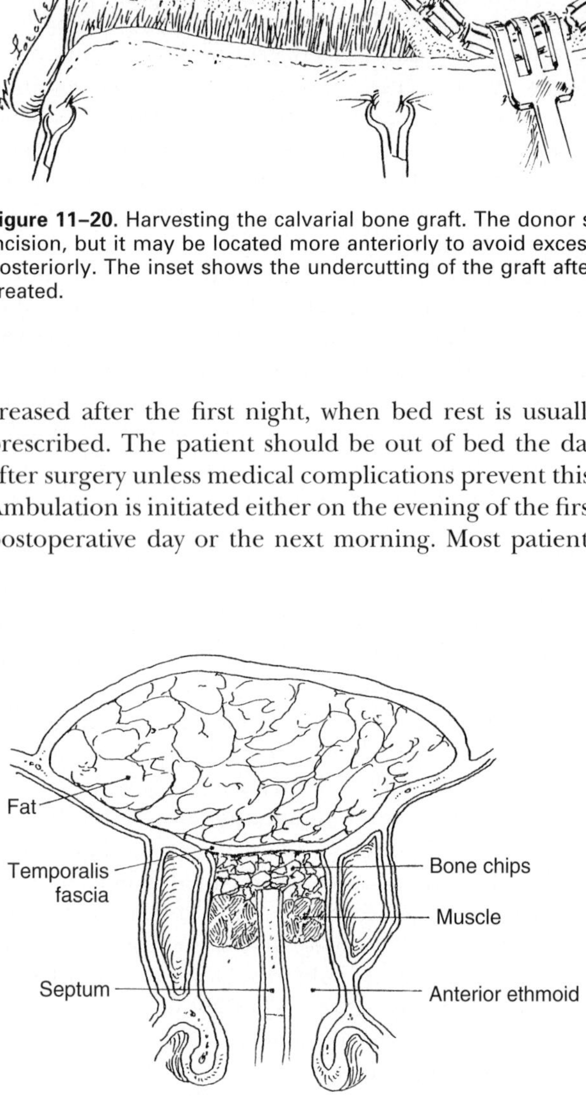

Figure 11–21. Final obliteration of the cavity. The four layers are (1) temporalis muscle, (2) calvarial bone chips, (3) temporalis fascia, and (4) abdominal fat. Agger nasi cells are shown lateral to the nasal cavity at this level.

Long-term follow-up evaluation of these patients is essential. The possibility of late complications is low but significant; therefore, vigilance must be maintained in order to detect and treat these problems as soon as they arise. A CT scan is routinely done 3 months after the surgery to confirm healing and absence of aeration and also to provide a baseline scan for later comparison. Early detection of postoperative recurrent infection or mucocele is very difficult, so this benchmark examination is invaluable in that respect. After that, annual follow-up scans are recommended for the first 3 years. If, at this point, no problems have been detected, further scans should be obtained only every 2 to 3 years.

Complications

In the author's experience, the osteoplastic flap procedure has been a safe and effective operation. Indeed, only two complications have occurred in the author's series. The first was a grand mal seizure, attributed to intravenous imipenem, on the second postoperative night. The patient had cystic fibrosis and a documented resistant Pseudomonas infection necessitating treatment with imipenem. Subsequent evaluation documented normal cerebrospinal fluid (CSF) and no intracranial complications on CT scan. Imipenem is well known to be associated with seizures and, after withdrawal of the antibiotic, no further problems were observed. The second complication was a postoperative seroma. This was noted in the temporal area 2 weeks after surgery at the time of a follow-up visit. Simple aspiration proved sufficient to resolve the problem.

Results have been excellent to date. According to follow-up data obtained over a period of up to 6 years, no incidence of mucocele or recurrent infection has been reported. One patient still has persistent headaches 3 years after surgery, but these were present before the operation. Migraine therapy has been somewhat successful in treating the headaches, but it is possible that they represent postoperative headache related to the surgery.

The list of potential complications is long, which is the reason that this operation has been so controversial. The list includes intracranial entry with hemorrhage, CSF leak, brain damage, and death. These theoretical risks should, in all cases, be avoidable. However, Hardy and Montgomery (1976)[46] reported a 19% incidence of intraoperative CSF leak. By contrast, in the author's series of 25 procedures involving osteoplastic flaps, no intraoperative CSF leaks have been reported. Other contemporary series have also not reported a high incidence of intracranial penetration.[47] Perhaps the availability of preoperative CT scans and modern microsaws have helped to avoid this problem. Theoretically, as long as the template is carefully made and applied and the flap is created using a steeply beveled cut, the risk should be acceptably low.

Other short-term complications include wound problems (hematoma, infection, or flap necrosis), blood transfusion, orbital injury, and medical complications. Among these problems, the medical complications would be the most important and most common. Like all operations of 4 or more hours' duration, there is a risk of cardiovascular problems, pulmonary infection, and thrombophlebitis. However, with careful anesthesia and awareness of these problems, these can be avoided in most cases. Most patients will develop some degree of orbital swelling from the creation of an osteoplastic flap. To date, this has not led to any lasting edema or any change in visual acuity. However, like the intracranial complications, intraorbital hematoma is possible so the surgeon must guard against this possibility during both the procedure and the postoperative period. A blood transfusion is rarely needed for the osteoplastic flap. Control of the scalp, as outlined in this chapter, is the most important factor is preventing the need for transfusion.

Wound complications are the most common acute problems seen with this operation. Flap necrosis is generally avoidable. However, technical errors, involving injury to both supraorbital arteries or straying from the surgical plane while elevating the scalp flap, may result in loss of blood supply to the flap. Hematoma and seroma may also occur. Failure to control a galeal blood vessel or the superficial temporal artery could lead to hematoma. However, maintaining the suction drains on wall suction until the bleeding stops should prevent this complication. Late occurrence of seroma is also rare, but may occur if the drains are removed while the wound is still weeping serous fluid. In the one patient who did have this problem, a small, 10-cc seroma developed over the temporal area. This resolved after a single aspiration. Wound infection should also be an unusual occurrence. By definition, this operation is a clean contaminated or grossly contaminated procedure. This class of cases is known to benefit from prophylactic antibiotics and, with appropriate antibiotics, the expected risk of infection should be less than 5%. Infection should be treated promptly with drainage and culture, as well as antibiotic therapy effective against the infecting organism.

Late complications of the osteoplastic flap with obliteration include recurrent infection, mucocele, chronic headache, frontal numbness, and cosmetic alterations. The most important problems with this procedure have been related to recurrent infection or mucocele secondary to reaeration from graft absorption or residual mucosa within the sinus. Many technical adaptations have been developed to overcome these problems, usually focusing on different ways to obliterate the sinus.[48, 49] However, the key to this operation is not the nature of the obliterating material, but the complete removal of all mucosal elements in the sinus, removal of all adjoining loculations and cells, and application of an adequate technique to obstruct the frontal recess. If these components of the procedure are correct, then there will be no long-term complications. In the series by Hardy and Montgomery, the incidence of reoperation for long-term complications was 10% and occurred up to 20 years later.[46] For this reason, long-term follow-up evaluation is recommended even if no problems arise early after the surgery.

Postoperative headache is a contentious and serious problem with this operation. It is always difficult to know the exact cause of a headache. Postoperative chronic headache is no exception to this dilemma. However, there does seem to be a true clinical entity of headache in patients undergoing craniotomy or other procedures on the skull. Perhaps this is related to periosteal reaction, damage to osseous nerves, or injury to the supraorbital nerves. The expected incidence will be about 5%. For this reason, if no other, the osteoplastic flap should be reserved for patients in whom there are no other alternatives or for those with life-threatening disease.

Persistent forehead numbness or paresthesia is related to injury to the supraorbital or supratrochlear nerves. Anatomic variations involving an abnormally superior position of the supraorbital foramen may rarely be encountered. Otherwise, injury only occurs if a technical error is made in the plane of dissection. As long as the nerves are anatomically preserved, even if there is temporary numbness, recovery can be expected. However, in the series by Hardy and Montgomery, 35% of patients had persistent problems after 3 years.[46] This complication rate is probably related to the large number of patients with mid-forehead incisions in this series. In the author's series, as well as in that of others, this high incidence has not been observed.[47]

Cosmetic alterations can occur if there is absorption of the bone flap or if excessive periosteal reaction leads to bone thickening. If a burr hole technique is used, this can lead to focal mid-forehead depressions. This can be avoided by simply using the technique described in this chapter. To date, these late cosmetic alterations have not been seen in the author's series. Such problems are unusual and require long-term follow-up evaluation to detect.

REFERENCES

1. Jacobs JB. 100 Years of frontal sinus surgery. Laryngoscope 107(S83):1, 1997.
2. Kennedy DW. Sinus surgery: A century of controversy. Laryngoscope 107:1, 1997.
3. Goodyear HM. Surgery of the frontal sinus. Laryngoscope 57:340, 1947.
4. Bergara AR, Itoiz AO. Present state of the surgical treatment of chronic frontal sinusitis. Arch Otolaryngol 61:616, 1995.
5. Sessions RB, Alford BR, Stratton C. Current concepts of frontal sinus surgery: An appraisal of the osteoplastic flap-fate obliteration operation. Laryngoscope 82:918, 1972.
6. Wells R. Abscess of the frontal sinus. Lancet 1:694, 1870.
7. Ogston A. Trephining the frontal sinus for catarrhal diseases. Med Chronicle No. 3 3:235, 1884.
8. Luc H. Lecons Sur Le Suppurations de L'Oreille Moyenne et des Cavities Accessoires des Fosses Nasales et leurs Complications Endocraniennes. Paris: Baillere, 1990.
9. Coakley CG. Frontal sinusitis: Diagnosis, treatment, and results. Trans Am Laryngol Rhinol Otol Soc 11:101, 1905.
10. Ritter RN. The Paranasal Sinuses: Anatomy and Surgical Technique, 2nd ed. St. Louis: CV Mosby, 1978.
11. Weymuller EA Jr, Rice DH. Surgical management of infectious and inflammatory disease. In Cummings CW (ed). Otolaryngology Head and Neck Surgery, 2nd ed., Vol. 1. St. Louis: Mosby Year Book, 1993, pp. 955–964.
12. Suonpaa J, Sipila J, Aitasalo K, et al. Operative treatment of frontal sinusitis. Acta Otolaryngol [Suppl] 529:181, 1997.
13. Ramadan HH. Endoscopic treatment of acute frontal sinusitis: Indications and limitations. Otolaryngol Head Neck Surg 113: 295, 1995.
14. Turner WJ, Davidson TM. Endoscopic management of acute frontal sinusitis. Ear Nose Throat J 73:594, 1994.
15. Thawley SE, Deddens AE. Transfrontal endoscopic management of frontal recess disease. Am J Rhinol 9:307, 1995.
16. Bent JP III, Spears RA, Kuhn FA, et al. Combined endoscopic intranasal and external frontal sinusotomy. Am J Rhinol 11: 349, 1997.
17. Sharp HR, Spraggs PD, Mackay IS. Combined approach intranasal endoscopic and external Lothrop procedure in chronic frontal sinus disease. J Laryngol Otol 111(7):635, 1997.
18. Bent JP III, Cuilty-Siller C, Kuhn FA. The frontal cell as a cause of frontal sinus obstruction. Am J Rhinol 8:185, 1994.
19. Wide K, Sipila J, Suonpaa J. The value of computerised rhinomanometry and a simple manometry with saline in predicting the outcome of patients with acute trephined frontal sinusitis. Rhinology 34(3):151, 1996.
20. Sipila J, Suonpaa J, Wide K, et al. Prediction of the clinical outcome of acute frontal sinusitis with ventilation measurement of the nasofrontal duct after trephination: A long-term follow-up study. Laryngoscope 106(3 Pt. 1):292, 1996.
21. Lynch RC. The technique of a radical frontal sinus operation which has given me the best results. Laryngoscope 31:1, 1921.
22. Sewell EC. External frontoethmo-sphenoid operation: New mucosal flap for controlling frontonasal drainage and granulation tissue—review of sphenoid technic. Arch Otolaryngol 20:57, 1934.
23. Boyden GL. Surgical treatment of chronic frontal sinusitis. Ann Otol Rhinol Laryngol 61:558, 1952.
24. McNally WJ, Stuart EA. 30-Year review of frontal sinusitis treated by external operation. Ann Otol Rhinol Laryngol 63:651, 1954.
25. Ogura JH, Watson RK, Jurema AA. Frontal sinus surgery: The use of a mucoperiosteal flap for reconstruction of a nasofrontal duct. Laryngoscope 70:1229, 1960.
26. Neel HB, McDonald TJ, Facer GW. Modified Lynch procedure for chronic frontal sinus diseases: Rationale, technique, and long-term results. Laryngoscope 97:1274, 1987.
27. Boyden GL. Chronic frontal sinusitis: End results of surgical treatment. Trans Am Acad Ophthalmol Otolaryngol 61:588, 1957.
28. Neel HB, Whicker JH, Lake CF. Thin rubber sheeting in frontal sinus surgery—Animal and clinical studies. Laryngoscope 86: 524, 1976.
29. Baron SH, Dedo HH, Henry CR. The mucoperiosteal flap in frontal sinus surgery. Laryngoscope 83:1266, 1973.
30. Anthony DH. Use of Ingals' gold tube in frontal sinus operations. South Med J 33:949, 1940.
31. Scharfe ED. The use of tantalum in otolaryngology. Arch Otolaryngol 58:133, 1953.
32. Amble FR, Kern EB, Neel HB III, et al. Nasofrontal duct reconstruction with silicone rubber sheeting for inflammatory frontal sinus disease: Analysis of 164 cases. Laryngoscope 106:809, 1996.
33. Sewell EC. External operation on the ethmosphenoid-frontal group of sinuses under local anesthesia: Technique for removal of part of optic foramen wall for relief of pressure on optic nerve. Arch Otolaryngol 4:377, 1926.
34. Goodale RL. Some causes for failure in frontal sinus surgery. Ann Otol Rhinol Laryngol 51:648, 1942.
35. Goodale RL. Trends in radical frontal sinus surgery. Ann Otol Rhinol Laryngol 66:369, 1957.
36. Boyden GL. Surgical treatment of chronic frontal sinusitis. Ann Otol Rhinol Laryngol 61:558, 1952.
37. Goodale RL. Montgomery WW: Experiences with osteoplastic anterior wall approach to frontal sinus. Arch Otolaryngol 68:271, 1958.
38. Montgomery WW. Osteoplastic frontal sinus operation. Ann Otol Rhinol Laryngol 74:821, 1965.
39. Montgomery WW. Surgery of the Upper Respiratory System. Philadelphia: Lea & Febiger, 1971.
40. Goodale RL, Montgomery WW. Technical advances in osteoplastic frontal sinusectomy. Arch Otolaryngol 79:522, 1964.
41. Zonis RD, Montgomery WW, Goodale RL. Frontal sinus disease: 100 cases treated by osteoplastic operation. Laryngoscope 76: 1816, 1966.
42. Kennedy DW, Josephson JS, Zinreich SJ, et al. Endoscopic sinus surgery for mucoceles: A viable alternative. Laryngoscope 99: 885, 1989.
43. Schaefer SD, Close LG. Endoscopic management of frontal sinus disease. Laryngoscope 100:155, 1990.

44. Hoffer ME, Kennedy DW. The endoscopic management of sinus mucoceles following orbital decompression. Am J Rhinol 8:61, 1994.
45. Beasley NJP, Jones NS. Paranasal sinus mucoceles: Modern management. Am J Rhinol 9:251, 1995.
46. Hardy JM, Montgomery WW. Osteoplastic frontal sinusotomy. An analysis of 250 operations. Ann Otol 85:523, 1976.
47. Weber R, Draf W, Keerl R, et al. Aspects of frontal sinus surgery. III: Indications and results of osteoplastic frontal sinus operation. HNO 43(7):414, 1995.
48. Wide K, Sipila J, Suonpaa J. Report on results of frontal sinus obliterations in Turku University Central Hospital 1977–1994. Acta Otolaryngol [Suppl] 529:184, 1997.
49. Shumrick KA, Smith CP. The use of cancellous bone for frontal sinus obliteration and reconstruction of frontal bony defects. Arch Otolaryngol Head Neck Surg 120:1003, 1994.

SECTION THREE

Plastic and Reconstructive Surgery

CHAPTER 12

Nasoseptal Surgery

In this chapter, surgical correction of a deviated septum, repair of nasoseptal perforation, and nasoseptal dermoplasty are discussed. Surgery to correct a deviated septum is variously referred to as nasoseptal reconstruction, septoplasty, and submucous resection of the nasal septum, depending on the authority quoted and the technique used.[1–6] Commonly, submucous resection is defined, according to the procedure ascribed to Killian, as resection of most of the septal cartilage and bone while preserving the mucosal envelopes.[1, 4] Nasoseptal reconstruction refers to procedures that resect portions of the septal bone and cartilage and then straighten and replace the bone and cartilage as free grafts.[2, 7] By contrast, septoplasty, as described by Cottle, attempts to preserve but alter the septal structures to achieve straightening.[3, 5, 6, 8]

The operation to correct a deviated nasal septum is among the most basic operations in the practice of otolaryngology. The intriguing aspect of this procedure is the wide variety of techniques available to achieve a straightened septum. It seems that every otolaryngologist has his or her own technique for correction of a deviated septum, with good results reported for almost every variation. Some of these techniques, reported in recent years, have been described as extracorporeal,[9] limited,[10] back-and-forth,[11] endoscopic,[12] sagittal section,[13] mini,[14] and hemostatic suture techniques.[15, 16] It is not the goal of this chapter to describe all or even most of the common techniques available. Rather, in this chapter, one technique will be presented that has been used successfully by the author and taught to numerous residents. This technique is an amalgamation of techniques learned from numerous teachers during residency and adapted through practice and repetition.

SEPTOPLASTY

Indications

Nasal Obstruction

In patients with deviated septum, there are several reasons for proceeding to surgery. The most common indication is symptomatic nasal obstruction. Deviated septum by itself, if minimal, may be totally asymptomatic. However, in patients with severe deviation, an increasing degree of nasal obstruction may develop. In most such patients, a prolonged trial of medical therapy is offered before resorting to surgery. The purpose of this therapeutic trial is to provide the patient with a firsthand understanding of the alternatives to surgical correction. Merely discussing medical therapy as an alternative to septoplasty does not truly inform the patient as to its potential benefits.

A complicating factor is that many patients have a combination of chronic rhinitis and deviated septum. It is common for such patients to be asymptomatic for much of the year and to have problems from the deviated septum only during periods of exacerbation of the chronic rhinitis. Medical management of the chronic rhinitis, usually with antihistamine-decongestant combinations and nasal steroid sprays, often alleviates the symptoms, obviating the need for septal surgery.

Whether or not rhinitis is a factor, the initial approach to management in most patients is medical therapy. After treatment with appropriate medication, many patients experience significant improvement and will want to defer or avoid the surgery. Other patients will choose to proceed with surgery, either because the medication incompletely relieves the symptoms or because the patient decides that they prefer not to remain on medication.

Prior to performing septoplasty, it is advisable to document the septal deviation. This may be undertaken for medicolegal reasons, insurance justification, or documentation of a research study. Several alternatives for evaluation are available. Both sinus radiographs and computed tomography (CT) scans can demonstrate the anatomy of the septum, but CT scans are preferred owing to their superior detail and capacity to differentiate cartilaginous and bony anatomy. CT scans also allow full evaluation of the sinuses and any possible interaction between the turbinates and the septum.

Two other tests are available that measure the nasal airway: rhinomamometry and acoustic rhinometry. Rhinomamometry is the measurement of nasal resistance using a pressure probe placed in the front or back of the nose.[17] Acoustic rhinometry uses a reflective ultrasonic wave to measure the cross-sectional anatomy of the nose; it can be used to measure either total nasal volume or that of a minimal cross-sectional area.[18] Both techniques have been used repeatedly in scientific studies of the nose. However, despite the fact that they are easy to perform and are well-established methods, these tests have not entered the realm of standard practice in otolaryngology. In the everyday practice of rhinology, objective documentation of increased resistance or decreased volume or cross-sectional area has not been necessary to diagnose or treat disease. However, over the next few years, perhaps these tests will become standard as means of documenting the preoperative problem and establishing the quality of the outcome.

Several common circumstances may prompt the decision to recommend surgery for an obstructing septal deviation without a prolonged trial of medical therapy. One is if the patient has a total or near-total obstruction. Medical therapy cannot relieve this type of problem and, unless there is associated rhinitis or sinusitis, medical therapy is not indicated. Despite the presence of total or near-total nasal obstruction, some patients will maintain that they are unaffected by the deviated septum. In these cases it is still appropriate to offer septoplasty. Total or near-total nasal obstruction is a markedly nonphysiologic circumstance that may have a bearing on later development of sinus or respiratory complications. In addition, correction of such a problem may result in unexpected benefits in terms of vitality, energy level, and quality of life. Indeed, patients often state that they did not realize how bad they felt not being able to breathe through their nose until they had regained that function.

The other situation in which medical therapy can be bypassed is in young patients with symptomatic septal deviation. These patients face a choice of relatively minor surgery versus life-long medical therapy with periods of symptomatic relapse. Patients in their 30s and older may have already learned to live with the problems caused by deviated septum. For these older patients, the benefits of medical therapy may provide substantial relief and may be sufficient for their needs. Conversely, patients in their teens or early 20s who are symptomatic have usually not adapted to the condition. Although these young patients may benefit from medical management, early surgical intervention may be able to prevent years of discomfort and possible progression to sinusitis.

Headache

Septoplasty for headache is a controversial but often successful procedure.[19] There seems to be little question that some patients get recurrent headaches from contact points within the nose.[20–25] The difficulty is to establish the diagnosis accurately. Headache can be classified into several categories, including classic and atypical migraine, tension, cluster, and various forms of atypical facial pain. Identifying the cause of headache as a pressure point in the nose that is the result of a deviated septum requires a suggestive history, supportive examination, and a positive localization test.

The history of a patient with so-called rhinogenic headache is one of recurrent headache or pain, usually described as a pressure sensation or a sharp, penetrating pain over the nasal dorsum. The headaches arise during periods of nasal congestion or during the congestive phase of the nasal cycle. There may be a relationship to changes in weather or body position. Often, the patient will report obtaining relief from nasal decongestants. Most often, the headache is unilateral and located over the area of the pressure point, but it may be bilateral or midline.

The examination that is suggestive of rhinogenic headache should demonstrate at least one significant contact point. Most often, this is a septal spur that juts into the middle turbinate. The second most common finding—impaction against the inferior turbinate—is more common, but is usually not associated with severe headache. Other possibilities causing pressure points include bowing of the superior part of the septum, which creates a broader area of contact against lateral wall structures, and abnormally large turbinates. It has also been reported that a pneumatized or enlarged superior turbinate can cause a severe headache syndrome.[26]

If both the examination and history suggest rhinogenic headache, then testing is necessary to confirm the diagnosis. This is accomplished during a period of headache. The nose is decongested and then the area of the contact point is anesthetized with either topical lidocaine or cocaine or injectable lidocaine.[27] The headache should resolve within the first few minutes after the local anesthetic is applied and should return after the anesthesia resolves. Later, direct palpation of the contact point should simulate the experience of the headache.

In cases when the rhinogenic headache cannot be confirmed by testing, surgery should not be performed for headache alone until after a complete neurologic evaluation and a trial of specific non-nasal treatment. However, if the history, examination, and testing all suggest rhinogenic headache, then septoplasty is a reasonable step and can be offered to the patient. In such cases, the patient should be advised that failure to relieve the headache is possible despite a highly suggestive clinical picture and adequate surgery. With carefully selected patients, the chance of success is good. In some series, success rates as high as 80% to 90% have been reported.[19] The key to achieving these excellent results is to select patients carefully and not rush to surgery as the first alternative.

Epistaxis

Management of epistaxis is covered in detail in a later chapter. There are patients with recurrent epistaxis, however, who may benefit from a septoplasty. Usually, these patients have pronounced septal spurs in the inferior airway where excessive airflow leads to drying, crusting, and recurrent epistaxis. Most of the time, conservative measures, such as humidification, moisturization, and judicious use of cautery, will control the problem. Rarely, a patient will develop either refractory bleeding or numerous recurrences of bleeding in which case a septoplasty can be considered as an alternative to other surgical procedures.

Surgical Access

Patients undergoing endoscopic sinus surgery or the more traditional intranasal ethmoidectomy require a clear path from the nares to the middle meatus. If this path is blocked by a deviated septum, then a septoplasty must be performed to facilitate the sinus procedure. Management of the deviated septum in this situation will depend on the severity of the deviated septum. Well-delineated spurs in the middle meatus can simply be resected through a limited incision over the spur itself.[10, 12] If the septum bows widely toward the middle turbinate, a formal septoplasty may be required to create exposure.

A more difficult clinical decision must be made in the case of mild deviation. In such cases, surgery may still be performed with excellent topical anesthesia and careful technique to avoid trauma to the septum. However, these patients are likely to have a difficult time with postoperative care and may not tolerate the cleaning necessary to prevent synechiae and ostial stenosis. In this situation, the surgeon must use judgment and experience to weigh whether the nasal passageway is sufficiently blocked to prevent the degree of postoperative care needed.

Pediatric Septoplasty

A long-standing controversy in otolaryngology has centered around the advisability of performing septoplasty in children. As a result of birth trauma, blunt nasal trauma in childhood, or unequal growth of the septum, many children do manifest septal deviation. As with adults, this may be the cause of significant symptoms or the cause of sinusitis. A septal deviation may also block access to the sinus for surgery in this population, as in adults. Traditional guidelines suggest that surgery be delayed until the age of 16 years or older to avoid interference with nasal growth. Closed nasal reduction has been suggested as an alternative that would not interfere with nasal growth.[28] Studies have suggested that septoplasty in children is typically successful in improving nasal air flow.[29] However, other studies have documented some undesirable surgical effects, especially on nasal length.[30] The safest recommendation is to defer septoplasty, if at all possible, until the patient is an adult, or at least until the age of 16 years.

Anatomy

Septoplasty, as an operation, is an exercise in anatomy. The details of the normal anatomy of the septum are covered in Chapter 1. It is important to emphasize certain aspects, however. The rigid structure of the septum is a joining of the anterior quadrilateral cartilage to the posterior vomer and perpendicular plate of the ethmoid. A tongue of cartilage interdigitates between the vomer and perpendicular plate of the ethmoid. This posterior tongue of cartilage varies widely in shape and length. It is this part of the septum that often becomes displaced, resulting in significant spurs. The quadrilateral cartilage sits in a groove of the maxillary crest and joins to the maxillary crest by dense, tendinous fibers. Posteriorly, the cartilage joins to the vomer and perpendicular plate in an end-to-end fashion without overlap or fibrous attachments. These relationships are critical in the development of methods to separate these structures. The nerve and blood supply to the septum are also critical, and delineate the location of injected local anesthetic.

Septal deviation can be classified by the shape of the septum, the cause of the deviation, or the elements of the deviation. The causes include trauma, congenital deviation, overgrowth of the septum, and enlargement of the inferior or middle turbinate. The elements of deviation may include cartilaginous bowing or spurs, bone spurs or fractures, or combinations of these. To best understand the septoplasty operation, one needs to understand the anatomy or shape of the deviation. There are several common shapes of septal deviation found in practice (Fig. 12–1). These include linear unilateral, C-shaped, or S-shaped deviation, and unilateral or bilateral spur.

Experience has shown that most septal deviations are caused by deviations in the bone. Bony deviations will push the cartilage along with it, whereas cartilaginous deviations will not affect the underlying bone. Correction of the septal deviation, therefore, demands that the surgeon address the bony aspects of the deviation, as well as the cartilaginous portions. Accordingly, correction of the bony deviation will allow straightening of the septum with only minimal resection of cartilage.

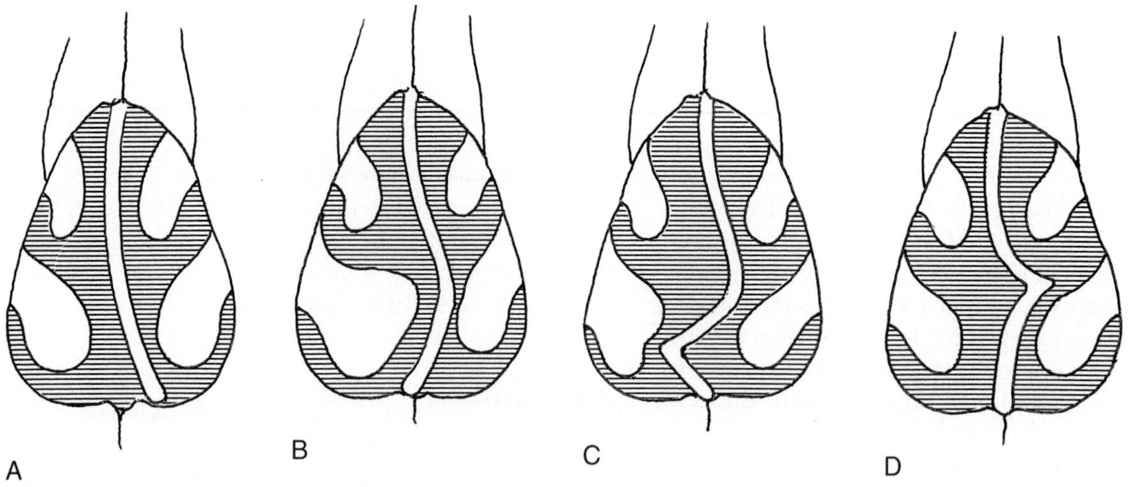

Figure 12–1. Anatomy of common septal deviations. *A*, Septal displacement from the maxillary crest. *B*, Bowing of the septum (C-shaped septum). *C*, Bilateral deviation (S-shaped septum). *D*, Unilateral spur (in this case, affecting the middle meatus, but any level can be affected).

Preoperative Considerations

Several issues must be addressed before the patient goes to the operating room for septoplasty. The first is the selection of which procedure to perform. Many surgeons use several different techniques tailored to the type of deviation present. The author utilizes a single, universal approach to septoplasty that involves complete exposure and correction of all aspects of deviation. This eliminates the concern or deliberation about which technique to perform.

A second consideration is whether or not to include turbinate resection. In most patients, the side opposite the septal deviation will have an enlarged inferior turbinate. On the side of the deviation, the turbinate is usually compressed by the septal deviation. This may result in a portion of the inferior aspect of the turbinate bulging into the nasal passage. Several studies have attempted to evaluate the benefit of turbinate surgery at the time of septoplasty. Most have shown that turbinectomy in some form does improve the subjective[31, 32] and objective[33] surgical outcome, at least in the short term. However, one randomized prospective trial with long-term follow-up evaluation failed to document significant benefit from turbinoplasty.[34] This study postulated that the turbinate hypertrophy on the side opposite the deviation eventually resolves without resection. This issue remains controversial. A more complete discussion of the controversy is presented in Chapter 7. However, owing to the low risk of complications and short-term benefits derived by the patient, the author usually performs conservative resection of the turbinate by inferior turbinoplasty or submucous resection at the time of septoplasty.

Occasionally, a septal deviation will be caused by an enlarged middle turbinate, usually due to a large concha bullosa. In such cases, resection of the lateral lamella and a partial ethmoidectomy will be necessary to achieve septal straightening.

There is significant controversy concerning the need for prophylactic antibiotics for septoplasty. The incidence of soft tissue infection of the nose and septal abscess is minimal, and there are no studies that definitively address this issue. One study of 1040 patients undergoing nasal surgery without surgical prophylaxis or skin preparation reported only a 0.48% rate of infection (5/1040).[35] A second study demonstrated that bacteremia is rare following nasal surgery.[36] The other important infectious complication is toxic shock syndrome.[37–40] This syndrome is caused by the liberation of a toxin by a staphylococcal species that infects the postoperative packing or splints. Antibiotics have not been shown to completely eliminate the risk of this syndrome. However, to minimize the risk, antistaphylococcal antibiotics are routinely prescribed by many surgeons while packing or splints are in place. Despite the lack of objective evidence that antibiotics reduce either the rate of postoperative soft tissue infection or toxic shock syndrome, the author routinely prescribes antistaphylococcal antibiotics for all patients with nasal packing for the duration of the packing.

Anesthesia

The first decision in septoplasty is whether to use general anesthesia or sedation. To the author, this is really not a significant issue. The operation can be equally well performed using either anesthetic technique. The difference is that the sedated patients may experience momentary discomfort during the procedure; however, they wake up faster and have less anesthesia-related nausea and emesis. Patients who receive general anesthesia are completely unaware of the operation and feel no discomfort, but require longer to wake up from the operation and experience more anesthesia-related complications. The ultimate decision for or against a particular method of anesthesia is left up to the patient and the anesthesiologist. The patient's preference in this decision should be the determining factor.

If sedation anesthesia is selected, the choice of agents is important. The only time during the procedure that significant pain would be expected is during the administration of the local anesthetic. At this time, a bolus of sedative is given to achieve deep sedation. Thereafter, the level of sedation is allowed to lighten progressively to the end of the operation, at which point the patient is essentially awake. Sodium Pentothal and propofol are two intravenous general anesthetic agents that tend to cause patients to become dysphoric and disoriented. This may result in the patient reacting to sensations during the surgery by withdrawing or turning the head away from the surgeon. These agents also tend to induce hypoventilation, thus requiring the anesthetist to support the airway, which may interfere with the surgery. For these reasons, the preferred anesthetic agents are a combination of a short-acting benzodiazepine and a narcotic. This combination achieves the appropriate sedation without loss of airway control or the patient's cooperation.

Regardless of the type of sedation or general anesthetic used, the same topical and local anesthetic agents are applied. The first step is to apply a topical decongestant. Either 1% oxymetazoline or 4% cocaine solution serves equally well. For patients with hypertension or cardiac disease, the oxymetazoline is preferred, but otherwise, cocaine is normally used. The key to hemostasis and anesthesia during the surgery is not the topical agent but the injected local anesthetic. For most patients, 1% lidocaine with 1 : 100,000 epinephrine is used, but for cardiac patients, the epinephrine can be diluted to 1 : 200,000. Using the rule of 7 mg/kg as the theoretical maximum dose of lidocaine, the typical 70-kg adult man can receive up to 49 cc of local anesthetic, which is more than sufficient. Typically, no more than 15 cc is used for a septoplasty when sedation is used.

The local anesthetic is administered using a 25-gauge needle and a control syringe. The injections are placed in multiple sites, achieving a blanching of the mucosa with each injection and attempting to instill the local agent into the subperiosteal plane. The locations of the injections are shown in Figure 12–2. It is important to achieve excellent infiltration in several key areas, including the columella, the floor of the nose anteriorly, along the dorsum of the septum, and as far posteriorly as possible. With rhinoplasty and other soft tissue procedures, excessive infiltration will lead to distortion and interference with assessment of the cosmetic result. For septoplasty, this is not a concern. Increased infiltration of local anesthetic results in improved anesthesia and hemostasis without distorting the anatomy. In fact, with accurately placed injections, it may be possible to hydrodissect the subperichondrial and subperiosteal planes, thereby facilitating the dissection.

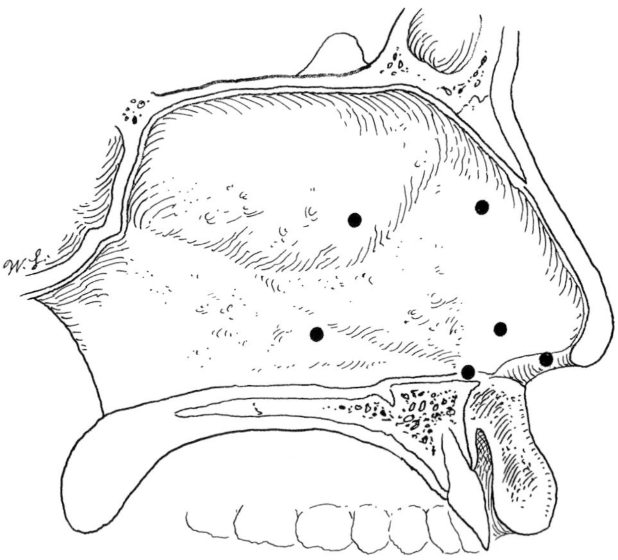

Figure 12–2. Injection points for local anesthetic prior to septoplasty. The black dots indicate injection points in the columella, along the floor, in the anterior cartilaginous septum, along the dorsal cartilaginous septum, against the vomer, and in the perpendicular plate of the ethmoid.

Instrumentation

Many instruments have been designed and produced for use during septoplasty. The following illustrations demonstrate those used by the author. Three sizes of nasal specula (Vienna, Cottle, Killian) are needed, as shown in Figure 12–3. During injection of local anesthetic and initial flap elevation, the Vienna speculum is used. The intermediate length and the narrow tips of the Cottle speculum are favored for most of the procedure. The narrower tips of this speculum allow better visualization at the end of the instrument than the wider-tipped specula. The longest speculum, the Killian, is used to visualize the posterior septum and sphenoid rostrum. It is used primarily in patients with deep or long noses or those with far posterior bony spurs.

Several different elevators are used (Fig. 12–4). These include the standard Cottle elevator, an inferior tunnel elevator or curved Cottle, a hockey stick elevator, and a Freer cartilage knife (also known as a D-knife or a half-round knife). Included in the set are a number of miscellaneous instruments. Figure 12–5 demon-

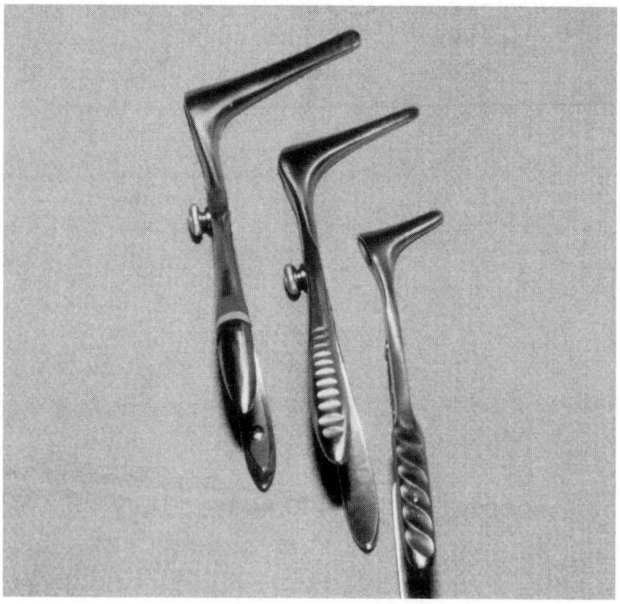

Figure 12–3. Nasal specula used during septoplasty, including the Vienna, Cottle, and Killian types.

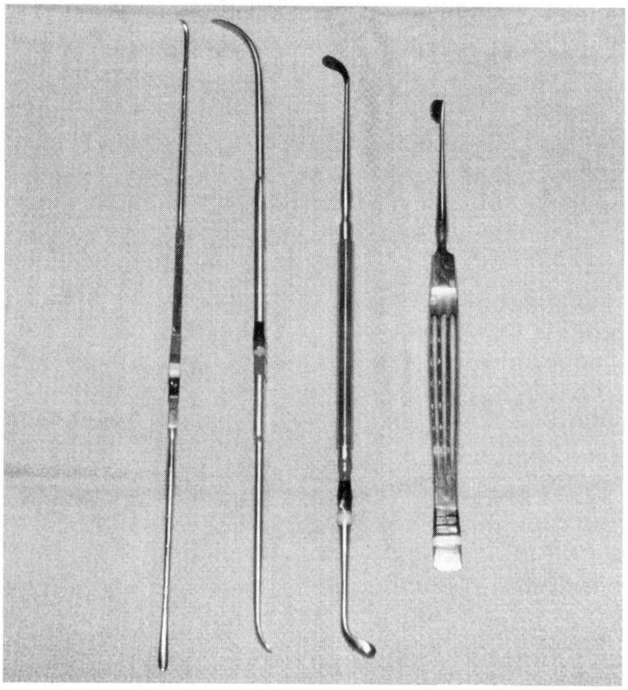

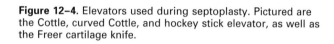

Figure 12–4. Elevators used during septoplasty. Pictured are the Cottle, curved Cottle, and hockey stick elevator, as well as the Freer cartilage knife.

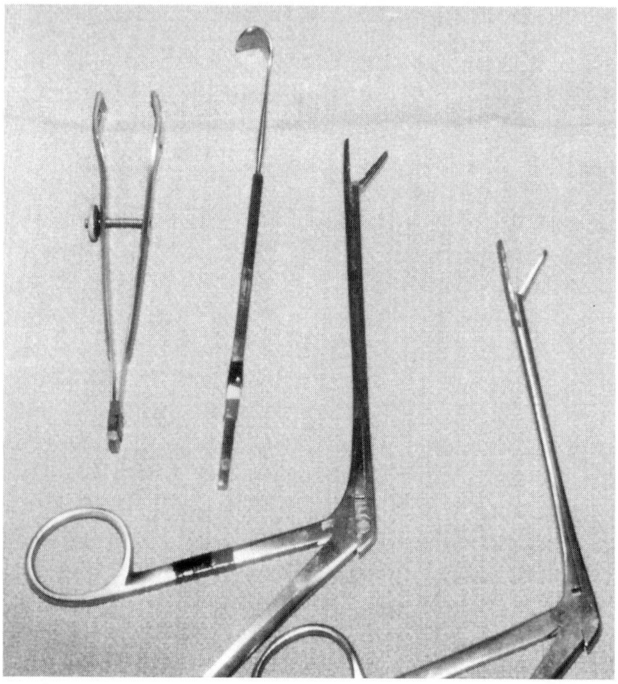

Figure 12–5. Miscellaneous instruments used during septoplasty, including the columella retractor, alar protector, Takahashi forceps, and Ferris Smith forceps.

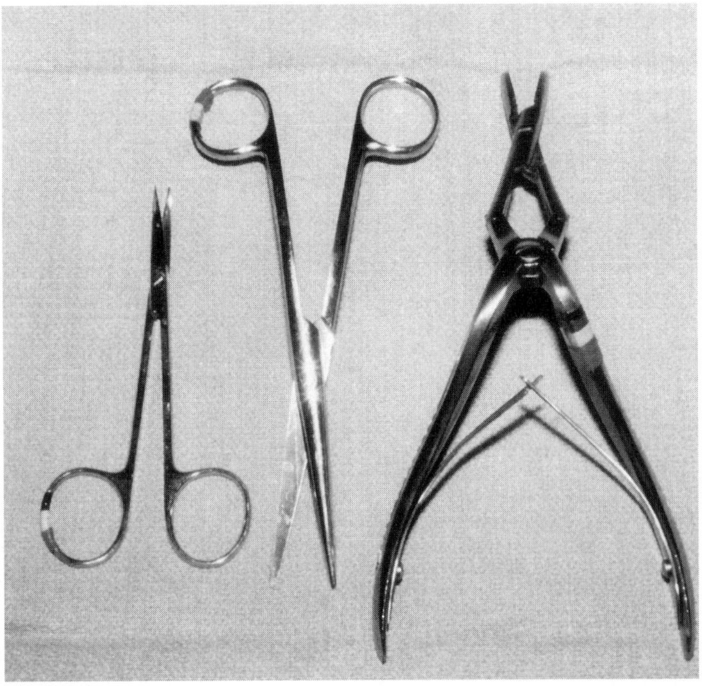

Figure 12–6. Cutting instruments used during septoplasty. Pictured are dorsal bone scissors, Jansen-Middleton forceps, and curved iris scissors.

strates the columella retractor, alar protector, Takahashi forceps, and Ferris Smith forceps. Finally, the instrument set includes cutting instruments, such as dorsal bone scissors, Jansen-Middleton rongeurs, and curved iris scissors (Fig. 12–6). Each of these instruments is used for a specific step in the operation, as discussed later in this chapter. The set also includes several standard surgical instruments, such as small double hooks, suture scissors, a knife handle, and a needle driver. The use of these instruments is self-explanatory and requires no further comment. This simple set of 18 instruments is sufficient to perform virtually all septoplasty operations. There are, however, numerous other instruments that many surgeons find useful or even essential. This discrepancy is indicative of the wide variety of techniques that have been proposed for this basic operation over a century of surgical development.

Technique

The procedure described in this section is the technique performed by the author. The operation is adapted from the swinging door technique. The principle of this technique is to completely free up the quadrilateral cartilage from all bony attachments, elevate the mucosa from the entire bony septum, and then preserve as much of the cartilage as possible. The bone of the septum is liberally removed, as needed, to achieve a straight septum. Free grafts are avoided. The reason for this is that these grafts are unpredictable in the degree of reabsorption and vascularization and have a tendency to drift during healing. Also, free grafts tend to encourage fibrosis and thickening of the septum over the area in which they are placed.

A final introductory remark is offered about handedness of the septoplasty procedure. This operation, as described in this chapter, is applicable for right-handed surgeons. The techniques utilized have been selected partially because they favor the angles experienced by a right-handed surgeon. A left-handed surgeon must switch sides to avoid clumsy, cross-handed manipulations. This may necessitate turning the table to the left, turning the patient's head to the left, and standing to the left of the patient.

Incision

For the standard septoplasty, three basic incisions are used: hemitransfixion, complete transfixion, and the Killian incision. The complete transfixion incision is used when the caudal end of the septum is completely resected and reimplanted. This incision is also favored during septorhinoplasty when the delivery technique is employed (see Chapter 13). A Killian incision directly over the cartilage on the side of elevation of the flap is favored by some. Its disadvantage is that it restricts vertical height of the incision and does not expose the caudal end of the septum. In the technique presented here, a right hemitransfixion incision is made (Fig. 12–7). The columella retractor is applied and the columella is displaced to expose the caudal edge of the septum. The superiolateral ala is retracted with an alar retractor. The incision is made on the right side of the columella

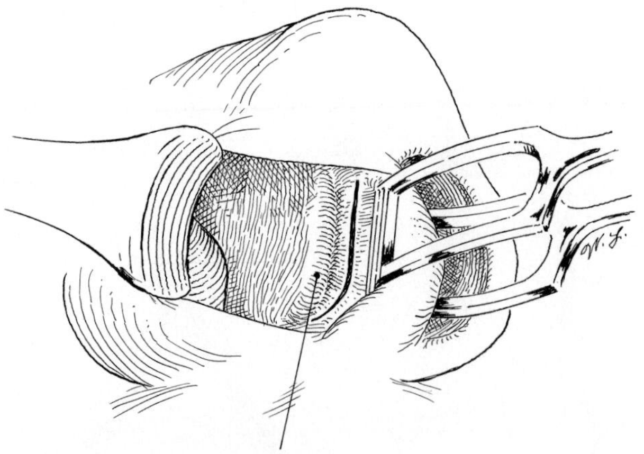

Figure 12–7. Right hemitransfixion incision. The incision is made in the patient's right nares on the left edge of the caudal end of the septum, extending from the floor of the vestibule to the dorsum of the columella.

but the left side of the caudal edge of the septum. The incision is started at the upper edge of the caudal edge of the septum and carried inferiorly about two thirds of the way to the base, cutting just through the epidermis and dermis. The incision is completed by moving the alar protector to the inferior nasal sill and retracting it inferiorly. The knife is turned to face superiorly and an incision is made starting from the pyriform aperture and continuing superiorly to join the initial incision.

With the incision completed, the alar protector is removed and a 2- or 3-mm double hook is placed on the caudal edge of the septum and retracted to the right. Using the curved iris scissors perpendicular to the cartilage, the soft tissues are spread down to the layer of the cartilage on the left side of the cartilage (Fig. 12–8). At this point, it is only necessary to expose a few millimeters of cartilage. However, it is important to be sure that true cartilage is exposed through the perichondrium.

The sharp side of the Cottle elevator is then used to develop the perichondrial dissection. The perichondrium is elevated posteriorly onto the septum for a few millimeters and then superiorly and inferiorly to undermine the remaining attachments of the incision. The remaining attachments can then be cut by the iris scissors.

Left Side Exposure

The next step is to completely expose the septum. This is begun with elevation of the left-sided mucosal flap, the so-called anterior and posterior tunnels. A small nasal speculum is then used to expose the septal dissection. By holding the speculum upside down, the handle is turned out of the way and the blades are oriented horizontally, optimally exposing the surgical dissection. The sharp side of the Cottle elevator is then used to elevate the perichondrium from the quadrilateral cartilage. The dissection should be performed under direct vision, switching to the Cottle speculum when needed to maintain direct vision. The sharp edge of the elevator should be kept firmly applied to the cartilage, and short, 1-mm steps should be used to elevate the perichondrium (Fig. 12–9).

The dissection is continued in this way until the bony cartilaginous junction is crossed. The Cottle elevator is then reversed, and the blunt end is used over the bone of the septum. Rather than a short, choppy motion, a sweeping motion is used on the bone. The elevation is extended superiorly to the nasal roof, posteriorly to the

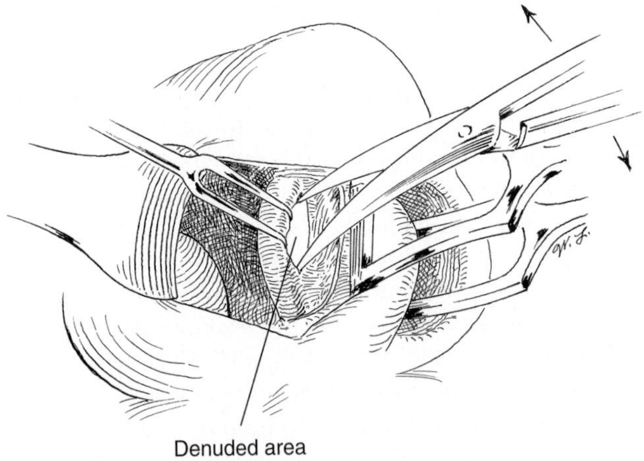

Figure 12–8. Initial exposure of the caudal end of the septal cartilage. The scissors are kept perpendicular to the cartilage and the tissues are spread through the perichondrium to the cartilage.

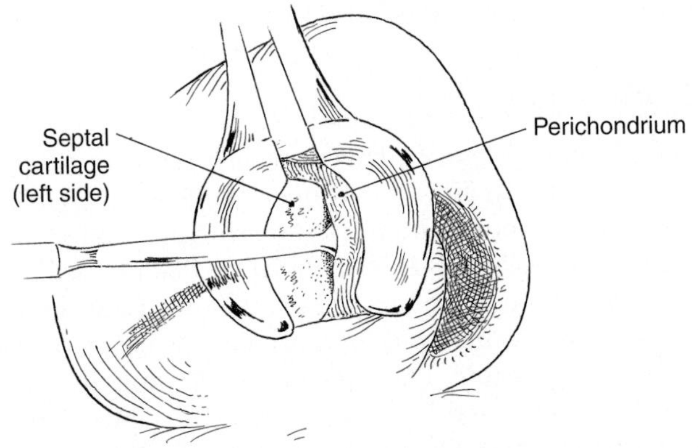

Figure 12–9. Elevation of the mucoperichondrial tunnel (anterior tunnel) on the left side. The sharp end of the Cottle elevator is held firmly against the cartilage while the perichondrium is scraped from the underlying cartilage.

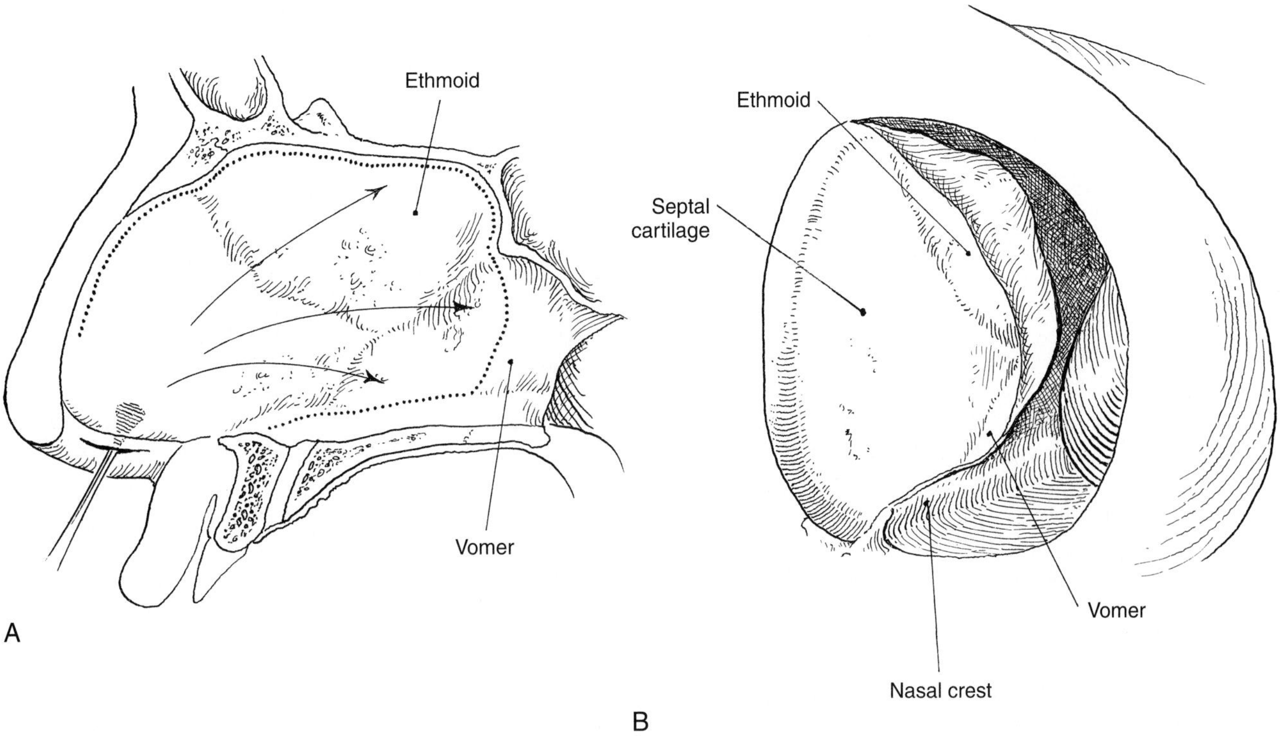

Figure 12–10. Completed exposure of the left side of the septum (anterior and posterior tunnels). *A,* The dotted line indicates the extent of exposure achieved at this point in the operation. The arrows indicate the direction of elevation. *B,* Surgical view of the exposure. The mucosal flap is folded back to show the quadrilateral cartilage, perpendicular plate, and vomer. In life, this exposure is possible only with a speculum. Note that the elevation has not yet extended down over the maxillary crest to the floor of the nose.

sphenoid rostrum, and inferiorly to the maxillary crest (Fig. 12–10).

The next step is to elevate the left-sided flap over the maxillary crest to the floor of the nose. There are three techniques that can be used to achieve this step. The first technique applies to cases when the deviation is to the right and there is no overhang on the left side. In such cases, a hockey stick elevator is used to elevate the flap. The hockey stick is firmly but gently worked toward the floor of the nose, posterior to the maxillary crest (Fig. 12–11). When the floor is reached, the hockey stick is worked anteriorly along the crest between the

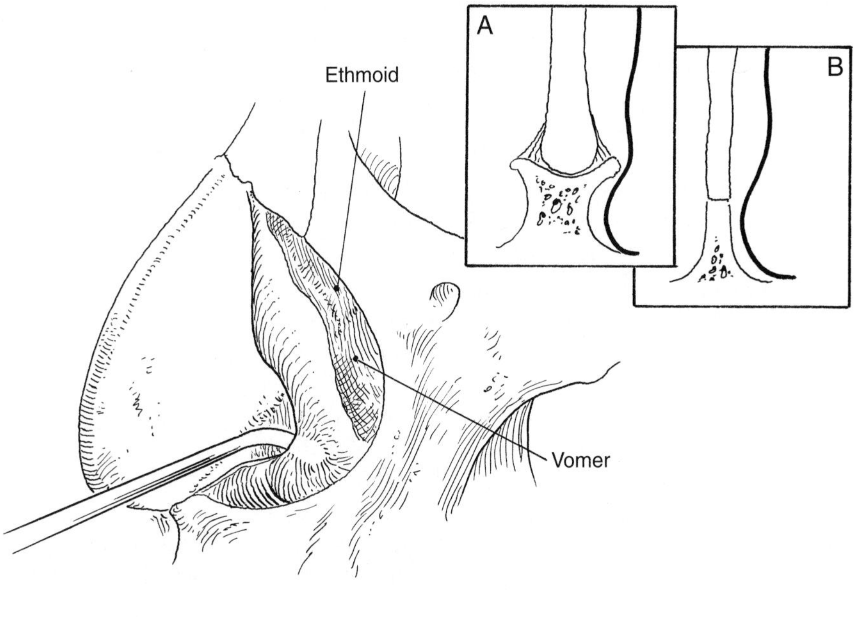

Figure 12–11. Type 1 exposure over the crest to the floor of the nose. This applies only to cases of deviation to the patient's right. The hockey stick elevator is used to dissect down to the floor behind the crest at the level of the vomer. The instrument is then worked forward, separating the mucosa from the crest. *A,* Anatomy of the septum at the maxillary crest. The cartilage sits in a tongue-and-groove position between two wings of the crest attached by fibrous bands. *B,* Anatomy of the septum at the level of the vomer. The cartilage (or perpendicular plate) joins directly to the vomer without fibrous attachments or tongue-and-groove configuration.

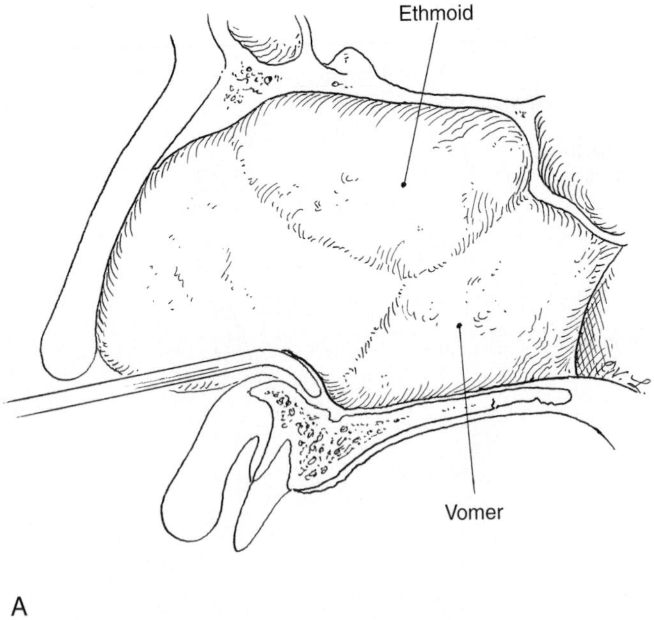

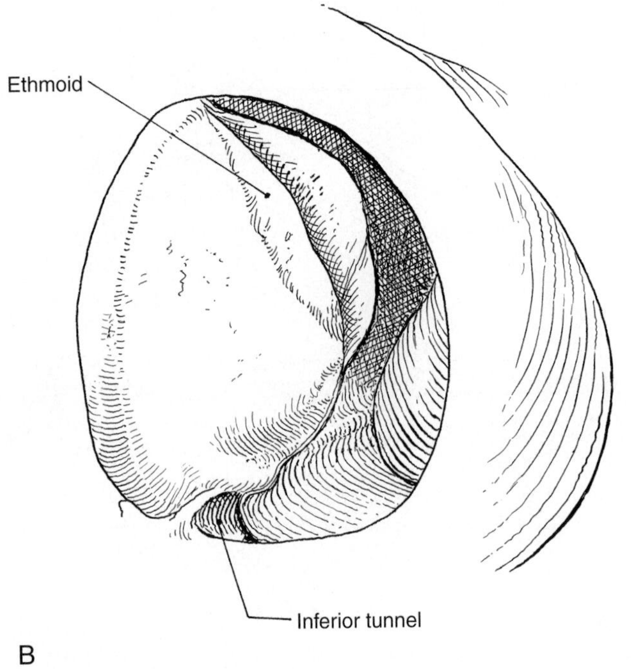

Figure 12–12. Type 2 exposure of the floor of the nose (inferior tunnel). This applies to cases of deviation to the left or those involving a pronounced inferior spur or crest. *A,* The curved end of the curved Cottle is used to begin the direct elevation over the pyriform aperture onto the floor of the nose. *B,* Surgical view of the inferior tunnel. Elevation of the mucosa from the floor has left the mucosa attached to the septum only along the septal spur.

bone and the periosteum until the maxillary crest is completely exposed.

The second technique is useful in cases when there is a deviation or spur to the left side or a significant horizontal projection of the maxillary crest. In this situation, the direct approach invariably results in perforation of the flap. Therefore, an inferior tunnel is created. The base of the septum is exposed at the level of the premaxilla and the pyriform aperture is exposed (Fig. 12–12). The curved Cottle elevator is then used to elevate the periosteum over the pyriform aperture down to the floor of the nose. The elevator is reversed and the flatter end of the curved Cottle is then used to extend the elevation posteriorly to the back of the nose, thereby completing the inferior tunnel. Working from an anterior position, the inferior and anterior tunnels are connected using the hockey stick elevator to lift the flap from the edge of the maxillary crest. When the spur is reached, elevation from below to the tip of the spur is followed by elevation from above down to the tip of the spur.

The third technique for elevating down to the floor over the maxillary crest is used in cases of extreme anterior cartilaginous deviations to the left, in which it is impossible to see the floor of the nose. In these cases, after the initial flap elevation down to the anterior tip of the deviation, the cartilage is incised anterior to the deviation, crossing over to the right side of the cartilage (Fig. 12–13). Subperichondrial elevation is continued on the right side, down over the maxillary crest to the floor of the nose. This portion of the cartilage is separated from the maxillary crest, vomer, and ethmoid bones. At this point, the cartilaginous spur should be completely detached from surrounding bone. This allows the spur to be displaced to the right and facilitates elevation of the mucosa over the sharp end of the spur (Fig. 12–14). With the cartilage removed and the maxillary crest exposed, either one of the other two techniques can be used to complete the elevation over the crest to the floor. If the bony aspect of the spur is so severe that neither technique can be used, an osteotome is used to detach the bone spur, allowing it to be displaced to the right in a similar fashion to that described for the cartilage. The mucosa on the left side of the spur can then be elevated under direct vision.

Right Side Exposure

In routine surgical cases, following completion of left side exposure, the next step is to cross over to the right side of the septum through the septal cartilage. In most cases, this is done at the bony cartilaginous junction.

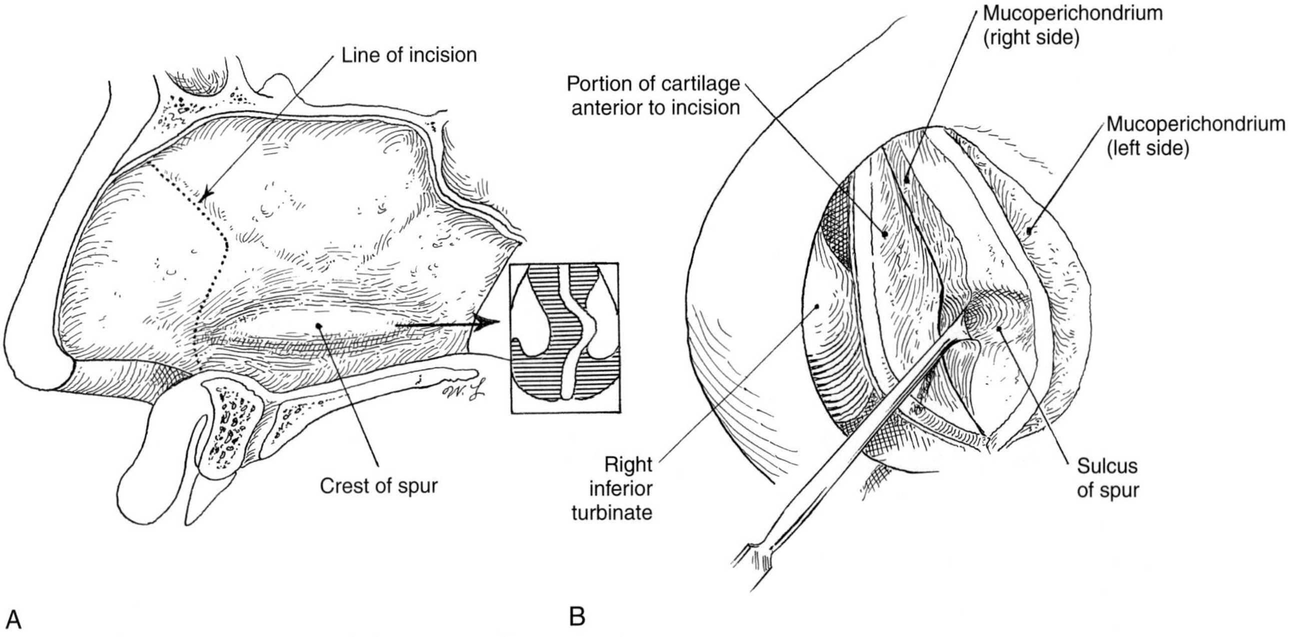

Figure 12–13. Type 3 exposure of the floor of the nose (in situ resection). This applies to the worst cases of deviation when the tip of the spur cannot be reached to elevate the mucosa. *A,* The dotted line demonstrates the site of incision through the cartilage from left to right in front of the spur. *B,* Surgical view. After the cartilage is incised, the mucosa is elevated from the right side of the spur. The exposed cartilage surface anterior to the incision is on the left side. The exposed cartilage surface posterior to the incision is on the right side. The mucosa is elevated from the concave side of the spur (sulcus). An inferior strip of cartilage is excised to free the cartilage from the crest, the dorsal bone scissors are used to cut above the spur, and a chisel is used to cut the bone below the spur.

One exception to this is in cases in which there is a sharp cartilaginous spur just anterior to the junction. In such instances, the crossover will be just anterior to the spur. To identify the junction, the sharp end of the Cottle elevator is pulled across the left side of the septum from posterior to anterior. The transition from bone to cartilage is easily appreciated by the change from a rough to smooth texture. The elevator is gently sawed through the junction until separation is achieved. It is important to make sure that the right side mucosal flap is not perforated at this point. Once the initial separation is developed, the elevator can be placed through this gap and the remainder of the bony cartilaginous junction separated with a careful sweeping motion

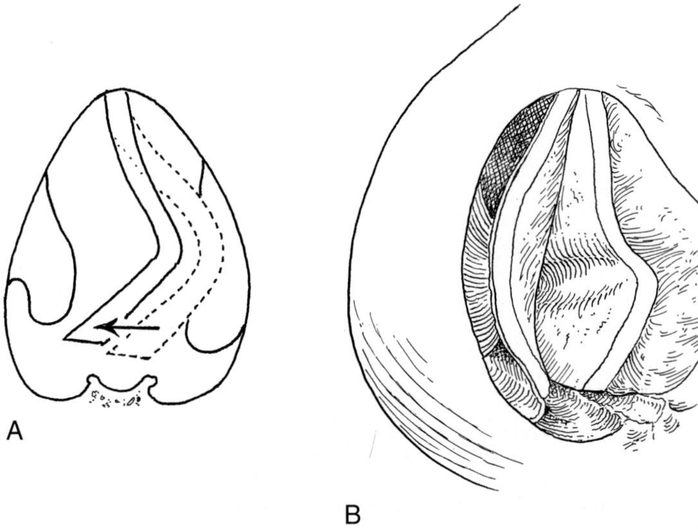

Figure 12–14. Completion of in situ resection. *A,* Conceptual drawing demonstrating displacement of the septum to the right. *B,* Surgical view showing the septum displaced to the right. After the spur is freed from the bony and cartilaginous attachments, it is displaced to the right. The mucosa can then be directly elevated from the left side of the spur without risking injury to the mucosa.

(Fig. 12–15). The separation should be continued superiorly to the nasal dorsum and inferiorly to the maxillary crest.

After the separation is completed, the mucosa is elevated from the bone of the septum on the right side. This is again easily achieved using a sweeping motion and the blunt end of the Cottle elevator. When this step is finished, the vomer and perpendicular plate of the ethmoid will both be completely exposed.

To complete the exposure, the mucosa must be elevated from the maxillary crest and the floor of the nose on the right side. The first step to accomplish this is to incise and remove a strip of cartilage from the maxillary crest (Fig. 12–16). This excision is performed with the Freer cartilage knife (D-knife or half-round knife). The strip is designed to extend from the vomer forward, to the anterior edge of the maxillary crest. It is important that at least 1 cm of the caudal end of the septum be preserved to maintain support to the nasal tip.

Once the inferior strip is removed, there is access to the right side mucosa, which needs to be elevated from the maxillary crest. Two techniques are available. If there is no spur to the right and no significant bony overhang, elevation can be achieved directly using the hockey stick elevator. The fibrous attachments to the crest are divided on the surface of the maxillary crest and then slowly worked laterally to the edge of the crest. The hockey stick is then worked between the periosteum and the vomer posterior to the crest. When the elevation is complete to the floor posteriorly, the instrument is drawn forward within the plane to continue the separation to the pyriform aperture (Fig. 12–17).

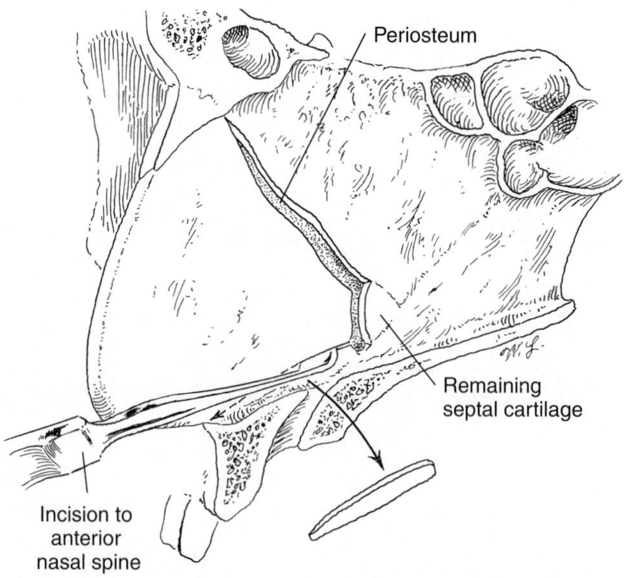

Figure 12–16. Removal of an inferior strip of cartilage. After the bony cartilaginous junction is completely separated, the Freer cartilage knife is used to remove the inferior 2-mm strip of cartilage above the maxillary crest. The inferior strip is extended anteriorly only to the anterior nasal spine.

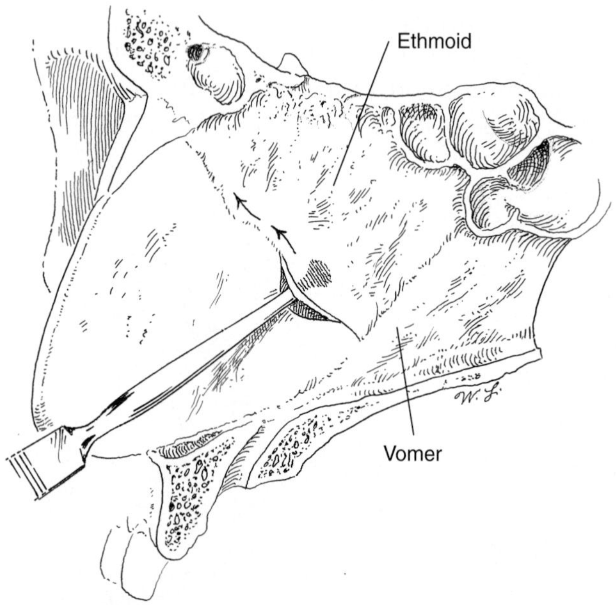

Figure 12–15. Separation of the septal cartilage from the vomer and perpendicular plate of the ethmoid. The sharp end of the Cottle elevator is used to cut through at the junction. This separation is extended to the nasal dorsum and the maxillary crest.

A second technique for exposure over the maxillary crest onto the right floor of the nose is useful in cases in which a significant spur arises from the crest and extends into the right side of the nose. In such cases, direct elevation over the spur from above will cause perforation in the flap. To avoid this problem, an inferior tunnel is created. The area of the pyriform aperture is exposed through the hemitransfixion incision, and the periosteum is elevated up to the aperture. The curved Cottle elevator is used to lift the mucosa from the floor of the nose back to the posterior choanae. The elevation is completed working from anterior to posterior, as described earlier for left side exposure, using the hockey stick elevator from above and below the spur.

This completes the exposure of the septum. At this point, the entire bony septum is exposed and the quadrilateral cartilage is attached to the mucosa on the right side and superiorly at the nasal dorsum.

Resection

Septal resection is performed in several stages. In the first stage, any significant bony septal spurs are resected. This is accomplished by first making a bone cut superior to the spur. This should always be performed sharply to avoid torsion on the cribriform plate. The preferred

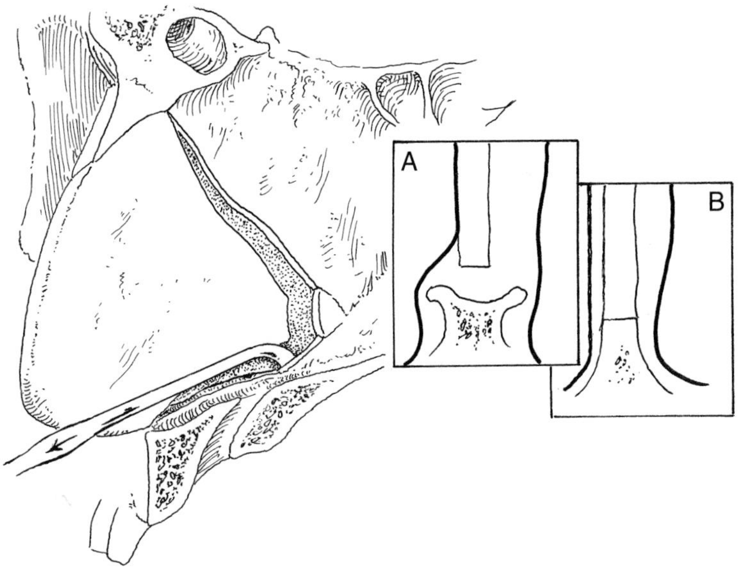

Figure 12–17. Elevation over the maxillary crest to the floor of the nose on the right side. The hockey stick elevator is used to dissect between the periosteum and the vomer behind the maxillary crest and down to the floor of the nose. The instrument is worked forward within this plane to elevate the mucosa from the crest. *A,* The relationship of the mucosa to the cartilage at the level of the crest. Note that the mucosa remains attached to the cartilage on the right side. *B,* The relationship of the mucosa to the perpendicular plate of the ethmoid and vomer in the posterior septum. Note that the mucosa is elevated bilaterally.

instrument is the dorsal bone scissors. The bone cut is extended from the cartilaginous junction posteriorly to the sphenoid rostrum. The vomer is then cut below the spur. This bone is usually too thick to be cut by scissors. Therefore, the cut is made using a 4-mm straight osteotome. The cut is started at the junction of the maxillary crest and the vomer and angled posteriorly and inferiorly. With the cuts completed, the spur is then grasped with Ferris Smith forceps, given a gentle twist, and removed. Residual deviated bone can be removed with Takahashi forceps.

The next step is to narrow the maxillary crest. The crest is evaluated by looking in the nose and displacing the septum first to one side and then the other with the Cottle speculum. With the cartilaginous septum displaced, significant lateral wings on the maxillary crest can be seen overhanging the floor of the nose. The crest is then narrowed by performing a sagittal osteotomy using a 4-mm straight osteotome (Fig. 12–18). Careful placement and control of the osteotome are important to avoid accidental resection of the entire crest. The crest is important for preserving support to the nasal tip, but it is not necessary that the lateral wings on the crest be present to hold the septum in the midline. Once healing is complete, the cartilaginous septum will form a secure union with the central aspect of the crest as long as good contact is preserved.

The final step is to address the dorsal septum. This area is often bowed to one side or the other and is typically very thick just at the junction of the bone and cartilage. This part of the septum is resected using Jansen-Middleton forceps. It is essential that small, 1-mm bites be taken one at a time. The forceps will not cleanly take bigger pieces without the risk of avulsing the perpendicular plate of the ethmoid or the quadrilateral cartilage.

This completes the resection of the bony septum. At this point, the septum behind the quadrilateral cartilage should be perfectly straight. Any residual bone that distorts or indents the septum can be resected using the Takahashi forceps. There should be residual bone in the perpendicular plate of the ethmoid superiorly and posteriorly, the central portion of the maxillary crest, and the inferior and posterior aspects of the vomer.

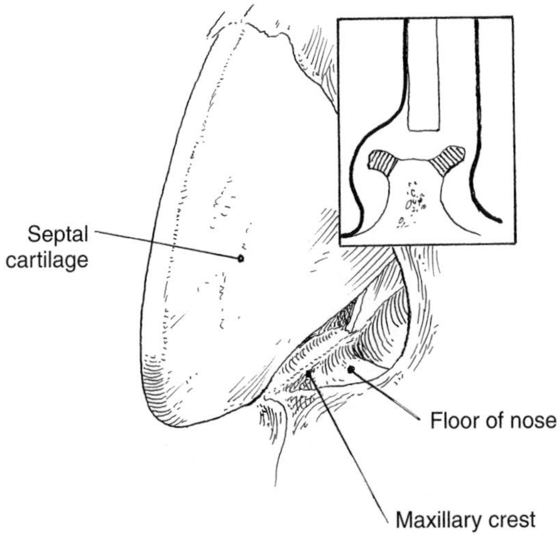

Figure 12–18. Narrowing the maxillary crest. The figure shows an idealized view of the septum after the inferior strip is removed, highlighting the lateral wings of the maxillary crest. The inset demonstrates the bone removed from the crest. This is performed using sagittal osteotomies.

Usually, a large amount of bone from the central part of the septum is resected. This bone is never replaced. Although many surgeons favor straightening and replacing the septal bone, the author does not use this technique. The grafted bone tends to drift, and even if it remains stable, it will widen the septum and lead to new bone growth.

Cartilage Contouring

Using the technique described in this chapter, the bulk of the cartilaginous septum is preserved. Deviations in the cartilage are dealt with by recontouring the cartilage in situ. Experience has shown that, by completely detaching the cartilage from the septal bone, most deviations of the cartilage can be managed by recontouring. Severe cartilaginous spurs adjacent to the bone are resected with the inferior strip or with the vomer resection. Severe anterior deviations, such as right-angle deflections of the caudal end of the septum, must be excised and reimplanted. Other than these exceptions, bowing and minor mid-cartilaginous spurs can be scored and recontoured. The technique involves multiple, parallel, horizontal and vertical incisions in the cartilage. Severe bowing to the left is overcome by bidirectional deep incisions, effectively achieving an in situ morselization (Fig. 12–19). Less severe bowing to the left or right can be dealt with using the same technique to whatever extent necessary.

Closure

Closure is achieved easily by simply reapproximating the hemitransfixion incision with two interrupted 4-0 chromic sutures. Significant mucosal tears should be repaired by reapproximating the edges using 4-0 chromic suture on a small cutting needle. Rather than using plicating mattress sutures or other techniques to set the septum, nasal splints are preferred. The author uses Doyle II airway splints (Xomed Corporation, Jacksonville, FL). These splints are made of pliable Silastic and contain a side-channel airway. The side channel serves two purposes: it provides a breathing passage to help maintain nasal airflow during the recovery period, and it fills the nose so that there is pressure on the septum. This helps to stabilize the septum in the midline and helps ensure hemostasis. The splints are secured with a single 3-0 nylon mattress suture through their anterior ends.

Some degree of nasal packing is often required. In patients undergoing simultaneous turbinate surgery, packing is always necessary. The only time that packing is not placed is when no turbinate surgery is performed in a patient with a small nose, in which case splints alone will create sufficient pressure to maintain hemostasis. The packing of choice is a rolled Telfa pad. The pad is usually coated with antibiotic ointment and placed along the floor of the nose between the splint and the inferior turbinate. The Telfa roll can be formed to any size desired to create the appropriate amount of pressure.

Postoperative Care

Following surgery, most patients are discharged to home within a few hours. On average, patients remain in the recovery area for about 1 hour and in the discharge area for an additional 1 to 2 hours. Overnight observation for routine septoplasty is generally only necessary in the presence of severe underlying medical conditions or some other factor that would increase the risk of airway problems after surgery, including severe obstructive

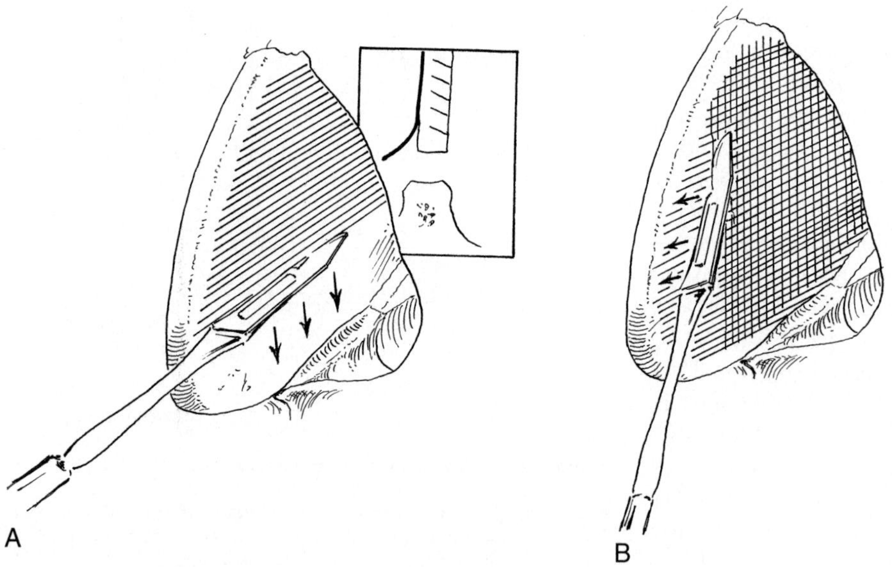

Figure 12–19. Cross-hatching of the quadrilateral cartilage. *A,* Horizontal cuts. *B,* Vertical cuts. The inset shows the ideal depth of the cuts. This complete unilateral cross-hatching results in an in situ morselization of the cartilage.

sleep apnea syndrome (OSAS). Occasionally, a patient with OSAS will have nasal obstruction from a septal deviation and will require septoplasty to facilitate continuous positive airway pressure (CPAP) ventilation. In this circumstance, a minimum of an overnight stay is warranted. Otherwise, the indications for prolonged observation include the onset of anesthesia-related complications, such as nausea and vomiting; cardiac or pulmonary complications; or surgical complications, including bleeding and uncontrolled pain. In the author's practice to date, all patients undergoing scheduled outpatient septoplasty have been able to be discharged on the day of surgery.

Patients normally experience some degree of bleeding in the first few days after the surgery. Until this bleeding subsides, a dressing sponge is folded and taped under the nose as a mustache dressing. The typical amount of bleeding will require a frequency of dressing changes that ranges from once after surgery to once per hour for the first night. A continuous stream of blood into the throat or anteriorly from the nose should not occur. If it does, this should alert the patient and physician that further intervention is warranted.

Postoperative pain with septoplasty is usually mild to moderate. Most patients experience a disturbing sense of fullness and pressure from the splints and packing, if any is used. Pain is usually manifested as headache, but some throbbing pain in the nose is not unusual. Rarely is more than a mild narcotic combination, such as acetaminophen with codeine, required. However, as with all surgery, there is a wide range of pain sensation, so the appropriate level of analgesic to prescribe is the amount necessary for the individual patient.

Activity levels should be kept to a minimum for the first night, with bed rest or reclining on a couch recommended with the head elevated to at least 30 degrees. This minimizes venous congestion in the septum and decreases bleeding. Once bleeding has completely stopped, the patient is free to resume normal activity, except that exercise or carrying of heavy objects is discouraged for the first 10 to 14 days postoperatively. Diet is restricted to clear liquids the night of surgery to help prevent emesis. Thereafter, the diet is liberalized to whatever is tolerated.

The only medication other than pain medication that should be prescribed for all patients is at least a 1-week course of antibiotics. As discussed earlier in this chapter, there is no good evidence that this is necessary or scientifically supported; however, the risk of toxic shock syndrome from the splints and packing is considered by some to be a mandate for the use of antibiotics. If a particular facility's standard does not require such prophylaxis, then theoretically, antibiotics can be omitted. If an antibiotic is prescribed, the drug should have activity against staphylococcal species. Examples include first-generation cephalosporins, erythromycin, and augmented penicillins.

The first return visit after surgery is usually within 5 to 7 days. Some patients do not tolerate the splints and packing well and require early removal, which can be considered after 48 hours. The optimal duration of splinting will vary with the nature of the surgery and the presence of mucosal tears. In patients with perfectly intact mucosal envelopes and relatively straight cartilage with minimal or no scoring, the splints can be safely removed after only 2 days. However, the more damage to the mucosal flaps and the more cartilaginous contouring that was done, the longer the duration of splinting needed.

At the first visit, packing, if any is present, is removed, after which the nylon stitch holding the splint is cut and the splints removed. Packing removal can cause significant discomfort, but the splints usually slide out with minimal pain. The nose should then be carefully inspected and suctioned clear of secretions and clots. If any bleeding is present, the nose can be sprayed with Neo-Synephrine or another topical decongestant.

For the next few weeks, the patient should rigorously adhere to the recommended care regimen, using saline nasal spray frequently and carefully cleaning the anterior nose with a cotton-tipped applicator to remove any crusting or clots. During the remainder of the first month, continued crusting may occur, especially if turbinate surgery has been performed as part of the procedure. For this reason, a second follow-up appointment is scheduled for 2 to 3 weeks after packing and splint removal.

For the first few months after surgery, patients should be instructed not to use nasal steroid sprays. The mucosa will be fragile during this period, and there is a possibility of septal perforation with use of these sprays. Any decision to reinstitute such sprays at a later date should be carefully considered, and the patient should be monitored closely. With close attention, septal damage may be detected before a perforation occurs. It has been theorized that, by preserving the quadrilateral cartilage in the area of impact of the steroid spray, the risk of subsequent perforation owing to the sprays can be minimized. Techniques that resect the central septal cartilage, leaving only an anterior strut for support, probably predispose the individual to septal perforation from nasal sprays and other forms of chronic trauma, such as digital trauma. This is another reason to favor the cartilage-preserving technique.

Complications

Septoplasty is one of the most successful operations, with one of the lowest complication rates, in the practice of otolaryngology. Perhaps the most important consideration in septoplasty is the success rate of the operation. This can be measured in two different ways: (1) the creation of a straight and intact septum and (2) patient satisfaction. Articles in the literature have documented the fact that achieving a straight septum is easier than satisfying the patient.[41–43] Nasal symptoms are related to a number of independent factors, including septal anatomy, presence of turbinate hypertrophy, rhinitis, and sinusitis. Addressing only the symptom of nasal airflow, as documented objectively, septoplasty alone is initially successful in most cases. Long-term problems associated with turbinate congestion and mucosal hypertrophy result in a significant percentage of patients having recurrent symptoms of obstruction. The results of septoplasty vary with the technique used,[44] the experience of the surgeon,[45] and the inclusion of turbinate surgery.[32, 33]

The most important complication associated with septoplasty is septal perforation. This risk varies significantly depending on the technique, skill of the surgeon, and length of follow-up evaluation. Perforation rates have been reported to range from 2% to 9% for the older submucous resection techniques,[41, 42, 46] whereas modern septoplasty techniques have yielded rates as low as less than 1%.[47] Using the technique described in this chapter, the author has not detected any septal perforations in a series of about 300 patients. Admittedly, the follow-up period in this series is not optimal, and the possibility of late-onset perforation cannot be excluded. However, all patients in this series have achieved primary healing of the septum after surgery.

The reasons for this success can be ascribed to three factors. The first is the preservation of the entire quadrilateral cartilage in almost every patient. With the natural cartilage preserved without grafting and attached to the natural blood supply on the right side of the septum, ischemia does not occur and the right-sided mucosa is not at risk. The second factor is the use of the septal splints. By shielding the mucosa during early healing, the edges of mucosal tears are held in approximation without extensive suturing, and septal hematoma is prevented. The final factor is the application of careful and skillful technique. It is believed that the technique described in this chapter is inherently stable and should provide any surgeon using it with a reproducible method that consistently avoids the possibility of severe complications.

Septoplasty may result in cosmetic alteration. Careful analysis of the appearance suggests that some effect can be detected in up to 21% of patients.[48] Significant changes resulting in deformity are rarer, described in only 1% to 9%.[42, 48, 49] Other significant complications include medical problems, bleeding, and infection. The medical problems may be associated with the topical and local anesthesia and with general anesthesia. Reports of cardiac complications caused by cocaine mixed with epinephrine have been found in the literature.[50] Guidelines for the combined use of these agents are detailed in Chapter 8. The risks associated with any form of anesthesia include heart attack, stroke, and death, as well as other reactions to the agents used. The author's series included one patient who had a minor myocardial infarction (MI) 1 week after surgery. The patient was an otherwise healthy 45-year-old woman without previous cardiac history. One week after the operation, she experienced chest pains and sustained a minor anterior MI. An angiogram demonstrated high-grade occlusion of the left main coronary artery. This was treated with angioplasty, resulting in renewed patency of the vessel. It is unlikely that the surgery caused the coronary disease, but the stress of the surgery may well have accelerated the onset of the MI.

In the author's series, postoperative bleeding has not, in general, been a problem with septoplasty, possibly because of the routine use of splints. Approximately 1% of patients undergoing turbinate procedures will, however, develop significant bleeding requiring additional postoperative care. This should be kept in mind when the combination surgery is performed.

The risk of infection, as discussed earlier, is very low. The types of infection that can occur include sinusitis, septal abscess, cellulitis of the nose, and toxic shock syndrome. The incidence of sinusitis in patients undergoing septoplasty is unknown. The possibility should be considered in patients who have suggestive symptoms after packing and splint removal. Septal abscess is probably always related to septal hematoma. This condition occurs rarely, regardless of technique, but is especially rare with the technique described in this chapter. If a septal hematoma is detected after splint removal, a small incision in the mucosa over the hematoma should be made and the hematoma evacuated. Following this, a piece of Gelfoam should be placed against the area of the hematoma, compressing the mucosal flap. Healing is usually prompt and complete. Nasal cellulitis is also a rare complication not seen in the authors' experience. However, if either abscess or cellulitis occurs, then prompt treatment with drainage and intravenous antibiotics is mandated.

Toxic shock syndrome is a rare but important complication following septal surgery. The author has seen one case associated with the use of Silastic splints. Prompt recognition of nausea, vomiting, purulent nasal secretions, hypotension, and rash establishes the diagnosis. The treatment is to remove the splints or packing, hydrate the patient, and support the blood pressure as needed. The one case in the author's practice was minor and resolved within 24 hours without sequelae.

Olfaction is at risk during any nasal surgery.[51] However, with septoplasty, olfactory function should not be affected unless significant scarring blocks the olfactory cleft. Gustatory rhinorrhea is an unusual complication of nasal surgery in which the nose is stimulated to secrete serous mucus on mastication.[52] The incidence of this is extremely low. Finally, numbness of the upper teeth and palate can occur after septoplasty.[53] This is relatively common in the first weeks after surgery, but should almost always resolve by 2 to 3 months after the operation.

REPAIR OF SEPTAL PERFORATION

Septal perforation is a surprisingly common finding. The principle cause is previous septal surgery. Other etiologies include trauma, recurrent digital trauma and major external blunt trauma, nasal steroid sprays, and the illegal use of cocaine. Other causes include tumors and intentional resection, as well as midline granulomatous diseases, including Wegener's granulomatosis and polymorphic reticulosis (nasal lymphoma).

Repair of septal perforation has traditionally been a difficult and challenging procedure in otolaryngology. As evidenced by the great number of techniques that have been developed, no single operation is perfect or ideal. The most popular techniques have utilized bipedicled septal advancement flaps.[54–60] Other surgeons prefer buccal or sublabial flaps.[61–64] Inferior turbinate flaps have also been described.[65, 66] Some authors have applied unique and creative techniques to this surgical problem, including mucosal expansion,[67] microvascular free tissue transfer,[68] and cross-septal mucosal flaps.[69] In this chapter, the technique that is described is borrowed and adapted from that described by Fairbanks.[60] With this technique, the success rate of the primary repair approaches 90%. Failure may be technical, or it may result from ischemia to the flap. In the author's experience, every case that has been successful has achieved complete closure of the perforation on both sides of the septum. Less than ideal closure has uniformly resulted in ultimate failure. In order to achieve success, virtual perfection in performing the operation is necessary. Unwanted perforations or trauma to the mucosal flaps will usually result in ischemia to the mucosal closure and failure to heal.

Indications

The mere presence of a septal perforation is not an absolute indication for repair. Some patients have no symptoms or knowledge that they have a perforation until it is discovered during an examination. The truly asymptomatic perforations are usually posterior and out of the area of peak airflow of the nose.

Symptoms of septal perforation typically include crusting, bleeding, and whistling of the nose during breathing. These symptoms can be very disturbing and significantly impair the patient's well-being. In severe cases, the patient may develop atrophic rhinitis secondary to the loss of mucociliary activity and chronic infection from the perforation. Other patients may experience headaches or pain from irritation at the edges of the perforation. In some patients, especially those who have had previous ethmoid sinus surgery, the perforation may contribute to recurrent sinusitis from abnormally turbulent airflow.

Patients who benefit from the operation are those who have some or all of these symptoms and whose symptoms cannot be controlled by routine nasal care using saline sprays, irrigations, and proper humidification of the home environment. Before electing to proceed with surgery, a septal obturator or button should be considered. In general, these devices help minimize the crusting, bleeding, and pain associated with septal perforation. In some patients, they may be the best option. However, the buttons require constant care and monitoring and can be associated with all of the problems that may arise with any foreign body in the nose. They are usually recommended only in patients who are deemed poor candidates for repair or who are medically unable to undergo surgery.

The main consideration in recommending repair is the size and anatomy of the perforation. The most important aspect is the height of the perforation (inferior to superior), not its length (anterior to posterior). The flap technique borrows from the septum above the perforation and the floor of the nose, so the height of the perforation is the critical issue. The maximum height that can be closed will be determined based on the height of the residual mucosa above and below the perforation. For most patients, this is about 2 cm. Another consideration is the condition of the septal mucosa. The healthier the mucosa, the more viable the flaps will be and the greater one's chance of success. Excessive granulation tissue around the perforation should be cleaned up and healed before embarking on surgery. Finally, the amount of residual bone and cartilage is important. The ideal situation is that the bone and cartilage are completely preserved except in the perforation. The more bone and cartilage that are missing, the more adherent the flaps will be and the higher the risk of perforation during elevation.

When recommending surgery, all of these considerations are taken into account. For the most part, surgical repair of septal perforation is appropriate for any symptomatic patient with a perforation measuring 2 cm or less in height with sufficient residual mucosa above and below the perforation.

Technique

Perioperative and anesthetic considerations are identical to those for septoplasty, as detailed earlier. The only difference in this procedure is that a temporalis fascia graft is harvested. This is routinely done before the nasal surgery is started. The area above the right ear is shaved over a 1.5 × 5 cm rectangular area. The hair is taped back out of the way and the incisional area is prepped with iodine solution according to the hospital policy for sterile surgery.

Graft Harvest

The incision is marked out in the transverse plane and injected with a combination of local anesthesia and epinephrine. The incision is made with a No. 15 scalpel blade through the dermis. Hemostasis is secured by cautery on the dermis of the scalp. A curved iris scissors is used to spread and expose the level of the true fascia of the temporalis muscle. Once in the correct plane of dissection, a finger can be used to widely dissect this plain. The graft is outlined in the fascia to the size required and incised with the scalpel. The free edge of the fascia is picked up with a forceps and the graft is elevated with the curved iris scissors using a spreading motion under the fascia. This should allow development of a large piece of thin fascia without attached muscle or fat. The graft is spread out on a flat, dry surface and allowed to air-dry until the time it is needed. The donor site is closed in two layers with 3-0 Vicryl sutures for the dermis and 4-0 nylon sutures for the skin.

Exposure

There are two approaches used for this procedure: the transnasal approach through a hemitransfixion incision and the external rhinoplasty approach. The transnasal technique is used for small, anterior perforations, whereas the external rhinoplasty technique is used for larger perforations. The hemitransfixion incision has been described in detail in the earlier section on septoplasty; the external rhinoplasty incision is discussed in Chapter 13.

The initial steps in exposure of the septum are identical to those involved in septoplasty. However, there are minor variations from the septoplasty technique in elevation of the flaps. It is advisable to stay out of the perforation as long as possible, working above and below it, until this becomes limiting. In accessing the floor of the nose, the inferior tunnel technique is always used on both sides of the septum. This is important as elevation needs to extend laterally to the lateral nasal wall in the inferior meatus.

When the right side of the septum is addressed, instead of crossing over at the bony cartilaginous junction, the elevation proceeds from anterior to posterior from the caudal end of the septum. This accomplishes complete bilateral exposure of the septum, ideally with an intact mucosal envelope from the dorsum to the lateral wall of the inferior meatus.

Relaxing Incisions

The mucosal flaps are created by making relaxing incisions in the attachment zones of the flaps superiorly and inferiorly (Figs. 12–20 and 12–21). This creates bipedicled mucosal flaps that slide superiorly or inferiorly as advancement flaps (see Fig. 12–20). If possible, it is best to have only one relaxing incision on each side with those incisions being opposite. For example, the incision on the right can be superior, with the incision on the left being inferior. This protects the blood supply to the closure and assists in healing. However, it is imperative that closure is tension-free, so if necessary, both superior and inferior incisions can be made bilaterally.

Rarely, the sliding flaps will fail to close the perforation without tension. In this circumstance, either the superior or inferior flap can be released from the anterior attachment, creating a single-pedicle, random-patterned, axial rotation flap. The vascularity of this flap is marginal, though, and is associated with a high risk of tip necrosis. Thus, it should be reserved only for situations when the initial flaps will not suffice.

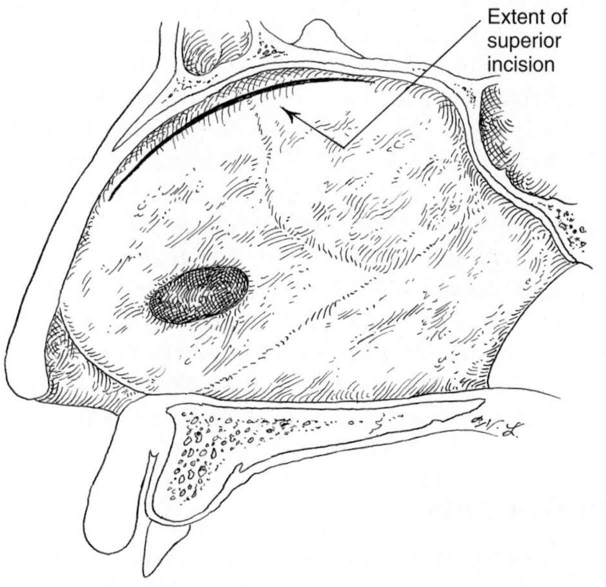

Figure 12–20. Superior relaxing incision for closure of septal perforation. The incision is high on the nasal septum and extends down to bone or cartilage; it may be extended anteriorly to the caudal end of the septum, if necessary.

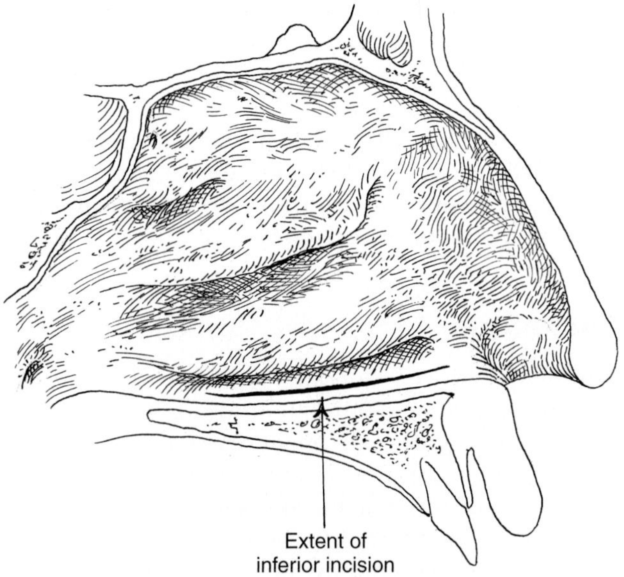

Figure 12–21. Inferior relaxing incision. The incision is at the junction of the floor of the nose and the lateral nasal wall under the inferior meatus. The incision is extended down to bone and may extend as far posteriorly as the choana and as far anteriorly as the pyriform aperture.

Closure

The actual suturing of the flaps to close the perforation is difficult and requires patience and a gentle, precise touch. The best needle to use is a small cutting needle, the preferred suture is chromic catgut. A bayonet-type needle driver is helpful in placing the sutures, although a fine, long, standard needle driver may be used as an alternative. The sutures should be placed through the inferior flap first and then brought out and regripped before sewing through the superior flap. This two-pass technique is important to avoid loosing the needle or creating torsion on the flap. To facilitate suture placement, the needle should be gripped along the end of the needle like a fishhook (Fig. 12–22). The needle is placed beyond the edge of the flap toward the back of the nose and drawn forward, hooking the flap edge. When the suture is tied, the needle driver grasps the suture and is pushed to the back of the nose in order to tighten the suture down squarely. Sutures should be placed at 1-cm intervals. Excessive suturing carries the risk of pulling the previous sutures out and does not add stability, as the goal of the suturing is to align the flaps and hold the edges together.

After the flaps on both sides of the septum are approximated, the graft is placed. The graft should be trimmed to size to span the area of cartilaginous defect. It is then set in place and smoothed out to prevent folds or creases.

The septal incisions are closed using 4-0 chromic sutures as for the septoplasty or 6-0 nylon as for external rhinoplasty. The septum is supported using the same Doyle II airway splints (Xomed Corporation, Jacksonville, FL) used for septoplasty and is secured using 3-0 nylon. Nasal packing is always required to support the septum and provide hemostasis for the relaxing incisions. Rolled Telfa pads coated with antibiotic ointment are preferred, with one or two used per side.

Postoperative Care

The initial postoperative care is the same as for septoplasty. The exceptions to this are that the packing can be removed in the first 48 hours; however, the splints should be maintained for a minimum of 5 days in all

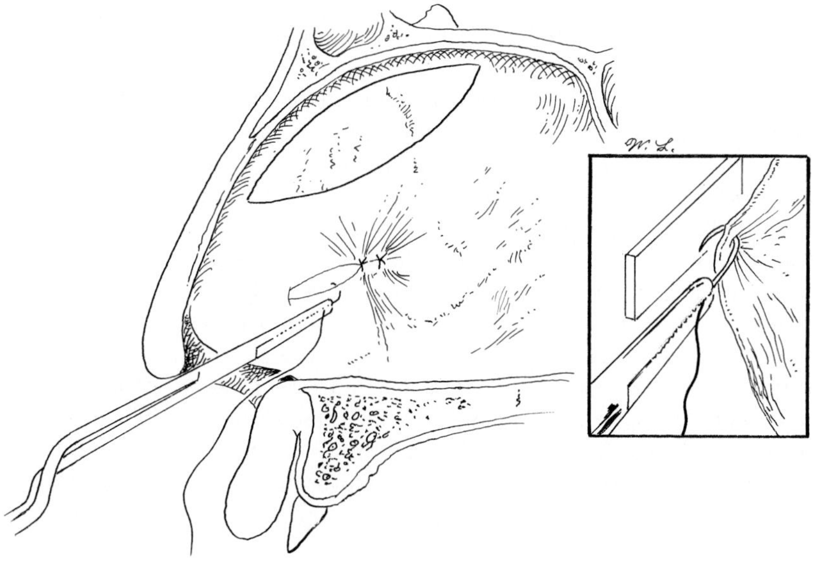

Figure 12–22. Suturing the septal mucosal flaps. Sutures are placed through one side of mucosal flap with each suture placed with two passes. The incision should close without tension. The inset demonstrates the fishhook technique of passing sutures.

cases. If the closure was difficult or the perforation large, the splints may be left in for an additional week. The benefit of this is improved stabilization during healing and protection from drying and crusting until the wound is stabile.

After splint removal, the closure may be tenuous or weak and will require several weeks before complete healing. Crusting over the septum should be removed very gently; the area may be soaked with decongestant before attempting to dislodge adherent crusts. The nose should be moistened every 2 to 3 hours with saline mist and an antibiotic ointment should be applied twice each day.

Complications

The complications for this procedure are the same as for septoplasty with the exception of the increased risk of failure with repair of septal perforations and the complications associated with the graft donor site. Donor site complications are uncommon, but are identical to those for any soft tissue surgery.

SEPTAL DERMOPLASTY

Septal dermoplasty is a unique, little-used procedure for the treatment of refractory bleeding from the anterior septum. It involves elevation of unilateral or bilateral mucosal flaps and placement of dermal or fascial grafts between the flaps and the septal cartilage and bone so as to prevent further bleeding. This operation has not gained wide recognition, and the evidence for its utility over septoplasty alone is lacking. However, for completeness, a brief description of the procedure is included here.

Indications

The only real indication for septal dermoplasty is in the treatment of refractory epistaxis from the septum. The traditional and original indication is hereditary hemorrhagic telangiectasia (HHT), also known as Osler-Weber-Rendu syndrome. This condition is marked by the presence of innumerable punctate telangiectases over the mucous membranes of the upper aerodigestive tract. These vascular malformations have a tendency to bleed, especially on the anterior septum, where digital trauma, airflow, and nose blowing cause constant irritation. Although telangiectases are primarily associated with HHT, other conditions are associated with these same vascular malformations and have the same clinical picture of recurrent epistaxis. In the author's practice, one patient with systemic lupus erythematosus had scattered telangiectases which led to recurrent epistaxis.

Patients with this problem are notoriously difficult to manage. Repeated bouts of epistaxis often lead to frequent transfusions and constant medical intervention. The initial management follows the algorithm for epistaxis, which is discussed in detail in Chapter 22. With HHT, there is a need to attempt some type of procedure to prevent recurrent bleeding. Septal dermoplasty is one of the options.

Technique

The preoperative considerations and anesthesia for septal dermoplasty are identical to those for septal perforation and septoplasty. The main decision is whether to use temporalis fascia or dermis as the graft source. Either is acceptable, but the dermal graft is somewhat thicker and, therefore, may be more efficacious. The approach and exposure for this procedure is through a hemitransfixion incision, with elevation of the mucosal flaps performed bilaterally just as for the repair of septal perforation described earlier.

Once the flaps are elevated, the dermal grafts are trimmed to size to line the entire septal surface. The flaps are laid back down into their natural positions and the incision is closed. Septal splints and packing are used to prevent hematoma and ensure normal healing.

Postoperative Care

Postoperative care is also identical to that provided the post-septoplasty patient. The only important difference is that the hemoglobin level of these patients should be monitored closely as their risk of bleeding is probably increased. The splints can usually be removed after 48 hours with minimal risk of hematoma after that point.

Complications

Septal dermoplasty is associated with an increased risk of failure of the graft to take. This may result in septal abscess and the need for removal of the graft. Although unlikely, this possibility should be considered during the follow-up period.

The risk of recurrent epistaxis in these patients is significant. As a result, subsequent devascularization procedures may need to be performed.

Following septal dermoplasty, the septum is significantly thickened. This is unavoidable. To prevent nasal obstruction and congestion, some treatment of the inferior turbinates may become necessary. Close follow-up evalution is required to determine whether, with time, the reabsorption of the graft will be sufficient to overcome this problem without surgical intervention.

REFERENCES

1. Killian G. Die submucose Fensterresektion der Nasenscheidewand. Arch Laryngol Rhinol 16:362, 1904.
2. Freer OT. The correction of defections of the nasal septum with a minimum of traumatization. JAMA 38:636, 1902.
3. Cottle M, Loring R. Corrective surgery of the external nasal pyramid and the nasal septum for restoration of normal physiology. EENT Monthly 26:147, 1947.
4. Bernstein L. Early submucous resection of nasal septal cartilage. Arch Otolaryngol 97:273, 1973.
5. Edwards N. Septoplasty: Rational surgery of the nasal septum. J Laryngol Otol 89:875, 1974.
6. Goldman IB. New techniques in the surgery of the deviated nasal septum. Arch Otolaryngol 64:183, 1956.
7. Metzenbaum M. Replacement of the lower end of the dislocated septal cartilage versus submucous resection of the dislocated end of the septal cartilage. Arch Otolaryngol 9:282, 1929.
8. Pearson B, Goodman W. SMR septoplasty and the surgical relief of nasal obstruction. Can J Otolaryngol 2(3):238, 1973.
9. Senyuva C, Yucel A, Aydin Y, et al. Extracorporeal septoplasty combined with open rhinoplasty. Aesthetic Plast Surg 21(4): 233, 1997.
10. Cantrell H. Limited septoplasty for endoscopic sinus surgery. Otolaryngol Head Neck Surg 116(2):274, 1997.
11. Mantovani M, Mazzola RF, Cioccarelli MG. The back-and-forth septoplasty. Plast Reconstr Surg 97(1):40, 1996.
12. Giles WC, Gross CW, Abram AC, et al. Endoscopic septoplasty. Laryngoscope 104(12):1507, 1994.
13. Godfrey NV. Sagittal section septoplasty: An intrinsically stabilized septoplasty. Plast Reconstr Surg 93(1):188, 1994.
14. Mayer B, Henkes H. Mini-septoplasty—For function and form. Laryngorhinootologie 69(6):303, 1990.
15. Lee IN, Vukovic L. Hemostatic suture for septoplasty: How we do it. J Otolaryngol 17(1):54, 1988.
16. Courtiss EH, Goldwyn RM. The effects of nasal surgery on airflow. Plast Reconstr Surg 72(1):9, 1983.
17. Pallanch JF, McCaffrey TV, Kern EB. Evaluation of nasal breathing function. In Cummings CW, Fredrickson JM, Harker LA, Krause CJ, Schuller DE (eds), Otolaryngology: Head and Neck Surgery, 2nd ed. St. Louis: Mosby Year Book, 1993, pp. 665–686.
18. Hilberg O, Jackson AC, Swift DL, et al. Acoustic rhinometry: Evaluation of nasal cavity geometry by acoustic reflection. J Appl Physiol 43:523, 1977.
19. Chow JM. Rhinologic headaches. Otolaryngol Head Neck Surg 111:211, 1994.
20. McAuliffe GW, Goodell H, Wolff HG. Experimental studies on headache pain from the nasal and paranasal structures. Am Res Nerve Ment Dis Proc 23:185, 1942.
21. Hansen RM. Pain of nasal origin. Laryngoscope 78:1164, 1968.
22. Ryan SE Sr, Ryan SE Jr. Headache of nasal origin. Headache 19:173, 1979.
23. Koch-Henriksen N, Gammelgaard N, Hvidegaard T, et al. Chronic headache: The role of deformity of the nasal septum. Br Med 288:434, 1984.
24. Gerbe RW, Fry TL, Fischer ND. Headache of nasal spur origin: An easily diagnosed and surgical correctable cause of facial pain. Headache 24:329, 1984.
25. Schonsted Madsen U, Stoksted P, Christensen PH, et al. Chronic headache related to nasal obstruction. J Laryngol Otol 100:165, 1986.
26. Clerico DM. Pneumatized superior turbinate as a cause of referred migraine headache. Laryngoscope 106:874, 1996.
27. Landrigan GP, Kirkpatrick DA. Intranasal xylocaine: A prognostic aid for pre-operative assessment of facial pain of nasal origin. J Otolaryngol 21(2):126, 1992.
28. Sooknundun M, Kacker SK, Bhatia R, et al. Nasal septal deviation: Effective intervention and long-term follow-up. Int J Ped Otorhinolaryngol 12(1):65, 1986.
29. Risavi R, Pisl Z, Sprem N, et al. Rhinomanometrical findings after septoplasty in children. Int J Ped Otorhinolaryngol 16(2):149, 1988.
30. Bejar I, Farkas LG, Messner AH, et al. Nasal growth after external septoplasty in children. Arch Otolaryngol Head Neck Surg 122(8):816, 1996.
31. Samad I, Stevens HE, Maloney A. The efficacy of nasal septal surgery. J Otolaryngol 21(2):88, 1992.
32. Grymer LF, Illum P, Hilberg O. Septoplasty and compensatory inferior turbinate hypertrophy: A randomized study evaluated by acoustic rhinometry. J Laryngol Otol 107(5):413, 1993.
33. Marais J, Murray JA, Marshall I, et al. Minimal cross-sectional areas, nasal peak flow and patients' satisfaction in septoplasty and inferior turbinectomy. Rhinology 32(3):145, 1994.
34. Illum P. Septoplasty and compensatory inferior turbinate hypertrophy: Long-term results after randomized turbinoplasty. Eur Arch Otorhinolaryngol [Suppl] 1:S89, 1997.
35. Yoder MG, Weimert TA. Antibiotics and topical surgical preparation solution in septal surgery. Otolaryngol Head Neck Surg 106(3):243, 1992.
36. Silk KL, Ali MB, Cohen BJ, et al. Absence of bacteremia during nasal septoplasty. Arch Otolaryngol Head Neck Surg 117(1):54, 1991.
37. Fishman G, Ophir D. Toxic shock syndrome. Harefuah 132(9): 622, 1997.
38. Allen ST, Liland JB, Nichols CG, et al. Toxic shock syndrome associated with use of latex nasal packing. Arch Intern Med 150(12):2587, 1990.
39. Huang IT, Podkomorska D, Murphy MN, et al. Toxic shock syndrome following septoplasty and partial turbinectomy. J Otolaryngol 15(5):310, 1986.
40. Wagner R, Toback JM. Toxic shock syndrome following septoplasty using plastic septal splints. Laryngoscope 96(6):609, 1986.
41. Bohlin L, Dahlqvist A. Nasal airway resistance and complications following functional septoplasty: A ten-year follow-up study. Rhinology 32(4):195, 1994.
42. Low WK, Willatt DJ. Submucous resection for deviated nasal septum: A critical appraisal. Singapore Med J 33(6):617, 1992.
43. Jessen M, Ivarsson A, Malm L. Nasal airway resistance and symptoms after functional septoplasty: Comparison of findings at 9 months and 9 years. Clin Otolaryngol 14(3):231, 1989.
44. Fjermedal O, Saunte C, Pedersen S. Septoplasty and/or submucous resection? 5 years nasal septum operations. J Laryngol Otol 102(9):796, 1988.
45. Haraldsson PO, Nordemar H, Anggard A. Long-term results after septal surgery—Submucous resection versus septoplasty. ORL J Otorhinolaryngol Relat Spec 49(4):218, 1987.
46. Bewarder F, Pirsig W. Long-term results of submucous septal resection. Laryngol Rhinol 57(10):922, 1978.
47. Courtiss EH, Goldwyn RM. The effects of nasal surgery on airflow. Plast Reconstr Surg 72(1):9, 1983.
48. Vuyk HD, Langenhuijsen KJ. Aesthetic sequelae of septoplasty. Clin Otolaryngol 22(3):226, 1997.
49. Min YG, Chung JW. Cartilaginous incisions in septoplasty. ORL J Otorhinolaryngol Relat Spec 58(1):51, 1996.
50. Littlewood SC, Tabb HG. Myocardial ischemia with epinephrine and cocaine during septoplasty. J La State Med Soc 139(5):15, 1987.
51. Kimmelman CP. The risk to olfaction from nasal surgery. Laryngoscope 104(8):981, 1994.
52. Guyuron B, Michelow B, Thomas T. Gustatory rhinorrhea—A complication of septoplasty. Plast Reconstr Surg 94(3):454, 1994.
53. Rettinger G, Engelbrecht-Schnur S. Palatal sensory impairment after septoplasty. Laryngorhinootologie 74(5):282, 1995.
54. Schultz-Coulon HJ. Nasal septum repair-plasty with pedicled flap technique in 126 patients—An analysis. Laryngorhinootologie 76(8):466, 1997.
55. Morre TD, Van Camp C, Clement PA. Results of the endonasal surgical closure of nasoseptal perforations. Acta Otorhinolaryngol (Belg) 49(3):263, 1995.
56. Schultz-Coulon HJ. Experiences with the bridge-flap technique for the repair of large nasal septal perforations. Rhinology 32(1):25, 1994.
57. Kridel RW, Appling WD, Wright WK. Septal perforation closure utilizing the external septorhinoplasty approach. Arch Otolaryngol Head Neck Surg 112(2):168, 1986.

58. Younger R, Blokmanis A. Nasal septal perforations. J Otolaryngol 14(2):125, 1985.
59. Goodman WS, Strelzow VV. The surgical closure of nasoseptal perforations. Laryngoscope 92(2):121, 1982.
60. Fairbanks DN, Fairbanks GR. Nasal septal perforation: Prevention and management. Ann Plast Surg 5(6):452, 1980.
61. Meyer R, Mayer B, Perko D. Concept and technique for closure of septum defects. Handchir Mikrochir Plast Chir 23(6):296, 1991.
62. Ohlsen L. Closure of nasal septal perforation with a cutaneous flap and a perichondrocutaneous graft. Ann Plast Surg 21(3): 276, 1988.
63. Rettinger G, Masing H, Heinl W. Management of septal perforations by rotationplasty of the septal mucosa. HNO 34(11):461, 1986.
64. Tardy ME Jr. Practical suggestions on facial plastic surgery—how I do it. Sublabial mucosal flap: Repair of septal perforations. Laryngoscope 87(2):275, 1977.
65. Hussain A, Kay N. Tragal cartilage inferior turbinate mucoperiosteal sandwich graft technique for repair of nasal septal perforations. J Laryngol Otol 106(10):893, 1992.
66. Vuyk HD, Versluis RJ. The inferior turbinate flap for closure of septal perforations. Clin Otolaryngol 13(1):53, 1988.
67. Romo T III, Jablonski RD, Shapiro AL, et al. Long-term nasal mucosal tissue expansion use in repair of large nasoseptal perforations. Arch Otolaryngol Head Neck Surg 121(3):327, 1995.
68. Delaere PR, Guelinckx PJ, Ostyn F. Vascularized temporoparietal fascial flap for closure of a nasal septal perforation. Report of a case. Otorhinolaryngolica 44(1):47, 1990.
69. Mladina R, Heinzel B. "Cross-stealing" technique for septal perforation closure. Rhinology 33(3):174, 1995.

CHAPTER 13

Rhinoplasty

Defined as an operation to alter the appearance of the nose, rhinoplasty is perhaps the most challenging and complex procedure in facial plastic surgery. Numerous excellent textbooks are available that cover the entire field of rhinoplasty.[1–4] A comprehensive review of the field of rhinoplasty is beyond the scope of this text and, in fact, the author cannot compete with the masters of rhinoplasty in terms of experience, reputation, or technical nuance in the performance of rhinoplasty. However, rhinoplasty is an operation that the average otolaryngologist or plastic surgeon should feel comfortable performing and be able to produce consistently good results. It is in this context that this chapter on rhinoplasty is presented. This chapter provides a description of the most common variations used in rhinoplasty that the average practicing otolaryngologist should know and master. Emphasis is placed on assessment and decision making and the application of specific techniques to create certain effects.

INDICATIONS

Cosmesis

The most common indication for rhinoplasty is cosmetic improvement. This includes alteration of anatomically normal but unappealing nasal appearance, post-traumatic deformities, and congenital abnormalities. The decision to offer a primarily cosmetic rhinoplasty to a patient, whether post-traumatic or purely cosmetic, should be based on a careful assessment of the patient's anatomy and what can be done to alter the anatomy. Almost any deviation from the theoretical aesthetic ideal could be considered an indication for rhinoplasty. It is important, though, in considering rhinoplasty, for both the patient and the surgeon to have clear and realistic goals for the procedure. Some patients have unreasonable expectations about what the procedure can do physically, and how the change may affect their life. If a patient's psychological stability is in doubt, then surgery should be deferred until such stability is assured. However, almost any patient who has appropriate and well-reasoned goals can be considered a potential candidate for rhinoplasty.

It is convenient to classify cosmetic deformities as either nasal pyramid problems or nasal tip problems. Of course, many patients have abnormalities in both the pyramid and the tip, and some have deformities, such as a twisted nose, which combine these considerations as a single deformity.

Abnormalities of the nasal pyramid are more limited in number and simpler to deal with than those of the tip. They can be classified into several different types, including dorsal deviation, overprojection, underprojection, and excessive width. The deviated dorsum is most commonly seen following nasal fracture and can be found in many different shapes. Some of the most common variations include angled to one side, C-shaped, and S-shaped.

The overprojected nasal dorsum or dorsal hump is extremely common and is, perhaps, the most frequent reason patients present for cosmetic alteration of the nontraumatic nose. This finding is especially common in certain ethnic groups, but can be found in any patient population. The severity or height of the hump can vary from a few millimeters to more than 1 cm. The surgical technique used to remove the hump will depend on the height of the dorsum in excess of the aesthetic ideal, as discussed later in this chapter. The opposite problem of underprojection is almost always caused by trauma or previous rhinoplasty surgery involving excessive reduction of a dorsal hump. A related abnormality, known as saddle nose deformity, is usually caused by loss of septal support to the supratip area. Saddle nose can be caused by septoplasty or septal necrosis from Wegener's granulomatosis, septal abscess, or other related inflammatory conditions.

An overly wide nasal dorsum can be the result of nasal trauma or may be a normal variation in some ethnic groups. Eastern Asian populations and people of African descent commonly have a wide, flat, nasal dorsum, but this is rarely an indication for cosmetic rhinoplasty.

Nasal tip anatomy and deformities are more complicated and varied. The tip structure can be analyzed in terms of several interacting dimensions. These include the projection of the tip, which is the height of the tip from the subnasale; the rotation of the tip, which refers to the angle formed by the line from the nasal tip to the subnasale and the plane of the premaxilla; and the width of the nasal tip. Other factors include the shape and symmetry of the tip, the columellar show, the width of the alar base, and the supratip angle. These factors are covered in greater detail later in this chapter.

Some of the most common nasal tip abnormalities that prompt patients to request surgery include a deviated tip, a hanging tip, a bulbous or wide tip, and a bifid tip. The deviated tip usually results from nasal trauma and is normally accompanied by a deviated dorsum. One common variation that includes a deviated tip is the twisted nose. This deformity consists of a dorsal deviation in one direction and a tip deviation in the opposite direction.

The hanging nasal tip or hooked nose has a rotation of less than 90 degrees. This type of deviation is usually acceptable in men, but is a common reason cited for cosmetic rhinoplasty in women. Bulbous and bifid tips are both normal variations, but are also reasonable indications for cosmetic rhinoplasty. The bulbous tip usually occurs because of large, poorly defined, lower lateral cartilages. The bifid tip occurs with prominent but well-separated lower lateral cartilages, creating a crease between the medial aspects of the nasal domes.

Nasal Obstruction

A second indication for rhinoplasty is to improve nasal breathing. Rhinoplasty can be combined with septoplasty to correct a deviated nasal septum associated with a deviated nasal dorsum or twisted nose. The so-called septorhinoplasty operation is indicated for nasal obstruction when the deformity is such that correction of the dorsal deformity is necessary to straighten the deviated septum. This most often occurs when the dorsal deviation is so severe that the straightened septum would continue to obstruct one side of the nose owing to the lateral attachment to the nasal dorsum. Severe depression of the nasal dorsum can also lead to collapse of the nose, compressing the airway. In this case, straightening the septum alone may result in a nasal airway that is shortened in the vertical dimension. Most patients with this type of problem have post-traumatic deformities.

The second nasal airflow problem amenable to rhinoplasty is nasal valve collapse. This can occur after trauma, previous surgery, or from natural weakness of the nasal valve cartilages. In this condition, the nasal valve lacks sufficient rigidity, which leads to inward collapse and nasal obstruction during inspiration.

Reconstructive Rhinoplasty

The reconstructive indications for rhinoplasty relate to the rebuilding of the nose after severe trauma, cancer ablation, or congenital deformity. These topics are covered in detail in Chapter 14.

Revision Rhinoplasty

Approximately 10% to 20% of patients undergoing primary rhinoplasty are dissatisfied with the results of the surgery and request revision.[5–10] When considering the possibility of revision rhinoplasty, it is important to precisely delineate the goals of the surgery in terms of the abnormality to be corrected and the result desired. It is imperative that the prior surgery be understood, especially in regard to the previous treatment of the nasal tip. When performing revision surgery, extra time and care must be taken to avoid surgical errors. Scar tissue and abnormal tissue planes will be encountered and must be recognized. The specific abnormalities to be corrected in revision surgery are widely varied but include the "pollybeak" deformity, inadequate nasal hump removal, dorsal deviation, and tip asymmetry.

PREOPERATIVE CONSIDERATIONS

Aesthetic Ideal

Since the beginning of modern civilization, humans have attempted to define human beauty and normal anatomy. More pertinently, rhinoplastic surgeons have struggled for centuries with these same concepts. The aesthetic ideal is so important because, within the limits of surgical technique, the form that is achieved depends greatly on the form that is desired to be achieved. The surgeon must have a clear idea, not only of the patient's desires, but what best fits the patient's face.

From the many attempts to define the ideal aesthetic nose, several underlying principles have come to be well accepted. The first aesthetic concept is symmetry. Symmetry should exist along the entire length of the nose, from the dorsum to the tip and alar base. The surgeon should always attempt to preserve and create side-to-side symmetry, as even minimal asymmetry is noticeable and draws attention to the nose.

The second concept is proportion. The nose should be proportionate to the rest of the face in both height and width at the dorsum and base. The ideal proportions, though, have been the subject of significant research and debate.[11–16] The ideal width of the dorsum, defined as the intercanthal distance, is usually said to be equal to the width of the eye from the medial to the lateral canthus. The width of the base should be the same as the intercanthal distance (Fig. 13–1).[17–19] The ideal vertical height can be appreciated by dividing it into thirds. Thus, the height of the trichion to the glabella should ideally be the same as the height of the nose from the glabella to the subnasale, and the same as the distance from the menton to the subnasale (Fig. 13–2).[16] The base of the nose should also be properly proportioned. The base can likewise be divided into thirds, with the lobule, middle portion, and alar base ideally being of equal heights (Fig. 13–3). However, these guidelines have been disputed, challenged, and modified by dozens of authors over the years. The nearest truth for the concept of proportion is that the perfectly proportionate nose is in the eye of the beholder.

The third aesthetic concept is projection (Fig. 13–4*A*), or the height of the nose. Both the dorsum and the tip can be described in terms of projection. Ideally, the dorsum should be 1 to 2 mm below a line from the nasal tip to the nasion in women, and should be even with this line in men (Fig. 13–4*B*). The proper projection of the tip is highly dependent on the overall proportion of the face and the ethnic background of the individual. One method for evaluating tip projection is to consider the angle formed by imaginary lines drawn from the nasion to the tip and from the nasion to the subnasale. This angle should measure 35 to 40 degrees. Another method for evaluating tip projection is to determine the ratio of the height of the nose from the alar groove to the nasal tip compared to the length of the nose from the alar groove to the nasion. This ratio should be from 0.55 to 0.60, with the smaller ratio being preferred in women.[16] Once again, however, the aesthetic ideal is in the eye of the viewer, so the goal should be to create a natural, proportionate nasal projection that is satisfying to the patient.

The next aesthetic concept to consider is rotation (Fig. 13–5). This is the angle created by the intersection of a line from the subnasale to the upper lip and a line from the subnasale to the tip, also known as the nasolabial angle. The ideal angle in men is usually thought to be 90 to 95 degrees, whereas in women, it usually ranges from 100 to 115 degrees.[17, 18, 20, 21]

The final aesthetic concept to consider is nasal tip shape. This quality cannot be measured. It includes all the components already discussed, but also includes the curve of the lateral crura of the lower lateral cartilages, the degree of pointedness of the tip, the presence of a

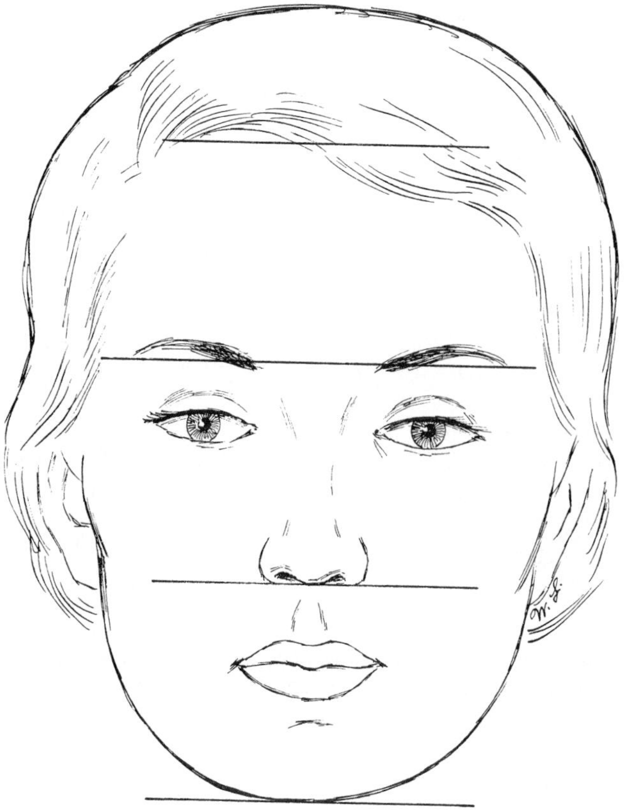

Figure 13–2. Ideal proportions of the vertical dimensions of the face. The face is divided into equal thirds extending from the trichion to the glabella, from the glabella to the subnasale, and from the subnasale to the menton.

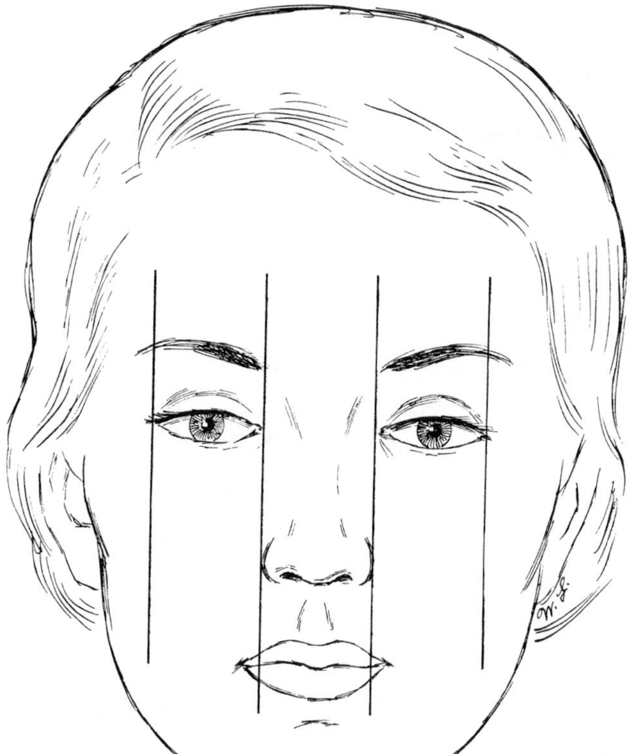

Figure 13–1. Ideal proportions of the horizontal dimensions of the face. The intercanthal distance and nasal base are equal to the width of the eye from the medial to the lateral canthus.

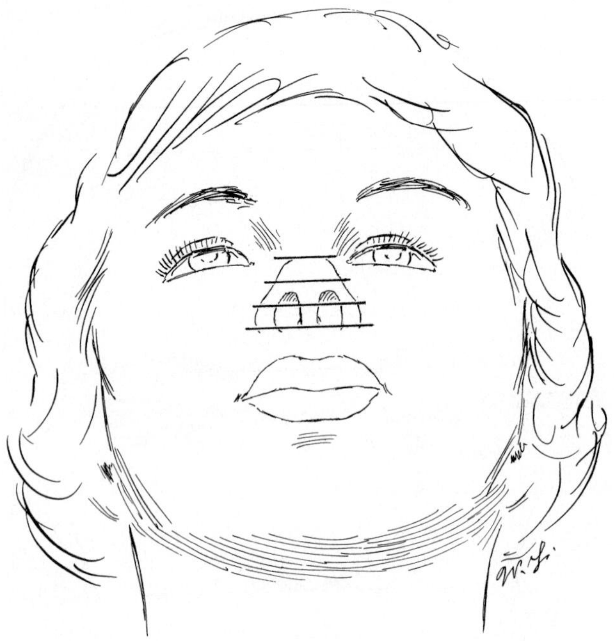

Figure 13–3. Ideal proportions of the base of the nose. The alae are equal in height to the tip and midportion of the base.

double break in the tip, and the presence of a supratip depression. The total effect of these factors defines the shape of the nasal tip.

Photography

All patients undergoing rhinoplasty should have preoperative and postoperative photographs taken. This is an essential part of the medical record, not only for medicolegal documentation, but also for preoperative patient analysis and intraoperative recall of the baseline anatomy.

All photographs should be taken with the same camera under standard lighting conditions and camera settings. The author prefers a 35-mm, single lens reflex (SLR) camera with a 105-mm lens and a camera-mounted, standard-type flash. A lens with variable or fixed focal lengths can be used, but the same magnification should always be used. In this way, the pictures are always the same. A ring flash, which is ideal for intraoperative photography, is actually less desirable than the traditional mounted flash for portrait photography, as the ring tends to cause undesirable reflections.

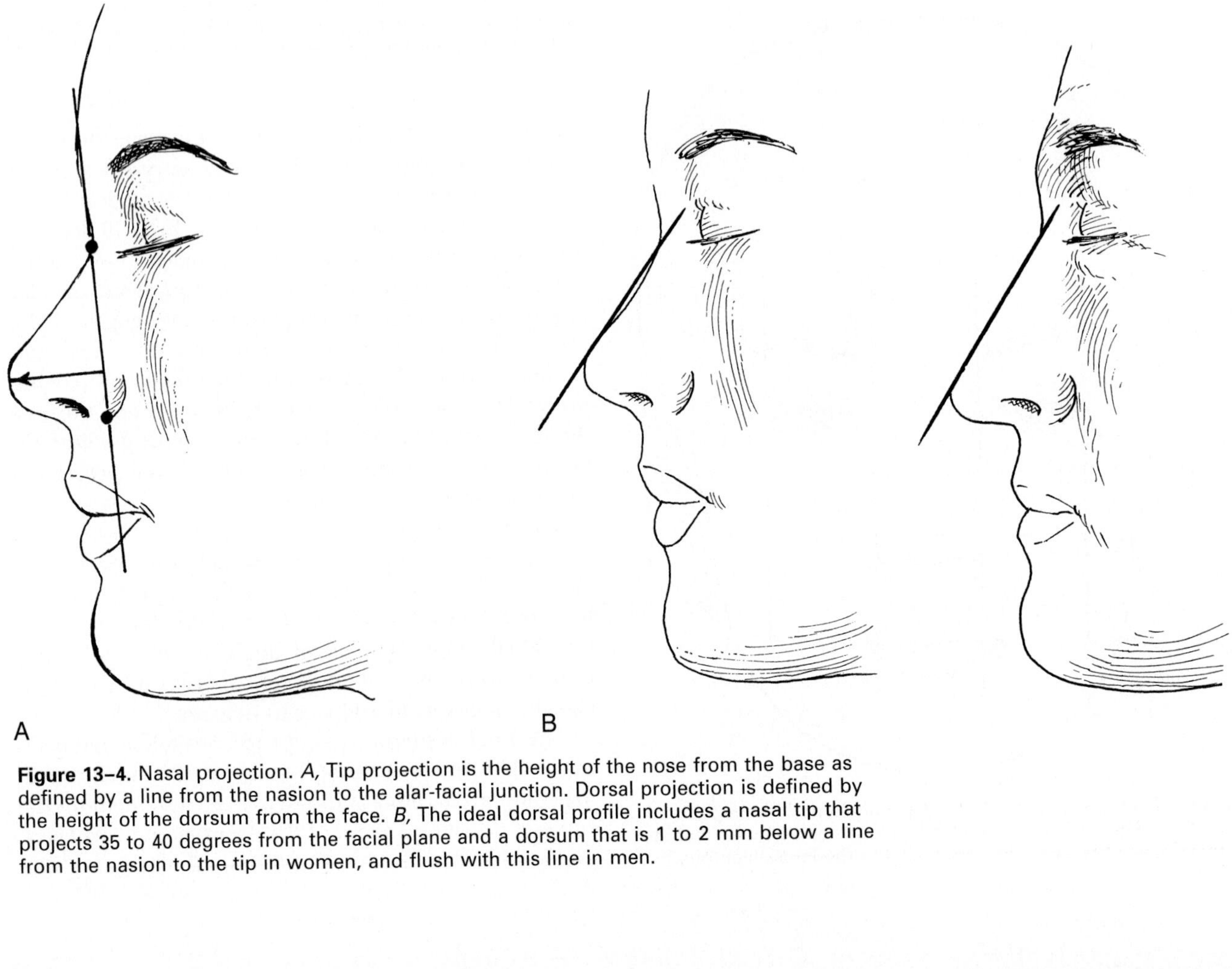

Figure 13–4. Nasal projection. *A,* Tip projection is the height of the nose from the base as defined by a line from the nasion to the alar-facial junction. Dorsal projection is defined by the height of the dorsum from the face. *B,* The ideal dorsal profile includes a nasal tip that projects 35 to 40 degrees from the facial plane and a dorsum that is 1 to 2 mm below a line from the nasion to the tip in women, and flush with this line in men.

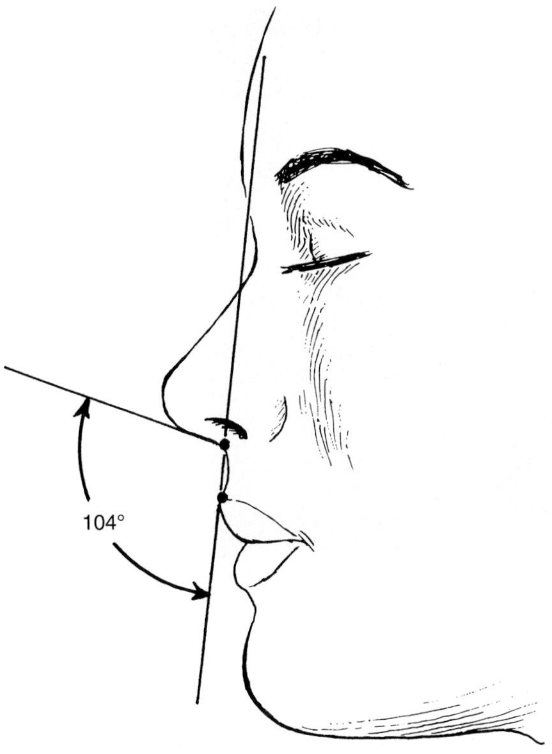

Figure 13–5. Tip rotation. Rotation is the angle between the plane of the face in the premaxilla and the nose. The ideal angle ranges from 100 to 115 degrees in women and from 90 to 95 degrees in men.

The traditional standard photographic views are the frontal view, right and left lateral, and the basal view (Fig. 13–6).[22, 23] Other valuable views include right and left oblique, and oblique or lateral smile views. The frontal view should be taken with the hair pulled back away from the face and with the frame extending from the hairline to the mentum and including the full width of the face. The patient should be looking directly into the camera with eyes open and face relaxed without smile. In the lateral views, the head should be positioned so that the Frankfurt line (from the inferior orbital rim to the top of the ear canal) is parallel to the floor. The tip of the nose should be centered in the frame. The basal view should reveal the nasal base fully, which is achieved by extending the head back. The nose should again be centered in the frame. The oblique views are taken with the Frankfurt line parallel to the floor and the head positioned 45 degrees to the side.

For economic reasons, a complete set of eight pictures is often not obtained. At a minimum, the author commonly obtains photographs of the frontal, basal, left lateral, and right oblique views to demonstrate the pertinent anatomy.

Patient Analysis

Before the actual operation is performed, a detailed analysis of the patient must be undertaken. Ideally, this should occur on at least two occasions prior to surgery. At the time of the first office visit, when the possibility of rhinoplasty is considered, it is important to perform both an anatomic and a psychological evaluation of the patient. The anatomic evaluation is clearly important, but it is equally important to assess the patient's suitability for cosmetic surgery from a psychological perspective. The primary concern is the motivation of the patient to have the operation, and this should be explored and documented. It is also worthwhile to find out about the patient's social situation and what external factors may be contributing to the decision to have surgery. Although this exchange usually takes only a few minutes, it helps in establishing a working relationship with the patient and allows any indication of abnormal psychology to be identified early.

Numerous studies have been conducted to clarify the psychological profile of patients seeking rhinoplasty, the effect of these psychological factors on the outcome of surgery, and the effect of surgery on the psychological profile of these patients. In general, patients considering rhinoplasty have not been found to harbor severe psychiatric disturbances.[24] However, patients seeking rhinoplasty often have a high degree of narcissism[25] and low self-esteem.[26, 27] Male patients tend to be more anxious and depressed,[24] and patients without a history of trauma who are seeking a cosmetic rhinoplasty tend to be more anxious and to show signs of neurosis more often than post-trauma patients.[28] Several studies have documented the overall beneficial effects of rhinoplasty on self-esteem and self-confidence.[26, 29, 30] Interestingly, these studies indicate that men seem to benefit less than women from rhinoplasty and express a generally higher degree of dissatisfaction with the surgical results.[30–32]

Also during this first office visit, a complete head and neck examination and an initial anatomic evaluation of the patient's nose are conducted. Purposely, photographs are not taken at this juncture for two reasons: this avoids wasting resources on patients who are not going to go through with the surgery and provides a convenient excuse for the patient to return for a second evaluation and discussion. At the completion of the first evaluation, the surgeon should discuss, in detail, the patient's desires for actual changes. Some rhinoplastic surgeons predominantly use a single approach that achieves a standard appearance for the patient. In this case, it is imperative that the patient be informed of this and be accepting of that aesthetic ideal. Otherwise, the surgeon should decline to perform the surgery. Most surgeons, however, utilize a variety of techniques designed to achieve different goals for different patients. In order to assist patients in understanding the proposed alterations in the nose and the ultimate effect of these changes on their appearance, some surgeons utilize computer graphics. These programs allow the surgeon to transfer a video image into the computer

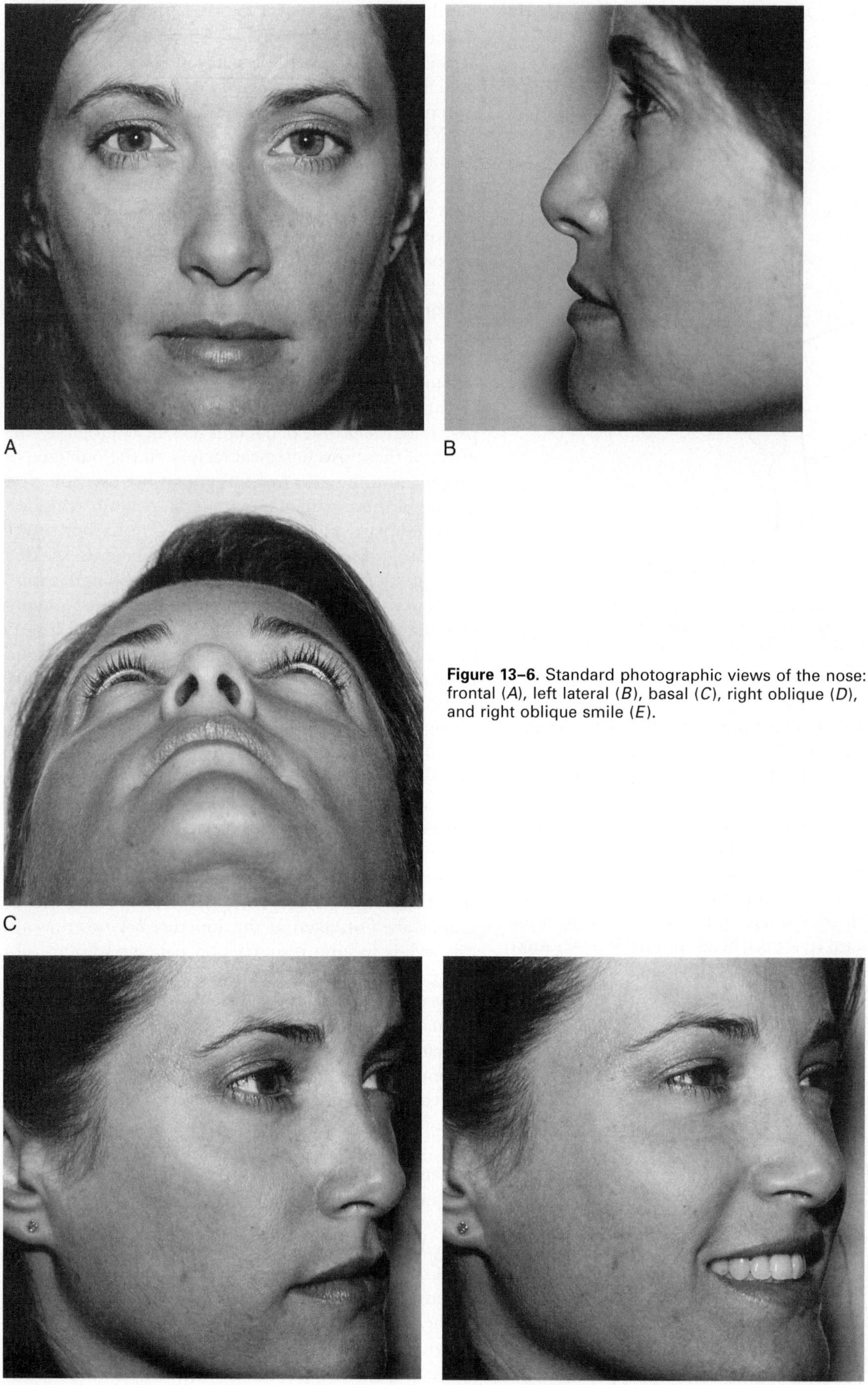

A B C D E

Figure 13–6. Standard photographic views of the nose: frontal (*A*), left lateral (*B*), basal (*C*), right oblique (*D*), and right oblique smile (*E*).

and then alter the image. This helps to inform patients about the possibilities of surgery, but it has also been criticized as a misleading, potentially fraudulent use of technology that can give the patient false expectations. Other surgeons prefer to use measurements taken from photographs, or cephalometric radiographs, as aids to evaluating and informing their patients. These types of precise data are often not that informative for the patient, but may assist the surgeon in setting realistic goals for the actual surgery.

At the second meeting with the patient, preoperative photographs are taken and the goals of the surgery are refined. It is also appropriate at this juncture to have a detailed discussion pertaining to informed consent. Some surgeons prefer to document this discussion by videotaping it. Other surgeons utilize an office version of informed consent which requires the patient to sign the consent after the discussion, attesting to the points discussed. This critical discussion is essential in today's litigious society and should be well documented. It is important to explain the risks, benefits, and alternatives to surgery, and to include information about poor cosmetic outcomes and the chances that revision surgery will be necessary. The best measure of the need for revision surgery can usually be garnered from the surgeon's own experience. However, in the absence of such data, an estimated revision rate of 10% to 20% is probably applicable for most surgeons.

When assessing the physical characteristics of the rhinoplasty candidate, there are many aspects to consider. The first consideration is the overall appearance of the individual. This includes hairstyle and hair coloration, shape of the face, and general body habitus. These characteristics help to define the nose that will best fit the individual patient. For example, a tall, thin person with straight hair would not be likely to look right with a small upturned nose, just as a short, heavy-set individual would not look right with a thin, projecting nose. The shape and projection of the forehead, cheeks, and chin are also important. A patient with a prominent chin will require more projection from the nose than a patient with a weaker or retrognathic mandible. This aspect of analysis is the least well defined and most subjective, and so requires careful consideration of the patient's preferences and a strong aesthetic sense.

The first specific area to evaluate is the nasal dorsum. This area should be assessed for all of the characteristics defined earlier in relation to aesthetic ideal, including symmetry, proportion, and projection. The most common variations include the dorsal hump and dorsal deviation. As a surgeon evaluates this aspect, the implications of the findings in terms of surgical techniques are also registered in his or her mind's eye. Specific issues, such as whether to use a rasp or chisel, or to perform medial and lateral osteotomies or multiple lateral osteotomies, are considered at this time.

The next and, perhaps, the most important characteristic to evaluate is the nasal tip. All of the previously detailed measures are assessed. This includes the width, rotation, projection, symmetry, and shape of the nasal tip. Careful attention should be directed not only to the shape of the structures, but also to the feel of the cartilages. The rigidity of the cartilages has significant implications in terms of the effectiveness of certain techniques to achieve the alterations desired. Soft, pliable cartilage is better suited to suturing than most rigid, inflexible cartilages, as sutures tend to pull through the latter. However, rigid cartilage is less likely to require grafting for adequate support. The characteristics of the tip shape will largely determine the approach used in surgery, as well as the technique used to sculpt the tip.

A final consideration is the quality of the patient's skin. The thickness, texture, and oiliness of the skin will have a significant impact on the results of surgery and the techniques performed. Thin, dry skin tends to contract around the nasal tip over time and is most likely to reveal irregularities in contour. However, this type of skin also shows off a good result better. By contrast, thick, sebaceous skin tends to mask and minimize the alterations achieved, especially in the short term. However, thick skin also hides any imperfections in the surgical result and thus can be beneficial as well.

Selection of Technique

During the initial evaluation, surgeons develop their own concept of what the nose should look like after surgery. However, in the final analysis, the desires of the patient take precedence. At this stage, it is necessary to create a surgical plan to achieve the goals agreed upon with the patient. By the end of the evaluation, a complete understanding of the anatomy, the patient's desires, the goals of the surgery, and the techniques that will be used during the procedure should be formulated.

Approach

The first decision is what basic approach will be used. The choices include the intercartilaginous, transcartilaginous, cartilaginous delivery, and external rhinoplasty approaches. The intercartilaginous approach, which is reserved for patients who do not require any nasal tip work, is used only to change the nasal bone structure. The transcartilaginous approach is infrequently used as it applies only to patients with a desire for only minimal tip refinement. With this approach, the incision allows excision of a dorsal strip from the lower lateral cartilage, but otherwise, the tip is not exposed for any further alterations. The patients who benefit from this technique have symmetrical, well-formed nasal tips that require only a small degree of rotation and narrowing of the tip. No other changes should be expected.

For most patients, the choice will be between cartilage delivery and the external approach. The cartilage delivery approach has the advantage of avoiding the small columellar incision. The external approach has the advantage of complete exposure and visualization of the tip. This choice has sparked a fiery controversy, with internationally known experts taking diametrically opposite views. The advocates of the delivery technique believe that this incision provides adequate exposure to allow any desired adjustments to be made without the necessity of the columellar incision. The advocates of the external approach counter that the precision that is possible with the external exposure allows greater accuracy, better access for grafting, and improved flexibility of technique. In addition, advocates of the external technique have achieved consistently good cosmetic results with the columellar incision, with most patients demonstrating undetectable scars.

The author uses the external approach for most rhinoplasties. The decision depends on whether nasal tip work is necessary. Whenever tip alterations are needed, the external approach is performed. In cases when only bony pyramid work is desired, the intercartilaginous approach is utilized. Essentially, the delivery technique is not used.

Nasal Pyramid

The second consideration in choice of technique is in the management of the nasal pyramid. Nasal hump removal may be achieved using an osteotome or rasp. Although either technique can be used in any situation, large humps are best excised with an osteotome, whereas minor alterations are best achieved with rasping alone.

The need to perform medial and lateral osteotomies is determined by a simple algorithm. Medial osteotomies are required when straightening a deviated dorsum that does not have a hump or when narrowing a wide dorsum without a hump. In both cases, hump removal would achieve the same effect as medial osteotomies by detaching the nasal bones medially. However, in cases when hump removal is not needed, in order to mobilize the nasal bones, medial osteotomies will be required.

Lateral osteotomies are required in most cases. This includes cases when nasal hump removal results in a flattened nasal dorsum. Lateral osteotomies are needed in such cases to prevent the open roof deformity. Other cases requiring lateral osteotomies include patients with a deviated or wide nasal dorsum. In cases of severe dorsal deviation or a twisted nose, multiple lateral osteotomies may be helpful. In these cases, an intermediate osteotomy will allow manipulation of the fragments into proper alignment to achieve a straight, symmetrical, nasal dorsum.

Nasal Tip

In addressing the nasal tip, the choice of technique will vary depending on the degree of narrowing, rotation, and projection that will be needed. The first step is to excise a dorsal strip of cartilage from the lateral crura of the lower lateral cartilages. This step narrows the tip and increases rotation. The greater the extent of resection, the greater the effect achieved. The limit of this resection is that at least 5 mm of the caudal strip must be preserved. Some surgeons have suggested that the cephalic strip technique never be used as it leads to loss of support for the nasal valve and potential functional problems with the airway. Most experienced rhinoplasty surgeons would agree, however, that conservative cephalic resection is both safe and beneficial. If greater narrowing and rotation is required, a dome division can be performed. Division, followed by suturing of the domes together, will increase rotation and projection and narrow the tip. In some cases, well-placed sutures may take the place of the dome division technique.

In addition to the previous techniques, many patients may benefit from grafting. Two basic types of grafts are utilized. The first is a columellar strut. Usually fashioned from septal cartilage, this strut can be used to support the nasal tip, increase projection, and increase columellar show. The second graft is the tip graft. This graft is typically used to improve the tip shape, help effect the desired double break, and increase rotation.

Finally, there are specialized techniques for special situations. In order to reduce projection, the feet of the medial crura can be trimmed. When this is done, it may also be desirable to trim the lateral ends of the lateral crura to maintain balance and proportion. To increase the height of the nasal dorsum, a dorsal onlay graft of bone, cartilage, or alloplastic materials can be placed. The ideal grafting material has yet to be determined, but if possible, autogenous materials should be used, of which cartilage is preferred. Among the alloplastic materials, Gortex is the implant material currently favored.[33]

Widening of the nasal valve area is also occasionally desired. Again, the best technique for this goal has yet to be determined. However, spreader grafts between the septum and the upper lateral cartilages are often used. Suturing techniques can also be applied to achieve the same effect.

In summary, the selection of technique should be made after thoughtful evaluation, and a plan should be designed before the actual surgery takes place. At the time of surgery, adaptations may be necessary, but these should represent only minor adjustments to a comprehensive plan.

Preparation

Preparation of the patient for surgery should include proper cleansing of the skin of the face. The risk of infection of the septum or soft tissues of the nose and face is minimal for rhinoplasty. However, especially for external rhinoplasty, it is customary to prepare the face by thoroughly cleansing it before making an incision. This can be accomplished either with antiseptic soap or iodine-containing solution. No preference has been noted.

Prophylactic antibiotics are not needed for rhinoplasty. This is a clean surgery contaminated by nasal bacteria, but infection rates, with or without antibiotics, are acceptably low. For this reason, preoperative antibiotics are optional.

In draping the patient for surgery, it is important that the face be well exposed. The eyes, nose, and mouth should be visible. This ensures that any anatomic alterations will be oriented to the remainder of the face. If general anesthesia is administered, the eyes should be taped with small, sterile, adhesive strips in the lateral corners of the eyelids.

Anesthesia

The choice of general anesthesia or sedation has little effect on the course of surgery. The advantage of general anesthesia is that patients avoid intraoperative discomfort. Its disadvantages include possible increased blood loss during surgery, potentially difficult emergence from anesthesia, and a slight increase in cardiovascular risk. Among these disadvantages, the most important are problems related to emergence from anesthesia. Often, patients will buck against the endotracheal tube, causing very high intranasal venous pressure. This can lead to bleeding and increased swelling. Also, patients may be severely disoriented after surgery and may attempt to rub their nose, possibly displacing the splint or the nasal pyramid. These problems are generally avoidable with careful anesthetic technique and the use of hand restraints during the first few minutes after the surgery.

Among the disadvantages of sedation are that the patient may experience discomfort during the procedure or become overly sedated, compromising the airway. Discomfort can usually be avoided by appropriate local anesthesia and judicious use of sedation. There is a fine line between adequate sedation and excessive sedation. The balance is best achieved using a combination of midazolam and fentanyl. Propofol as a continuous infusion is also popular. The problem with propofol anesthesia, as well as Pentothal anesthesia, is that patients can become disoriented and uncooperative. The midazolam-fentanyl combination avoids this problem.

Regardless of the choice of general or sedation anesthesia, the patient should receive the same topical and local anesthesia. For topical anesthesia, either 4% cocaine solution or a combination of oxymetazoline with lidocaine works well. The advantages of cocaine flakes, as discussed in Chapter 8 with regard to endoscopic sinus surgery, also apply to this surgery. However, nerve blocks of the sinuses are not necessary for this surgery, and the most important effect of the topical anesthetic is thorough decongestion.

The key to hemostasis and analgesia during rhinoplasty is accurate placement of the local anesthesia. Usually, a combination of 1% lidocaine and 1 : 100,000 epinephrine is used. A dose of up to 7 mg/kg can be used. For a 70-kg individual, this amounts to 49 mL of local anesthetic. In no case, however, should this amount be used. Rather, the goal should be to achieve infiltration of key areas with as little local anesthetic as possible. Typically, only 5 to 10 mL is required. The local anesthetic should be infiltrated through the intercartilaginous area along the nasal dorsum medially and laterally in the nasal facial groove (Fig. 13–7). With infiltration of the septum, columella, and dorsum, the nose should be numb. Direct infiltration of the tip should be avoided to prevent distortion of the structures.

TECHNIQUE

Intercartilaginous Approach

The intercartilaginous approach is used in patients who require bony pyramid work without any nasal tip work. The goal is to mobilize the soft tissues of the nasal dorsum to allow the underlying bones to move freely after osteotomies are performed. Exposure of the intercartilaginous area is best achieved using a small nasal speculum to spread the ala while pushing the lower lateral cartilages superiorly. This maneuver places the inferior edge of the upper lateral cartilage in relief (Fig. 13–8). The incision is made with a No. 15 blade just superficial to the free edge of the upper lateral cartilage. After the incision is made, a curved iris scissors is used to spread the incision open and to elevate the soft tissues over the upper lateral cartilages onto the nasal dorsum.

The iris scissors are then used to elevate the tissues in a blind fashion. The scissors are opened and closed using a short, firm, and slow motion (Fig. 13–9). Over the upper lateral cartilage, the proper plane is on the surface of the perichondrium, whereas over the nasal bones, the plane should be subperiosteal.

At the end of the procedure, the incision is closed with two, simple, interrupted 4-0 chromic sutures on each side. Tip-supporting dressings are not needed, but tape should be applied over the dorsum to help force the soft tissues against the underlying nasal bones.

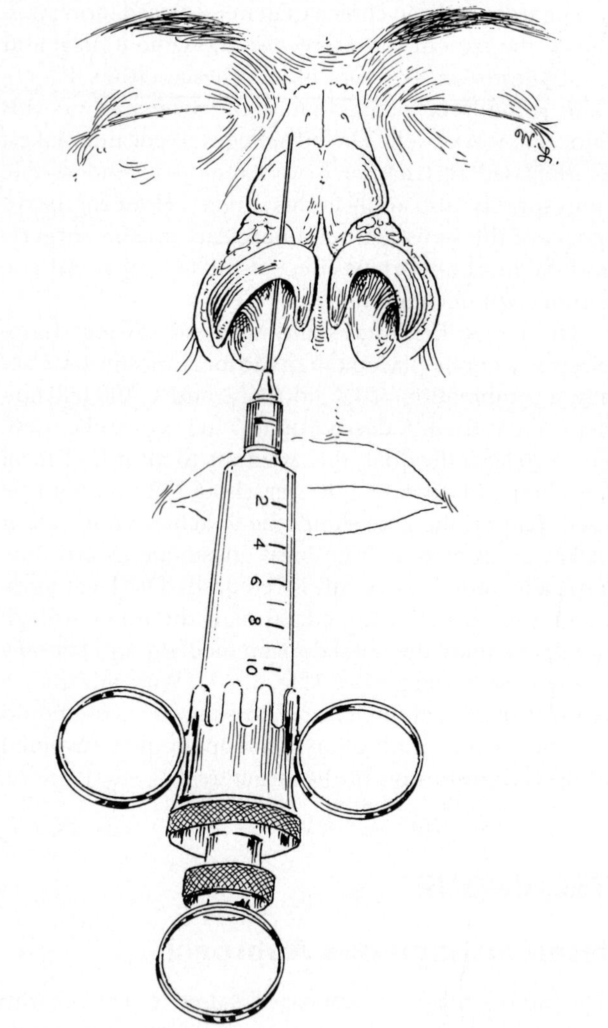

Figure 13–7. Injection of the nasal dorsum. The needle passes ventral to the lower lateral cartilage and dorsal to the upper lateral cartilage through the intercartilaginous space.

Transcartilaginous Approach

The transcartilaginous approach is used when the only nasal tip work required is simple excision of a dorsal (cephalic) strip from the lateral crura of the lower lateral cartilages. To visualize the area of the incision, the ala is retracted using either a double-ball hook retractor or a small nasal speculum. The incision, which is made with a No. 15 blade, extends through the skin overlying the lateral crura. The vestibular skin is elevated from the overlying cartilage cephalad to the superior edge of the cartilage. The appropriate amount of cartilage can then be excised under direct vision, preserving the perichondrium of the dorsal surface. At a minimum, a 4- to 5-mm strip on the caudal edge of the lower lateral cartilage must be maintained (Fig. 13–10). The cartilage is incised in situ through the full thickness of the cartilage, with care being taken to preserve the overlying perichondrium. The dorsal surface of the cartilage to be excised is followed superiorly and the soft tissues are retracted (with an Aufrict retractor) to the intercartilaginous space where the upper lateral and lower lateral cartilages meet. The upper portion of the cartilage that has been incised is then removed. Further elevation over the upper lateral cartilages and onto the nasal dorsum can easily be accomplished at this point.

At the completion of the operation, the incision is closed. Two simple, interrupted, 4-0 chromic sutures per side are all that are needed. After surgery, a standard nasal tip dressing is placed to apply pressure to the skin over the tip.

Cartilage Delivery Approach

The cartilage delivery technique is the approach favored for nasal tip work by surgeons who do not use the external approach. This technique employs three separate incisions: the complete transfixion incision, the intercartilaginous incision, and the marginal incision. The first incision is the complete transfixion incision. Initially, this incision resembles the hemitransfixion incision described in Chapter 12. The incision is made, using a No. 15 blade, along the caudal end of the septum through the skin of the columella. An iris scissors is used to spread the soft tissues over the caudal end of the septum. The counterincision on the opposite side of the columella is made in a similar fashion. With simple spreading, the incisions are joined together (Fig. 13–11).

The next incision is the intercartilaginous incision. This is accomplished by first using a small nasal specu-

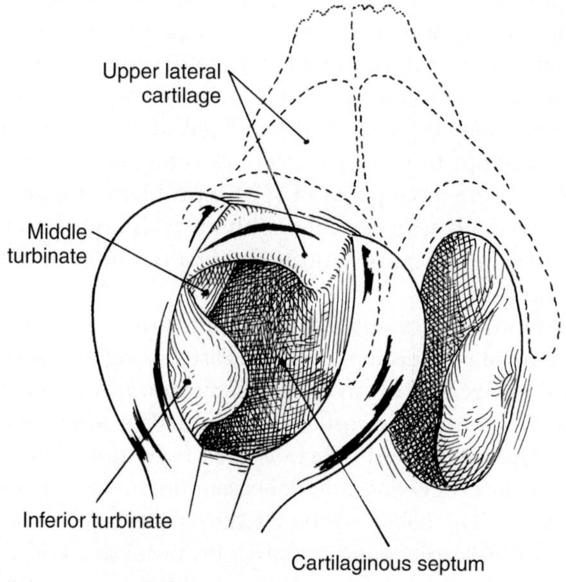

Figure 13–8. Intercartilaginous incision. By pushing the lower lateral cartilage upward, the inferior edge of the upper lateral cartilage is projected into the nasal vestibule. The incision is made on the dorsal surface of the upper lateral cartilage.

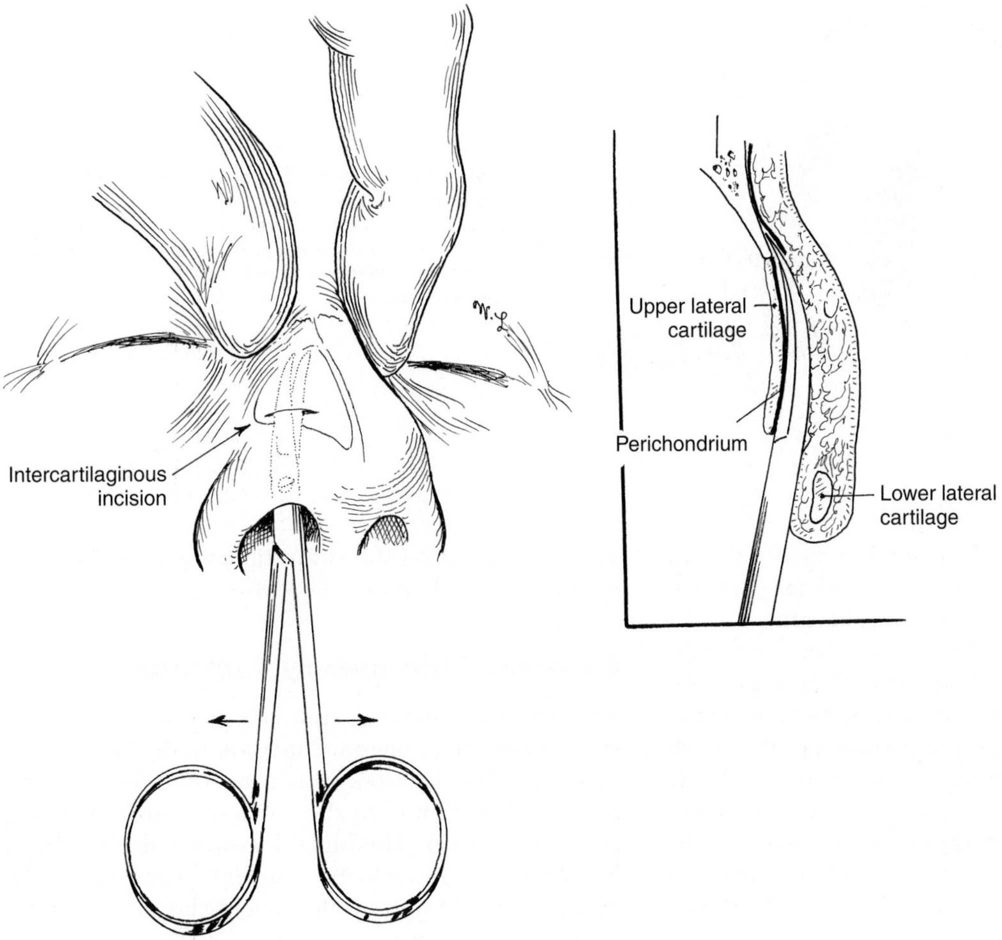

Figure 13–9. Elevation of the nasal dorsum. The scissors are placed through the intercartilaginous incision and spread open to dissect the plane. The plane of dissection should be over the perichondrium of the upper lateral cartilage and under the periosteum of the nasal bones.

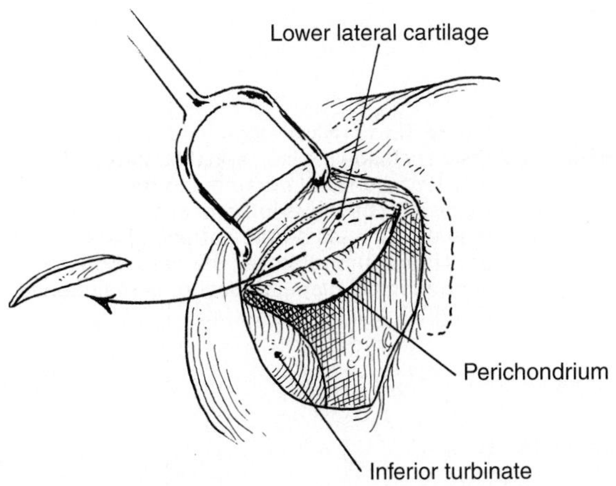

Figure 13–10. Transcartilaginous incision. The incision is made over the ventral surface of the lower lateral cartilage with elevation of the vestibular skin on the surface of the perichondrium up to the intercartilaginous area. The desired amount of cephalic strip is then excised.

lum to push the lower lateral cartilage cephalad over the caudal end of the upper lateral cartilage. An incision is then made with a No. 15 blade just dorsal to the caudal end of the upper lateral cartilage (see Fig. 13-8). This incision can then be connected medially to the transfixion incision, although some surgeons believe that this results in an unacceptable incidence of vestibular stenosis. Careful closure can avoid this problem, and the resultant improved exposure facilitates the ease and accuracy with which surgery of the upper lateral cartilages and nasal bones is performed. Using the iris scissors, the intercartilaginous incision is then spread open to expose the nasal dorsum. The dorsal exposure is completed using a Cottle elevator or Freer elevator to elevate the nasal dorsum in the subperiosteal plane. When the dissection is complete, the soft tissues of the nose should be freed from the nasal bones, upper lateral cartilages, and septum (Fig. 13–12).

The third incision is the marginal incision. The incisional site is exposed with a double-hooked retractor. An incision is then made which follows the inferior edge

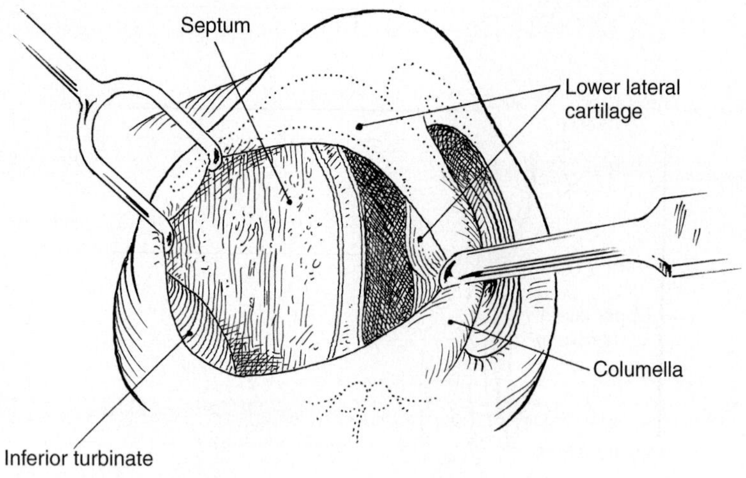

Figure 13–11. Complete transfixion incision. The columella is incised from the floor of the nose up to the septal angle between the caudal end of the septum and the medial crura of the lower lateral cartilages bilaterally to expose the caudal end of the septum.

of the lower lateral cartilage, extending medially from the columella and laterally to the end of the cartilage (Fig. 13–13). As the incision extends laterally, it drifts dorsally away from the rim of the ala to follow the margin of the lateral crus of the lower lateral cartilage. The dorsal surface of the cartilage is carefully followed cephalad right on the surface of the periosteum. When the dorsal surfaces of the cartilages have been completely exposed cephalad to the superior margin of the cartilage, the lower lateral cartilages can be delivered by sliding the cartilages inferiorly. If desired, the cartilages can be dissected free across the midline on the dorsal surface. This allows the entire tip complex to be delivered into a single nares (Fig. 13–14).

External Rhinoplasty Approach

The external rhinoplasty approach combines a columellar incision with a marginal incision to deglove the entire nose. The incision, which incorporates a central notch, is first drawn on the columella with a marking pen (Fig. 13–15). The initial incision is made using a No. 15 blade through the skin only. Care should be taken to avoid injury to the underlying medial crura,

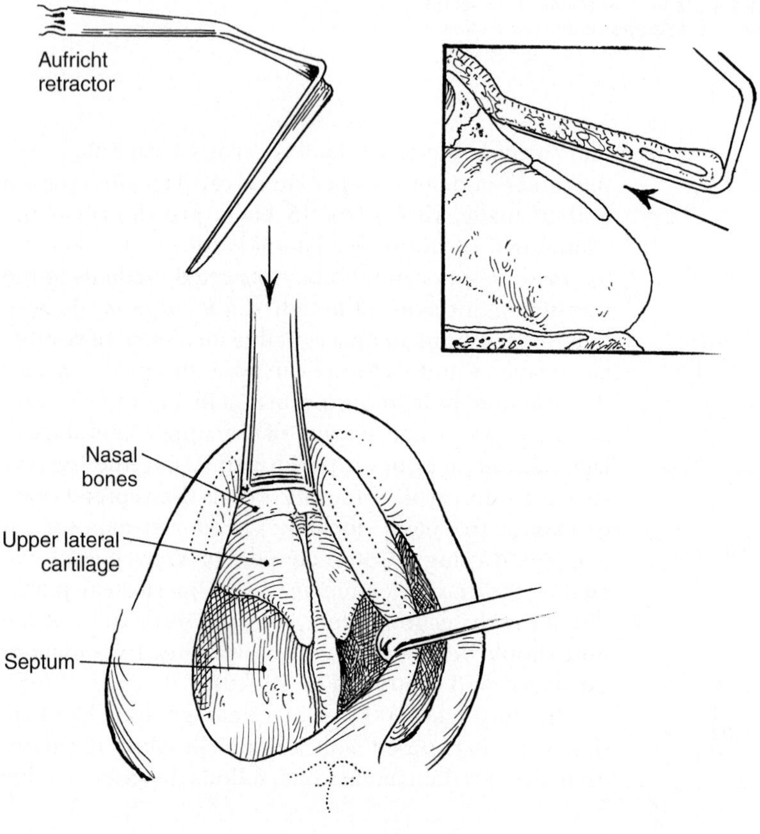

Figure 13–12. Nasal degloving. By connecting the transfixion incision and the intercartilaginous incision, the nasal dorsum can be completely exposed. The elevation proceeds over the upper lateral cartilages on the surface of the perichondrium and over the nasal bones in the subperiosteal plane. Exposure is maintained using an Aufricht retractor.

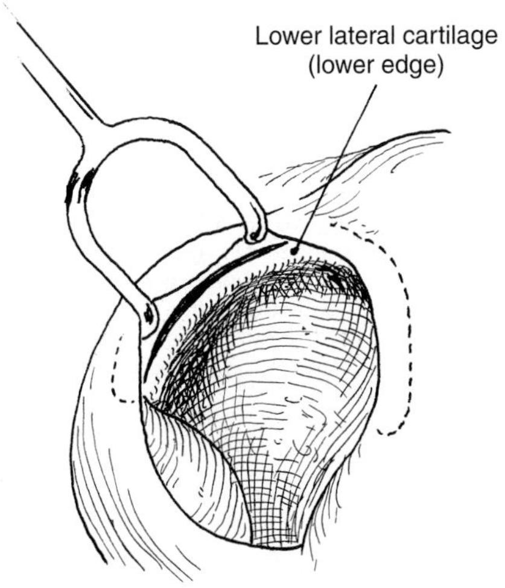

Figure 13–13. Marginal incision. This incision follows the caudal end of the lower lateral cartilage. The incision can extend medially around the alar rim and anterior to the medial crura, making sure to avoid incising the area of the soft triangle.

which are immediately deep to the skin. The incision is extended superiorly along the columella, just on the inside of the columella. The columellar incision extends to the medial aspect of the marginal incision, which is created similarly to the cartilage delivery technique described earlier.

With the initial incision made, the skin is then elevated over the nasal skeleton. A small double hook is used on the inferior edge of the skin flap, and an iris scissors is used to slowly spread and divide the fascial connections between the skin and the cartilage (Fig. 13–16). The best plane of dissection is on the surface of the periosteum. The skin flap is elevated over the nasal tip, maintaining this same plane of dissection. As the elevation proceeds, the area is expanded laterally to expose the entire tip and cephalad to expose the nasal dorsum (Fig. 13–17). As the elevation proceeds across the supratip area, it is important to maintain the proper plane of dissection. The lower lateral cartilages curve away from the skin and, in some cases, under the inferior edge of the upper lateral cartilages. The tendency is to either follow the lower cartilages under the upper lateral cartilages, or to cut across the soft tissue of the supratip area, leaving excessive soft tissue on the nasal dorsum. The ideal plane of dissection is immediately on the surface of the perichondrium, which leaves all of the soft tissue on the under surface of the skin. This preserves blood supply to the nasal tip skin and avoids bleeding.

Tip Sculpting Techniques

In this section, techniques commonly used to modify the nasal tip are addressed. During this part of the procedure, the surgeon is called upon to use experience and judgment to match the technique and degree of resection/alteration to the desired effect. There are no precise guidelines for determining how much of the cephalic strip to take or how large a graft to place. Pertinent variables include the thickness of the patient's cartilage and skin, the shape of the cartilage, and the overall appearance of the nose, all of which must be taken into account in the final decision of how to shape the tip. Thus, available techniques are described in this section, but the way in which they are applied must be determined on a case-by-case basis.

Cartilage Scoring

A minimal technique for altering the shape of the lower lateral cartilages involves the use of cartilage scoring. This technique softens the cartilage, making it more susceptible to contouring. Contouring can then be achieved through judicious use of tape during dressing application or by careful placement of sutures. Also, the depth and direction of the cartilage scoring can directly affect the shape of the cartilage by causing it to bow in a particular direction. These effects are subtle but can be meaningful. The goal is to make partial-thickness cuts in the surface of the cartilage. This causes the dorsal surface to bow away from the cut, thereby increasing the degree of convexity of the cartilage. This technique can be used in conjunction with the cephalic strip, dome division, or suturing techniques.

Suturing Techniques

There are many imaginative and useful ways to use suturing to modify the nasal tip. These techniques are best applied through an external approach for accurate

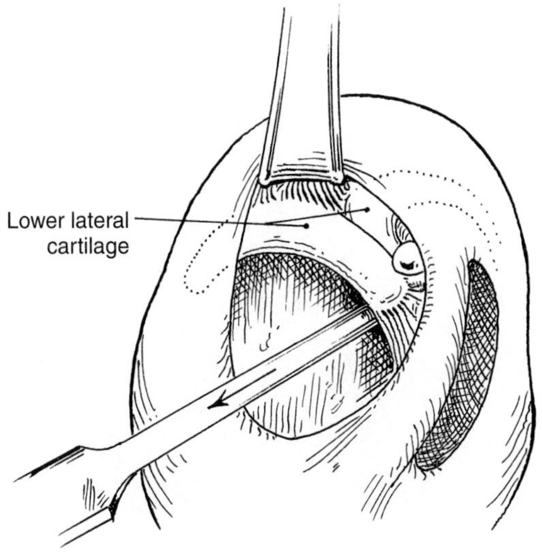

Figure 13–14. Cartilage delivery. After completing all of the incisions and elevating on the surface of the cartilages across the midline, the entire tip complex is delivered into a single nares.

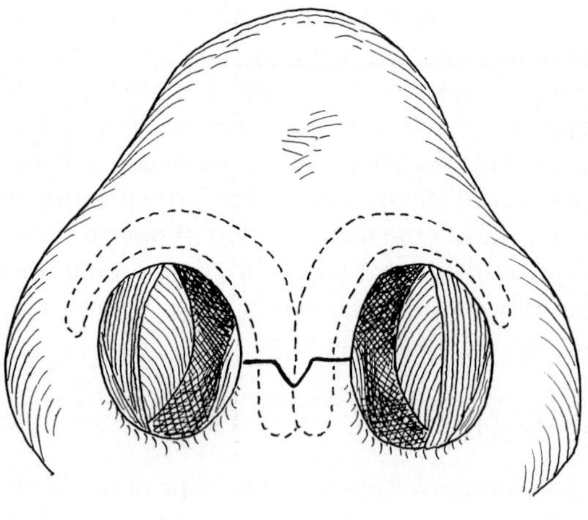

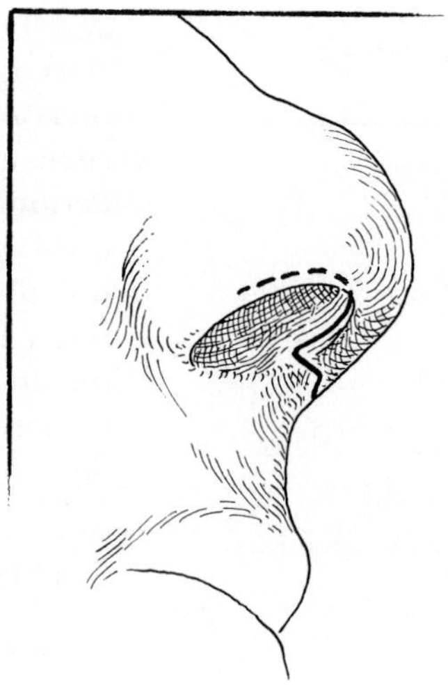

Figure 13–15. Incision for the external rhinoplasty approach. The incision is designed with a notch to help camouflage the incision. The position of the incision should be just below the midpoint of the columella.

placement. One possible drawback of relying on sutures to effect cosmetic improvements is that sutures can break, pull through, or slip. To combat this problem, permanent sutures are always used during rhinoplasty. Theoretically, the sutures must remain intact for the life of the patient to maintain their effect. However, in all probability, once healing is complete, little or no change should be expected from failure of the sutures.

Many suturing techniques have been described in the literature, and many others are used in practice by rhinoplasty surgeons. In this section, only a few of the most commonly used suturing techniques are described. When performing an external septorhinoplasty procedure, the medial crura and domes are separated to access the nasal septum. The most commonly used suturing techniques are horizontal mattress sutures that reapproximate the medial crura and domes (Fig. 13–18).

The medial crural sutures can be used to increase or decrease the amount of columellar show. By imbricating the septum between the medial crura to a varying extent, the amount of columellar show is controlled. Suturing the medial crura with the end of the septum in between will minimize columellar show, whereas suturing the medial crura together in front of the septum will maximize columellar show. This can be achieved, using the cartilage delivery technique, by exposing the medial crura and then separating them.

At the conclusion of the external rhinoplasty, sutures can be placed to bring the domes together. Depending on the placement of the suture, different effects can be achieved. In most cases, a horizontal mattress suture is placed to narrow the nasal tip and help create the tip-

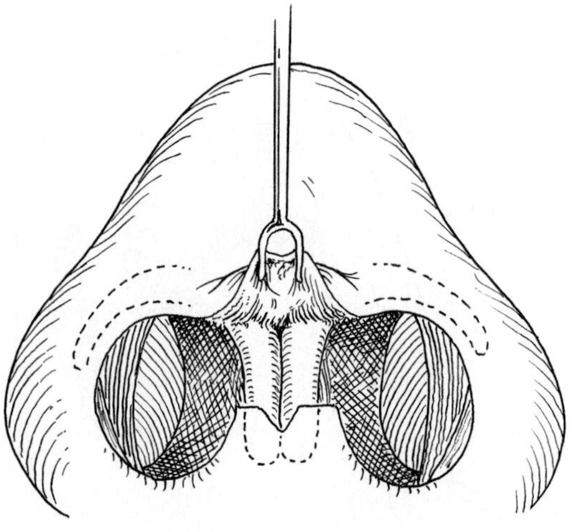

Figure 13–16. Elevation of the columellar skin. The elevation should be on the surface of the perichondrium. A small double hook is used to retract the skin during elevation.

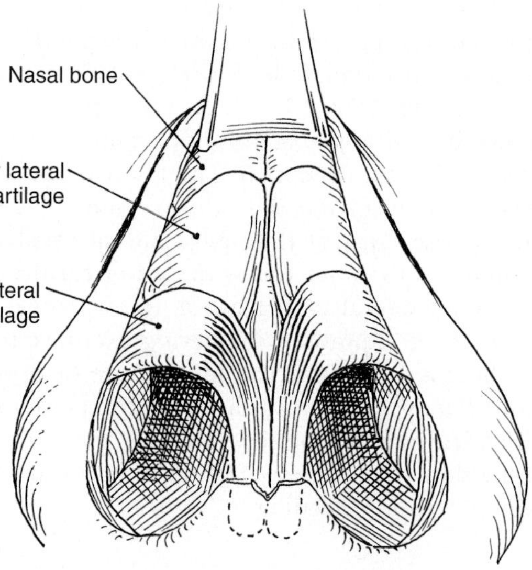

Figure 13–17. Completed exposure for the external rhinoplasty. The soft tissues are retracted by an Aufricht retractor. The plane of dissection is on the surface of the perichondrium and under the periosteum.

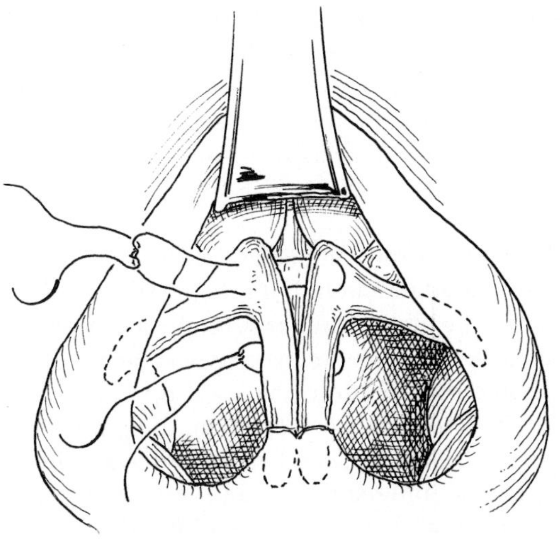

Figure 13–18. Horizontal mattress suture. After tip sculpting is completed, the cartilages are reapproximated with two horizontal mattress sutures. The first suture is placed at the midpoint of the columella. This sets the position of the medial crura. The caudal end of the septum can be interposed between the medial crura to decrease the columellar show or the medial crura can be set in front of the septum to increase columellar show. The last suture is used to pull the domes together. The positioning of this suture will determine the final shape of the nasal tip and the position of the tip-defining points.

defining points. A supratip suture increases rotation. A lateral suture that extends from the upper end of the lateral crura to the lower end of the upper lateral cartilage can help increase rotation and decrease valve collapse.

With the delivery technique, suturing is used to help sculpt the nasal tip. Combining cartilage scoring with a transdomal suture can help narrow the nasal tip in minimally wide noses. Alternatively, sutures can be combined with the cephalic strip or a vertical dome division to alter the nasal tip dramatically.

Cephalic Strip

The cephalic strip is a simple resection of the cephalic border of the lateral crus of the lower lateral cartilage. The best method is to first draw the intended resection directly on the cartilage with a marking pen (Fig. 13–19). To achieve symmetry, it is not so important that the resections be exactly the same, but that the remaining cartilages be the same. The cartilages are excised with a scalpel, cutting just through the cartilage and preserving the ventral periosteum. The cephalic strip is removed by elevating the cartilage from the underlying periosteum. It is important to preserve at least a 4- to 5-mm border of the caudal edge of the cartilage. A good guideline is never to resect more than 50% of the height of the lower lateral cartilage. Excessive resection may lead to contracture of the nasal tip, resulting in a pinched-in appearance and nasal valve collapse.

In general, the cephalic strip technique will narrow the nasal tip and cause it to rotate cephalad. The greater the degree of resection, the greater these anticipated effects will be. The final effect of this alteration on nasal appearance will take many months, if not years, to be realized. It is also generally true that the thicker the skin over the dorsum, the longer the final result will take to manifest and the less effect will be seen initially.

Dome Division

Dome division is a technique used to narrow a wide, bulbous, nasal tip when the cephalic strip with scoring and sutures would be insufficient to achieve the desired outcome. This technique is usually combined with a cephalic strip and may be combined with grafting as well. The principle of the technique is to make a vertical incision through the full height of the lower lateral cartilages, subsequently suturing the cartilages into a tripod to push up and narrow the central tip.

The first step in dome division is to decide on the location of the vertical incision. The more medial the incision, the narrower the nasal tip will be. Typically, the site of the incision will be a few millimeters lateral to the tip-defining points (Fig. 13–20). If desired, some of the lateral crura can be excised vertically to narrow the tip further. After the incisions are made, the medial tips of the lateral crura are sutured back to the medial crura under the domes (Fig. 13–21). Typically, two hori-

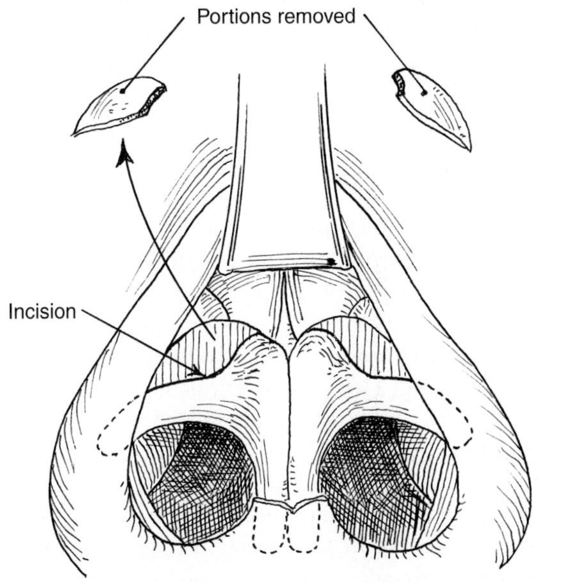

Figure 13–19. Cephalic strip. A cephalic strip can be excised from the lateral crura to narrow and rotate the nasal tip. The exact shape of the excision will vary depending on the effect desired. At least half of the height of the cartilage should be preserved to avoid loss of tip support.

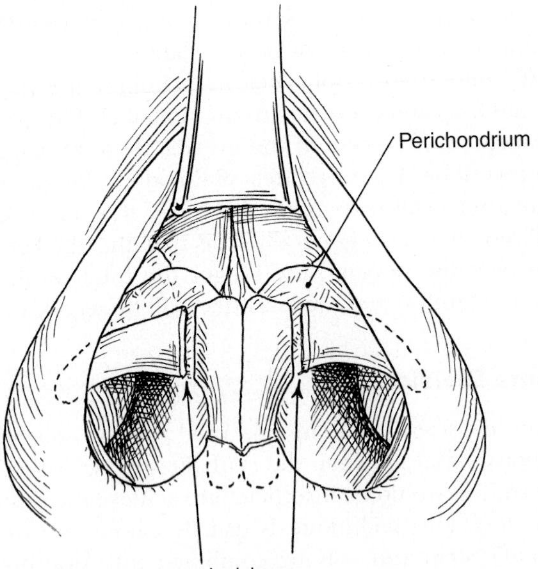

Figure 13–20. Dome division. After the cephalic strip is excised, a dome division may be performed to further narrow the nasal tip. The location and shape of the cartilaginous incision depends on the desired effect.

zontal mattress sutures are placed that extend from one lateral crus across the medial crura through the opposite lateral crus. The position of the cartilages can be adjusted to either increase or decrease projection of the tip. The higher under the domes the cartilages are sutured, the less projection this imparts. Conversely, the lateral crura can be sutured lower on the medial crura, thereby pushing the nasal tip up and increasing projection. In extreme cases, a vertical segment of the lateral crus can be resected prior to resuturing the lateral crura to the domes. This will accentuate the degree of tip narrowing.

Grafting Techniques

There are two basic grafting techniques that are commonly used in rhinoplasty: the columellar strut and the shield-shaped tip graft. In addition to these standard grafts, other grafts may be used to augment the nasal dorsum, fill in contour defects, or augment the lower lateral cartilages. The source of grafting materials varies. In almost all cases, the quadrilateral cartilage of the septum is utilized for columellar and tip grafts, whereas auricular cartilage is used for contour defects and lower lateral cartilage augmentation. The material used for dorsal augmentation has varied through the years, as discussed in detail in the later section on bony pyramid procedures.

The columellar strut is the most common graft used in rhinoplasty. This graft can achieve multiple effects, including an increase in tip support, tip projection, and columellar show. The graft is harvested from the septum using a Freer knife. The best location for obtaining the graft is from the area of the septum lying in the maxillary crest. This is usually removed during a septoplasty as the so-called inferior strip. As the thickest, most rigid cartilage in the septum, it is ideally suited for this purpose.

The length of the columellar strut will vary depending on its intended function. If it is to provide nasal tip support only, the graft should rest on the anterior ledge of the maxillary crest, between or against the medial crura, and should extend up to the nasal tip (Fig. 13–22). If the intent is to increase projection, the graft should lie against the caudal end of the septum, deep to the medial crura, and should extend up and into the tip, pushing the tip outward. If the intent is to increase columellar show, the graft can be laid over the medial crura or deep to the crura. Conversely, locating the graft between the crura will prevent changes in columellar show.

The strut is generally fixed to the medial crura or septum using two or three sutures. Clear 5-0 nylon sutures are preferred, and the sutures should be placed to hide the knots deep to the graft. After the graft is secured in place, the skin must be redraped over the nose to assess the effect of the graft. Adjustments should be made to ensure optimal positioning before contemplating closure.

Tip grafts are also commonly used in rhinoplasty when contouring of the existing cartilages alone will be inadequate to achieve the desired result. Tip grafts can increase rotation and projection somewhat, but are primarily used to help create the tip shape desired. The tip can be asymmetric, bifid, or have a rounded, plump appearance. In these circumstances, using a carefully

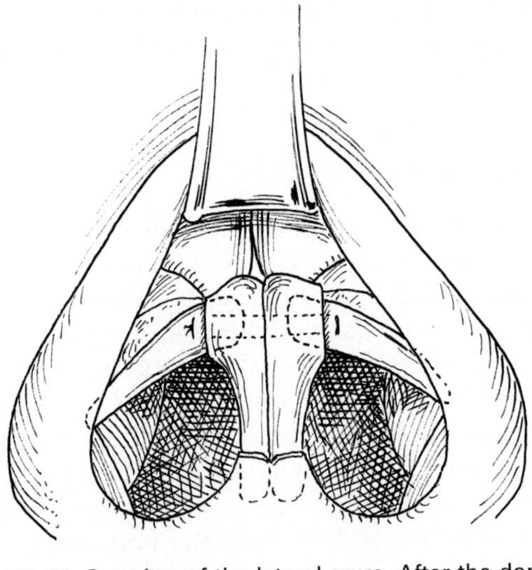

Figure 13–21. Suturing of the lateral crura. After the dome division, the medial ends of the crura are sutured together to narrow the nasal tip. A horizontal mattress suture is used to pull the cartilages together. The exact position of the suture will greatly affect the final result.

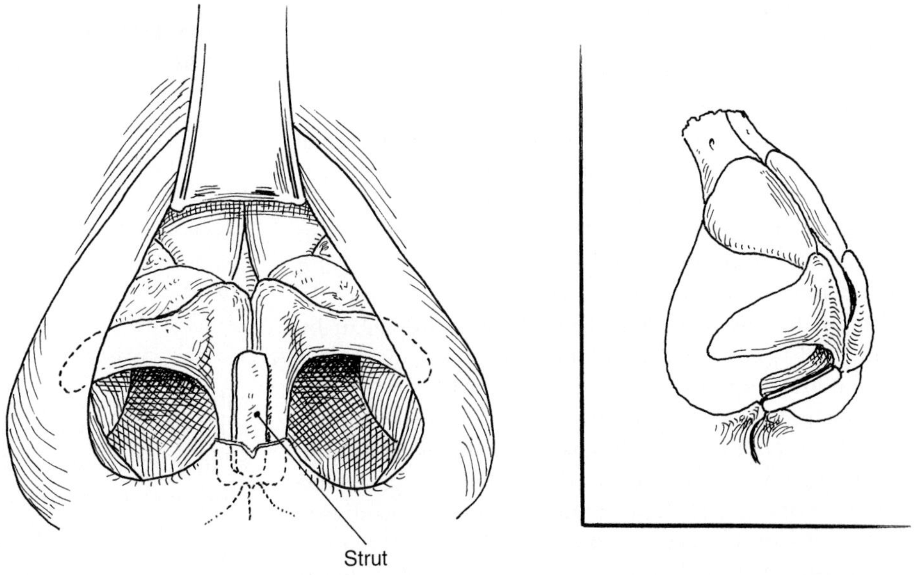

Figure 13–22. Columellar strut. To improve nasal tip support and projection, a columellar strut is placed. This can be positioned in front of the medial crura or between the crura, depending on the columellar show desired.

shaped tip graft can hide underlying problems by creating symmetrical, well-demarcated, and rounded tip-defining points. The graft enhances the alterations already made and smooths and proportions the tip.

The graft is best formed from septal cartilage and can be sculpted from any flat area of the septum. Generally, the cartilage is harvested from a posterior area of the septum that will not affect septal form or function. The graft is carved slowly and carefully into a shield shape using a scalpel (Fig. 13–23). The exact shape and size of the graft will vary with the configuration of the nose. The surgeon must use both judgment and experience in fashioning the graft and should assess the appearance by redraping the skin over the nose. Optimal graft placement can only be determined by trial and error, but generally tends to be approximately flush with the dorsum of the tip. If the graft sticks out too much, it will create a ridge across the tip. Conversely, underprojection of the graft will result in a failure to achieve the desired result. Once positioned, the graft is fixed in place with clear 5-0 nylon sutures with the knots buried beneath the graft.

Narrowing the Nasal Tip

It is useful to apply an algorithm for decision making when considering narrowing the wide or bulbous nasal tip. In progressing from the ideal nasal tip, which re-

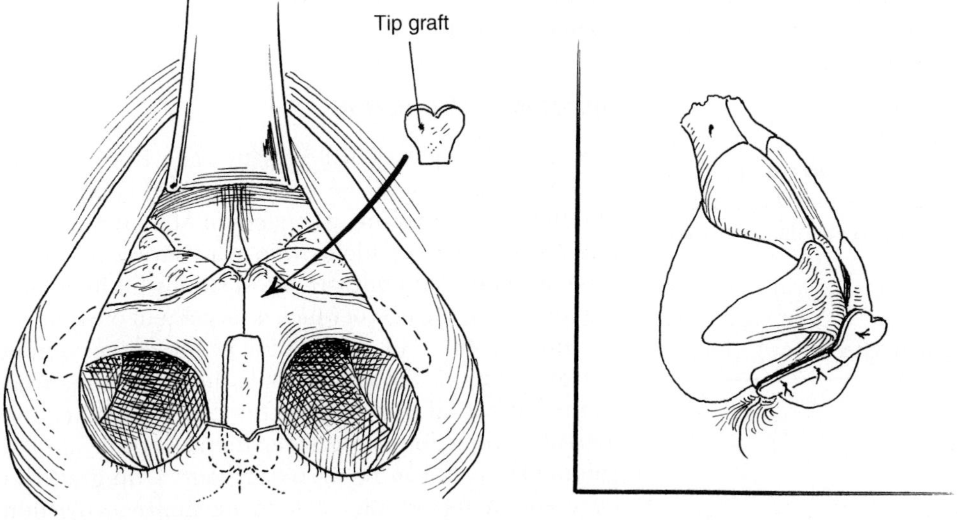

Figure 13–23. Nasal tip graft. To help improve tip shape and position, a shield-shaped tip graft may be placed. The inset shows the final position of the graft sutured in place.

quires no narrowing, to the widest tip, which requires dramatic narrowing, the techniques become additive in their effect (Table 13–1). In each patient undergoing cosmetic rhinoplasty, the surgeon will encounter some degree of soft tissue in the nasal tip and intradomal areas. When attempting to narrow the tip, it is frequently necessary to remove this soft tissue or to defat the tip. This is easily accomplished by grasping the tissue and dissecting it from the underlying cartilages or overlying skin using tenotomy scissors or curved iris scissors. In addition to this basic step, the following steps can be employed to narrow the widened tip progressively.

The first step involves scoring the cartilages with intradomal sutures. This technique, which achieves a modest refinement in the width of the nasal tip, is applicable to those patients with a properly rotated and projected tip who nonetheless desire minor changes in tip shape. The next step used to narrow the nasal tip is creation of a cephalic strip. The degree of narrowing achieved is proportional to the amount resected. This procedure also adds rotation. This technique is most applicable to patients with a moderately wide nasal tip that requires significant but not dramatic refinement. Combining the cephalic strip with intradomal suturing is the next step. This may be accompanied by scoring of the cartilage, either in one direction or bidirectionally, to weaken the domes. The combination of cephalic strip and intradomal suture with cartilage-relaxing incisions will significantly narrow the nasal tip. In most situations, these procedures will suffice to achieve the desired outcome.

However, in patients with the widest, most bulbous nasal tips, overaggressive suturing may impart a squared-off or angled unnatural appearance to the tip. In these cases, the vertical division or dome division technique is applied. Depending on where along the dorsum of the dome the vertical division is placed, the nasal tip will be more or less narrowed. The more medial the division, the more narrowing will be achieved. In the most extreme cases, dome division can be combined with cartilage-relaxing incisions, intradomal sutures, and vertical resection of the lateral crus.

Increasing Rotation

As with the considerations for tip width, tip rotation can be increased incrementally using a graduated approach (Table 13–2). Again, the initial step is cartilage scoring with placement of intradomal sutures. This procedure will increase rotation slightly. The next step is creation of a cephalic strip. This predictably rotates the tip a modest amount. The next level of rotation is achieved by combining the cephalic strip with supradomal sutures, which can pull the tip upward to a significant extent when performed in combination with the cephalic strip. The optimal application of this method, though, is when the nasal tip starts out at about the horizontal plane or 90 degrees of rotation. In such cases, this combination will usually be sufficient to create the 95- to 105-degree angle desired.

For patients with a hanging nasal tip that hooks downward, additional rotation is required. In these cases, the columellar strut and then the tip graft procedures are added. The strut is placed first and is combined with the cephalic strip and supradomal suture techniques. Often, however, with the hanging tip, a tip graft must be added to support the tip in the new position and create a rounder, smoother appearance. In such cases, the surgeon should be certain that the patient in fact desires the tip to be rotated to this extent. Many people with a hanging nasal tip fear that overrotation of the tip will yield too dramatic a change. In such patients, the use of the strut alone, possibly without supradomal sutures, may be adequate to rotate the tip to a 90- or 95-degree angle.

TABLE 13–1
Techniques for Narrowing the Nasal Tip

Cartilage scoring
Cartilage scoring with intradomal suture
Cephalic strip
Cephalic strip with intradomal suture
Vertical dome division

TABLE 13–2
Techniques for Increasing Tip Rotation

Cartilage scoring with introdomal suture
Supratip suture
Cephalic strip
Cephalic strip with supratip suture
Cephalic strip with supratip suture, columellar strut, and tip graft

Increasing Projection

Occasionally, a patient will present who wishes the projection of the nose to be increased. This is primarily, although not exclusively, a concern of African American and Eastern Asian patients who may have a flat, wide nose. Several techniques are most successful in achieving this result, the first of which is placement of columellar sutures. When placed just below the domes and at the midpoint of the columella as horizontal mattress sutures, these sutures will push the domes together and increase projection. To further increase projection, a columellar strut can be placed. Finally, a tip graft can be used on top of the strut to maximize projection and support. It is imperative that the patient be well informed of the extent of modification to be performed in this case, as the most dramatic alterations may be aesthetically pleasing to the surgeon but too pronounced for the patient.

Decreasing Projection

Decreasing nasal projection may be a concern for other patients. Most patients who think that their nose is too big generally are unhappy with the width of the nose, the length of the nose, and the height of the nasal dorsum. Only occasionally is a true decrease in the projection of the nose desired. The techniques available to achieve this goal are either to trim height from the septum or to lower the tip by trimming from the medial crura. Trimming from the septum is, in fact, the less desirable technique because it is associated with the formation of a hanging nasal tip. Trimming the caudal edge of the septum causes the tip to hang over the edge of the septum, resulting in a curvature to the profile and a hanging nasal tip. To avoid this, supratip sutures or a columellar strut must be used. The preferred technique is to combine dorsal septal resection and trimming of the medial crura at the nasal spine. These two steps will drop the nasal tip toward the maxilla. To avoid decreasing the rotation, a columellar strut is usually placed, and a supradomal suture is used to make fine adjustments in the tip position.

This procedure may cause lateral bowing of the ala. To compensate for this effect, either the lateral ends of the lateral crura will need to be trimmed or the alae will need to be brought inward using alar base excision. It is preferable to trim the lateral ends of the lateral crura first, before committing to alteration of the alar base.

Great care should be taken before deciding to proceed with decreasing the projection of the nose. In most cases, it is not the aspect of the patient's nose that truly bothers them, and the risk of poor outcomes with these techniques is higher than with more conservative techniques.

Narrowing the Alar Base

Occasionally, a narrowing of the alar base is required as part of an overall restructuring of the nose. This should always be done in the context of other changes taking place during the procedure, and it is not a bad idea to consider delaying this step to a later time if it has not been discussed thoroughly with the patient before surgery. The general principle upon which the technique is based is the creation of a triangular excision in the floor of the nose at the attachment of the ala to the face, with subsequent mobilization and reapproximation of the edges to narrow the width of the alar base (Fig. 13–24).

The versatility of this approach is evidenced by the fact that the location of the excision and the size of the excision can be varied to create different effects. Orienting the excision vertically just inside the ala, in combination with trimming of the lateral edge of the lateral crura, will lower the height of the lateral flare of the ala without narrowing the base. Orienting the excision on the floor of the nose will tend to narrow the base but not decrease its height. Alternatively, by combining trimming of the lateral crura with an excision on the floor and vertical alar rim, both lowering the height and narrowing the base can be accomplished.

Bony Pyramid

Almost every rhinoplasty procedure involves some alteration of the bony pyramid. This step is always saved for

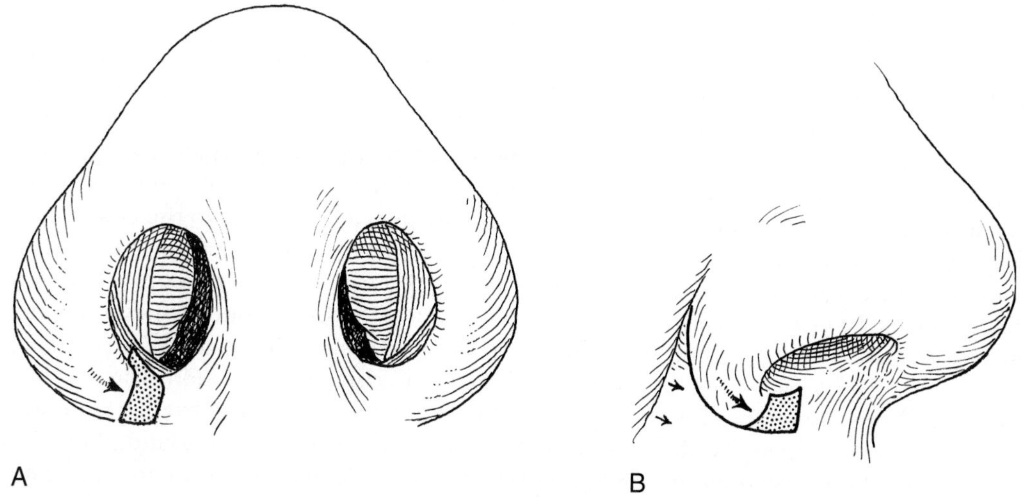

Figure 13–24. Alar excision. To narrow the alar base, an alar excision may be performed. The shape and location of one variation is demonstrated. The exact excision is tailored to the desired effect.

last and is performed immediately before ending the surgery. The reason for this is that the osteotomies always cause bleeding and swelling, and the sooner the nose is packed and dressed after the osteotomies are done, the less bleeding and swelling will occur. There has been considerable discussion in the literature concerning strategies for minimizing the swelling and bruising that result from bony pyramid work in rhinoplasty. Some surgeons advocate the use of perioperative intravenous and postoperative oral steroids to help minimize swelling. Others have touted the benefits of adequate local anesthesia and still others have proposed the use of smaller and sharper osteotomes, with or without guides.

The author believes that several steps may be useful in minimizing swelling, as discussed later. However, the most important factor is accurate and skillful use of selected instruments, with gentle, precise, and controlled technique. In this procedure, as in so many in surgery, the skill of the surgeon is paramount in minimizing tissue trauma and maximizing the benefits of surgery.

Nasal Hump Reduction

Among the most popular goals in rhinoplasty is the reduction of a dorsal nasal hump. This basic and essential step in rhinoplasty is performed first after the completion of the nasal tip work. It is important to realize that most dorsal humps are a combination of nasal bone and septal and upper lateral cartilages. The goal of nasal hump removal is to achieve a smooth dorsum that, in men, lies flush with a line from the nasion to the tip and that, in women, lies 1 to 2 mm below the line. A second general rule in hump removal is to overresect the hump slightly. Owing to periosteal reaction and new bone formation, a proportion of the bone excised will be replaced by either soft tissue reaction, scarring, or new bone. This overresection should not take on major proportions, but instead, should approximate 0.5 to 1.0 mm.

The cartilaginous portion of the nasal hump is removed first. A variety of techniques have been described to achieve cartilaginous hump removal. The author prefers to use the dorsal cartilage scissors. Through either the external or endonasal approach, the instrument is angled tangentially to the dorsum of the nose. The upper lateral and septal cartilages are excised in a single cut. It is best to underestimate the excision at this point to avoid excessive hump removal that would require free-graft augmentation.

Removal of the bony portion of the nasal hump follows the cartilage excision and can be achieved with either rasps, saws, or osteotomes. The decision as to instrumentation is largely individual; however, a good rule of thumb is to remove a small hump with a rasp and a large hump with an osteotome or a combination of instruments. When a rasp is used, short, unidirectional, scraping motions are preferred. The rasp should be intermittently cleaned of bone dust and, if a great deal of rasping is needed, it may be helpful to alternate between two rasps with different cutting surfaces to maintain good contact between the bone and the rasp.

When using an osteotome, a flat, wide blade is preferred. The osteotome is held firmly but not tightly with a backhanded grip in the tangential plane desired (Fig. 13–25). It is always advisable to underestimate the amount of bone to be removed so that one does not resect too much. If this were to occur, then a dorsal bone graft would be necessary to correct the deformity.

After the bulk of the nasal hump has been removed with the osteotome, the rasp is usually applied to smooth out the contours and complete any additional hump removal. Once the bony hump removal is complete, the cartilaginous hump is further trimmed with either scalpel or scissors to match the new bony dorsum. Again, a gradual reduction of the cartilaginous hump is recommended rather than attempting complete removal with the first cut. It is easier and better to lower the dorsum to the correct height gradually than to overresect and have to place grafts.

Medial Osteotomies

Medial osteotomies are necessary whenever lateral osteotomies are planned to alter the nasal dorsum, but a dorsal hump removal is not performed. In all cases, medial osteotomies are performed before lateral osteotomies. This can be done through either an endonasal or external approach. With the endonasal technique, the osteotome is impacted against the inner aspect of the caudal end of the nasal bones (Fig. 13–26*A*). With the external approach, the osteotome is placed against the outer or dorsal aspect of the nasal bones under direct vision (Fig. 13–26*B*).

Ideally, the osteotome should have a straight, 3- to 4-mm blade. Firm but gentle taps are applied to the blunt end of the osteotome by an assistant while the surgeon holds the osteotome in one hand while guiding the tip between the thumb and index finger of the other hand. The osteotomy is advanced up to the attachment of the nasal bones to the frontal bones at the nasion. The surgeon will feel the transition in resistance between the nasal bones and the frontal bone. Also, the impact produced by the osteotome cutting through the nasal bones will create a crisp, hollow sound, whereas the impact of the osteotome against the frontal bone will cause a dull thud. Both by feel and by sound, then, the surgeon will be able to detect the precise instant when the osteotome completes the nasal bone cut and contacts the frontal bone. The cut should be stopped at this point.

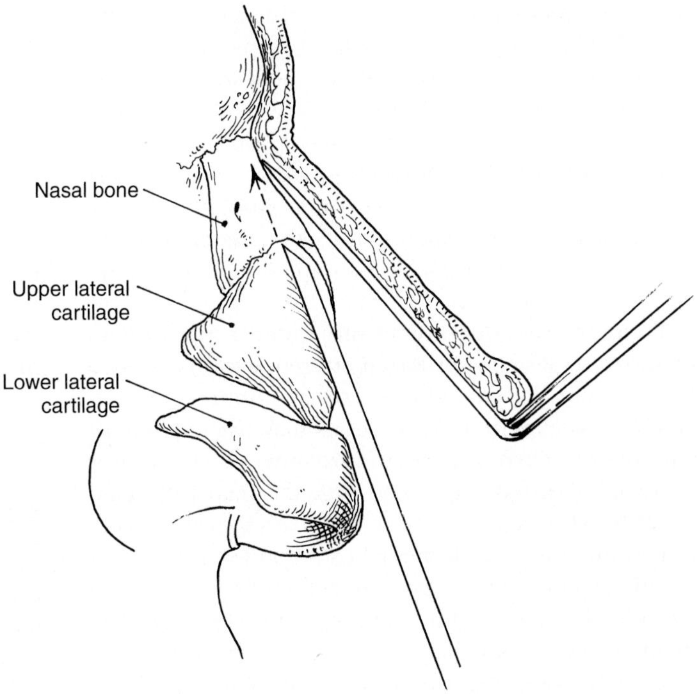

Figure 13–25. Nasal hump reduction. A lateral view of the position of the osteotome is demonstrated through the external approach. A wide, flat blade is required for a smooth resection. Typically, the cartilage resection precedes the bony resection.

The right and left nasal bones should each be incised in a similar fashion, with the two cuts parallel and separated by the desired amount of intact bone. This amount of bone is determined by the goals of the surgery. If the dorsum is merely wide and not deviated, a wider strip of bone can be preserved between the medial osteotomies. This will allow medial displacement of the lateral aspects of the nasal bones without disturbing an otherwise normal dorsal contour. Conversely, if the dorsum is deviated, the medial osteotomies may need to be immediately adjacent to each other to avoid preserving a deviated central strip.

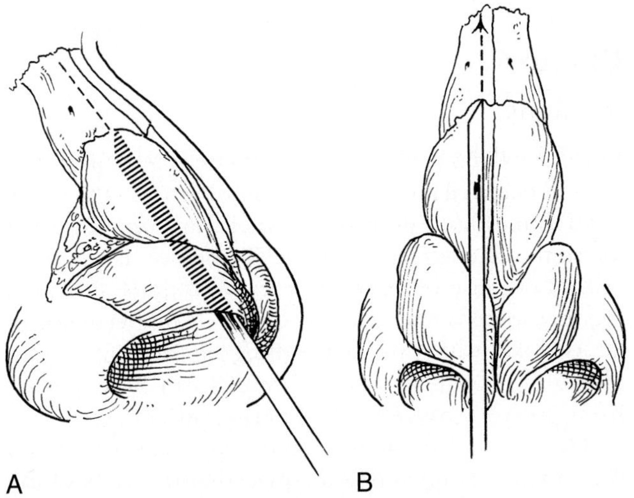

Figure 13–26. Medial osteotomy. A small, straight osteotome is used to make a paramedian cut through the nasal bones. *A,* Transnasal technique. *B,* External technique.

Lateral Osteotomies

Lateral osteotomies are almost always required in rhinoplasty unless the nasal bones are ideal and no alterations are needed. Lateral osteotomies are indicated to realign a deviated dorsum, to narrow a wide dorsum, or to prevent an open roof defect after removal of a nasal hump. Lateral osteotomies are always the last step performed before completion of the rhinoplasty. Whether done via an external or endonasal approach, lateral osteotomies are always performed through a small incision in the nasal vestibule overlying the lateral aspect of the pyriform aperture (Fig. 13–27). The area of the incision is usually injected with local anesthetic and a short interval allowed to elapse for anesthetic effect

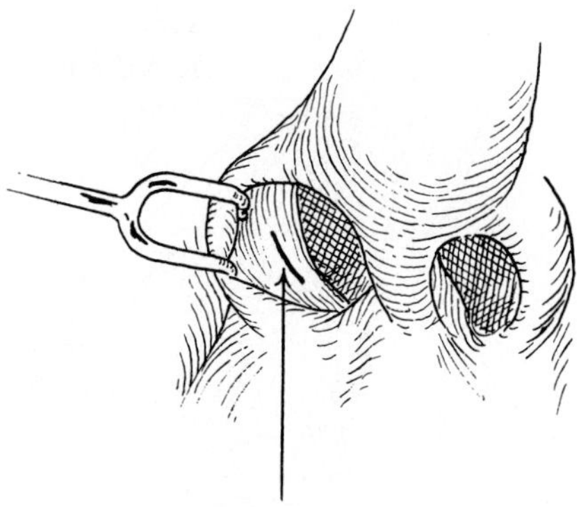

Figure 13–27. Vestibular incision for lateral osteotomy. This is made in the skin of the vestibule anterior to the inferior turbinate.

before the incision is made. The incision is made with a No. 15 blade. The incision is spread open with an iris scissors down to the bone of the pyriform aperture. An elevator (usually, a Cottle elevator) is then used to elevate the periosteum over the nasal bones in the line of the osteotomy. This is done to avoid tearing of the periosteum and excessive bleeding. Also, this lateral periosteal elevation helps to ensure that the nasal bones will be able to move freely after completion of the osteotomies.

Preferences in osteotomes vary widely from surgeon to surgeon. Very experienced surgeons prefer a 2- to 3-mm straight or curved osteotome without a guide or guard. Less experienced surgeons may use any one of a number of curved, guarded instruments. The author prefers a guarded osteotome with the guard directed laterally so the guard can be felt beneath the skin during osteotome use. As with medial osteotomies, the recommended technique is to have an assistant apply the mallet to the blunt end while the surgeon holds the instrument firmly in one hand and directs the tip of the osteotome using the thumb and index finger of the opposite hand.

The initial move is to engage the osteotome with the instrument angled perpendicular to the pyriform aperture (Fig. 13–28, a). After the osteotome is advanced a few millimeters, the angle is slowly dropped until the plane is horizontal (Fig. 13–28, b). The line of the osteotomy follows the nasal facial groove superiorly up to the level of the medial canthus of the eye. The angle then

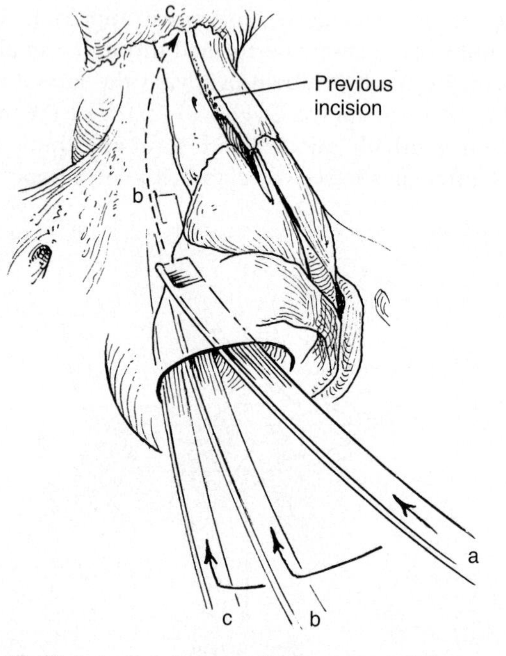

Figure 13–28. Lateral osteotomy. As the bone incision proceeds, the angle of the osteotome progressively flattens out from position *a* to *b* to *c*. The exact path of the incision varies according to the desired effect.

curves medially toward the medial osteotomies (Fig. 13–28, c). The superior extent of the lateral osteotomy is reached when the bone instrument reaches the level of the nasion. The osteotome is then rolled medially, with pressure applied to the nasal bones to complete the mobilization by fracturing the superior attachment. At this point, the ipsilateral nasal bone should be fully mobilized and should be supported only by the internal periosteum. Care should be taken to ensure that the nasal bone is completely mobilized without residual attachments to the surrounding bones. If residual attachments persist, this can lead to the so-called greenstick fracture or rocker, with subsequent healing leading to a rebound of the bone to its original position.

Intermediate Osteotomies

In patients with a twisted nose or a severely deviated dorsum, an intermediate osteotomy—sometimes referred to as multiple lateral osteotomies—may be required. When there is a significant bulge in the nasal bones to one side, classic medial and lateral osteotomies will result in mobilization of a markedly bowed nasal bone which, upon displacement, will remain bowed, preventing creation of a smooth, straight nose. An intermediate osteotomy midway between the medial and lateral osteotomies allows the curve to be broken into two smaller, flatter pieces that can separately be manipulated into position to create the desired contour (Fig. 13–29).

Intermediate osteotomies are usually only done on the convex side of the nasal dorsum, and they are always done after the medial osteotomy or nasal hump removal but before the lateral osteotomies. This avoids the situation of trying to cut a mobile bone. The technique is essentially the same as that described for medial osteotomies.

Closure

Incisions

In the external rhinoplasty procedure, there are internal and external incisions to repair, whereas in the endonasal rhinoplasty procedures, there are only internal incisions. The external columellar incision is the most critical because of its cosmetic ramifications. Provided the incision is made carefully with a clean, perpendicular cut and with careful handling of the flap during elevation, excellent cosmetic results can be expected from precise closure of the external incision.

The external incision is closed using 6-0 nylon suture. The initial sutures should be placed at the apex of the notch and the lateral margins of the columella. Subsequent sutures are placed at intermediate points as necessary to achieve adequate alignment. The remaining as-

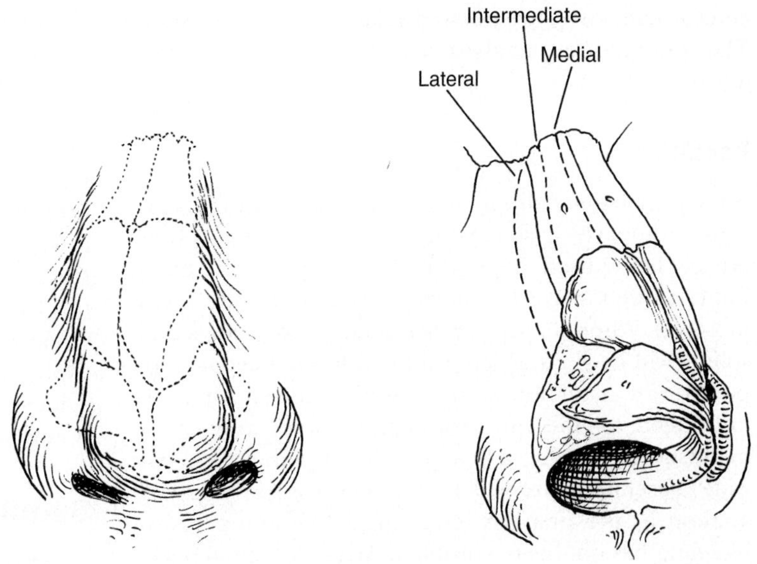

Figure 13–29. Intermediate osteotomy. In patients with a twisted nose, intermediate osteotomies are required to straighten the dorsum. The positions of the medial, intermediate, and lateral osteotomies are shown.

pects of the incision, which extend vertically toward the tip and along the margin of the lateral crura, are closed with a minimum number of 5-0 or 6-0 chromic catgut sutures. This part of the incision will generally line up well, and will heal without discernible scar with only a few sutures.

The internal incisions used for the cartilage delivery technique have the potential to lead to excessive scarring and vestibular stenosis. To avoid this complication, careful closure is required. A 4-0 chromic catgut suture is typically used throughout this closure. The initial stitch should be placed at the apex of the incision. The transfixion incision is then closed with two or three interrupted sutures on each side. An equal number of sutures is used to close the intercartilaginous incision. The marginal incisions can be approximated as needed to align and stabilize these incisions.

Taping

An essential step in the performance of rhinoplasty is to tape and splint the nose after surgery. The goals of taping are to stabilize the nose, facilitate the desired contouring, apply the skin to the underlying framework, and limit postoperative swelling. The tape should be applied as soon as the incisions are closed. The skin should be cleaned and prepared with an adhesive material. During placement of the tape, it is important to make sure that the nasal dorsum is not displaced from the desired position.

Tape is applied from a superior to inferior direction, with each piece cut to specifications. After a basal layer of tape is applied, supporting strips are wrapped around the nasal tip (Fig. 13–30). It is important that this strip not be too tight around the nasal tip, as it is possible for additional swelling to cause the tape to cut into the columellar skin. Finally, additional tape can be applied over the first layer to reinforce the initial layer at critical points, such as the supratip area.

Splinting

Following application of tape, an external nasal splint is placed. There are many types of splints available, including plaster casts, metal, and plastic. The goals of splinting in each case are the same: stabilization, compression, and protection. The ideal splint should achieve these goals, be light, moldable, and easy to apply. The author prefers the Thermoplast splint (Xomed-Treace Inc., Jacksonville, FL). This plastic mesh has adhesive on one side and is softened by immersion in 180° F water. After 30 to 45 seconds, the plastic becomes soft and moldable. The splint is then applied

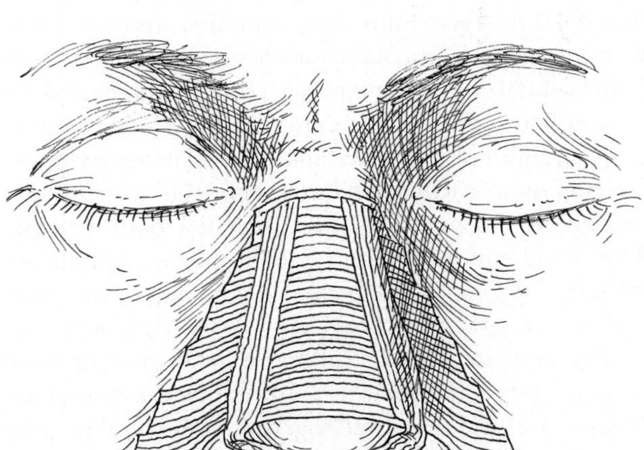

Figure 13–30. Taping the nose. After surgery is completed, the nose is taped. The style of taping will help determine the postoperative result.

carefully, making sure not to displace the nasal dorsum. The splint hardens in about 5 minutes at room temperature.

Packing

Nasal packing is traditionally used following rhinoplasty. If no septoplasty has been performed and septal splints are not being used, the packing must support the nasal bones as well as control hemostasis and line the nasal incisions. When septoplasty has been performed, septal splints will be used which will provide the needed support for the nasal bones. In this setting, the packing will only need to line the vestibular incisions and effect hemostasis. Usually, a few lengths of standard, 1-cm wide, Vaseline gauze will suffice. This can be removed as soon as the first day after surgery if postoperative bleeding has not been a problem. When full nasal packing is required, either traditional gauze packing or a Merocel sponge can be used.

SPECIAL PROCEDURES

The Twisted Nose

The twisted nose is defined as one in which the nasal dorsum deviates to one side and the tip deviates to the opposite side. This relatively common deformity is challenging to correct and has been the subject of numerous articles throughout the literature. The goal of this operation is to improve breathing, straighten the nasal profile, and provide desired cosmetic refinements to the nasal tip. The techniques to achieve these results are a combination of the steps outlined above. The preferred approach for these cases is the external rhinoplasty. This approach allows optimal exposure of the areas involved in this procedure.

The incision and degloving of the nose proceeds as described for the routine case. The first step is to separate the medial crura of the lower lateral cartilages down to the caudal end of the septum. Through this exposure, a complete septoplasty is performed. To achieve complete straightening of the septum, it is necessary to detach the septal cartilage from the upper lateral cartilages bilaterally, the maxillary crest, and the bony septum. The blood supply and the stability of the septum are preserved by maintaining the attachments of the cartilage to the mucoperichondrium on the right side.

The next step is to modify the nasal tip. Attention should be directed toward ensuring that the domes are symmetrical and resutured together in the midline. Any cosmetic alterations in the shape of the tip are performed at this time. It is advisable not to attempt too much during this procedure. Complex alterations of the nasal tip, when combined with adjustments to straighten the nose, can yield unpredictable results.

When the nasal tip has been modified, the next step in the procedure is to perform the osteotomies. In addition to the medial and lateral osteotomies, an intermediate osteotomy on the convex side of the dorsal deviation is required. This allows the bowed segment to be flattened. Usually, this will complete the operation. However, if there is extreme deformity of the upper lateral cartilages, this would be addressed at this point. Rather than resecting the upper lateral cartilage that is bowed, the cartilage can be cross-hatched with a scalpel and weakened to the extent required for reshaping. Alternatively, it may be necessary to graft the concave side to achieve symmetry. The preferred source for this graft is auricular cartilage.

Saddle Nose Deformity

Patients who lose the dorsal aspect of the quadrilateral cartilage have a deformity referred to as saddle nose. The saddle nose deformity is marked by a pronounced supratip depression, shortening of the nose, and overrotation of the tip (Fig. 13–31). This can occur as a result of destructive diseases of the septum, such as Wegener's granulomatosis, polymorphic reticulosis, or nasal lymphoma, or it may be iatrogenic, resulting from overly aggressive or accidental resection of the dorsal aspect of the septum during septoplasty.

The goals of repair are to lengthen the nose, decrease rotation, support the nasal tip, and fill in the dorsal depression. If possible, repair of any septal perforation should be done during a separate surgery at a later

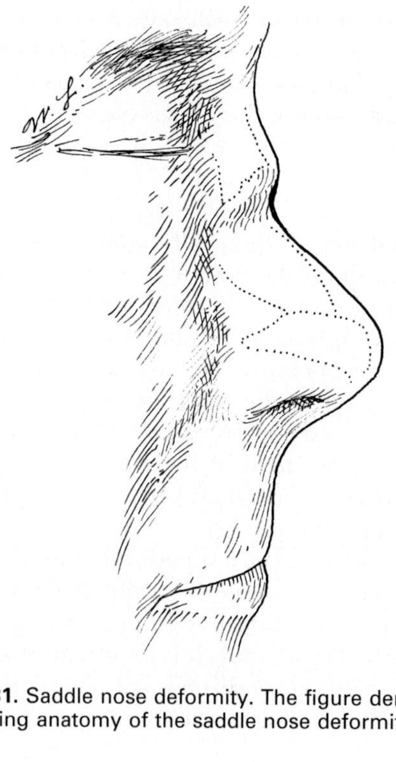

Figure 13–31. Saddle nose deformity. The figure demonstrates the underlying anatomy of the saddle nose deformity.

date. The operation is best performed using the external approach for accurate placement of grafts and release of any scar tissue along the dorsum. The first step in the procedure, after the exposure is complete, is to lyse any scar bands on the dorsum. Alterations in the tip cartilages are performed next. These may include any of the techniques described earlier. In most cases, only minimal changes in tip appearance should be attempted in this setting. The most important goals of this procedure should not be compromised by too ambitious an attempt at perfection. The same principle applies to alterations of the bony dorsum.

When the preliminary steps are completed, the dorsal graft is placed (Fig. 13–32). The graft material may be septal or auricular cartilage, calvarial bone, or synthetic materials. Selection of the optimal graft material will depend on the severity of the defect being repaired. In the worst cases, calvarial bone is the best choice. In the case of a minimal defect, cartilage can be used. In both situations, the graft must serve two purposes: (1) to fill in the dorsal defect and (2) to push the nasal tip down to reduce rotation. The final step before closure is to support the nasal tip with a columellar strut to avoid creating a hanging tip.

Valvular Collapse

One of the less common but most problematic causes of nasal obstruction is valvular collapse. This occurs when the nasal valve area of the airway collapses inwardly during inspiration. This may be because of lack of rigidity of the alar cartilages or overresection during a previous surgery. Valvular collapse can be diagnosed by a simple examination of the nasal valve area during inspiration and sniffing. The condition may be symptomatic if the valve occludes during either normal inspiration or light sniffing. Most people can induce some degree of collapse during maximal sniffing. This should not be construed as significant. However, in situations in which light sniffing or simple normal inspiration leads to significant collapse, surgical correction may be indicated.

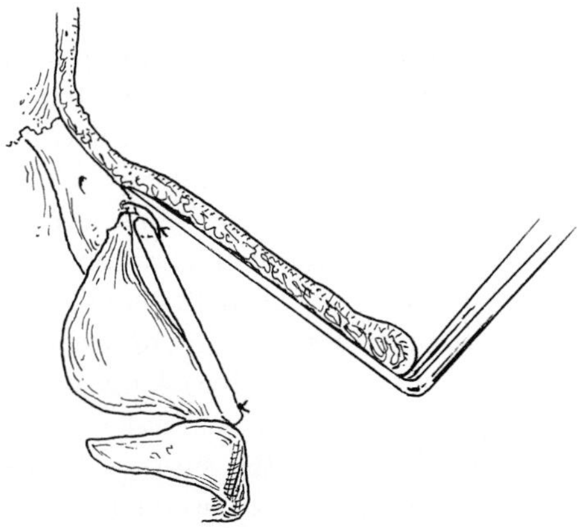

Figure 13–32. Dorsal onlay graft. A piece of calvarial bone is placed over the dorsum and sutured to the nose through small drill holes in the bone.

The main alternative to surgery is the use of the BreatheRight strip (C.N.S., Inc., Minneapolis, MN). This product is a simple piece of light metal with adhesive on one side. When applied to the nose, the metal band pulls the valve open. This is a good solution to valvular collapse that is mainly symptomatic during deep inspiration, such as occurs in athletic competition or during sleep.

For those who elect surgical intervention, there are three main alternatives: suturing the valve, valve implants (alar onlay or batten grafts), and spreader grafts. The valve suture is a relatively new technique in which a buried suture is attached to the inferior orbital rim to pull the valve open.[34] This procedure has not yet stood the test of time, but it is a relatively simple, rapid method to effect the desired result. A small, conjunctival incision is placed on the inside of the medial aspect of the lower eyelid (Fig. 13–33). The suture is placed either through the periosteum of the inferior orbital rim or a small drill hole in the bone of the rim. A straight needle is then used to pass a 3-0 nylon suture into the nose above the valve. The needle is then passed back below the valve into the conjunctival incision (Fig. 13–33). The suture is tied in such a way as to exert the desired amount of pull on the valve. The suture will create a slight bulge in the nasal facial groove, but should not be palpable.

A more traditional technique involves placement of direct cartilage implants into the valve.[35, 36] This is indicated in cases when the problem is lack of rigidity of the upper and lower lateral cartilages. Auricular conchal cartilage is the preferred grafting material for this procedure. An intercartilaginous incision is placed. The area of the valve is elevated over the upper and lower lateral cartilages to create a pocket. The cartilage is then placed into the pocket and the incision is closed. This technique imparts a slight fullness to the external nasal contour.

For patients with a narrow nasal valve area, spreader grafts can be considered.[37] This technique, which is performed through an external rhinoplasty approach, involves insertion of a cartilage graft between the septum and upper lateral cartilages (Fig. 13–34). The area of the nasal dorsum is incised and the attachments of the upper lateral cartilage to the septum are divided. Septal cartilage grafts are then inserted and sutured in place. This should widen the valve area. There will be a minimal widening of the nasal dorsum from this technique.

POSTOPERATIVE CARE

Rhinoplasty in contemporary medicine is always performed as an outpatient procedure. Unless there has

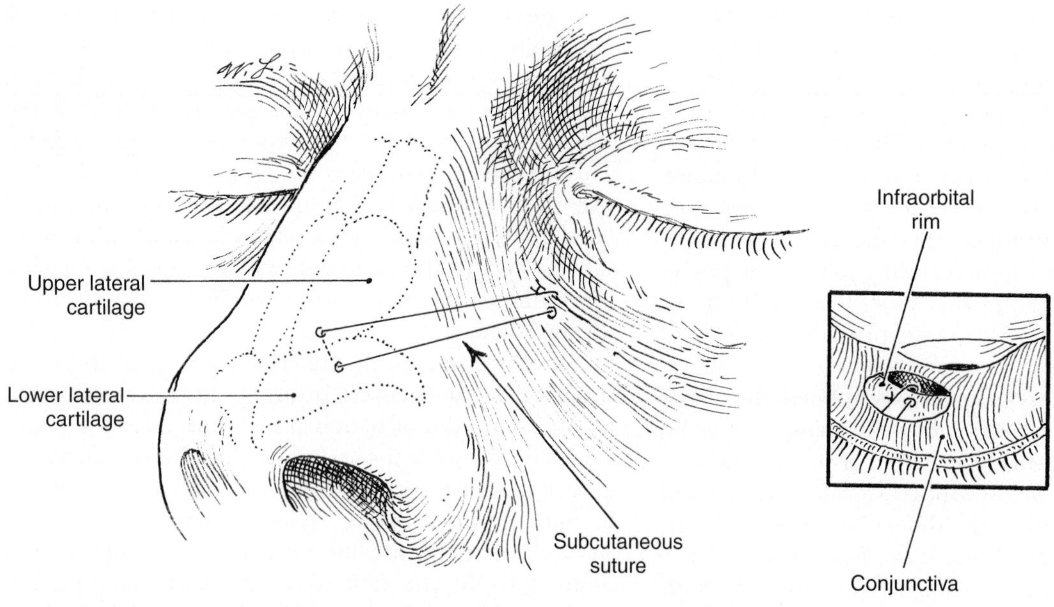

Figure 13–33. Nasal valve suture. The conceptual location of a suture placed to open a collapsed nasal valve is shown. The inset demonstrates the purchase of the suture through a small drill hole in the orbital rim.

been an intraoperative medical or surgical complication, the patient will be discharged within 1 to 2 hours after surgery. Only minimal care is required before the first postoperative visit. Ice is applied to the dorsum and eyes immediately after surgery, with application continued for the first 24 to 48 hours. A gauze pad is kept under the nose for the first day or so until bleeding has resolved.

Activity is restricted to bedrest with bathroom privileges the first night and advanced to walking the next morning. Exercise should be avoided for the first 10 days, and activities that involve physical contact or balls should be avoided for 6 weeks. This conservative approach protects the healing nasal bones from the chance of accidental injury, which could jeopardize the results of the surgery. In the case of competitive athletes who wish to return to competition as soon as possible, a special clear mask can be worn to protect the nose. However, formal cosmetic rhinoplasty should be deferred until after the individual has retired from competition. A temporizing closed nasal reduction can be offered in the case of acute trauma.

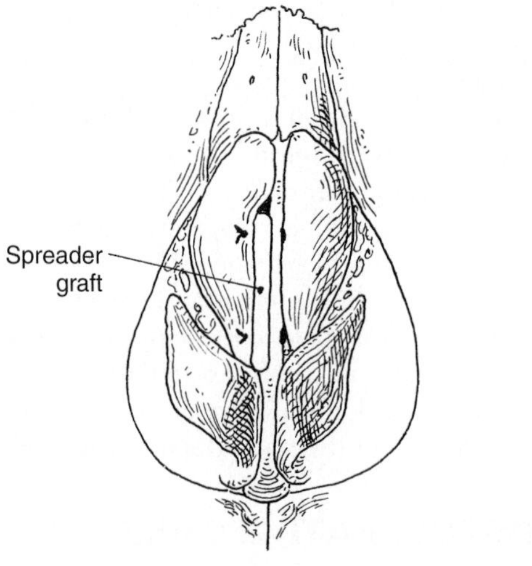

Figure 13–34. Spreader graft. A cartilaginous strut from the septum or auricle is placed between the septum and upper lateral cartilage to widen the nasal valve.

Diet is restricted only on the night of surgery to avoid inducing emesis. Prophylactic antibiotics are not typically prescribed unless packing or intranasal splints are used, in which case a 1-week course of a suitable antistaphylococcal antibiotic is prescribed, theoretically to prevent toxic shock syndrome. Pain medication is always prescribed. Most patients derive adequate pain management from a combination of acetaminophen and codeine. Most patients do not require more than 1 week of analgesics. Oral steroids and intraoperative intravenous steroids have been advocated by some to help minimize swelling and edema.[38] The definitive answer to this minor controversy has not yet been clarified.

The first follow-up visit is usually scheduled for 5 to 7 days after the operation. At this time, the external splint and internal splints and packing are removed. Subsequent appointments are scheduled 2 to 3 weeks after surgery and 3 months after surgery. At the second postoperative visit, the acute swelling and bruising should be nearly completely resolved. This is the surgeon's first opportunity to critically assess the results of the surgery. At this point, a noticeable deviation of the nasal dorsum may still be able to be corrected by external manipulation of the nasal bones. Also, significant fullness in the supratip area can be recognized and treated with an injection of triamcinolone. Major deformities at this stage almost always indicate the need for revision surgery. The timing of such surgery will need to be individualized. At the 3-month follow-up visit, a further assessment of the results of surgery can be done. At this stage, problems may be treated with steroid injections, massage, or consideration of the possibility of revision.

The results of the surgery will begin to take shape at this time, but the long-term results of rhinoplasty will not be known for many years. Subtle changes continue to occur for several years. For this reason, long-term follow-up evaluation is recommended. Photographs demonstrating the results of the surgery should be obtained at least once after the operation. The earliest point at which these photographs are meaningful is 3 months postsurgery; however, 1 year after surgery is a more optimal time if only one set of pictures will be taken.

COMPLICATIONS

Rhinoplasty is similar to septoplasty in terms of the risks of nonspecific complications, such as anesthetic and medical complications, bleeding, and infection. None of these problems is common, and rhinoplasty poses no significantly increased risk for these problems compared to other nasal surgeries. Soft tissue infection of the nose following rhinoplasty is a potentially serious problem, possibly resulting in abscess, tissue necrosis, or graft loss.[39–43] Evidence of infection warrants an immediate response with drainage of any purulent material, if present, and intravenous antibiotics. Medical complications have been reported, but are rare.[39, 44, 45] Postoperative epistaxis is one of the most common problems associated with rhinoplasty.[46–48] This may be caused by bleeding from the osteotomies, incisions, septum, or turbinates. Management of this condition is discussed in detail in Chapter 22.

The potential specific complications of rhinoplasty are numerous. Postoperative pain is present in some degree in all patients undergoing rhinoplasty. For most patients, the postoperative pain is moderate and well controlled by mild narcotic agents, such as acetaminophen with codeine, hydrocodone, or propoxyphene. Pain usually resolves by the end of the first week, but residual tenderness may persist for several months.

Ecchymosis and edema are related to the performance of osteotomies. However, the degree of edema and ecchymosis is strongly tied to the technique used during the operation. Several factors are critical in minimizing these unwanted effects. Local anesthesia should be accurate and sufficient and timed to ensure maximal potency at the correct point in the operation. The periosteum should be carefully elevated from the osteotomy site to avoid tearing of the periosteum with the osteotome. Additionally, a small, 2- to 3-mm, unguarded osteotome can be used to sharply cut the bone with as little soft tissue trauma as possible. After the surgery, ice should immediately be placed over the nasal dorsum to help limit swelling and ecchymosis.

There have been a number of reports of complications associated with nasal implants of various types.[33, 49–51] Probably, there is no completely safe foreign substance that can be placed into the nose. However, it appears that, based on a relatively short-term follow-up period of less than 10 years, Gore-Tex implants may be the safest yet described, being associated with only a 2% risk of implant-related problems.[33]

Nasal valve obstruction has been one of the most commonly debated complications of rhinoplasty. Various experts have expressed strong views on the avoidance[52–55] and correction of the problem.[35, 36, 53, 56] Several factors seem to be clearly associated with this nasal valve collapse. These include overresection of the lower or upper lateral cartilages, resection of the internal mucosal lining of the nose, and imprecise closure of intranasal incisions. Avoiding these errors will go a long way toward preventing nasal stenosis or collapse.

Neurologic injuries resulting in permanent numbness to the nasal tip[57] or face[58, 59] have been described and are attributable to nerve injuries. Other neurologic complications include a numb or dead tooth,[60, 61] olfactory disturbance,[46, 62] and intracranial injuries.[63] Blindness is a special problem that is rarely associated with rhinoplasty.[59, 64, 65] The cause of most such cases is either retrobulbar hematoma or direct mechanical injury to the optic nerve from extension of bony fractures during osteotomy. Prompt recognition of retrobulbar hematoma with orbital decompression and control of the bleeding source may save the eye. Careful performance of the osteotomy using sharp osteotomes should prevent direct extension into the optic canal.

Periodically, the development of postoperative tumors and cysts of the nose has been reported.[66–74] These masses have included epidermoid cysts, mucoid cysts, vascular malformations, and cartilage implant proliferation. These conditions are unpredictable and difficult to avoid. Most are attributable to bad luck, but certainly, infolding of tissue from either the nasal or skin side can result in the late development of such masses.

The most common complications of rhinoplasty are the cosmetic deformities that can occur following surgery. Patients must be carefully counseled about this possibility. A reasonable estimate of the need for revision is 10% to 20%.[5, 6, 8] Most revision surgeries are related to failure to achieve a straight nose,[75] which may result from a crooked septum, imbalanced osteotomies, or misalignment of the nasal bones. Revision rhinoplasty is required to correct these deformities. The external approach is favored for most revision surgeries undertaken to repair a crooked nose.

An imperfect aesthetic result in the nasal tip is another common problem requiring revision surgery.[76] The causes of this are numerous and include polly beak deformity, tip asymmetry, projection problems, pinched tip, tip ptosis, and columellar problems. The successful correction of these deformities lies in proper identification of the underlying anatomic abnormality and appropriate surgical revision. The polly beak deformity describes a fullness or rounding of the supratip area. This may be caused by inadequate resection of cartilaginous dorsal humps, excessive resection of the domes, or excessive scarring in the supratip area. The latter problem can be related to poor draping of skin, unremoved tissue debris, or poorly applied compression dressings.[75] Correction is best achieved by identification of the underlying cause and specific correction, either by excising excess cartilage or soft tissue in the supratip area or reinforcing the columella with a strut graft.[75, 77] If early development of supratip fullness becomes apparent during the first weeks to months after rhinoplasty, injection of triamcinolone suspension into the area may help prevent the formation of a polly beak deformity.

Other nasal tip problems, such as asymmetry and projection problems, can be corrected by careful preoperative and intraoperative assessment of the underlying cause and precise surgical technique. These revisions are best achieved using the external rhinoplasty approach so as to maximize visualization of the structures and appropriate analysis of the deformities. Overresection of one lateral crura should be treated by grafting, whereas underresection of a lateral crura is appropriately treated by additional resection. Placement or adjustment of tip and columellar grafts is necessary to correct most projection problems.

Finally, dorsal irregularity or asymmetry is a potential problem. It is common for the patient to be able to feel a degree of irregularity over the nasal dorsum. However, there are cases when the irregularity becomes noticeable. One such situation is if one of the lateral osteotomies is incomplete. This is also known as a greenstick fracture. The fracture may pull back into the preoperative position, creating a marked irregularity or even a visible point or ridge along the lateral dorsum. This can be corrected with revision osteotomies or by rasping down the irregularity. In other cases, the patient may develop periosteal thickening resulting in a nasal bossa.[78] This can be treated with either triamcinolone injection or revision surgery.

REFERENCES

1. Rees TD, LaTrenta GS. Aesthetic Plastic Surgery, 2nd ed. Philadelphia: WB Saunders, 1994.
2. Sheen JH. Aesthetic Rhinoplasty. St Louis: Mosby-Year Book, 1985.
3. Berman W. Rhinoplastic Surgery. St Louis: Mosby-Year Book, 1989.
4. Tardy ME. Rhinoplasty. Baltimore: Williams & Wilkins, 1984.
5. Cvjetkovic N, Lustica I. Secondary rhinoplasty (analysis of failures over a 5-year period). Lijec Vjesn 119(2):68, 1997.
6. Gubisch W. Causes of failures of rhinoplasty and therapeutic attitudes. Rev Laryngol Otol Rhinol (Bord) 112(3):255, 1991.
7. Busca GP, Amasio ME, Sartoris A. Complications of rhinoplasty. Acta Otorhinolaryngol Ital 10(Suppl 31): 1, 1990.
8. Gilain L, Bossard B, Juvanon JM, et al. Failure and complications of esthetic rhinoplasty. Apropos of 30 reoperations. Ann Otolaryngol (Paris) 106(6):310, 1989.
9. Holt GR, Garner ET, McLarey D. Postoperative sequelae and complications of rhinoplasty. Otolaryngol Clin North Am 20(4):853, 1987.
10. Tardy ME Jr, Cheng EY, Jernstrom V. Misadventures in nasal tip surgery. Analysis and repair. Otolaryngol Clin North Am 20(4):797, 1987.
11. Powell N, Humphreys B. Proportions of the Aesthetic Face. New York: Thieme-Stratton, 1984.
12. Seltzer AP. Plastic Surgery of the Nose. Philadelphia: JB Lippincott, 1949.
13. Gonzalez-Ulloa M. Planning the integral correction of the human profile. J Int Coll Surg 36:364, 1961.
14. Ricketts RM. Divine proportions in facial esthetics. Clin Plast Surg 9:401, 1982.
15. Dingman RO, Natvig P. Surgical anatomy in aesthetic and corrective rhinoplasty. Clin Plast Surg 4:111, 1977.
16. Powell NB. Aesthetic evaluation of nasal contours. In Cummings CW (ed). Otolaryngology Head and Neck Surgery, 2nd ed. Baltimore: Mosby-Year Book, 1993, pp. 687–701.
17. Bernstein L. Esthetics in rhinoplasty. Otolaryngol Clin North Am 8:705, 1975.
18. Denecke HJ, Meyer R. Plastic Surgery of the Head and Neck. Corrective and Reconstructive Rhinoplasty. New York: Springer-Verlag, 1967.
19. Krugman ME. Photoanalysis of the rhinoplasty patient. Ear Nose Throat J 60:56, 1981.
20. Aufricht G. Rhinoplasty and the face. Plast Reconstr Surg 43:218, 1969.
21. Wright WK. Surgery of the bony and cartilaginous dorsum. Otolaryngol Clin North Am 8:575, 1975.
22. Farkas LG, et al. Is photogrammetry of the face reliable? Plast Reconstr Surg 66:346, 1980.
23. Krugman ME, Lopez R, McKenzie P. Facial series of photographs as viewed by the plastic surgeon with special emphasis on the nose. J Biol Photogr 47:201, 1979.
24. Slator R, Harris DL. Are rhinoplasty patients potentially mad? Br J Plast Surg 45(4):307, 1992.
25. Marcus P. Some preliminary psychological observations on narcissism, the cosmetic rhinoplasty patient and the plastic surgeon. Aust NZ J Surg 54(6):543, 1984.
26. Sheard C, Jones NS, Quraishi MS, et al. A prospective study of the psychological effects of rhinoplasty. Clin Otolaryngol 21(3): 232, 1996.
27. Bonne OB, Wexler MR, De-Nour AK. Rhinoplasty patients' critical self-evaluations of their noses. Plast Reconstr Surg 98(3):436, 1996.
28. Meyer L, Jacobsson S. Psychiatric and psychosocial characteristics of patients accepted for rhinoplasty. Ann Plast Surg 19(2):117, 1987.
29. Klassen A, Jenkinson C, Fitzpatrick R, et al. Patients' health-related quality of life before and after aesthetic surgery. Br J Plast Surg 49(7):433, 1996.
30. Goin MK, Rees TD. A prospective study of patients' psychological reactions to rhinoplasty. Ann Plast Surg 27(3):210, 1991.
31. Guyuron B, Bokhari F. Patient satisfaction following rhinoplasty. Aesthet Plast Surg 20(2):153, 1996.
32. Meyer L, Jacobsson S. The predictive validity of psychosocial factors for patients' acceptance of rhinoplasty. Ann Plast Surg 17(6):513, 1986.
33. Godin MS, Waldman SR, Johnson CM Jr. The use of expanded polytetrafluoroethylene (Gore-Tex) in rhinoplasty. A 6-year experience. Arch Otolaryngol Head Neck Surg 121(10):1131, 1995.

34. Paniello RC: Nasal valve suspension. An effective treatment for nasal valve collapse. Arch Otolaryngol Head Neck Surg 122: 1342, 1996.
35. Toriumi DM, Josen J, Weinberger M, et al. Use of alar batten grafts for correction of nasal valve collapse. Arch Otolaryngol Head Neck Surg 123(8):802, 1997.
36. Constantian MB. Functional effects of alar cartilage malposition. Ann Plast Surg 30(6):487, 1993.
37. Gunter JP, Rohrich RJ. Correction of the pinched nasal tip with alar spreader grafts. Plast Reconstr Surg 90(5):821, 1992.
38. Berinstein TH, Bane SM, Cupp CL, et al. Steroid use in rhinoplasty: An objective assessment of postoperative edema. Ear Nose Throat J 77(1):40, 1998.
39. Lawson W, Kessler S, Biller HF. Unusual and fatal complications of rhinoplasty. Arch Otolaryngol 109(3):164, 1983.
40. Cabouli JL, Guerrissi JO, Mileto A, et al. Local infection following aesthetic rhinoplasty. Ann Plast Surg 17(4):306, 1986.
41. Abifadel M, Real JP, Servant JM, et al. Apropos of a case of infection after esthetic rhinoplasty. Ann Chir Plast Esthet 35(5):415, 1990.
42. Moscona R, Ullmann Y, Peled I. Necrotizing periorbital cellulitis following septorhinoplasty. Aesthet Plast Surg 15(2):187, 1991.
43. Rettinger G, Zenkel M. Skin and soft tissue complications. Fac Plast Surg 13(1):51, 1997.
44. Dubost J, Kalfon F, Roullit S, et al. Giant subcutaneous emphysema, pneumomediastinum and bilateral pneumothorax following rhinoseptoplasty. Can Anesthesiol 34(2):161, 1986.
45. Russo C, Corbanese U, Della Mora E. Nasocardiac reflex during rhinoseptoplasty. Description of a clinical case. Minerva Anestesiol 58(1–2):63, 1992.
46. Padovan IF, Jugo SB. The complications of external rhinoplasty. Ear Nose Throat J 70(7):454, 1991.
47. Churukian MM, Zemplenyi J, Steiner M. Postrhinoplasty epistaxis. Role of vitamin E? Arch Otolaryngol Head Neck Surg 114(7): 748, 1988.
48. Teichgraeber JF, Russo RC. Treatment of nasal surgery complications. Ann Plast Surg 30(1):80, 1993.
49. Stoll W. Complications following implantation or transplantation in rhinoplasty. Fac Plast Surg 13(1):45, 1997.
50. Raszewski R, Guyuron B, Lash RH, et al. A severe fibrotic reaction after cosmetic liquid silicone injection. A case report. J Craniomaxillofac Surg 18(5):225, 1990.
51. Berbis P, Lebeuf C, Vaisse C, et al. Pyodermatitis of the nasal pyramid disclosing a complication of rhinoplasty with silicone implant. Ann Dermatol Venereol 116(3):233, 1989.
52. Adamson JE. Constriction of the internal nasal valve in rhinoplasty: Treatment and prevention. Ann Plast Surg 18(2):114, 1987.
53. Adamson P, Smith O, Cole P. The effect of cosmetic rhinoplasty on nasal patency. Laryngoscope 100(4):357, 1990.
54. Constantinides MS, Adamson PA, Cole P. The long-term effects of open cosmetic septorhinoplasty on nasal air flow. Arch Otolaryngol Head Neck Surg 122(1):41, 1996.
55. Broker BJ, Berman WE. Nasal valve obstruction complicating rhinoplasty: Prevention and treatment. Pt. I. Ear Nose Throat J 76(2):77, 1997.
56. Chait LA, Fayman MS. Treatment of postreconstructive collapsed nasal ala with a costal cartilage graft. Plast Reconstr Surg 82(3):527, 1988.
57. Thompson AC. Nasal tip numbness following rhinoplasty. Clin Otolaryngol 12(2):143, 1987.
58. Meyer M, Moss AL, Cullen KW. Infraorbital nerve palsy after rhinoplasty. J Craniomaxillofac Surg 18(4):173, 1990.
59. Thumfart WF, Volklein C. Systemic and other complications. Fac Plast Surg 13(1):61, 1997.
60. Sykes JM, Toriumi D, Kerth JD. A devitalized tooth as a complication of septorhinoplasty. Arch Otolaryngol Head Neck Surg 113(7):765, 1987.
61. Bergmeyer JM. Death of a tooth after rhinoplasty. Plast Reconstr Surg 93(7):1529, 1994.
62. Fiser A. Changes of olfaction due to aesthetic and functional nose surgery. Acta Otorhinolaryngol (Belg) 44(4):457, 1990.
63. Marshall DR, Slattery PG. Intracranial complications of rhinoplasty. Br J Plast Surg 36(3):342, 1983.
64. Wind J. Blindness as a complication of rhinoplasty. Arch Otolaryngol Head Neck Surg 114(5):581, 1988.
65. Cheney ML, Blair PA. Blindness as a complication of rhinoplasty. Arch Otolaryngol Head Neck Surg 113(7):768, 1987.
66. Shulman Y, Westreich M. Postrhinoplasty mucous cyst of the nose. Plast Reconstr Surg 71(3):421, 1983.
67. Anderson R, Sprinkle PM, Bouquot J, et al. Complication of septoplasty. Benign or malignant? Arch Otolaryngol 109(7):489, 1983.
68. Guyuron B, Licota L. Arteriovenous malformation following rhinoplasty. Plast Reconstr Surg 77(3):474, 1986.
69. Grocutt M, Chir B, Fatah MF. Recurrent multiple epidermoid inclusion cysts following rhinoplasty—An unusual complication. J Laryngol Otol 103(12):1214, 1989.
70. Harley EH, Erdman JP. Dorsal nasal cyst formation. A rare complication of cosmetic rhinoplasty. Arch Otolaryngol Head Neck Surg 116(1):105, 1990.
71. Zijlker TD, Vuyk HD. Nasal dorsal cyst after rhinoplasty. Rhinology 31(2):89, 1993.
72. Rettinger G, Steininger H. Lipogranulomas as complications of septorhinoplasty. Arch Otolaryngol Head Neck Surg 123(8): 809, 1997.
73. Kotzur A, Gubisch W. Mucous cyst—A postrhinoplasty complication: Outcome and prevention. Plast Reconstr Surg 100(2):520, 1997.
74. Reiter D, Peters B, Amsberry J, et al. Tumefactive cartilage proliferation after rhinoplasty. A newly reported complication. Arch Otolaryngol Head Neck Surg 123(1):72, 1997.
75. van Olphen A. Complications of pyramid surgery. Fac Plast Surg 13(1):15, 1997.
76. Sulsenti G, Palma P. Complications and sequelae of nasal base and tip surgery. Fac Plast Surg 13(1):25, 1997.
77. Tardy ME Jr, Kron TK, Younger R, et al. The cartilaginous pollybeak: Etiology, prevention, and treatment. Fac Plast Surg 6(2): 113, 1989.
78. Kramer FM, Churukian MM, Hansen L. The nasal bossa: A complication of rhinoplasty. Laryngoscope 96(3):303, 1986.

CHAPTER 14

Nasal Reconstruction

Nasal reconstruction after destructive surgery or trauma of the nose is one of the most challenging and rewarding fields of rhinology. This specialty is often considered to be primarily part of facial plastic surgery, rather than rhinology. However, the rhinologic surgeon should be well versed in the anatomy and able to understand these procedures, if not perform them. This chapter is primarily authored by Richard Arden, M.D. He is an accomplished facial plastic surgeon who has performed hundreds of nasal reconstructions in affiliation with a Mohs dermatologic surgeon. The techniques and options for reconstruction of the more common nasal defects are described, as well as details of how to perform these procedures. These operations are applicable not only to defects after resection of skin cancer, but also to all cases of nasal deformity.

PREOPERATIVE ASSESSMENT

Decisions regarding nasal reconstructive surgery must consider the patient's desires rather than the surgeon's desires, and must focus the evaluation process on what should be done, not what can be done. Ultimate satisfaction is achieved, and ethical responsibility served, when patients' goals are met in the context of their general physical and mental health. Clearly, an 80-year-old recluse with multi-organ system disease or poor insight into his/her disease process should be managed differently than a healthy 40-year-old socialite. Whereas healing by secondary intention or primary skin grafting may be chosen for the former patient, consideration of staged-flap reconstruction may be most appropriate for the latter.

Age, as a criterion, is not an absolute and so should be defined biologically, not chronologically. Regardless of age, there are several factors that increase the risk of microcirculatory problems leading to tissue loss or flap failure. These include a history of diabetes mellitus, local irradiation, prior surgery, and smoking. Another factor affecting the quality of wound healing is skin type. Patients with thicker, coarse, sebaceous skin, often associated with underlying inflammatory conditions (e.g., rhinophyma), are at increased risk for wound dehiscence and hypertrophic scar formation. As skin grafts applied to this type of skin often do poorly, such patients are better served by local or regional flap reconstructions.

Once the surgeon's and patient's goals are defined in the context of these extrinsic and intrinsic factors, a surgical plan can be formulated. The first step is to define the defect, both anatomically and physiologically. For instance, it is not enough simply to replace the soft tissue cover for an alar lobule cutaneous defect. The alar lobule is both an aesthetic anatomic unit and a critical part of the nasal respiratory system. Without cartilaginous reinforcement, the forces of wound contraction will distort the alar rim and base and may alter breathing mechanics. On the other hand, the same size of defect, when located over the nasal dorsum or sidewall, can simply be replaced without physiologic implication. For each patient, the surgeon must systemically determine what are the lining, support, and coverage requirements.

The second step in creating the surgical plan is to formulate options for repair. For every defect, there are usually several reasonable options for reconstruction. These options must be framed in the context of the patient's medical history, as discussed earlier, and the skill and experience of the surgeon. Some techniques are technically demanding and require extensive experience for good results to be achieved.

Finally, the options must be presented to the patient. During this discussion, the patient's wishes are incorporated to arrive at the final surgical plan. Some surgeons ask the patient to sign the informed consent at this time. Regardless, this discussion should be carefully documented in the patient's medical record.

SURGICAL PRINCIPLES

Subunit Principle

The concept of aesthetic units of the face was first espoused by Gonzalez-Ulloa.[1] Burget and Menick have since extended these principles to the nasal subunit.[2] These subunits include the columella, tip, and dorsum, and the paired sidewalls, alar lobules, and soft tissue triangles (Fig. 14–1). By virtue of their convex and concave surfaces, light is reflected or casted as shadows, thereby defining regional borders of the nose. These topographic landmarks do not necessarily relate one-to-one with the defined borders of the underlying nasal substructure. For instance, two individuals possessing a supportive nasal framework of similar size, shape, and consistency, but vastly discrepant skin thicknesses, may have markedly different subunit borders. The nasal subunit, therefore, typically varies between individuals and is not of a fixed size or configuration.

In addition to the subunit principle, there are two basic tenets that affect the placement of incisions and excisions. These are segmental facial composition and prioritization of contour over scars. These tenets maintain that excision of tissue should incorporate an entire subunit, and that best cosmetic results are obtained by prioritizing contours and placing the scars at the borders of anatomic subunits. In this way, trapdoor deformities are better camouflaged, and scars can be positioned aesthetically. As a corollary to this, defect borders can be undermined and advanced into subunit lines, or skin electively excised to complete a subunit defect (Fig. 14–2). In general, additional excision to complete a subunit resection is justified when 50% or more of a nasal subunit has been lost. This is particularly important when the defect involves convex subunits, such as the tip, ala, and dorsum. This intentional sacrifice of tissue for the sake of aesthetics represents one of the few exceptions in plastic surgery to the principle of conservation of tissue.

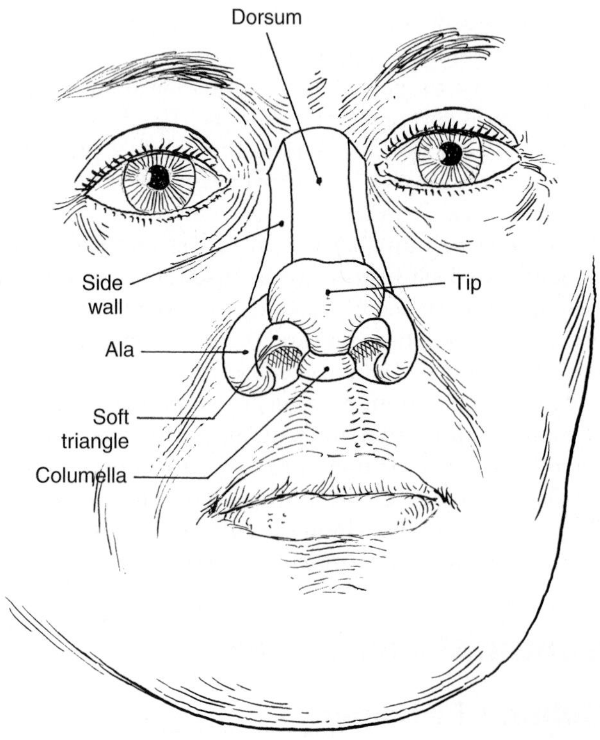

Figure 14–1. The aesthetic border lines that define the nasal subunits are delineated.

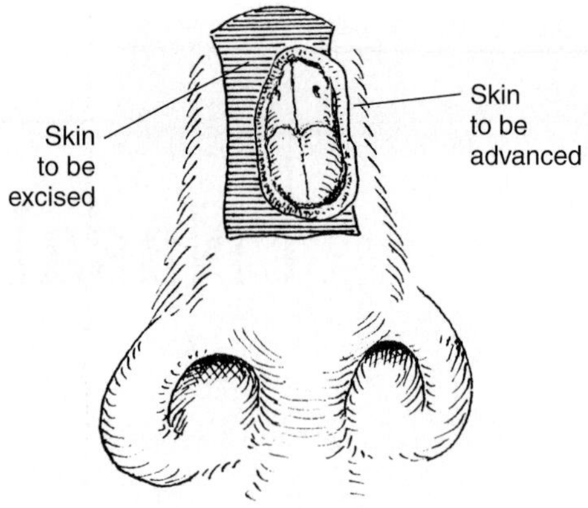

Figure 14–2. This off-center defect can be advanced and further excised to complete subunit excision.

Healing by Secondary Intent

In selected cases, allowing a wound to heal by secondary intent may be the most efficacious and optimal method of management. This technique allows the wound to heal naturally without reconstruction. Both patient-related issues (age, underlying medical health, expectations, ability to care for an open wound) and wound-related issues (location, size, depth) must be considered when choosing this option. Several factors favor healing by secondary intention. Smaller, mainly superficial defects, as well as those located on planar or concave surfaces and those that lack the potential to distort anatomic landmarks (e.g., the alar rim, eyelid, or upper lip) are most likely to yield favorable outcomes. The quality of the adjacent skin (i.e., its porosity, thickness, and color) becomes a factor in the lower one third of the nose. In this area, skin features may contrast sharply with the pale, shiny, atrophic scar developing from a contracted wound. Specifically, superficial wounds of the nasal sidewall and small wounds straddling the alar groove are ideal for healing by secondary intention. Deep wounds of the nasal tip and ala are, in contrast, poor candidates for nonreconstruction.

Several other factors may favor healing by secondary intention or reconstruction. The presence of exposed bone or cartilage, or both, represents a relative contraindication to healing by secondary intention. This is because of the potential for osteitis/chondritis and the predictably unfavorable aesthetic results associated with this situation. Prolonged recovery from an open wound may cause problems in the immunocompromised patient due to infection. Therefore, in the immunocompromised patient, wounds generally warrant some form of primary repair. By contrast, in the elderly, infirm patient, or in individuals who lack insight into their recovery process, healing by secondary intention should be strongly considered.

Specific instances may justify a delayed reconstructive approach or healing by tertiary intent. An intermediate-depth excision in the subcutis, in which skin grafting is contemplated, can often be better served by allowing maturation of granulation tissue prior to grafting. This can enhance surface contour and make the wound more shallow. Similarly, enhanced "take" of a skin graft can be afforded over bare bone or cartilage by allowing granulation tissue time to fill in the wound. Finally, delayed reconstruction following wound contraction (assuming that there are no adjacent landmarks that could be displaced) can minimize tissue requirements for resurfacing.

RECONSTRUCTIVE OPTIONS

When the surgeon considers a nasal defect for reconstruction, several factors need to be considered. The first is the completeness of the excision and the need for further excision. Presuming that the excision is complete, specific reconstruction must then be planned. Defects should be analyzed in terms of the subunits missing and the structures that require replacement. This analysis includes an evaluation of the nasal lining defect, structural support defect, and nasal covering defect. In the following sections, each of the components of the defect is discussed, with special attention to the options for reconstruction.

Intranasal Lining Options

In choosing options for intranasal lining, the location and size of the recipient defect, as well as the status of the adjacent tissue, must be considered. Usually, either local tissue or free grafts will be sufficient. Rarely is it necessary to resort to regional flaps (i.e., forehead or pericranial flaps) or free flaps (i.e., radial forearm flaps) to provide internal lining. The exceptions are in certain cases of subtotal or total nasal loss when the septum is not available as a donor source. The authors' bias is to select thin, vascularized, pliable flaps whenever possible. Donor sites meeting these criteria include the vestibule, middle vault, and nasal septum.

For the sake of discussion, it is convenient to consider the reconstructive nasal lining options for the lower one third, middle one third, and upper one third, and to consider total intranasal loss separately. In the following sections, these situations are analyzed and discussed, with the options for each situation considered separately.

Lower Third

Lower one-third losses involve primarily stratified squamous epithelium of the nasal vault caudal to the valve area. Limited defects measuring up to several millimeters in size can usually be closed by undermining the residual vestibular skin and advancing the tissue toward the alar rim. Owing to the tendency of such a flap to retract back during wound healing, reinforcement of the rim with a cartilage graft should be employed.

If the size or shape of the defect or the anticipated degree of tissue release is not likely to permit adequate advancement, consideration may be given to local hinge flaps for alar margin losses (Fig. 14–3). These flaps are only applicable in cases in which a skin graft or flap lies adjacent to the defect, or when healing by secondary intention has achieved reepithelialization of the leading edge. Owing to the tenuous nature of their blood supply, which must cross a scarified junction zone, hinge flaps should be limited to 5 to 10 mm in height. Desic-

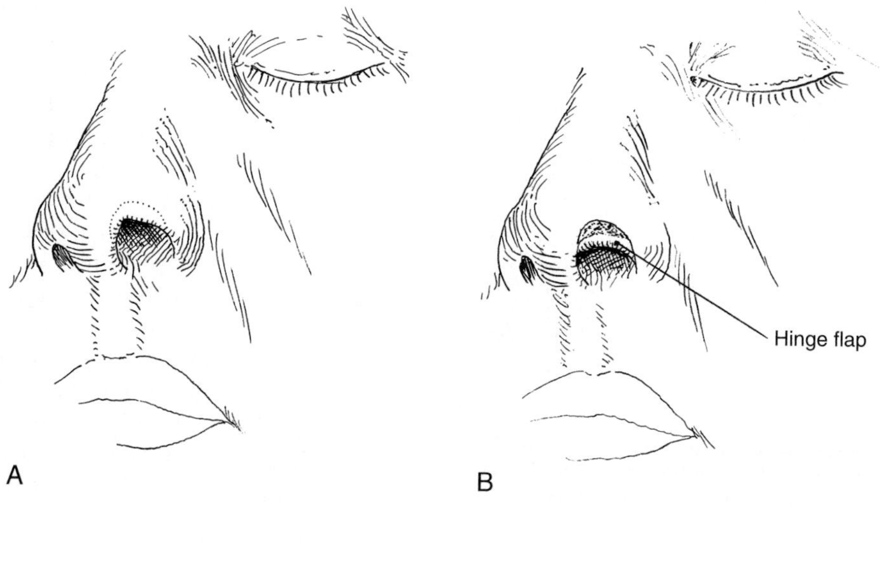

Figure 14–3. Limited retraction of the alar rim repositioned with a hinge flap provides the necessary internal lining. The secondary defect can be closed with a local flap.

cated, inflamed, ulcerated, or previously irradiated tissue should be considered contraindications to hinge flaps. Because of the stiffness and limited tendency for contraction of hinge flaps, alar batten grafts are typically not required to maintain rim position. Extreme care in the handling and development of these delicate flaps is essential to avoid penetrating the hinge area, which would devascularize the flap.

More extensive lining losses of the lower one third of the nasal vault are best replaced with an anteriorly based, septal, mucoperichondrial, turn-over flap (Fig. 14–4). As mobilization of this flap requires transection of branches of the ethmoidal and sphenopalatine arteries, hemostasis must be assured. Preparation of the nasal mucosa with 4% topical cocaine and infiltration of the mucosa with a local anesthetic will help minimize bleeding. For patients receiving local/sedation anesthesia, passage of a No. 14 French red Robinson catheter through the contralateral nares into the nasopharynx and attachment to suction effectively controls bleeding into the pharynx. After the flap is mobilized, suction cautery can be used carefully along the cut mucosal edges. After surgery, a Merocel sponge (Xomed, Jacksonville, FL) is usually sufficient to maintain hemostasis.

To preserve the blood supply, the flap pedicle must capture the septal branch of the superior labial artery as it enters the nasal septum, lateral to the nasal spine. A pedicle width of 1.2 to 1.5 cm should be maintained caudally. Expansion of the flap width is allowable further posteriorly within the septum. By not extending the flap length beyond the midseptal position, a length : width ratio of 3–4:1 results. Following the horizontal and vertical mucosal cuts, retrograde submucoperichondrial elevation toward the external nares is carried out. Elevation should be carried far enough anteriorly to allow for tension-free insetting of the mucosal flap into the recipient vestibular defect. Septal cartilage grafts, if required, can be obtained through the flap incisions.

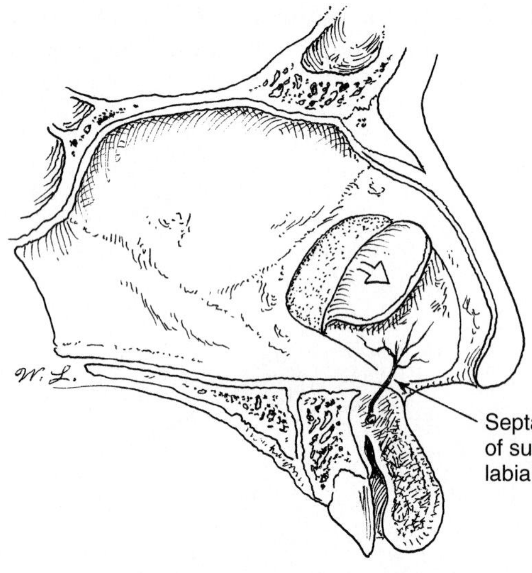

Figure 14–4. An anteriorly based septal mucoperichondrial turn-over flap can be used to reconstruct lining defects of the lower one third of the nasal vault.

Middle Third

Lining losses of the middle nasal vault typically require cartilage grafts to avoid inspiratory collapse at the valve area. The preferred coverage is, once again, septal mucosal flaps. Unilateral defects can be closed by a superiorly based septal hinge flap (Fig. 14–5). This is based off the anterior ethmoidal artery, as originally described by deQuervain.[3] The incisions include two vertical cuts and one inferior transverse cut. Quadrangular cartilage cuts are created several centimeters apart after the ipsilateral mucoperichondrium is elevated up to the dorsum and removed. The cartilage component is developed and then the flap elevation is completed by incising across the contralateral mucosa. Removal of a thin cartilaginous strip dorsally allows for the composite chondromucosal flap to swing laterally into the recipient defect. The reflected ipsilateral mucosa can then be folded over the raw cut edges, trimmed, and sutured to promote healing of the permanent septal perforation. For more extensive losses of the lower two thirds of the nasal vault, initial elevation of an anteriorly based, septal, mucoperichondrial, turn-over flap can be combined with the deQuervain flap, as they derive their blood supplies from separate source arteries.

When bilateral lining losses are encountered in the lower two thirds of the vault, a septal pivot flap can be used (Fig. 14–6). This is also based off the septal branch of the superior labial artery. Depending on the size and location of the defect, long, angled, or whole septal composite flaps can be created and stabilized above the remaining nasal infrastructure. In this way, bilateral mucosal flaps can be turned downward, toward the nasal cavity, to provide the necessary lining requirements. The remaining osseocartilaginous septal component can then be trimmed and used as an autograft for the subsurface framework.

Because the surface area requirements for lining the lateral nasal wall are greater for the lower one third than the upper one third, septal pivot flaps can be tapered distally during harvest. The use of local hinge flaps at the nasofacial junction can offset tissue shortages in this area and can be combined with the mucosal component of the pivot flap to complete the closure.

When the septum is unavailable for use, local, regional, or even free flaps may be employed to provide internal reconstruction. A superiorly based nasolabial flap is one regional option. This flap can be rolled over onto itself to create a tubular lining for the lower third of the nasal vault (Fig. 14–7). Typically, these flaps are bulky, fail to create the desired kidney-bean configura-

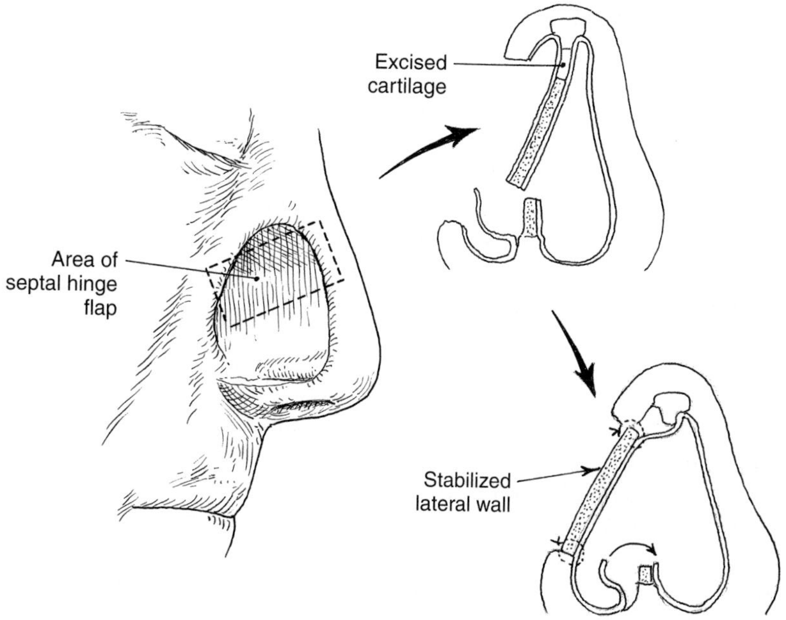

Figure 14–5. A superiorly based septal hinge flap is used to reconstruct lateral wall defects of the middle one third of the nasal vault. Note the submucoperichondrial excision of the dorsal septal attachment, which allows mobilization of the composite flap. The external mucoperichondrium is denuded prior to soft tissue coverage.

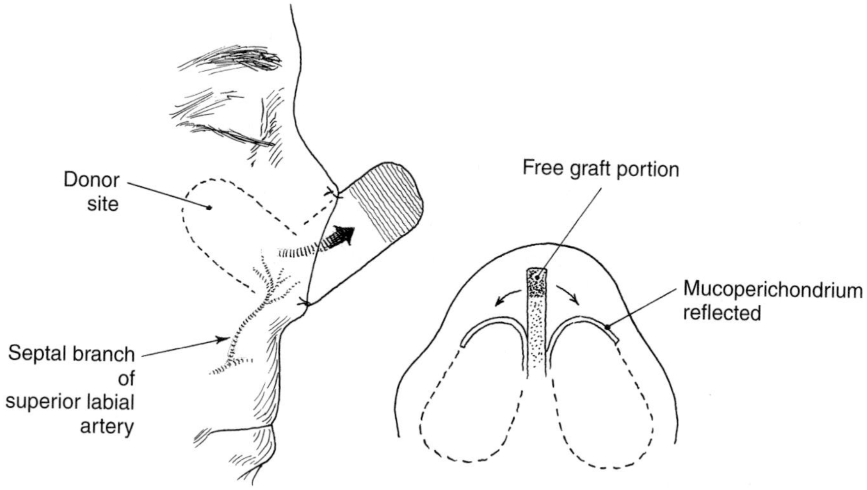

Figure 14–6. Anteriorly based septal pivot flap. This is a full-thickness septal flap that is secured to the anterior nasal spine and the dorsal nasal remnant. This provides subsurface framework and reestablishes nasal length and projection. Reflection of the overprojected mucosal flaps provides internal lining. Excess cartilage and bone can be trimmed and used as a batten, strut, or sidewall brace.

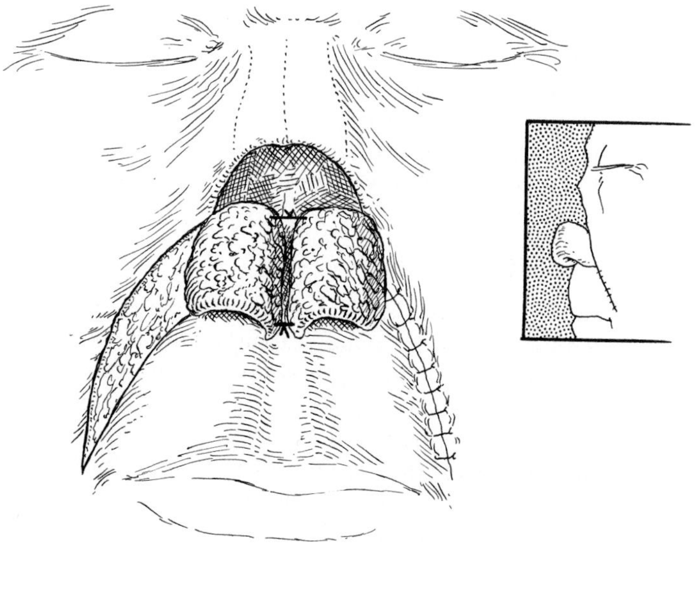

Figure 14–7. Superiorly based nasolabial turnover flaps may be used for internal reconstruction of the lower one third of the nasal vault. Subsequently, a columellar strut and cartilage onlay grafts are placed to provide stability and maintain form.

tion of the external nares, and maintain an alar-facial junction point that is lateral to the aesthetic norm. Subsequent debulking, structural grafting with cartilage battens and struts, and alar base narrowing are necessary to provide support, shape, and position. Nonetheless, superiorly based nasolabial flaps are reliable, have good vascularity, and are capable of supporting primary graft placement (columellar strut). Tissue is adequate to provide ample surface area for complete vestibular replacement.

Upper Third

Isolated upper-third lining defects are almost never seen. This is because lesions that require bony dorsum removal are typically larger and involve multiple areas of the nose. For combined upper and middle vault reconstruction, several options exist. Skin grafting of the undersurface of a forehead flap has been described for external-internal lining. However, this does not permit primary cartilage placement (unless prefabricated at the forehead donor site as a staged procedure) owing to the problems with a "graft-on-graft" interface. Although the forehead flap is vascularized, the skin graft and cartilage would not take against each other. The preferred alternative is to suture a buccal mucosal or split-thickness skin graft to the undersurface of a pericranial flap. This can be developed contralateral to the paramedian forehead flap to be used for external coverage. Access for both flaps can easily be gained through the traditional harvest incisions for the paramedian flap without imparting additional morbidity.

Pericranial flaps are thin, vascularized, fascial flaps that can support free grafts on both surfaces. To ensure reliable transfer, the vascular base of the flap should capture the supratrochlear-supraorbital arterial axis. Secondary debulking of the fullness in the glabellar area created by folding the flap on itself can be addressed at the time of subsequent recontouring procedures.

When these options are not available, it may become necessary to rely on free tissue transfer (typically a radial forearm free flap). Owing to the conspicuous donor scar, the need to skin graft the forearm, and the sacrifice of a major artery to the extremity, this technique is reserved as a last option in very rare circumstances.

Support Options

A commonly held axiom in nasal reconstruction is that nasal contour supersedes nasal scarring. This means that achieving the desired shape is the primary goal, and that scarring is a secondary consideration. To this end, the delicate contours and highlights that define the various subunits of the nose must be restored while still maintaining airway patency. A second guiding principle is to "replace like tissue with like tissue." Typically, cartilage autografts are used in reconstruction of the lower two thirds of the nose, whereas bone or cartilage can be used in the upper third to one half. In general, conchal cartilage is preferred for restoring the natural convexity of the alar and tip subunits, whereas the more rigid septal cartilage is well suited to provide support in nasal sidewall or extensive lower lateral cartilage losses. In either case, if nasal obstruction secondary to septal deviation coexists, it is advisable to harvest septal cartilage to achieve the dual benefits of a graft source and improvement in nasal airflow.

As a third choice, if auricular or nasal septal cartilage is unavailable, costal cartilage can be utilized. However, it is more frequently applied as a compound osseocartilaginous graft for dorsal nasal support. Figure 14–8 illustrates the use of an osseocartilaginous graft cantilevered off the anterior nasal spine as an L-graft. These grafts can also be easily shaved cross-sectionally to serve as a supportive framework for the nasal sidewall. To use rib cartilage for lower lateral cartilage replacement requires creating thin, longitudinal, split grafts and releasing interlocked stresses (Gibson's principle). Owing to a more conspicuous scar, increased donor site pain, and the potential for pneumothorax, costal cartilage grafts remain a last resort.

In cases of subtotal or total nasal loss, where dorsal support is required, the preferred technique is to utilize a precisely contoured, split-calvarial bone graft. The graft is rigidly fixed at the nasofrontal angle with microplates to provide support and projection from the radix to the supratip. To avoid the unwanted rigidity and

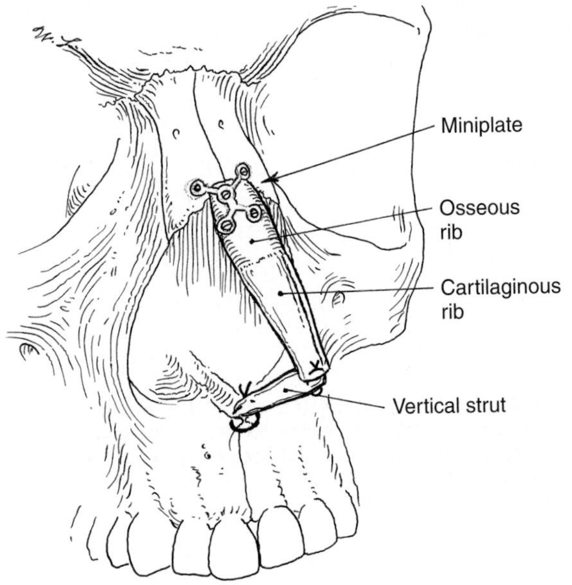

Figure 14–8. An L-frame construct derived from osseocartilaginous rib components provides dorsal support and projection. The graft is divided into dorsal and vertical struts, which are rigidly fixed to the nasal dorsum and anterior nasal spine.

potential for pathologic fracture at the tip, cartilaginous reconstruction is performed, with stabilization afforded by transosseous sutures. The iliac crest donor site is a poor second option, mainly because of increased postoperative discomfort.

Harvest of the concha can be performed through either anterior or posterior incisions. The anterior approach is slightly quicker (5 to 10 minutes), involves less undermining of skin, and results in a shorter external incision. However, the scar is more visible. To achieve an acceptable scar, care must be taken in reapproximating the skin edges to avoid ridging or a step-off. The posterior approach is favored for most cases, particularly in younger patients with short hairstyles.

With any cosmetic or reconstructive procedure, the results seen on the operating table are not necessarily static over time. The dynamic forces of wound healing, initiated by myofibroblastic activity beginning at 2 to 3 weeks after surgery, must be accounted for in the primary surgery to optimize the outcome. Secondary revisions to reposition key anatomic landmarks and reexpand skin lost to tissue contraction can rarely achieve results that can be obtained through accurate primary stabilization. This stabilization is best achieved through judicious use of contoured cartilaginous battens and struts over the entire reconstructive surface. It is not enough to replace anatomically what has been lost; rather, it is essential to brace those areas that are physiologically unstable. This is particularly true for the alar lobule, alar rim, and soft tissue triangle, which are normally devoid of skeletal support.

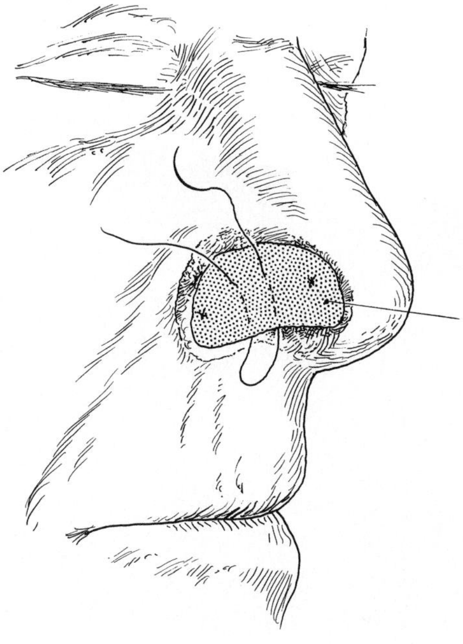

Figure 14–9. A conchal cartilage free graft is used to reconstruct the ala. Vertical mattress sutures coapt the internal mucoperichondrial layer to the cartilage onlay graft, thereby facilitating revascularization of the graft.

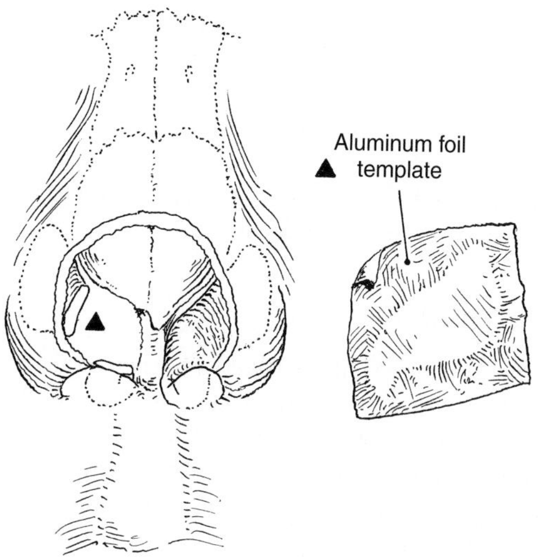

Figure 14–10. A foil template of lower lateral cartilage on the intact side is used to guide fabrication of a replacement graft on the resected side.

In order to properly accommodate the overlying soft tissue cover and replicate the thinner native cartilaginous skeleton of the nose, the size of the replacement cartilage must be reduced by several millimeters, and the graft thinned to 1.0 to 1.5 mm. The flatter, more rigid hyaline cartilage of the septum is more conducive to this than the flexible, curved, elastic, conchal cartilage. Once appropriately sized and shaped, it is imperative that the grafts be stabilized with sutures. Vertical mattress sutures (4-0 chromic) provide good apposition of the thin, vascularized, lining layer to the undersurface of the cartilage graft (Fig. 14–9).

Whenever possible, replication of the size, shape, and geometry of the nasal cartilages should be patterned after the contralateral intact structures (Fig. 14–10). This can be achieved by direct exposure through the wound, or when visible, by contouring an aluminum foil wrap about the external surface. When bilateral losses are present, a best-guess estimate must be made based on existing nasal landmarks and a knowledge of standard nasal proportions. Occasionally, prior photographs of the patient may be useful in planning the reconstruction. The basic concepts of aesthetic rhinoplasty relative to nasal length, tip shape, projection, and rotation remain applicable.

Coverage Options

In considering coverage options for the nose, arbitrary division into upper, middle, and lower thirds assists in the treatment planning. For cutaneous defects of the lower third, both surface area and subunit involvement may dictate use of any one of six reconstructive techniques described in the following section. Because the lower third of the nose is primarily defined by convex contours with a thicker, more sebaceous skin quality, flaps are preferred over skin grafts. Options for coverage include the subcutaneous melolabial island flap, bilobe flap, nasalis flap, axial frontonasal flap, J-flap, and the paramedian/oblique forehead flaps.

Lower Third

Subcutaneous Melolabial Island Flap. Defects confined in whole or in part to the nasal ala are well suited for reconstruction with adjacent cheek tissue. For these situations, the medially based subcutaneous melolabial island flap is preferred. Superior color match, texture, and wound healing response (convex bulging) result from the melolabial island flap. The alternative is a superiorly based nasolabial flap. However, this flap is limited by the frequent occurrence of alar rim retraction and trapdoor deformities, particularly with partial subunit losses. With either flap, subunit defects of more than 50% should be converted to a whole subunit resection for aesthetic continuity.

To prepare for the reconstruction, a template of the ala is fabricated from the contralateral intact side by ink-marking a Telfa pad. Owing to the transposition of the flap, the outline must be marked out on the skin 180 degrees with respect to the nasal alar defect. The flap is placed just lateral to the melolabial crease (Fig. 14–11). An allowance of 1 mm greater than the defect dimension is planned to account for wound contraction. The distance from the alar-facial groove to the medial aspect of the flap should be approximately 2.5 to

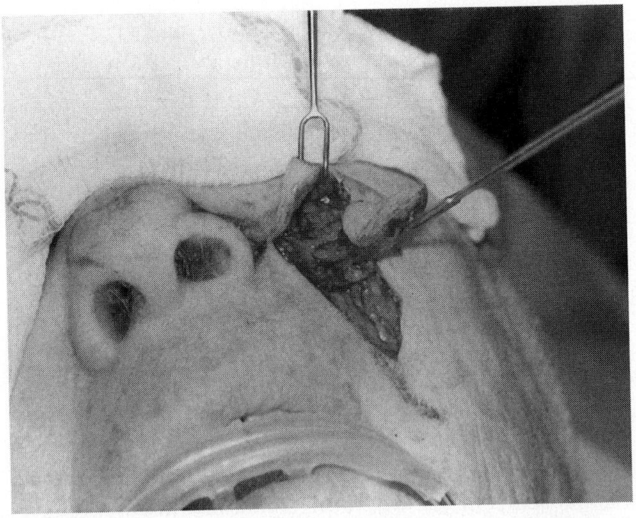

Figure 14–12. Intermediate step in subcutaneous melolabial island flap. The dissection of the island flap proceeds from skin to superficial subcutaneous tissue to deeper tissue plane to capture the facial vessel perforators.

3.0 cm. This allows sufficient flexibility in the subcutaneous pedicle to provide tension-free insetting of the flap.

Dissection proceeds from inferolateral to superomedial, initially in the superficial subcutaneous plane. Ultimately, the level of dissection is directed to the supramuscular plane to capture the vertically oriented facial vessel perforators (Fig. 14–12). Loupe magnification and blunt hemostat dissection of the medial flap provide a safe means of mobilization. After complete elevation, the flap is rotated 180 degrees along the axis

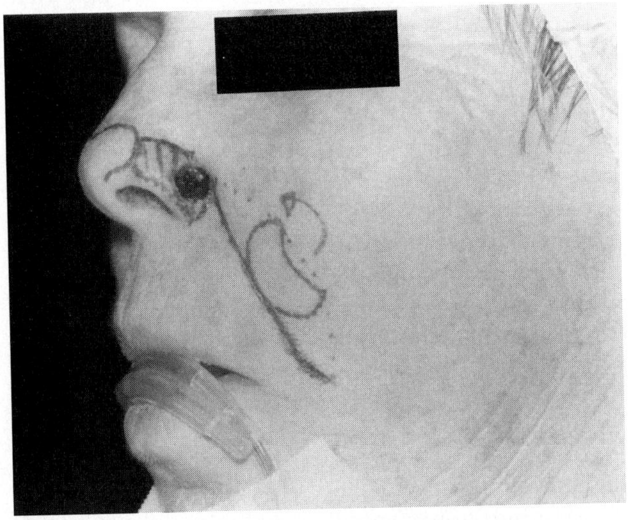

Figure 14–11. Subcutaneous melolabial island flap. The design uses a reverse template from the contralateral intact side. Note the lines of the intended alar subunit skin excision and the outlined melolabial crease.

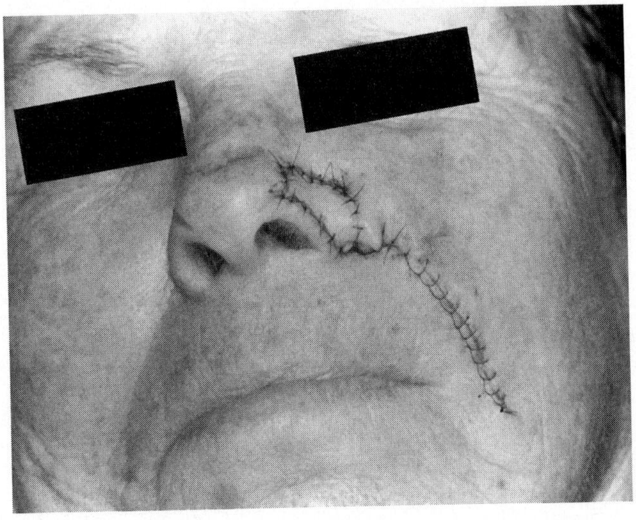

Figure 14–13. Appearance after first-stage melolabial island flap transfer. Note that the triangular skin flap from the medial cheek (just lateral to the ala) is used to provide coverage for the subcutaneous pedicle.

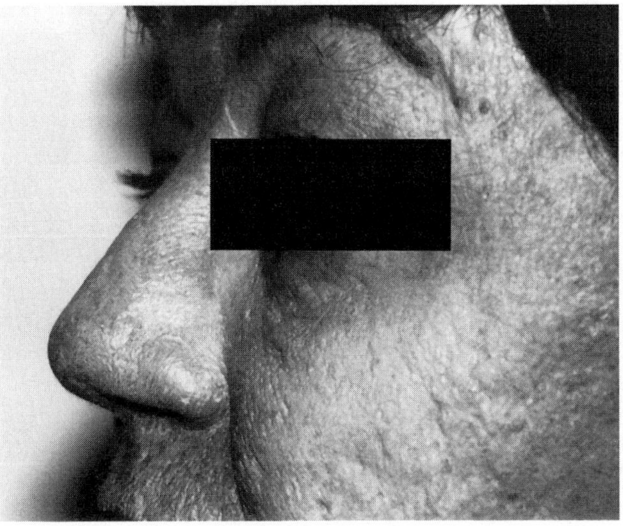

Figure 14–14. Lateral view (of a different patient than in Figure 14–13) 3 months after melolabial island transfer.

of the pedicle to place the skin paddle into the defect. Flap insetting and closure is achieved with 5-0 interrupted subcuticular and 6-0 cutaneous sutures (Fig. 14–13). The donor site in the cheek is closed by initially mobilizing inferiorly based subcutaneous fat and rotating it into the defect. This avoids a contour deformity that could occur with skin closure alone. Wide undermining of the medial cheek with advancement into the melolabial crease line provides for anatomic restoration of the cheek facial unit. Suction drainage is unnecessary.

Three weeks later, second-stage division and inset may be performed. Reincision along the lateral ala and superior aspect of the melolabial crease line allows access for defatting and reestablishment of the alar-facial junction (Figs. 14–14 to 14–16). Redundant medial cheek skin is advanced medially, trimmed, and closed

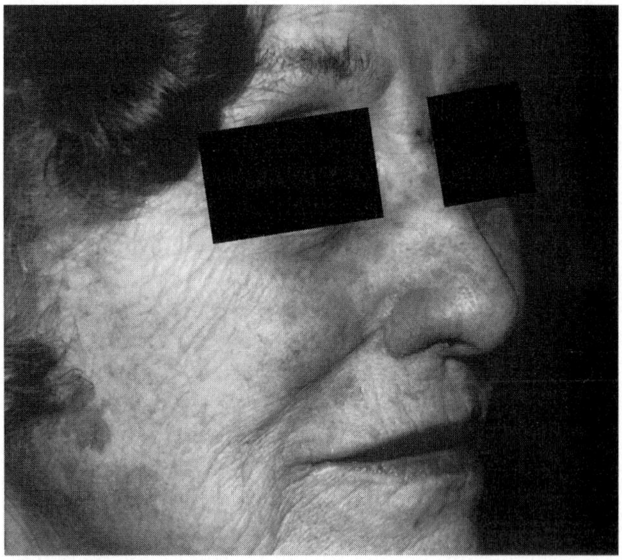

Figure 14–16. An oblique view (of a different patient than in previous figures) 4 months after reconstruction of the right ala using a melolabial island flap. The flap remains somewhat rubrous secondary to neovascularization. The convex alar contour and the alar-facial and alar-labial junctions are well preserved.

into the melolabial crease line. Final-stage alar rim thinning may be required. If so, it is performed 3 to 4 months later through a wedge excision along the leading edge of the alar rim (see nasal refinement section).

Forehead Flaps. Forehead flaps are indicated for lower nasal coverage, primarily for large defects exceeding 1.5 to 1.75 cm in diameter. In these cases, local nasal flaps would result in too much distortion. The forehead flaps are also indicated for multiple subunit reconstruction. Additionally, under special circumstances, the forehead may be the donor site of choice for whole alar subunit losses. This is the case for patients possessing a shallow

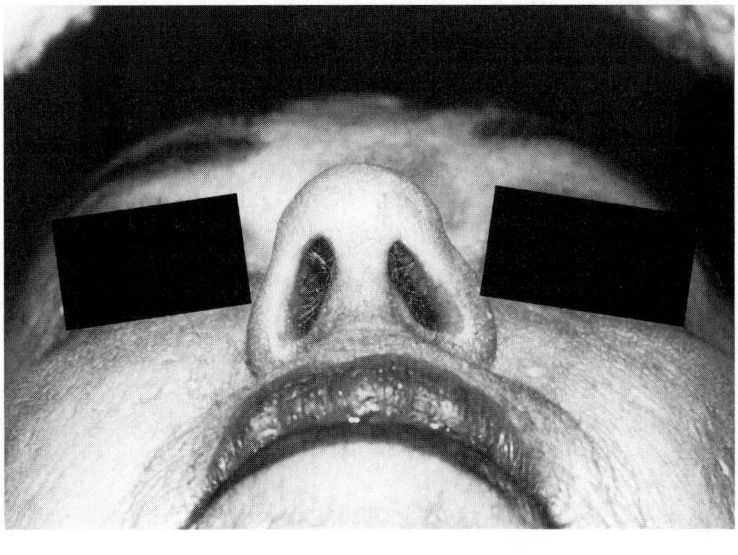

Figure 14–15. Basal view of the same patient as in Figure 14–14. This view shows preservation of the alar-facial junction angles and nostril symmetry.

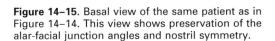

melolabial sulcal depth or those who are at high risk for flap-related complications (i.e., smokers, diabetics, and those with a prior history of irradiation).

Compared to the melolabial island flap, the forehead flap is less pliable, coarser in texture, and does not heal with any significant contraction at the recipient site. However, the forehead flap provides a larger tissue volume with greater flexibility of design and has a more reliable vascular supply.

Forehead flaps can be designed as paramedian or obliquely oriented flaps. The decision to use an oblique forehead flap design over a paramedian design is determined strictly by the vertical distance of the hairless portion of the frontal scalp. The oblique flap provides a longer pedicle length without crossing the frontal hair line. It is possible to remove hair by epilation or with subsequent laser treatments to expand the length of the paramedian flap across the hairline. However, this is tedious, requires multiple treatments, and generally results in transfer of skin with inferior quality and texture. The pedicle length can be extended by 1.0 to 1.5 cm by careful dissection into the superomedial orbit to mobilize the supratrochlear vessels. If, after measuring an arc of rotation from this point to the most distal point of the recipient defect, inadequate length of forehead skin is determined, an oblique design is selected. The oblique flap requires an extra procedure to delay elevation so as to ensure enhanced viability to the distal-most nonaxial skin. To do this, one simply incises skin along the entire flap design down to the pericranial layer without any flap elevation. After reapproximating the skin, and after an interval of 2 weeks, the flap is ready for second-stage transfer.

The paramedian flap is designed by centering a 1.2- to 1.5-cm pedicle base over the corrugator crease (Fig. 14–17). It is not necessary to use a Doppler to identify the vessels unless there is a question of their integrity secondary to prior surgery or trauma. The flap length is determined by measuring the distance from the flap base to the distal-most point of the recipient defect and adding 1 cm. This ensures tension-free insetting and accounts for the distance lost through flap rotation at its base. The distal flap design can be determined by making a template of the defect. At this point, the flap is incised and undermined in the subgaleal plane inferiorly, to the level of the supraorbital rims (Fig. 14–18). Further inferior release toward the orbit is done sharply with curved iris scissors. This extension should be in the subperiosteal plane, parallel to the axis of the supratrochlear vessels. After identifying the vessels, more extensive subcutaneous skin release is performed. In a nonsmoker, distal thinning to the axial subdermal vessels is allowable to create a more pliable flap.

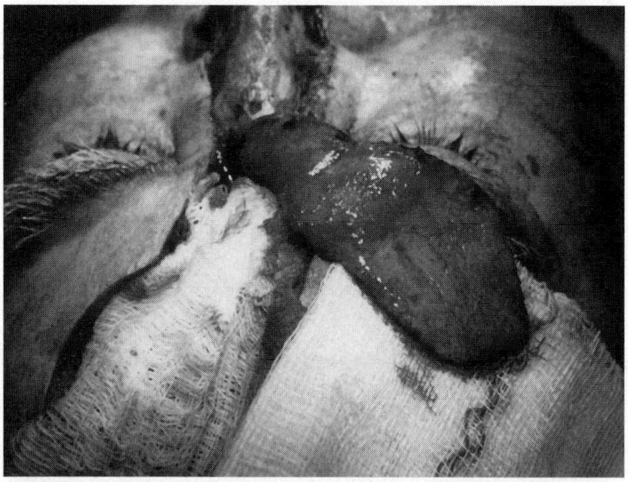

Figure 14–18. Intermediate stage of the development of the paramedian forehead flap. The flap has been dissected to the superomedial orbital rim in the subgalleal plane. The flap has been thinned under the skin intended for transfer to the axial vessels within the superficial subcutaneous tissue plane.

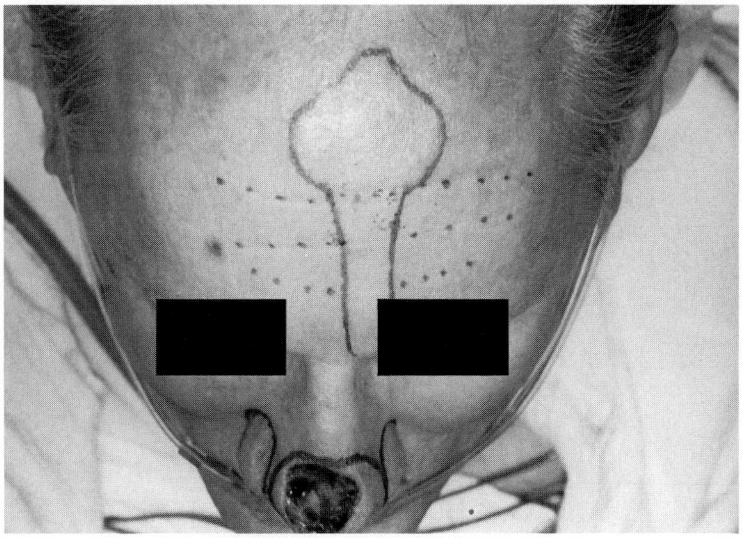

Figure 14–17. A left paramedian forehead flap is used for reconstruction of a nasal tip defect. The flap is centered over the corrugator crease and designed to replace the entire nasal tip subunit skin. Transverse forehead creases are dotted to assist in realignment of skin edges following flap transfer.

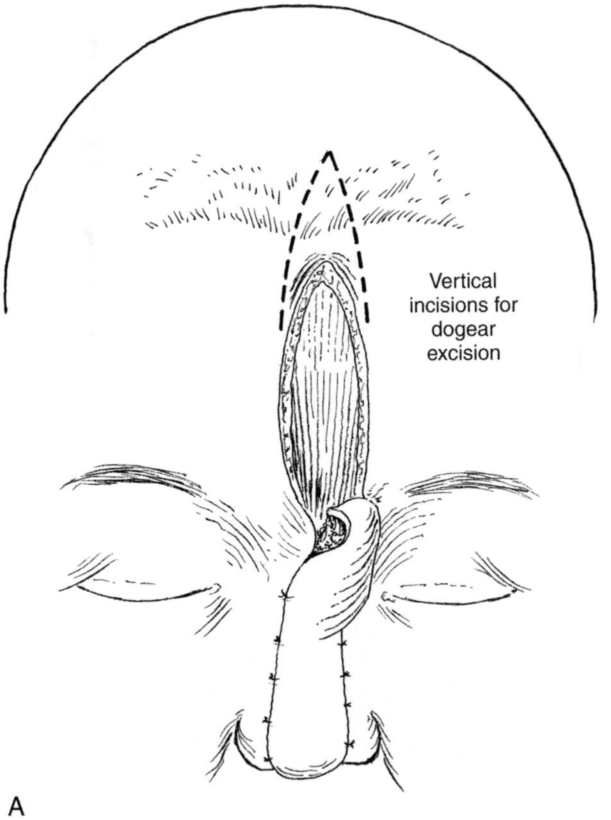

A

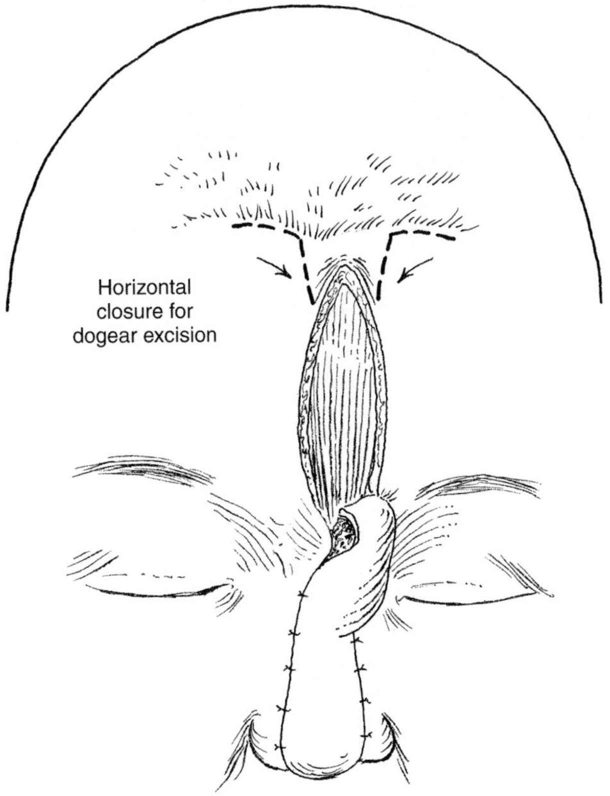

B

Figure 14–19. Two methods of correcting a dogear formation in the upper forehead created by wide skin excisions. *A,* Fusiform excision at the upper apex of the flap skin paddle (along the dashed lines) allows primary closure with a smooth contour. *B,* O-to-T closure. Additional incisions are indicated by the dashed lines. The lateral tissue flaps are rotated into the defect to close the wound. This places the transverse scar along a pretrichial line or along a relaxed skin tension line.

After the flap is elevated and inset, complete forehead closure is usually achievable. This is facilitated by several measures, including wide undermining, vertical galeotomies, and rapid intraoperative tissue expansion. In large, distal forehead defects, a simple pretrichial O to T closure (i.e., bilateral rotation flaps) can be used (Fig. 14–19). For those rare defects that will not close without excessive tension, partial closure is performed, and the distal aspect is allowed to heal by secondary intention. This allows for autocontraction and reepithelialization, which can be revised later. Figures 14–20 to 14–23 highlight the utility of this flap for convex surface repairs.

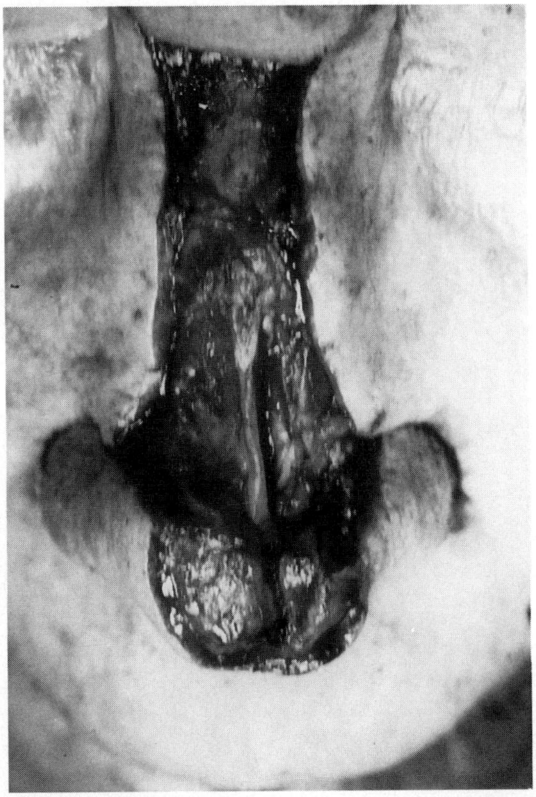

Figure 14–20. Completed nasal excision for a basal cell carcinoma. The dorsal nasal and nasal tip subunits are completely excised, and the nasal sidewalls are advanced to the dorsal nasal subunit lines to limit the flap width. Note that the dorsal cartilaginous resection has created an open middle-vault deformity.

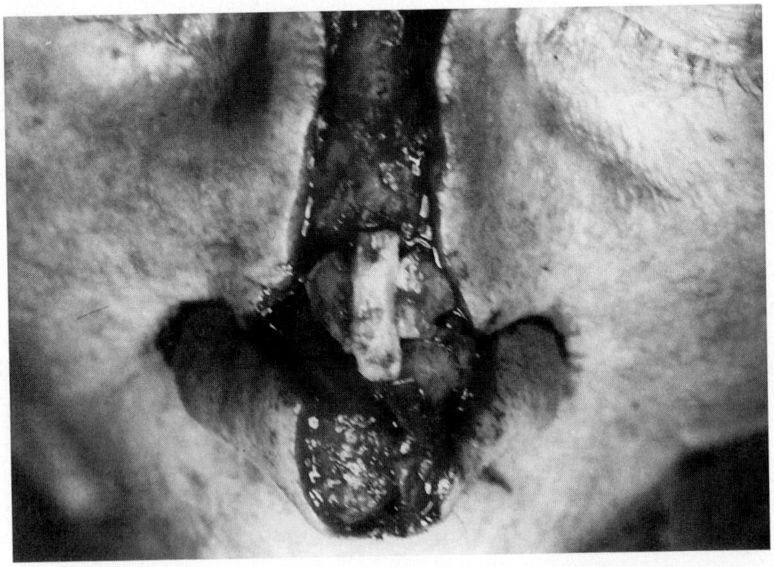

Figure 14–21. Reconstruction of the middle nasal vault (same patient as in Figure 14–20). The middle vault mucosa has been reapproximated. A conchal cartilage butterfly graft is used to reestablish dorsal nasal relationships.

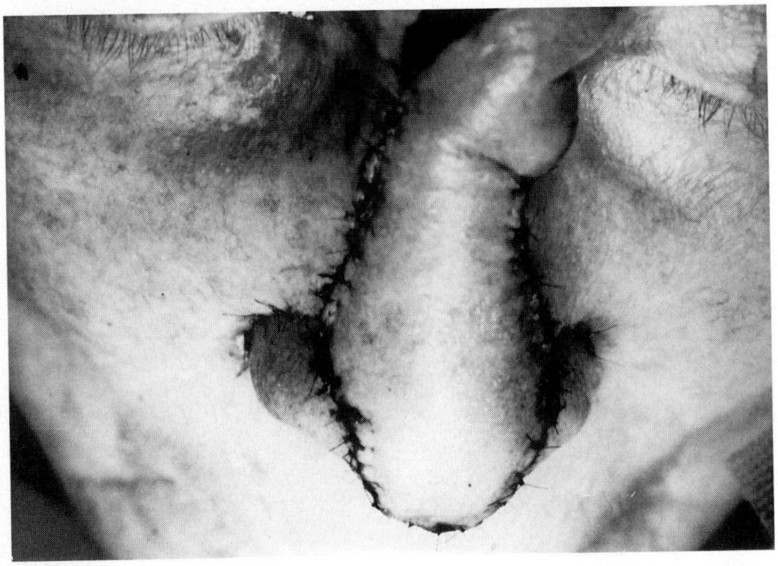

Figure 14–22. Skin resurfacing of the nasal tip and dorsum (same patient as in Figures 14–20 and 14–21). A paramedian forehead flap has been transferred. No grafting of the raw edges of the flap pedicle will be used. Instead, petroleum-iodine strip gauze (1 × 8 inches) is circumferentially wrapped to keep the edges moist.

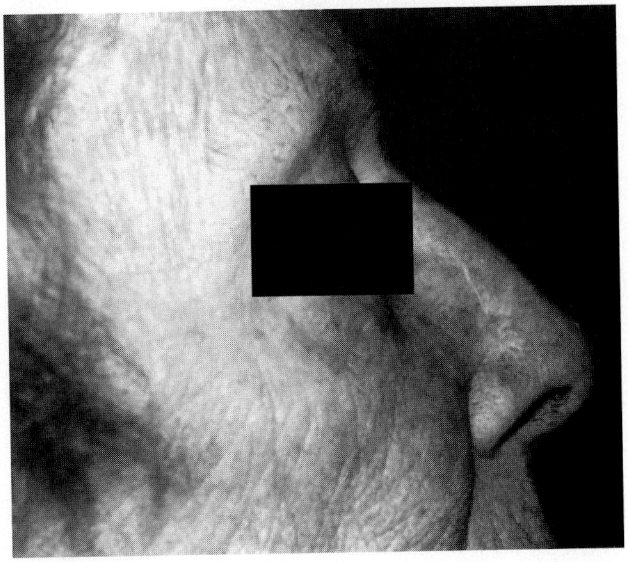

Figure 14–23. Lateral view showing the healed result 6 months after nasal reconstruction (same patient as in Figure 14–22). The dorsal contour and scar camouflage are acceptable.

Bilobe Flap. The bilobe flap was inially described by Esser[4] and later modified by Zimany[5] and Zitelli.[6] It is appropriate for smaller (<1.5 cm) skin defects in thick skin zones of the nose (i.e., tip, supratip, ala). Depending on the defect location, either a medially based or laterally based design may be used. In general, medial defects (tip) require laterally based flaps, whereas lateral defects (ala) require medially based flaps. The basic principle is that a primary flap is first elevated to close the original defect; a smaller secondary flap is then elevated to close the primary flap defect, and the secondary flap defect is closed on itself (Figs. 14–24 and 14–25). The Zitelli design specifies 45- to 50-degree arcs of transposition of the primary and secondary lobes (i.e, a total arc ≤ 100 degrees). The primary flap width should equal the defect width, and the secondary flap width should be one half to three fourths the width of the primary flap. The dissection should be in a submuscular plane. Tissue distortion is minimized when the secondary flap is planned to lie in the looser skin of the nasal dorsum or sidewall. The pivot point for the primary lobe is planned one defect radius away and should be positioned away from the alar rim to avoid distortion following transposition.

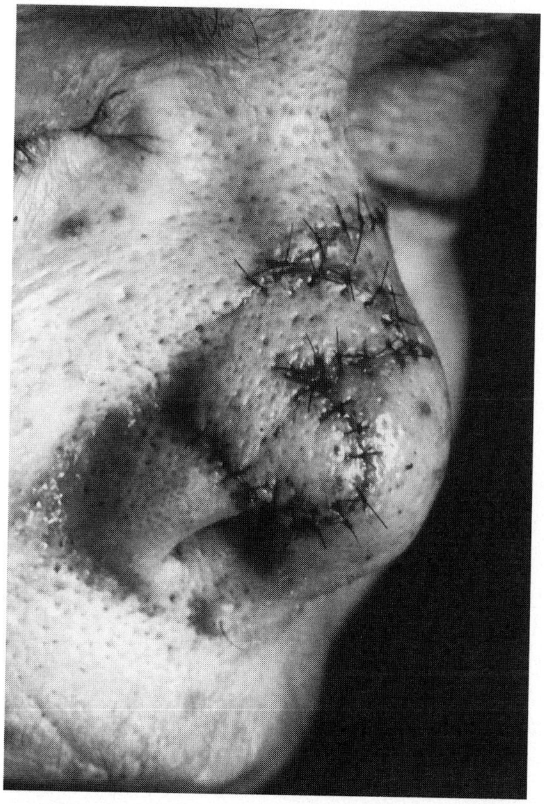

Figure 14–25. Appearance after flap closure (same patient as in Figure 14–24). Note that tension-free insetting is achieved by exploiting the laxity of the skin along the upper nasal sidewall.

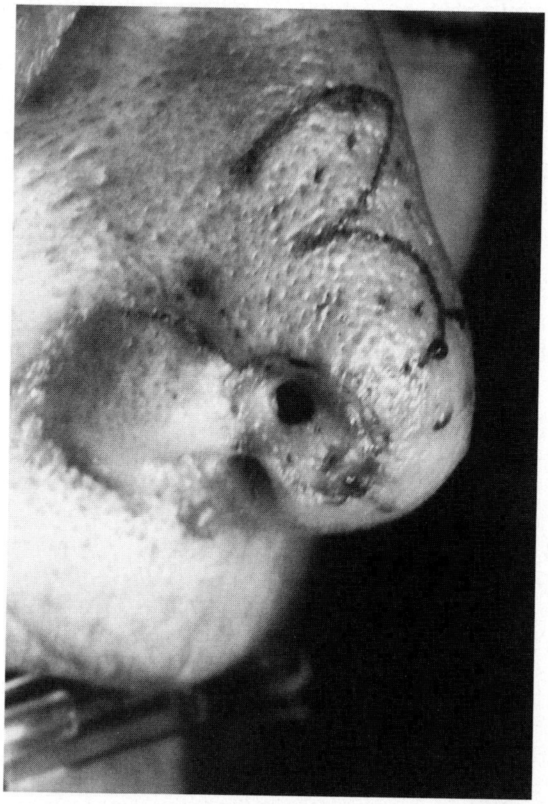

Figure 14–24. Alar defect measuring 1.3 cm with a full-thickness skin defect involving the soft tissue triangle and right nasal tip. Reconstruction is outlined with a laterally based bilobe flap using the Zitelli design. The small lining defect was repaired by a bipedicled mucosal advancement flap prior to bilobe flap transposition.

Disadvantages of this flap include a need for extensive undermining to distribute tissue tension, scar lines that do not follow the relaxed skin tension lines of the nose, and a tendency for trapdoor deformity of the primary lobe of the bilobe flap. Additionally, when the recipient site defect lies close to the alar rim, inferior and inward bulging of the alar margin is frequently seen and often requires subsequent revision. Despite proper planning, it is not uncommon for a slight, standing, cutaneous cone to develop at the pivot point and a transverse depression to occur at the base of the secondary lobe. Despite these minor shortcomings, this is a reliable and versatile flap that affords superior color and textural match for small cutaneous defects in the thick-skinned zones of the nose.

Nasalis Flap. Technically, the nasalis flap is an axial-pattern myocutaneous flap. The blood supply is derived from the multiple branches of the alar branch of the facial artery as it passes around the pyriform aperture. The perforating cutaneous branches about the alar base ramify extensively through the nasalis muscle to course dorsolaterally and interconnect with the opposite side.

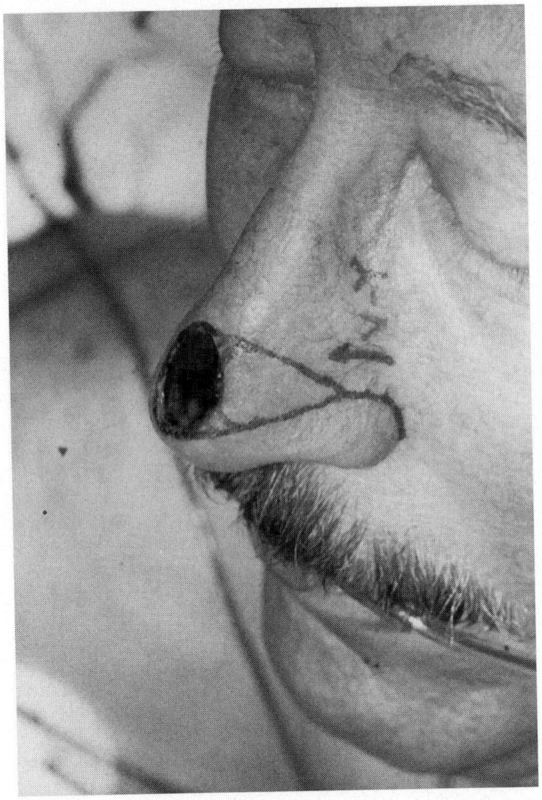

Figure 14–26. Central tip skin defect. Reconstruction is planned with a nasalis myocutaneous flap. Note the ice cream cone shape and the relationship of the lower limb to the alar groove.

With a vascular base located at the alar-facial junction, and movement limited to approximately 1.25 cm along its longitudinal axis, this flap is well suited for reconstruction of small, full-thickness skin defects of the lower lateral nasal sidewall, supratip, or upper ala. When bilateral flaps are employed, midline tip–supratip defects of 2 cm can be reconstructed. There are several major advantages of the nasalis flap over the bilobe flap. Because tissue movement is directed from lateral to medial via V-Y advancement, there is little, if any, tendency for alar rim retraction. Moreover, the incisions that are used run roughly parallel to the relaxed skin tension lines, one of which is usually placed along the alar groove. Unlike the bilobe transposition flap, there is no tendency for trapdoor contraction and prolonged flap edema. The advantages of the nasalis flap over rotational flaps are that long incisions are not required to achieve tissue movement, and "dogear" formation does not occur.

To design the nasalis flap, two incisions must be created that form an apex near the alar base (Fig. 14–26). Typically, the lower incision is drawn from the inferolateral aspect of the defect and follows the alar groove as much as possible. The superior incision begins at the uppermost aspect of the defect and curves convexly upward. This incision should parallel much of the alar groove, finally tapering laterally at the alar-facial junction. Undermining of skin above the nasalis musculoaponeurotic layer is extended 1 cm cephalically and 5 mm caudally from the flap. Submuscular dissection over the perichondrium of the lower lateral cartilage is directed from medial to lateral (Fig. 14–27). The flap is mobilized at the alar base by releasing the deep nasalis attachments to the pyriform aperture and canine fossa. Medial advancement can then be achieved and the flap can be inset into the defect. The donor wound is closed in a V-Y fashion (Fig. 14–28). Often, the triangulated ends of the medial flap must be rounded to accommodate the shape of the recipient defect at the time of insetting.

J-flap. The J-flap is a rotational flap with a pivot point that lies along the nasal dorsum cephalad to the defect and utilizes a peripheral arc along the alar groove. Simi-

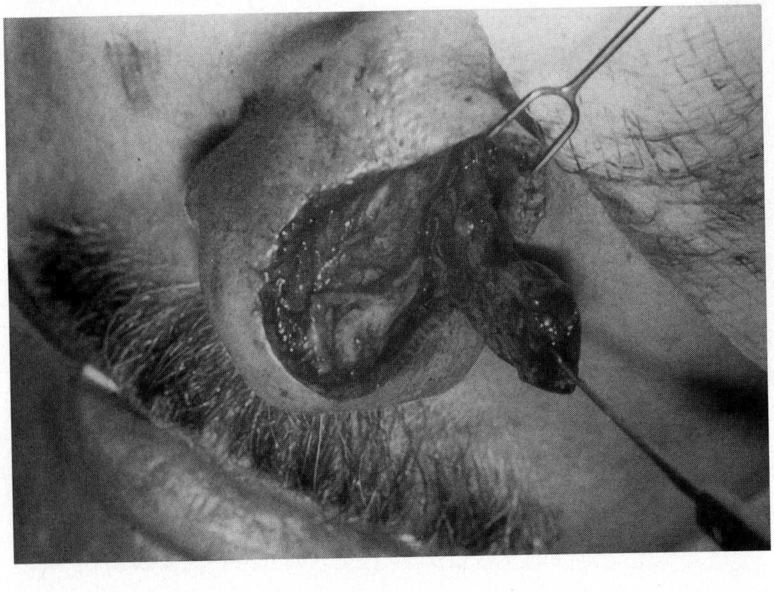

Figure 14–27. Intermediate stage of nasal tip reconstruction using a nasalis flap (same patient as in Figure 14–26). Supraperichondrial-submuscular dissection from medial to lateral is used to elevate the nasalis flap. Note the wide musculoaponeurotic base maintained laterally, despite tapering of the cutaneous component.

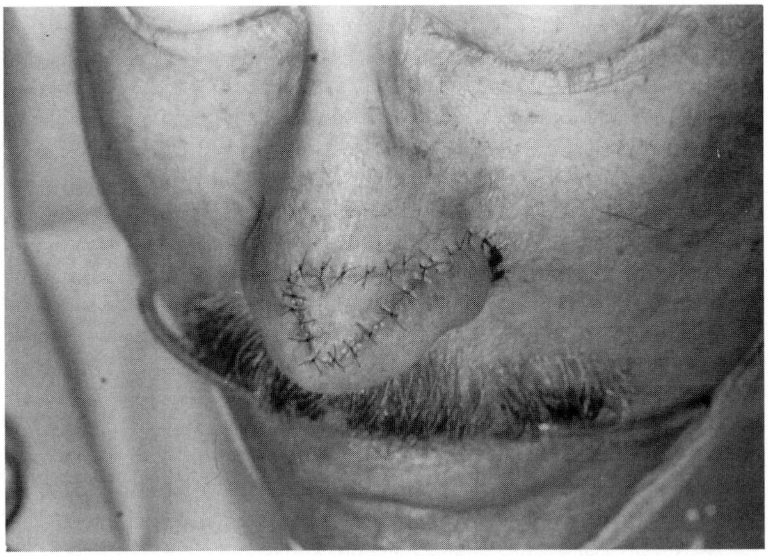

Figure 14–28. Final closure of the nasal tip defect using the nasalis flap is achieved by V-Y advancement (same patient as in Figures 14–26 and 14–27).

lar to the nasalis flap, tissue movement is directed from lateral to medial. However, rather than mobilizing tissue as an axial-based island flap from a deep bony attachment, this random-based flap recruits tissue from the medial cheek in the superficial subcutaneous tissue plane. This flap is ideally suited for median or paramedian full-thickness skin defects with a fusiform shape that have their long axis oriented vertically. The principal advantage of the J-flap over the nasalis flap in this situation is that a transverse scar is avoided, which would be more conspicuous with longer defects.

To effect movement around the alar lobule and to avoid dogear formation over the nasal dorsum, two triangular skin incisions must be created (Fig. 14–29). Initially, the base of an isosceles triangle is marked out at the alar-facial junction with the transverse width 1.5 times the width of defect. A second triangle, with its base oriented caudally, is marked just above the dorsal nasal defect. Incisions along the alar groove and base are made, and wide lateral undermining is performed in the superficial subcutaneous tissue plane. The now-mobilized lateral nasal and medial cheek tissue is advanced superiorly and rotated medially into the recipient defect. The Burrow's triangle is then excised to prevent dogear formation. To avoid excessive fullness along the nasofacial junction at the time of closure, conservative defatting of the flap is performed. Blunting of the nasofacial junction and alar-facial groove is further avoided by the use of buried tacking sutures along these junctional landmarks. Half-buried mattress sutures within the alar groove help to prevent obliteration of this important aesthetic boundary. As in tip rhinoplasty, Steri-strip tape reinforcement is used to support the newly positioned skin envelope.

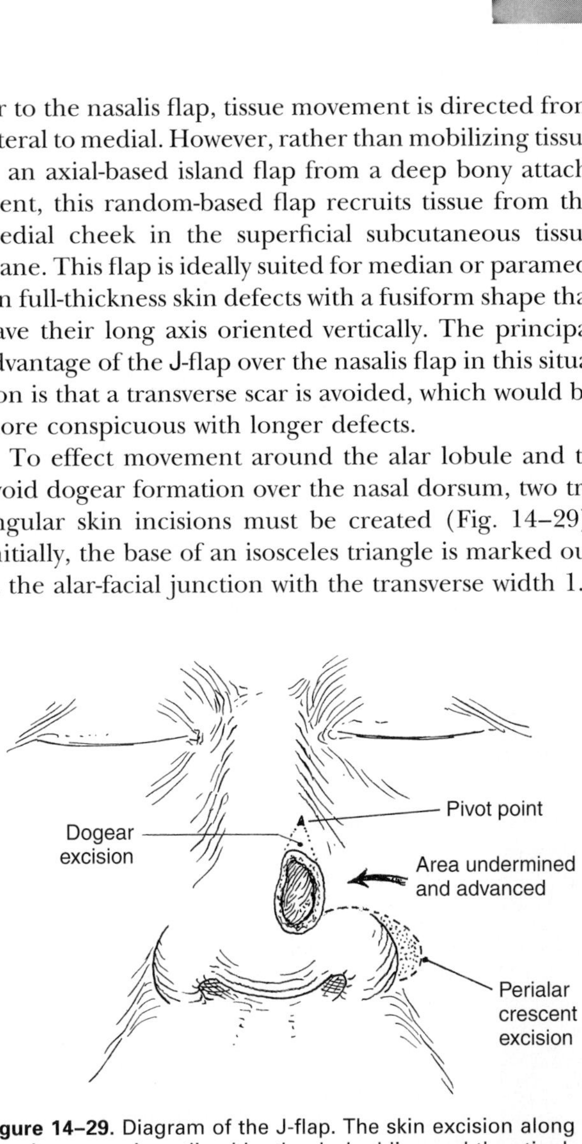

Figure 14–29. Diagram of the J-flap. The skin excision along the alar crease is outlined by the dashed line and the stippled area. The skin excision outlined by the dotted line prevents a dogear on the nasal dorsum. This flap is ideally suited for paramedian supratip defects in which the long axis lies vertically.

Axial Frontonasal Flap. The axial frontonasal advancement-rotation flap (modified Rieger flap)[7] is a flap of second choice for midline defects (tip, supratip, dorsum) of the lower half of the nose that are greater than 1.5 cm in diameter. It has the advantage over a paramedian forehead flap of achieving closure in one stage, with adjacent tissue possessing similar qualities of thickness, color, and texture. It is often the procedure of choice for elderly or infirm patients who are not so concerned with achieving aesthetic ideals. Transfer of tissue can be achieved quickly, reliably, and without concern for the status of the recipient bed (unlike skin grafts). The major disadvantages of this flap are threefold: (1) long incisions are required for seemingly small tissue gains; (2) the incisions do not follow relaxed skin tension lines; and (3) tissue thickness discrepancies must be accounted for as the thicker, more sebaceous glabellar skin is transferred onto the thinner, smoother skin of the medial canthal region.

The blood supply of the flap is derived from contributions of the angular and supraorbital arteries that join at the level of the medial canthal tendon. Based on the axial pattern of this flaps' blood supply, an island flap from either side may be developed, encompassing the remaining dorsal and lateral nasal skin cephalad to the defect. Usually, a long back-cut toward the vascular axis is not required to achieve the necessary tissue movement for a tension-free closure. Lax glabellar skin is advanced in a V-to-Y fashion to achieve closure of the caudal flap. Medial flap movement results from rotation along a peripheral nasal arc with the pivot point centered at the medial canthal level.

In designing this flap, the pedicle is planned to lie contralateral to the defect. For a truly midline lesion, either side may be chosen. A curvilinear incision is extended from the defect to a point just lateral to the nasofacial junction (contralateral to the pedicle). The incision is then extended toward the naso-orbital line into a glabellar frown line. An inverted V-shaped incision in the glabella is completed with an apex situated 1 to 2 cm above the brow line. The second limb of the V on the pedicle side should be symmetrical to the first limb and placed in a frown line (Fig. 14–30). This incision stops approximately 1 cm superior to the pedicle. Wide undermining is performed on the nasal portion of the flap in the supraperichondrial and supraperiosteal planes. In the glabellar portion, elevation is performed in the superficial subcutaneous plane to allow for better thickness matching of the medial canthal skin. After the flap is released and rotated into the defect, a Burrow's triangle is marked out distally and excised ipsilateral to the pedicle. This is done to avoid a dogear at the pivot point. In this way, the smallest possible scar necessary for reestablishing contour is achieved. Meticulous two-layer closure is necessary to avoid step-offs and contour imbalances, especially along the upper nasal sidewalls. Owing to the exposure afforded by elevation of this flap, consideration is usually given to certain rhinoplastic procedures (i.e., tip modification, hump reduction) that may be performed concurrently. Should medial and lateral osteotomies be performed, more prolonged packing (5 days) is generally required for internal stabilization as the lateral sidewall support from the skin has been lost secondary to flap elevation.

Middle Third

Full-Thickness Skin Grafts. As a general rule, split-thickness skin grafts have a very limited role in external resurfacing of the nose. Full-thickness skin grafts afford superior color and textural properties, more closely approximate the thickness match required, are more durable, generally resist contraction, and have the potential to grow in children. Although the requirements for graft "take" are somewhat more stringent, proper timing of graft application and preparation of the recipient bed should result in desirable outcomes (Figs. 14–31 to 14–33). The criteria for optimal graft take are a wound devoid of fibrinous debris or foreign body material (i.e., Gelfoam, Surgicel, etc.), less than 10^5 organisms per gram of tissue, and a supportive vascular base and edges. Although the "bridging phenomenon" may allow graft take for defects of less than 1 cm^2 over bare cartilage or bone, it is often advisable to delay grafting until granulation tissue has grown over the bone or cartilage to provide a more reliable nutrient base. This option may also be chosen, even when a vascular base is present, for the deeper defect in order to optimize surface contour prior to grafting. By allowing granulation tissue to build up in the wound base, the depth of the wound is decreased to better match the thickness of a skin graft.

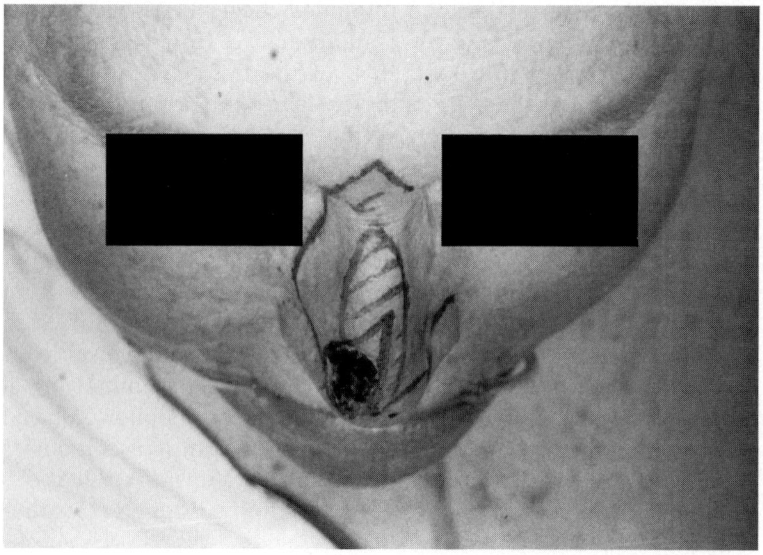

Figure 14–30. Design of the axial frontonasal advancement-rotation flap. With this flap, tissue is rotated from the lateral nasal wall into the defect. Note the dogear excision outlined at the superior edge of the defect. The apex of the triangular excision defines the pivot point for the rotational component of the flap. The hatched area is undermined to improve rotation. An inverted V incision in the glabellar area defines the advancement component and is closed by V-to-Y advancement. Extension of the lateral incision just beyond the nasofacial junction is done intentionally to allow for medial scar migration.

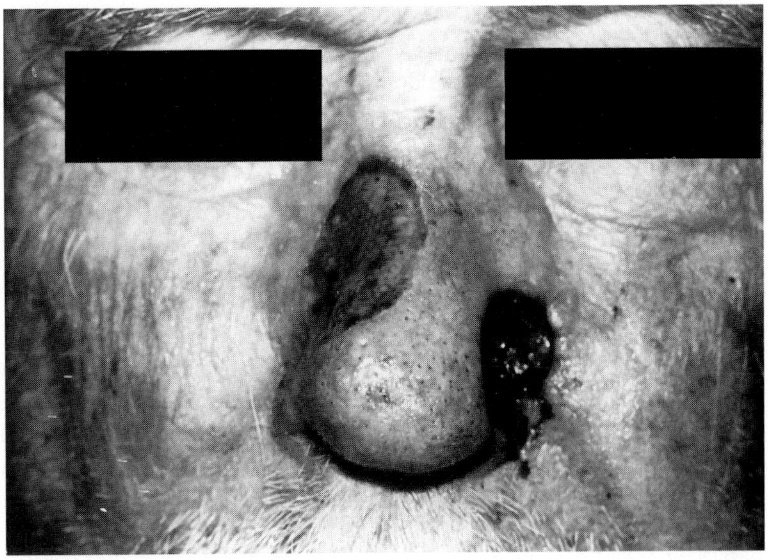

Figure 14–31. A patient with two subunit defects, one involving the left ala and the second involving the right nasal sidewall. The sidewall defect is through the full-thickness of skin and has a granulating base.

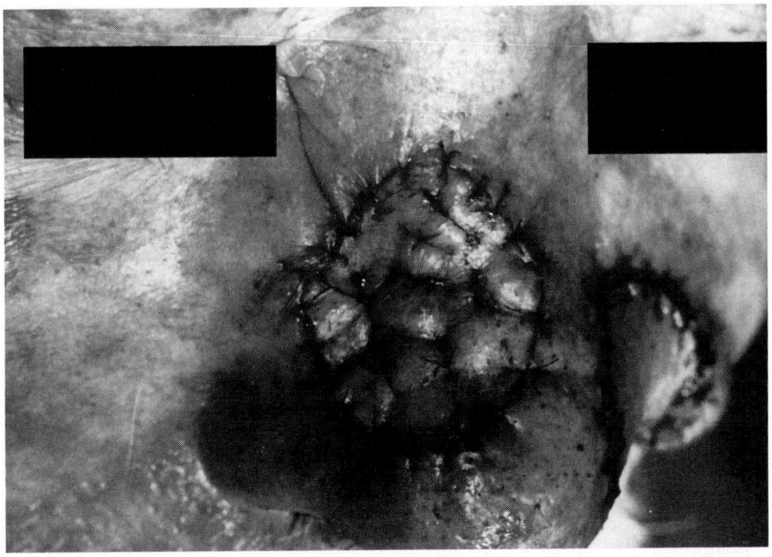

Figure 14–32. A full-thickness skin graft from the preauricular donor site is transferred to the right sidewall defect (same patient as in Figure 14–31). The graft is secured with several basting sutures.

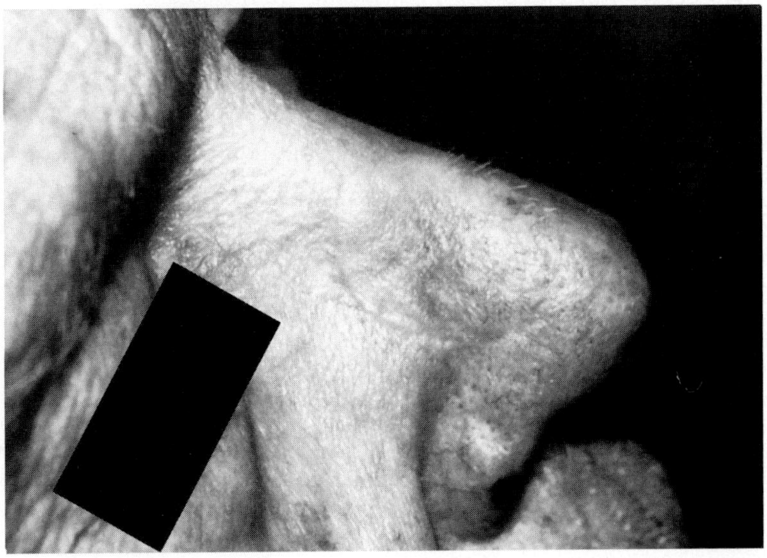

Figure 14–33. Lateral view of the healed full-thickness skin graft (same patient as in Figures 14–31 and 14–32). The contour is good and the scar borders are relatively inconspicuous.

Unlike local nasal flaps, which bulge as they contract, full-thickness skin grafts do not, and so are well suited to reconstruct the superficial planar or concave surfaces of the upper two thirds of the nose (i.e., dorsum or sidewalls). This is in contrast to the lower third of the nose. When applied to the thicker, more sebaceous subunits of the ala, tip, and supratip, a sharp contrast in texture and a conspicuous, patch-like appearance are often seen. This is especially notable over prominent or sharply angulated domal arches.

The size of the graft is limited only by the ability to primarily close the donor site and the subunit principle need not be applied. The choices for donor site typically include preauricular or postauricular skin, the supraclavicular area, or the melolabial sulcus. Before selecting a site, one should carefully examine the features of each with respect to thickness, color, texture, and content of hair follicles and sebaceous glands. The postauricular donor site affords a well-hidden scar, but its skin is thin, smooth, photo-protected, and has fewer adnexal structures. It has a tendency to retain a rosy hue following engraftment, and this may persist. However, the postauricular site is often the preferred choice in young patients with fair features and without well-formed creases in the preauricular or melolabial regions. By comparison, the preauricular skin is thicker and usually closely matches the color of nasal skin owing to similar actinic exposure. Depending on the size of the graft obtained, preauricular skin has the potential to displace the sideburn hair in a man, creating visible asymmetry. The preauricular site is ideal when a formed preauricular crease is present with posterior cheek redundancy. The melolabial sulcus is usually a second choice to the preauricular area, mainly because of its more conspicuous position in the midface. Color match and thickness are generally very good, but selection is driven by the ability to conceal the scar and avoid asymmetry. The supraclavicular area provides the most abundant donor site for grafting. The skin here is usually thinner than that of the central or posterior cheek. However, owing to variable exposure to the sun, the supraclavicular skin may present a color mismatch. A shiny, brown, wrinkled surface may result after graft maturation.

With all donor sites, optimal revascularization of the graft is promoted by thinning the undersurface down to the dermis. Hemostasis in the recipient bed should be ensured prior to graft placement to prevent hematoma formation and allow for a nutrient interface. Both tie-over bolster and basting suture techniques have been used with equal success to stabilize the graft. The goal following graft application is to immobilize the graft and prevent sheer forces that could disrupt the processes of inosculation and neovascularization.

Superiorly Based Melolabial Flap. The superiorly based melolabial flap is an alternative for defects in the middle third of the nose. The application of this flap to lower-third or upper-third defects typically results in disruption of aesthetic junction lines. When inset into the ala, obliteration or blunting of the alar-facial junction and alar groove can occur. Because of the design, this flap results in loss of continuity of the melolabial sulcus at the point at which the upper extension of the lateral incision is advanced medially into the nose. This can be secondarily corrected, but the resulting contour is never as good as reconstructions that avoid incisions and dissection into these key anatomic landmarks. For this reason, melolabial interpolation flaps for single subunit alar defects, or paramedian forehead flaps for multiple subunit losses involving the ala, are preferred. A second reason to avoid the superiorly based melolabial flap for alar reconstruction is that there is a tendency for this flap to cause trapdoor deformities. For middle-third skin losses occurring over the nasal dorsum, use of this flap necessitates extension of the lateral incisions and excision of otherwise intact skin along the sidewall subunit. This seems unwarranted. In these situations, depending on the orientation and size of the defect, preference is given to a modified axial frontonasal flap or paramedian flap. For thinner surface losses, full-thickness skin grafts are a reasonable alternative. Finally, this flap should never be applied for upper-third nasal reconstructions because of the proximity to the lower eyelid skin and the potential for medial ectropion.

The primary indication for use of the superiorly based melolabial flap is for deeper defects that would otherwise be treated with full-thickness skin grafts occurring in the lateral midnasal region. When applied in this way, thickness and color match requirements are optimized. In addition, this avoids distortion of the superior triangular extension of the lateral labial subunit. Although alar-facial distortions are avoided, blunting of the nasofacial sulcus can occur during transposition and must be addressed.

In designing the flap, a length : width ratio of up to 4 : 1 is usually well tolerated owing to the robust blood supply from the facial vessels. A flap width of 1.5 to 2.5 cm is typically chosen to allow for primary closure of the donor site without significant visible distortion (Fig. 14–34). The thickness of the flap may be adjusted, but it is best to keep the flap thin distally to minimize the tendency for pincushioning. A guide is to retain 1 to 2 mm of subdermal fat distally and 2 to 3 mm proximally.

Owing to the angular movement of tissue at the pivot point that is inherent to all transposition flaps, the actual flap length required must exceed the apparent length needed. One should plan for an additional 1.0 to 1.5 cm of flap length to allow for tension-free insetting. A short flap or a flap that just reaches its recipient site exerts an upward and outward pull on the ala. The width of the flap should be 1 to 2 mm greater than the width of the defect to account for the natural tendency of these flaps to contract. Should a trapdoor deformity

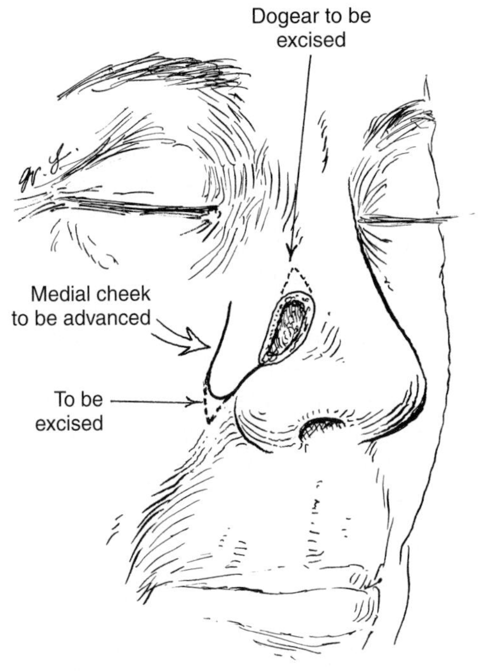

Figure 14–34. Superiorly based melolabial flap. The flap is rotated into the defect and the medial cheek skin is advanced to close the flap defect. Burrow's triangles are excised both proximally and distally to avoid dogears. This flap may be used to repair defects of the lower lateral sidewall or ala.

occur, intralesional steroid injections (i.e., Kenalog-20) may be initiated 3 to 6 weeks postoperatively and repeated at 4-week intervals as needed. If this is unsuccessful, surgical correction by wide undermining, cross-hatching of the undersurface of the flap (micro Z-plasty), and debulking may offer further improvement.

Bilobe Flap. The laterally based bilobe flap, which capitalizes on the skin laxity in the glabellar area, may be considered for small (<1.5 cm) central defects of the middle third of the nose. Used in this way, there is a natural tendency for contraction of the primary flap. This creates a desirable outward bulge. As a local flap largely confined to the nose, the color and textural matches afforded are superior. The major disadvantage lies in the scars created, which do not follow the ideal relaxed skin tension lines or aesthetic junction lines.

Axial Frontonasal Flap. The axial frontonasal flap can be used for central defects of the midnose measuring up to 4 cm^2. The application of this flap to the middle third of the nose, however, is more restricted than if it were being used for a lower-third reconstruction. This is mainly due to the limitations encountered in extending the peripheral arc laterally. Superiorly, the medial canthus and lower eyelid limit the available width in the lower portion of the flap, unlike in the lower third of the nose, where some extension laterally onto the medial cheek is tolerated.

Paramedian Flap. For large defects, or those spanning multiple nasal subunits, the paramedian flap is preferred. When reconstructing a middle-third defect, the flap length required for insetting relative to the flap base is short. This minimizes the donor scars on the forehead. The ability to thin this flap to the axial subdermal vessels allows for adjustments in flap thickness according to the depth of the defect. Owing to the natural tendency of these flaps to contract and bulge outward, this flap lends itself well to reproduction of the natural dorsal nasal convexity desirable in reconstruction of the middle third of the nose. Adjustments in defect dimensions and position by excision or advancement allow for flap positioning into natural contour lines or anatomic junction zones.

Upper Third

Surface reconstructions of the upper third of the nose must take into account several factors. The first is that there is a differential skin thickness and quality that exists between the thicker, coarser, and more sebaceous skin of the glabellar/nasofrontal region and the thinner, smoother, glabrous skin of the upper sidewall. A second important factor is that tissue movement created during flap elevation and insetting should not significantly distort the medial brow position. Finally, key anatomic landmarks, such as the medial canthus or lid margin, must not be displaced.

Primary Closure. Limited tissue losses in this area may allow for primary closure. This can be achieved by vertical advancement of adjacent nasal and glabellar skin. As long as this can be done without blunting the nasofrontal angle or distorting medial brow position, this is the simplest option. Wide, central undermining; deep tacking sutures; and adjustments in tissue thickness can be used to help achieve closure. If successful, this may result in normal nasal contours and a limited transverse scar that parallels the relaxed skin tension lines.

Full-Thickness Skin Grafts. Owing to limited skin thickness, a scant subcutaneous tissue layer, and a concave surface profile, lateral defects of the upper third of the nose are well suited to reconstruction with full-thickness skin grafts. Limited superficial defects that are not juxtaposed to the medial canthus heal well by secondary intention and do not require grafting. Defects that are large, deep, or very close to the medial canthus should be grafted (assuming at least a viable periosteal layer is present). This will prevent distortion that could occur during wound contraction. For defects devoid of periosteum, flap options are considered.

Glabellar Flap. Limited central or combined central and lateral defects of the upper third of the nose are well suited for single-stage reconstruction with glabellar flaps. Depending on design, these flaps may be random or axially based (supratrochlear vessels), and may be classified as advancement, rotational, or transpositional flaps, based on their tissue movement. Furthermore, the incisions used in the design of these flaps may be median or paramedian depending upon the size and location of the primary defect. Unlike skin grafts, flexibility in adjusting tissue thickness and the ability to cover raw, bony defects provide decided advantages. Transposition and rotational glabellar flaps are primarily limited by glabellar width and the degree of medial displacement of the eyebrows. Advancement glabellar flaps are relatively more limited by the potential for inferior displacement of hair-bearing skin. With all glabellar flaps, blunting of the nasofrontal angle, asymmetry of brow position, epicanthal webbing, and surface contour disturbances must be avoided. To preserve segmental facial composition and to optimize aesthetic outcome, glabellar flaps should be restricted to nasal and epicanthal defects. Although extended flaps have been described for reconstruction of medial cheek and lower eyelid defects, alternative methods (i.e., cheek flaps, full-thickness skin grafts) are preferred for these subsites when possible.

The superiorly based advancement glabellar flap is best designed so that the vertical incisions follow the dorsolateral naso-orbital contour lines. The incisions should flow into the supraciliary margin of the superomedial brow (Fig. 14–35). Following advancement, the medial brow skin redundancy may be excised as a Burrow's triangle to reestablish glabellar contour. The inferior transverse closure line should optimally follow the relaxed skin tension lines of the nasal dorsum. Depending on the height and location of the defect, tissue thickness should be adjusted to account for the transition in soft tissue volume overlying the nasion and rhinion.

Glabellar rotation flaps using V-to-Y advancement are best suited for dorsolateral defects (Fig. 14–36). With the base of the flap and, therefore, its pivot point, oriented medially, dogear correction is often required in the nasofrontal region (particularly for circular defects). The inverted V incision should follow the glabellar frown lines as closely as possible. The upper extension of the V incision can be roughly estimated by anticipating that the vertical component of the Y limb following closure will equal the height of the defect. The height of the vertical extension of the incision above the defect would, therefore, equal the height of the defect. Insetting near the base of the flap should be done first, with trimming of any redundant tissue near the tip and excision of Burrow's triangles done last.

Single-lobe transposition flaps have the greatest potential for disturbing naso-orbital and nasofrontal contours and so are the least preferred option. Blunting of the nasofrontal angle opposite the flap base is a frequent occurrence and difficult to correct secondarily. Vertical designs, with the long axis of the flap oriented 90 degrees to the defect, result in considerable redundancy at the pivot point, requiring undesirable back-cuts for correction.

USE OF THE SEPTUM IN RECONSTRUCTIVE RHINOPLASTY

The nasal septum is a potential graft source that can provide composite tissue for both lining and support.

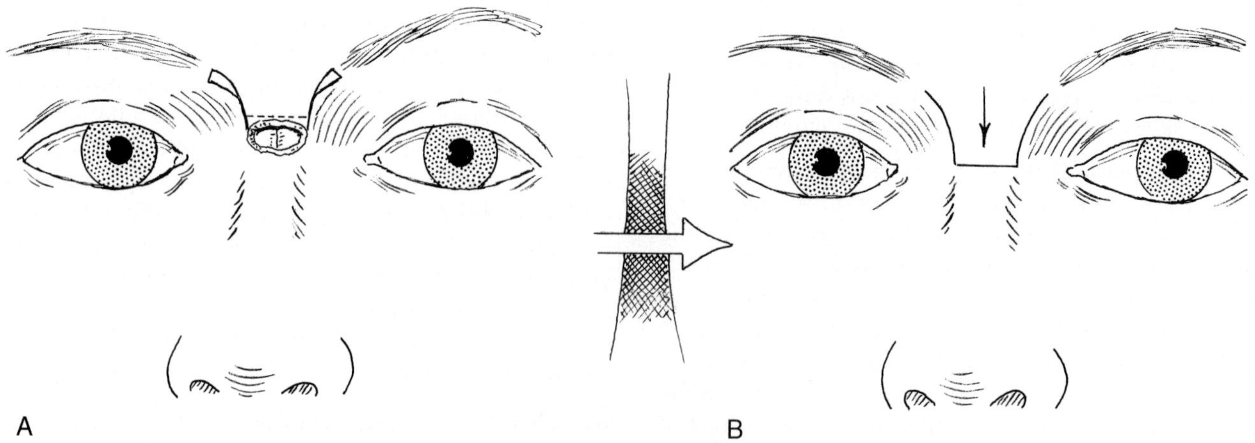

Figure 14–35. Superiorly based glabellar advancement flap. This flap exploits the laxity in the nasofrontal region. *A,* Design of the flap. Well-placed Burrow's triangles can lead to optimal closure along the orbitofrontal and transverse nasal crease. *B,* Final result.

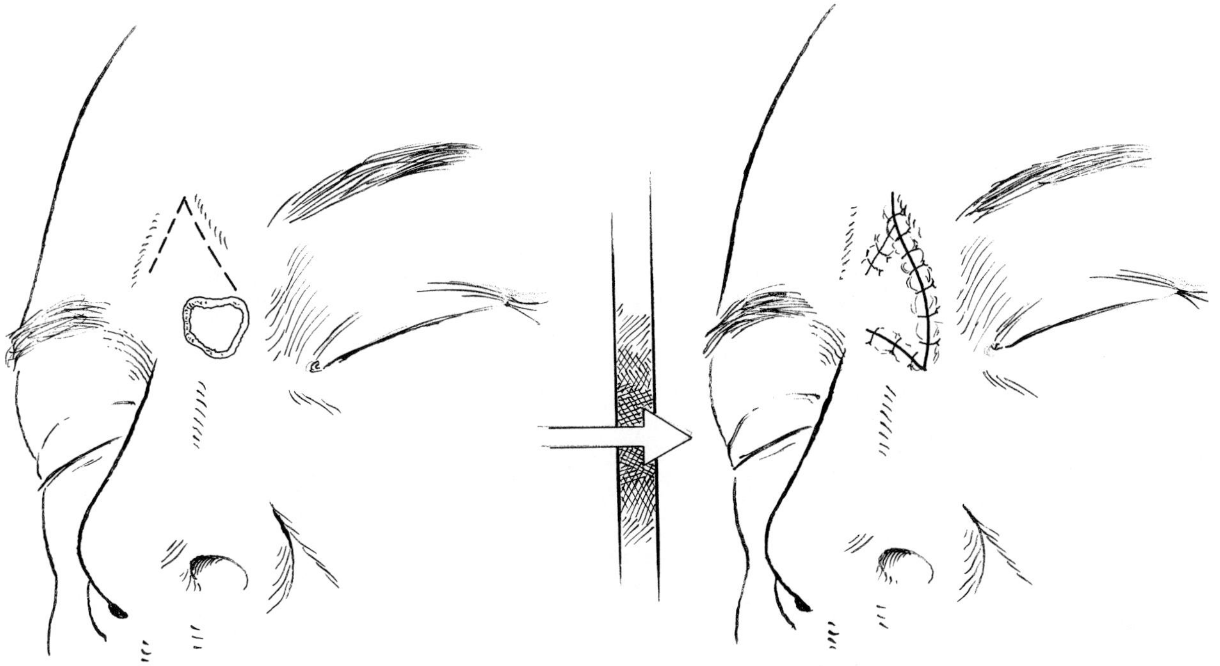

Figure 14–36. Glabellar rotation flap with V-Y advancement. If possible, the incision should be made in skin folds. The defect is closed by a V-to-Y advancement. This flap is well suited for defects in the lateral upper one third of the nose.

Prior discussion highlighted its application in middle vault reconstructions when harvested as a septal hinge (de Quervain) flap. Emphasis has also been placed on reinforcing the entire subsurface framework with structural grafts (septal and/or conchal cartilage) that will resist the contractile forces of wound healing. Cartilaginous and bony free grafts from the septum, applied as struts, battens, and braces, provide support to maintain inspiratory function.

When surgical resection has sacrificed key supportive structures of the nasal base (columella, medial crura, membranous septum, caudal cartilaginous septum), the reconstructive surgeon is faced with the challenge of reestablishing nasal mechanics and aesthetic form. Thin, reliable, vascularized, lining flaps, either integrated as a composite chondromucosal flap or capable of supporting structural free grafts, are desirable. Composite flaps are preferred owing to their increased intrinsic stability.

For reconstructions of the lower half of the nose, there are two commonly applied septal flap techniques. Both of these create obligatory septal perforations, but differ in their indications. The septal pivot flap is indicated when the vascular entry zone between the piriform aperture and skin of the upper lip near the philtrum is intact. This flap is based on the septal branch of the superior labial artery. As part of the flap, the entire anterior septum (quadrangular cartilage, portions of the perpendicular plate of ethmoid) can be rotated dorsally and caudally (Fig. 14–37). This septal flap can be anchored to the remaining dorsal nasal skeleton to provide an L frame for the nose. Following an initial healing period of 4 to 6 weeks, the mucosal flaps may be divided in the midline and turned over to provide internal lining for the middle and lower nasal vault. Depending on the degree of internal lining loss, local hinge flaps from the remaining nasal sidewall may be combined with the mucosal turn-over flaps to complete the internal reconstruction. The osseocartilaginous component of the septal flap above the dorsum may be removed and applied as a structural free graft.

If nasal length, dorsal height, and/or structural stability remain inadequate following the septal pivot flap, an additional stage can be added. After the initial septal pivot flap is created and before the mucoperichondrial turn-over flap stage is performed, a dorsal nasal strut (typically, a costal cartilage graft) can be placed. In this procedure, the cartilage graft is secured proximally to the nasal bones and rests dorsally over a tunneled segment of the pivot flap. The graft is inserted into a submucosal pocket of the pivot flap that will provide nourishment and support during engraftment (Fig. 14–38). The tunnel is created by submucosal resection of bone/cartilage at a 30-degree angle, corresponding to the nasofacial plane. Because graft dimensions and shape can vary, dorsal nasal height, length, and width are easily controlled. Once a stable septal framework has been established, nasal tip projection and rotation can be defined through precisely carved cartilage autografts.

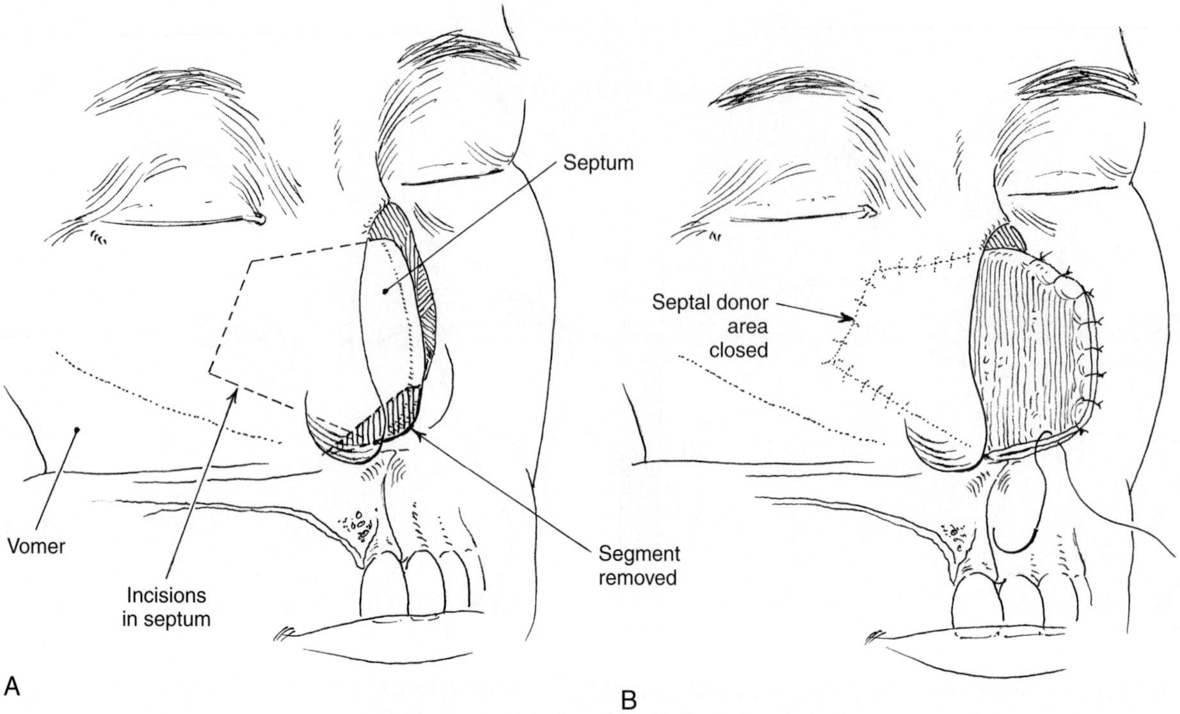

Figure 14–37. Septal pivot flap. This flap rotates the entire septal cartilage anteriorly and inferiorly. It is used for lining and subsurface framework support in dorsal-caudal nasal reconstruction. *A,* The dashed line marks out the full-thickness incisions through the septum. The cartilage of the hatched area at the anterior base is removed by a submucosal excision through an incision in the anterior mucosa. This allows forward movement of the composite septal flap. *B,* The flap is rotated into position. The mucosa is sutured over the cut edge of the cartilage at both the donor site and on the composite flap.

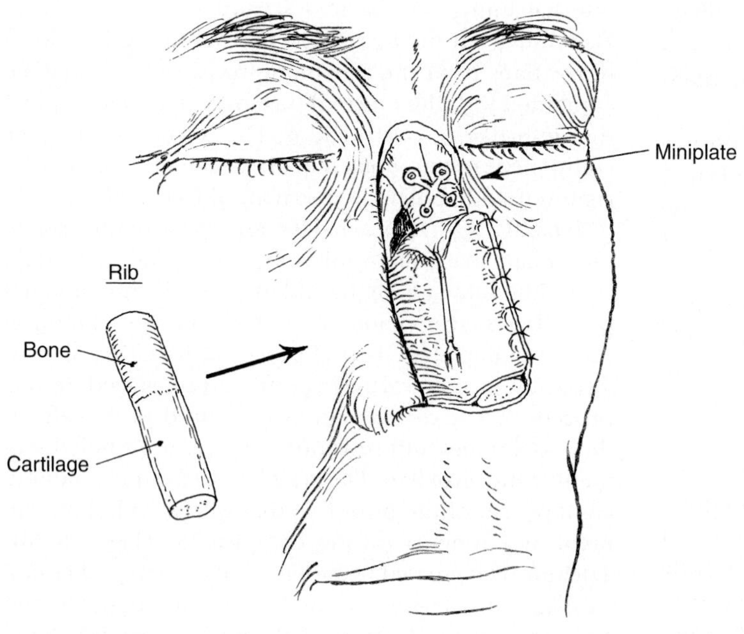

Figure 14–38. Dorsal strut in conjunction with a septal pivot flap. After a suitable interval for healing (several months), a rib graft is tunneled through the dorsal aspect of the septal pivot flap and fixed proximally to the nasal bone remnant.

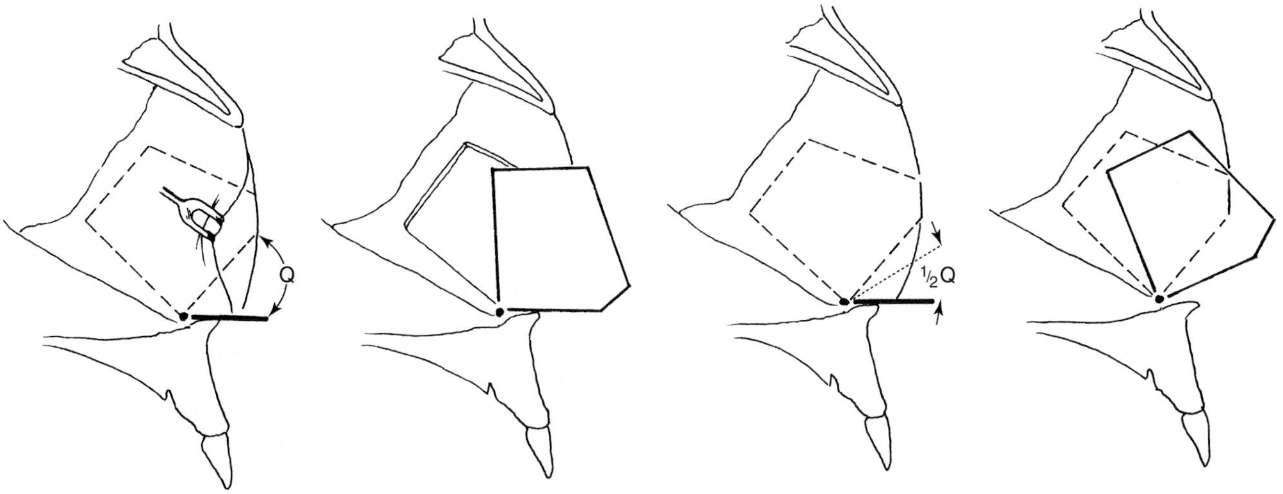

Figure 14–39. Illustration of the angle of rotation for a septal pivot flap. The angle of the wedge resection (Q) determines the degree of forward rotation. In the first two illustrations, the rotation achieved is maximized by a large excision. In the second two illustrations, the angle or rotation is reduced by a smaller wedge excision. The pivot point of the flap is at the apex of the wedge excision.

An alternative septal technique, described by Millard,[8] involves advancement of a superiorly based L-shaped composite chondromucosal flap. Despite a non-axial blood supply, this flap has been successfully used. It is particularly applicable to patients with a flat nasal tip resulting from caudal septal resection. In those cases where violation of the vascular entry zone of the septal branch of the superior labial artery exists, it remains the technique of choice. Despite sharing a similar ability to provide support as a tip scaffold, this flap cannot provide any substantial lining material owing to the narrow cuts (1.0 to 1.5 cm) required for its intranasal rotation. Additionally, because of concerns about compromising the vascular base of the septal flap with transmucosal fixation sutures, a more tenuous, single-point fixation at the anterior nasal spine is required with this technique.

Regardless of the septal flap chosen, the key to successful application lies in the submucosal release of the quadrangular cartilage to allow caudal movement of the leading edge of the septum. In the case of the septal pivot flap, a wedge resection, with its triangular base situated just above the anterior nasal spine, allows for forward rotation (Fig. 14–39). The degree of movement is controlled by the height of the triangular base and the posterior position of the pivot point. Typically, the pivot point is planned near the junction of the anterior extension of the vomer and quadrangular cartilage. For the Millard L flap, stellate releasing incisions are created at the base of the chondromucosal flap in order to allow it to rise high enough to rest its distal tip on the anterior nasal spine (Fig. 14–40). Both flaps are secured in this region by sutures fixating the cartilaginous septum to the periosteum.

Figure 14–40. Chondromucosal flap of Millard. Full-thickness incisions release the front of the septum to rotate forward, thereby augmenting the nasal dorsum. The L-shaped design of this flap is supplied through the subdermal plexus of the upper septum, not a defined axial arterial blood supply. This is a more tenuous blood supply for the composite flap and does not allow for mucosal turn-over flaps.

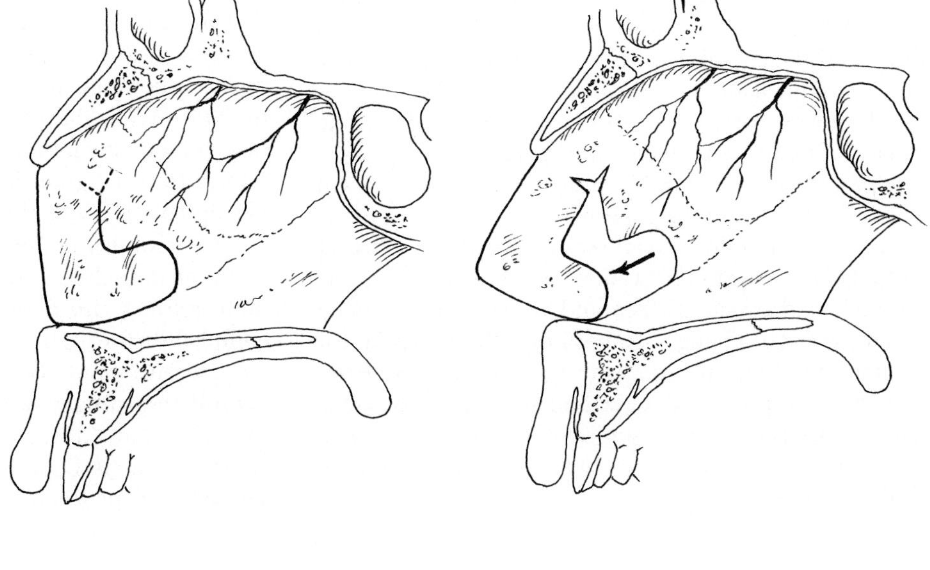

NASAL REFINEMENT

Despite the most meticulously planned soft tissue flap or free graft transfers to the nose, reestablishment of ideal aesthetic form often requires secondary or tertiary refinements. The range of revisional procedures is diverse, but most involve debulking and recontouring, recreation of an anatomic junction line or boundary (i.e., alar groove, alar-facial groove), repositioning of a displaced landmark (i.e., alar rim, alar base), and surface enhancement (i.e., dermabrasion, epilation). In most cases, these refinements are delayed for 3 to 4 months following final tissue transfer or insetting to allow time for wound maturation. In the case of trapdoor deformities or displaced landmarks secondary to wound contraction, a longer interval is recommended, particularly if progressive improvements are noted with intralesional steroid injections.

Debulking and Recontouring

A knowledge of topographic nasal anatomy and aesthetic ideals is a key element for reestablishing proper surface contour. Maintaining symmetry does not guarantee form. The subtle highlights and depressions defined by the skeletal composition of the nose and the varying thickness of its overlying skin are what distinguishes the nose. Therefore, the key is differential thinning of the subcutaneous layer, typically accessed through established external scars. In doing this, the surgeon must account for the thicker soft tissue zones of the nasal tip, ala, and nasion and the thinner tissues over the dorsum and sidewalls. More extensive subcutaneous sculpting along the nasal dorsum and sidewalls is necessary to fully define the naso-orbital and dorsal profile lines.

In preparation for this procedure, the amount of injected local anesthetic should be minimized, with adequate time allowed for absorption to avoid distorting the tissues. A marking pen is used to outline essential topographic landmarks, such as the tip-defining points, alar grooves, dorsal profile lines, nasofacial junction lines, and the curvilinear naso-orbital lines. When present, the contralateral, uninvolved landmarks are used as references. Surface templates can be created to accurately define the matched counterparts on the opposite side. Existing scars should be used for incisions. Skin flaps are elevated in the superficial subcutaneous tissue plane. Volume reduction is accomplished with a No. 11 scalpel blade in a graded fashion by removing thin layers parallel to the skin surface and repetitively assessing surface contour change. To minimize the potential for dermal dimpling, subcutaneous atrophy, and excessive scar tissue response, cauterization should be conservative. Temporary basting sutures, Steri-strip reinforcement, and external splints are helpful for skin redraping in these cases.

Re-Creation of the Alar Crease

The alar crease represents an important visual transition between two anatomically distinct subcomponents of the nose: the nasal ala and the lateral sidewall. When the nasal defect involves both of these regions, flap reconstruction typically obliterates the alar crease. Reestablishing this landmark is best done by a direct incision, rather than by subcutaneous thinning and burying deep sutures. To determine the position and length of the crease, the contralateral alar groove is ink-marked onto a Telfa pad, along with the alar rim and the alar-facial junction. The template is then reversed and tattooed on the side to be sculpted. After incising skin along the alar crease line, a superficial skin flap is elevated caudally for about 5 mm and then cephalically for whatever distance is necessary to provide access for subcutaneous debulking (Fig. 14–41). At this point, subcutaneous tissue is thinned along the lower lateral sidewall and immediately deep to the alar crease, near the level of the lower lateral cartilage (or its graft replacement). Following hemostasis, a three-point suture technique is used that captures both skin edges and the deeper tissue along the alar crease (Fig. 14–42). In this way, a controlled depression (groove) is created that varies with the degree of subcutaneous thinning along the alar crease. As the depth of the crease lessens from the alar-facial junction toward the nasal tip, differential thinning must be employed to achieve symmetry and balance with the contralateral side.

Re-Creation of the Alar-Facial Junction

The alar-facial junction may be blunted following certain procedures for alar reconstruction, including the melolabial island flap. In order to recreate the alar-facial junction, the subcutaneous pedicle must be debulked and the free alar and upper lip skin edges invaginated. Prior to this refinement, however, it is essential that the alar base be positioned properly. Calipers can be used to measure the columellar-alar angle and the distance between the alar base and vermillion border to aid in determining the amount of correction necessary. It is equally important to preserve the proper position of the triangular junction of the superiormost upper lip subunit with the alar base.

After mobilizing the alar subunit skin from its attachments to the cheek and upper lip skin, subcutaneous undermining and debulking of the alar lobule are accomplished through lateral exposure (Fig. 14–43). Caliper measurements of alar rim thickness, based on a contralateral intact side (if present), may help guide the dissection. Closure, as described for alar crease reconstruction, is begun at the apex of the upper lip subunit and proceeds inferomedially around the alar

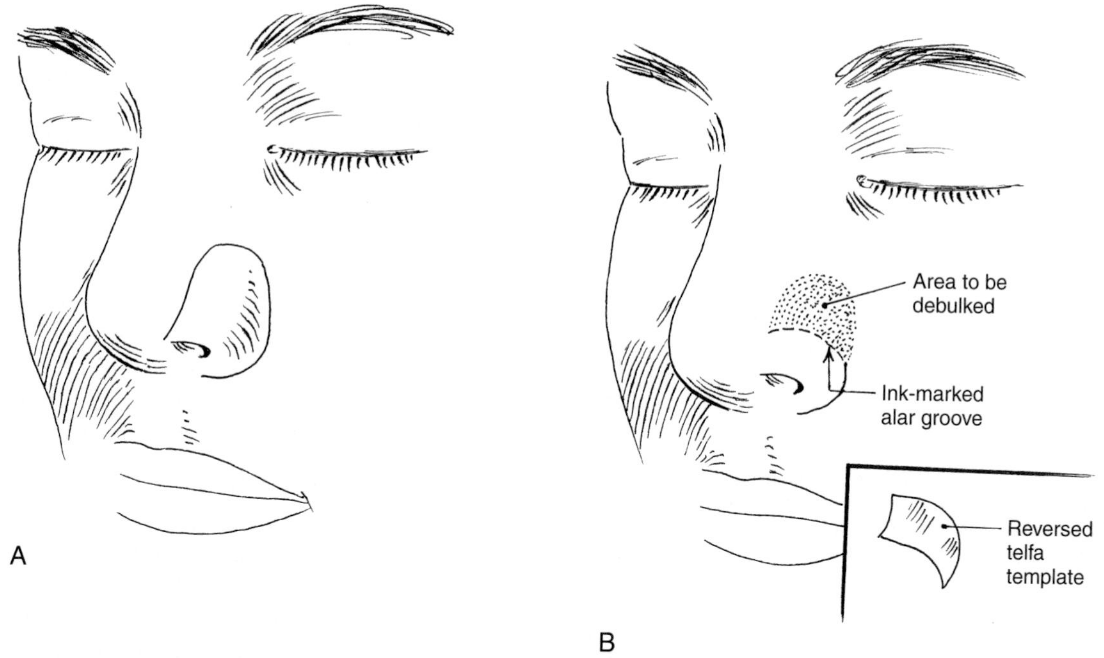

Figure 14–41. Re-creation of the alar crease with debulking and recontouring of the nasal sidewall. *A,* A bulky alar subunit without a defined crease following flap reconstruction. *B,* A template from the contralateral side is reversed to define the alar subunit anatomy and crease position.

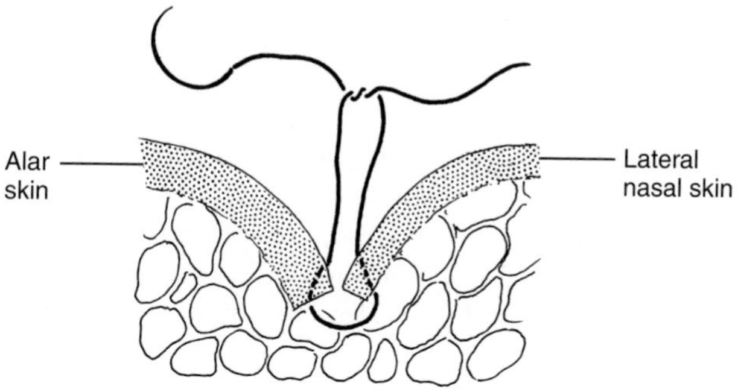

Figure 14–42. Creating a skin crease. The three-point suture technique is used to invaginate the skin edges along an anatomic junction line to create the skin crease.

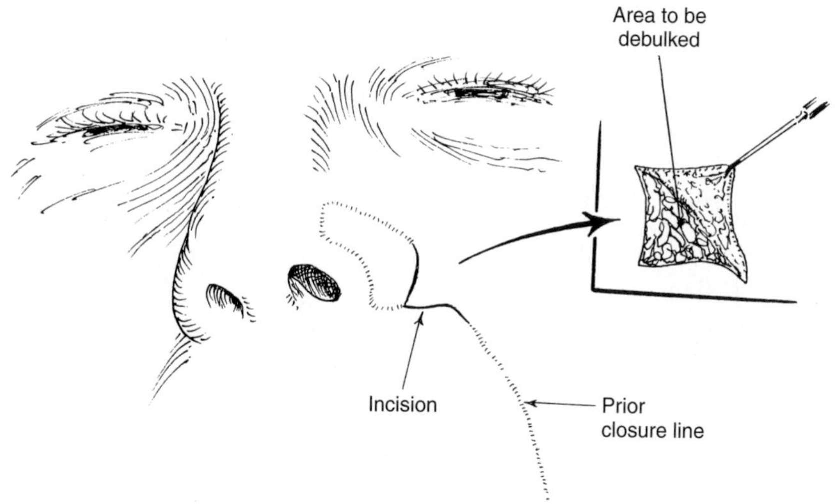

Figure 14–43. Second-stage division and inset following melolabial island transfer. The first step is to elevate the triangular skin paddle at the alar-facial incision. The subcutaneous tissue is then debulked to create the proper alar-facial contour. The cheek tissue is then advanced to the alar crease and the triangular skin paddle trimmed to lie in the alar crease.

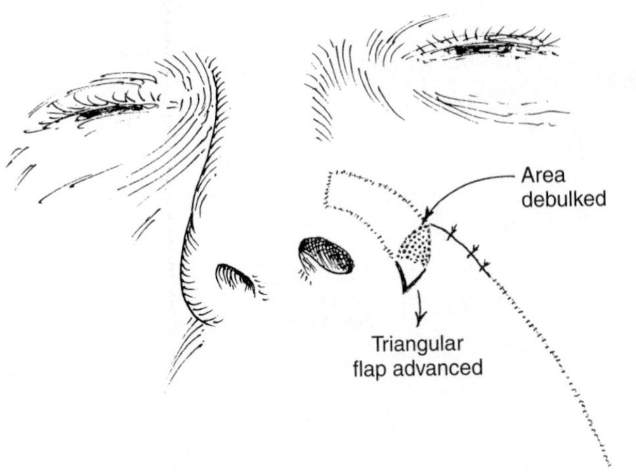

Figure 14–44. Second-stage division and inset following melolabial island flap. The final steps in the procedure are to advance a second triangular skin flap at the inferior margin of the ala near the nasal sill and to resect redundant tissue.

lobule. Upon reaching a point close to the nasal sill, skin redundancy is created on the alar rim. To correct this, a short back-cut is made along the free edge of the alar rim near its base (Fig. 14–44). Skin edges are next overlapped, a wedge excision is made of the redundant tissue, and the rim edges are closed with 6-0 nylon suture. Finally, the skin edges of the medial cheek are approximated along the melolabial crease using a similar technique as described for alar groove closures.

Correction of the Alar Notch

The most common cause of alar notching is inadequate or unreliable lining flaps. It may also result from inadequate bracing of the alar rim with cartilage grafts or poorly designed cover flaps. To correct this deformity, skin and cartilage must be added to the ala to counterbalance the forces of wound contraction. Chondrocutaneous composite grafting of the nasal vestibule, following internal release of the alar rim, has been described by Ellenbogen[9] (Fig. 14–45). Although frequently successful in a postrhinoplasty revision, application of this approach to an already reconstructed nose is less predictable. An alternative approach, described by Millard[10] (Fig. 14–46), involves transposition of a caudally based chondromucosal flap from the contralateral nasal vestibule. Following wide tunneling over the anterior septal angle and cartilaginous release at the base of the flap, tension-free insetting into the recipient bed becomes possible.

Occasionally, enough skin cover and internal lining are present that, following alar debulking and undermining (via rim incision), both flaps can be advanced caudally to compensate for the retracted distance. Cartilaginous bracing of the alar rim, between the nasal tip and alar base, will be necessary to prevent recurrence of the deformity. Gently tied transcutaneous sutures that capture the alar batten are helpful in maintaining rim contour, particularly at the original notched position.

Thinning of the Alar Rim

Commonly, following either melolabial island or paramedian forehead flap reconstruction involving the alar subunit, an alar thinning procedure must be performed to reestablish symmetry. Through a marginal incision along its free border, the alar rim may be thinned or lifted. If rim position is good but simply too thick, an internal wedge excision, determined by caliper measurement, is made (Fig. 14–47). Excision of the excess subcu-

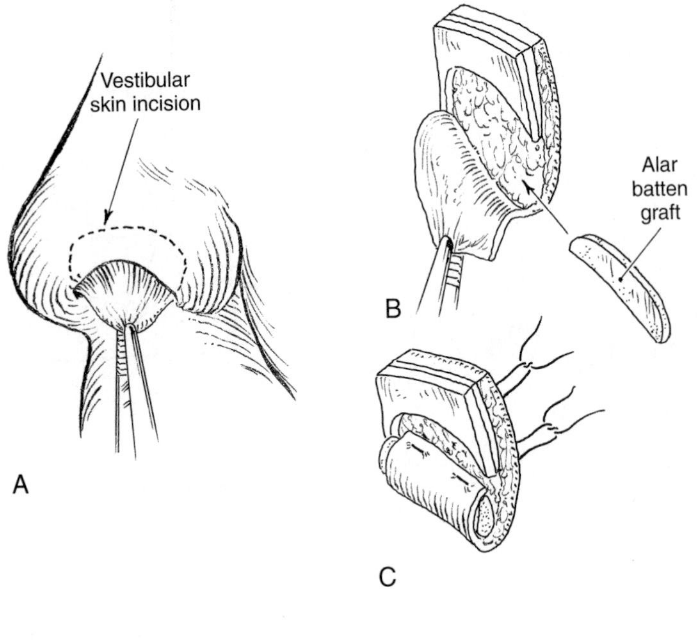

Figure 14–45. Correction of a retracted alar rim. The internal lining is released and an alar batten graft is placed. The graft is secured with transcutaneous mattress sutures.

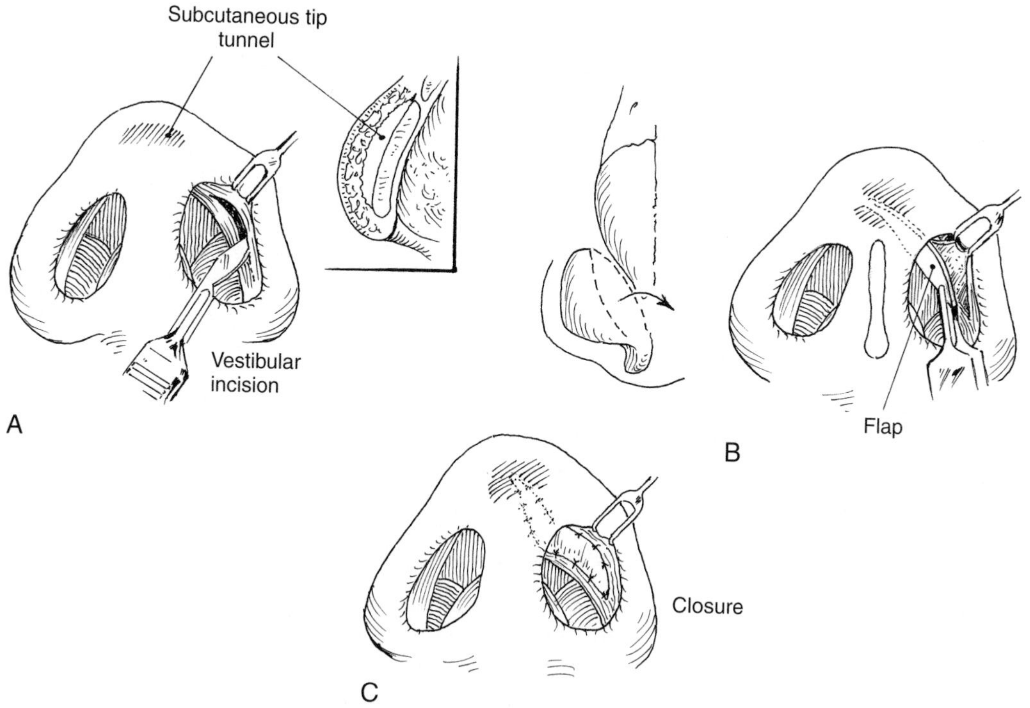

Figure 14–46. A chondromucosal lower lateral cartilage flap may be used to correct a vestibular lining shortage. *A,* An incision is made in the vestibular skin and the soft tissues are separated. A pocket across the nasal tip is tunneled. *B,* The caudally based composite skin and cartilage flap are developed contralaterally and transposed over the anterior septal angle into the recipient site. *C,* Final appearance after closure.

taneous tissue is accomplished with a No. 11 blade. This should proceed over, and not through, previously placed cartilaginous grafts so as not to compromise supportive function. Meticulous and conservative hemostasis is critical in avoiding the undesirable sequela of hematoma.

If the intent is to elevate the rim, as well as to thin it, an external wedge excision should be marked out using the contralateral kidney-bean shape of the intact nostril as a guide (Fig. 14–48). The intended position of the apex of the reconstructed nostril and the width

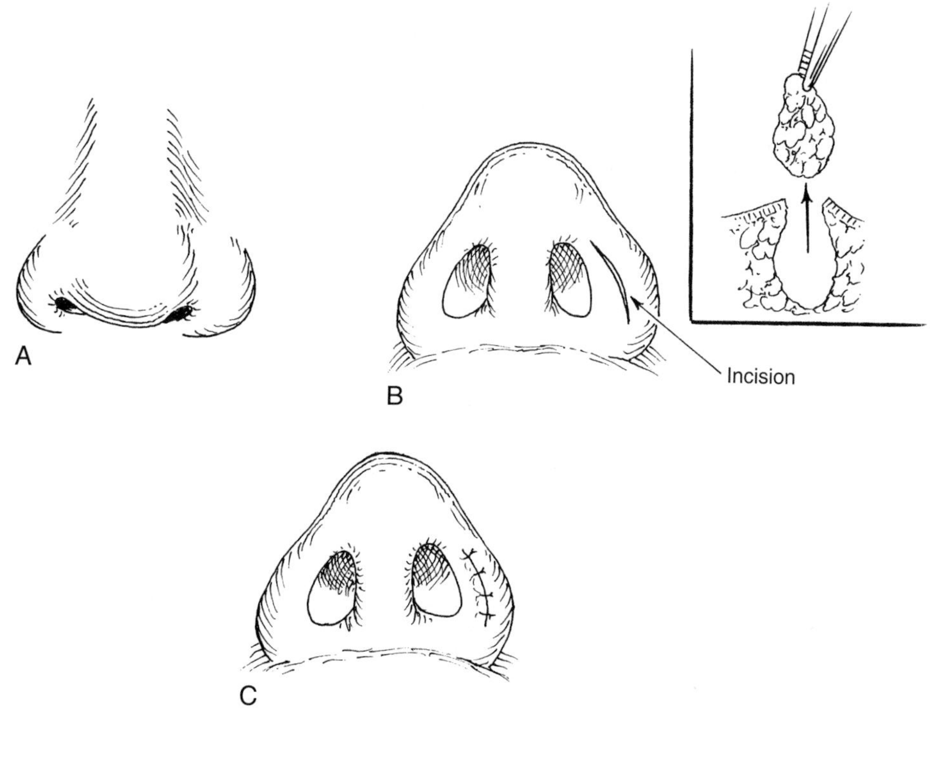

Figure 14–47. Correction of alar rim thickness asymmetry when the rim position is acceptable. *A,* An overly thick alar rim can be seen on the left side. *B,* A linear skin incision is made on the inferior edge of the rim and an internal soft tissue wedge is excised. No skin is excised. *C,* Final result after closure.

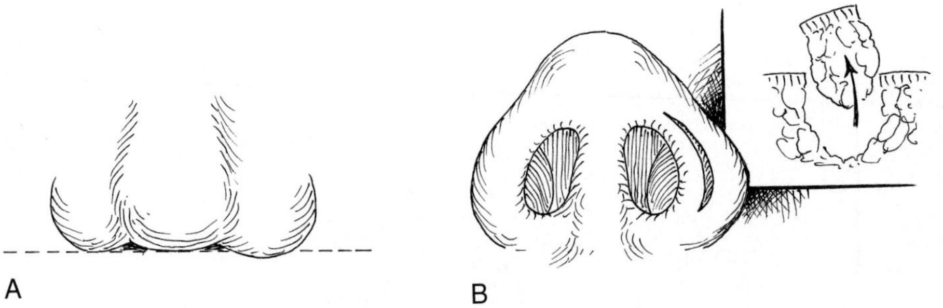

Figure 14–48. Correction of alar rim thickness asymmetry when the alar rim position is too low. *A,* Demonstration of an overly thick and inferiorly positioned alar rim. *B,* Removal of a crescent-shaped wedge of skin and soft tissue simultaneously thins and elevates the rim following closure.

of the nostril at the midpoint are determined. Basal and profile views from both sides are helpful in planning the reconstruction. A 6-0 nylon suture is used for skin closure, after which internal packing and external tape splinting is maintained for 1 week.

Correction of Alar Base Malposition

The appropriate position of the alar base can easily be determined by taking measurements. The distance from the midline to the alar-facial junction determines the alar base width. The distance from the vermillion-cutaneous junction to the alar-labial groove defines the vertical alar base position. The latter reference point assumes there has been no distortion of the upper lip. A template obtained from an intact contralateral upper lip is a useful reference in determining the alar base relationships.

Medial or lateral repositioning of the ala can be achieved by applying the Z-plasty principle. For the medially displaced ala, an inferiorly based skin flap can be transposed from a position lateral to the alar base into the nasal sill (Fig. 14–49). The raw area from which the flap was transposed then becomes the platform for the newly positioned ala. The width of the flap created determines the transverse distance acquired in the repositioning. Conversely, for the laterally displaced ala, an inferiorly based flap from the nasal sill can be transposed lateral to the alar base. Given the narrow flap widths and random blood supply to these flaps, precise and atraumatic handling of these tissues is essential.

Surface Enhancement

Despite one's best efforts at flap closure, surface contour irregularities along closure lines can develop. These may result from partial wound dehiscences, suture granulomas, stitch abscesses, or wound contraction. These problems tend to occur most often in patients with thick, sebaceous, or dark skin. Following a 4- to 6-month period of wound maturation, either spot dermabrasion or CO_2 laser resurfacing can be offered to improve surface aesthetics. Owing to the risk of hyperpigmentation, it is recommended that patients use sunscreens (SPF 30 or greater) and avoid unprotected direct sun exposure for 3 months.

COMPLICATIONS

Complications following nasal reconstruction can result from errors of commission, omission, or underlying comorbid factors that cannot be controlled. Wound healing, as it relates to local tissue perfusion, is influenced by smoking, atherosclerotic vascular disease, dia-

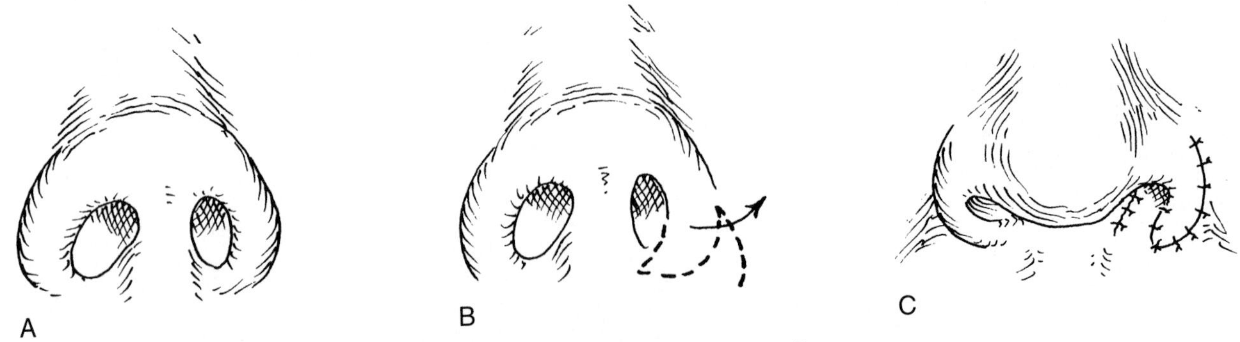

Figure 14–49. Alar base repositioning. *A,* A medially displaced left rim with small nares. *B,* Design of a double Z-plasty with the medial transposition of the skin lateral to the alar base. *C,* The final result after closure shows expansion of the vestibule and lateralization of the alar-facial attachment.

betes mellitus, a history of irradiation to the tissue bed, and certain collagen vascular disorders. Protein malnutrition, as well as trace metal and ascorbic acid deficiencies, can delay the quality and extent of collagen formation and maturation. Prior surgeries at the sites of graft or flap harvest, existing fistulas, or areas of prior trauma may lead to tenuous, unreliable tissues for reconstruction. Careful preoperative planning is essential if one is to minimize the risk of operative failure. At the very least, smoking should be discontinued 3 or more weeks before and after surgery, hypertension should be controlled, and nutritional status should be optimized to the extent possible. To minimize the risks of intraoperative/postoperative bleeding, aspirin therapy should be discontinued 10 to 14 days prior to surgery, most nonsteroidal anti-inflammatory agents (i.e., ibuprofen, naproxen) should be discontinued 3 to 5 days preoperatively, and coumadin should be discontinued 3 to 4 days prior to surgery. Delicate tissue handling, conservative use of cauterization, layered closures, obliteration of dead space, preparation of recipient sites, and thoughtful selection of donor tissues are all important aspects of the surgical plan. Some aspects of postoperative complications relative to specific flaps have already been discussed in earlier sections of this chapter. The following is a more general discussion of some of the most common problems.

Hematoma

Hematoma formation is most likely to occur in patients with labile or poorly controlled hypertension, those receiving anticoagulants or platelet inhibitors, and patients in whom flap harvesting has resulted in extensive undermining. The use of epinephrine with the local anesthetic may camouflage areas of expectant bleeding. Hematomas are often heralded by progressive pain, swelling, skin discoloration, and bleeding at the suture margins. Large hematomas require urgent reexploration to identify and control the source of bleeding. Afterward, a drain may be placed and a pressure dressing applied if feasible. Small hematomas that are confined and not expanding can often be evacuated by removing several sutures, by making a stab incision over the hematoma, or possibly, by aspiration.

Infection

The uncommon occurrence of localized infections following nasal reconstruction is classically attributed to the robust blood supply of the face. Nonetheless, in those patients with poorly controlled diabetes, poorly prepared recipient beds with retained foreign body material, or extensive localized tissue trauma (i.e., overzealous cauterization), this risk factor increases. Patients with oily, sebaceous, and thick skin are at increased risk for cellulitis following surgery. This condition may be attributable to increased surface colonization with gram-positive and anaerobic bacteria. For these patients in particular, the author's preference is to administer perioperative prophylactic antibiotics. Appropriate management of infection involves draining any purulence, instituting saline irrigation, prescribing culture-directed antibiotic therapy, and applying warm compresses. If the patient fails to improve within 48 to 72 hours, or if there are clinical signs of disease progression, consideration of intravenous antibiotics is warranted.

Partial Flap Losses

Partial flap losses most commonly result from localized ischemia with progression to necrosis. They may be attributable to either poor flap design, excessive closure tension, infection, or overly aggressive or untimely recontouring procedures. Flap design problems may be related to one of several technical errors. These include failure to incorporate the vascular base of an axial-patterned flap (e.g., a paramedian flap with supratrochlear vessels), failure to delay the random component of an axial flap (e.g., an oblique forehead flap), failure to capture sufficient perforating vessels supplying a directionally oriented random flap (e.g., a subcutaneous melolabial island flap), or direct injury to the dermal plexus of any pedicled flap (e.g., overaggressive thinning of the distal end of paramedian flap).

Excessive closure tension can usually be recognized intraoperatively when loss of capillary refill is seen over a broad portion of the flap. The use of epinephrine, however, may mask this finding. The safest course of action in this case is to remove the necessary number of sutures and mobilize the flap further, or to consider delayed secondary closure. Infectious complications leading to partial flap loss should be treated conservatively by delaying debridement until demarcation between viable and unviable tissue is clear. The degree and extent of debulking and recontouring at the time of second-stage flap division and inset are inversely proportionate to donor-recipient edge contact (the surface area supporting the dermal plexus). That is, the larger the area of the flap that has healed in, the smaller the portion of the devascularized pedicle that must be resected after division. Conversely, the smaller the flap area that is healed in, the greater the portion of the pedicle that must be excised. In all cases of recontouring, it is imperative that the closure lines from original flap insetting remain undisturbed.

Management of partial tissue losses for a given flap will depend on the extent of loss, the location of the loss, the potential for secondary deformities consequent to wound contraction, and the tissues available for repair. In general, these problems are approached conservatively, allowing 3 to 4 months to elapse before revision procedures. This allows sufficient time for reepithelialization of the defect, establishment of collateral blood flow, and tissue recovery from surgical trauma.

Total Flap Loss

Total flap loss is exceedingly rare; when it does occur, it is almost always a result of technical error. The following are examples of how this might occur. The most common cause of total flap loss is failure to capture the vascular axis of the flap. During the harvest of a nasalis flap, another cause may be injury to the alar arterial branches as they enter the nasalis muscle. This can occur from aggressive submuscular mobilization and cauterization. Also, extensive back-cuts in the medial canthal and distal aspects of the axial frontonasal advancement-rotation flap can compromise the supportive vasculature (infratrochlear or angular artery) at the point of flap attachment.

In the case of a total flap loss, it is best to debride the flap completely and proceed with a second flap option. For instance, in the case of a paramedian flap, the contralateral side may be used, with the same tissue quality advantages. A nasalis flap could likely be salvaged with a bilobe flap, or a frontonasal flap with a paramedian forehead flap. Under these circumstances, surgeons should avoid the natural tendency of "cutting their losses" by using a technique that is simpler or "less risky" (e.g., a skin graft) for fear of another bad outcome. The patient will be grateful for a properly executed technique that affords optimal reconstruction, even at additional donor site morbidity. Proper patient counseling, patience, and thoughtful delivery of an alternative flap are likely to yield the greatest degree of satisfaction for both patient and surgeon.

Unsightly Scars

Given that the patients who undergo nasal reconstruction are most commonly elderly people with skin cancer, most scars heal quite acceptably. Elderly patients have increased skin laxity, deep skin creases and furrows, and are, in general, less critical of the scarring. However, in younger patients, in those with thick, oily, sebaceous complexions, or when excessive closure tension is required, hypertrophic scar formation is possible. In these cases, conservative efforts using intralesional steroid injections, silicone gel sheeting or cream, massage, and passage of time are usually helpful. After an appropriate interval (6 to 9 months), if the patient is still dissatisfied, scar revision can be undertaken. In the forehead, a regular W-plasty, which maximizes placement of the majority of the scar close to the ideal relaxation skin tension lines, is preferred. Scars on the nose usually respond to direct excision, readvancement, and planned dermabrasion at a later date. Every scar revision should attempt to place closure lines along anatomic junction lines, subunit excision lines, or relaxed skin tension lines.

Stitch Abscesses

Stitch abscesses are most commonly seen in thick, excessively oily skin, and theoretically should be associated more often with the use of multifilamentous suture material, which can trap bacteria within the interstices. Suture material that has a slow resorption rate, and is, therefore, likely to elicit a foreign body reaction, may also carry this risk. Proper skin preparation, consideration of prophylactic antibiotics for those with higher-risk skin types, and early stitch removal should help minimize the risk of stitch abscess. When such an abscess does occur, treatment involves removing the stitch, if possible, evacuating any purulent contents, and applying topical antibiotic ointment.

Suture Granulomas

Suture granulomas can often be recognized by a "string of beads" appearance along the closure line several weeks to months after surgery. Intralesional steroid injections (Kenalog-20), massage, and time often lead to improvement. When resolution does not occur, consideration can be given to direct excision and reclosure using a deep layer closure material that can be absorbed rapidly.

Wound Dehiscence

Wound dehiscence may occur from suture breakage (excessive tension, expanding hematoma, etc.), flap-edge necrosis, or comorbid effects that compromise wound healing. Treatment strategy should focus on correcting identifiable causes and reclosing the wound. Specific attention should be given to freshening the edges to healthy tissue, deep layer support favoring eversion, and gentle tissue handling.

Contour Imbalance

The most commonly encountered contour imbalances in nasal reconstruction are trapdoor deformities and excessive bulging of convex subunits reconstructed with regional flaps. The preferred treatment for these entities is to wait 3 to 4 months and then revise by wide undermining, liposculpturing, and placement of basting sutures. Trapdoor deformities may also benefit from careful cross-hatching of the undersurface of the flap (micro Z-plasty) and planned postoperative steroid injections.

REFERENCES

1. Gonzalez-Ulloa M. Restoration of the face covering by means of selected skin in regional aesthetic units. Br J Plast Surg 9:212, 1957.
2. Burget GC, Menick FJ. Nasal support and lining: The marriage of beauty and blood supply. Plast Reconstr Surg 84:189, 1989.
3. de Quervain F. Ueber Partielle Sietliche Rhinoplastik. Zentralbl Chir 29:297, 1902.
4. Esser JFS. Gestielte lokale Nasenplastik mit Zweizipfligem lappen Deckung des Sekundaren Detektes vom ersten Zipfel durch den Zweiten. Dtsch Z Chir 143:385, 1918.
5. Zimany A. The bilobed flap. Plast Reconstr Surg 11:424, 1953.
6. Zitelli JA. The bilobed flap for nasal reconstruction. Arch Dermatol 125:957, 1989.
7. Rieger RA. A local flap for repair of the nasal tip. Plast Reconstr Surg 40:147, 1967.
8. Millard DR. Various uses of the septum in rhinoplasty. Plast Reconstr Surg 81:112, 1988.
9. Ellenbogen R. Alar rim lowering. Plast Reconstr Surg 79:50, 1987.
10. Millard DR. The versatility of a chondromucosal flap in the nasal vestibule. Plast Reconstr Surg 50:580, 1972.

CHAPTER 15

Trauma

GENERAL CONSIDERATIONS

Evaluation of the Trauma Patient

Most patients who sustain a fracture of the nose or sinuses will initially present to an emergency room for evaluation. In the emergency department, the patient will undergo an initial assessment that will include stabilization of the airway, breathing, and circulation. Facial trauma, when severe, may cause significant airway compromise. Owing to loss of support of the facial skeleton, blood in the airway, and altered mental status, immediate control of the airway may be necessary. In this situation, the patient is invariably also at risk for cervical spine injury, intracranial injury, thoracic and abdominal injuries, and circulatory collapse from blood loss.[1, 2] Complete coverage of the management of the acute phase of trauma is beyond the scope of this book. However, this is a vitally important consideration in the management of the severely injured patient with facial trauma, and a specific protocol to manage this situation should be part of every emergency department's preparations.

In addition to emergency management of the patient, patients with facial trauma may have need of urgent management for bleeding, cerebrospinal fluid (CSF) leak, and facial lacerations. Epistaxis from acute facial trauma usually stops spontaneously within the first minutes to hours after the injury. However, in severe cases, bleeding may be profuse, flowing into a compromised airway, or affecting a patient with altered mental status. In these cases, acute management may be achieved with either a large nasal tampon or a transnasal Foley catheter with an anterior nasal pack. Detailed discussion of control of epistaxis will be covered in Chapter 22.

Management of CSF rhinorrhea will be covered in Chapter 20. In summary, the acute management of this problem in a trauma patient is usually conservative. Initially, bed rest with the head of the bed elevated, stool softeners, and antitussives are recommended. If, after 5 to 7 days, the leak is persistent, lumbar drainage can be considered. Surgical intervention is reserved for refractory cases and is never done in the first days after diagnosis.

Facial lacerations should, whenever possible, be repaired immediately in the emergency room. The basic principle for repair of these lacerations is to conserve tissue when possible and to perform primary closure.[3] Careful technique should be used to ensure accurate realignment of the skin edges and avoidance of trapdoors and step-offs. Secondary revision of poor outcomes is always possible, but in most circumstances, will not be necessary.

After the initial evaluation of the patient is completed, a secondary screening is conducted. At this time, it is appropriate to begin the evaluation of the facial injury. In many circumstances, the facial injury will be the only significant injury or the most significant injury. In this situation, the evaluation of the facial trauma can take priority. In cases when associated injuries are present, the facial trauma evaluation will have to be coordinated with the remainder of the patient's care. Two of the most important associated injuries to assess before prioritizing the facial trauma are intracranial injury and injury of the cervical spine. Any patient who has been hit hard enough to sustain a facial fracture is at risk for these more life-threatening injuries. Often, a computed tomography (CT) scan of the brain and a cervical spine series are performed before the facial trauma specialist is called to evaluate the patient. If this has not been performed, the patient should at least be questioned and examined to determine the likelihood of these associated injuries.[4–6]

Once the facial injuries are evaluated, a routine history and examination may be performed. Important historical points that may affect the management of the patient should be discussed, including previous facial trauma, serious medical illnesses, bleeding tendency, and history of sinusitis. The physical examination should document obvious visible deformities, swelling, ecchymosis, and lacerations. Careful palpation of all facial bones is performed, locating any areas of tenderness or step-offs. A systematic, complete head and neck examination should be also performed. Attention should also be given to the ophthalmologic examination, including an evaluation of visual acuity, extraocular motions, pupillary responses, and ocular adnexa. The presence of abnormal findings on the screening eye examination should prompt urgent ophthalmologic consultation. A complete examination of the condition of the dentition, occlusion, jaw opening, and mobility of the maxilla should also be done. Finally, an assessment of the cranial nerves, including an evaluation of facial motion and sensation, is necessary.

Following the examination, it is usually possible to predict the presence and pattern of facial fractures. However, radiologic evaluation is routinely used to diagnose the injury and plan treatment. Emergency room physicians often request plain radiographs. However, traditional plain radiographs offer little more than a screening examination in the modern practice of facial trauma surgery. By identifying blood in the maxillary sinus, the Waters view can suggest an acute fracture. Similarly, blood or opacification in the frontal sinus suggests a fracture. Conversely, plain radiographs are notoriously unreliable in diagnosing acute nasal fracture.

By contrast, CT scanning is extremely useful.[7–10] To be of maximal use, the scan is performed in both axial and coronal planes with bone and soft tissue algorithms. The scan should be obtained as early as possible, before traumatic edema sets in. CT scans will accurately delineate the pattern of fracture and the degree of comminution. For this reason, it has become the standard of care in most communities to obtain a CT scan before repairing almost any facial fracture. Three-dimensional reconstructions of CT scans have become available in recent years.[11] These scans depict the facial skeletal anatomy in a three-dimensional format that allows the surgeon to view the fractures as if holding the skull in their hands. The value of these costly and high tech scans is difficult to ascertain. However, in certain cases, the three-dimensional image can enhance the physician's understanding of the fracture. The most likely scenario in which three-dimensional reconstructions would be helpful is in patients with complex fracture patterns with significant comminution.

Surgical Timing

After a significant fracture requiring surgical intervention is identified, the operation needs to be scheduled. The timing of surgical repair is flexible for most facial fractures. One notable exception, however, is the open frontal sinus fracture, which implies a combination of a full-thickness laceration in communication with an anterior wall fracture. In this situation, there is a risk of severe contamination of the sinus. The laceration should be repaired immediately in the emergency department. The repair of the frontal sinus fracture can then be performed when the patient is stabilized, fully evaluated, and cleared for surgery. If there is a significant delay in repairing the fracture, it is important to evaluate the laceration before proceeding. Local infection in the forehead flap can lead to a high risk of postoperative complications. In this instance, the surgery should be postponed until soft tissue healing is complete.

For most fractures, delayed elective repair is preferred. This allows the acute swelling to subside. The advantage of delay is that facial symmetry and normal contours can be better assessed when the edema is minimal. Also, these cases may be lengthy, and delaying the procedure facilitates scheduling. The theoretical disadvantage to delayed repair is an increased incidence of infectious complications. Facial fracture repairs, as a general class of operations, are associated with a low infection rate. It has never been clearly established that prophylactic antibiotic therapy or early surgery is beneficial. With the possible exceptions of mandible fractures and open frontal sinus fractures, early repair is an elective option.

Despite the advantages of delaying surgery to allow edema to resolve, the natural healing of the injury may prompt the surgeon to consider prompt intervention. The longer the delay, the greater the amount of fibrosis that will set in, and this can impair the operative mobilization of the fracture fragments. A general guideline is that surgery should be performed within 3 weeks of the date of injury; otherwise, osteotomies may need to be performed to mobilize the fractures.

Fixation Systems

Recent advances in fixation technology have greatly improved the management of nasal and sinus trauma. Today, the surgeon has the choice of utilizing traditional wiring techniques, mesh, or a variety of plating systems. Wiring is now used only rarely. It can be applied to virtually any fracture repair. However, the only cases when wiring is preferred are comminuted fractures or when precise alignment is not possible and postoperative manipulation may be necessary. Comminuted fractures may be best pieced together using wires. When the fracture segments are particularly small and numerous, they may become free floating. Plating will not allow stabilization of these types of bone fragments. However, thin-gauge wire threaded through small drill holes can be used to align and stabilize even the smallest fragments. With wires in place, it may also be possible to achieve some degree of postsurgical closed reduction to refine the result. If the alignment is not completely satisfactory, some manipulation of the wired bone fragments may be performed. In practice, however, postoperative manipulation is not a common occurrence.

Mesh and fixation plates are, by far, the most common materials used for fracture repair today. Both the mesh and plates are available in stainless steel and titanium. Of the two, titanium is the newer product and is favored because of its increased malleability and biocompatibility. The malleability is the most important advantage, as this allows the plate or mesh to be molded to the desired shape easily and rapidly. Mesh comes in various thicknesses, screw sizes, and mesh sizes. The best to use in a particular case will depend on the size and thickness of the bone fragments. The larger and thicker the fragments, the larger the mesh size and screw size applicable. The mesh systems are preferred mainly for comminuted fractures of the anterior wall of the maxillary or frontal sinuses.

A variety of plating systems are also available. Each system comes with a variety of plate shapes and sizes. Several manufacturers have marketed plating sets that include three different sizes of plates in a single system, each with an assortment of shapes. The plate sizes are classified as micro (1.0 mm), mini (1.5 mm), and standard (2.0 mm). The size measurement refers to the diameter of the screw. These modern systems come with self-tapping screws that do not require the drill holes to be prethreaded with a tapping device. Because of the versatility and ease of application of these systems, plating has become the preferred technique for almost all facial fractures.

NASAL FRACTURE

The nasal bones are the most commonly fractured bones in the face.[12, 13] Owing to their projection from the face, the nasal bones are a natural target for all manner of accidental injuries. The nature of the object causing the injury, the force applied, and the direction of the blow to the nose will determine the specifics of the individual fracture. The physics of the mechanism of injury can be described in detail in terms of the mass, velocity, size, and hardness of the object causing the injury. Regardless of the mechanism, though, management will be based on careful diagnosis of the extent of injury in the individual patient. The fracture may be managed by a variety of techniques, including closed nasal reduction, closed nasal reduction with buttresses, open reduction, and delayed secondary reconstruction (rhinoplasty).

The specific nature of an individual fracture will vary greatly from one patient to the next. As described earlier, there are numerous variables contributing to the end result. A broad, flat object will tend to spread the force of impact over a larger surface area, causing the bones to break at areas of weakness along the suture lines. Conversely, small, sharp objects transfer force to a smaller area, leading to fractures directly under the area of impact. The degree of comminution will be related to the amount of force applied during the injury. Any factor that increases the force of impact will tend to increase the degree of comminution.

During an injury, the nasal bones will be fractured away from the object causing the injury. For example, a straight-on impact to the nasal dorsum will fracture the bones inward, flattening the nasal dorsum. Blows from the side will displace the dorsum to the side opposite the impact. As the force of the impact increases, the amount of displacement and degree of comminution will increase. In certain situations, such as altercations or car accidents, multiple blows to the nose are possible, resulting in compound or combination injuries. However, because most fractures involve a single impact, the two most common patterns of injury are the flattened dorsum and the deviated dorsum.

Diagnosis

The diagnosis of acute nasal fracture is suggested by appropriate history, but is made on physical examination. The history of a severe blow to the nose followed by epistaxis usually denotes an acute nasal fracture. Patients often describe "seeing stars," but actual loss of consciousness is unlikely. On examination, the patient will usually manifest swelling of the nose and orbit, ecchymosis, and tenderness. These findings are nonspecific. The presence of fracture is indicated by detection of step-offs, mobility, or gross deformity of the nasal bones. Initial examination must also assess the associated facial trauma and internal nasal injuries. The most likely associated injuries include orbital fractures and nasal orbital ethmoid fractures. Orbital fractures should be considered when there is orbital rim step-off, abnormal ophthalmologic examination, or suggestive radiographic findings. Nasal orbital ethmoid fractures are suggested by blunting of the medial canthus or apparent telecanthus.

The first goals of intranasal examination are to remove blood clots, decongest the nose, and control epistaxis. The nose should be evaluated for septal lacerations, deviations, protruding fragments, CSF leak, and septal hematoma. Acute injuries to the septum are usually managed by nasal packing or decongestants. The exception to this is a septal hematoma.

The presence of septal hematoma must be definitively excluded. Hematoma is suggested by edema or enlargement of the septum which, on palpation with an applicator, is soft and compressible.[14] If septal hematoma is present, immediate drainage of the blood is essential. This is accomplished through an incision in the mucosa over the hematoma.[15] The blood is suctioned out and the cavity is compressed with intranasal splints or packing. Alternatively, the hematoma space can be drained with a wick of strip gauze. The consequences of failure to treat the septal hematoma can include septal abscess, perforation, and saddle nose. The key to prevention of these complications is recognition at the time of injury and prompt adequate treatment.

After completing the physical examination, the nature of the injury should be well delineated. Simple nasal fractures without associated injuries do not require further evaluation, and a decision on repair can be delayed until some of the swelling has resolved. Typically, patients in this category will be seen back in the office or clinic for follow-up examination after 5 to 7 days. At this point, the swelling should be largely resolved and an assessment of the need for operative repair can be made.

In the case of complicated nasal fracture with possible associated fractures, additional information can be helpful in planning the course of management. In this setting, radiographic studies are typically requested. Plain radiographs, including a classic sinus series with a specific lateral nasal view, will provide only limited information and lack precision and specificity. The alternative is CT scanning. Although not usually required for nasal fracture evaluation, in cases of complex fractures or suspected associated fractures CT studies will best demonstrate the anatomy of the injuiry.

Indications for Surgery

The indications for surgery are fairly straightforward in the case of nasal fracture. Repair is recommended whenever there is a functional or cosmetic deformity. Except in the case of the nondisplaced nasal fracture, this includes virtually all other injuries. The issues surrounding nasal fracture can usually be considered separately in deciding whether corrective intervention is warranted. When nasal fracture results in nasal obstruction, either from deviation of the septum or collapse of the lateral nasal wall, correction of the problem is indicated. Straightening of the nasal septum is most effectively achieved by traditional septoplasty. This can be accomplished as soon as the swelling from the acute injury subsides, generally 7 to 14 days after the injury. The alternative is to attempt closed reduction.

Closed reduction of septal deviation has been described and supported by various surgeons.[16–18] In the author's experience, though, this has proven unsatisfactory for several reasons. Firstly, the degree of correction is often not as good as can be expected from septoplasty. Second, preexisting septal deviations are cause for some uncertainty as to what can and cannot be bluntly corrected. Finally, the act of forcing the septum back into the midline with blunt manipulation is very rough on the nasal mucosa and can lead to abrasions, lacerations, and adhesions in the nose. For these reasons, a septal deviation is usually repaired by septoplasty. The technique is described in detail in Chapter 12.

The cosmetic alterations that result from nasal fracture range from subtle to overt. The most important factor in evaluating these injuries is to allow sufficient time for the acute edema to resovle before judging the extent of the disfigurement. Edema may accentuate the injury, causing a nondisplaced fracture to appear asymmetrical, or it may minimize a significant deformity by hiding the bony deflection under a swollen soft tissue covering. For this reason, repair should not be scheduled before a second evaluation at least 5 days after the injury. An exception to this would be patients with severe open fractures in which bone fragments are protruding through the skin. In these patients, immediate reduction and skin closure are necessary to avoid infection. In the more common case, when a laceration overlies a fracture but no bone is extruded, the skin should be closed initially and the fracture addressed in a delayed fashion as otherwise indicated.

The final decision as to whether to repair a nasal fracture for purely cosmetic reasons will always rest with the patient. In most situations, the patient will want the fracture reduced. However, some individuals may not be concerned about their appearance, in which case surgery is not indicated. Alternatively, individuals may decide to await final healing to determine the effect on their appearance, preferring a formal rhinoplasty to an immediate reduction. This latter approach should be discouraged, as the chances of achieving a good surgical result from immediate repair are better than from rhinoplasty correction of a deformed nose.

Once the decision to undergo repair of the nasal fracture is finalized, the surgeon must decide between closed and open reduction of the fracture. Closed reduction involves manipulation of the nasal skeleton through intact skin and mucosa. Open reduction involves manipulation of the nasal bone fragments through incisions that expose the fragments directly. The latter approach also affords the opportunity for rigid internal fixation. For most cases of nasal fracture, the closed technique is preferred. This has the advantage of avoiding incisions and allows the periosteum of the nasal bones to help hold the fragments in alignment. Also, closed reduction minimizes the risk of resorption from loss of blood supply that may occur after open reduction.

The open reduction technique is reserved for cases when the closed technique fails to achieve good results. If, during the closed nasal procedure, the surgeon is unable to reduce the fragments owing to impaction, the open approach can be considered. In addition, in cases when the reduction cannot be maintained because of loss of support, open reduction with internal fixation can be undertaken. Some surgeons suggest that the most comminuted fractures benefit from the open approach. However, treatment with open reduction and internal fixation may rigidly fix the bones in malalignment. In such cases, revision requires first removal of the internal fixation and then secondary rhinoplasty. A closed reduction avoids this problem. If rhinoplasty is necessary because of persistent deformity, this can be done without reopening the nasal incisions. In addition, secondary manipulation of the fragments in the first weeks after the surgery is possible with closed nasal reduction. For these reasons, the closed nasal reduction is favored for all nasal fractures. Open surgical procedures are reserved for cases when closed reduction fails.

Preoperative Considerations

Anesthesia

Closed nasal reduction can be performed using general anesthesia, local anesthesia with sedation, or no anesthesia at all. Open reduction is typically performed with administration of general anesthesia, but it can be accomplished using local anesthesia with sedation. The choice of anesthesia is based on the convenience and comfort of the patient. In patients with lateral deviation of the dorsum without septal deviation, the reduction can be achieved with a single quick pop. In such cases, some patients prefer to have this done as an office procedure without anesthesia. The advantages of this approach are immediate reduction without injection of local anesthesia and avoidance of hospitalization and operating room time. The disadvantage is the pain this procedure causes. However, as long as the reduction requires only a single adjustment without subsequent manipulation, the degree of pain should not be prohibitive. For depressed fragments, comminution, septal deviation, or in simple cases when the patient prefers, the reduction can be performed in the operating room. The choice between sedation and general anesthesia will be made by the patient after discussion of the pros and cons of each option. Sedation has the advantages of rapid recovery, decreased nausea, and, theoretically, a lower risk of anesthesia-related complications. General anesthesia has the advantage that the patient will be completely pain free during the procedure, allowing unrestricted manipulation of the fragments.

If the patient is to receive general anesthesia, local anesthetic agents are necessary only if septoplasty is to be done. It is preferable not to inject local anesthetic over the nasal bones to avoid the distortion and swelling that can result from the injection. However, it is worthwhile and advantageous to decongest the nasal mucosa thoroughly before reduction is performed. Either 4% cocaine solution or 0.5% oxymetazoline will equally suffice. For patients undergoing sedation anesthesia, both topical and local anesthetics are required. The topical agent in such cases should be 4% cocaine, rather than oxymetazoline, as the former helps to anesthetize the mucosa. Intranasal injection of the septum, columella, and nasal dorsum will help minimize the discomfort of the procedure. The dorsal injections are made through the intercartilaginous space, as described in Chapter 13. Efforts should be made to inject the least amount of anesthetic possible over the dorsum to avoid distortion of the natural contours of the nasal bones.

Technique

Closed Nasal Reduction

The simplest form of closed nasal reduction is performed in patients with laterally displaced nasal bones without depression or comminution. In such cases, simple, firm, digital pressure will suffice to reduce the fracture (Fig. 15–1). The physician's thumbs are placed on the side of the deviation with the index fingers on the brow and cheek. A quick firm push is then applied to the nasal dorsum, which usually results in the bones popping back into place. If alignment is not ideal at this point, the fracture segments can be further manipulated by applying pressure with one thumb on either side of the nose (see Fig. 15–1). If this technique does not result in acceptable reduction, then an intranasal technique can be attempted.

Patients with more complex fractures with depression of fragments or significant comminution will require a combination of intranasal and surface manipulations. In this setting, complete anesthesia is usually required, both intranasally and over the dorsum (if sedation anesthesia is used). After the anesthesia has taken effect, either a unilateral or bilateral nasal instrument is inserted into the nose. The favored unilateral instrument is the Boise elevator, whereas the favored bilateral instrument is the Ashe forceps. With the instrument on the inside of the patient's nose, the physician's other hand is used to apply counterpressure on the nasal dorsum to control the manipulations. The bones are lifted up and pulled inferiorly to disimpact the fragments; lateral pressure is then applied to move them into alignment (Fig. 15–2). The decision of whether to use the Boise or Ashe forceps will depend on whether the fracture is unilateral or bilateral. After the fragments are reduced, they can be rocked back and forth gently to ensure precise alignment.

Closed Reduction with Buttresses

This procedure is a simple extension of the closed nasal reduction technique whereby the nasal bones are supported with external splints fixed by a transnasal wire. It is indicated in cases when reduction is possible with-

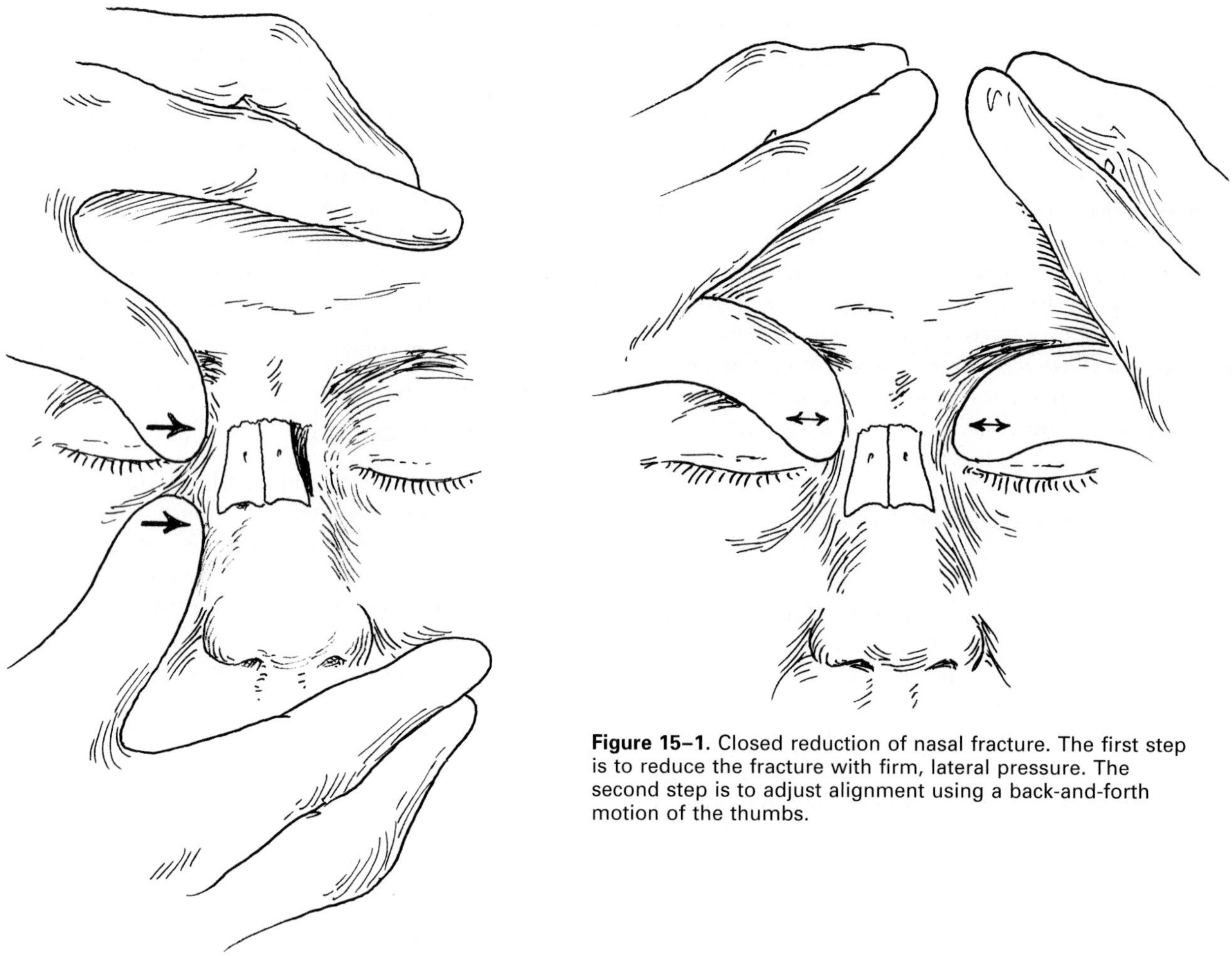

Figure 15–1. Closed reduction of nasal fracture. The first step is to reduce the fracture with firm, lateral pressure. The second step is to adjust alignment using a back-and-forth motion of the thumbs.

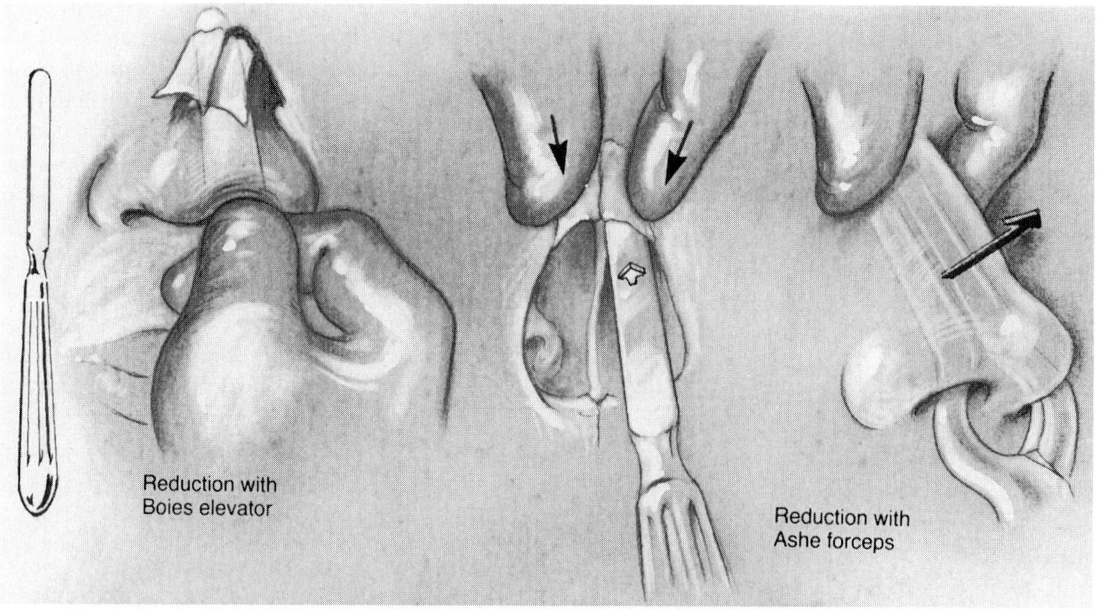

Figure 15–2. Closed reduction of a nasal fracture using internal leverage. A smooth, rigid instrument is used to create outward forces to elevate depressed nasal bones or disimpact fractured bones. (Reprinted with permission from Mathog RH (ed). Atlas of Craniofacial Trauma. Philadelphia: WB Saunders, 1992, p. 232.)

out an open approach, but alignment cannot be maintained. Usually, these cases involve a significant depression of the nasal dorsum that will not maintain projection after reduction. In such instances, external buttresses can be affixed to support the bone stabilizing the projection.

After completion of the closed nasal reduction, the splints are prepared. Either lead or silicone can be used. Holes are created in the splints and the wire is passed through one hole on one side and then across the nose (Fig. 15–3). The wire is then passed through the splint on the opposite side, then back through the splint on that same side, then back through the nose and through the splint on the first side. The wire is tightened down until the splints compress the nasal bones into the alignment desired.

Open Reduction

Rarely, fractures may be so severe that the nasal bones become impacted into the nose and cannot be dislodged using the closed technique. Also, there may be rare cases in which the nasal bones protrude through the skin. In these situations, open reduction is required. This is performed through standard, Lynch-type, medial canthal incisions to gain exposure to the fracture lines. If necessary, bilateral incisions can be used. When internal fixation is required, it may be advisable to make a transverse incision across the nasal dorsum, connecting the medial canthal incisions. This allows direct exposure of the fractures for optimal repair. The medial canthal incision is described in detail in Chapter 9 in connection with the external ethmoidectomy procedure. The only difference in this case is that, rather than elevating laterally into the orbit, the dissection moves medially over the nasal dorsum. The dissection should be performed carefully with a Freer elevator, being sure to stay on the external surface of the nasal bones in the plane between the bone and periosteum so as not to inadvertently dissect on the internal side and completely devascularize the bone fragments.

The exposed nasal bones are grasped with either a bone clamp or a towel clip and gently rocked until the fragment is disimpacted. Once all of the impacted fragments are mobilized, it is worthwhile to insert an intranasal instrument, such as the Ashe forceps, to help manipulate the bones, as with closed nasal reduction. After adequate reduction has been achieved, a decision about whether or not to apply internal fixation must be made. Patients who benefit from fixation are those in whom the bones do not stay in alignment with nasal packing and an external nasal splint. Some judgment will be necessary to make this determination. It is preferable not to use rigid fixation for the reasons stated earlier (i.e., malalignment and the inability to adjust the positions of the bones after surgery). However, in certain cases, only rigid fixation will hold the bones in position.

When fixation is used, the preferred technique is microplating. Now widely available, these 1.0-mm size plates contour easily, achieve rigid fixation, and have a low profile, which prevents the plates from being palpable or visually apparent. The main alternative is to use fine-gauge surgical wire (26 or 28 gauge) to secure the fragments (Fig. 15–4). The disadvantage of the wire is that it is harder to apply, more time consuming, and may leave more of a palpable foreign body. The shape of the plate used will depend entirely on the fracture pattern. A general rule is to use as few screws as possible and as few plates as possible to achieve the goal of stabilization.

The plate is applied by first contouring it to the surface of the nasal bones. The plate is held in position using either digital pressure or a bone clamp. Using a minidriver or other suitable drill, the first hole is drilled into the solid bone of the glabella or orbital rim. The

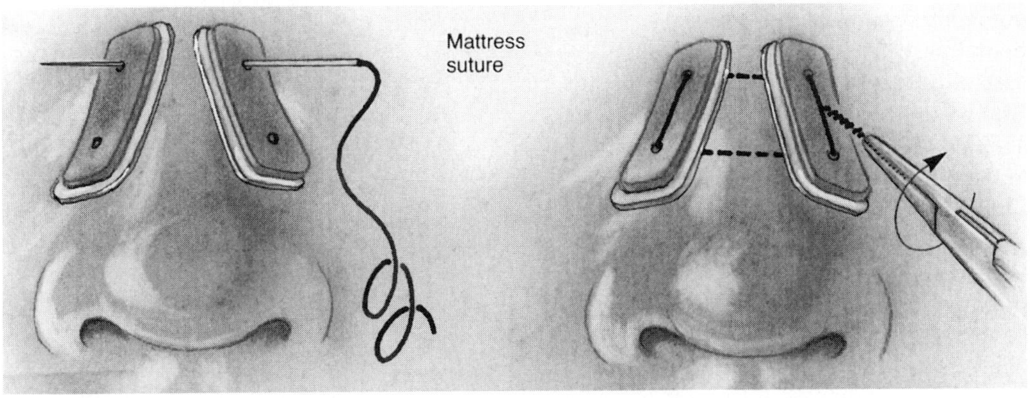

Figure 15–3. Use of external stabilization for an unstable nasal fracture. Lead plates, in combination with Silastic, are used to bolster a transnasal wire holding unstable nasal bones in the reduced position. (Reprinted with permission from Mathog RH (ed). Atlas of Craniofacial Trauma. Philadelphia: WB Saunders, 1992, p. 235.)

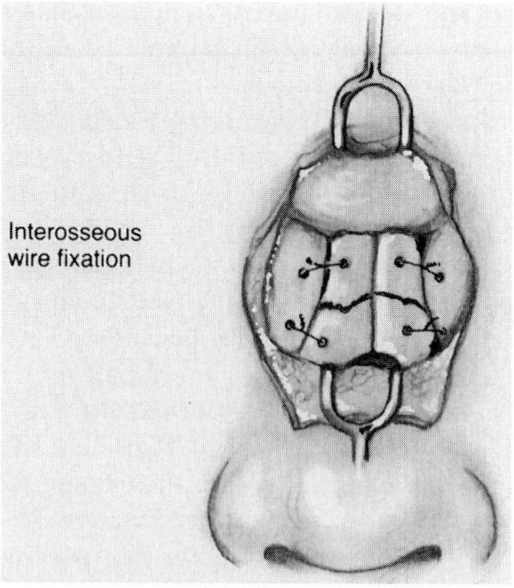

Figure 15–4. Wire osteosynthesis of a comminuted nasal fracture through an "open sky" incision. (Reprinted with permission from Mathog RH (ed). Atlas of Craniofacial Trauma. Philadelphia: WB Saunders, 1992, p. 243.)

depth of the hole can be measured or estimated; usually, it is 3 to 5 mm. The superior end of the plate is fixed with the first screw. The fragments are then sequentially secured from superior to inferior using 2- or 3-mm screws (Fig. 15–5). After the plate is in position, the skin should be redraped over the nose and the result evaluated. It is usually possible to manipulate the fragments slightly after microplate fixation to improve the result. Care should be taken at this stage, though, as undue pressure or torque will break these delicate plates.

Closure

When the final reduction has been achieved, the incisions, if present, are closed, and packing and splints are applied. The incisions are closed with 6-0 nylon suture with a minimal number of subcutaneous sutures to align the edges. Drains are not typically used as the external dressing will apply sufficient pressure to ensure hemostasis. Nasal packing is used only if required for hemostasis or support of the nasal bones. In this case, the best packing is the standard strip gauze with antibiotic ointment. This can be layered in carefully and symmetrically to achieve the desired effect.

An external nasal dressing is required in all but the simplest closed nasal reductions. As with dressings for rhinoplasty, there are many options. The author uses adhesive strips over the skin and a Thermoplast splint (Xomed-Treace, Inc., Jacksonville, FL) for the nasal bones over the tape. The skin is first prepared with alcohol to cleanse and dry the skin. A skin glue is then applied and allowed to dry. The adhesive strips are cut to size and carefully laid over the nasal dorsum extending from superior to inferior. The final step is to heat the splint in hot (>180°F) water, which softens the splint and allows it to conform to the nasal dorsum. The splint is then held in position until cooled and firm.

Postoperative Care

With closed nasal reduction, patients can be expected to have only minimal pain or discomfort. Open reduction with internal fixation, however, is usually associated with more significant pain. In either case, acetaminophen with codeine should suffice as an analgesic. If packing is used internally, a postoperative antibiotic is normally prescribed that covers routine gram-positive organisms, including staphylococcal species. Other medications are not routinely prescribed.

Diet is advanced to regular as tolerated by the patient. For patients receiving general anesthesia, clear liquids are usually advised the night of surgery to avoid emesis. Activity after reduction of a nasal fracture should be limited the first night to rest, with resumption of normal ambulatory activities thereafter. Aerobic physical activity is delayed for about 10 days to make sure that the elevated blood pressures experienced during exercise do not induce epistaxis. Contact sports, such as football, basketball, wrestling, or hockey, should be delayed for 3 months after reduction of the fracture unless the athlete can be equipped with a special mask for protection. Boxing is a sport in which the participants are expected to take blows to the nose, however, and protection is not allowed. In this case, a severely broken nose should give the participant pause to consider retirement from

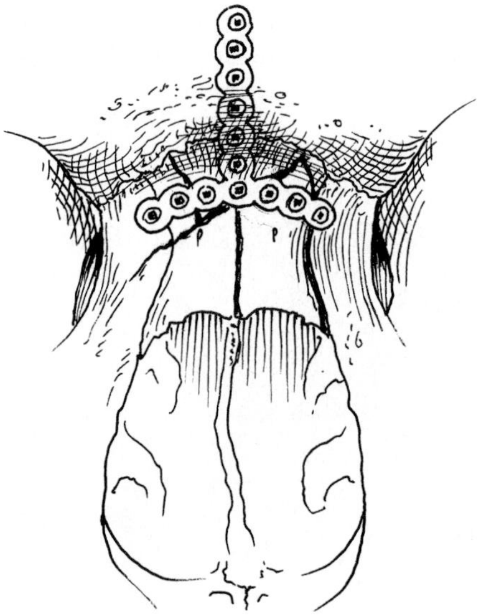

Figure 15–5. Open fixation of a comminuted or unstable nasal fracture. A T-shaped microplate is shaped to fit the contours of the nasal dorsum. At least one screw is placed in each fragment.

the sport; routine fractures should be allowed to heal for up to 6 months before resuming competition.

The first postoperative visit should be scheduled within 5 to 7 days for removal of the nasal splints. If internal nasal packing has been placed, this may be removed as early as 24 to 48 hours after the surgery. Following the removal of the external nasal splint, the nose should be carefully examined to assess the alignment. If the alignment is off significantly, some manipulation in the office can be attempted. Further follow-up visits should be individualized. At least one visit should be scheduled 2 to 3 weeks after the procedure to make a final assessment of the results of the reduction after the swelling has resolved. This is the last chance to take corrective action using further closed nasal reduction.

Complications

The complications of this procedure are similar to those associated with other nasal operations. They include anesthesia-related medical complications, bleeding, infection, and unsatisfactory cosmetic or functional results. If a septoplasty was performed, the complications of this operation would include additional risks. The medical complications associated with anesthesia have been covered elsewhere in this text.

Bleeding over the nasal dorsum that causes hematoma can be prevented by the proper application of an external nasal splint or cast. In the worst case, severe ecchymosis and swelling occur, which typically resolve in 2 to 3 weeks. Following reduction of a nasal fracture, epistaxis in the absence of septoplasty or turbinate surgery is unusual. When it does occur, the most likely source of the bleeding is the branches of the anterior ethmoidal artery. The bleeding can usually be controlled by repacking the nose. However, if necessary, an external or intranasal ligation of the anterior ethmoid artery will result in control of the bleeding.

Infections after closed nasal reduction for nasal fracture without associated injuries are very rare. Because there has not been any violation of skin or mucosal barriers, theoretically, there is not a source of contamination to cause an infection. However, infection caused by the packing, including sinusitis or toxic shock syndrome, is a concern. The effectiveness of antibiotic prophylaxis in preventing these problems has not been documented, but the author routinely prescribes antibiotics in these cases. After open nasal reduction, the risk of infection increases greatly. The infection class for this surgery is rated as clean if no internal nasal connections occur, or as clean contaminated if internal nasal contamination does occur. The risk of soft tissue infection in these classes of surgery is typically less than 5%. No documented role for antibiotic prophylaxis has been established for this class of surgeries. However, local practices may dictate that, for medicolegal safety, at least a 24-hour course of antibiotic prophylaxis be administered.

Unsatisfactory cosmetic results are the most common problems associated with both open and closed nasal reduction. Except in the case of the simplest, laterally displaced fractures for which a single pop reduction is generally effective, an ideal result is difficult to achieve. Once the nasal bones are fractured, return to the exact premorbid appearance is unlikely. Most of the time, an acceptable result is obtained. Commonly, however, a noticeable deviation or hump persists. The patient may accept the result or may pursue delayed secondary rhinoplasty after a minimum of 3 months of healing.[19, 20]

NASO-ORBITAL ETHMOID FRACTURES

Naso-orbital ethmoid (NOE) fractures are much less common than the other forms of nasal and sinus trauma described in this chapter. The inciting injury must be a severe blow to the nasal dorsum or medial canthal area. Typically, this fracture is found in association with other facial fractures, particularly of the inferior orbital rim, maxillary sinus, and frontal sinus. Naso-orbital ethmoid injuries can be conveniently classified into three distinct patterns (Fig. 15–6).[21] Type I is defined as an injury that either cuts across or avulses the medial canthal tendon, with or without a single piece of bone attached. Type II fractures are unilateral, with comminution of the medial canthal area resulting in displacement of the medial canthal tendon. Type III fractures are true NOE fractures and involve injury to the nasal bones, medial orbital walls, and ethmoid sinus. These fractures are always comminuted and bilateral and result in bilateral displacement of the medial canthal tendons.

Diagnosis

Naso-orbital ethmoid fractures are suggested by the presence of blunting of the medial orbital fissure. Normally, the medial canthus has an angled appearance with a sharp acute angle formed by the junction of the upper and lower eyelids. When the medial canthal tendon is displaced, the fissure is rounded or blunted, and the angle between the lids becomes more obtuse (Fig. 15–7). In addition, the lower eyelid sags, resulting in increased scleral show between the limbus and the lid margin. The rounding of the medial canthus should not be confused with the webbing or swelling of the lateral nasal dorsum that can be seen normally or after nasal fracture. The presence of true displacement of the medial canthal tendons can be assessed objectively by taking measurements of the various orbital dimensions. In most people, the intercanthal distance is equal

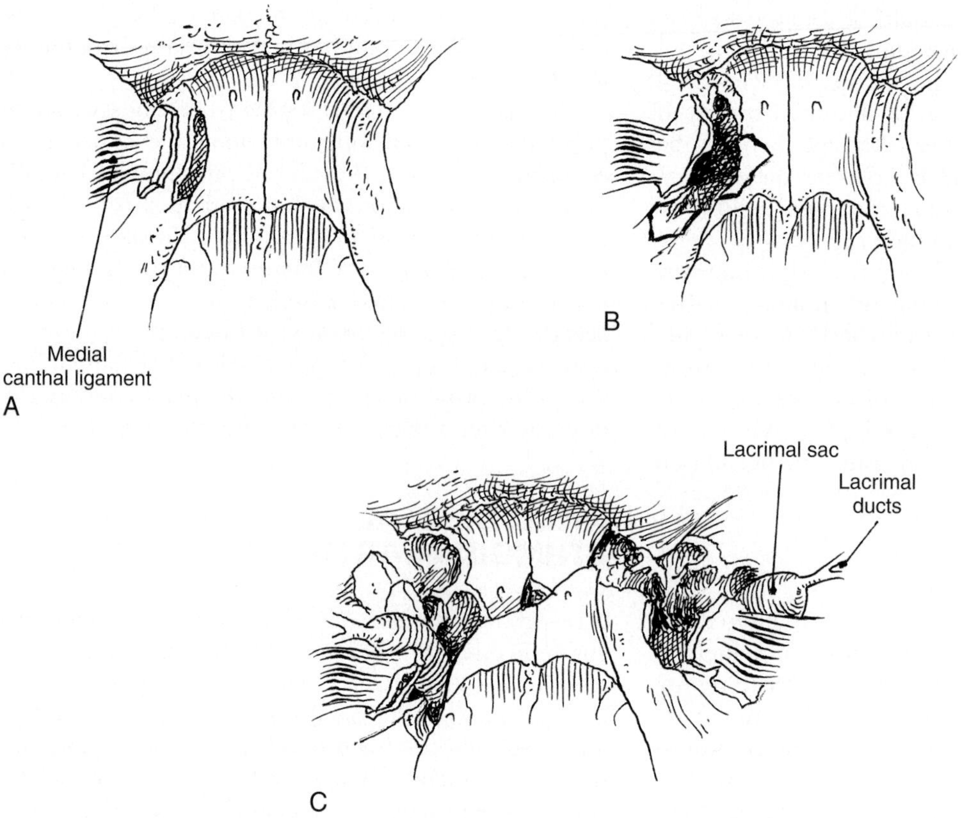

Figure 15–6. Anatomy of naso-orbital ethmoid fractures. *A,* Type 1: avulsion or single fragment attached to the medial canthal ligament. *B,* Type 2: comminution of a unilateral fracture involving the medial canthal ligament. *C,* Type 3: bilateral fractures involving the medial canthal ligament.

to the palpebral fissure width, with the nasal canthal width being equal to one half of the palpebral fissure width. An increase in the nasal canthal width is indicative of an NOE fracture (see Fig. 15–7). Bilateral NOE fractures can be inferred by bilateral increases in the nasal canthal width.

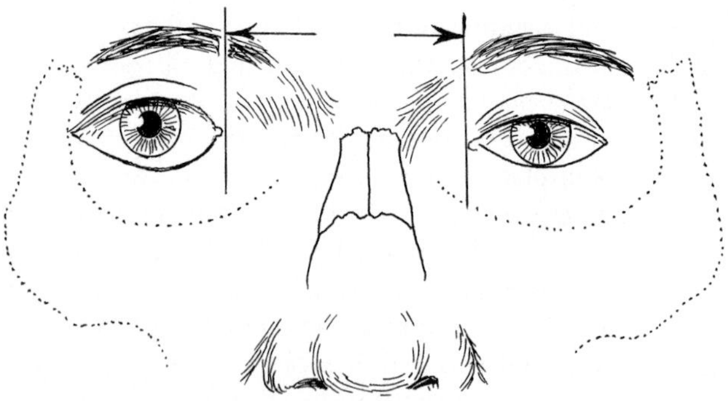

Figure 15–7. Change occurring with a right naso-orbital ethmoid fracture. Detachment of the medial canthal ligament leads to pseudotelecanthus, demonstrated by increased nasal canthal distance, rounding of the medial orbital fissure, and drooping of the lower eyelid.

In addition to the blunting of the medial canthus that defines an NOE fracture, these fractures often are associated with epiphora and injuries to the eye itself. Epiphora is caused by either transection of the lacrimal apparatus or loss of the lacrimal pumping system secondary to displacement of the lacrimal adnexa. The patient with an NOE fracture is at high risk for injuries to the eye.[22, 23] For this reason, a complete eye examination should be performed. An immediate ophthalmology consultation should be requested if there is any evidence of decreased visual acuity.

Other common associated findings include epistaxis, nasal obstruction, and CSF rhinorrhea. Patients with type III injuries are at especially high risk for these complications. An assessment for CSF leak is important in all patients with severe midface trauma, especially those with more advanced NOE injuries. These fractures, by definition, involve the ethmoid bone, and extension into the cribriform plate or ethmoid roof is not unusual. CSF rhinorrhea is suggested by the presence of clear fluid from the nose or the double-ring sign if the nasal discharge is bloody. This sign occurs when bloody drainage from the nose is allowed to run onto a piece of filter paper or a bedsheet and the CSF diffuses farther out than the blood, leaving a clear ring around a central bloody spot. Management of CSF leak is discussed in detail in Chapter 20.

When a naso-orbital ethmoid fracture is suspected, an orbital maxillofacial CT scan is required. This will help define associated injuries, as well as assist with staging the type of naso-orbital ethmoid fracture present. This information is essential in planning the repair. The scan should be performed in the coronal and axial planes with both soft tissue and bone windows. In most cases, contrast medium is not required. However, if orbital hematoma or intracranial injury is suspected, administration of contrast material will improve the diagnostic quality of the scan.

Indications

Virtually all naso-orbital ethmoid fractures, once diagnosed, should undergo timely surgery for repair.[24–26] The best results are almost always achieved with early intervention, as failure to correct a naso-orbital ethmoid fracture will result in permanent deformity and chronic epiphora. The operation can, however, be delayed for 5 to 7 days to allow the acute edema from the injury to subside. This time frame is the preference of many surgeons. The surgical approach is almost always through a medial canthal (Lynch) incision, as outlined in Chapter 9. The specifics of the repair will vary depending on the type of naso-orbital ethmoid fracture. The combination of naso-orbital ethmoid fracture with other fractures, such as of the frontal sinus, orbital rim, or maxillary, will alter the approach and order of repair. For example, a naso-orbital ethmoid fracture combined with a fracture of the anterior wall of the frontal sinus could be approached through a bicoronal incision, with the frontal sinus repair being performed first and the NOE repair after. If the repair can be performed through the bicoronal exposure, it may be possible to avoid medial canthal incisions. In general, the rule is to proceed from superior to inferior in facial trauma surgery, anchoring the repair to stabile bone from above. In this way, the order of repair is normally frontal sinus, naso-orbital ethmoid, orbital rims, malar eminence, and maxillary alveolus. In some centers, the mandible, if fractured, is repaired last, whereas in others, it is repaired first. This decision will be based on one's general philosophy as to which technique is better able to achieve occlusion and to manage the airway.

Preoperative Considerations

Anesthesia

Although it may be possible to perform repair of an NOE fracture with administration of local anesthesia with sedation, in practice, all patients receive general anesthesia. Oral tracheal intubation is used unless the patient has a pre-existing tracheostomy. If the procedure is to repair an NOE injury alone, the operation will not be expected to last more than 2 to 3 hours, and bladder catheterization and invasive monitoring are not indicated. Conversely, if frontal sinus, Le Fort, or complex orbital fractures coexist, the operating time may extend up to 8 hours or more. In these cases, invasive monitoring is worthwhile and usually, a bladder catheter, arterial line, and central venous line are used. Prophylactic antibiotics are indicated for type II and III fractures, as they involve communication of the wound with the internal contents of the nose and sinuses.

Technique

The following descriptions of surgical repairs have been largely adapted from the work of Robert H. Mathog, as presented in the text *Atlas of Craniofacial Trauma.*[27]

Type I

The type I NOE fracture is approached through a medial canthal incision unless there is an existing laceration or alternative. The site of incision is marked on the skin, the area is injected with local anesthesia, and the incision is made exactly as described in Chapter 9 for external ethmoidectomy. A second incision in the inferior margin of the lateral brow is marked and infiltrated with local anesthetic to prepare for a lateral canthal release, but the decision to proceed is deferred until the need for this adjunctive approach is assessed. Once the bone is exposed, elevation of the periosteum and orbital contents proceeds as with external ethmoidectomy. The anterior and posterior lacrimal crests are identified, and the orbit is elevated posteriorly to the level of the anterior ethmoid artery. During this elevation, the area of the fracture is exposed and the exact nature of the injury is delineated.

The area of attachment of the medial canthal tendon is evaluated at this point. Fractures involving the anterior lacrimal crest should have been identified by the preoperative CT scan, but these are confirmed at this point. The bony attachment of the medial canthal tendon is identified and reduced to its normal position. The bone is then fixed in position using either wire or a microplate (Fig. 15–8). A figure-of-eight or horizontal mattress suture using a 30-gauge wire is the preferred technique. The wound edges are approximated and the patient is examined. If the reduction results in restoration of normal intercanthal and nasal canthal dimensions, the procedure is complete and the incision can be closed. If the result is not adequate, several steps can be taken.

To create greater pull on the medial canthal tendon, it can be detached from the bony fragment and fixed

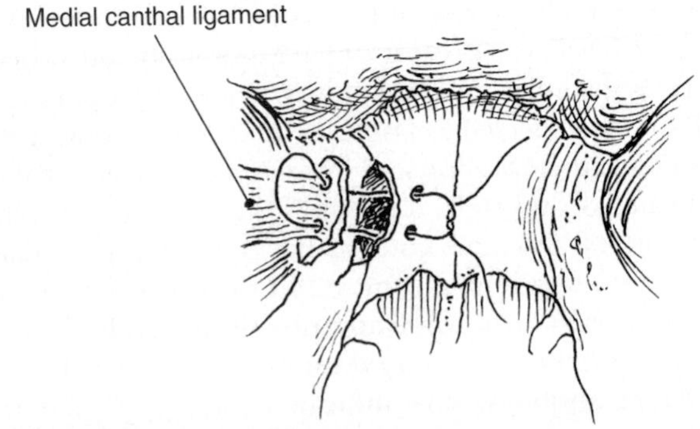

Figure 15–8. Repair of a right, type I, naso-orbital ethmoid fracture. A horizontal mattress suture is placed through the medial canthal ligament using either 30-gauge wire or 4-0 nylon suture.

to the superior aspect of the posterior lacrimal crest. This increases the tension on the tendon and holds it in closer approximation to the orbital wall. A drill hole is placed through the posterior lacrimal crest and a suture is passed though the hole and the medial canthal tendon (Fig. 15–9). It may be necessary to dissect the soft tissues to locate the tendon precisely. It will be recognized as a thickening of the subdermal layers in the area of the periosteum of the anterior lacrimal crest.

At this point, the result is again assessed. Failure to achieve adequate medial displacement of the medial canthus may be related to restriction by the lateral attachments. In this situation, the lateral canthus is released from its attachments by performing a lateral canthotomy to allow resuturing and overcorrection of the medial position of the eyelids. This is simply achieved by incising the lateral brow and dissecting down to the bone of the lateral orbital rim. An elevator is used to elevate the periosteum from the lateral orbit. In doing this, the lateral canthal attachments should be released.

Type II

With the type II NOE fracture, there is usually not sufficient stabile bone in the region of the medial canthus to support local fixation. If it is attempted, it usually results in slippage of the medial canthal tendon and recurrence of the telecanthus. The preferred technique utilizes fixation by a transnasal wire through the contralateral lacrimal fossa or crest. The incisions used are the same as for the type I repair with the addition of a contralateral medial canthal incision. The incisions are marked and injected with local anesthetic as previously described. The ipsilateral dissection is performed, identifying the fracture fragments and the medial canthal tendon. It is important to assess the surrounding bone for stability to determine if, by chance, the bone of the posterior lacrimal crest is stabile enough to support the repair. Typically, this will not be the case with the type II fracture.

The contralateral incision is made and the anterior and posterior lacrimal crests are identified, along with the anterior ethmoid artery. A 30-gauge wire on a large curved needle is passed through the medial canthal tendon and then through the nose and lacrimal fossa on the opposite side. The wire is released from the needle and the opposite end of the wire is rethreaded onto the needle. The needle is then passed back through the nose, coming out posterior to the first pass

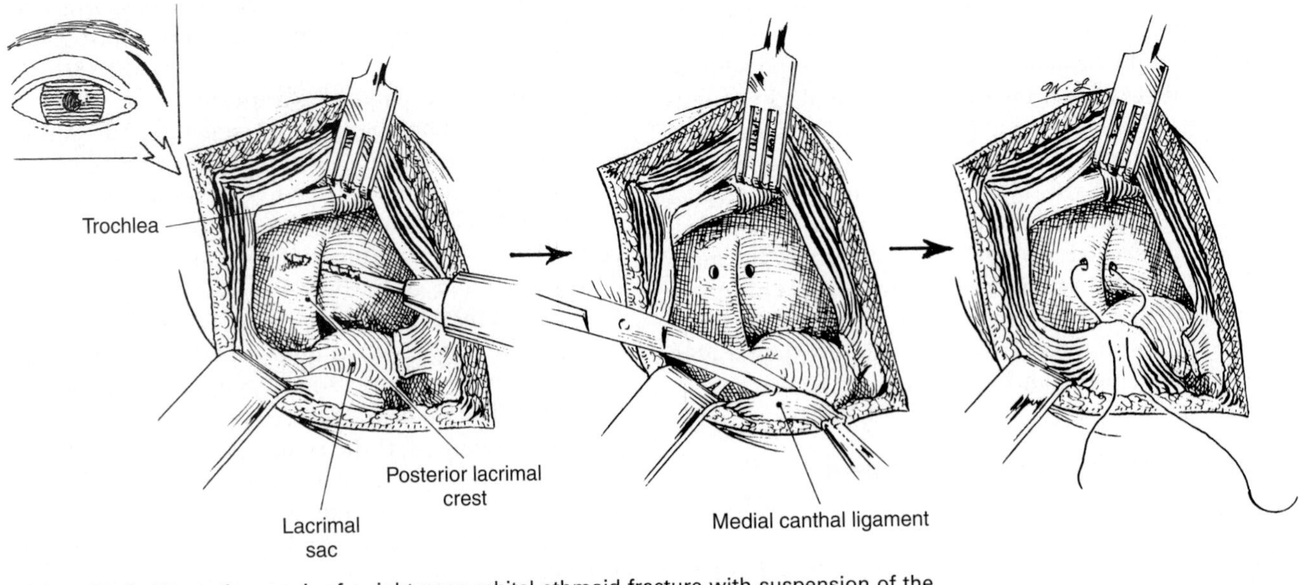

Figure 15–9. Alternative repair of a right naso-orbital ethmoid fracture with suspension of the medial canthal ligament to the posterior lacrimal crest. The medial canthal ligament must be carefully dissected away from the lacrimal sac before suturing.

(Fig. 15–10). The wire is twisted down against lacrimal fossa and posterior lacrimal crest on the opposite side. As the wire is twisted, the medial canthal tendon on the injured side is pulled medially. As with the type I repair, if the lateral attachments of the orbit prevent sufficient medial pull to achieve overcorrection, a lateral canthotomy can be performed.

Type III

The type III NOE fracture, by definition, is bilateral and will probably not have sufficient stabile bone in the area of the posterior lacrimal crest and lacrimal fossa to allow the type II repair to be performed bilaterally. However, if this is the case, and stabile bone is present along the superior aspect of the medial canthal area, the type II repair is done bilaterally. In most cases, this will not be applicable, and the medial canthal tendons will have to be sutured to each other. In such cases, lateral canthotomy should always be performed to prevent excessive tension on the tendon.

The approach is as outlined for the type I and II repairs with the exception that bilateral medial and lateral canthal incisions are required. During the dissec-

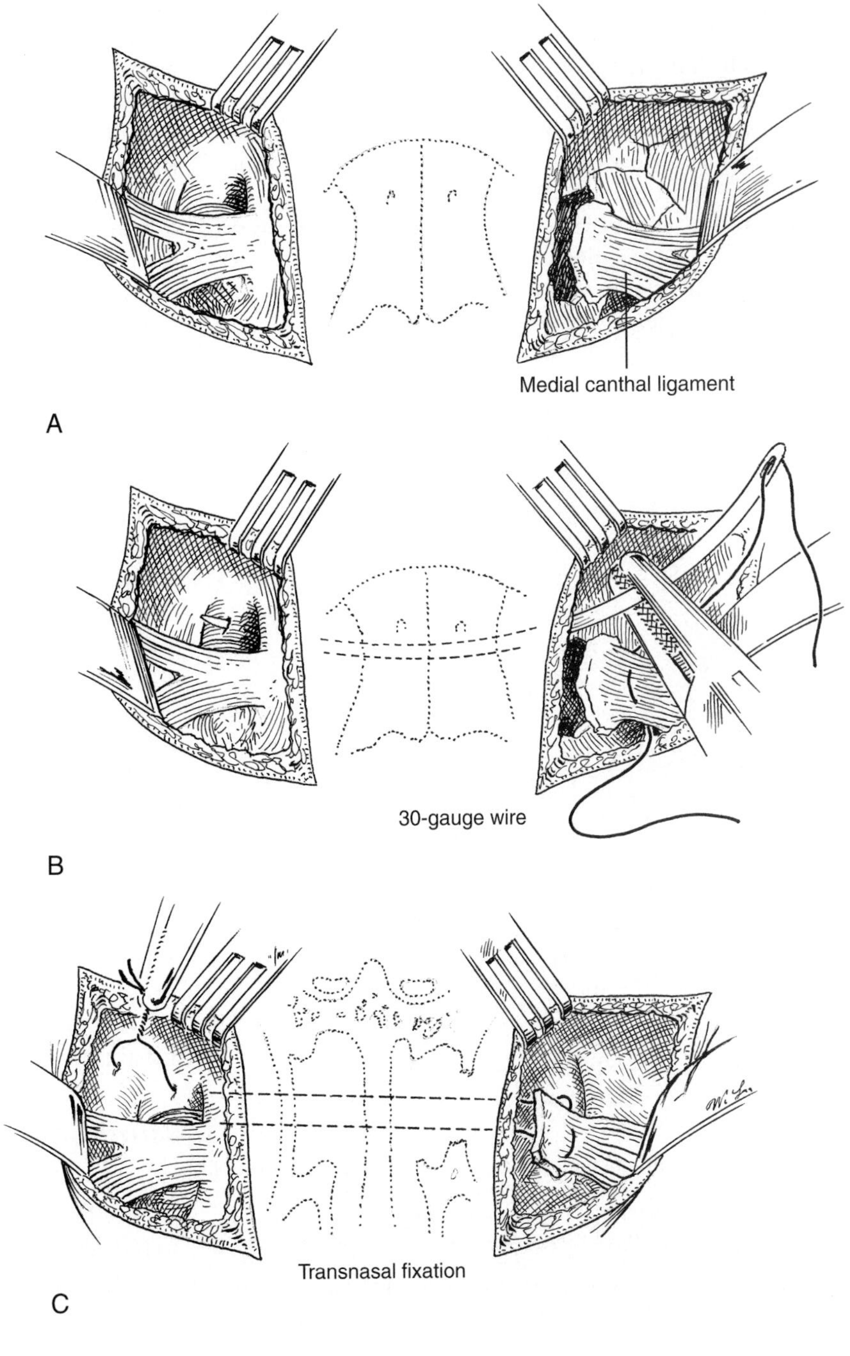

Figure 15–10. Repair of a left, type II, naso-orbital ethmoid fracture using a transnasal wire. *A,* The medial canthal ligament fragment is identified. *B,* A 30-gauge wire is passed through the medial canthal tendon and then across the nose and out through the lacrimal fossa. *C,* The needle is attached to the second end of the wire and passed through the nose, exiting posterior to the posterior lacrimal crest. The wire is then twisted down to secure the fracture.

tions, the medial canthal tendons of both eyes should be identified. A transnasal wire is then passed through both medial canthal tendons. It is desirable to pass the transnasal wire through solid bone if any is available. This will help to stabilize the transnasal wire. Assuming that no solid bone is locally available, the wire is passed through one tendon, and each end of the wire is, in turn, passed through the nose and brought out on the opposite side. Both ends of the wire are then passed through the opposite tendon. Before the wire is tightened down, bilateral lateral canthotomy is necessary. The wire is then tightened until the tendons are pulled together (Fig. 15–11).

One problem with the type III repair is that the tendons may pull anterior to the ideal location. This results in the eyelids and the medial canthus establishing an abnormally anterior position, which causes an undesirable cosmetic and functional result. To avoid this, the transnasal suture should be placed through the nose as far posterior as possible. Even if there is not any bone present in the medial wall to anchor the suture, the nasal septum will provide some resistance to anterior dislocation. The positions of the medial canthi can be reinforced after skin closure with medial nasal buttresses, as described for the repair of nasal fractures.

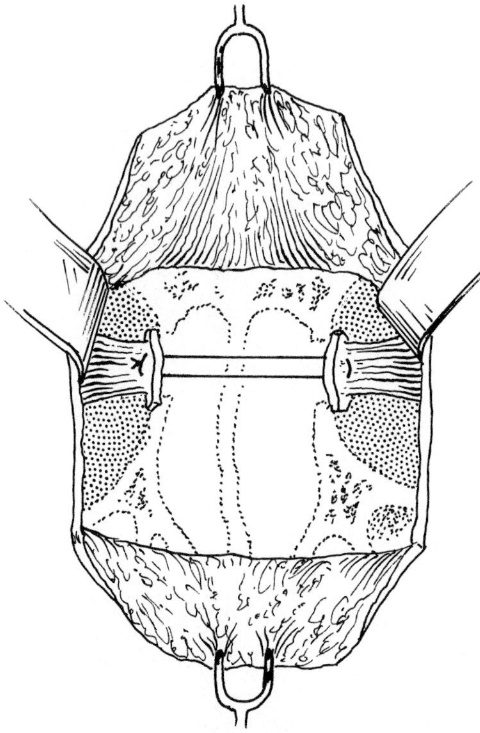

Figure 15–11. Repair of a type III, naso-orbital ethmoid fracture using an "open sky" incision. A transnasal wire is passed through the medial canthal ligament on one side and then across the nose and out through the opposite medial canthal ligament. The other end of the wire is then passed across the nose and out though the opposite medial canthal ligament; it is then twisted down to pull both ligaments medially.

Eventually, with healing, the positions of the medial canthi will stabilize and the buttresses and even the canthal sutures may be able to be removed.

Postoperative Care

Owing to the risk of orbital complications from repair of an NOE fracture, a minimum of one night's hospital stay is necessary. During the observation period, the eye should be examined every 2 to 4 hours to assess for visual acuity and pupillary reactions. Provided the postoperative recovery is uneventful and the orbital edema is minimal, the patient may be discharged the morning after surgery. Before release, a complete eye examination is essential to ensure that acute orbital problems are not present. In the event that there is any question about the safety of the eye, the patient should be kept in the hospital until the eye examination demonstrates stability. In addition, any other postoperative problem that requires monitoring or treatment is handled before discharge.

While hospitalized, the postoperative pain can be managed by parenteral narcotics. By the time of discharge, the patient should be converted to oral medications, most often, acetaminophen with codeine. Prophylactic antibiotics are generally prescribed, but unless nasal packing is used, the patient need not be treated with antibiotics after the surgery. Activity should be limited to bed rest the night of surgery, but ambulation is initiated the next morning and advanced to full activity over the first few days. The diet is limited to clear liquids the night of surgery and then advanced to a regular diet as tolerated.

Following discharge from the hospital, the patient should return for suture removal 5 to 7 days after the procedure. At this time, the surgeon can make the initial assessment of the result of the repair. The cosmetic appearance of the naso-orbital complex is evaluated in the same way as before the operation. Attention should be paid to the nasal airway, extraocular motions, and lacrimal system. Abnormalities are not necessarily indicative of permanent problems. Often, edema from the surgery will cause initial difficulty with these functional outcomes, but these may resolve once the edema subsides. The main course of action if an abnormality is found is to follow the problem closely. Revision surgery can be contemplated as early as 2 to 3 weeks after the initial repair if significant problems are identified.

Complications

There are many potential complications associated with surgery to repair naso-orbital ethmoid fractures. These include the usual risks of anesthesia, bleeding, infection, scarring, and pain, but also include deformity, such as persistent telecanthus or deviated nasal dorsum; orbital complications, including lacrimal obstruction and orbital hematoma; and intracranial complications, such as CSF leak or intracranial hemorrhage.

The most likely of the serious complications are injuries to the eye or orbit.[28] Orbital hematoma is a risk of any procedure that involves elevation of the orbital periosteum. By controlling the anterior ethmoid artery early in the procedure and avoiding unnecessary orbital penetration, this can be minimized. The diagnosis and management of orbital hematoma are covered in Chapter 21. The risk of direct injury to the extraocular muscles is minimal, as there is generally no indication to explore inside the orbital periosteum. If, however, penetration with significant bleeding occurs during elevation of the medial orbit, an injury may occur. Altered lacrimal function is one of the most common problems after these fractures.[29] This may result from injury to the lacrimal puncta or collecting ducts, lacrimal sac, or the nasolacrimal duct. Evaluation and management of these problems are covered in detail in Chapter 21 as well.

Intracranial injuries are possible but uncommon sequelae of naso-orbital ethmoid fractures. The most common problem is CSF rhinorrhea. This can occur from the initial fracture, but usually can be controlled with conservative therapy, and postoperative leaks are not expected. The possibility of a leak should always be considered, however, and if suspected, managed accordingly. Intracranial hemorrhage from manipulation of fracture segments should not occur. This can happen, though, if fragments of bone are sticking through the dura and are reduced without considering the situation. Craniotomy may need to be considered to control reduction if displacement is very severe. This should be able to be determined before surgery on the basis of the preoperative CT scan.

The most likely of all complications of repair of an NOE fracture is a poor cosmetic result, especially in the case of comminuted fractures. The nasal dorsum may be malaligned; the medial canthus may slip after surgery, pulling away from the orbital wall; or the original repair may underestimate or overestimate the degree of tendon pull required to achieve the desired result. The steps described in this chapter are designed to prevent this from happening, but errors or imprecision are possible. In the event that the result is truly unacceptable, a secondary revision can be attempted.[30, 31]

The risk of the routine complications is equivalent to that of other facial trauma procedures. There should be a low incidence of serious problems, but occasionally, minimal complications can be seen. The most common of these would be epistaxis. Either as a result of direct mucosal laceration from the injury or surgical manipulation, raw surfaces are created, and often some bleeding does occur. Significant bleeding requiring intervention is more unusual. The risk of acute infection from NOE fracture repair should be less than 5%, as for any clean or clean contaminated case. The risk of late-onset sinusitis or mucocele secondary to ethmoid trauma is unknown. Certainly, these complications do occur, but there are no long-term prospective studies available to help estimate the true incidence of this problem. If they occur, the management will most likely be surgical owing to the need to correct the underlying anatomic cause of the sinusitis.

FRONTAL SINUS FRACTURES

One of the least common facial fractures, frontal sinus injuries are nonetheless among the most important in terms of the short-term and long-term effects on the patient. Frontal sinus fractures are rare in children younger than 13 years of age owing to the late development of the frontal sinus.[32, 33] Conversely, the frontal area of the face is often the zone of maximum impact in children because of the relative increase in the proportion of the skull compared to the face. With increasing age, the face elongates in relation to the frontal bone, changing proportions to deemphasize the frontal area. Thus, with increasing age, the facial trauma victim becomes more likely to sustain impact to the lower face or midface. These factors combined keep the incidence of frontal sinus trauma to a minimum. A final factor in the low incidence of frontal sinus trauma is the resistance of the frontal sinus to injury. The thick outer table over the brow provides a major deterrent to fractures. The force of injury required to fracture the frontal sinus is the highest of the facial bones.

Frontal sinus fractures can involve the anterior table, root of the sinus, or posterior table. In addition, the fractures may be variably comminuted, displaced or nondisplaced, depressed, or in open communication with a skin laceration. All combinations are possible depending on the nature of the blow to the face and the aeration of the sinus. Repair of the fractures may be through a bicoronal, mid-forehead, or brow incision, or through an existing laceration. The repair can involve reduction and internal fixation, obliteration, or cranialization of the frontal sinus. In this section, these options are covered in detail.

Diagnosis

At the time of injury, it is essential to fully evaluate the patient with frontal sinus fracture for the possibility of acute intracranial injury and cervical spine injury. Owing to the tremendous forces required to fracture the frontal sinus, most patients with this type of injury will suffer loss of consciousness and be at risk for intracranial injury.[6] On arrival at the hospital, the patient will initially be evaluated by the hospital's trauma service and will normally undergo a neurosurgical evaluation and CT scans of the head. Diagnosis and management of the frontal sinus injury must take second priority.

Once the extent and management plan for any intracranial and cervical injuries are established, the frontal sinus injury can be addressed. The suggestive history is any severe blow to the frontal region of the head. The initial examination may reveal an obvious depression or swelling, hematoma, ecchymosis, or lacerations. Neurologic evaluation may show sensory deficits over the frontal region from injury to the supraorbital or supratrochlear nerves. Extreme tenderness of the area is expected. Motor deficits from injuries to the frontal branch of the facial nerve are not expected, but transient dysfunction may occur from direct injury to the muscle or hematoma.

The critical step in the diagnosis of frontal sinus fractures is obtaining an appropriate CT scan. Both coronal and axial sections with bone windows are necessary to delineate the full extent of the fracture. In some cases, sagittal reconstructions are also very helpful. On the CT scan, the exact nature of the fracture pattern should be evident. Plain radiographs of the frontal bones using lateral and anteroposterior views may be helpful in establishing the presence of a frontal sinus fracture, but for accurate diagnosis and operative planning, a CT scan is necessary.

Indications for Surgery

The decision to proceed with operative repair of a frontal sinus fracture and the type of repair required are dependent on several factors. These include the pattern of the fracture, the presence of associated injuries, and the presence of cosmetic deformity. There are three basic indications for repair of the frontal sinus fracture. The first is the presence of cosmetic deformity. This only occurs when there is depression of fragments of the anterior wall of the sinus. Nondisplaced anterior wall fractures do not require fixation to prevent late deformity. With displaced fractures, the early deformity may be masked by acute reaction. When the edema resolves, the deformity becomes more evident. In the case of an isolated anterior wall fracture, some patients may elect not to undergo repair, choosing instead to accept the cosmetic alterations. The more severe the displacement, the more likely the patient will desire surgical intervention. Anterior wall fractures are repaired with reduction and internal fixation. The options for fixation include wires, microplates, and micromesh. Cases with significant comminution can be reconstructed accurately with mesh. Less severe fractures may be able to be fixed adequately with wires or microplates.

The second indication for surgery is to prevent late complications, including frontal sinusitis and mucocele.[34] It is unclear in any individual case whether a displaced fragment will lead to mucosal entrapment and late onset of mucocele or cyst. For this reason, surgery to reduce and repair minimally displaced fractures to prevent late complications is controversial. Convincing prospective studies addressing this issue are lacking. The lack of quality prognostic information is compounded by the long time frame over which these complications can arise and the difficulty in obtaining long-term follow-up evaluation of facial trauma patients. When repair is elected, the fragments are reduced, entrapped mucosa is excised, and the fragments are aligned and stabilized with internal fixation. The alternative is frontal sinus obliteration or cranialization. Owing to the risk of late complications from entrapment of mucosa, even patients that do not undergo the operation should be monitored long-term to detect complications early in their course.

It has been widely accepted that, when the fracture extends through the frontal sinus ostium, the patient is at high risk for development of ostial obstruction and mucocele.[35–37] Past experience has shown that fractures extending through the internal os are associated with a high risk of late complications. Fractures that involve the floor of the sinus or anterior and posterior tables are highly likely to extend into the frontal sinus ostium. In these cases, the sinus should be obliterated or cranialized.

The final indication for surgery is the presence of CSF leak.[38, 39] Regardless of whether the leak is through the anterior wall of the sinus, into the nose, or into the pharynx, CSF leak is an indication for surgery. If the leak persists after appropriate conservative management, surgery is indicated. In these cases, either cranialization or obliteration should be performed.

The decision as to whether to perform cranialization or obliteration is of minimal importance. The sinus ostium is blocked the same way in both cases, and the sinus cavity is filled with fat in either case. The only difference is in the handling of the posterior wall of the sinus. In cranialization, the posterior wall is removed. This is preferred primarily when the posterior wall is either badly displaced with dural penetration or severely comminuted. Neurosurgical assistance in disimpacting the fragments is important and should be arranged in advance of the surgery. If only comminution is present, the posterior wall can be drilled down with a diamond burr and the sinus obliterated.

Technique

Approach

The frontal sinus can be approached through three basic incisions or through a preexisting laceration in the forehead from the initial trauma. When a small laceration is present in the forehead overlying the frontal sinus fracture, this should be closed and the repair of the fracture should be delayed 1 to 2 weeks until the laceration is healed. This allows a full realm of surgical options to be considered. A unique problem develops in the case when the laceration becomes infected. In this situation, the repair should be postponed until full healing of the wound has occurred. A large laceration in continuity with the fracture is an indication for immediate repair. In this situation, the fracture can be repaired directly through the laceration, avoiding a second incision. Alternatively, the laceration can be closed in the emergency room and the fracture repair delayed until the laceration has healed.

The incisions available for repair of a frontal sinus fracture are the same as for osteoplastic frontal sinusectomy, described in detail in Chapter 11. For most patients, a bicoronal incision is preferred. The exception to this is in a balding man without hair to cover the incision. In this case, the patient may opt for a mid-forehead incision if there is a deep forehead crease, or a brow incision if the forehead is smooth.

The bicoronal flap is the preferred approach in cases of frontal sinus fractures associated with orbital and malar fractures. In patients with fractures requiring frontal, malar, nasal, orbital, and maxillary reduction and fixation, the bicoronal flap is extended inferiorly to the zygomatic arches and the nasal dorsum. Several additional steps are required beyond those presented in Chapter 11. The first is releasing the supraorbital nerves. The supraorbital nerve is usually encased at the supraorbital foramen by a thin rim of bone. This bone is removed on the orbital side by carefully incising the foramen with a 2-mm osteotome. The nerve is then elevated from the canal with a Freer elevator.

The other extension is laterally, where the flap is extended down to the zygomatic arch. The frontal branch of the facial nerve will cross through this field just superficial to the temporalis fascia. To avoid injury to the facial nerve, the plane of dissection must change from superficial to the surface of the temporalis fascia to deep to the temporalis fascia. This transition should occur about 2 to 3 cm above the zygomatic arch (Fig. 15–12). This incision enters the fatty layer of the temporal fossa and is not an avascular plane. Dissection requires careful control of bleeding during elevation to

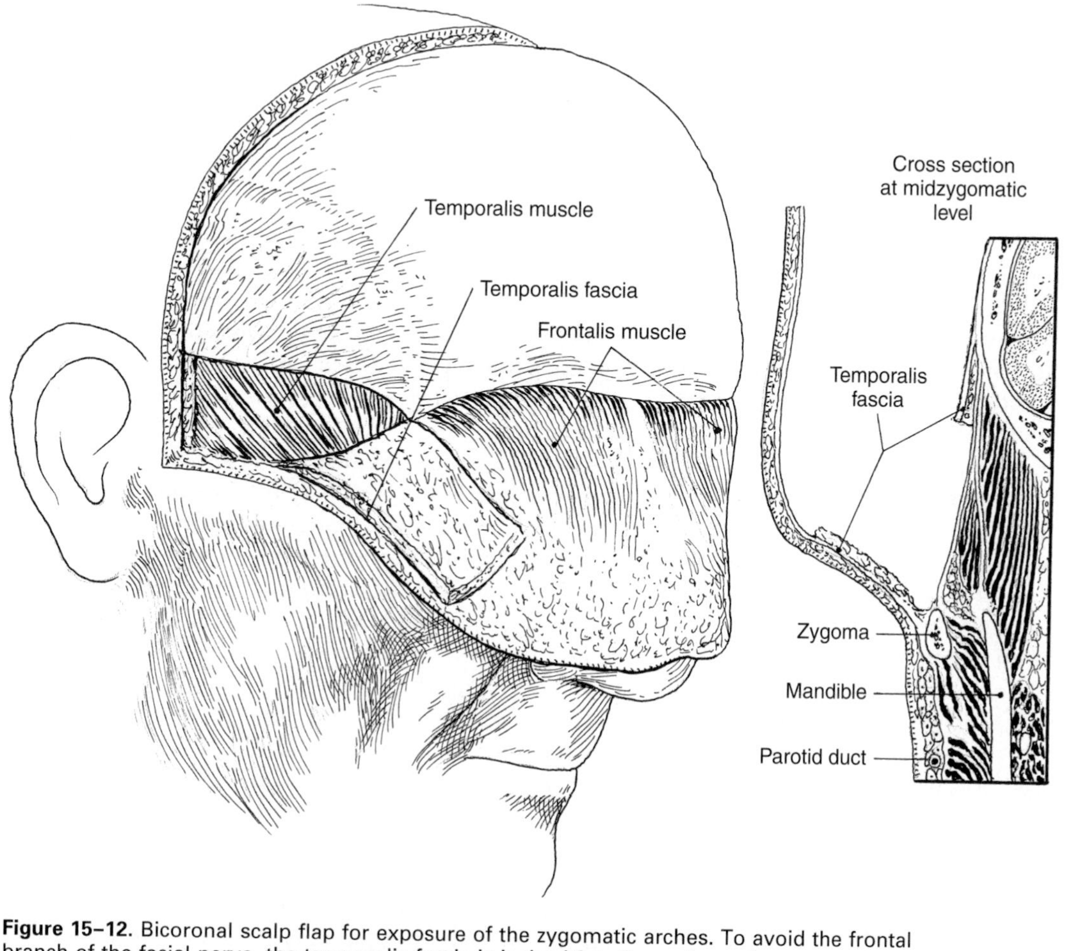

Figure 15–12. Bicoronal scalp flap for exposure of the zygomatic arches. To avoid the frontal branch of the facial nerve, the temporalis fascia is incised 2 to 3 cm above the zygomatic arch, with subsequent dissection proceeding in a deeper plane on the surface of the muscle. A cross-sectional view demonstrates the shift in dissection level to the surface of the muscle.

maintain a bloodless field. Bipolar cautery is preferred for this. When the zygomatic arch is reached, the periosteum is incised and a periosteal elevator can be used to expose the entire arch.

Fracture Repair

The first step in repair of the fracture is to examine and assess the extent of the fracture. Specific questions to answer relate to the condition of the posterior table, the floor of the sinus, and the internal ostium. This exploration can usually be accomplished by removing the largest fragments of the anterior table. If access is limited, the sinus can be explored through an osteoplastic flap, formed as described in Chapter 11. Alternatively, if the CT scan suggests an isolated anterior wall fracture, the repair can be performed without exploring the sinus. The order of the repair will be removal of the mucosa of the inside of the sinus, repair or removal of the posterior wall, blockage of the ostia, obliteration of the sinus, and repair of the anterior wall. If the ostia are intact, then the procedures for removal of the mucosa, blockage of the sinus, and obliteration are omitted, and the only procedures performed are repair of the posterior and then anterior tables.

Repair of the Anterior Table

Depressed fractures of the anterior table require reduction and fixation to avoid cosmetic deformity. The best technique to achieve this goal depends on the severity and degree of comminution of the fracture. When there are only one or two large fragments, the preferred method is to use microplates. A straight, curved, L-shaped, or square plate can be used. Because there are no active stresses on the repair, alignment and fixation alone are adequate to successfully treat these fractures. This is in contrast to malar, maxillary, and mandible fractures, which must bear significant muscle and masticatory forces. Each fragment should be supported by at least two screws, with two screws anchored in the surrounding intact bone (Fig. 15–13).

The first step in placing the plate is to align the fragments in the desired orientation. The plate is selected and contoured to smoothly span the fracture fragments. The plate is secured to the stable intact bone initially. To accomplish this, the plate is held in place and the drill hole placed. It is best to use a drill bit with an automatic stop on the shaft to prevent inadvertent intracranial penetration. If the drill bit does not have a stop, then the surgeon should carefully support the drill with both hands, applying slow, gentle pressure until the outer table of the skull is passed and the softer, diploic space is entered. It is not necessary to drill beyond this level.

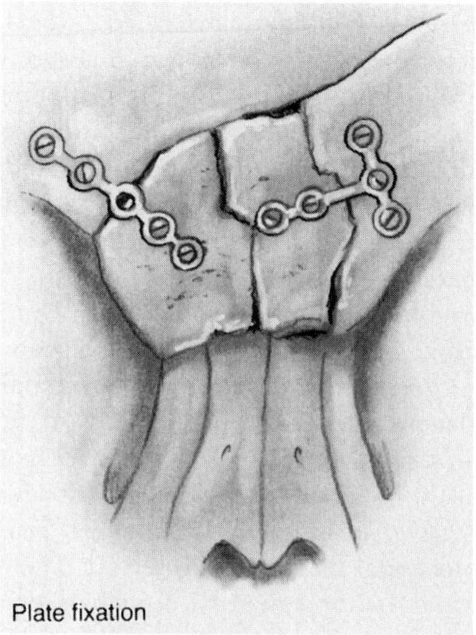

Figure 15–13. Miniplate fixation of the anterior wall of the frontal sinus. At least two screws are placed in each fracture segment and on the stable bone. (Reprinted with permission from Mathog RH (ed). Atlas of Craniofacial Trauma. Philadelphia: WB Saunders, 1992, p. 359.)

After the initial screws are placed in the adjacent skull to stabilize the plate, the fracture fragments are addressed. The fragments can be supported with a small, single hook through an opening between fracture fragments. Each screw should be slowly but firmly turned to avoid stripping the head or breaking the screw. Each screw should be tightened down flush to the plate. It is possible to use the force of the screw during tightening to bring the fragment up to the plate. Once the final screws are in place, the contour should be assessed and, if inadequate, minor adjustments may be made by bending the plate in place. Great care should be taken if this is done because it is possible to fracture the plate during such maneuvers.

In patients with significant comminution, the use of titanium micromesh is suggested.[40] The titanium mesh is preferred over stainless steel mesh because of improved biocompatibility and ease of contouring the mesh. After the posterior table and internal sinus are addressed, the fracture pattern is assessed. The fragments may be removed and reassembled on the back table with the mesh overhanging the superior and lateral edges of the reassembled fragments. Alternatively, the mesh can be aligned over the frontal bone with the fragments left in place and secured to the mesh by supporting the fragments with a small hook through the mesh.

With either of these techniques, there may be gaps in the anterior wall of the frontal sinus covered only by the mesh and superficial soft tissues. This has not been a problem to date, as patients are generally unaware of the gaps, either by change in contour or feel. Ultimately, the mesh will be covered by fibrous tissue and incorporated into the overlying periosteum. The mucosa will regenerate over the fibrous tissue or, in the case of obliteration, the sinus will fill in with fat and fibrous tissue.

If the anterior wall is being reassembled off the surgical field, it is important to maintain the orientation of the fragments to each other as they are removed. Each fragment is cleaned of mucosa and then carefully placed on a sterile surface in the exact orientation as originally in the patient (see Fig. 15–15B). When all of the fragments to be assembled are in place, the mesh is placed over the frontal bone, cut to size, and contoured to the patient. A finger is pressed over the mesh as it is held against the bone to achieve the desired contour (Fig. 15–14). This will usually be sufficient to mold the mesh to the approximate shape desired. It is important when doing this to remember to keep the inferior edge of the mesh at about the level of the supraorbital ridge so that it does not protrude into the orbit. Also, the surgeon must allow adequate overlap onto the frontal bone so that the mesh can be securely anchored to the stabile bone.

Beginning with the inferior fragments, the anterior wall is reconstructed against the mesh off the surgical field. The inferior fragments should overlap the inferior edge of the mesh to maintain the relationship between the mesh and the orbits (Fig. 15–15C). The wall is then sequentially reassembled against the mesh, proceeding from inferior to superior (see Fig. 15–15C). As the fragments are added, it is possible to refine the contour of the mesh to maintain the desired relationships between the fragments. Each of the fragments should be secured by at least two 1.0-mm screws. However, some fragments may be too small to allow this. For these small fragments, a single screw can suffice as there will not be any forces applied to distract the fragments during healing. When all of the fragments are secured, the complex is placed into the frontal bone defect and the mesh anchored to the surrounding stabile bone with several screws (Fig. 15–15D). As the final screws in the stabile frontal bone are placed, the complex of mesh and fragments will tend to pull into the proper alignment with the natural contour of the forehead. It is also possible at this late stage to adjust the contour of the mesh to fit the natural contour.

The alternative technique is to maintain the fragments in position during repair. This is usually done only when the posterior wall and floor are intact and the sinus is not to be obliterated or cranialized. In this situation, the first step is to contour the mesh to the frontal bone as before (see Fig. 15–14), but the mesh is then securely anchored to the surrounding stabile bone with several screws (usually at least 10). The largest fragments are next secured to the mesh by holding the fragments up against the mesh using a small hook placed through the mesh and between the fragments. As the larger fragments are secured, some of the smaller fragments may become dislodged and may not be able to be realigned. In this circumstance, it is better to remove these small fragments rather than allow them

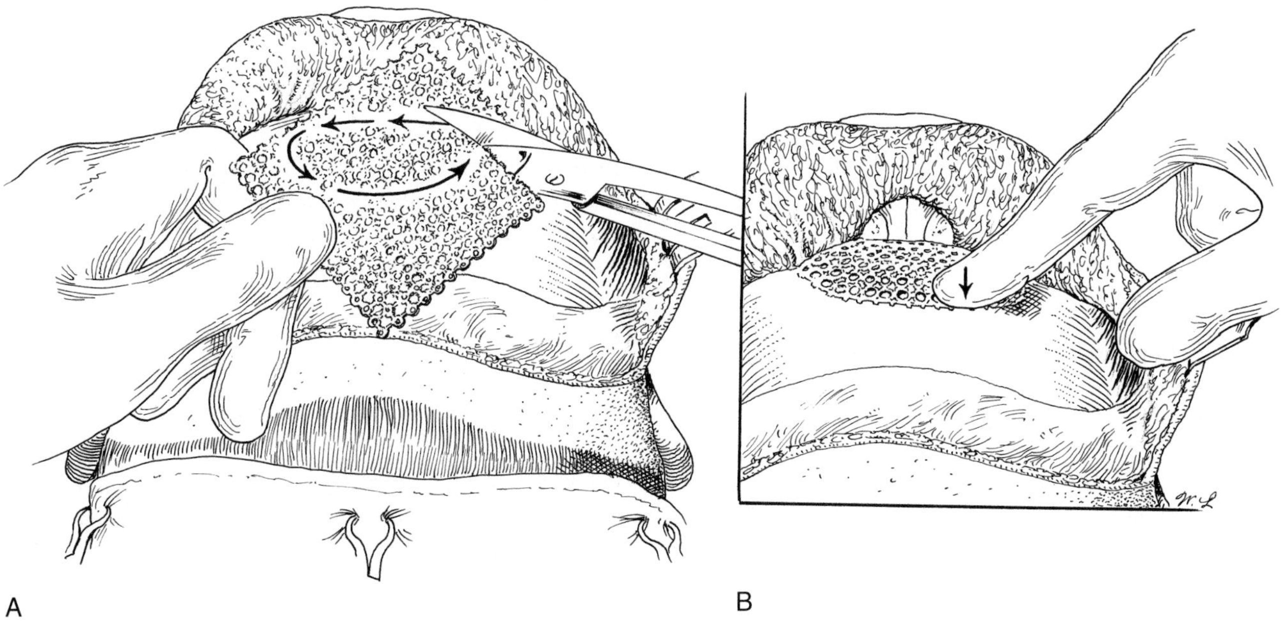

Figure 15–14. Micromesh fixation of the anterior wall of the frontal sinus. *A,* The mesh is cut to the appropriate size and shape. The mesh must overlap onto the stabile frontal bone sufficiently to allow coverage of all fragments to be fixed. Care should be taken to make sure the mesh does not contact the orbital tissues. *B,* The mesh is contoured to the shape of the frontal bone by applying firm pressure while holding the mesh in the desired position.

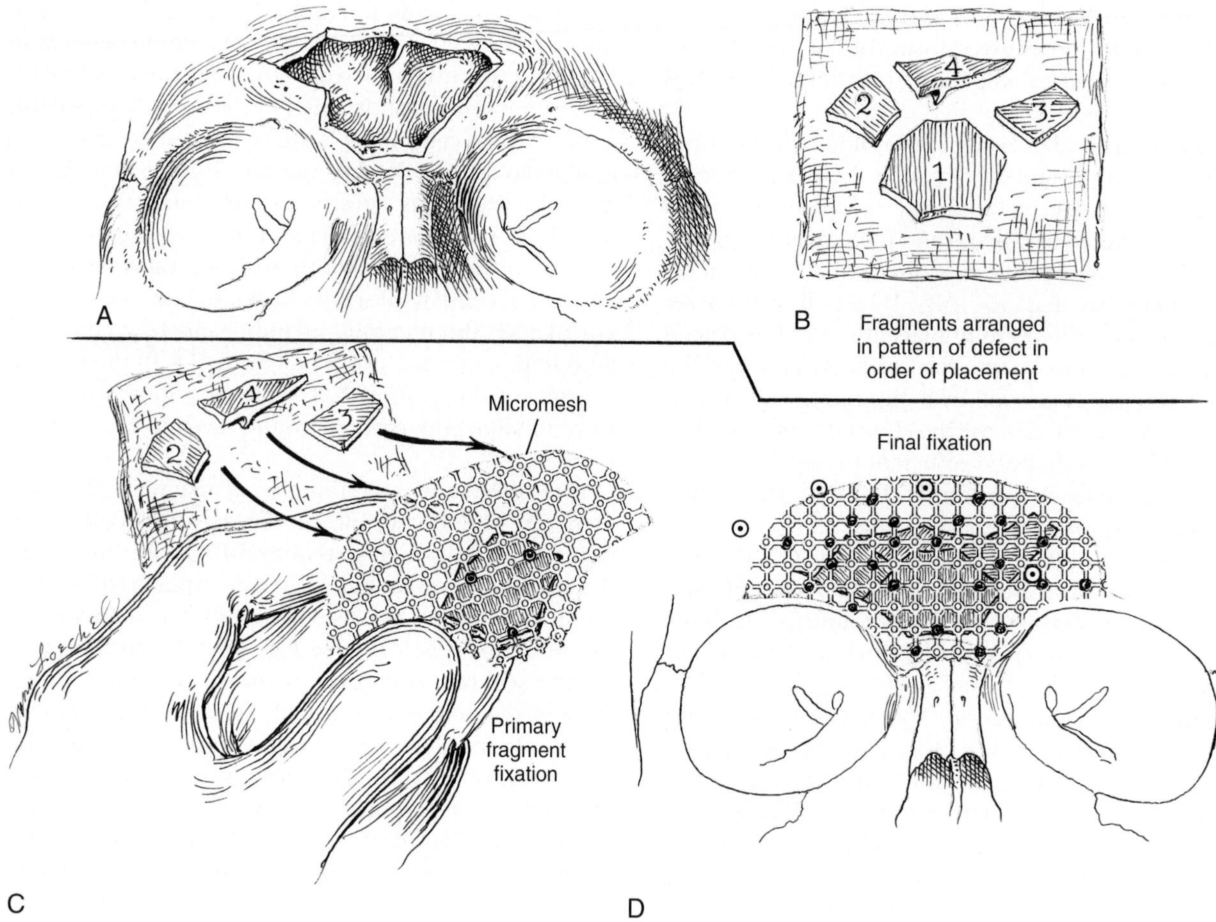

Figure 15–15. Micromesh fixation using the back table method. *A,* Anterior wall defect of the frontal sinus. *B,* The removed fragments are carefully lined up in their natural positions on a working area off the surgical field. *C,* The fragments are fixed in place in their relative positions. The lowest fragment should be placed first and the alignment checked against the defect before proceeding to subsequent fragments. Each adjacent fragment is then fixed to the mesh, reconstructing the defect like a puzzle. *D,* The completed repair shows numerous screws holding the mesh to the stabile bone that is placed last.

to fall into the sinus or remain unsecured with the potential for mucosa to be trapped between the fragments.

To date, both of these techniques for applying micromesh for frontal sinus fractures have been successful. The back table technique is used primarily when the sinus is obliterated or cranialized, and the in situ technique is used primarily when the sinus is preserved. However, the back table technique can always be used if the in situ technique is not yielding adequate results during an individual case. The postoperative results with the use of titanium micromesh are excellent. The contours and stability achieved and the ease of application are unmatched by older, more traditional techniques. During the repair, every attempt is made to achieve the best reconstitution of the anterior wall as possible. In practice, however, it is probably not critical that exact reassembly be accomplished. Reasonable approximation is usually sufficient, and even large, 1- to 2-cm gaps in the anterior wall do not cause problems. The mesh will maintain rigidity and cover up imperfections in the repair. For this reason, it is highly favored except in the simplest cases, as detailed earlier.

Obliteration

Whenever the ostial area of the frontal sinus is involved in the fracture, obliteration of the sinus is indicated. To perform the obliteration, the anterior wall of the sinus should be completely removed to expose the entire interior of the sinus. In most cases, the anterior wall will have a displaced fracture. Here, the fragments are removed, cleaned of mucosa, and placed on a sterile table in the exact relationship as originally in the patient. After the loose fragments are all removed, the remainder of the anterior wall is developed into an osteoplastic flap. With a clear view into the sinus, this is easily accomplished. The saw blade is traced around the outer extent of the sinus with the cut evaluated from inside the sinus. If possible, the entire remainder of the anterior wall should be elevated as a single, inferiorly pedicled, bone flap. However, multiple pedicled or free bone fragments may result, depending on the fracture pattern.

Once the anterior table is completely elevated, the interior mucosa of the sinus should be completely removed. Usually, a Freer elevator is used initially to remove the mucosa. The entire internal surface of the sinus must then be carefully drilled down using a diamond burr on an otologic drill. All internal septations should be completely taken down, and supraorbital ethmoid cells must be unroofed and cleaned out. The posterior table of the sinus should be relatively intact for obliteration, without significant comminution or displacement. If comminution or displacement is noted, the sinus should be cranialized rather than obliterated. Care must be taken when drilling over fracture fragments on the posterior wall. A microscope, medium to large diamond burrs, and relatively low drill speeds with copious irrigation are recommended.

The sinus ostia are obstructed exactly as described in the procedure outlined in Chapter 11 for obliteration of the sinus for chronic infection or mucocele. Multiple layers, including temporalis muscle, parietal bone, and temporalis fascia, are placed in order from inferior to superior. The sinus lumen is packed with fat from a sterile secondary incision in the abdomen or thigh. The procedure is completed by repairing the anterior wall using the titanium mesh assembled on the back table described above.

Cranialization

For patients with comminution or displacement of the posterior wall of the frontal sinus, the preferred management approach is cranialization. The anterior table, floor, orbital surfaces, and ostia are handled exactly as in the obliteration procedure. The only differences between obliteration and cranialization are the creation of a pericranial flap and complete removal of the posterior wall of the sinus in the latter. The pericranial flap is developed from the periosteum of the frontal bone. Instead of incising the periosteum 1 to 2 cm above the apex of the sinus, the incision is placed about halfway up the frontal bone. The periosteum is then elevated down to the nasal root and the osteoplastic flap is removed as a free bone flap. During obstruction of the sinus ostia, the pericranial flap will be used instead of a free temporalis graft to cover the upper end.

The principle difference between cranialization and obliteration is the handling of the posterior wall. In simple cases in which there is not significant displacement or impaction of bone into the dura, the fragments can simply be elevated from the dura with a Freer elevator and discarded. After the loose fragments are removed, the dura is elevated from the remaining posterior wall with either a Freer or Woodson elevator and the bone removed with a Kerrison or other bone rongeur.

It is easy to remove the posterior wall superiorly to the apex of the sinus. It is more difficult (and unnecessary) to remove the bone flush to the floor of the cranial fossa. However, the lower the bone resection, the further the frontal lobe will be able to come forward to fill the defect. If a small, 2- to 3-cm opening into the back of the sinus is left, the brain will not expand into the sinus to fill the cavity.

In cases in which there is either clear-cut or suspected dural penetration by bone, the fragments must be removed from the dura and underlying brain parenchyma. Assistance from a neurosurgeon is highly recommended for this intervention. Whoever disimpacts this bony fragment must be prepared to handle the possibility of intradural bleeding from either the brain itself, a meningeal vessel, or a dural sinus. Most otolaryngologists do not have the experience or competency to handle such an occurrence.

Management of the potential space of the sinus after removal of the posterior wall remains controversial. Some surgeons maintain that the space can be left alone and allowed to fill in with fluid and that, eventually, the brain will come forward to collapse the space. However, others have suggested that the space never really collapses and it is best to fill the space with an inert substance, such as a free fat graft. The local neurosurgeon should be included in this decision. In the author's experience, the local custom is to place the fat graft.

At the time of closure, the initial steps in blockage of the sinus ostia are the same as for obliteration. However, instead of placing a free temporalis graft over the bone chips in the ostia, the pericranial flap is folded down into the sinus to line the floor and posterior wall. The fat graft is then placed over the flap, and the anterior table is reconstructed as for the obliteration technique using titanium mesh and assembling the fragments on the back table. As described previously, it is worthwhile forming the initial contour of the mesh over the frontal bone before the anterior table is disassembled and placed on the back table.

Closure

After the frontal sinus fracture repair is completed, the wound is closed. Closure is performed exactly as detailed for frontal sinus obliteration in Chapter 11, with repair of the periosteum, placement of drains, and two-layered closure of the scalp. The exception is when cranialization is performed and the pericranial flap is turned into the sinus. In this situation, there will not be a periosteum to close over the anterior wall. In circumstances in which there is not coverage of the anterior wall and there are gaps in the anterior wall reconstruction, care must be taken not to place a drain directly over the gap, as this could result in suctioning of the fat graft.

Otherwise, the periosteum is closed with interrupted 3-0 Vicryl (Johnson & Johnson, Inc., Somerville, NJ). Drains are placed over the supraorbital ridges and across the vertex of the skull behind the incision and secured with an anchoring suture. The skin is closed in two layers with a galeal layer of 3-0 undyed Vicryl and staples for the skin.

Postoperative Care

The postoperative course will depend on the extent of the procedure. The need for close observation after surgery is greatest when cranialization is performed. The status of these patients should be monitored according to a postcraniotomy protocol, including intensive care monitoring, measures to minimize intracranial pressure, and invasive monitoring. Presuming that the patient awakens normally without altered mental status or neurologic deficits, transfer out of the intensive care unit may occur as early as the morning after surgery. Management of the patient with intracranial complications is beyond the scope of this discussion, but would include continued intensive care observation, probably hyperventilation, and possibly lumbar drainage. The exact treatment plan would be individualized.

The duration of hospitalization varies according to the output from the frontal drains. The drains are removed when the fluid accumulation is serosanguinous and less than 20 cc per day. Typically, this is on the third or fourth day after surgery, with discharge from the hospital usually possible on the fourth or fifth day. Other criteria for discharge include stable vital signs, ambulatory status, and adequate oral intake.

Postoperative medications include antibiotics and analgesics. The antibiotics should cover routine skin flora with no need for prophylaxis for sinusitis bacterial flora. Unless there has been gross contamination of the sinus following the injury, only minimal prophylactic therapy is necessary. Pain management will require parenteral narcotics for the first 2 to 4 postoperative days, with oral medications thereafter.

Activity is usually restricted until the patient is out of the intensive care unit. Ambulation is encouraged as early as the first postoperative day. Diet is also restricted early after the surgery, with advancement to a regular diet as tolerated by the patient.

Long-term follow-up evaluation is essential for these patients. If the sinus is preserved, long-term success is likely if a Caldwell view of the sinus 3 months after the surgery demonstrates aeration. Conversely, if the sinus is not aerated, endoscopic sinusotomy or trephination should be considered. In cases of an obliterated or cranialized sinus, a CT scan should be obtained 3 months after surgery as a baseline and then again after 1 and 2 years. Thereafter, periodic scans every 2 to 3 years are recommended for up to 20 years after the operation.[41,42]

Complications

It is important to distinguish between complications of the injury and complications of the surgery to repair the injury. The potential associated injuries that can occur with frontal sinus fractures have been discussed earlier in this chapter. In this section, complications associated with the repair of the injury are presented. The most serious complications associated with repair of frontal sinus fractures are intracranial, including hemorrhage, pneumocephalus, infection, and CSF leak.[43,44] All of these complications are rare. Because of this, it is difficult to accurately predict the risk of these complications as only a few individual surgeons have had a large enough series of these cases to report more than one patient with any of these complications.

Several possible complications are associated with the function of the sinus, including chronic or recurrent sinusitis if the sinus is preserved.[43–45] Mucocele and reabsorption of the sinus packing with reaeration of the sinus are considerations if the sinus is not preserved.[43,46,47]

The most common complication is residual cosmetic deformity after the repair. This can occur either from malalignment of the fracture or postoperative slippage. Using the techniques outlined in this chapter, the surgeon should be able to avoid these acute problems. In the long term, the patient may develop cosmetic deformity from frontal bossing or reabsorption of the bone flap. This has been estimated to occur in 5% to 10% of cases.[48]

MAXILLARY SINUS FRACTURES

Fractures of the maxillary sinus include a diverse group of injuries. They can be classified as isolated anterior or lateral wall fractures, orbital floor fractures, trimalar and orbital rim fractures, sagittal fractures, and Le Fort fractures.[49] The Le Fort fractures are subclassified as type I, II, and III depending on the highest level of fracture present (Fig. 15–16).[50] In practice, the Le Fort fractures are often mixed and comminuted, and may be combined with other fractures, such as naso-orbital ethmoid, frontal sinus, and mandibular fractures.

All maxillary sinus fractures involve one or more of the walls of the maxillary sinuses, but typically involve some of the surrounding structures as well, including the orbit, malar eminence, dentition, nasal wall, and pterygoid plates. The importance of the injury is related more to the surrounding structures than to the sinus itself. During repair, the goals of surgery will be related to which functional and cosmetic units are injured, but

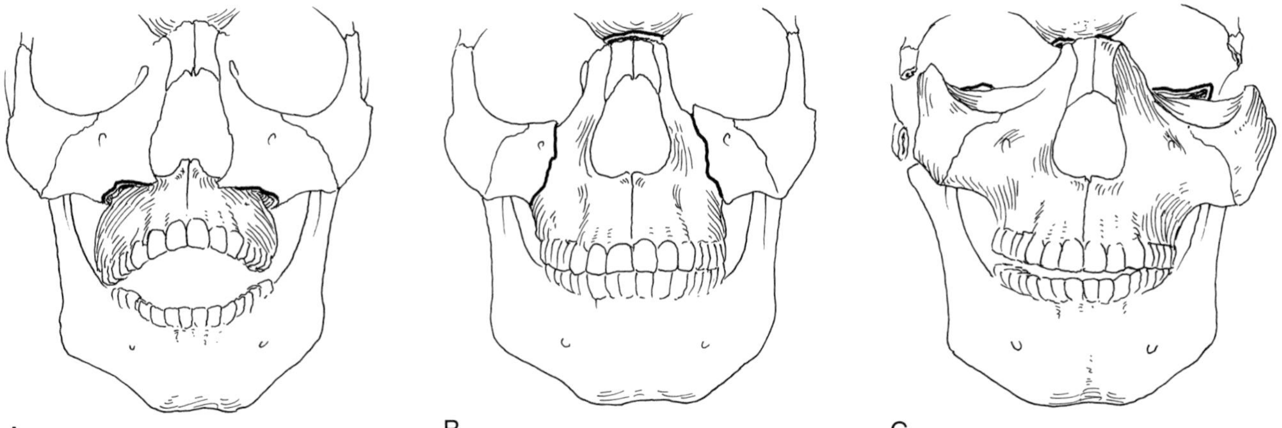

Figure 15–16. Pattern of classic Le Fort fractures. *A,* Type I. The fracture crosses the maxilla above the alveolar ridges, extending into the pyriform aperture and through the septum, medial walls of the maxillary sinuses, and the pterygoid plates. *B,* Type II. The fracture crosses vertically through the anterior wall of the maxilla, through the orbital rims, and across the floor of the orbits, lamina papyracea, root of the nose, and the pterygoid plates. *C,* Type III. The fracture crosses the zygomatic arches, the frontozygomatic suture lines, the floor of the orbits, the lamina papyracea, the nasal bones, and the pterygoid plates.

will include cosmetic correction, restoration of dental occlusion, maintenance of the nasal airway, and reconstruction of the orbit.

Diagnosis

The patient with maxillary sinus fracture typically demonstrates signs of obvious facial injury with swelling, ecchymosis, and epistaxis. The presence of a fracture of the maxillary sinus, whether isolated or not, is suggested by a finding of either opacification or air-fluid level on a Waters view radiograph of the sinuses. Further delineation requires a CT scan.[10, 51] The important aspects of the injury to understand before determining a treatment approach are the presence of comminution, the degree of displacement, and the involvement of the surrounding structures. Other associated injuries to rule out include orbital, nasal bone, and alveolar ridge involvement. During examination, the orbital rim should be palpated carefully to assess for step-offs, the alveolar ridge should be grasped and rocked to determine whether it is mobile, and a complete ophthalmologic examination should be performed to rule out ocular injury.

When dealing with maxillary sinus fractures, particularly the Le Fort fractures, special attention must be given the dentition. Careful inspection of the teeth is performed, with identification of occlusion and any nonviable teeth. A panoramic radiograph or other specific dental x-ray studies help to determine if any of the teeth are involved in the fracture. The condition of the dentition will have a major impact on the techniques involved in the repair. In situations when the dentition is inadequate to support intermaxillary fixation (IMF), the surgeon should consult a prosthodontist for fabrication of interdental or occlusal splints.

Indications for Surgery

The isolated anterior wall fracture will not need to be repaired for cosmetic reasons if the orbital rim, malar eminence, and pyriform aperture are all intact. These critical buttresses maintain the facial projection and contours. This is the reason that the Caldwell-Luc operation, with removal of the anterior wall of the sinus but preservation of the buttresses, does not cause deformity. There is some risk that the patient may develop a mucocele or cyst from mucosa being trapped between the fracture fragments. For this reason, if the patient is unlikely to be available for long-term follow-up evaluation, these complications can be avoided by treatment at the time of injury.

The main indication for repair of the anterior wall of the maxillary sinus is involvement of the pyriform aperture with medial displacement.[52] This results in narrowing of the nasal valve on the ipsilateral side, with the possibility that the nose will retract in that location, resulting in loss of projection and lateral rotation of the nasal tip. In this situation, the goal of surgery will be to elevate the pyriform aperture and fix it in place in the natural anatomic position.

The indications for repair of orbital floor fractures have been the subject of considerable controversy over the last decades. Prevailing surgical preferences have shifted from mandatory repair of all fractures, to repair of only those fractures associated with entrapment or enophthalmos, to a middle-ground approach. The difficulty is in trying to predict which fractures will result in late complications, specifically, enophthalmos. It is clear that patients without displacement of the orbital floor are at no risk for late enophthalmos, whereas patients with significant prolapse into the maxillary sinus are at high risk for this difficult complication.[53] The controversy is fueled by the technical difficulty of secondary repair of enophthalmos.[54–56] If the patient is unfortunate enough to develop diplopia secondary to late enophthalmos, it can be extremely difficult to overcome this problem in secondary repair. For this reason, some surgeons have advocated repair of all but nondisplaced fractures. Other surgeons have cited the ultimately low incidence of these complications as their rationale for operating for entrapment or measurable enophthalmos after the acute swelling has resolved.

The author takes the middle ground on this controversy and suggests repair for entrapment, measurable enophthalmos, and identifiable prolapse of orbital contents into the maxillary sinus on coronal CT scan.

There are several indications for repair of orbital rim and trimalar fractures.[57–61] The first is when the trimalar fracture is associated with depression of the zygomatic arch, resulting in trismus. Trismus is caused by compression of the temporalis muscle and blockage of the opening of the temporomandibular joint. A second reason for repair of a trimalar fracture is to prevent orbital expansion. In severe cases, the lateral and inferior orbit may expand enough to result in displacement of the globe and diplopia. The most common indication for repair of the trimalar and orbital rim fractures is to prevent cosmetic deformity. Both of these fractures can result in expansion of the orbital rim. This gives the perception of an enlarged, hollow orbit. The trimalar fracture can also result in malar flattening. Gravity tends to pull down on these fractures over time, and may cause distraction of the fracture fragments. This is very difficult to reconstruct secondarily. For this reason, reduction and internal fixation is indicated for all but the completely nondisplaced fractures. The truly nondisplaced fracture may be observed for 2 weeks and reexamined at that point. If the fracture remains nondisplaced and the malar eminence is not mobile after 2 weeks, surgery can be avoided.

Le Fort fractures are always repaired so as to avoid malocclusion, elongation of the face, and retrusion of the face. Le Fort I fractures may be repaired with IMF alone if they are not comminuted. Alternatively, internal fixation can be applied, which will shorten the duration of IMF required. Le Fort II and III repairs are usually complex and require both IMF and internal fixation. As noted earlier, these injuries are often associated with significant comminution and other facial fractures. The approach to these injuries will be discussed in detail later in the chapter.

Technique

Isolated Anterior Wall Fracture

Isolated anterior wall fractures of the maxillary sinus are uncommon injuries. They usually result from a hard blow to the face with a small object or a gunshot wound to this area. As stated previously, the anterior wall fractures that extend into the pyriform aperture (medial maxillary fractures) are the ones that require repair. The two cases of this type of injury in the author's experience were the result of a boot kick to the face and a gunshot wound from a small-caliber handgun. Higher-impact injuries and injury from larger objects tend to cause a larger area of injury and will result in combination fractures, rather than isolated anterior wall injuries.

The approach to this fracture repair is through a simple sublabial incision. The technique is identical to that outlined in Chapter 10 for surgery of the maxillary sinus in the presence of inflammatory disease. The only difference is that, when repairing the anterior wall fracture, it is necessary to achieve complete exposure of the medial aspects, including the pyriform aperture. For this reason, the incision should be extended medially at least to the midline, and it can be extended as far laterally on the contralateral side as necessary.

After the incision is completed down through the periosteum to the bone, the periosteum is elevated. Final exposure should extend up to the infraorbital nerve and frontal process of the maxilla superiorly, the pyriform aperture medially, and the malar eminence laterally (Fig. 15–17A). It is important during elevation to make sure that small fragments are not lifted with the cheek flap. Careful and slow dissection should be able to detect these small fragments as they are approached.

The fracture, once exposed, must be reduced to the premorbid alignment. This is accomplished by using an instrument in the nose to push outwardly and laterally on the pyriform aperture. Rather than trying to preserve the entire anterior wall, it is best to resect the smaller, loose fragments. As noted earlier, these fragments are not necessary to maintain cosmetic or functional integrity. Larger fragments are levered into position using either a hook or an elevator. It is advisable to make sure that mucosa is not trapped in between fragments of bone before beginning the fixation.

The usual choices for fixation are applicable to anterior wall fractures. Plate size is important over the pyriform aperture area, as 2.0-mm plates and larger will definitely be palpable. If the fracture is simple, a curved microplate (1.0 to 1.2 mm) is preferred. If the fracture is comminuted, micromesh is selected. The repair proceeds with alignment of the fragments, contouring of the plate or mesh, and careful fixation. The plate or

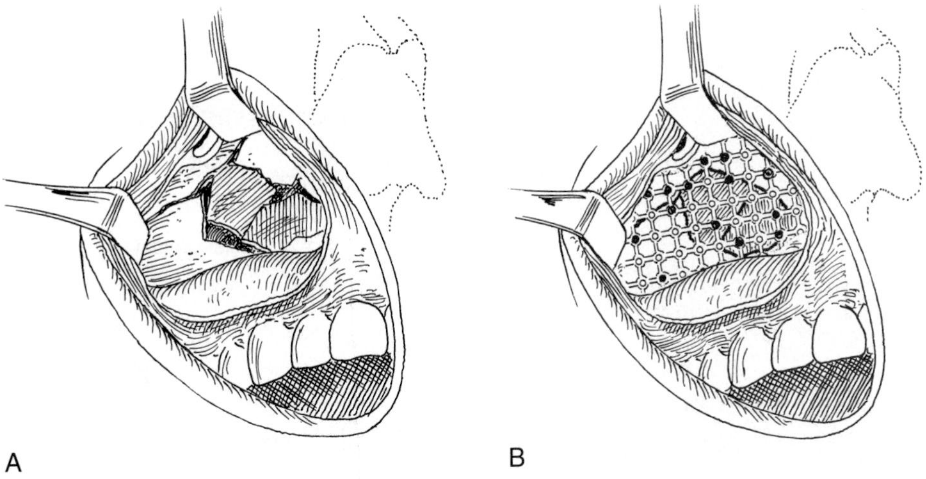

Figure 15–17. Repair of a medial maxillary fracture using titanium micromesh. *A,* The area of the fracture is exposed through a sublabial incision and subperiosteal dissection. *B,* The mesh is contoured and fixed in place, securing each fragment with two or more screws.

mesh should be secured to stable surrounding bone first and then to the loose fragments (Fig. 15–17B). The procedure is completed with closure of the sublabial incision using simple interrupted sutures.

Orbital Floor Fracture

Orbital floor fractures can be repaired by numerous different techniques using a variety of implants or grafts. The basic approach is either through a subciliary or transconjunctival incision.[62–65] More complicated cases may require a sublabial incision to enter the maxillary sinus, in addition to the orbital incision. The decision to use the transconjunctival or the subciliary incision will depend on previous experience, training, and the results achieved by a particular surgeon. Both incisions are acceptable. The subciliary incision typically heals very well without perceptible scar. The main disadvantage of the subciliary incision is an increased incidence of postoperative ectropion. This results from scarring and contracture, which pull the lid margin inferiorly. The incidence of ectropion with this incision will vary with the degree of exposure, the exact location of the incision relative to the lid margin (the greater the proximity to the lid, the higher the risk of ectropion), and the skill of the surgeon in avoiding trauma to the underlying orbital septum and orbicularis muscle.

The transconjunctival incision has the disadvantage of less exposure to the orbital rim and the medial and lateral extent of the orbits. For this reason, it is primarily used for isolated orbital floor fractures with a moderate degree of fracture displacement. The subciliary incision is preferred when there is a combination of orbital rim with orbital floor, or when an extensive floor fracture is present, requiring wider exposure.

The subciliary incision is placed 2 to 3 mm below the lash line. It is marked out and then injected with local anesthetic containing 1:100,000 epinephrine (Fig. 15–18A). The incision is carried through the subcutaneous layers and the orbicularis muscle (Fig. 15–18B). Once the orbicularis muscle is incised, the orbital septum should be easily identifiable immediately deep to the muscle. The inferior edge of the muscle is grasped with a fine forceps (such as a Bishop-Harmon) and the lid margin is stabilized superiorly for countertraction. The muscle is dissected from the underlying septum inferiorly to the orbital rim using curved iris scissors. Another technique that works well for this is to use two cotton-tipped applicators, one holding the lid margin superiorly, the other applying tension on the developing plane. When the orbital rim is reached, the orbit is retracted with a malleable retractor while the lid is retracted over the orbital rim using a Senn retractor (Fig. 15–18C). This stretches the tissues over the orbital rim, allowing palpation of the superior edge.

The superior edge of the inferior orbital rim is exposed by incising the stretched tissues with a scalpel down to the bone on the facial side of the rim. The orbital floor can then be exposed by elevating the orbital periosteum using a Freer elevator.

Similar techniques are applied using the transconjunctival incision. The initial incision is placed about 5 mm below the lid margin (Fig. 15–19). The incision is carried through the orbital fat to the septum. The internal surface of the septum is followed inferiorly a few millimeters before incising the orbital septum. This is to ensure that the crossover point is inferior to the tarsal plate. The external surface of the orbital septum is then followed inferiorly to the orbital rim. The remainder of the procedure is performed as for the subciliary incision.

The orbital periosteum is elevated from the rim onto the floor with the Freer elevator. A headlight will be necessary for visualization. The orbital contents are then retracted with a malleable and the lid retracted as necessary with a Senn or Army-Navy retractor. During eleva-

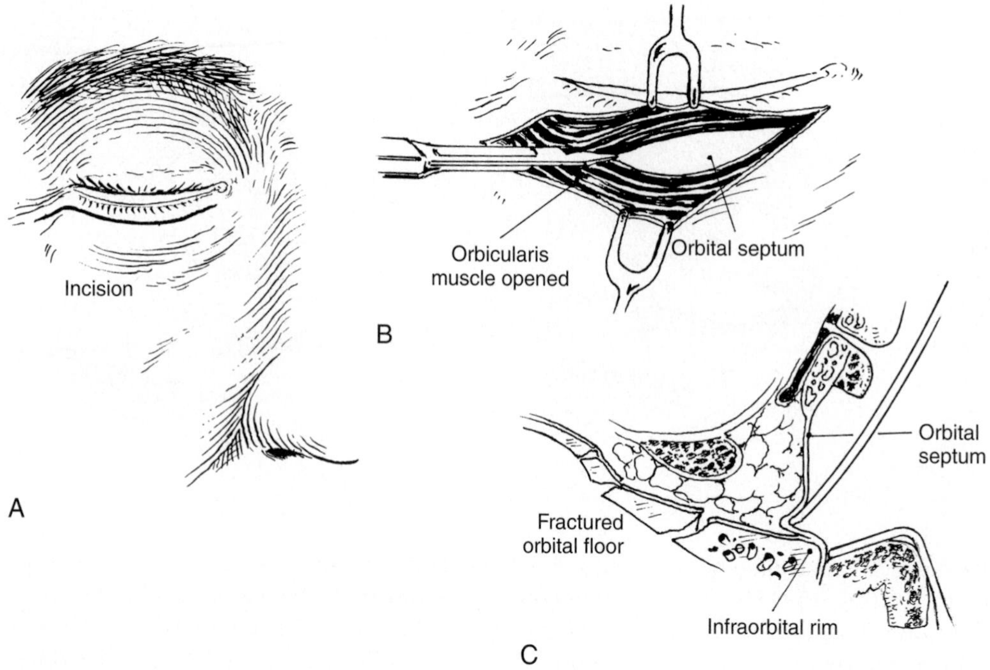

Figure 15–18. Subciliary incision for exposure of the orbital floor. *A,* The incision parallels the eyelid 2 to 3 mm below the lash line. If lateral extension is needed, this follows a natural skin crease. *B,* The incision is carried through the skin, subcutaneous tissues, and orbicularis muscle to the level of the orbital septum. *C,* After the lid is dissected on the surface of the orbital septum down to the level of the orbital rim, a malleable is used to retract the orbit and a Senn retractor in used to pull the periosteum tight against the underlying muscle.

tion, care should be taken to avoid trauma to the infraorbital nerve and vessels. As the dissection proceeds, the inferior orbital fissure will be reached laterally in the floor. If it is necessary to achieve exposure posterior to this point, the contents of the fissure may be divided. When the defect in the floor is identified, it is best to elevate completely around the defect to establish the level of the orbital floor. This also helps to gain leverage on the tissues prolapsed into the defect. The tissues of the orbit are then slowly teased out of the defect. The goal is to completely elevate the orbital structures circumferentially around the defect in the floor. Extreme care must be exercised when elevating posterior to the defect, as this is invariably close to the optic nerve.

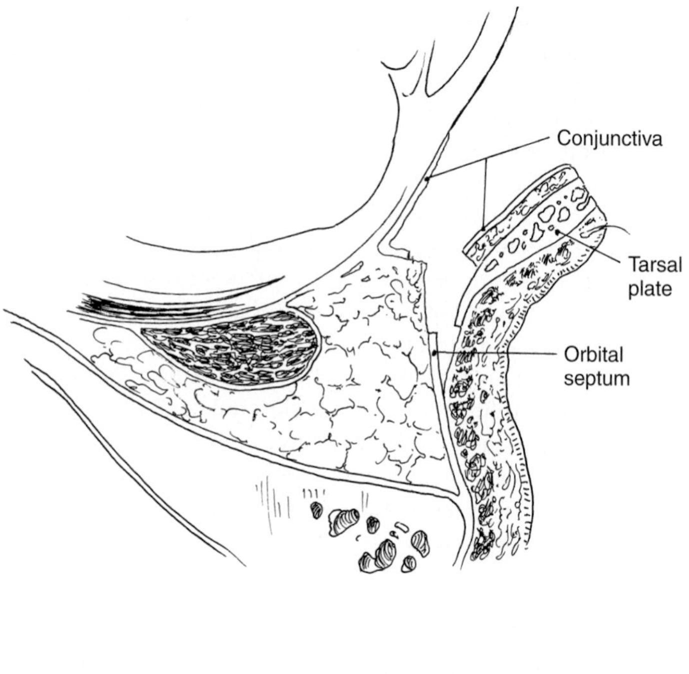

Figure 15–19. Conjunctival incision for exposure of the orbital floor. The incision is made about 5 mm below the lid margin. The tarsal plate is followed down to the orbital septum. The orbital septum is incised, and the remainder of the dissection proceeds on the outer surface of the septum, as for the subciliary incision.

Once the defect is completely exposed, a decision on the nature of the repair must be made. Usually it is possible to elevate the fragments back into position, but they will not be stable and will not hold. For that reason, some means of supporting the floor and orbital contents must be identified. One possibility is to support the floor using packing or a balloon catheter in the maxillary sinus. This has not proven to be necessary or preferable in most cases. A variety of implants and grafts have been proposed to support the orbit.[66–72] The author uses Marlex mesh (Davol, Inc., Cranston, RI) for most cases, and split calvarial bone grafts when the Marlex is not sufficient. Marlex is a synthetic polymer (polyethylene) that bends but has good rigidity and strength. It is easily trimmed and slides nicely into the orbit (Fig. 15–20). Normally, it does not need to be secured, as it will be held in place by the pressure of the orbit.

When there is a large defect that cannot be bridged stably by Marlex mesh, the split calvarial graft is used. In most cases, this is decided prior to surgery based on the CT scan findings. In this way, the graft can be harvested before the orbit is opened. This minimizes the trauma to the orbit and the amount of edema present at the time the graft is placed. The graft is notched posteriorly to allow it to rest against the posterior bone ledge (Fig. 15–21). The graft is typically not secured, but can be plated or wired anteriorly to prevent slippage.

In rare cases, it is necessary to approach the orbital floor through both the orbit and the maxillary sinus. In such cases, severe prolapse of the orbit into the sinus makes it difficult to elevate the periosteum from the orbital bone owing to the severe angle. A Caldwell-Luc approach is used to expose the fracture from below. In this way, the plane between the bone and periosteum can be identified and the dissection begun. Once the orbital contents are freed from the bone, the eye can be easily elevated back into the orbit and the floor can usually be reduced. It is always necessary to support the floor in this situation, usually with a bone graft.

The subciliary incision is closed with a running subcuticular 5-0 Prolene suture (Johnson & Johnson, Inc., Somerville, NJ). The periosteum is intentionally not closed, as this will increase the risk of ectropion. The transconjunctival incision is reapproximated with interrupted 6-0 chromic sutures. Unless the incision has been placed too far toward the lid margin, these sutures should not irritate the cornea.

Trimalar and Orbital Rim Fracture

The trimalar fracture is one of the most common fractures caused by facial trauma.[57–61, 73, 74] Typically, there are four fractures: the frontozygomatic suture line, the zygomatic arch, the lateral wall of the maxillary sinus, and the inferior orbital rim (Fig. 15–22). Frequently, there will be comminution, especially in the inferior orbital rim, and there may be associated adjacent fractures, most commonly in the orbital floor. Adequate repair of this fracture requires, at a minimum, fixation of two fracture lines to avoid rotation about any single fracture site repair.

The most common deformity associated with trimalar fracture is for the malar eminence to be rotated inferiorly and depressed or flattened. The inferior orbital

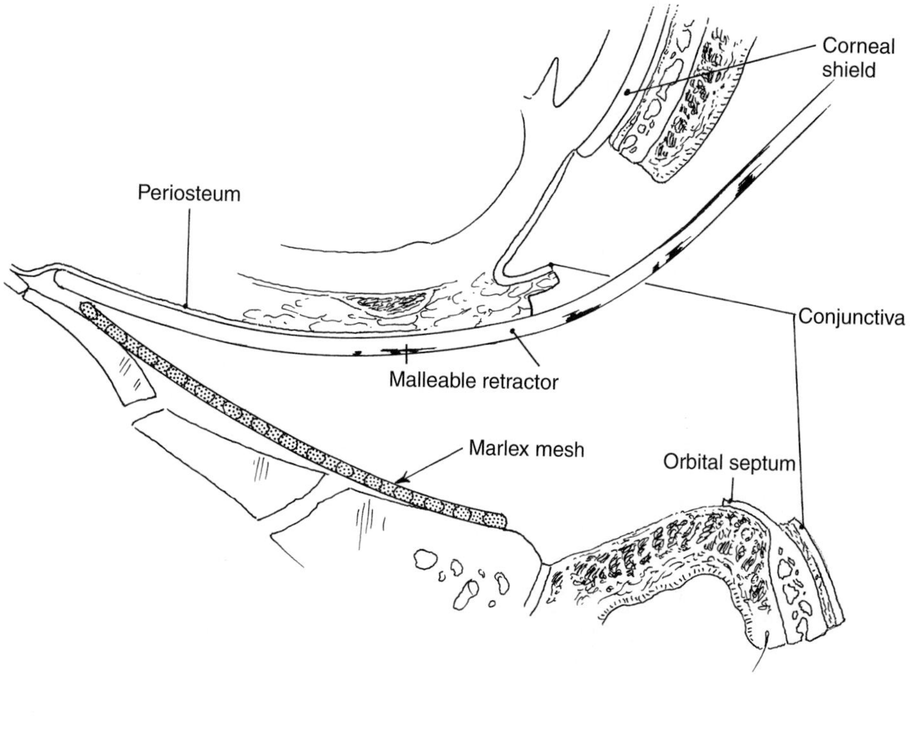

Figure 15–20. Repair of an orbital floor fracture with Marlex mesh. The orbital contents are dissected from the orbital floor in a subperiosteal plane. The subluxed contents are elevated, the bone fragments are elevated into position, and the mesh is placed over the defect resting on stabile bone completely around the defect.

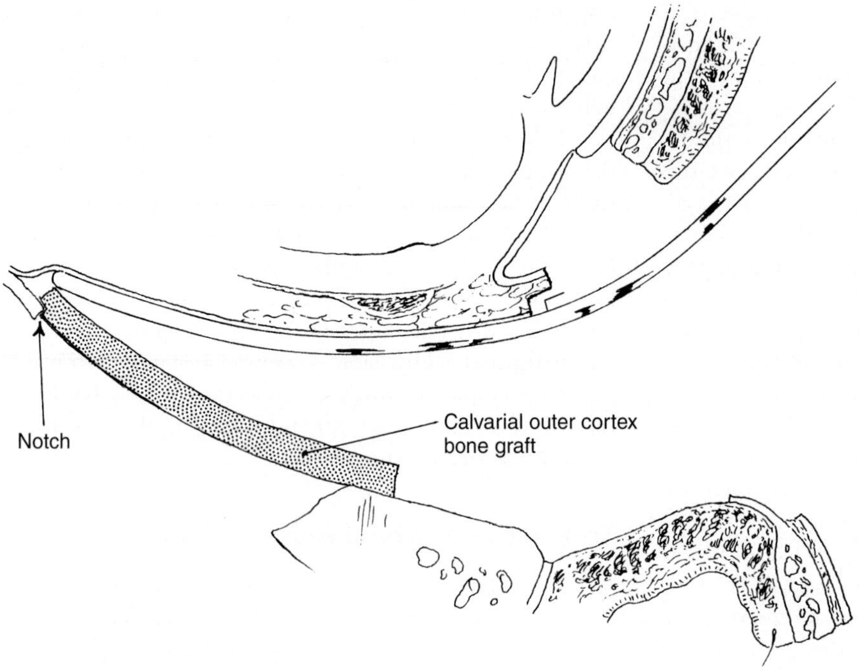

Figure 15–21. Repair of an orbital floor fracture using a split calvarial bone graft. The approach is identical to that used for the mesh repair. The defect is spanned by a polished graft trimmed to the best shape. If the graft cannot easily lay on the stabile bone behind the defect, a notch in the graft can be carved to rest against the posterior ledge of bone.

rim is usually also inferior and depressed. The goals in this procedure are to recreate the premorbid malar projection, restore the inferior orbital rim contour, and reduce the zygomatic arch to avoid trismus. The most difficult aspect of this repair is to achieve the appropriate malar projection. The surgeon must use premorbid photographs and the contralateral side as guides to gauge the proper position.

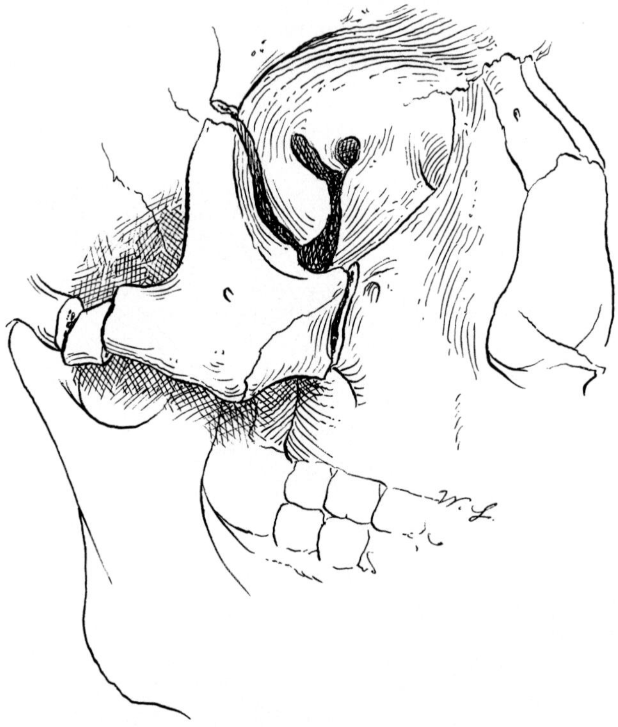

Figure 15–22. Trimalar fracture. The fractures extend through the zygomatic arch, frontozygomatic suture, anterior wall of the maxilla and orbital rim, orbital floor, and lateral wall of the orbit.

There are a variety of approaches to achieve this repair. The orbital rim can be approached through a sublabial incision, transconjunctival incision, or subciliary incision. The frontozygomatic fracture is typically approached through a lateral brow incision. The zygomatic arch is normally approached through a Gillies' incision behind the temporal hairline.[75] However, as an alternative to the brow and Gillies' incisions, a bicoronal incision with maximal inferior and lateral extension can expose the lateral orbital rim and zygomatic arch.

The preferred approach is to combine the subciliary, lateral brow, and Gillies' incisions. This maximizes exposure for both reduction and fixation without unacceptable cosmetic alterations. The subciliary incision has been described earlier. The lateral brow incision is oriented in the lateral aspect of the eyebrow along the upper border of the brow (Fig. 15–23A). When making this incision, it is advisable to bevel the incision to parallel the hair shafts. This will avoid cutting across the follicles. The incision is continued through subcutaneous layers of fascia, muscle, and periosteum to the lateral orbital rim. The periosteum is elevated from the bone in all directions until both the fracture and sufficient bone on either side are exposed (Fig. 15–23B).

The Gillies' incision is used to approach the zygomatic arch. The temporal hairline should be marked out and then shaved back about 3 cm; alternatively, a

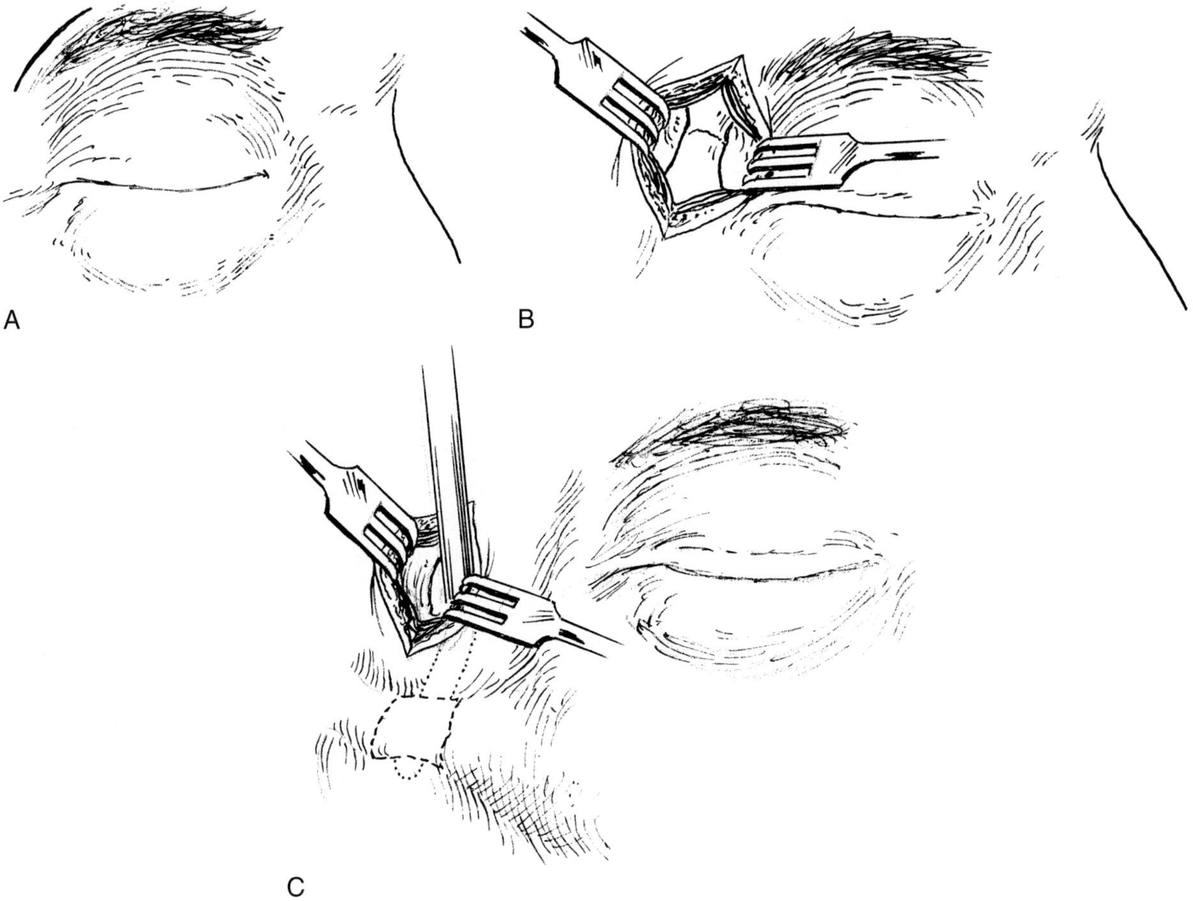

Figure 15–23. Exposure of trimalar fracture. *A,* A lateral brow incision allows exposure of the frontozygomatic suture. *B,* Exposure of the frontozygomatic suture. The mobile skin of the lateral brow is pulled down to the lower orbital rim at the suture. *C,* Gillies' incision and dissection. The incision is in the bicoronal incision behind the hairline. The elevator is directed deep to the temporalis fascia and below the depressed fragments of the zygomatic arch.

small patch of hair at the incision site can be shaved. The incision is made parallel to the line of a bicoronal incision. The incision need only be 2 or 3 cm in length. The incision is carried down through the temporalis fascia to the surface of the temporalis muscle. A curved blunt elevator (Gillies' elevator) can then be dissected on the undersurface of the temporalis fascia deep to the zygomatic arch (Fig. 15–23C).

Before the first fracture is plated, all fracture sites should be fully exposed. In most cases, this includes the inferior and lateral orbital rims. The orbital floor is normally explored to rule out blow-out fracture. The zygomatic arch is only exposed if there is a significant depression of the arch that requires elevation. Once all the incisions have been completed, the first step is to reduce the zygomatic arch. The elevator is worked into place and lateral pressure is applied to the fractured arch. Usually, reduction will be accompanied by a palpable pop or click, and the mobilized arch can be felt to elevate into position.

The next goal is to rotate the malar eminence into position. An elevator is placed through the lateral brow incision and along the lateral orbital rim deep to the root of the zygomatic arch (Fig. 15–24). A second elevator is directed through the subciliary incision under the inferior orbital rim. Simultaneous rocking pressure should mobilize the malar eminence. If this fails, a towel clip or bone clamp can be applied to the orbital rim to apply increased force. If this is still not sufficient, the fracture can be approached through a sublabial incision through the maxillary sinus. An instrument is pushed outward on the lateral superior aspect of the sinus. With a combination of these techniques, it should be possible to mobilize the fracture and achieve alignment. If a significant delay has occurred between the injury and repair, the bones may already have begun to heal. In

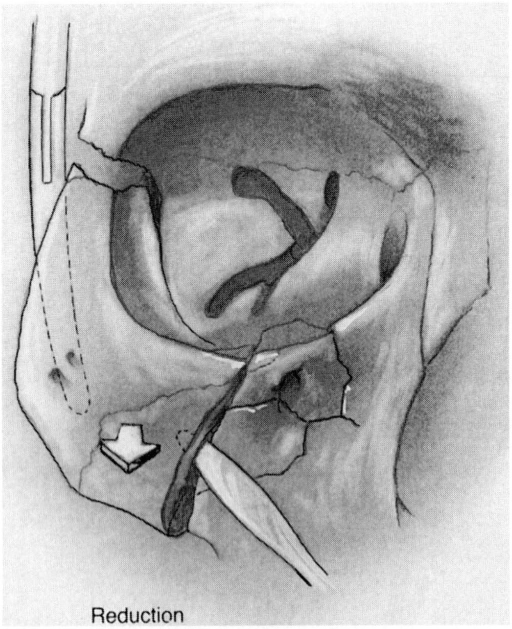

Figure 15–24. Reduction of the trimalar fracture. Elevators through the lateral brow and subciliary incision exert leverage against the zygoma from two directions. (Reprinted with permission from Mathog RH (ed). Atlas of Craniofacial Trauma. Philadelphia: WB Saunders, 1992, p. 272.)

this case, osteotomies may be necessary to loosen the fracture segments.

Fixation is achieved using a 4-hole, 1.5-mm plate on the lateral orbital rim. The plate in this location usually needs little or no contouring and is normally placed first. The inferior orbital rim is reconstructed with a curved, 1.5-mm plate (Fig. 15–25). This can be trimmed to the size needed, but may need to extend from the lateral orbital rim to the nasal bones to achieve stability. Generally, a minimal amount of contouring is required to match this plate to the desired shape. The most stabile point is secured first, and the opposite end is then secured before any central comminuted fragments are secured. In the case of an isolated unilateral trimalar fracture, the nasal bone should be stabile and would, therefore, be attached to the plate first. However, with combination fractures, this may not be the case and the plate may need to be secured to the lateral orbital rim first.

Le Fort Fractures

Le Fort fractures are variable and are almost always associated with other facial fractures. The exact procedure, therefore, is dependent on the unique circumstances of each case. The basic principles are always the same, however: disimpact the maxilla, achieve IMF, and stabilize the fractures beginning from the lowest stabile point and proceeding inferiorly.[76–78] For example, if a patient has bilateral Le Fort I, II, and III fractures in addition to frontal sinus and type III naso-orbital ethmoid fractures, the frontal sinus is secured first, the NOE second, the malar eminence and zygomatic arches next, the inferior orbital rims next, and the alveolar ridges to the malar eminences last.

Before the fracture can be addressed, it is necessary to decide on the management of the airway.[79] Two options are commonly available. The simplest approach is to perform a tracheostomy. This removes the endotracheal tube from consideration and allows both nasal packing and IMF. Another option is to first orally intubate the patient. The maxilla is then disimpacted as described below. The oral tracheal tube is then switched to a nasotracheal tube to allow IMF. After the Le Fort fracture is stabilized, the IMF can be released, and the tube switched to the oral cavity, thus allowing the nasal injuries to be addressed. Alternatively, an armored endotracheal tube can be passed behind the teeth to allow IMF and nasal manipulation. The decision of which technique to use depends on the severity of the injuries and the difficulty in obtaining an airway through repeated intubation. If the intubation is difficult or the injuries are severe and suggest the need for long-term IMF, the tracheostomy is always available. The tracheostomy can be decannulated as early as the patient is able to control the airway.

The first step in repairing the fracture is to disimpact the maxilla, which is often pushed back and rotated (Fig. 15–26). Several instruments are available specifically for this purpose. These instruments resemble tongs; a flat tine is positioned inside the nose against

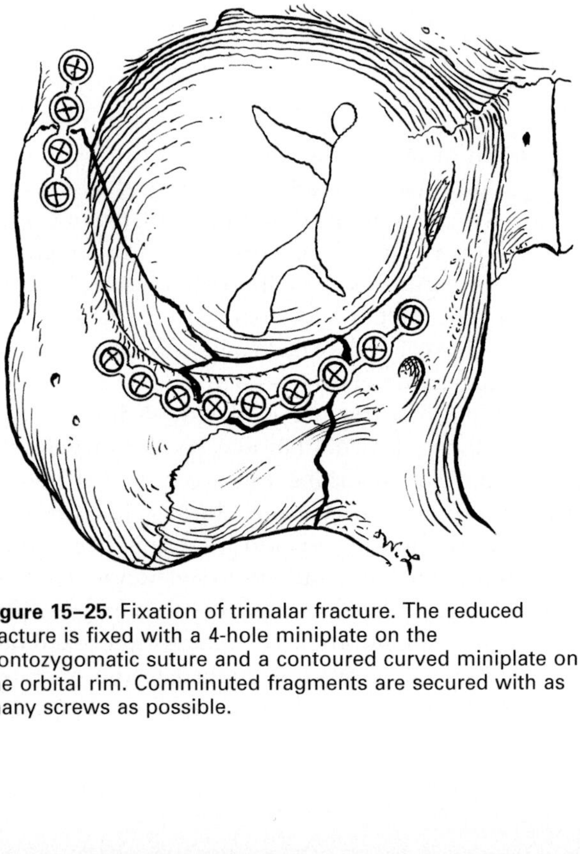

Figure 15–25. Fixation of trimalar fracture. The reduced fracture is fixed with a 4-hole miniplate on the frontozygomatic suture and a contoured curved miniplate on the orbital rim. Comminuted fragments are secured with as many screws as possible.

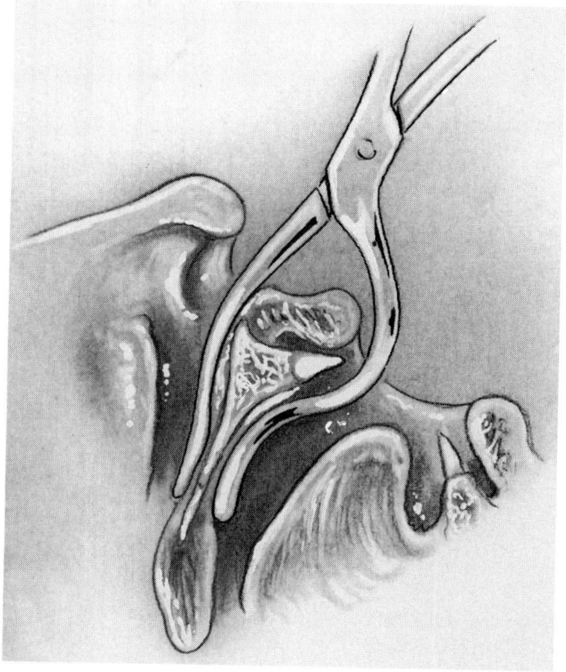

Figure 15–26. Disimpaction of the maxilla using Rowe forceps. The forceps are placed through the nose and around the teeth to grasp the palate from both sides. The maxilla is then rocked down and pulled forward. (Reprinted with permission from Mathog RH (ed). Atlas of Craniofacial Trauma. Philadelphia: WB Saunders, 1992, p. 153.)

the floor of the nose and a curved tine extends around the maxillary teeth into the mouth to grasp the palatal side. With one of these instruments on each side of the nose, the maxilla can be rocked anteriorly and pulled forward into position.

The next step is to secure the occlusal relationships. The two most common techniques include Erich arch bars and Ivy loops. The Ivy loops are faster and easier, but do not achieve the degree of stabilization that arch bars create. Ivy loops may be used when there is inadequate dentition to support full arch bars or if only minimal stabilization is needed. Usually, a 25-gauge wire is used. A small loop is created in the middle of the wire. The two loose ends are passed through the same interdental space from outside to inside the mouth. The wires are then passed around the distal and mesial teeth, respectively, through the interdental spaces and back to the buccal surface (Fig. 15–27). The two ends are then twisted together to tighten the loop to the adjacent teeth. Loops from the maxillary and mandibular teeth are wired together to hold the jaws in occlusion.

Erich arch bars are applied to the entire dental arch. Typically, the bars are secured to four teeth on each side for both the maxillary and mandibular arch. The preferred pattern is to use the first molar, both premolars, and the canine on each side. Each wire is passed on the side of the bar away from the occlusal surface through the interdental space from outside to inside the mouth. The wire is then turned and passed back from inside to outside of the mouth on the side of the bar closest to the occlusal surface of the tooth (Fig. 15–28). The ends of the wire are then twisted together in a clockwise direction to tighten the loop to the bar and tooth.

For the canine teeth, a special technique called a Dingman loop is used to avoid slippage against the smooth crown of the canine. The wire is passed from outside to inside the mouth on the side of the bar away from the occlusal surface, as with the normal situation, but is passed back on the same side of the bar. The wire is then looped around the arch bar and tightened. After eight teeth on the maxillary and mandibular arches have been secured, the arch bars are wired together to bring the teeth into occlusion. The teeth should be placed in the same alignment as the premorbid occlusion. This can be ascertained using dental models, if available, or by examining the wear facets on the teeth. In most cases, the relationships are not hard to determine.

After the occlusion is stabilized, the fractures are exposed through a variety of incisions. The exact incision used will depend largely on the associated injuries present. For pure Le Fort I fractures, bilateral sublabial incisions are sufficient. For pure Le Fort II fractures, the sublabial incision will need to be augmented by some technique to access the inferior orbital rim (either a subciliary or transconjunctival incision). For Le Fort III fractures, these incisions can be combined with lateral brow incisions and Gillies' incisions, or a bicoronal incision can be used. The presence of accompanying fractures, such as a naso-orbital ethmoid, orbital floor, or frontal sinus fractures, may require that an alternative approach be considered.

The Le Fort I fracture may be repaired using a variety of methods. If the fracture is simple and not comminuted, IMF with circumzygomatic wires alone may suffice. Alternatively, direct plating, using either 1.5-mm plates or mesh, may be performed. After IMF, this is achieved through the sublabial approach. The fractures are carefully exposed to avoid elevating the fragments during periosteal dissection. Once the fractures are adequately exposed, plates are placed from the alveolar segment across the fracture line to stabile bone (Fig. 15–29). A plate with at least three screws on each side of the fracture is recommended to achieve optimal stability.

The Le Fort II fracture requires some form of rigid fixation. Both the sublabial and subciliary incisions should be performed bilaterally before beginning the repair. The orbital floor should be explored and significant defects repaired first, as described earlier. The orbital rim is repaired next, using a curved minifixation plate, as shown in Figure 15–25. The last step is to secure the alveolar ridge to the malar eminence. In most cases,

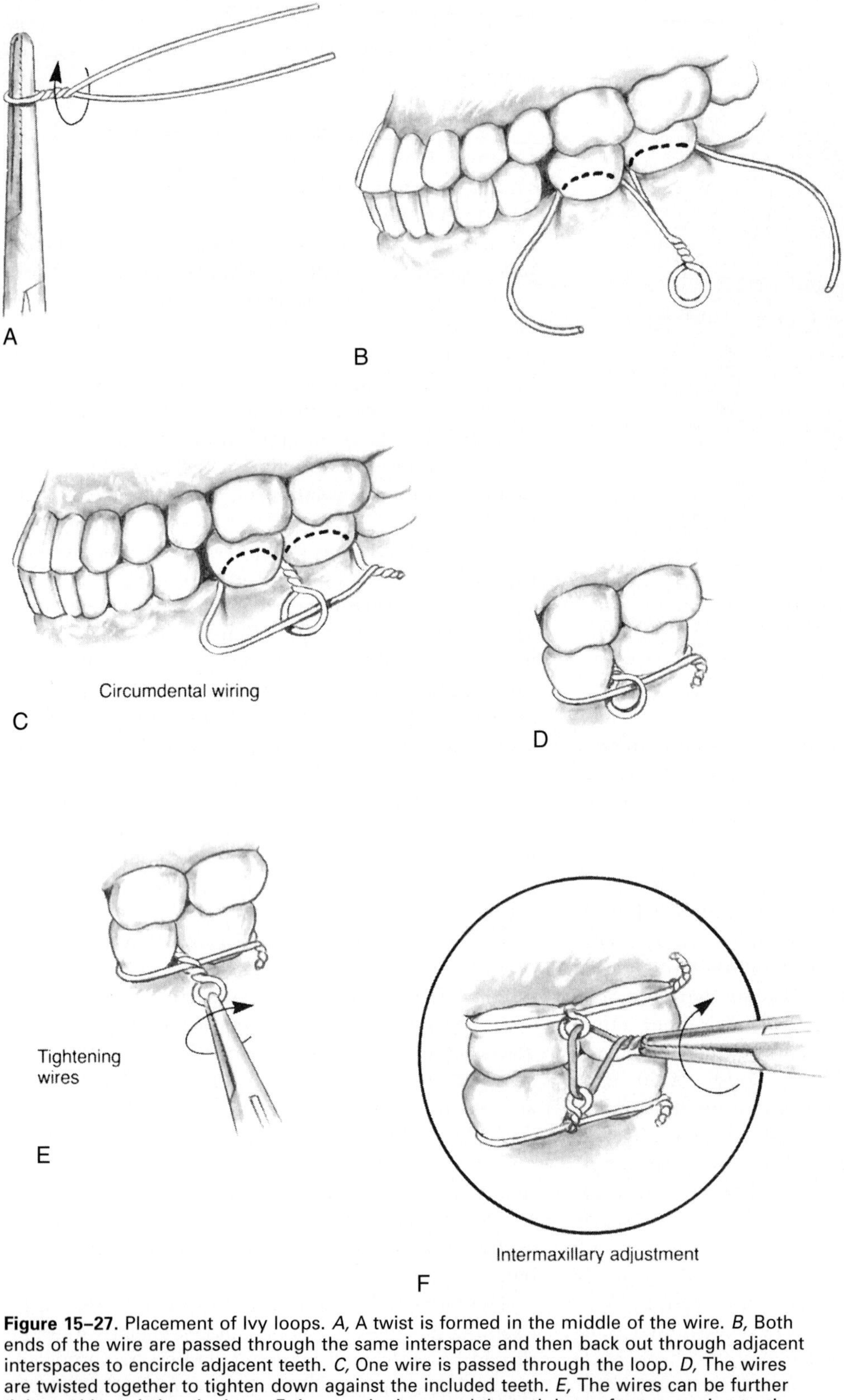

Figure 15–27. Placement of Ivy loops. *A,* A twist is formed in the middle of the wire. *B,* Both ends of the wire are passed through the same interspace and then back out through adjacent interspaces to encircle adjacent teeth. *C,* One wire is passed through the loop. *D,* The wires are twisted together to tighten down against the included teeth. *E,* The wires can be further tightened by twisting the loop. *F,* A new wire is passed through loops from opposing teeth and tightened down to hold the teeth in occlusion. (Reprinted with permission from Mathog RH (ed). Atlas of Craniofacial Trauma. Philadelphia: WB Saunders, 1992, p. 42.)

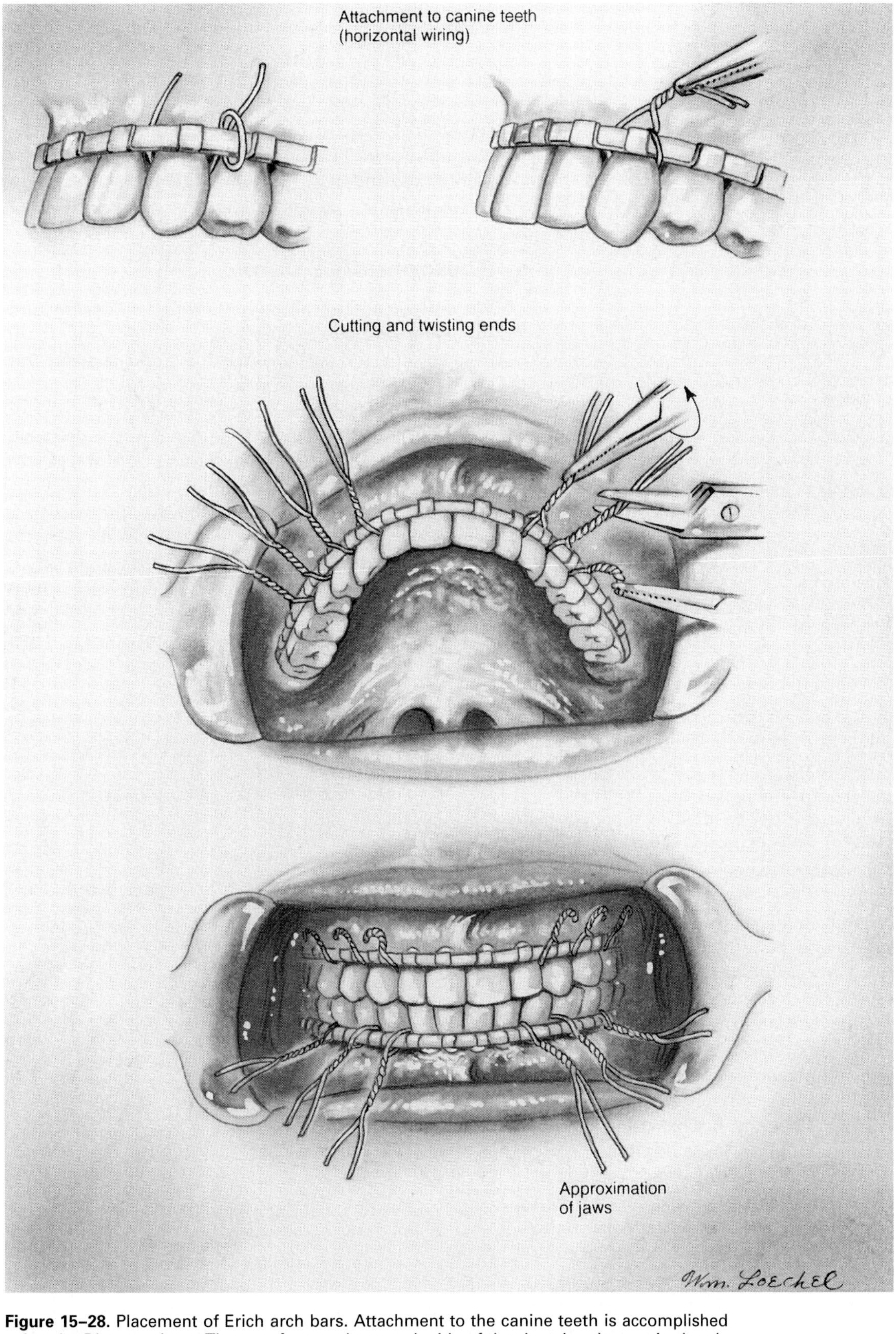

Figure 15–28. Placement of Erich arch bars. Attachment to the canine teeth is accomplished using the Dingman loop. Three or four teeth on each side of the dental arch are wired and the wires are tightened. The wires are then trimmed and turned in to avoid catching on the mucosa. (Reprinted with permission from Mathog RH (ed). Atlas of Craniofacial Trauma. Philadelphia: WB Saunders, 1992, p. 39.)

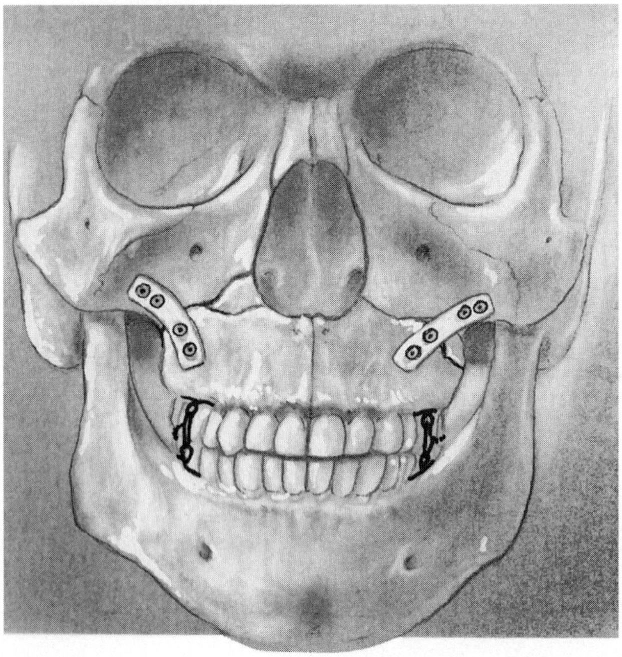

Figure 15–29. Repair of a Le Fort I fracture using Ivy loops and compression plate fixation. The plate extends from the mobile alveolar ridge segment to the stabile malar bone. (Reprinted with permission from Mathog RH (ed). Atlas of Craniofacial Trauma. Philadelphia: WB Saunders, 1992, p. 157.)

this is done with a plate that extends from the alveolar segment onto stabile bone of the malar eminence across the fracture. In cases in which there is severe comminution or bone loss from the anterior wall, bone grafts, using split calvarial strips, can be used to stabilize the fracture (Fig. 15–30). Alternatively, titanium micromesh can be used in this instance.

Le Fort III fractures are repaired by securing the facial bones to stabile bone of the skull, proceeding from the lowest point of stability to the alveolar segment. The most popular approach is through the bicoronal flap, as this exposes the zygomatic arches and lateral orbital rims optimally. The key to a good cosmetic result with Le Fort III fractures is to ensure that the facial projection from the zygomatic arches is correct. For this reason, this is usually the first step in repair. The arches can be plated on the superior surface using 4-hole, 1.5-mm plates. If comminution is present, a longer plate will be required. The next step is to secure the lateral orbital rim where the fracture usually extends through the frontozygomatic suture line. As described for the trimalar fracture, this is usually adequately accomplished with a 4-hole, 1.5-mm plate. The last step is to evaluate the position of the nasal bones. If these bones are in reasonable alignment, direct rigid fixation is not necessary. However, if the nasal bones are depressed or if there is subluxation, fixation may be necessary. The nasal bones are usually plated with 1.0-mm microplates.

In most patients, the classic Le Fort III fracture is accompanied by severe comminution and, often, a combination of all three types of Le Fort fracture. If this is the case, the repair begins, as described earlier, with disimpaction, IMF, and repair of the Le Fort III level repair first. Once this is completed, the lower fractures are addressed. The inferior orbital rims are then repaired, and the final step is to plate the alveolar ridge fragments to the malar eminence.

Postoperative Care

Without exception, all patients with Le Fort fractures should be hospitalized after surgery. Other patients with isolated anterior wall, orbital floor, and trimalar fractures may be operated on as outpatients if all factors are favorable. The most critical issues for these patients center around the status of the eye and the degree of swelling of the face. The patient may be discharged if postoperative swelling is minimal and not increasing and if the eye edema is mild, allowing the patient to keep the eye open. However, if the eye swells closed or if the facial swelling is severe, the safest approach to management is to keep the patient under observation, at least overnight. In the case of Le Fort fractures, most patients will stay at least 2 nights after the surgery. These

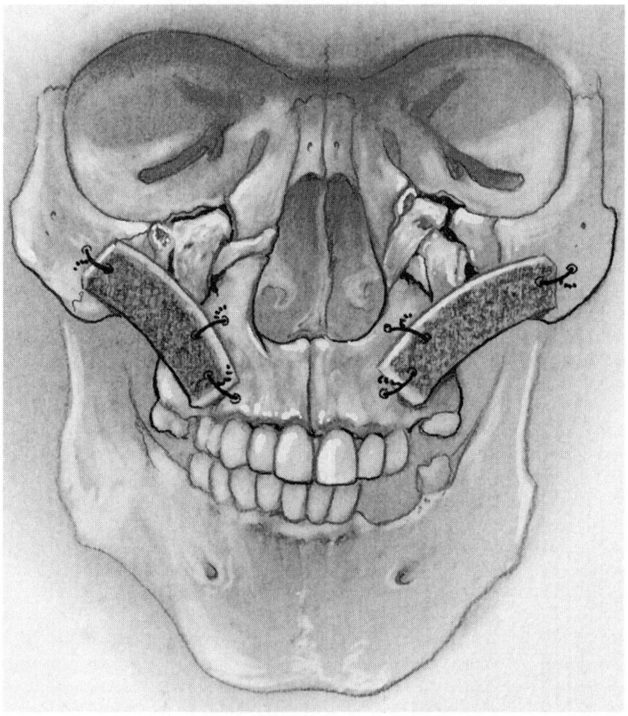

Figure 15–30. Repair of a comminuted Le Fort II fracture using calvarial bone grafts. The grafts are wired or plated and span from the mobile alveolar ridge segment to the stabile malar bone. (Reprinted with permission from Mathog RH (ed). Atlas of Craniofacial Trauma. Philadelphia: WB Saunders, 1992, p. 165.)

patients are generally in rigid IMF, have undergone prolonged anesthesia, and will have severe swelling of the face and eyes. Intensive care unit monitoring may be advisable in patients undergoing the most complex procedures, which may take 6 to 8 hours to perform, or in those with associated injuries dictating this level of observation. If a tracheostomy has been performed, decannulation can occur as early as the second or third postoperative day. Otherwise, the patient will need to be trained in tracheostomy care. Home care and follow-up evaluation will need to be arranged before discharge from the hospital.

Intravenous prophylactic antibiotics have not been clearly demonstrated to be beneficial for most maxillary sinus fractures.[80] The exceptions are when the dentition is involved or when there is an associated mandibular or frontal sinus fracture. If prophylactic antibiotics are prescribed, the minimal perioperative course is all that is indicated. Other medications routinely prescribed include analgesics and antiemetics. Systemic steroids may be considered for the treatment of postoperative facial and orbital edema, but remain controversial.

Ice should be applied to the face for the first 24 hours after surgery, and the head of the bed should be kept elevated for the first several days. Early ambulation is encouraged after facial trauma surgery. However, exercise and sports should be restricted until at least the 10th postoperative day. Contact sports should be avoided for at least 6 weeks to allow adequate bone healing. The patient is restricted to a diet of clear liquids the night of surgery, but thereafter, the diet may be advanced as tolerated. The exception to this is the patient with a Le Fort fracture. In such cases, chewing is restricted to soft foods only, such as mashed potatoes and pudding, for the first 6 weeks. Harder food is then introduced gradually, with an assessment made to ensure that the fracture is stabile.

For the patient undergoing IMF, a special set of postoperative instructions applies. Patients with rigid wire bridges holding arch bars in occlusion should have a wire cutter taped to their chart when they are moved to the recovery room and then to an inpatient bed. This wire cutter should be kept at the bedside and sent home with the patient as long as the rigid IMF is in place. Patients undergoing IMF will be unable to take solid food until the IMF is released. During this time, nutritional supplementation with high-calorie formulas or homemade milkshakes is essential to avoid weight loss. It is imperative that the patient be cautioned about the high risk of alcohol intake while in IMF. Intoxication impairs judgment and puts the patient at considerable risk should emesis or sedation occur.

Before discharge, postreduction x-ray studies of the repair should be performed for two reasons. First, the repair should be assessed to determine whether revision will be necessary as soon as possible. The second reason is for medicolegal purposes. Documentation of the exact condition of the repair prior to discharge can be invaluable should subsequent injury or problems arise.

After discharge from the hospital, the patient will need to return 5 to 7 days after surgery for suture removal. At this time, the IMF is also checked to make sure the wires have not slipped and that the teeth are still in good occlusion. Subsequent follow-up evaluation will be determined on a case-by-case basis. Typically, if adequate rigid internal fixation has been used for the Le Fort fracture, the IMF can be released within 2 weeks. The arch bars are usually left on for another 1 to 2 weeks in case the occlusion slips after release. In this case, the IMF can be reestablished without delay using rubber bands. The upper arch bar is usually left in place for 6 weeks to help stabilize the upper arch during healing, especially if any sagittal fractures are present.

Complications

In addition to the routine risks of surgery that include anesthesia-related problems, medical complications, bleeding, and infection, there are a number of cosmetic and functional complications associated with fractures of the maxillary sinus.[81–88] The functional problems include epiphora secondary to ectropion, diplopia secondary to enophthalmos, nasal obstruction from external deformity and septal deviation, malocclusion, trismus, sinusitis, and mucocele. The cosmetic complications include bad scarring of the incisions, nasal deformity, malar flattening, widening of the orbit, and facial elongation.

Ectropion is one of the most common complications associated with subciliary incisions. This will usually be evident beginning 1 to 2 weeks after surgery. Early management should consist of massage. After 2 weeks, an injection of triamcinolone into the incision may be tried. If these measures do not resolve the condition within 6 weeks after facial repair, surgical correction of the ectropion should be considered. Several techniques are available for this, including a lateral tarsal strip with lysis of scar tissue.

Significant enophthalmos is usually related to unsuccessful correction of an orbital floor fracture. This is usually not detected early after surgery because of swelling around the eye. As soon as the swelling resolves, enophthalmos may be detected. If so, this should be repaired as soon as possible with revision of the orbital floor fracture. Late detection of enophthalmos can also be corrected surgically. The best technique for correction of late enophthalmos is by placement of split calvarial or iliac crest bone grafts in three positions within the orbit. The grafts are placed inferiorly, superolaterally, and medially within the orbit.

Nasal deformity and obstruction are handled by secondary open septorhinoplasty, as described in detail in

Chapter 13. The procedure should be delayed for a minimum of 3 months after the initial surgery to allow adequate healing of the fractures. Earlier intervention may result in unpredictable fracture patterns when creating medial and lateral osteotomies.

Malocclusion can be a difficult problem to deal with, and revision within the first few days should be considered if significant malocclusion is present. If this is not discovered until the fractures have healed, then management will require secondary procedures. If minimal malocclusion is present, orthodontic appliances can be considered to achieve realignment. In the worst cases involving crossbite or gross malocclusion, orthognathic surgery will be required.

Trismus is usually the result of inadequate reduction of zygomatic arch fractures or prolonged IMF. In the case of continued entrapment from a healed zygomatic arch fracture, direct repair by osteotomies through a bicoronal approach should be considered. Most patients with trismus, though, will respond to physical therapy involving stretching exercises for the jaw.

The incidence of sinusitis and mucoceles following maxillary sinus trauma is unknown. Most of these patients can be managed by endoscopic sinus surgery. There are some patients with maxillary sinus fractures who develop lateral or anterior mucoceles inaccessible by endoscopic means. These patients will require a Caldwell-Luc procedure or, in some cases, a Weber-Furgusson incision for resection.

Cosmetic deformities after surgery can be revised at the discretion of the patient. Scar revision should, in all cases, be delayed for at least a year to allow final healing and fading of the scar before determining the need for revision. Malar flattening is best handled with either a bone graft or implant. Several synthetic, prefabricated, cheek implants are commercially available for this purpose. Facial elongation and orbital widening are difficult to correct, but this can be attempted in severe cases. Usually, removal of the previously placed plates and osteotomies is necessary to mobilize the desired bones.

REFERENCES

1. Davidson JSD, Birdsell DC. Cervical spine injury of patients with facial skeletal trauma. J Trauma 29:1276, 1989.
2. Ruskin JD, Tu HK. Integrated management of the maxillofacial trauma patient with multiple injuries. Oral Maxillofac Surg Clin North Am 2:15, 1990.
3. Latoni JD, Shibuya T, Arden RL. Soft tissue trauma. In Mathog RH, Arden RL, Marks SM (eds). Trauma of the Nose and Paransal Sinuses. New York: Thieme Medical Publishers, 1995, pp. 1–20.
4. Roberge RJ, Wears RC, Kelly M, et al. Selective application of cervical spine radiography in alert victims of blunt trauma: A prospective study. J Trauma 28:784, 1988.
5. Lewis VL, Manson PN, Morgan FG, et al. Facial injuries associated with cervical fractures: Recognition, patterns and management. J Trauma 25:90, 1985.
6. Sinclair D, Schwartz M, Gruss J, et al. A retrospective review of the relationship between facial fractures, head injuries, and cervical spine injuries. J Emerg Med 6(2):109, 1988.
7. Johnson DH Jr, Colman M, Larsson S, et al. Computed tomography in medial maxillo-orbital fractures. J Comput Assist Tomogr 8(3):416, 1984.
8. Gentry LR, Manor WF, Turski PA, et al. High-resolution CT analysis of facial struts in trauma: Osseous and soft-tissue implications. AJR 140(3):533, 1983.
9. Laine FJ, Conway WF, Laskin DM. Current problems in diagnostic radiology. Curr Probl Diagn Radiol 22(4):145, 1993.
10. Rowe LD, Miller E, Brandt-Zawadzki M. Computed tomography in maxillofacial trauma. Laryngoscope 91(5):745, 1981.
11. Levy RA, Edwards WT, Meyer JR, et al. Facial trauma and 3-D reconstructive imaging: Insufficiences and correctives. AJNR 13(3):885, 1992.
12. Facer GW. A blow to the nose. Postgrad Med 70:83, 1981.
13. Schultz RC, DeVillers YT. Nasal fractures. J Trauma 15:319, 1975.
14. Fry H. The pathology and treatment of hematoma of the nasal septum. Br J Plast Surg 22:331, 1969.
15. Smith D, Mathog RH. Diagnosis and management of acute nasal fracture. In Mathog RH, Arden RL, Marks SM (eds). Trauma of the Nose and Paranasal Sinuses. New York: Thieme Medical Publishers, 1995, pp. 21–38.
16. Murray JAM, Maran AGD. The treatment of nasal injuries by manipulation. J Laryngol Otolaryngol 94:1405, 1980.
17. Murray JAM, Maran AGD, MacKenzie IJ, et al. Open vs closed reduction of the fractured nose. Arch Otolaryngol 110:797, 1984.
18. Harrison DH. Nasal injuries: Their pathogenesis and treatment. Br J Plast Surg 32:57, 1979.
19. Gilbert JG. Treatment of posttraumatic nasal deformity. NZ Med J 100(836):713, 1987.
20. Courtiss EH. Septorhinoplasty of the traumatically deformed nose. Ann Plast Surg 1(5):443, 1978.
21. Mathog RH. Classification and pathophysiology of naso-orbital fractures. In Mathog RH (ed). Atlas of Craniofacial Trauma. Philadelphia: WB Saunders, 1992, pp. 317–320.
22. Gruss JS, Hurwitz JJ, Nik NA, et al. The pattern and incidence of nasolacrimal injury in naso-orbital-ethmoid fractures: The role of delayed assessment and dacryocystorhinostomy. Br J Plast Surg 38:116, 1985.
23. Jabaley ME, Lerman M, Saunders HJ. Ocular injuries in orbital fractures. Plast Reconstr Surg 56:410, 1979.
24. Duvall AJ, Banovetz JD. Nasoethmoid fractures. Otolaryngol Clin North Am 9:507, 1976.
25. Gruss JS. Naso-ethmoid-orbital fractures. Classification and role of primary bone grafting. Plast Reconstr Surg 75:303, 1985.
26. Beyer CK, Smith B. Naso-orbital fractures, complications and treatment. Ophthalmologica 163:418, 1972.
27. Mathog RH. Chapters 63–65. In Mathog RH (ed). Atlas of Craniofacial Trauma. Philadelphia: WB Saunders, 1992, pp. 321–332.
28. Balle VH, Andersen R, Siim C. Incidence of lacrimal obstruction following trauma to the facial skeleton. Ear Nose Throat J 67:66, 1988.
29. Stranc MF. The pattern of lacrimal injuries in naso-ethmoid injuries with increased intercanthal distance. Br J Plast Surg 23:8, 1970.
30. Whitaker LA, Schaffer DB. Severe traumatic oculo-orbital displacement. Diagnosis and secondary treatment. Plast Reconstr Surg 59:352, 1977.
31. Furnas DW. The pulley canthoplasty for residual telecanthus after hypertelorism repair or facial trauma. Ann Plast Surg 5:85, 1979.
32. Weber SC, Cohn AM. Fracture of the frontal sinus in children. Arch Otolaryngol 103(4):241, 1977.
33. Messinger A, Radkowski MA, Greenwald MJ, et al. Orbital root fractures in the pediatric population. Plast Reconstr Surg 84:213, 1984.
34. Larrabee WF Jr, Travis LW, Tabb HG. Frontal sinus fractures—Their suppurative complications and surgical management. Laryngoscope 90(11):1810, 1980.
35. Stanley RB, Becker TS. Injuries of the nasofrontal orifices in frontal sinus fractures. Laryngoscope 97:728, 1987.
36. Rohrich RJ, Hollier LH. Management of frontal sinus fractures. Adv Craniomaxillofac Fracture Mgmt 19:219, 1992.

37. Harris L, Marano GD, McCorkle D. Nasofrontal duct: CT in frontal sinus trauma. Radiology 165:195, 1987.
38. Calcaterra TC. Exracranial surgical repair of cerebrospinal fluid rhinorrhea. Ann Otol Rhinol Laryngol 87:108, 1980.
39. Donald PJ, Bernstein L. Compound frontal sinus injuries with intracranial penetration. Laryngoscope 88:225, 1978.
40. Marks SC. Titanium mesh plating for frontal sinus fractures. Oper Tech Otolaryngol Head Neck Surg 6(2):133, 1995.
41. Montgomery WW. The fate of adipose implants in a bony cavity. Laryngoscope 74:816, 1964.
42. Catalano PJ, Lawson W, Som P, et al. Radiographic evaluation and diagnosis of the failed frontal osteoplastic flap with fat obliteration. Otolaryngol Head Neck Surg 104:225, 1991.
43. Wilson BC, Davidson B. Comparison of complications following frontal sinus fractures managed with exploration with or without obliteration over 10 years. Laryngoscope 98:516, 1988.
44. Wallis A, Donald PJ. Frontal sinus fractures: A review of 72 cases. Laryngoscope 98:593, 1988.
45. Nadell J, Kline D. Primary reconstruction of depressed frontal skull fractures including those involving the sinus, orbit and cribiform plate. J Neurosurg 41:200, 1974.
46. Donald PJ. The tenacity of the frontal sinus mucosa. Otolaryngol Head Neck Surg 87:557, 1979.
47. Bordley JE, Bosley WR. Mucoceles of the frontal sinus: Causes and treatment. Ann Otol Rhinol Laryngol 82:696, 1973.
48. Hardy JM, Montgomery WW. Osteoplastic frontal sinusotomy: An analysis of 250 operations. Ann Otol Rhinol Laryngol 85:523, 1976.
49. Robinson KL, Marks SC. Maxillary trauma. In Mathog RH, Arden RL, Marks SC (eds). Trauma of the Nose and Paranasal Sinuses. New York: Thieme Medical Publishers, 1995, pp. 50–64.
50. Le Fort R. Experimental study of fractures of the upper jaw. Rev Chir Paris 23:208, 360; 1901. Reprinted in Plast Reconstr Surg 50:497, 1972.
51. Laine FL, Conway WF, Laskin DM. Radiology of maxillofacial trauma. Curr Prob Diagn Radiol 22(4):151, 1993.
52. Hillstrom R, Moore GK, Mathog RH. Medial maxillary fractures. Otolaryngol Head Neck Surg 104:270, 1991.
53. Koutroupas S, Meyerhoff WL. Surgical treatment of orbital floor fractures. Arch Otolaryngol 108(3):184, 1982.
54. Kawamoto HK Jr. Late posttraumatic enophthalmos: A correctable deformity? Plast Reconstr Surg 69(3):423, 1982.
55. Converse JM, Smith B. Enophthalmos and diplopia in fractures of the orbital floor. Br J Plast Surg 9:265, 1975.
56. Mathog RH, Archer KF, Nesi FA. Posttraumatic enophthalmos and diplopia. Otolaryngol Head Neck Surg 94:69, 1986.
57. Covington DS, Wainwright DJ, Teichgraeber JF, et al. Changing patterns in the epidemiology and treatment of zygoma fractures: 10-year review. J Trauma 37(2):243, 1994.
58. Champy M, Lodde JP, Kahn JL, et al. Attempt at systematization in the treatment of isolated fractures of the zygomatic bone: Techniques and results. J Otolaryngol 15:39, 1986.
59. Shaw GY, Khan J. Precise repair of orbital maxillary zygomatic fractures. Arch Otolaryngol Head Neck Surg 120(6):613, 1994.
60. Freeman LN, Seiff SR, Aguilar GL, et al. Self-compression plates for orbital rim fractures. Ophthalmic Plast Reconstr Surg 7(3):198, 1991.
61. Bosniak SL, Tizes BR. Trimalar fractures: Diagnosis and treatment. Adv Ophthalmic Plast Reconstr Surg 6:403, 1987.
62. Wray RC, Holtmann B, Ribaudo JM. A comparison of conjunctival and subciliary incisions for orbital fractures. Br J Plast Surg 30(2):142, 1977.
63. Heckler FR, Songcharoen S, Sultani FA. Subciliary incision and skin-muscle flap for orbital fractures. Ann Plast Surg 10:309, 1983.
64. Martinez-Lage JL. Reconstruction of the orbital region. Ann Plast Surg 7:464, 1981.
65. Converse JM, Firmin T, Wood-Smith D, et al. The conjunctival approach in orbital fractures. Plast Reconstr Surg 52:656, 1973.
66. Burres SA, Cohn AM, Mathog RH. Repair of orbital blowout fractures with Marlex mesh and Gelfilm. Laryngoscope 91(11): 1881, 1981.
67. Raz S. Gelfilm and blowout fractures. J Laryngol Otol 90(7): 699, 1976.
68. Kummoona R: Chrome cobalt and gold implant for the reconstruction of a traumatized orbital floor. Oral Surg Oral Med Oral Pathol 41(3):293, 1976.
69. Antonyshyn O, Gruss JS, Galbraith DJ, et al. Complex orbital fractures: A critical analysis of immediate bone graft reconstruction. Ann Plast Surg 22:220, 1989.
70. Converse JM, Smith B. Reconstruction of the floor of the orbit by bone grafts. Arch Ophthalmol 44:1, 1950.
71. Parkin JL, Stevens MH, Stringham JC. Absorbable gelatin film versus silicone rubber sheeting in orbital fracture treatment. Laryngoscope 97:1, 1987.
72. Polley JW, Ringler SL. The use of Teflon in orbital floor reconstruction following blunt facial trauma: A 20-year experience. Plast Reconstr Surg 79:39, 1987.
73. Stanley RB, Mathog RH. Evaluation and correction of combined orbital trauma syndrome. Laryngoscope 93(7):856, 1983.
74. Karlan MS, Cassisi NJ. Fractures of the zygoma. Arch Otolaryngol 105:320, 1979.
75. Gillies MD, Kelner TP, Stone D. Fractures of the malar-zygomatic compound. Br J Plast Surg 14:651, 1927.
76. Kelly KJ, Manson PN, Vander Kolk CA, et al. Sequencing Le Fort fracture treatment (organization of treatment for a panfacial fracture). J Craniofac Surg 1:168, 1990.
77. Markowitz BL, Manson PN. Panfacial fractures: Organization of treatment. Clin Plast Surg 16:105, 1989.
78. Lee ST. Management of severe maxillo-facial injuries. Ann Acad Med Singapore 12(S2):446, 1983.
79. Thompson JN, Gibson B, Kohut RI. Airway obstruction in Le Fort fractures. Laryngoscope 97(3 Pt 1):275, 1987.
80. Mathog RH, Crane LR, Nowak GS. Antimicrobial therapy following head and neck trauma. In Johnson JT (ed). Antibiotic Therapy in Head and Neck Surgery. New York: Marcel Dekker, 1987, pp. 31–49.
81. Weymuller EA Jr. Blindness and Le Fort III fractures. Ann Otol Rhinol Laryngol 93(1 Pt 1):2, 1984.
82. Reynolds JR. Late complications vs. methods of treatment in a large series of mid-facial fractures. Plast Reconstr Surg 61(6): 871, 1978.
83. Mathog RH, Rosenberg Z. Complications in the treatment of facial fractures. Otolaryngol Clin North Am 9:533, 1976.
84. Kristensen S, Tveteras K. Zygomatic fractures: Classification and complications. Clin Otolaryngol 11:123, 1986.
85. Lederman IR. Loss of vision associated with surgical treatment of zygomatico-orbital floor fracture. Plast Reconstr Surg 68:94, 1981.
86. Martin BC, Trabue JC, Leech TR. An analysis of the etiology, treatment and complications of fractures of the malar compound and zygomatic arch. Am J Surg 92:920, 1956.
87. Nordgaard JO. Persistent sensory disturbances and diplopia following fractures of the zygoma. Arch Otolaryngol 102:80, 1976.
88. Schiffer HD, Austerman KH, Busse H. Ophthalmological long-term effects of malar fractures. Klin Monatsbl Augenheilkd 71:567, 1977.

SECTION FOUR

Tumors

CHAPTER 16

Surgical Approaches for Tumors of the Nose, Sinuses, and Anterior Skull Base

Tumors of the nose, sinuses, and anterior skull base are surgically challenging because of the relatively inaccessible location of these structures within and behind the face. Approaches need to account for the surrounding critical structures, functional considerations of the sinuses and nose, and the cosmetic appearance of the face. Pioneers in head and neck surgery have developed many innovative and effective techniques to overcome these problems, and today, the surgeon treating tumors of this area has a variety of approaches from which to access the tumor to allow complete oncologic excision. In this chapter, the most important of these approaches will be covered in detail. Subsequent chapters cover the techniques of tumor resection and reconstruction after ablation.

LATERAL RHINOTOMY

Indications

The lateral rhinotomy approach is the traditional and standard technique for tumor surgery of the nose and sinuses.[1–4] The excellent exposure from this incision allows almost any surgery to be performed. This incision is often considered the gateway to the nose, sinuses, and anterior skull base. The great advantage of this incision is the tremendous exposure it affords, allowing tumors to be resected under direct vision without the impediment of overlying soft tissues. The lateral rhinotomy approach can be adapted to include orbital surgery, ethmoid sinus surgery, and access to the maxillary sinus. The extended incision has become known as the Weber-Fergusson incision. Using the Weber-Fergusson incision, the lateral rhinotomy approach has become the standard technique for treating tumors of the nose and sinuses.

The limitation of this exposure is that structures on the contralateral face cannot easily be accessed through this one incision. If such exposure is required, the lateral rhinotomy incision will need to be combined with a secondary incision, such as a medial canthal incision or a degloving incision of the contralateral face.

The principle disadvantage of the approach is that it leaves a long facial scar. With careful incision and suturing, however, the scar can largely be hidden in the natural skin creases and shadow areas of the face. However, the scar is always evident to the careful observer and, on occasion, can leave a cosmetically poor result. For this reason, the lateral rhinotomy incision is reserved for cases that cannot be handled by one of the other available techniques. Cases that are normally performed through this approach include both maxillectomy and craniofacial resection when these procedures include orbital exenteration. Other indications for this approach are tumors that require significant skin resection owing to direct extension of the tumor into the face and cases of skull base tumors that are approached through the maxillary swing technique.

Preoperative Considerations

When a lateral rhinotomy is planned, the patient should be examined carefully prior to surgery to determine the optimal placement of the incision. This should be determined with the patient awake and upright. General anesthesia and supine posture combine to change the facial appearance, possibly altering the ideal location of the incision. If it would be helpful, the incision can be marked onto the skin in the preanesthesia care unit.

Other preoperative considerations are similar to those for any patient undergoing general anesthesia and major surgery. Careful medical evaluation is imperative, and adequate monitoring should be arranged, which may include a urinary catheter, an arterial line for blood pressure monitoring, a central venous catheter, or a Swan-Ganz catheter. Prophylactic antibiotics should be administered to all patients. The optimal choice of antibiotic will depend on individual patient factors.

The patient's position and the equipment needed for the surgery will depend more on the nature of the subsequent resection than the fact that a lateral rhinotomy incision is planned. However, the entire surgical field should be prepared in a sterile fashion according to local hospital protocols. Despite the fact that potentially contaminated sinuses and the oral cavity will be in the wound, to avoid an increased incidence of soft tissue infections after surgery, the skin should be disinfected before making the incision.

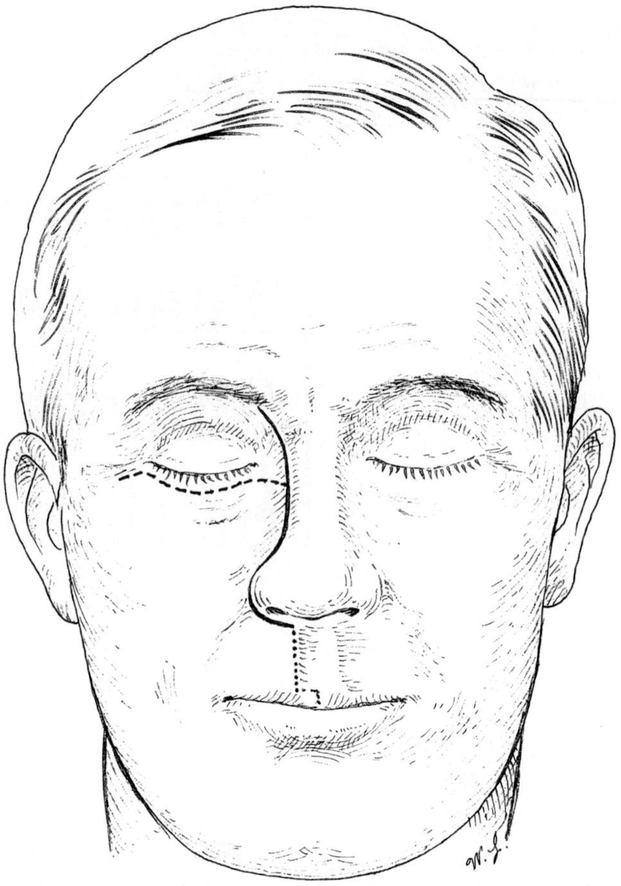

Figure 16–1. Lateral rhinotomy incision. The solid line is the basic incision used for access to the nasal cavity. The dotted lines indicate possible extensions to allow wider access (Weber-Fergusson incision). Note that the incisional line follows the crest of the filtrum to the vermilion border and then along the vermilion border to the midline. Alternatively, the incision can extend through the middle of the filtrum in the midline.

Technique

Before the initial incision is made, it should be marked out on the skin and injected with local anesthesia containing 1% lidocaine with 1 : 100,000 epinephrine. The exact location will depend on the exact nature of the procedure being performed. Figure 16–1 demonstrates the course of the basic incision with possible extensions. The basic incision starts at the lateral alar crease and extends in the crease superiorly to the nasal facial groove, continuing to the level of the medial canthus. Older patients with increased skin laxity will usually have a conspicuous crease in which to hide the incision. Younger patients may have no observable crease. In the latter cases, it is important to identify the best location for the incision before the operation, as indicated earlier. The basic incision is adequate for nasal surgeries, such as septectomy and medial maxillectomy.

In order to expose the maxilla, the basic incision must be extended inferiorly through the lip and laterally from the superior edge across the lower eyelid. Inferiorly, the incision curves around the alar crease to the base of the nose. The incision is carried inferiorly to the vermilion border. This can extend through the midline or paramedian if the patient has a prominent Cupid's bow. If a paramedian incision is used, the incision is directed medially along the vermilion border to the midline and then is extended through the lip in the midline. Otherwise, the midline incision through the lip extends directly through the vermilion border into the mucosa. The superior extension of the basic incision branches off the upper part of the incision at a right angle onto the lower eyelid. The incision should be angled up to the lid margin and should extend laterally in the subciliary line about 2 mm below the lash line.

If orbital exenteration is to be part of the resection, the incision will vary around the orbit. In addition to the subciliary lower lid extension, an upper lid extension is included that joins up to the lower lid incision laterally. The upper lid incision should course 2 to 3 mm above the lash line. The goal here is to preserve as much normal skin as possible while resecting all conjunctival and orbital elements and both lid margins.

When a lateral rhinotomy incision is combined with a bicoronal incision, the upper limb of the incision should stop below the eyebrow to make sure that the supraorbital vessels are not damaged. These vessels are the principle blood supply to the bicoronal flap, so their loss may lead to flap necrosis.

After the incision is marked out and injected with local anesthetic, the incision is made. A No. 15 blade should be used, and tension on the face should pull laterally. The incision is usually started inferiorly and carried superiorly. The lip is grasped with two fingers on either side, occluding the labial artery during the incision. Both ends of the transected labial artery should be identified and coagulated or ligated. As the incision is extended superiorly, rather than cutting straight down to bone, the tissues are cut in layers, with hemostasis confirmed after each layer. This minimizes blood loss and ultimately may save time.

At the eyelid, the incision should extend through the orbicularis muscle but stay superficial to the orbital septum (Fig. 16–2). The eyelid skin is elevated in this plane to the level of the inferior orbital rim, where the periosteum is incised to join the lid flap with the facial flap (Fig. 16–3). The next step is to incise the mucosa under the lip. This incision extends laterally from the lip splitting incision a few millimeters on the labial side of the gingival labial sulcus. The placement of the incision in this location will allow a more secure closure as the sutures will not pass through the relatively immobile gingiva. Sutures through the gingiva tend to pull through with minimal tension. The submucosal tissues are divided with either cautery or a knife down through the periosteum to the bone of the maxilla. It is important to make sure that the dissection stays inferiorly angling toward the teeth to avoid injury to the inferior branch of the infraorbital nerve as it enters the lip. Once this incision is complete, the entire facial flap is elevated from the maxilla in the subperiosteal plane using a periosteal elevator. The elevation continues laterally to the infraorbital nerve. The nerve is generally sacrificed at this point if complete maxillectomy is to be performed. The elevation of the flap can then be extended as far laterally as the malar eminence (Fig. 16–4).

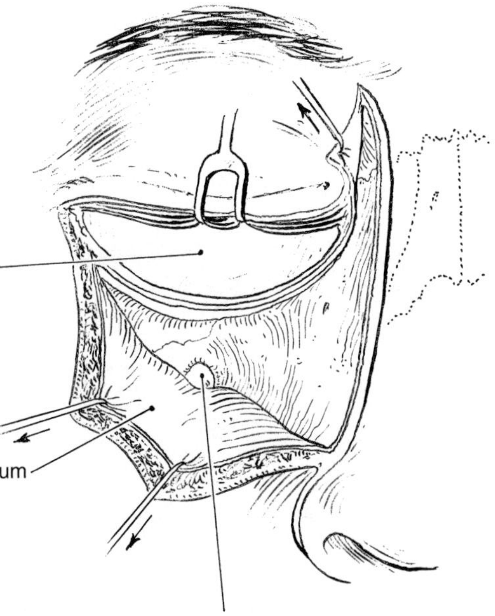

Figure 16–3. Development of the facial flap. The dissection extends on the surface of the orbital septum out to the orbital rim. At the orbital rim, the periosteum is incised; further elevation is in the subperiosteal plane.

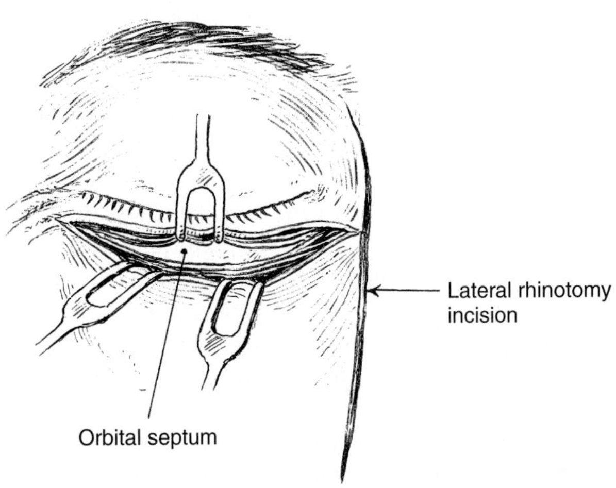

Figure 16–2. Subciliary extension of the lateral rhinotomy incision. The incision is carried down through the orbicularis muscle to the layer of the orbital septum.

Modifications of this technique are necessary if the tumor invades the overlying skin of the face. In this circumstance, the tumor-involved skin will have to be incorporated into the resection. To accomplish this, the area of desired resection is outlined before the incision is made. The lateral rhinotomy incision is drawn around this area as necessary to incorporate the excision (Fig. 16–5A). When the incision is made, the area outlined for skin excision is incised down to the bone. This allows the flap elevation to occur without violating the tumor (Fig. 16–5B).

The next step in the formal lateral rhinotomy technique is to enter the nose. In many procedures, this will not be necessary. When it is necessary, the actual rhinotomy can be accomplished in a number of ways. The simplest is to use an osteotome to cut the nasal bone where it attaches to the frontal process of the maxilla. A second fracture line can be created in the midline and at the nasal frontal suture to allow the nasal bones to fold open like a book. Alternatively, a Kerrison's rongeur can be used to simply remove the bone at the nasal maxillary suture, exposing the inside of the nose. Once this is complete, the soft tissues con-

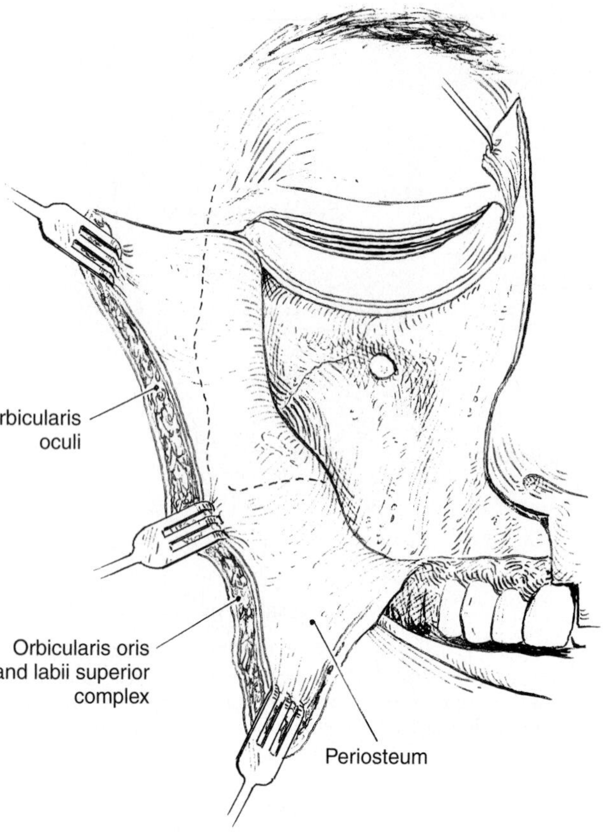

Figure 16–4. Completed facial flap using the Weber-Fergusson incision. Note that the inferior orbital nerve is transected. The exposure reaches the root of the zygomatic arch and the lateral canthus.

necting the nasal mucosa to the vestibule can be divided at the pyriform aperture to complete the exposure.

After the approach is complete, tumor exposure, resection, and reconstruction can proceed. These procedures are covered in Chapters 17 and 18. The final step in the surgery is always closure of the lateral rhinotomy incision. Closure requires different layers, depending on the portion of the incision being addressed. The lip is typically closed in three layers: a central muscular layer, a mucosal layer, and the cutaneous layer. The cutaneous and mucosal layers come together at the vermilion border. This landmark should be approximated first, before the remainder of the lip is sutured. For the muscle closure, interrupted 3-0 Vicryl (Ethicon, Inc., Somerville, NJ) mattress sutures are used. The mucosa is closed with interrupted 4-0 chromic gut on the lip. The vermilion border and the cutaneous portion of the lip between the vermilion border and the nose are closed using simple interrupted 6-0 nylon sutures.

The second area of concern is the gingival labial sulcus. This incision, like the Caldwell-Luc incision, is closed with chromic gut by many surgeons. However, the author prefers interrupted 3-0 Vicryl sutures, as these do not lose strength and pull out early. It is believed that their use results in a decreased rate of dehiscence of this closure. The lower eyelid subciliary incision is closed with running subcuticular 5-0 Prolene (Ethicon, Inc., Somerville, NJ). No subcutaneous or periosteal sutures are used, as these tend to increase the incidence of ectropion. Finally, the skin between the nasal base and the medial canthus is closed in two layers. A subcutaneous-dermal layer of interrupted 4-0 Vicryl sutures is used to approximate the skin edges and take tension off the closure. The skin is closed with 5-0 or 6-0 nylon sutures.

Dressings and/or butterfly bandages are not used, as they do not stick well to surfaces that are not flat. In any case, it is preferable to be able to visualize the incision after surgery to monitor the area for complications, such as hematoma and skin edge necrosis. Antibiotic ointment is routinely applied to the incision after surgery.

Postoperative Care

bMost postoperative care issues relate to the underlying tumor surgery and not to the incision itself, although the incision does require some care. Beginning with the day after surgery, the incision should be cleaned with a cotton-tipped applicator and hydrogen peroxide twice each day. After each cleaning, the incision is covered with a thin layer of antibiotic ointment. The sutures can be removed as early as 5 days after the surgery if healing appears to be progressing normally.

Complications

Complications from the incision itself are usually minor and easily managed. Hematoma is rare owing to the fact that, in most cases, the anterior wall of the maxilla is removed during tumor resection. Therefore, all bleeding seeps into the cavity and does not accumulate. For the same reason, skin infections are rare; however, cellulitis may be seen after lateral rhinotomy. This should be treated with drainage of any fluid collection and intravenous antibiotics. If culture results are not available, antistaphylococcal antibiotics are the first choices for empiric therapy.

Suture line dehiscence can occur in either the sublabial incision, the lip, or along the lateral aspect of the nose. This is most likely to occur in the area of the gingiva if the incision is too close to the sulcus. An unusual but significant problem is skin necrosis of the medial aspect of the flap. In certain cases, the distal skin edges are far from the arterial source and may become ischemic, especially if closed under tension. This typically occurs only if skin excision was necessary during the procedure. Otherwise, the blood supply to the face is sufficient to tolerate this procedure with little risk of problems.

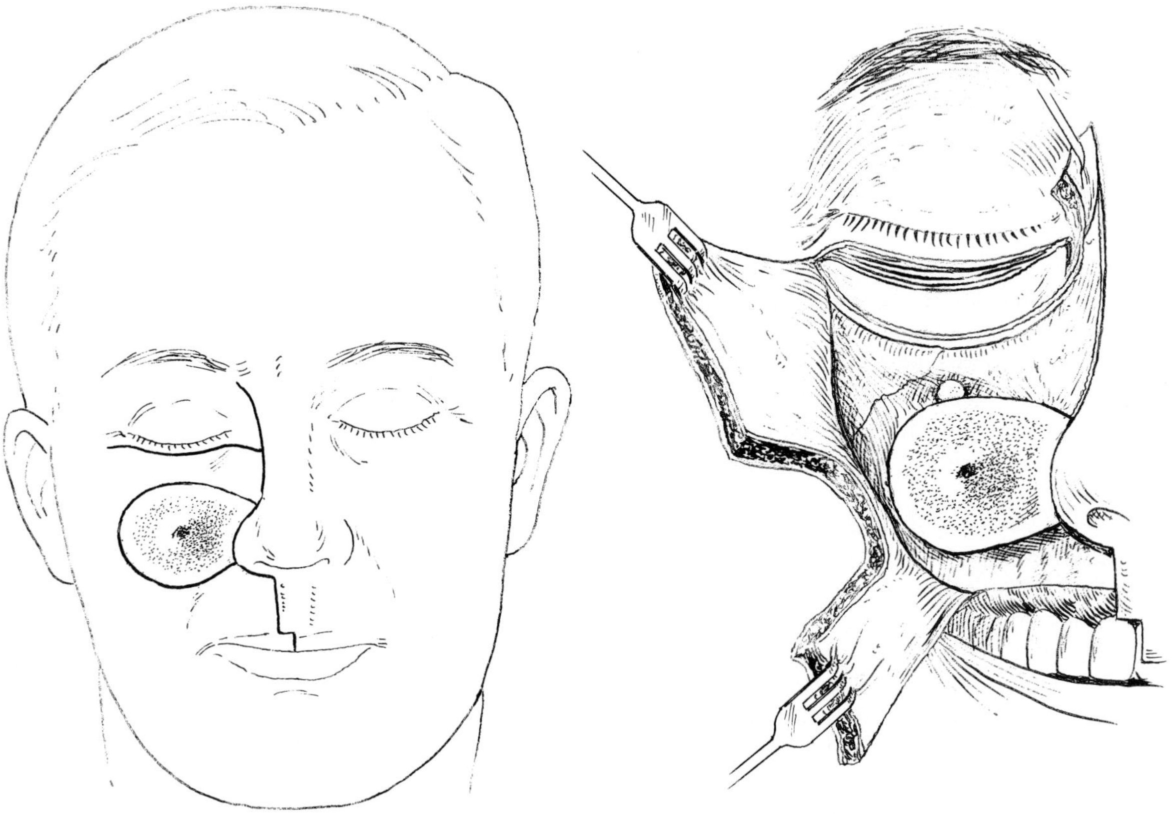

A B

Figure 16–5. Possible adaptation of the Weber-Fergusson incision, including excision of facial skin involved in direct extension of the tumor through the anterior wall of the maxillary sinus. *A,* The outline of the incision. *B,* Completed flap elevation.

Unsatisfactory cosmetic results may occur from either technical mistakes in placement of the incision, inaccurate closure, or from abnormal scarring. One area of concern is at the vermilion border, where notching of the lip is possible if careful suturing is not performed. The other main area of concern is the medial canthal area where scar contracture can occur, distorting the medial canthus and interfering with lacrimal function. The key to avoiding this problem is to make sure that the subciliary incision branches off the lateral rhinotomy incision at right angles and does not get too close to the medial canthus. The incision should be kept at least 1 cm inferior to the medial canthus before it is curved up to the subciliary line.

MIDFACIAL DEGLOVING

Indications

Midfacial degloving has become a popular approach for a wide variety of tumor operations.[5–7] This procedure has the advantages of completely avoiding facial incisions and allowing bilateral exposure. The exposure of the lower part of the midface, including the nose and maxillary sinuses up to the orbits, is excellent. The limitation of this technique is that it affords relatively poor access to the orbit, the lateral aspect of the maxilla, and the ethmoid sinus. However, these limitations are not critical and it is still possible, if the infraorbital nerve is sacrificed, to access all of these areas.

The midface degloving approach is utilized as the primary option for medial maxillectomy, radical maxillectomy, and uncomplicated craniofacial resection.[5–8] The main contraindications to this approach are when there is a need for orbital exenteration or if significant skin excision from the face is needed. In these circumstances, the cosmetic advantages of the midface degloving are lost and the straightforward lateral rhinotomy incision becomes the preferred option.

Preoperative Considerations

There are no specific preoperative considerations when planning midface degloving. The only technical concern is that the patient has an adequate nasal opening to allow the incisions inside the nose. Otherwise, all the considerations for this operation are the same as for any major surgery. These include the patient's medical condition, the assessment of anesthetic risk, perioperative monitoring, and prophylactic antibiotics. In terms of obtaining consent from the patient for the operation, it is important to inform the patient of the permanent numbness associated with sacrificing the infraorbital nerve if this is to be performed.

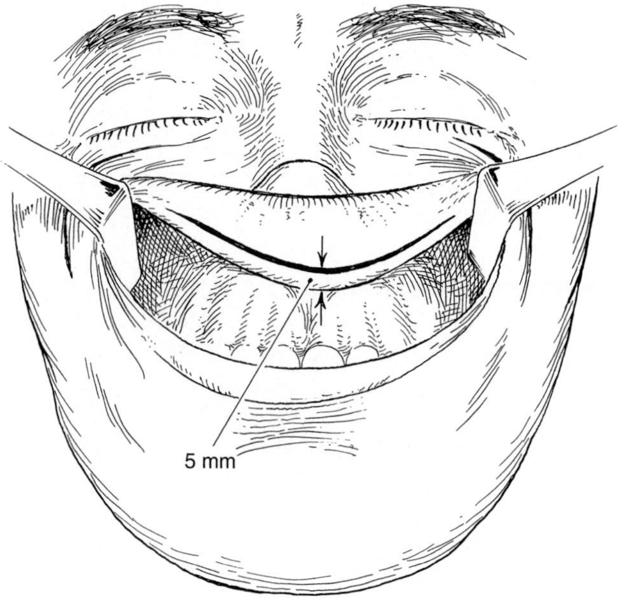

Figure 16–7. Sublabial incision. A 5-mm cuff of mucosa is preserved above the gingival labial sulcus. At a minimum, the incision extends from first molar to first molar.

Technique

The patient is positioned on the operating room table in the supine position with the neck slightly extended. The face is prepared with disinfectant as per the local hospital protocol. The eyelids are either taped closed with sterile tape oriented vertically over the lateral aspect of the eye or closed with a temporary tarsorrhaphy suture.

The nose is decongested with either oxymetazoline or 4% cocaine solution. The nose and sublabial incision are injected with local anesthesia using 1% lidocaine with 1:100,000 epinephrine. Injections are placed in the columella, intercartilaginous space, and nasal floor bilaterally. Local anesthetic is also administered through the intercartilaginous space over the nasal dorsum, medial and lateral to the nasal facial groove.

The first incision is a complete transfixion incision. This is performed exactly as in the rhinoplasty cartilage delivery technique. The transfixion incision is connected across the apex of the nasal vestibule to an intercartilaginous incision. This is also done in precisely the same way as in the rhinoplasty technique. At this point, the operation diverges from rhinoplasty. The incisions are extended laterally around the inside of the ala along the cephalic border of the lower lateral cartilage down to the floor of the nose. The incision is carried across the floor of the nose to the columella. Floor incisions should be placed about 2 mm inside the nasal sill, leaving enough room to suture without crossing the edge of the nares (Fig. 16–6). The floor incision should not be placed over the pyriform aperture as this could lead to scar contracture and vestibular stenosis.

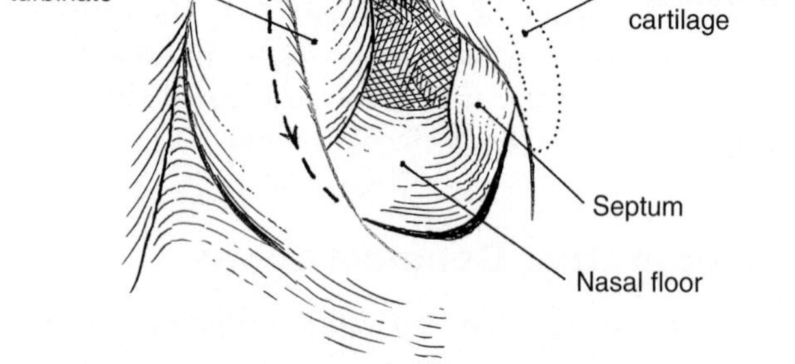

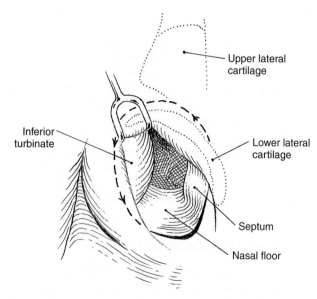

Figure 16–6. Intranasal incisions for the midfacial degloving approach. A complete transfixion incision is connected to an intercartilaginous incision and carried around the lateral ala onto the floor of the nose. Notice that the incision in the nasal floor should be anterior to the pyriform aperture.

After the initial incisions are completed, the tips of curved iris scissors are spread perpendicular to the incision to open the incisions more widely. The nasal dorsum is accessed by dissecting and elevating in the plane between the upper lateral and lower lateral cartilages, leaving the upper lateral cartilages attached to the nasal bones but elevating the lower lateral cartilages with the columella and nasal skin.

With the nasal structures mobilized, the sublabial incision can be made. This should extend from the end of the maxillary alveolus on the ipsilateral side across the midline to the contralateral canine area. If bilateral exposure is required, the incision can be extended as far laterally as necessary on each side. As with other sublabial incisions, it is best to keep the incision about 5 mm on the labial side of the gingival labial sulcus to facilitate closure (Fig. 16–7). The incision is then divided down to the maxilla, making sure that the direction of the dissection is angled inferiorly to avoid the infraorbital nerve.

The periosteum of the maxilla is then elevated with a Freer elevator up to the pyriform aperture. To connect the nasal incision to the sublabial incision, the scissors are used to spread the incision in the floor of the nose

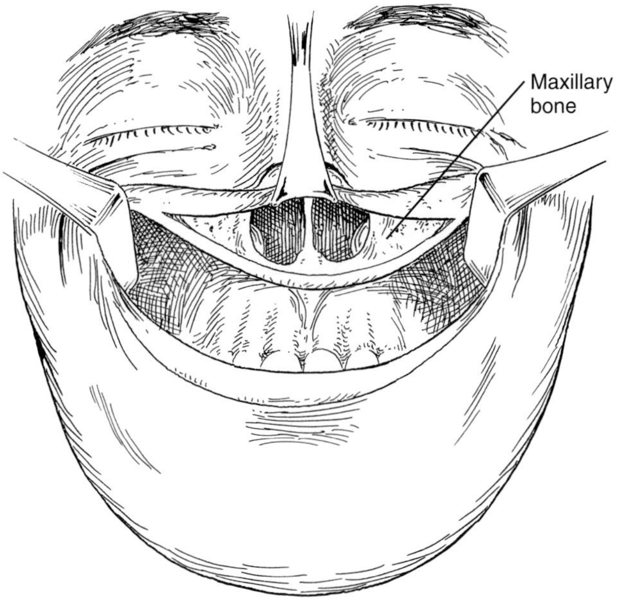

Figure 16–8. Initial elevation during the midfacial degloving approach. The intranasal incisions are made and a subperiosteal dissection is carried out. The anterior septum and nasal cavity are observed.

until this connects to the oral side. The incisions can then be easily merged across the length of the nose (Fig. 16–8). At this point, the periosteum over the maxilla should be elevated up to the infraorbital nerve. With a retractor placed under the lip in the midline and a second retractor positioned laterally under the lip at the level of the eye, a thick soft tissue bridge will be left holding the face down to the lateral pyriform aperture and nasal bones (Fig. 16–9). This tissue should be carefully dissected or cut with a cautery to avoid bleeding from the angular vessels that run in this area.

The typical exposure for the midfacial degloving procedure is demonstrated in Fig. 16–10. Note that the infraorbital nerve and the opposite side of the face limit the exposure. This basic minimal dissection will adequately expose the anterior maxillary wall, alveolar ridge, and unilateral nasal bones. This is primarily used for uncomplicated medial maxillectomy without the need for en block ethmoidectomy or access to the orbit or pterygomaxillary fissure. For more extensive exposure, the infraorbital nerve is sacrificed and full dissection is performed on the contralateral side (Fig. 16–11). This allows the elevation over the inferior orbital rim to expose the floor of the orbit, as well as the medial aspect of the orbit. With this degree of exposure, medial maxillectomy with en block ethmoidectomy, radical maxillectomy, and craniofacial resection is possible. It is possible, by making encircling incisions around the eyelashes, to include the orbital contents with this approach. However, the exposure of the optic foramen through this approach is never quite optimal, and for this reason, the lateral rhinotomy approach is preferred for resections that include orbital exenteration.

Accurate closure of the midface degloving approach is essential for optimal cosmetic results. The intranasal

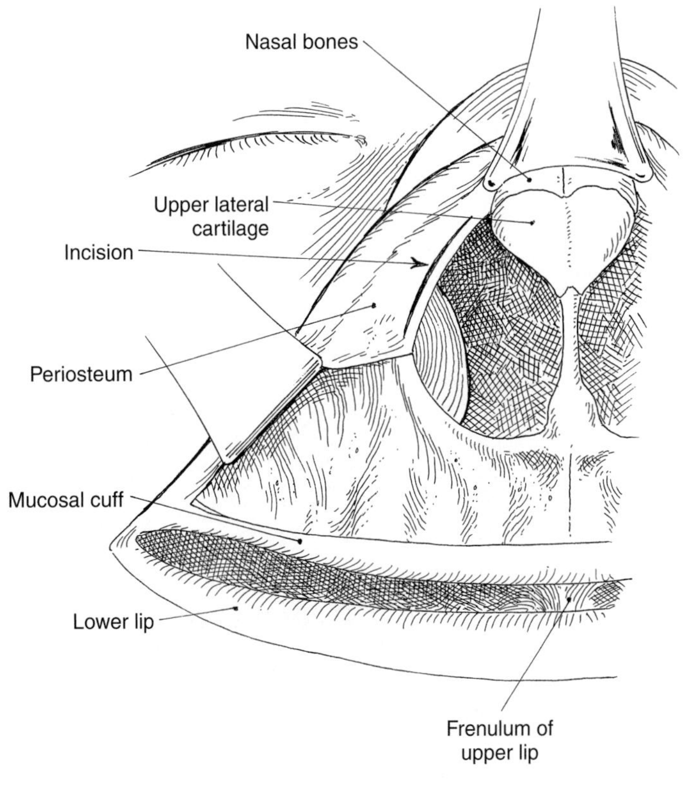

Figure 16–9. Development of the midfacial degloving approach. After exposure of the upper lateral cartilages and the inferior pyriform aperture, the periosteum of the lateral pyriform aperture must be incised to continue the subperiosteal dissection superiorly.

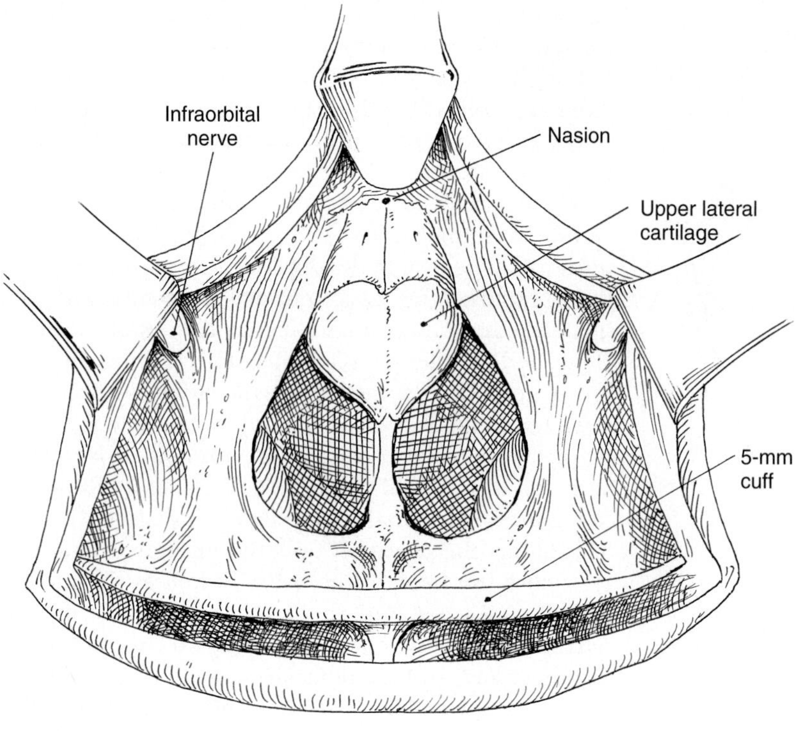

Figure 16–10. Completed initial exposure. The infraorbital nerves are identified bilaterally and the dissection extends up over the nasal bones to the nasion. Normally, there is a cuff of soft tissue around the pyriform aperture (not shown).

incisions are always closed first, followed by the sublabial incision. Nasal packing is placed and an external splint is applied. The intranasal incisions are the most critical and time-consuming. A 4-0 chromic suture is used throughout. The first sutures should approximate the apex of the vestibule at the junction of the columella and the intercartilaginous incision on either side of the nose. The base of the columella is sutured next. This sets the midline of the nose and is the most critical step in a good cosmetic result. The remaining sutures are placed as needed to complete the intranasal closure.

The sublabial incision is closed with interrupted 3-0 Vicryl in the same fashion as the Caldwell-Luc incision. This should approximate the midline first, then proceed from lateral to medial. The absolute midline should be carefully judged as inaccuracy will result in a poor cosmetic outcome. The gingival side can be identified by the labial frenulum, whereas the midpoint of the filtrum will identify the midpoint of the labial side of the incision.

Nasal packing is necessary only to stent the incisions. However, the maxillectomy cavity will generally be fully packed and the end brought out through the nose prior to initiating intranasal suturing. The external nose is dressed with adhesive strips in a single compressive layer. The Thermoplast nasal splint (Xomed, Jacksonville, FL) is preferred for external stabilization. It is easy to use and provides adequate compression.

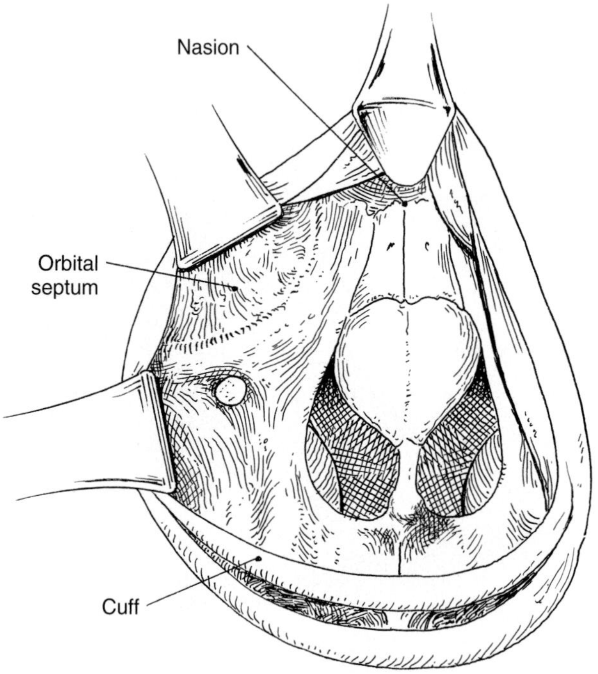

Figure 16–11. Extended midfacial degloving exposure. With transection of the infraorbital nerve, the inferior orbit and frontal process of the maxilla can easily be exposed.

Postoperative Care

Postoperative care in these patients is largely driven by the nature of the tumor surgery. Of particular importance is the care of the incisions, packing, and splints. The intranasal portion of the packing that lines the vestibule can be removed as early as the morning after surgery provided there is not overt bleeding. The nasal splints may be removed after 5 days to allow sufficient time for the periosteum to re-adhere to the nasal bones. The intranasal sutures are not removed, but are allowed to dissolve over the first weeks after surgery. The sublabial sutures can be removed as early as 2 to 3 weeks after the surgery, but generally they are allowed to dissolve and fall out on their own.

Complications

The midface degloving procedure is notable for its lack of complications. Owing to the avoidance of skin incisions, infections and cosmetic problems are not expected. Hematoma under the cheek flap is possible, especially on the side opposite the resection. If this does occur, the hematoma should be drained and the bleeding source controlled.

The most frequent complication of the midface degloving approach is nasal vestibular stenosis. This can occur as a result of the circumferential incision in the nose, and may lead to a contracting circular scar or a web, either across the floor or the apex of the vestibule. Stenosis is prevented primarily through careful closure and by avoiding placement of the incision directly over the pyriform aperture inferiorly. Alternatively, a notch in the incision in the nasal floor may also help to avoid stenosis.[9] The apical suture, if placed inaccurately, may lead to formation of a web at this location.

To become symptomatic, the stenosis would need to be quite severe on the resection side. This is because the nasal airway is dramatically opened if either medial or radical maxillectomy is performed. The biggest risk for symptomatic stenosis is on the side opposite the resection. Management of stenosis is necessary when it limits nasal breathing. To repair stenosis, dilatation, excision and splinting, or Z-plasty on the floor of the nose may be performed. The exact choice of technique will depend on the specific anatomy of the stenosis. In the author's series of approximately 30 cases of midfacial degloving, several patients have developed some degree of nasal stenosis, but none have required treatment.

MAXILLARY SWING PROCEDURE

Indications

A relatively new approach to the anterior skull base is to displace the maxilla by either rotating it laterally based on the greater palatine vessels or completely removing the maxilla as a free graft.[10–13] This unique approach was developed in the last 10 years as an alternative technique to gain access to tumors of the nasopharynx and middle cranial base. The procedure has certain advantages and disadvantages over existing alternative procedures.

The advantages of this surgical option are improved exposure and improved functional outcome. Performed through a Weber-Fergusson incision, wide displacement of the maxilla exposes the nasopharynx, infratemporal fossa, and skull base in the region of the sphenoid sinus and pterygoid plates. As originally described, the procedure also includes a temporoparietal craniotomy to increase exposure to the infratemporal fossa and skull base. With this extension, it is possible to access the cavernous sinus and cavernous carotid artery at the upper medial aspect of the field and the clivus and foramen magnum at the lower end of the surgical field. This exposure differs from the lateral subtemporal and infratemporal fossa approaches in that the angle of view is from the anterior. A second difference is that the exposure is potentially wider and the target surgical field is closer to the surgeon. These factors combine to minimize the functional consequences of this approach. The alternative lateral procedures may lead to injury to multiple cranial nerves and damage to the temporomandibular joint. The maxillary swing approach is also favored owing to the relatively acceptable cosmetic result. Once the surgeon has adapted to the change in orientation, the maxillary swing approach may become a preferred technique.

Specific surgical indications are not possible to enumerate. For each tumor in this region, the surgical team must carefully examine the available imaging studies, which should include computed tomography (CT) scanning, magnetic resonance imaging (MRI), and four-vessel angiogram, to determine the optimal surgical approach. The local spread of the tumor, tumor cell type, and past experiences of the surgical team will all have a bearing on the decision to utilize a particular approach.

Specific contraindications include extension into the temporal bone posterior to the carotid artery, anterior extension into the anterior cranial base, and extension across the midline into the contralateral skull base. Any or all of these factors make the anterior approach untenable owing to lack of exposure of critical structures during tumor removal.

Preoperative Considerations

The maxillary swing procedure poses the usual considerations of anesthetic risk, intraoperative monitoring, and prophylactic antibiotics during surgery. These factors are the same as for the previous two approaches discussed. Extensive preoperative evaluation is required before undertaking this operation, including a CT scan and MRI of the head and face and, usually, a four-vessel arteriogram. The arteriogram is necessary to study the vascular supply to the tumor, the involvement of the carotid arteries, and the quality of collateral blood flow from the opposite carotid artery. In addition, consideration of embolization of the tumor is made depending on the specific cell type, location, and arterial supply.

A critical decision in this procedure is whether to remove the maxilla or merely rotate the maxilla laterally. Removing the maxilla as a free bone graft improves the exposure, especially laterally, within the surgical field. It also increases the amount of room in the field to manipulate the instruments, a significant concern in skull base surgery. However, this does place the maxilla at risk for ischemic complications affecting the mucosa and dentition. These concerns must be addressed, especially in cases in which lengthy tumor dissection and removal is anticipated after the exposure is completed. For this reason, the maxillary swing procedure is usually preferred unless the additional exposure afforded by removal of the maxilla becomes paramount.

Whenever this operation is to be performed, consideration must be given to the possibility of tracheostomy. Without a tracheostomy, the endotracheal tube will be in the surgical field the entire procedure. Also, extubation becomes a concern owing to the swelling of the posterior pharyngeal wall and palate from the operation. Finally, without a tracheostomy the endotracheal tube will rub against the newly reconstructed palate, which may cause wound breakdown of the soft palate. With a tracheostomy in place, all of these problems are avoided. For these reasons, tracheostomy is preferred for most of these procedures, and it can be removed as early as several days after the surgery.

Technique

The procedure described here is the maxillary swing operation without craniotomy. For details on the more extensive procedure, the reader is referred to articles listed in the reference list. The maxillary swing procedure begins with a Weber-Fergusson incision, as described earlier. Unless the orbit is to be exenterated in the resection, it is probably advisable to keep the orbital extension of the incision in this procedure slightly lower than the usual subciliary incision to avoid ectropion and medial canthal contractures. The facial soft tissues are elevated in the subperiosteal plane from medial to lateral, and the infraorbital nerve is sacrificed to allow exposure of the malar eminence and the lateral orbital rim.

After the initial incisions are performed, the swing procedure is started in earnest. Before any bone cuts are made, reconstruction plates are aligned, contoured, and set in place (Fig. 16–12). At least two screws on each side of the bone cuts should be drilled to ensure proper alignment at the conclusion of the case. The minimal number of plates used is usually three: one along the midline anteriorly, one from the body of the maxilla to the frontal process of the maxilla, and the third from the body of the maxilla to the malar eminence.

The first surgical decision is whether to include the septum in the rotation. The advantage of doing this is that the medial exposure is extended across the midline to the contralateral side. If this is desirable, the palatal

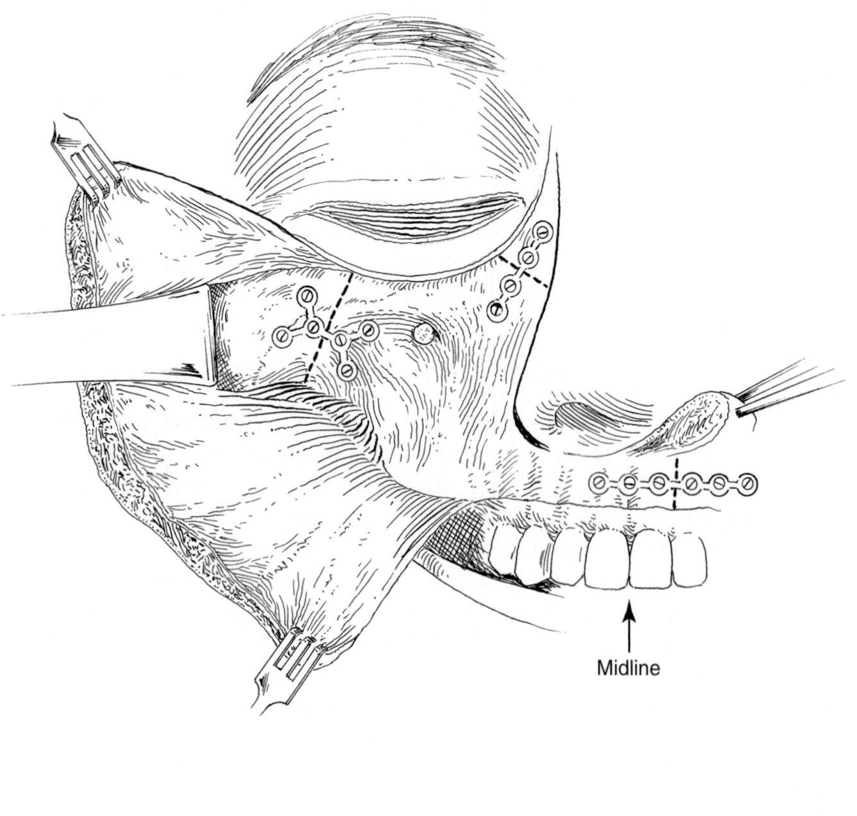

Figure 16–12. Preparation for the maxillary swing procedure. A Weber-Fergusson incision has been completed and the facial flap elevated. Microplates are placed over the areas in which osteotomy will be performed. This ensures accurate reconstruction at the end of the procedure.

incisions will be through the floor of the nose on the contralateral side. However, if the exposure is primarily unilateral, without the need for contralateral exposure, the incision can be across the floor of the nose on the ipsilateral side. In the event that the septum is to be included in the swing, an incision through the dorsum of the septum, disconnecting the septum from the nose and cribriform plate, will be needed (Fig. 16–13).

Assuming the septum will be included in the swing, the soft palate is first divided beginning on the contralateral side of the uvula and curving immediately back to the midline (Fig. 16–14). This facilitates closure, as incisions directly through the uvula tend to result in dehiscence. This incision should be made with a scalpel, not with cautery, to avoid excessive damage to the mucosa. However, either bipolar or unipolar coagulation can be applied to the underlying bleeding vessels to minimize blood loss. After elevation of the palatal mucosa, the hard palate is cut, using an oscillating saw with a thin blade, through the contralateral floor of the nose from posterior to anterior (Fig. 16–15). The cut can angle back to the midline anteriorly to emerge between the central incisors so that neither tooth need be sacrificed. A complete transfixion incision is performed to detach the septum from the columella anteriorly. Dorsal bone scissors are then used to cut through the septum, hugging the nasal dorsum all the way to the nasopharynx.

The next step is to make the bone cuts on the anterior face (Fig. 16–16). The medial cut crosses from the pyriform aperture to the orbital rim. This cut can be inferior or superior to the origin of the nasolacrimal sac, as needed. Inferior to the lacrimal sac, the cut will transect the nasolacrimal duct. Superior to the lacrimal sac, the cut will tether the maxilla to the eye, limiting rotation. Usually, the cut is made inferior to the lacrimal sac, requiring lacrimal stenting at the end of the procedure. The bone cuts are performed with the oscillating micro-

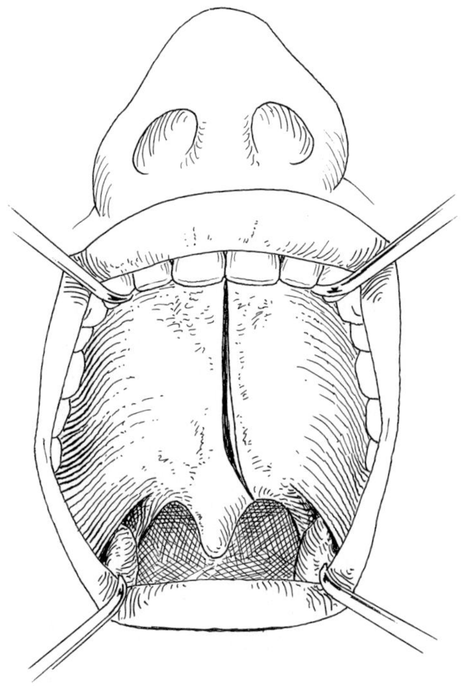

Figure 16–14. Palatal incision for maxillary swing procedure. The incision starts at the base of the uvula and curves back to the midline.

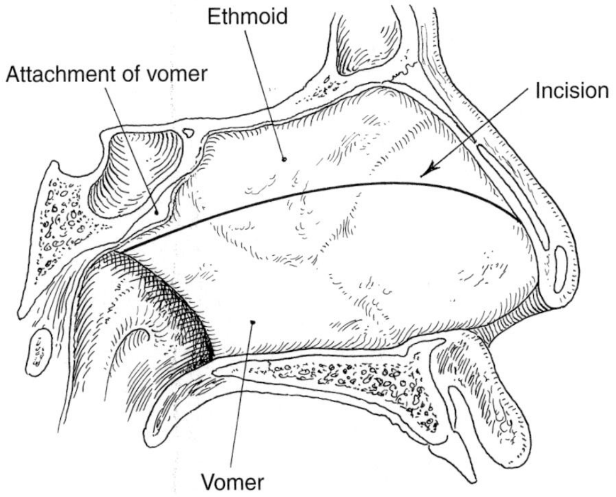

Figure 16–13. Septal transection. In certain cases, it may be desirable to translocate the septum with the maxilla. In this case, a high transection across the upper part of the septum, keeping below the cribriform plate, is performed.

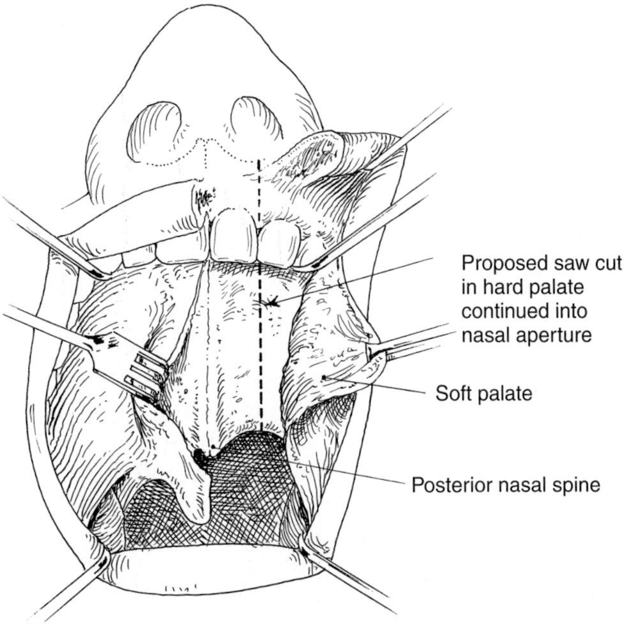

Figure 16–15. Palatal osteotomy for the maxillary swing procedure, including septal translocation. Palatal flaps are elevated. The dotted line extends through the hard palate into the floor of the nose on the side opposite the maxillary swing.

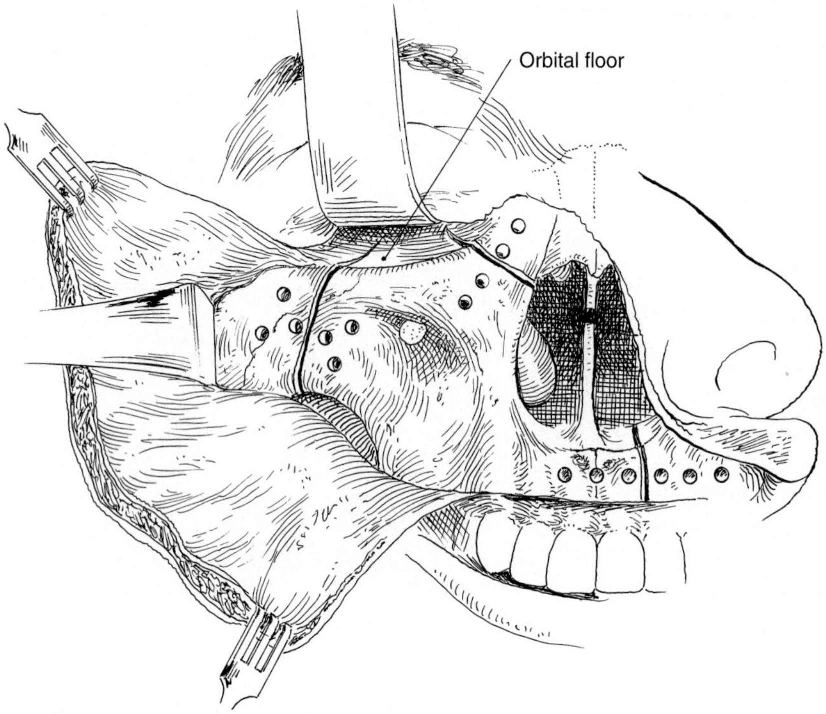

Figure 16–16. Completed osteotomies for the maxillary swing procedure. The palatal cut extends through the floor of the nose opposite the swing. The septal cut is high, but below the cribriform plate. The superior cut extends across the orbital rim to include the floor of the orbit. This cut can be above the lacrimal sac, thus maintaining the integrity of the nasolacrimal duct, or below the sac, transecting the duct. The lateral cut may be inferior to the zygomatic arch or posterior and superior if the lateral orbital wall will be included in the swing.

saw. The upper cut will angle laterally to the orbit and either go through the inferior orbital rim or enter into the maxillary sinus just inferior to the rim. The decision will hinge on whether the orbital rim is to be included in the swing or not. Including the orbital rim and floor will increase the exposure of the superior aspect of the infratemporal fossa and the skull base by allowing retraction of the eye superiorly. The lateral facial cut can either be made inferior to the zygomatic arch or superior to the arch. As with the previous decisions, the more superior level provides increased exposure, in this case, laterally in the infratemporal fossa. The lateral cut, when made above the arch, crosses the lateral orbital rim just above the arch and also must cut through the arch just lateral to the malar eminence. The inferior option of the lateral cut crosses the malar eminence inferior to the arch and crosses the orbital rim inferior to the arch.

At this point, the orbital cuts are performed (Fig. 16–17). The orbital periosteum is elevated from the floor of the orbit, extending from the rim anteriorly to the inferior orbital fissure posteriorly. When the floor of the orbit is included in the swing, the inferior orbital nerve must be transected at the point that it enters the maxillary sinus. The medial and lateral facial cuts are then extended from where they cross the orbital rim into the orbital floor posteriorly. The floor cuts extend posteriorly to the orbital fissure to include the entire roof of the maxillary sinus.

If all of the cuts have been made correctly, at this point, the only attachments of the maxilla are the mucosa of the lateral soft palate and the posterior wall to the pterygoid plates and pterygomaxillary fissure. These attachments contain the main blood supply to the sinus and should be maintained unless the maxilla is to be

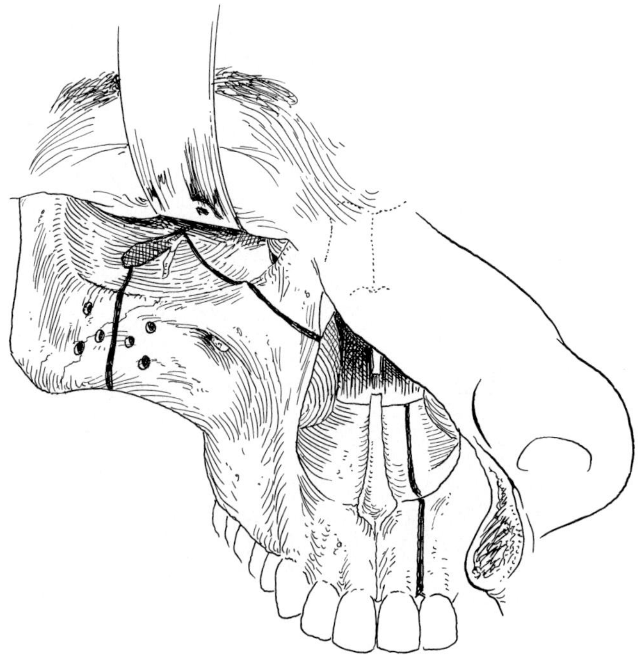

Figure 16–17. Orbital floor osteotomies. The cuts extend back to the inferior orbital fissure to include the entire floor of the orbit. The lateral cut may include the lateral wall of the orbit if it is placed above the zygomatic arch.

delivered as a free graft. The maxillary free graft is not recommended in most patients, especially those with viable dentition. Complete devascularization of the dentition will result in tooth loss. However, the greater palatine artery, superior alveolar artery, and the septal branch of the sphenopalatine artery should all remain intact and provide adequate blood supply to nourish the maxilla.

The flap is mobilized by applying gentle but constant lateral pressure on the maxilla. This should fracture the maxilla from the pterygoid plates atraumatically. The residual attachments are bluntly dissected from the posterior surface as necessary to mobilize the flap. The maxilla is then retracted laterally to the extent desired. A large, self-retaining retractor, such as a cerebellar retractor, can be positioned anteriorly between the nasal bones and the maxilla to keep the flap over (Fig. 16–18). Alternatively, a wide, flat retractor, such as a Deaver retractor, can be placed along the medial aspect of the flap to provide additional retraction posteriorly. When setting the retractors, it is important to remember that the blood supply is derived from the back, so too much retraction can damage the vessels, causing either intimal tears leading to thrombosis or frank avulsion with massive hemorrhage.

During reconstruction at the end of the procedure, attention should be paid to the lacrimal system. In most cases, the nasolacrimal duct will be transected. If the duct is violated, a dacryocystorhinostomy (DCR) should be performed by removing the medial wall of the lacrimal sac and placing Crawford lacrimal tubes through the superior and inferior punctum. Before replacing the maxilla, a large inferior nasal antral window is created. Maxillary rotation surgery may result in swelling of the mucosa and temporary dysfunction of the natural mucociliary clearance. The nasal antral window will help to ensure that the sinus drains properly.

The maxilla is rotated back into position and the bone plates are secured. A minimum of two screws on each side of each plate is recommended, but the preferred number is three on each side. Low-profile microplates are used in this setting and will normally suffice to reattach the maxilla securely. As stated earlier, three plates at the key buttresses should be adequate to anchor the maxilla. The orbital floor and palate are not plated or supported unless this is deemed necessary at the time of the closure.

Skin closure can proceed as previously described for the lateral rhinotomy incision. To reiterate, the lip is closed with 4-0 chromic sutures on the vermilion, 3-0 Vicryl on the muscle, and 6-0 nylon on the skin and vermilion-skin border. The sublabial incision is closed with 3-0 Vicryl, and the subciliary incision is closed with a running subcuticular 5-0 Prolene. The skin of the nasal facial groove is closed in two layers, using 4-0 Vicryl for the dermis and muscle and 6-0 nylon sutures on the skin surface.

A splint is placed on the septum if it was included in the rotation, and nasal packing is placed on the side of the incision along the floor of the nose. Finally, the palate is closed using 3-0 Vicryl sutures throughout to improve the strength and duration of the sutures. The soft palate is closed first. The inferior mucosal edges should be approximated with the first suture. The nasopharyngeal side is closed next with interrupted sutures up to the hard palate. The muscle should then be reap-

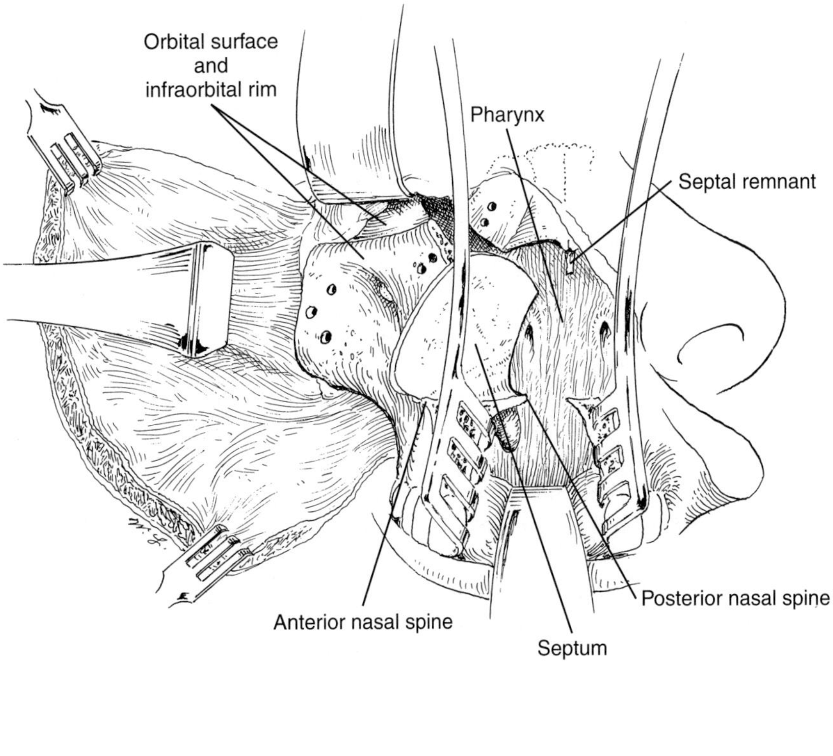

Figure 16–18. Completed maxillary swing. The nasopharynx and pterygomaxillary fissure are well exposed.

proximated with a second layer, and the oral mucosa is closed with a third layer. The hard palate mucosa is closed last. If the mucosa does not close well, palatal flaps will be necessary. To fashion the simplest palatal flap, one merely elevates the mucosa laterally to see whether this will result in tension-free closure. If this does not prove adequate, the mucosa can be advanced from the entire hard palate on the contralateral side as a rotation flap. This should be more than enough to achieve an adequate closure.

Postoperative Management

There are several aspects to consider in the postoperative care of patients undergoing the maxillary swing procedure in addition to those outlined for patients undergoing lateral rhinotomy. The first issue is airway management. If a tracheotomy has been placed, the care is the same as that for any tracheostomy. In cases in which oral intubation was maintained, the airway management is more individualized. The patient should be kept intubated and observed overnight in the intensive care unit or recovery room. Immediate postoperative extubation is risky because of the prolonged surgery time, the unknown degree of swelling of the palate and tongue, and the unpredictable amount of bleeding and secretions into the pharynx in the first hours after the operation. During this period of intubation, it is important to try and keep the tube from eroding through the soft palate closure. A ray tube is useful for this purpose; alternatively, the tube can be securely taped to the corner of the mouth, against the mandible on the side opposite the resection. The indications for extubation on the day after surgery are a fully awake patient with normal swallowing reflexes, absence of significant bleeding, and minimal to moderate palatal edema. If the patient is not ready for extubation within 24 to 48 hours of the completion of surgery, a tracheostomy should be considered.

The second consideration is oral dietary intake. The palatal closure is tenuous by nature, so early oral alimentation is likely to cause dehiscence of the suture line, resulting in cleft palate. During the first days after surgery, observation of the wound should be limited, especially if the patient has a significant gag reflex, as this may contribute to the risk of palatal breakdown. Despite withholding oral intake, a nasogastric or orogastric feeding tube must be avoided. These tubes constantly rub against the palatal closure and may lead to erosion of the suture line and dehiscence. There are three options for intravenous nutritional management in the first days until oral intake can be initiated: (1) 5% dextrose solution, which will supply about 500 calories per day; (2) peripheral parenteral nutrition using 10% dextrose and lipids, which can supply up to 1500 calories per day; or (3) total parenteral nutrition through a central venous catheter, which supplies full nutritional support. The alternative is to place a gastrostomy or jejunostomy tube for direct alimentation, which also can supply full nutritional support. Most patients will tolerate the caloric deficit associated with peripheral parenteral nutrition for the 5 to 7 days necessary to resume normal oral intake.

An additional concern for these patients is long-term management of dentition. If any of the teeth were damaged by the surgery, they can possibly be saved by adequate dental care. This may include excavating the pulp, permanent fillings, or root canal procedures.

Attention should also be paid to the possibility of chronic sinusitis. Ischemic damage to the sinus mucosa, entry into the maxillary sinus during the procedure, or trapping of mucosa during reconstruction may all lead to long term problems with sinus function. A plan for radiographic follow-up evaluation of the sinuses using CT scan at periodic intervals should be discussed with the patient and arranged during the early postoperative visits. Management of chronic sinusitis in these patients should follow the usual guidelines presented in earlier chapters in this book.

Complications

Complications relating to the incision have already been presented in the earlier section on lateral rhinotomy. The complications specifically associated with the maxillary swing procedure involve the components of the structures being rotated. In addition to the usual risks of hemorrhage, infection, and systemic problems, there are numerous potential problems with this surgery. The expected incidence of these complications is unknown, as the results of large series of these procedures have not been published in the medical literature. In addition, the literature that is available originates from those who originally described the procedure and have had success with it.

One set of complications relates to the patient's dentition. In addition to ischemic damage to the teeth from loss of blood supply, if the feeding vessels are injured, there can be direct damage to the central incisors during the initial bone cuts. Perhaps the most significant risk is malocclusion, which can occur when the fracture lines do not line up properly after surgery. This can be avoided by predrilling the reconstruction plates before the bone cuts are made. Trismus is also a possibility. When the maxilla is rotated, the pterygoid muscles are torn or stretched. This can result in contracture and postoperative trismus. This is usually treatable by physical therapy.

As mentioned earlier, the sinuses can also be injured during the procedure, leading to chronic sinusitis, mucous cyst formation, or mucocele formation. These complications can be prevented by careful placement of the osteotomies and creation of a nasal antral window to allow drainage after surgery. Nasal function may also be impaired secondary to damage to the septum, especially if the septum is included in the swing procedure. The cut across the dorsum may result in septal perforation or septal deviation. Anosmia is also a possibility.

Transection of the lacrimal collecting system may result in lacrimal duct stenosis and epiphora. DCR is, therefore, often a part of the operation. However, despite prophylactic DCR, lacrimal stenosis resulting in epiphora is always a concern. Secondary repair may be needed if the initial approach to management is not successful. Other injuries to the orbit are also possible, including orbital hematoma, corneal abrasion, and injury to the inferior rectus muscle. A more likely problem is enophthalmos, which can be caused by imperfect alignment of the bones of the floor of the orbit. In this instance, support of the orbital floor may be needed to avoid prolapse into the maxillary sinus. In all cases, this should be assessed during reconstruction. An alloplastic material, such as Marlex mesh, can be used to reinforce the floor if necessary.

Dehiscence of any part of the palatal closure will result in oronasal fistula or cleft palate. These two problems can be managed in the short term with a palatal prosthesis, provided the patient has adequate dentition to support the prosthesis. Definitive management may not be necessary if the wound is obturated by a prosthesis and given sufficient time to heal secondarily. Surprisingly, this strategy is often successful as long as the dehiscence is not complete. If a complete cleft palate is formed, surgical repair is the only option. In this case, the surgeon will need to evaluate the available tissue and design a method of closure. Complete discussion of management of cleft palate is beyond the scope of this chapter.

LE FORT I OSTEOTOMY

Indications

Another unique approach to the nasopharynx and middle skull base is the Le Fort I osteotomy.[14–16] This technique involves creating a transverse facial osteotomy along the lines of the classic Le Fort I fracture and inferiorly displacing the palate to expose the nasopharynx, clivus, and potentially, the sphenoid sinus. This approach can be combined with unilateral or bilateral medial maxillectomy and resection of the septum to increase the width and height of the exposure.

There are no circumstances when this approach is the only viable option. However, in the hands of its advocates, the Le Fort I osteotomy is an advantageous, even preferred approach to selected skull base tumors. With the addition of a medial maxillectomy, lateral exposure is extended to the pterygomaxillary fissure and infratemporal fossa. The limitation of the approach is that it cannot provide exposure anterior to the pituitary or posterior to the carotid artery.

Among the advantages of this option over other approaches to this area are the ease, rapidity, and safety with which it can be performed and its excellent cosmetic and functional results. There are no skin incisions or changes in the external facial appearance. The nose and sinuses are typically unaffected. The palate is not incised or injured, and the procedure itself takes much less time and is easier to reconstruct than the maxillary swing approach. The disadvantage of this operation is that it provides a limited surgical exposure, both in terms of visualization and introduction of instruments into the surgical field.

For these reasons, the best indications for this technique are midline tumors with minimal lateral and anterior extension, examples of which include clivus chordomas, juvenile nasopharyngeal angiofibromas, and nasopharyngeal carcinomas. Other, less common nasopharyngeal or clival lesions are potential indications for this procedure, including certain clival meningiomas and bony tumors of the clivus. The final decision to utilize this approach is made jointly with the participating neurosurgeon and is based on the specific circumstances of the patient and the tumor and the previous experience of the surgical team.

Preoperative Considerations

As with all skull base surgery, the patient will require careful medical evaluation and anesthetic planning. Prophylactic antibiotics and adequate invasive monitoring are routine measures. In contrast to the maxillary swing procedure, the airway in the Le Fort I osteotomy is not at risk. Orotracheal intubation is routine, with extubation performed when the patient is awake, breathing, and able to protect the airway from secretions.

The important considerations for this procedure are to decide the exact extent of the exposure required. This is helpful in limiting the number of changes of the surgical teams and can ultimately save operating time. Another important consideration is the patient's teeth. This operation has the potential for devascularizing the teeth if the blood supply is damaged and for causing malocclusion if the reconstruction is inaccurate. The condition of the teeth should be fully evaluated and any significant dental work completed before surgery.

Technique

The patient should be prepared for surgery with the head supported and the neck bent slightly forward. This will help to maintain the appropriate exposure and orientation during the operation. The face should be prepared and draped for sterile surgery even though the initial incision is through nonsterile mucosa. Lidocaine 1% with 1 : 100,000 epinephrine is injected into the gingival labial sulcus and upper lip to improve hemostasis.

The incision is similar to that for midfacial degloving except that it must extend laterally on both sides. The incision should be kept about 5 mm on the labial side of the sulcus to aid in closure at the end of the operation. The initial incision is made with a scalpel through the mucosa and then extended down through the periosteum with cautery. The angle of this dissection should be maintained as low as possible to avoid the inferior orbital nerve.

The facial soft tissues are elevated using a Freer elevator or any suitable periosteal elevator. Elevation should extend superiorly to the level of the infraorbital foramen, but the nerve itself should be preserved and protected throughout the operation.

Before the first bone cuts are made, the reconstruction plates should be aligned and contoured. The holes are drilled, and at least two screws are placed on each side of the planned osteotomy. An X-shaped, L-shaped, or straight plate can be contoured to the medial buttresses bilaterally (Fig. 16–19). Securing the plates with at least two screws on each side of the intended fracture line will ensure that, after reconstruction, the palate is in good position and the occlusion is maintained at preoperative alignment. The plates used can be either the 1.5 or 1.0 mm in size, depending on the thickness of the bones. For most patients, the lighter and thinner microplates are preferred.

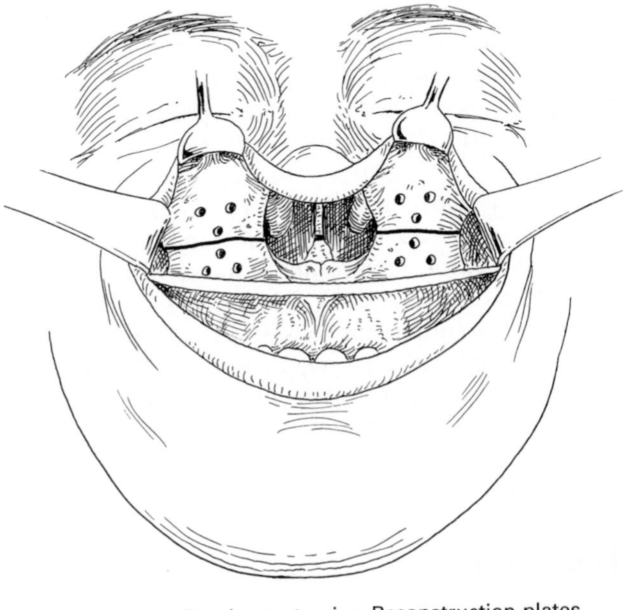

Figure 16–19. Le Fort I osteotomies. Reconstruction plates have been predrilled and removed. The anterior bone cuts extend across the maxilla from the pyriform aperture to the pterygoid plates.

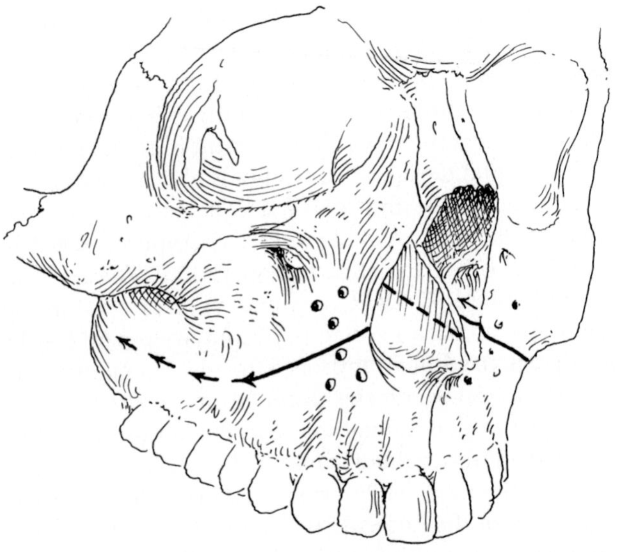

Figure 16–20. Le Fort I osteotomies. The anterior cut extends laterally to the pterygoid plates. The septum is transected along the floor of the nose. The medial maxillary cut is not shown.

The last step before the bone cuts are made is to elevate the mucosa from the floor of the nose. Under direct vision, this is not a difficult maneuver, and it will prevent damage to the mucosa and the subsequent scarring that could otherwise cause vestibular stenosis. The initial bone cuts are made anteriorly, extending from the pyriform aperture across the medial buttress at the level of the floor of the nose (see Fig. 16–19). A microsaw is preferred for this step to avoid unnecessary bone loss at the osteotomy sites. Using the same microsaw blade, the anterior cuts are extended around the lateral wall of the sinus to the posterior aspect of the alveolar ridge. The anterior cuts are completed by cutting across the root of the septum and through the anterior maxillary spine and the maxillary crest below the septum. The osteotomy is then extended posteriorly below the septum to the nasopharynx (Fig. 16–20). This can be accomplished using a 1-cm straight osteotome.

The bone cuts across the medial walls of the maxillary sinus are then made. The medial wall of the maxillary sinus is cut along the floor of the nose, from anterior to posterior, using a straight 1-cm osteotome (Fig. 16–21). An osteotome is preferred for this step as it is difficult to accurately cut with a powered instrument through the inside of the nose. This bone cut begins where the medial aspect of the anterior bone cut ends. Again, it is best to keep this inferior within the sinus. Next, a curved osteotome is directed around the back of the maxillary sinus above the alveolar ridge to disconnect the sinus from the pterygoid plates. The osteotome is guided into position by feel, as this area cannot be visualized during this bone cut.

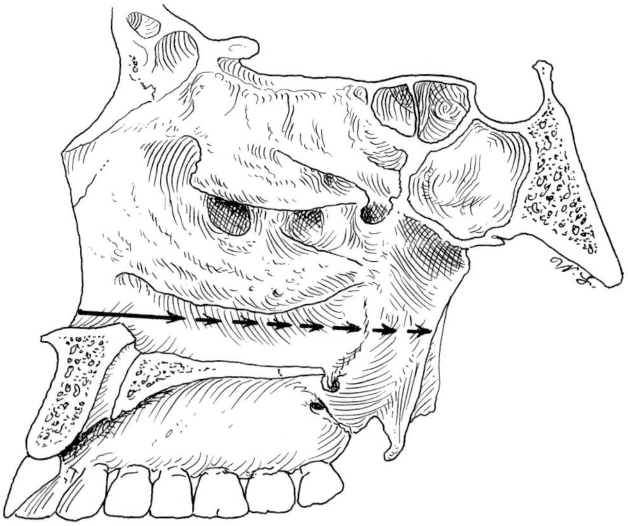

Figure 16–21. Medial maxillary osteotomy. The cut extends through the floor of the maxilla back through the medial pterygoid plate.

The last cut is through the posterior wall of the maxillary sinus. This is performed through the opening made by the combination of the anterior and medial cuts. The osteotome is wedged through this opening and up against the posterior wall, and the bone cut is made with gentle technique and firm control of the osteotome. Medially, this cut will cross thick bone near the sphenopalatine foramen. By being careful in this area, it is possible to make this cut without injuring the sphenopalatine artery or nerve.

The entire palate should be free of bony attachments at this point. It will remain attached by the soft tissues of the soft palate, the periosteum of the posterior wall, and the vessels of the pterygomaxillary fissure. It is essential to preserve these vessels to avoid making the palate a free devascularized flap. Moreover, loss of the blood supply could jeopardize the teeth.

The vertical dimensions of the exposure are determined by the degree of retraction applied to the palate in an inferior direction. The vessels will be the main limitation. Gentle handling of the palate is essential to avoid injury to the vessels. The anterior separation is greater than the posterior separation, causing the field to be cone-shaped, with the apex of the cone in the nasopharynx (Fig. 16–22).

As the bone cuts are made, various secondary blood vessels are transected, leading to significant blood loss. It is difficult to control the bleeding during this stage of the procedure. However, as soon as the palate is mobilized and dropped down, hemostasis can be achieved with a combination of cautery and bone wax.

If additional exposure is desired, the septum can be removed. The septum is approached after the Le Fort I osteotomies are completed. The caudal end of the septum is easily exposed by retraction of the lip superiorly. The mucosa of the septum is then easily elevated from anterior to posterior for the full length of the septum. Initially, the left side is elevated completely. Care should be taken to avoid tears in the mucosa during this elevation, as this will likely result in septal perforation. The bony cartilaginous junction is divided and the mucosa is elevated from the bone on the right side of the septum. At this point, the bone of the septum should be completely exposed and can then be easily removed to the extent required. A Hardy pituitary retractor can then be inserted to displace to the right the

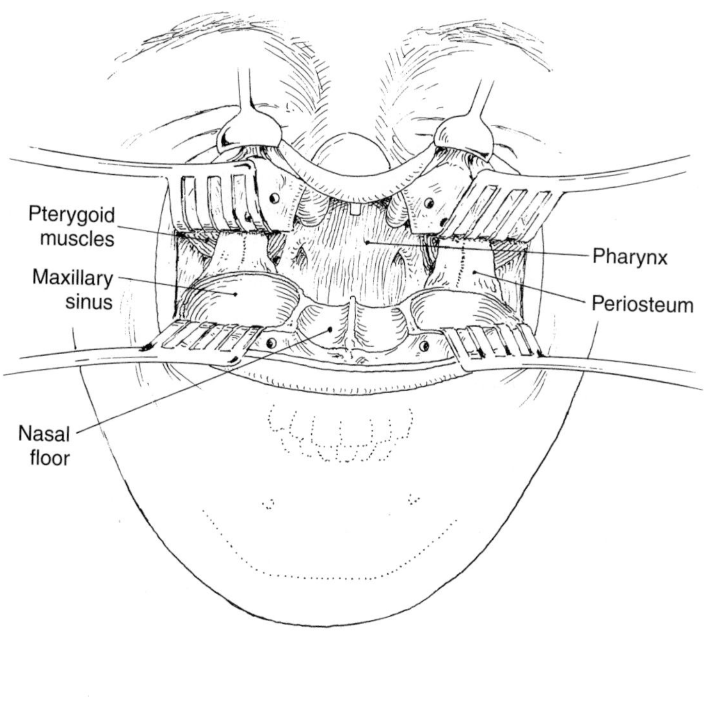

Figure 16–22. Completed Le Fort I exposure. The upper nasopharynx is well visualized. The septum can be resected to increase exposure superiorly. The blood supply to the palate is through the descending palatine arteries.

cartilaginous septum that is still attached to the mucosa on the right side.

Exposure is further enhanced by resection of the medial wall of the maxillary sinus. After the palate is dropped, the medial wall is removed by simply cutting across the wall from anterior to posterior, at the level desired, up to the floor of the orbit. The pyriform aperture can be preserved, but this will minimize the value derived from the additional exposure. The better technique is to remove the medial wall with the lateral border of the pyriform aperture. During reconstruction, this bone can simply be plated back into position to avoid distortion of the nasal-facial relationship. The final cut to remove the medial wall is from superior to inferior across the posterior attachment. This cut should not be carried into the pterygoid plates directly, but should be angled anterior to this plane to avoid injuring the blood supply to the palate.

After the tumor resection is completed, reconstruction is performed. The palate is rocked back into position and secured by placing the fixation plates that were aligned before the bone cuts were made. The sublabial incision is closed in routine fashion using interrupted 3-0 Vicryl sutures. Finally, the septum is splinted with Silastic splints to hold it in position. Nasal packing is optional, but should be used if significant bleeding is a possibility.

Postoperative Care

Postoperative care for patients undergoing the Le Fort I osteotomy will largely be based on the nature of the tumor resection. The unique aspects of care specific to this approach include management of the dentition and nasal packing. The dentition will need to be watched closely over the ensuing weeks for signs of devascularization. A dentist should be consulted and should participate in this aspect of observation. Oral intake can be started any time after the surgery as tolerated by the patient. However, the diet should be limited to liquids for the first 2 weeks, and to soft foods requiring no mastication for up to 6 weeks. The nasal packing can be removed as early as the first postoperative day if bleeding has not been a problem. Nasal splints should be left in place for a minimum of 5 days to allow the septum to stabilize.

Complications

The problems associated with this surgery are similar to those encountered with the maxillary swing operation, with several notable exceptions. If the blood supply to the palate is lost completely, the entire alveolar ridge and palate will exist as a free devascularized flap. This may result in all of the teeth undergoing root degeneration, as well as the palatal soft tissues becoming necrotic. This would lead to significant functional deficits requiring major reconstructive surgery or prosthetics to repair.

Less severe problems may arise as a result of bleeding and wound infection, but these are rare and can usually be treated easily by straightforward management. Long-term problems involving the sinuses, related either to mucocele or obstruction of the maxillary sinus, can occur and may require delayed intervention up to many years after the surgery.

Nasal problems, including deviation of the septum, perforation of the septum, or nasal stenosis, would be expected to be among the more common problems encountered. Cosmetic problems related to this surgery should be minimal, as there are no facial incisions. Removal of the medial buttress (lateral pyriform aperture) will result in contracture of the nose in this direction. This can be overcome by reconstructing this buttress. Loss of septal support may result in collapse of the nasal supratip and some degree of saddle nose deformity. This can be overcome with a dorsal onlay graft. Malunion or nonunion of one of the osteotomies can result in malocclusion, whereas multiple failed plates may result in facial elongation.

TRANSPALATAL APPROACH

Indications

The most commonly used technique for access to the nasopharynx is the transoral or transpalatal approach.[17–20] The transpalatal approach to the skull base is not, strictly speaking, a nasal or sinus surgery, but it is discussed here as a principle alternative to the Le Fort I osteotomy approach to the nasopharynx. For many types of pathologic disease of the nasopharynx and clivus, the transpalatal operation is the preferred alternative to other approaches owing to its simplicity and direct and rapid technique.

A number of variations of the basic procedure have been described according to the degree of exposure required and the type of pathologic process involved. In its simplest form, the transpalatal approach requires only retraction of the soft palate. This procedure is routinely used for adenoidectomy, as well as for excision of nasopharyngeal cysts, biopsy, and excision of some small tumors.

The second variation in the procedure involves a mucosal incision in the hard palate that allows the soft palate to be dropped away from the hard palate. This exposes the nasopharynx between the hard palate and soft palate and avoids a palate-splitting incision. This is the preferred technique for transpalatal repair of choanal atresia and choanal stenosis. In very young infants, this procedure allows the surgeon to avoid an incision in the soft palate that otherwise could result in velopharyngeal incompetence, a severe complication in an infant.

The variation used for most tumor surgery and for transpalatal approaches to the upper cervical spine is a straight, vertical division of the soft palate. With lateral retraction of the soft palate to either side, the nasopharynx is exposed from the lower third of the clivus to the base of the second cervical vertebrae. The superior extent of exposure can be further extended by removing the posterior aspect of the hard palate and vomer. This will improve the superior exposure, allowing visualization up to the superior aspect of the clivus and floor of the sphenoid sinus. The mandible and lower teeth limit further superior exposure.

Finally, the transpalatal approach may include a median labiomandibular glossotomy. By splitting the lip, mandible, and tongue through the midline, the posterior wall exposure can be extended superiorly to the top of the sphenoid sinus and inferiorly to the fourth cervical vertebrae. This degree of exposure is rarely needed, but may be used in patients in whom exposure is difficult owing to trismus or in those with very large tumors limited to the midline.

Because of the versatility and simplicity of the operation, it is the most common approach to the nasopharynx. Palatal retraction is used for adenoidectomy, nasopharyngeal biopsy, excision of cysts, and excision of small tumors. As stated earlier, the palatal drop procedure is the preferred technique for the transpalatal approach to choanal atresia and stenosis, and may be used for certain cases of angiofibroma. The palatal split procedures are most commonly used for orthopedic procedures of the upper cervical spine and clivus. They are appropriate for use in basilar impression, a condition in which the odontoid process projects posteriorly and superiorly into the brain stem, causing compression. Other spinal indications include resection of pannus secondary to rheumatoid arthritis. In advanced cases, arthritic pannus from C1 and C2 can lead to brain stem compression. The preferred technique for resection is through the palatal split procedure.

The palatal split approach may also be used to resect certain tumors. The most well documented of these are the juvenile nasopharyngeal angiofibroma and the clivus chordoma. Such lesions should be evaluated in detail by preoperative radiographic studies to make sure that this approach is suitable. Extension of the tumor into the cavernous sinus, intracranially through the dura, or laterally into the infratemporal fossa renders this approach less attractive than the lateral approaches. Other tumors that have been removed through this approach include schwanomma, sarcoma, and meningioma.

Finally, the transpalatal approach has been used for ligation of certain basilar artery aneurysms. This procedure is fraught with risk and difficulty, however, and a high incidence of morbidity and mortality has been reported, primarily associated with the inability to create a watertight seal of the wound. The result is secondary cerebrospinal fluid (CSF) leak and, ultimately, meningitis.

The principal limitation of these transpalatal/transoral approaches is that they are not appropriate for any case requiring intradural surgery. Reliable control of bleeding behind the lesion from this direction is difficult, and prevention of CSF leak is problematic. The mucosal flaps from the posterior wall of the nasopharynx that are raised during this surgery are heavily infiltrated with lymphoid tissue, making them friable and difficult to close in a watertight fashion. Furthermore, the flaps usually undergo significant retraction during the resection phase of the procedure, which may damage the flaps and further complicate watertight closure.

Additional limitations of the transpalatal approach to the nasopharynx relate to the anatomic limits of the exposure. With this approach, exposure anterior to the posterior choanae and sphenoid sinus, lateral to the eustachian tube, and posterior to the foramen magnum, spinal cord, and brain stem is impossible.

A final factor that limits the utility of the transpalatal approach is the need for anterior bone grafting. For certain spinal procedures, stabilization of the cervical spine using grafts is necessary following surgery. Because a watertight seal is difficult to guarantee with this approach, bone grafts placed through the incision may become contaminated, increasing the risk of subsequent infection and nonunion. In most patients, posterior fusion can be accomplished safely after the anterior resection and pharyngeal repair. However, the transpalatal approach should be avoided in those who require anterior grafting.

Preoperative Considerations

In addition to the usual preoperative considerations of antibiotics, anesthesia, and monitoring, this procedure does require significant planning before surgery. The first decision involves the degree of exposure required. As discussed earlier, the various modifications in the technique yield predictable results in terms of exposure. Knowing the full extent of the lesion before surgery allows a logical decision to be made regarding the exact choice of modification to use. Depending on the variation chosen, certain secondary problems may need to be considered.

When a vertical palatal split is used, the status of the airway and nutritional support after the surgery become significant issues. The airway can be compromised by blood and secretions from the wound, as well as by edema of the palate and the posterior wall of the pharynx. Tracheostomy is a possibility, but usually prolonged intubation will suffice. When a median labiomandibular glossotomy is performed, a tracheostomy becomes essential.

Owing to the risk of palatal dehiscence, the patient must not eat for several days after surgery. A nasogastric tube should never be placed for feeding, as the tube would rub against the line of closure. A gastrostomy is almost never necessary and would not be placed prophylactically. As a result, the surgeon must choose between various intravenous options, specifically, intravenous fluids, peripheral parenteral nutrition, or total parenteral nutrition.

Technique

The transpalatal procedure is always performed using general anesthesia. However, it is also a good idea to inject local anesthesia into the mucosa of the incision to minimize blood loss. As stated earlier, there are several variations in the technique of transpalatal surgery. In all cases, the oral cavity and oropharynx must be exposed using a self-retaining retractor. The options include the Crow-Davis mouth gag, devised for tonsillectomy; the Dingman mouth gag, initially designed for cleft palate repair; or the Crockard retractor set, which was specifically designed for transpalatal surgery of the skull base. This last device has the advantage of a variety of attachments that assist in retracting the palate and posterior wall flaps. The best choice of retractor for an individual case will depend on the procedure that is planned. The Crowe-Davis gag is ideal for adenoidectomy and simple cyst excision, as these procedures do not require palatal incision. The Dingman gag is especially useful for cases in which a hard palate incision is made, with operation through the soft palate–hard palate junction. The Crockard retractor set is the best option for cases requiring a palatal split incision. Regardless of the type of retractor chosen, all provide tongue retraction and oral opening. The tension on the tongue may cause ischemia to the tip of the tongue. To avoid problems, the gag should be released periodically. A sensible regimen would be retraction for 40 minutes, followed by 5 minutes of release time.

The simplest transpalatal method is to retract the soft palate with a red rubber catheter. After the oral cavity is exposed with the oral gag, a No. 8 or 10 French catheter is placed through the nose, grasped in the oropharynx, and brought out through the mouth. The two ends of the catheter are then pulled taught and clamped together at the nose to maintain retraction. Either unilateral or bilateral catheters can be used, depending on the degree of exposure desired.

Palatal Drop

The transpalatal approach for choanal exposure is best performed through the hard palate–soft palate junction. The incision in the mucosa incorporates both greater palatine arteries and most of the palatal mucosa (Fig. 16–23). The incision is made through the mucosa and periosteum down to the palatal bone with a No. 15 blade. The flap is developed back to the hard palate–soft palate junction using a periosteal elevator. At the palatal junction, cautery is used to divide the muscles of the soft palate from the hard palate and the nasopharyngeal mucosa at the junction. A malleable retractor can be used to push the flap down, exposing the nasopharynx. To increase the exposure of the posterior choanae, the posterior edge of the hard palate can be removed with a drill. An otologic cutting burr is preferred. As the hard palate is removed, the posterior aspect of the septum is visualized and can be removed to further increase exposure (Fig. 16–24).

Palatal Split

The next step in the progression of exposure is to use a palatal split. Either a direct midline or a paramedian incision can be used (see Fig. 16–23), but the paramedian incision is preferred because it avoids cutting into the uvula. The direct median split is more likely than the paramedian incision to result in dehiscence owing to the inherent lack of strength of the uvula. When the paramedian incision is used, the incision begins just lateral to the base of the uvula, curves immediately back to the midline, and then traverses the midline of the soft palate. The incision generally is extended for a few centimeters onto the hard palate to allow the soft palate to retract without tearing. The incision in the mucosa is always made with a scalpel, rather than cautery, to

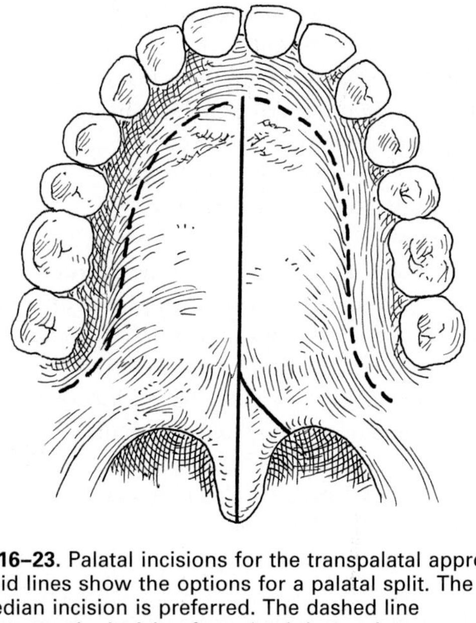

Figure 16–23. Palatal incisions for the transpalatal approach. The solid lines show the options for a palatal split. The paramedian incision is preferred. The dashed line demonstrates the incision for palatal depression, as preferred for choanal atresia.

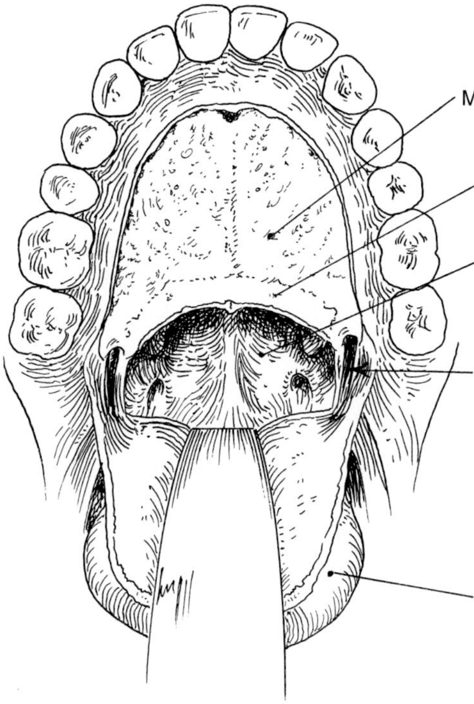

Figure 16–24. Completed exposure for the transpalatal approach using palatal depression. The posterior hard palate and vomer have been removed.

minimize damage to the mucosa. The muscle edges of the palatal mucosa will bleed and may be controlled with bipolar cautery.

The soft palate is divided vertically up to the junction with the hard palate. To allow retraction of the palate laterally, the soft palate can be detached submucosally from the hard palate at the junction. This is accomplished by extending the incision onto the hard palate. Instead of simply extending the incision in the midline, a curvilinear incision can be made to allow the palatal mucosa to be elevated as a flap (Fig. 16–25). The muscular attachments of the soft palate to the hard palate, as well as the nasopharyngeal mucosal surface, can then be divided using cautery or dissected free with an elevator. At this point, the soft palate is only attached laterally to the anterior tonsillar pillar and anteriorly to the hard palate mucosa. With maximal retraction, the entire nasopharynx and posterior edge of the hard palate can be visualized. The soft tissues of the palate can be retracted using either a large, self-retaining retractor, such as a Wheatlander or cerebellar retractor, or the palatal attachments of the Crockard set. The posterior aspect of the hard palate can then be removed using an otologic burr. This will expose the posterior aspect of the septum, which can also be removed, if desired, to maximize superior exposure in the direction of the sphenoid sinus.

After the palatal dissection is complete, the posterior pharyngeal wall may be incised to expose the clivus or upper cervical spine. Three basic options are available for incising the posterior wall: a vertical midline incision, a superiorly based flap, and an inferiorly based flap (Fig. 16–26). The two flap techniques are greatly preferred over the simple midline incision. This is because the midline incision does not create adequate side-to-side exposure without excessive retraction on the mucosal edges. Aggressive retraction of the mucosa may result in injury to the mucosa and subsequent difficulties in closure. Conversely, the U-shaped flaps expose the

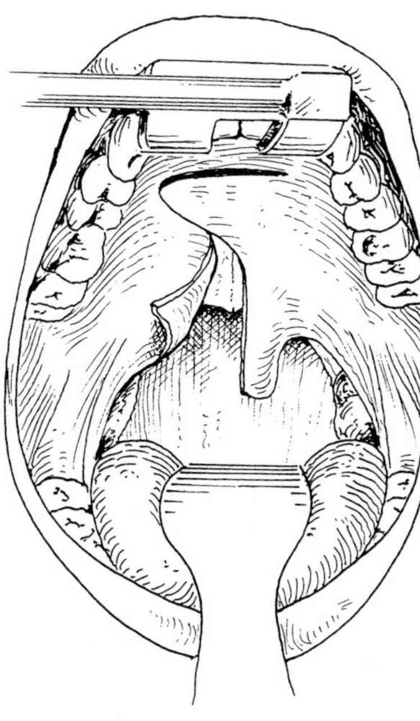

Figure 16–25. Palatal flap option for a palate-splitting incision.

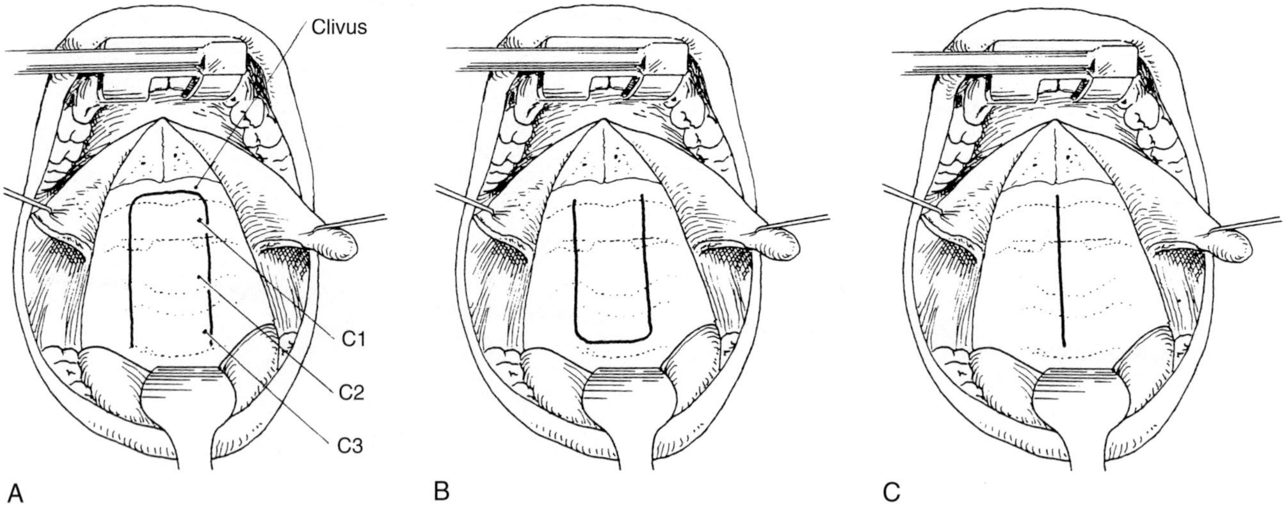

Figure 16–26. Pharyngeal wall incisions. *A,* Inferiorly based flap. *B,* Superiorly based flap. *C,* Midline linear incision.

entire width of the nasopharynx without retraction on the mucosal edges. This is a major advantage for closure at the end of the operation. The superiorly based flap provides excellent exposure from the base of the third cervical spine to the lower third of the clivus, but does not allow exposure to the top of the clivus or sphenoid sinus. The inferiorly based flap allows exposure from the floor of the sphenoid sinus superiorly down to the level of the base of the second cervical spine. For most cases, this is the preferred technique.

The flap is incised with a No. 15 blade fixed on a long scalpel handle. The distal tip of the flap is gently grasped with toothed forceps and retracted inferiorly so that long, curved, Metzenbaum scissors can be used to elevate the flap. The plane of elevation is at the level of the prevertebral fascia. Once the plane is entered, elevation proceeds easily with small spreading and snipping with the scissors. The inferiorly based flap is tucked down the lumen of the pharynx to keep it out of the way. The superiorly based flap is sutured to a red rubber catheter that is passed through the nose and retracted back up into the nose.

The tissues of the prevertebral fascia are very tough and do not elevate well as a flap. Typically, they are incised in the midline and elevated laterally as best as possible. Often, a cautery is used to excise the fascia, thereby improving exposure. However, if the fascia can be preserved as a flap, it creates an excellent deeper layer of closure. At this point, the neurosurgeon or an appropriately trained otolaryngologic skull base surgeon is called in to perform the definitive procedure.

The next and last level of progression in transpalatal surgery is the median labiomandibular glossotomy. This procedure involves a tracheostomy, midline lip incision, mandibular split, and division of the tongue. This technique uses a standard lip-splitting incision that incorporates a notch in the supramental crease. The lip is divided through the labial mucosa down to the submental surface of the mandible. A stair-step osteotomy is performed after reconstruction plates are aligned and predrilled. The tongue is then divided in the midline from the tip to the circumvallate papillae and even to the vallecula if necessary. With retraction, this will allow exposure from the fifth cervical spine to the sphenoid sinus.

Closure of the transpalatal approach proceeds in two stages. The first stage is repair of the posterior pharyngeal wall. Under most circumstances, a CSF leak will not have occurred during the operation, so closure can proceed rapidly without excessive concern that the closure be watertight. However, when a CSF leak does occur, the closure must be performed as carefully as possible to achieve a watertight closure. The surgical cavity can be packed with a combination of fat and fascia harvested from the abdomen or thigh. Fibrin tissue glue is helpful for sealing this graft in place. The fascia is next closed if available. Interrupted 3-0 Vicryl sutures on a tapered needle are used for this layer, as well as subsequent layers. Fast-dissolving gut and chromic gut sutures are not favored, as added time is beneficial to ensure healing. The mucosal layer of the flap is also closed with interrupted 3-0 Vicryl. These sutures on the posterior wall are difficult to place, requiring patience and slow, careful technique to avoid tearing of the fragile mucosa. Initially, the flap may appear not to reach to the end of the surgical defect. The flap must be slowly advanced from the base out to stretch it to the full length.

Palatal closure is performed in three layers: nasopharyngeal mucosa, muscle, and oral mucosa. The first suture should align the inferior free margin of the palate. The sutures should then proceed superiorly, along the nasal side first, to the hard palate junction. The muscle layer is next sutured, with the last on the oral side. These sutures, too, must be placed with extreme control and care to avoid tearing the tissues.

Postoperative Care

As alluded to earlier, the patient who has undergone transpalatal surgery of the skull base will not usually be able to be extubated in the early postoperative period. The risk of bleeding into the airway or obstruction from edema is sufficient to warrant at least overnight observation with the endotracheal tube in place. The possibility of bleeding is self-explanatory. By the morning after surgery, the wound is normally dry, and only normal secretions are present. The risk of airway obstruction is secondary to both palatal edema from the surgery itself and from tongue edema caused by excessive retraction. If significant edema is not present by the morning after surgery, it is unlikely that airway obstruction will occur. The patient should be examined the morning after surgery. If there is no bleeding, if the edema is minimal, and if the patient is fully conscious, the endotracheal tube can be safely removed. Failure to meet any of these criteria should prompt the surgeon to postpone extubation. To assist in resolving edema, intravenous dexamethasone can be administered, usually at a dosage of 10 mg every 6 hours for the first night after surgery. If criteria for extubation have not been met within 48 to 72 hours after surgery, a tracheostomy should be performed.

Oral intake should be delayed for at least 5 days after surgery. This minimizes the risk of palatal dehiscence and posterior pharyngeal wall infection. After 5 days, if everything is proceeding without complication, the patient may be started on a liquid diet. The diet is advanced slowly, with the first solid food being offered about 7 days after the procedure. During this interval, nutrition can be maintained either by peripheral parenteral nutrition or total parenteral nutrition through a central venous catheter. Wound complications that significantly delay oral intake are an indication for placement of a feeding gastrostomy. However, in no circumstance should a nasogastric tube be placed, as this will rub against the incision, leading to a high risk of breakdown.

Although it is important to inspect the palate and posterior pharyngeal wounds periodically in the postoperative period, it is advisable to avoid excessive examination. Depressing the tongue sufficiently to examine the palate and posterior pharyngeal wall completely may stimulate a gag reflex, resulting in maximal muscle pull on the healing incision. Before oral intake is begun, a fiberoptic laryngoscopy should be performed through the nose to examine the nasopharynx. This will allow careful inspection of the pharyngeal suture line to document the quality and degree of wound healing.

In the case of a CSF leak during the procedure, special postoperative care is in order. A lumbar drain is placed, and 20 cc of CSF is removed every 2 hours to keep the wound decompressed. A tracheostomy should also be placed to prevent airway difficulties from affecting the wound healing. The patient is kept on bed rest for the first 5 days after surgery, and the oral intake is delayed until at least 7 days after surgery. The lumbar drain is closed off on the fifth day and CSF pressure is allowed to return to normal. If no sign of CSF leak is present within 24 hours after the drain is closed off, the drain can be removed. If leakage is suspected, an intrathecal contrast study should be performed to document the leak. Confirmed CSF leak at this point is an indication for urgent reoperation to close the leak. Several possible techniques are available, including local mucosal rotation flaps, a sternocleidomastoid muscle flap, or a free vascularized radial forearm flap.

Complications

The most feared complication of this procedure is CSF fistula. This occurs only when intracranial penetration is combined with failure of a primary attempt to control the leak. The inevitable result of failure to close such a leak is meningitis, which will become recurrent until the leak is stopped or the patient fails to survive. The incidence of CSF leak depends on the nature of the procedure performed. Extradural procedures, such as removal of angiofibroma, chordoma, or odontoidectomy, are associated with a very low risk of CSF leak. By contrast, intracranial procedures, such as aneurysm clipping, resection of meningioma, or resection of other intracranial tumors, are associated with a risk of CSF leak of up to 25% to 33%. For this reason, only extradural procedures are recommended for the transpalatal approach.

Wound complications associated with the posterior pharyngeal wall are common, with partial breakdown of the incision being present in most cases. Usually, however, this will not be severe, and healing by secondary intention will result in a normal, functional nasopharynx. More severe problems, such as abscess and cervical vertebral bone infections, can occur, but fortunately are rare and not often described in the literature.

Palatal wound problems also occur frequently. Complete dehiscence occurs in approximately 10% of the cases, with minor problems reported more frequently. Small areas of breakdown may heal with time. A palatal prosthesis may assist in the healing process while preventing nasal reflux during the time of healing. In the case of palatal dehiscence, repair or prosthetic treatment is necessary. Repair can be effected by simple closure, with or without bolsters or flaps. A potential problem after initial breakdown is velopharyngeal incompetence, in which case reflux of fluids and solids, as well as decreased voice intensity from hypernasality of speech, may be reported. Rehabilitation with a palatal lift prosthesis or digital manipulation may help soften the palate enough to regain sufficient function to prevent the unwanted side effects.

REFERENCES

1. Lore JM. Partial and radical maxillectomy. In Meier AE (ed). An Atlas of Head and Neck Surgery, 3rd ed. Philadelphia; WB Saunders, 1988, pp. 157–168.
2. Close LG. Lateral rhinotomy. In Bailey BJ (ed). Atlas of Head and Neck Surgery Otolaryngology. Philadelphia: Lippincott-Raven, 1996, pp. 22–28.
3. Mertz JS, Pearson BW, Kern EB. Lateral rhinotomy. Arch Otolaryngol 109:235, 1983.
4. Saunders WH, Miglets A. Surgical techniques for eradicating far advanced carcinoma of the orbital-ethmoid and maxillary areas. Trans Am Acad Ophthalmol Otolaryngol 71:426, 1967.
5. Maniglia AJ. Indications and techniques of midfacial degloving: A 15-year experience. Arch Otolaryngol Head Neck Surg 112:750, 1986.
6. Price JC, Holliday M, Kennedy D, et al. The versatile midfacial degloving approach. Laryngoscope 98:291, 1986.
7. Maniglia AJ, Phillips DA. Midfacial degloving for the management of nasal, sinus, and skull-base neoplasms. Otolaryngol Clin North Am 28(6):1127, 1995.
8. Nishikawa K, Nishioka S, Aoji K, et al. Skull base surgery using the degloving technique—An approach without facial scarring. J Otorhinolaryngol Soc Jpn 96(9):1447, 1993.
9. Crockett DM. Midfacial degloving procedure. In Bailey BJ (ed). Atlas of Head and Neck Surgery Otolaryngology. Philadelphia: Lippincott-Raven, 1996, pp. 882–884.
10. Janecka IP, Sen CN, Sekhar LN, et al. Facial translocation: A new approach to the cranial base. Otolaryngol Head Neck Surg 103(3):413, 1990.
11. Schuller DE, Goodman JH, Brown BL, Frank JE, Ervin-Miller KJ. Maxillary removal and reinsertion for improved access to anterior cranial base tumors. Laryngoscope 102(2):203, 1992.
12. Arriaga MA, Janecka IP. Facial translocation approach to the cranial base: The anatomic basis. Skull Base Surg 1:26, 1991.
13. Wei WI, Lam KH, Sham JS. New approach to the nasopharynx: The maxillary swing approach. Head Neck Surg 13(3):200, 1991.
14. Nuss, DW, Janecka IP. Surgery of the anterior and middle cranial base. Otolaryngol Head Neck Surg 4:3318, 1993.
15. Brown DH. The Le Fort I maxillary osteotomy approach to surgery of the skull base. J Otolaryngol 18(6):289, 1989.
16. Dailey RA, Dierks E, Wilkins J, Wobig JL. Le Fort I orbitotomy: A new approach to the inferonasal orbital apex. Ophthalmic Plast Reconstr Surg 14(1):27, 1998.
17. Crockhard HA. The transoral approach to the base of the brain and upper cervical cord. Ann R Coll Surg Engl 67:321, 1985.
18. Fang HS, Ong GB. Direct anterior approach of the upper cervical spine. J Bone Joint Surg [Am] 44:1588, 1962.
19. Jenkins HA, Canalis RF. Transpalatal approach to the skull base. In Sasaki C, McCabe B, Kirchner J (eds). Surgery of the Skull Base. Philadelphia: JB Lippincott, 1984.
20. Kennedy DW, Papel ID, Holliday M. Transpalatal approach to the skull base. Ear Nose Throat 65:125, 1986.

CHAPTER 17

Maxillectomy

In this chapter, a group of procedures ranging from medial maxillectomy to radical maxillectomy with orbital exenteration is discussed. For nearly a century, maxillectomy has been in the clinical realm of the head and neck surgeon as the principal operation to control tumors of the nose and sinuses, and it has undergone few changes during that period. Maxillectomy may be performed through either the midface degloving or lateral rhinotomy approach, as discussed in Chapter 16, or as part of a craniofacial resection, as presented in Chapter 18. In the following sections, the indications and techniques for performing maxillectomy are covered in detail.

Maxillectomy is performed for treatment of tumors of the nose and sinuses and, rarely, for management of inflammatory conditions, in particular, rhinocerebral mucormycosis. The tumor type is not as important in the choice of the particular variation of maxillectomy as is the extent of the tumor. Certain tumor types, however, are more likely to be associated with particular procedures. The best examples of this are the use of medial maxillectomy for inverted papilloma and radical maxillectomy for squamous cell carcinoma. However, before getting into the details of the surgical indications, it is important to discuss the staging of sinonasal tumors and the classification of the surgical options for maxillectomy.

STAGING

Every year, the American Joint Council for Staging Criteria (AJCC) publishes a manual for staging of head and neck cancer with updates occurring every 5 to 10 years as mandated by advancements in the knowledge of cancer. The 1997 edition of the manual includes staging for cancer of the maxillary sinus.[1] The TNM system is used, with the cancer staged according to the size and extent of the tumor (T), any spread to the lymph nodes (N), and any distant metastases (M). Table 17–1 lists the details of the system. The TNM classification is combined to yield an overall stage of cancer (Table 17–2). This staging system is intended to provide the treating physicians with a means of communicating with other physicians about the nature of a tumor, as well as to help provide general guidelines for prognosis and treatment. However, the staging system was never meant to imply a cookbook-type approach to the management of cancer at any site. This is particularly true of maxillary sinus tumors. In this site, the nature of the treatment has little to do with the actual stage of the tumor. There is very little substantive information available that would support prescribing a certain treatment for a particular stage of disease. Rather, it is necessary to evaluate each patient fully and individually as to the extent of tumor and the particular surgery or other therapy applied to treatment.

INDICATIONS FOR AND CLASSIFICATION OF PROCEDURES

There are a number of variations of the maxillectomy procedure. In the following sections, the specific indications for each of these procedures are detailed.

Medial Maxillectomy

Medial maxillectomy is an operation that involves removal of the medial wall of the maxillary sinus from the floor of the orbit to the floor of the nose. In the anteroposterior dimension, the resection may either preserve or resect the pyriform aperture, and it may extend to just anterior to the posterior attachment of the inferior turbinate or through the attachment into the pterygoid plates. The medial maxillectomy can also be extended to include the lower ethmoid sinus and lamina papyracea. The most common indication for the operation is inverted papilloma.[2–6] This operation allows complete en block resection of the tumor while preserving the orbit, alveolar ridge, and nasal facial contours. Other potential indications include any tumor, benign

TABLE 17–1
Staging of Maxillary Sinus Cancer

Tumor Stage

T1: Tumor confined to the inferior aspect of the sinus below Ohngren's line

T2: Tumor extending to the superstructure of the sinus

T3: Tumor extending into the ethmoid sinus, nasal cavity, or oral cavity

T4: Tumor extending into the orbit, skull base, or soft tissues of the face

Nodal Stage

N0: No clinically detectable metastatic lymph nodes

N1: A single metastatic lymph node less than 3 cm in greatest dimension

N2A: A single metastatic lymph node greater or equal to 3 cm but less than 6 cm in greatest dimension

N2B: Multiple metastatic lymph nodes ipsilateral to the tumor, all less than 6 cm in greatest dimension

N2C: Contralateral metastatic lymph node; all nodes less than 6 cm in greatest dimension

N3: Single metastatic lymph node 6 cm or larger in greatest dimension

Distant Metastasis

M0: No clinically evident distant metastasis

M1: Any clinically evident distant metastasis

or malignant, that is fully limited to the medial wall of the sinus and lower portion of the ethmoid sinus. Larger tumors should be approached with more radical surgery.

The reason for opting for this technique over other choices is that the procedure allows complete resection of the benign but locally aggressive inverted papilloma without sacrificing form or function. The operation can easily be performed by the midface degloving approach with preservation of the pyriform aperture. Patients usually tolerate the procedure well and heal in 3 to 4 weeks. Cure rates with this procedure have been excellent, with various authors reporting recurrence rates of 0% to 30% with the initial surgery.[3, 4, 6–8] With these qualities, the medial maxillectomy has become the standard of care for management of localized inverted papilloma.

Posterior Maxillectomy

Posterior maxillectomy involves resection of the posterior aspect of the palate and maxillary sinus, with or without portions of the soft palate. This operation is generally performed transorally and is intended for tumors involving the soft palate that extend to the junction with the hard palate or just onto the hard palate.[9] Extensive involvement of the hard palate by tumor requires a more extensive operation. The usual indication for this procedure is a squamous cell carcinoma of the oropharynx that extends up to the margin of the hard palate. To provide a negative margin to the resection of such a tumor, the posterior part of the hard palate and maxillary sinus must be removed. This is only done when the patient has a reasonable chance for local control and cure.

The patient who undergoes a combination of soft and hard palate excision for tumor will be left with a large oronasal communication. Without reconstruction or prosthetic rehabilitation, the patient will never be able to swallow. Reconstructive techniques for large palatal defects rely on pedicled myocutaneous flaps or free tissue transfer. Prosthetic rehabilitation will depend on the patient's ability to retain an obturator. Preservation of the maxillary teeth is very helpful in this situation, as is an adequate shelf of bone on the palate to help support the obturator.

Before a decision is made to proceed with surgery, the risks and benefits of the surgery must be weighed and compared with those for nonoperative therapy. For most tumors in this location, combination therapy with surgery followed by irradiation will provide superior local control, if not superior disease-free survival. The combination of chemotherapy and irradiation for squamous cell carcinoma at numerous other sites has been established as a viable alternative therapy. Demonstration of benefit for this particular subsite, however, is still pending.

Inferior Maxillectomy

Inferior maxillectomy is an operation that is designed to remove all or part of the hard palate. This procedure is indicated for tumors of the palate that have not or have only minimally penetrated the inside of the maxillary sinus.[9] Significant involvement of the mucosa of the interior of the sinus is a contraindication for this procedure. There is some flexibility on this point, however, but once the cancer penetrates the submucosa of the sinus, it tends to spread widely in this layer, making determination of margins difficult from both a clinical and pathologic perspective. For most cancers that extend through the palate into the mucosa of the sinus, a radical maxillectomy is required.

TABLE 17–2
Overall Staging of Maxillary Sinus Cancer

Stage I: T1 N0 M0

Stage II: T2 N0 M0

Stage III: T3 N0 M0; T1,2,3 N1 M0

Stage IV: Any T4, N2, M1

The most common tumor types that would be resected by an inferior maxillectomy are squamous cell carcinoma and tumors of the minor salivary glands of the palate. These include high-grade and low-grade adenocarcinoma, mucoepidermoid carcinoma, adenoid cystic carcinoma, and pleomorphic adenoma.

For the minor salivary gland tumors of the palate, surgical resection is the usual treatment of first choice. For those limited to the oral side of the palate without significant penetration into the sinus, the inferior maxillectomy would be the best procedure. For those with deeper penetration, radical maxillectomy may need to be considered. Radiation therapy and chemotherapy remain adjuvant therapies and treatments of second choice for these tumors. If the tumor is unresectable because of extension into the nasopharynx, infratemporal fossa, or cavernous sinus, several other treatments are possible. Perhaps the most promising of the these are combined neutron radiation therapy and combined radiation therapy and chemotherapy. To date, though, sufficient information is not available to document the outcome of these alternatives as equivalent to that of surgical extirpation.

The current treatment of choice for squamous cell carcinoma of the oral cavity, whether involving the palate, tongue, or floor of the mouth, remains surgical resection. Adjuvant therapy is indicated in cases in which the tumor is of an advanced stage or there has been suboptimal resection. Organ preservation approaches, with induction chemotherapy followed by radiation or combined chemoradiation, have been demonstrated to be valuable options for laryngeal, oropharyngeal, hypopharyngeal, and nasopharyngeal tumors. However, for unknown reasons, cancers of the oral cavity do not tend to respond as well. This may be attributable to difficulties with the bone of the palate and mandible interfering with the radiation beam. Another theory is that it may be difficult to eradicate tumor cells that are within the bone. Another possibility for this failure of nonoperative therapy for oral cavity carcinoma may be a true difference in the tumor biology of this site. Unfortunately, at this time, the reasons remain a mystery.

Total Maxillectomy

Total or radical maxillectomy implies the complete removal of all elements of the maxillary sinus. This procedure is classically indicated for tumors of the maxillary sinus that are confined to the interior of the sinus without spread to the pterygomaxillary fissure, orbit, or ethmoid sinus.[9–12] Involvement of the facial soft tissues does not necessarily preclude the procedure, but does require extending the procedure to include the face. Likewise, extension into the orbit is not necessarily a contraindication to resection either, but does require inclusion of orbital exenteration if the tumor has penetrated the periosteum of the orbit into the orbital fat.[13–15] Spread into the optic canal or inferior or superior orbital fissure renders the patient's tumor unresectable. Spread of the tumor into the ethmoid sinus, cribriform plate, or anterior cranial fossa does not preclude complete resection. However, these findings would mandate a craniofacial approach to achieve negative margins.[16–18] Spread of the tumor into the pterygomaxillary fissure has traditionally been a contraindication for surgery for cancer of the maxillary sinus. However, a few surgeons have been challenging this dogma by resecting some of these tumors. The results have yet to validate this approach completely. Extension into the nasopharynx, sphenoid sinus, cavernous sinus, and middle cranial fossa is considered by most surgeons to be a sign of an unresectable tumor.[19–22]

Two tissue types dominate the differential diagnosis of maxillary sinus tumors: squamous cell carcinoma and adenocarcinoma. The squamous cell tumors are the most common and have been linked to cigarette smoking and certain industrial exposures, including heavy metals.[23] Adenocarcinomas of the maxillary sinus are also prevalent and have been associated with woodworking and carpentry.[24] These tumors are high-grade cancers and tend to spread rapidly to surrounding structures. Complete surgical removal with negative margins is the clear goal of operating on these tumors. Failure to achieve negative margins is almost always associated with rapid recurrence and, ultimately, death of the patient.

For adenocarcinoma, there are little data to suggest that nonoperative therapy has a significant chance of controlling the cancer or achieving cure. However, for squamous cell carcinoma, there are some studies that suggest that these tumors may be responsive to radiation therapy, especially when given concurrently with cisplatinum chemotherapy.[25–27] Unfortunately, there is still a lack of prospective randomized data to help determine the advisability of this approach for maxillary sinus cancer. For this reason, most surgeons continue to recommend maxillectomy for resectable squamous cell carcinoma of the maxillary sinus.

Inflammatory Conditions

The final indication for maxillectomy is treatment of inflammatory disease of the sinuses, most often rhinocerebral mucormycosis.[28, 29] This infection occurs predominantly in diabetics, but is also found in patients with other forms of immunosuppression. The syndrome is caused by the fungus Mucor. This exists usually as a nonseptated branching hyphal form that has a propensity to invade and thrombose blood vessels. This leads to an ischemic necrosis of the infected tissue and rapid spread through the sinuses and face. Once the diagnosis is suspected, the patient must be taken to the operating room for urgent, radical debridement of all involved tissues. This may be a limited partial maxillectomy if discovered early, but usually, Mucor entails a radical maxillectomy and may require orbital exenteration, facial resection, or rhinectomy.

PREOPERATIVE CONSIDERATIONS

Diagnosis and Evaluation

Patients with tumors of the walls or interior of the maxillary sinus may present with a wide variety of symptoms and physical findings. Tumors of the oral cavity cause ulceration or mass lesion that become detectable on routine intraoral inspection. Intranasal tumors usually lead to nasal obstruction, anosmia, or epistaxis and are observable by intranasal examination as unilateral nasal masses. Maxillary sinus tumors present later in most cases because the early tumors cause minimal or no symptoms. Early tumors of the interior of the maxillary sinus are almost always discovered during evaluation for inflammatory sinus disease. A computed tomography (CT) scan of the sinuses usually reveals a possible tumor recognized by the presence of bone erosion and tissue infiltration. More advanced tumors may present as a nasal mass or in association with epistaxis, headache, anosmia, and facial anesthesia from involvement of the infraorbital nerve.

Often, tumors of the nose and sinuses present initially as either otitis media with effusion or occasionally as an isolated neck mass. Middle ear effusion may develop because of direct involvement of the tumor with the eustachian tube or because of secondary sinusitis that leads to eustachian tube dysfunction. Metastatic disease of the cervical lymph nodes from cancer of the maxillary sinus is uncommon. Other intranasal tumors, such as nasopharyngeal carcinoma or esthesioneuroblastoma, are more likely to cause such metastasis. The primary tumor types, such as adenocarcinoma and squamous cell carcinoma of the maxillary sinus, can result in neck metastases, but usually do not until the tumor is far advanced or recurrent.

When a tumor of the nose or sinuses is suspected, it is important to obtain adequate imaging studies to delineate the extent of the tumor precisely. A CT scan of the sinuses, with direct axial and coronal cuts with bone windows, is essential to visualize the bony landmarks. In most cases, a magnetic resonance imaging (MRI) study of the sinuses is also performed. This not only aids in understanding the size and scope of the tumor but also allows detection of perineural spread into the skull base and central nervous system. Angiography may be useful in certain cases, especially for vascular tumors and those characterized by intracranial involvement. For routine cases, however, angiography provides little added benefit.

Finally, it is important to assess the patient for the possibility of distant metastasis. Although this is an uncommon finding in the original presentation of nasal and sinus tumors, it is imperative that metastases be diagnosed before treatment. The usual evaluation includes posteroanterior and lateral chest x-ray studies, a calcium level, and liver function tests. In patients with large or multiple neck metastases, a CT scan of the chest is warranted to confirm that the chest is clear before proceeding with treatment.

Once the imaging studies are completed, it is necessary to perform a biopsy of the tumor to establish a diagnosis. In almost all circumstances, this is possible using the transnasal route. If a nasal mass is present, this can be accomplished in the office using either traditional anterior rhinoscopy or nasal endoscopy. In the office setting, a small cup forceps biopsy sample is taken and sent for laboratory analysis. Larger biopsy samples should be avoided in this setting owing to the risk of bleeding. Minimal biopsy in the office can be performed prior to imaging studies if the examination clearly demonstrates the mass not to be an encephalocele or other lesion with direct intracranial connections. Usually, tumors will be irregular and polypoid, whereas encephaloceles will be smooth and firm.

In many cases, intraoffice biopsy will not be adequate. This may be due to the presence of a large polyp in front of the tumor, preventing easy access, or it may be because the tumor is not accessible in the nose. For example, biopsy of an intrasinus maxillary sinus cancer cannot be performed in the office using intranasal endoscopy. However, it is almost always possible to obtain the biopsy through the nose using endoscopic techniques, rather than a Caldwell-Luc approach. This has the advantage of not violating the tissue planes of the face prior to definitive resection.

Medical Evaluation

All maxillectomy procedures have the potential for periods of rapid blood loss. Once the bony cuts are started, bleeding is uncontrolled until the tumor specimen is removed. Additionally, either the internal maxillary artery or several of its major tributaries may be transected in the final stages of the resection. This can result in significant hemorrhage. Because of this fact, all patients need to be properly evaluated medically for this possibility. To prepare for this possibility, all patients should undergo a careful preoperative assessment by an internist, cardiologist, and anesthesiologist who are aware of the nature of the surgery. For patients with a significant cardiac history, an echocardiogram and a stress test should be considered.

A second medical concern is the long duration of some of these procedures. Although many can be completed in 3 to 4 hours, the more complicated surgeries may last up to 8 to 10 hours. For this reason, the pulmonary status of patients is also important to consider. After a long anesthesia, a patient with borderline pulmonary function may end up on long-term mechanical ventilation. Chest x-ray studies and pulmonary function tests are warranted in patients with a history of lung disease.

As a final consideration, all patients should be assessed for difficulties with bleeding and coagulation. Any possibility of coagulopathy should be investigated thoroughly. All patients should also undergo a routine complete blood count and have a blood sample sent to the blood bank for type and screen before surgery.

Intraoperative Monitoring

Patients undergoing maxillectomy should be considered candidates for maximal intraoperative monitoring during surgery. To begin with, large-bore intravenous catheters are necessary to allow rapid infusion of crystalloid or blood products should this become necessary. A central venous catheter for monitoring is necessary if the patient has a history of cardiac problems that may be associated with unusual atrial or ventricular filling pressures. For patients with marginal ability to undergo the procedure, a Swan-Ganz catheter for monitoring of left heart filling pressures and cardiac output can be very useful. An arterial catheter for monitoring of blood pressure and rapid sampling of the blood is also very useful in patients with significant medical history.

Other monitoring devices for prolonged surgery are now considered routine for all of these cases. These would include a pulse oximeter, temperature probe, and urinary bladder catheter.

TECHNIQUE

Approach

Chapter 16 presented the details of various approaches for maxillectomy. Maxillectomy can be performed through either the midface degloving or a lateral rhinotomy approach. The decision to use one or the other option is based on the experience and training of the surgeon and the extent of the tumor. The author uses the midface degloving approach for almost all maxillectomy procedures. The exposure is more than adequate and results in an improved cosmetic outcome owing to the absence of a large facial scar. The difficulty with this approach is in the final removal of the tumor and dissection of the pterygomaxillary fissure. Without the lateral exposure afforded by the open approach, the surgeon must rely on feel and experience which, for most, is not an impediment. Even when the surgery includes orbital exenteration, the midface degloving approach can still be used. However, the advantage of avoiding the facial incision is all but lost on a patient undergoing orbital exenteration. In this setting, the lateral rhinotomy approach is favored.

Medial Maxillectomy

Once the exposure of the anterior wall of the maxilla is completed, resection can begin. The first step is to remove the anterior wall of the maxillary sinus. An opening is made in the anterior wall using a 4-mm osteotome. Over the area of the canine fossa, a 1 × 1 cm window is created. A Kerrison's rongeur is used to complete removal of the anterior wall to the fullest extent possible. Attention should be paid to the infraorbital nerve which, in most cases of medial maxillectomy, can be preserved. After completion of this step, a wide exposure of the medial wall is gained (Fig. 17–1).

In some cases, the interior of the sinus will be filled with mucus; in others, it will be filled with edematous mucosa or tumor. If the mucosa is normal, it can be preserved. However, if there are any abnormalities, it is best to remove the mucosa at this step to be certain that there is no tumor involvement. This is accomplished by carefully elevating the mucosa from the bone with a Freer elevator. The mucosa is lifted from lateral to medial in an attempt to keep the mucosa attached to the

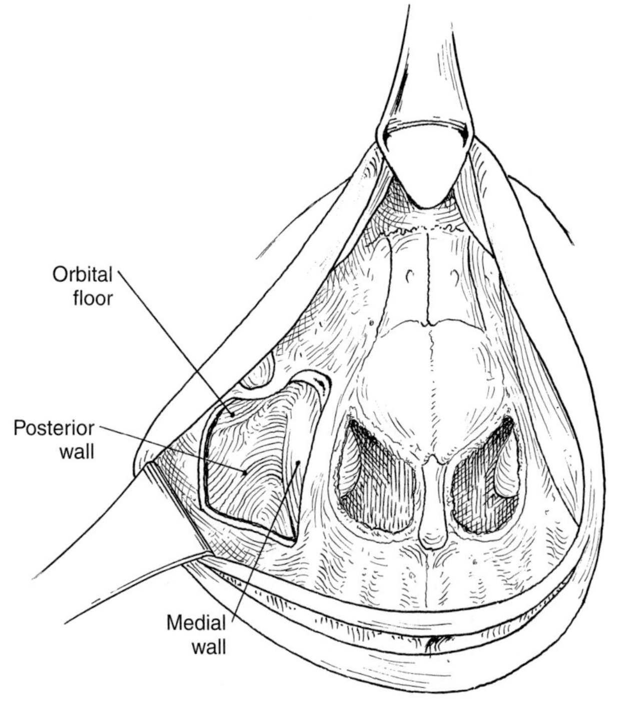

Figure 17–1. Midfacial degloving approach for medial maxillectomy. A wide anterior antrostomy exposes the inside of the maxillary sinus. The infraorbital nerve is preserved.

medial maxillary resection. If this is not possible, the contents of the sinus can be removed in a piecemeal fashion. At the completion of this step, all mucosal remnants from the areas of concern should be completely cleaned from the sinus. If necessary, a drill can be utilized to ensure complete removal.

Before beginning the bone cuts, it is advisable to inspect the wound for hemostasis. Soft tissue and bone bleeding points should be controlled. It is worth spending a few minutes at this time to avoid confusing the situation later, when the blood loss can become heavier. Also, it is worthwhile to warn the anesthesiologist at this point that the blood loss will begin to increase as the bone cuts are made. Once the initial bone cuts are made, the bleeding cannot be controlled until the tumor specimen is removed. Therefore, it is important to be prepared to move quickly and definitively to complete the resection once initiated.

For the purposes of this discussion, it will be assumed that the ethmoid sinus is not involved and will not need to be included in the resection. In this case, the first cut will be the anterior attachment of the medial wall. For most tumors, the pyriform aperture can be preserved as the tumor is almost never involved with this area. This does lead to restriction of the exposure, but the end cosmetic result is superior, so every attempt should be made to achieve preservation. Removal of the pyriform aperture will result in the nose retracting laterally to the side of the surgery. The degree of retraction depends on the size of the gap between the nasal bone and the alveolar ridge; large gaps result in increasingly severe retraction. If the pyriform aperture is to be resected, then there is no anterior cut to be made. Instead, the inferior and superior cuts are simply initiated at the pyriform aperture rather than inside the sinus.

When the pyriform aperture is preserved, the anterior cut is made just posterior to the pyriform aperture using a curved, 1-cm osteotome (Fig. 17–2). This cut will extend through the mucosa on the sinus side and the bone, but usually will not cut the vestibular skin on the nasal side. A cautery or knife can be used to cut through the anterior aspect of the inferior turbinate and vestibular skin to complete the anterior cut.

The second cut is made along the inferior edge of the medial wall using the same 1-cm, curved osteotome (Fig. 17–3). This cut is made just at the junction of the medial wall and the floor of the sinus, roughly equivalent to the junction of the floor of the nose and the lateral wall of the nose. The bone and mucosa are easily cut with the osteotome back to the level of the posterior wall of the sinus. At the posterior wall, the bone becomes very thick where the lateral and posterior walls join to the pterygoid plates. The mucosa along the floor of the nose may dissect away from the bone as the osteotome passes from anterior to posterior. If this occurs, it is simple enough to complete the mucosal cut with scissors or a knife.

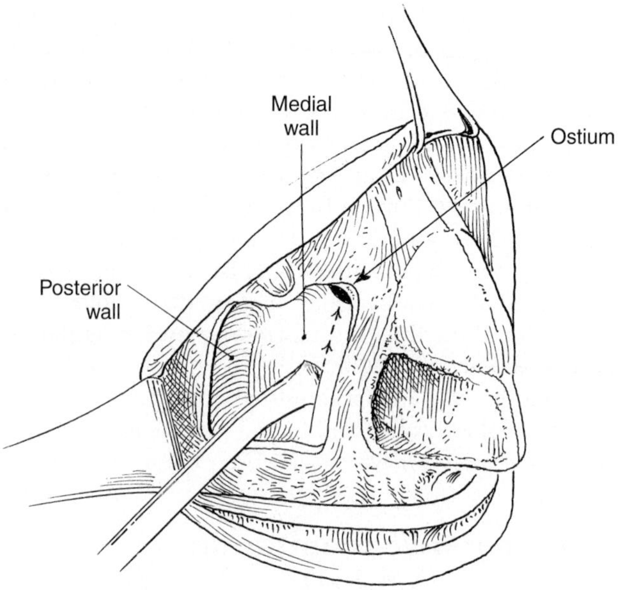

Figure 17–2. Medial maxillectomy in which the pyriform aperture is preserved. The first bone cut is made just inside the pyriform aperture from inferior to superior. The cut extends anterior to the sinus ostium and the nasolacrimal duct.

The superior cut is completed next. When the ethmoid is not involved, this cut is simply made at the junction of the medial wall and the roof of the sinus. The osteotome is angled, curve down, and driven through the superior attachment (Fig. 17–4). At the posterior end of this cut, the posterior fontanelle will be encountered. This is best cut with angled turbinate scissors. In making this cut, care should be taken to avoid cutting into the tumor and to avoid entering the orbit. The osteotome must be kept at just the proper angle to keep this cut in the correct plane. It is during this cut that the nasolacrimal duct will be transected. Normally, this is done with the scissors after the osteotome sections the bone. If a clean cut is made, it is not necessary to place a lacrimal stent to avoid stenosis and epiphora.

The final cut is through the junction of the medial wall with the posterior wall of the sinus. As long as tumor is not present is this area, the cut can be made just on the inside of the sinus anterior to the posterior attachment of the inferior turbinate. If there is tumor in the area, it is best to resect the junction of the posterior and medial wall by angling the osteotome through the posterior wall (Fig. 17–5). This will remove the posterior attachment of the inferior turbinate and will cross the medial pterygoid plate and the pterygomaxillary fissure, usually disrupting branches of the internal maxillary artery. The final muscular and mucosal attachments are then divided with scissors.

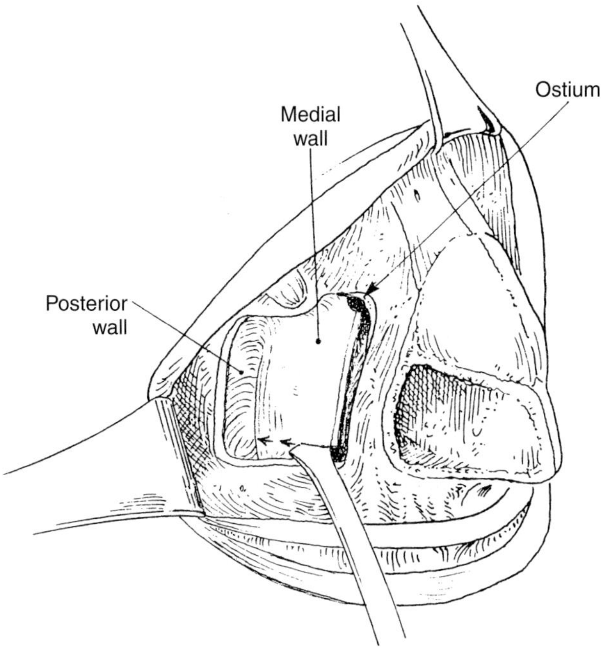

Figure 17–3. Medial maxillectomy. The second bone cut is along the floor of the nose from anterior to posterior. This cut stops short of the posterior wall and the attachments of the pterygoid plates.

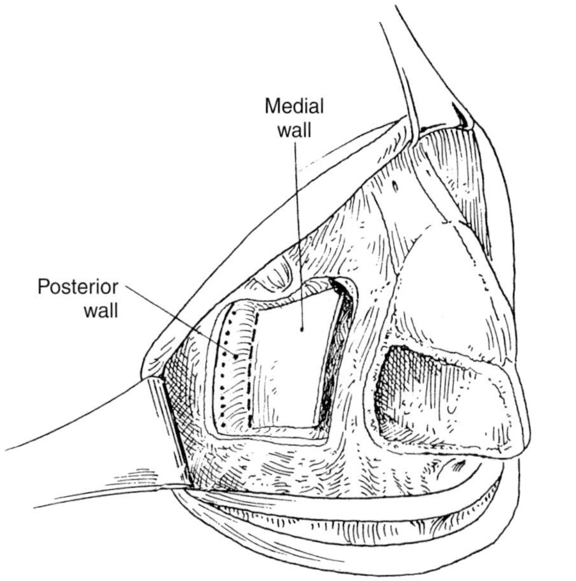

Figure 17–5. Medial maxillectomy. The fourth bone cut may be anterior or posterior to the junction of the medial and posterior walls. If the cut is anterior to the junction, it will cross the posterior aspect of the inferior turbinate. If the cut is posterior to the junction, it will enter the pterygomaxillary fissure. To complete the resection, the posterior cut must be connected to the superior and inferior cuts. This will require cutting across the attachment of the pterygoid plates and will transect the sphenopalatine artery and nerve.

Once the tumor is removed, a sponge should be placed into the cavity to create pressure and arrest any bleeding. A few minutes of pressure will help to minimize the bleeding by allowing the smaller vessels to thrombose. This "time out" is also important to allow the anesthesiologist to catch up with the blood loss and stabilize the patient. In most cases, the patient will not have lost more than a few hundred milliliters of blood. However, it is worthwhile to allow a few minutes at this point to assess the patient and to permit the surgeon's nerves to settle down. After this period of time, the branches of the internal maxillary artery should be identified, clamped, and ligated. This requires good lighting with a headlight and a well-functioning suction to evacuate the blood and reveal the bleeding vessels. Usually, it is possible to identify the vessel precisely, place a clamp, and ligate the vessel with a silk suture (Fig. 17–6). Other, smaller vessels can be controlled with a bayonet-type bipolar electrocautery forceps. Any resistant bleeders from the pterygoid muscles can be controlled using a prothrombotic material, such as oxidized cellulose (Surgicel, Johnson & Johnson, Arlington, TX) or microfibrillar collagen (Avitene, Davol, Inc., Boston, MA).

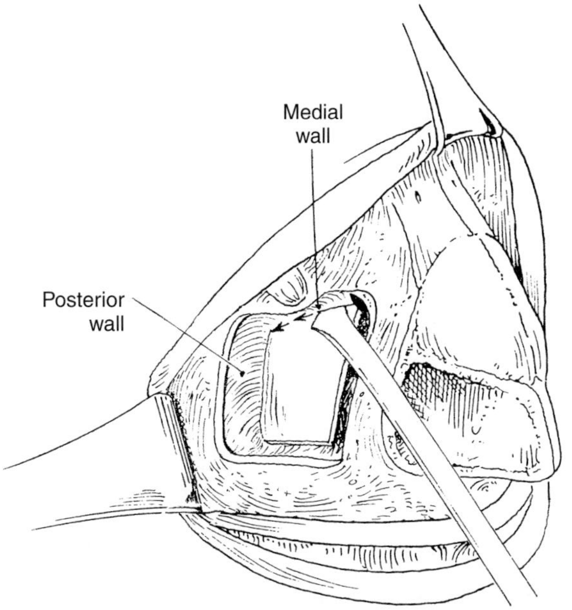

Figure 17–4. Medial maxillectomy. The third bone cut is along the superior aspect of the medial wall of the sinus. This extends from the superior end of the first cut, across the nasolacrimal duct, through the sinus ostium, to the posterior wall of the sinus. This cut should hug the floor of the orbit.

Medial Maxillectomy with Ethmoidectomy

When the tumor extends into the ethmoid sinus, middle turbinate, or lamina papyracea, it is necessary to extend the resection to include these structures. This is usually still possible through the midface degloving approach, without creating additional incisions. The proviso is that

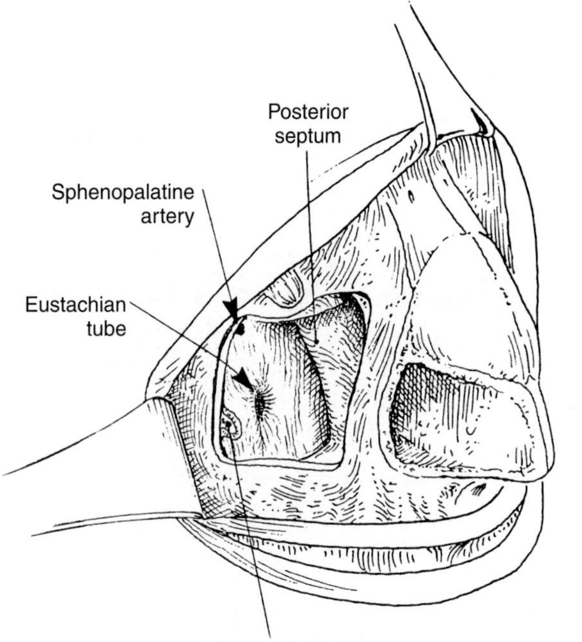

Figure 17–6. Medial maxillectomy. The appearance of the cavity after resection anterior to the posterior wall. The stump of the inferior turbinate is seen inferiorly, and a branch of the sphenopalatine artery is transected superiorly.

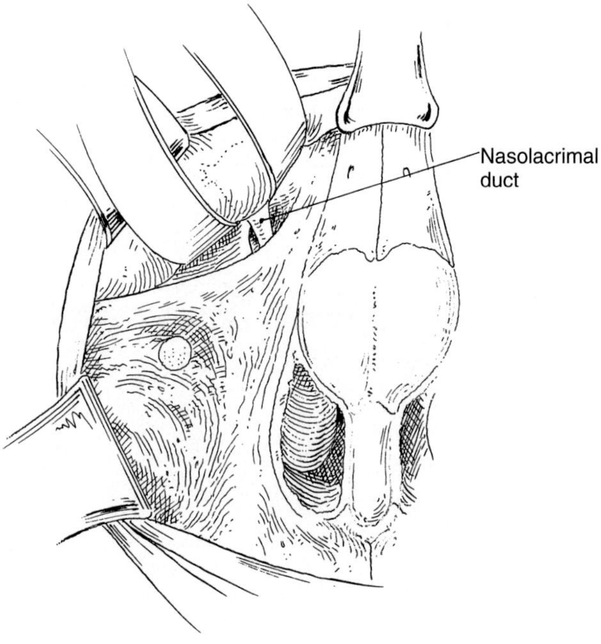

Figure 17–7. Extended medial maxillectomy. When including the ethmoid sinus in the resection, the nasolacrimal duct is divided on the orbital side of the floor of the orbit. This allows wide exposure of the medial and inferior walls of the orbit.

the inferior orbital nerve on the ipsilateral side should be sacrificed to allow adequate superior retraction of the lip to visualize the medial orbital structures. Conversely, if the tumor extends to the roof of the ethmoid, cribriform plate, or into the orbit, a standard medial maxillectomy is not possible and alternative strategies should be considered.

With transection of the inferior orbital nerve, it is usually possible to gain exposure to the level of the nasion and the nasofrontal and frontoethmoidal suture lines. The initial steps in the procedure are the same as described earlier. The sinus is entered and the inside cleaned out. Before starting the bone cuts, the medial orbital dissection is performed. A Freer elevator and a malleable for retraction are used to expose the medial orbital wall from the frontoethmoidal suture line superiorly to the lacrimal fossa inferiorly. The anterior and posterior ethmoid arteries should be cauterized and divided. The nasolacrimal duct is transected just as it exits the lacrimal fossa (Fig. 17–7). This allows the dissection to transition onto the floor of the orbit.

At this point, it is time to begin the bone cuts. The anterior and inferior cuts are made identically, as described earlier for standard medial maxillectomy. The next cut is made inside the medial orbital rim from the frontoethmoidal suture superiorly to the floor of the orbit inferiorly (Fig. 17–8). This cut can be made using either a curved osteotome or a microsagittal saw. The exact location of the cut in terms of its anterior-to-

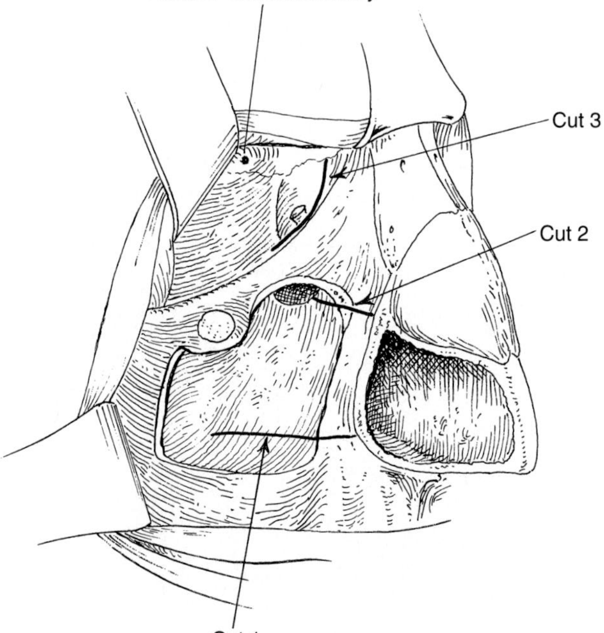

Figure 17–8. Extended medial maxillectomy. This procedure includes resection of the pyriform aperture. The first cut is through the pyriform aperture and the inferior attachment of the medial wall along the floor of the nose. The second cut is through the pyriform aperture posteriorly to the orbital floor. This cut should be above the ostium of the sinus. The third cut is from the frontomaxillary suture line superiorly to the floor of the orbit just anterior to the anterior lacrimal crest.

posterior dimension is determined by the individual tumor. It is not usually necessary to resect the orbital rim itself. More superiorly, the cut should be made just at the junction of the lamina papyracea and the frontal process of the maxilla. The cut extends inferiorly through the lacrimal bone to the floor of the orbit and into the maxillary sinus just posterior to the inferior orbital rim. This bone cut has to pass through thick bone to enter the nose anterior to the middle turbinate attachment and nasolacrimal duct.

The next cut is made along the superior edge of the lamina papyracea just inferior to the frontoethmoidal suture line, the ethmoidal arteries, and the skull base (Fig. 17–9). This cut is best made with the osteotome to maintain control and feel as the ethmoid is transected. The cut moves from anterior to posterior, one osteotome-width at a time, with each cut passing through the ethmoid and middle turbinate into the nasal cavity. The landmark for identifying the posterior end of the cut is the posterior ethmoid artery. Tumor extending posterior to this point should not be resected by this technique.

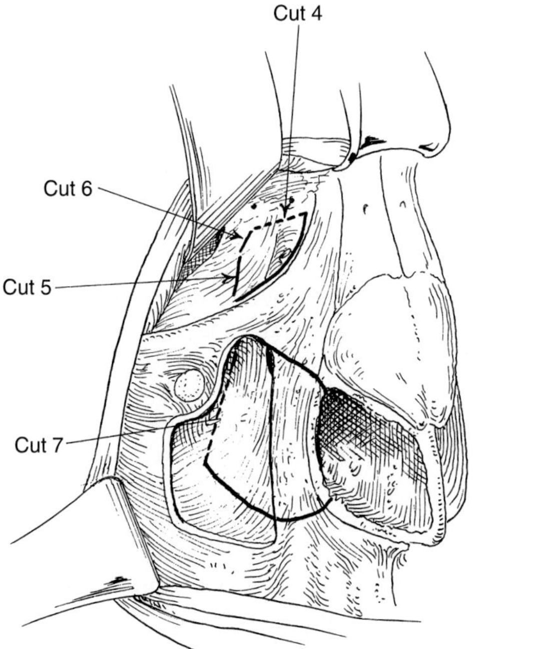

Figure 17–9. Extended medial maxillectomy. Completion of the bone cuts. The fourth cut is parallel to the frontoethmoidal suture line and just inferior to it. The fifth cut is from anterior to posterior along the floor of the orbit. This cut stops posteriorly at the level of the posterior wall of the maxillary sinus and posterior ethmoidal artery. The sixth cut connects the previous two orbital cuts posteriorly. This should free up the ethmoid sinus. The seventh and final cut crosses along the posterior wall of the maxillary sinus, as illustrated in Figure 17–5. This should be the final cut, allowing delivery of the specimen.

The inferior cut is then made. Beginning at a point just inside the inferior orbital rim, the orbital floor is cut with the osteotome from anterior to posterior to the level of the posterior ethmoidal artery (see Fig. 17–9). This bone is thin and will cut easily. When making this cut, it is important to protect the eye with a malleable. As this cut is made, the osteotome will enter the maxillary sinus connecting the ethmoid specimen to the medial wall of the maxillary sinus. The inferior orbital fissure is located posteriorly and laterally. The cut should not need to extend past this point.

Perhaps the most difficult cut in this procedure is the posterior ethmoidal cut. This must join the posterior ends of the superior and inferior cuts just described (see Fig. 17–9). This is accomplished by retracting the orbit laterally with a malleable and using a curved osteotome pointed medially. Ideally, the cut should extend through the full thickness of the ethmoid in a lateral to medial direction. In practice, this may be difficult. As long as the orbital bone is thoroughly cut, the last ethmoid attachments should break free easily when the specimen is delivered.

The last cut is made, once again, at the junction of the medial wall of the maxillary sinus and the posterior wall of the sinus (see Fig. 17–9). This cut is made, as described earlier for the standard medial maxillectomy, either anterior to the posterior wall or through the posterior wall. At this point, only mucosal attachments and the residual soft tissue attachment of the pterygomaxillary fissure remain. The specimen is rocked back and forth and delivered out through the nose. It is possible that the entire specimen will not be able to be delivered in one piece. If this occurs, it is only important that the final cavity reflect the complete resection intended.

After the resection, there will be a tendency for the orbit to prolapse into the ethmoid sinus. In most cases, as long as the periorbita has been preserved intact, the eye will maintain a satisfactory position. However, in some cases, reconstruction may be required to prevent enophthalmos and diplopia. The preferred technique is to use split calvarial bone grafts. Harvested as described in Chapter 11, the grafts can be trimmed to the size and thickness desired and placed into the defect to hold the orbit into position. As long as a good purchase is achieved, the grafts will not need to be wired or plated in position but will be held in place by pressure from the surrounding tissues. As an alternative, an alloplastic material can be used to reconstruct the orbit. In addition to orbital position, lacrimal function must also be considered. When the lacrimal sac is transected, as in this procedure, it is probably best to place a lacrimal stent to prevent stenosis. Crawford lacrimal tubes are preferred and may be easily placed through the upper and lower lid puncta, through the lacrimal sac, and into the nose to be tied off inside the nose.

Closure

The details of the closure of the midface degloving and lateral rhinotomy incisions are covered in Chapter 16. Before the closure is started, the cavity should be packed. Vaseline-coated strip gauze is one of the options. The gauze comes in prepackaged tubes containing 6 feet of ½-inch gauze impregnated with Vaseline (Sherwood Medical, St. Louis, MO). The packing material is layered in from back to front in the ethmoid sinus and from back to front and lateral to medial in the maxillary sinus. Normally, more than 6 feet of packing material is required. In this case, the strip gauze can be tied together to lengthen the pack. Often, as many as three or four full tubes are required to fill the cavity. One advantage of this technique is that the knots are easily recognized during removal, which helps to distinguish the amount of packing removed and the amount remaining.

After packing is complete, the incisions are closed as previously described. The external nose is dressed with adhesive strips over the skin and a nasal splint is placed to help keep the skin tightly applied to the underlying nasal bones.

Endoscopic Medial Maxillectomy

For small, inverted papillomas located on the medial wall of the maxillary sinus, endoscopic medial maxillectomy is an option.[30–34] This is a continuing controversy, but until long-term follow-up studies are available, it will remain a secondary option. The procedure, however, is attractive in principle, as it avoids any incisions and can be performed on an outpatient basis.

The procedure is performed under general anesthesia using the topical and local anesthesia described in detail in Chapter 8. Visualization is achieved with the 0-degree, 4-mm endoscope. The tumor is identified along the lateral wall of the nose, the middle turbinate is in-fractured, and the uncinate process is identified. The superior portion of the uncinate process is removed using back-biting forceps to expose the natural ostium of the maxillary sinus. At this point, if the tumor is found to involve the roof of the maxillary sinus or posterior wall of the maxillary sinus, or if it extends into the ethmoid sinus, the procedure should be aborted. In these situations, the tumor is not resectable endoscopically and an open approach is indicated. However, if the tumor is limited to the medial wall, complete endoscopic resection is possible.

To proceed, curved endoscopic scissors are used to incise the medial wall of the maxillary sinus from anterior to posterior, beginning from the natural ostium and extending through the posterior fontanelle. This cut needs to extend to the level of the posterior wall of the maxillary sinus. The next cut must extend inferiorly through the inferior turbinate into the inferior meatus. This is either accomplished using curved scissors or a down-biting forceps. When the turbinate is transected, brisk bleeding may occur. In this case, suction cautery can be used to stop the bleeding. Following this, the back-biter is used to cut from posterior to anterior through the inferior meatus. This cut should stop just at the level of the nasolacrimal duct. The resection should remain posterior to the nasolacrimal duct to avoid problems with epiphora. The final cut extends from superior to inferior through the anterior aspect of the inferior turbinate just posterior to the nasolacrimal duct. The specimen is then removed. Frozen sections can be taken from the surrounding mucosa to verify complete resection.

Posterior Maxillectomy

As described here, posterior maxillectomy is typically performed for squamous cell carcinoma of the oral pharynx involving the soft palate–hard palate junction. As such, it includes resection of the posterior aspect of the hard palate and part of the posterior wall of the maxillary sinus. This is performed using transoral exposure without need for either the midface degloving or lateral rhinotomy. The mouth is held open either with an oral gag, such as a McIvor, a bite block, or a self-retaining retractor, such as a Moltz.

Depending on the details of the individual tumor, it may be preferable to perform the posterior maxillectomy either at the beginning or end of the resection. In either case, it is possible and desirable to keep the palate pedicled to the remainder of the specimen. This helps maintain orientation of the resection specimen, which will assist in evaluating the resection margins. If the lesion is limited to the central part of the palate, it may be possible to preserve part of the soft palate. In most cases, the soft palate will be removed in its entirety during the resection. If part of the soft palate is to be preserved, it is advisable to make the posterior soft palate cuts first. These are made through the full thickness of the soft palate using a knife or electrocautery.

The hard palate is incised anterior to the discernible tumor, allowing at least a 2-cm margin of normal mucosa (Fig. 17–10). The mucosa can be cut with the cautery through the submucosal layers and periosteum to the bone. This incision is carried laterally across the alveolar ridge up to the gingival buccal line. The mucosa is then incised posteriorly from this point to the retromolar trigone and back onto the pharyngeal mucosa. The mucosa anterior to the incision is elevated for about 1 cm onto the anterior palatal bone. This will later be used to fold over the bone stump to help create a strong tissue layer to support the palatal obturator.

The bone is cut using a microsagittal oscillating saw. The bone cut is placed about 1 cm anterior to the

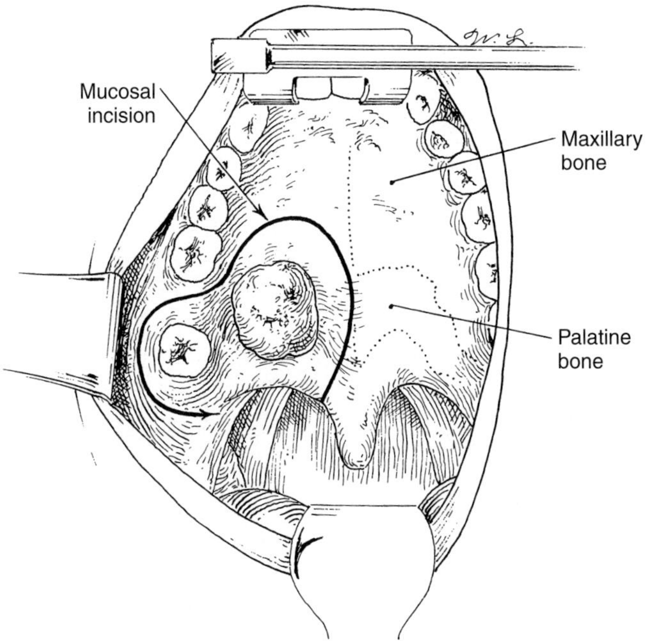

Figure 17–10. Posterior maxillectomy. Mucosal incisions around a palatal cancer include the posterior aspect of the alveolar ridge. Maintaining a 2-cm margin around the tumor is indicated.

mucosal cut through the hard palate into the maxillary sinus and nose. The cut is then directed posteriorly to the soft palate–hard palate junction (Fig. 17–11). If complete bilateral posterior maxillectomy is required, this bone cut can extend straight across the hard palate to the alveolar ridge on the opposite side. Laterally, the cut extends across the alveolar ridge. If the patient is fully dentulous, the tooth in the line of the cut is removed. It is better to sacrifice a tooth and cut through the socket than to attempt to cut between two teeth. In the gingival buccal sulcus, the bone cut is directed posteriorly in a horizontal plane (Fig. 17–12).

At this point, the specimen should be free of attachments except where the posterior wall attaches to the pterygoid plates and pterygomaxillary fissure. The anterior edge of the specimen is displaced inferiorly, opening up the inside of the maxillary sinus. The back of the sinus can then be visualized. A cut through the pterygoid plates and surrounding tissues will free up the specimen. Significant bleeding from branches of

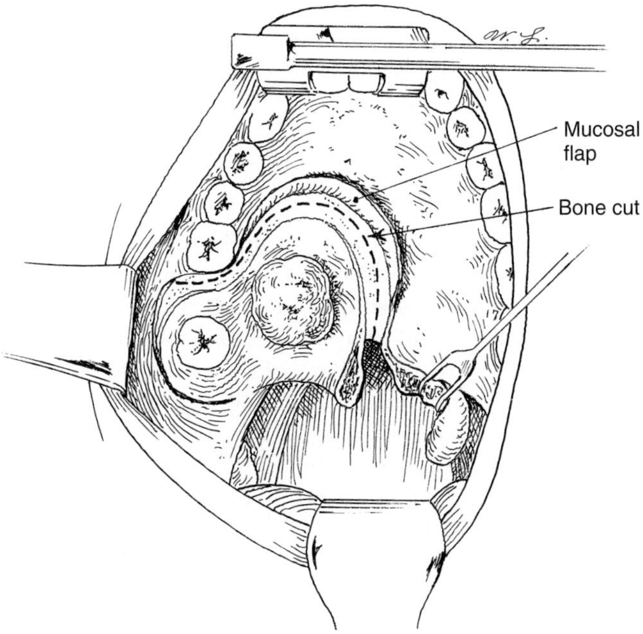

Figure 17–11. Posterior maxillectomy. The mucosa on the hard palate is elevated as a flap. The bone cut is indicated by the dashed line.

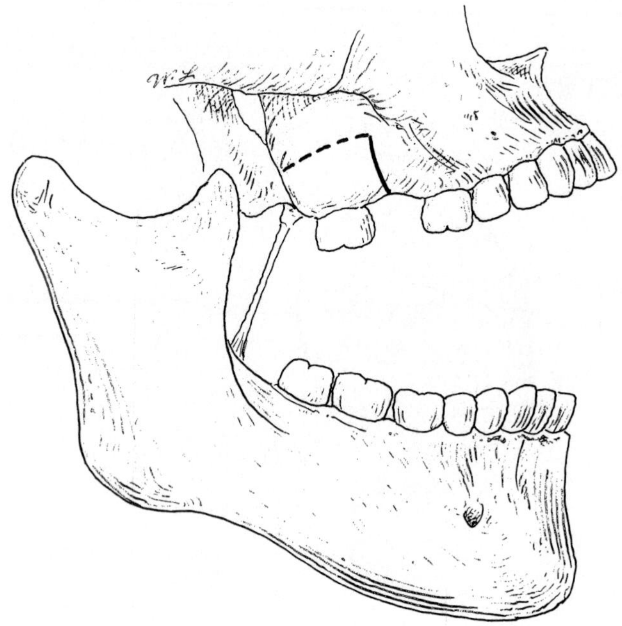

Figure 17–12. Posterior maxillectomy. Anatomic illustration of the lateral bone cuts in posterior maxillectomy performed for palatal cancer. The solid line indicates the first cut made on the palatal side. The dashed line indicates the second cut made on the gingival side.

the internal maxillary artery and vein and from the pterygoid plexus is expected at this point. A sponge should immediately be placed into the wound to tamponade the bleeding, allowing the remainder of the resection to be performed.

After the specimen is removed, there is usually sufficient room through the mouth to identify and control the major bleeding vessels. A good headlight and adequate suction are needed to make this step as easy as possible. The vessels should be identified and clamped and ligated with 3-0 silk suture. Smaller residual bleeders can usually be controlled with bipolar cautery, pressure, or prothrombogenic material.

Inferior Maxillectomy

Inferior maxillectomy can be a unilateral or bilateral procedure and can cross the maxilla at almost any level. In most cases, it is used for tumors of the hard palate, and therefore, the inferior maxillectomy usually crosses just above the level of the floor of the sinus. The operation can be performed through either the lateral rhinotomy or midface degloving approach. Because the exposure does not need to extend to the orbital rim, this procedure is almost always done through the midface degloving approach. If the tumor extends into the sinus and involves the mucosa of the interior of the sinus, the inferior maxillectomy is probably not the correct procedure.

The unilateral procedure is described here. After the initial exposure of the anterior maxilla, the sinus is entered through an anterior antrostomy, as described for the Caldwell-Luc operation. The opening in the anterior wall should be made sufficiently large to allow visualization of the entire interior of the sinus so that the surgeon can confirm that the sinus is free of tumor. The mucosal cuts on the palate are then made. The soft palate need be resected only if it is involved by tumor. As with most oncologic surgery, a generous 2-cm mucosal margin around the suspected border of the tumor is marked and then incised. When the tumor is confined to one side, the mucosal margin is generally at or just beyond the midline. The cuts through the soft palate can be made with cautery and incised completely through the full thickness of the palate (Fig. 17–13). The palatal soft tissue cut is extended around the retromolar trigone to join the gingival buccal incision.

The bone cuts are performed next. If possible, all or part of the alveolar ridge may be preserved. The exact cut made should be adequate to remove the tumor completely and to allow a safe margin. For some tumors, all palatal bone cuts may made be within the palatal arch, thereby preserving the entire alveolar arch and occlusal surface. In the case of a hemipalatectomy, the anterior cut will cross the alveolar ridge in the midline. This cut will extend posteriorly to the hard palate–soft palate junction, extending through the full thickness into the floor of the nose just to one side of the septum or the other. In other cases, a more limited resection

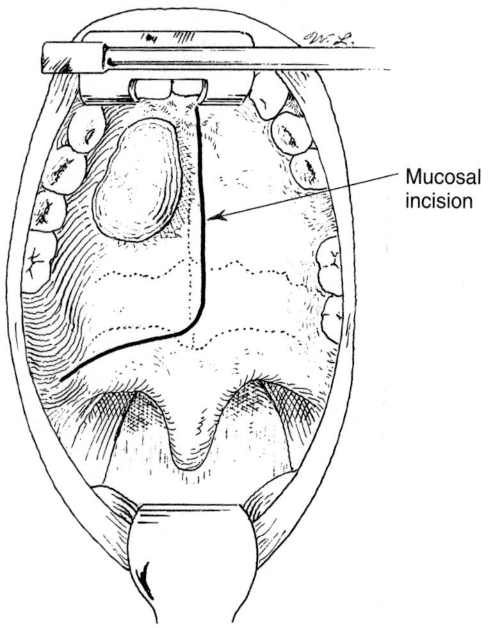

Figure 17–13. Inferior maxillectomy. Mucosal incision for inferior maxillectomy or hemipalatectomy. The incision allows at least 2-cm margins around the lesion but preserves the uninvolved soft palate.

is required, and the cut may curve around the tumor to cross the alveolar ridge a second time more posteriorly.

Once the palatal cuts are complete, the anterior wall cut is made. This will extend from the farthest lateral position on the contralateral side across to the posterior cut through the alveolar ridge on the ipsilateral side. In the case of a hemipalatectomy, the anterior wall cut will extend to the posterior edge of the alveolar ridge (Fig. 17–14). Anteriorly, the cut may cross into the pyriform aperture, extend across the septum, or through the contralateral pyriform aperture into the maxillary sinus to include the contralateral nasal floor and medial maxillary wall.

The vertical structures that hold the palate in place must then be divided. These may include the medial wall of the maxilla on the ipsilateral side, the septum, and the medial wall of the maxilla on the contralateral side, depending on where the palatal bone cut is located. These cuts can be made using a knife to incise the mucosa and an osteotome to cut the bone. Once this step is completed, the only attachments of the palate will be to the posterior wall.

To complete the resection, the palate is pushed down anteriorly to increase exposure of the posterior wall. The level of the cut through the posterior wall will again be determined by the exact location of the tumor. In most cases, the cut can be made just above the junction of the floor and the posterior wall. The mucosa is incised and the posterior wall cut with the osteotome. Medially, the pterygoid plates will attach and need to be cut with the osteotome; directly behind the posterior wall are the structures of the pterygomaxillary fissure. These contents are either divided or bluntly dissected from the posterior aspect of the specimen.

After delivery of the specimen, hemostasis is achieved. Bleeding from branches of the internal maxillary artery is controlled by clamping and ligation. Smaller vessels usually can be controlled using bipolar cautery. Diffuse bleeding from the pterygoid muscles can be stopped with a prothrombotic material or direct monopolar cautery at high levels of current. Bone edges that are bleeding are controlled with bone wax.

Total Maxillectomy

Total or radical maxillectomy is performed through either the midface degloving or the lateral rhinotomy approach. The midface degloving technique provides the better cosmetic result, but the lateral rhinotomy provides the better exposure. The operation represented here is the standard unilateral total maxillectomy. However, it can be modified to include as much of the adjoining structures as required.

Because this operation is most often performed for squamous cell carcinoma of the maxillary sinus, extension of the procedure beyond the standard procedure should be carefully considered in terms of oncologic soundness. Some of the more common extensions are to include the skin of the anterior face, the ethmoid sinus, the orbit, and the contralateral nasal cavity or maxillary sinus. If the ethmoid is involved with the cancer, the margin through the ethmoid needs to be one cell layer above the highest extent of the tumor. If the tumor goes into the upper cells, against the cribriform plate or against the skull base, a craniofacial resection is indicated. If the tumor erodes the orbital bone but the periorbita is clear, the orbital wall and periorbita are resected as the margin. However, if the tumor extends

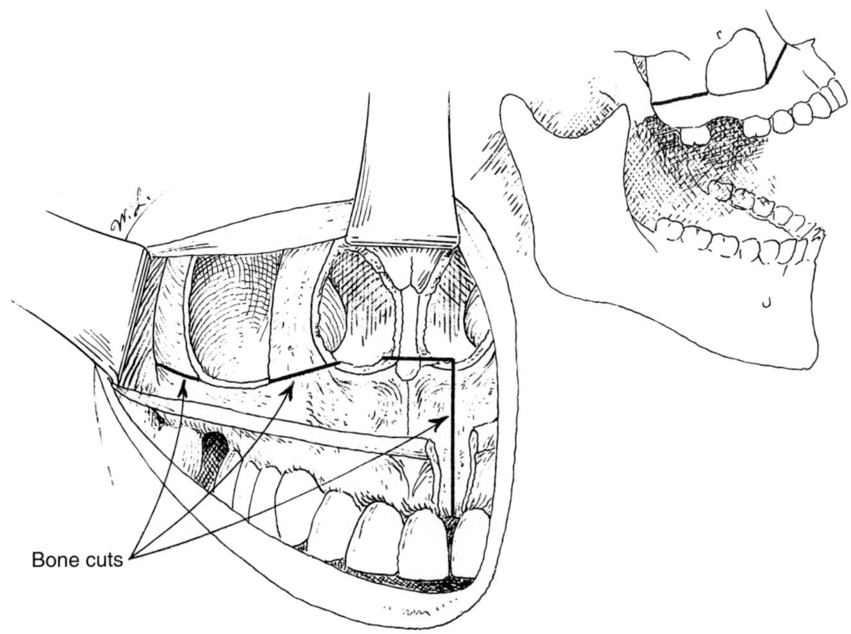

Figure 17–14. Inferior maxillectomy. The anterior bone cuts, as seen through a midfacial degloving approach. A large anterior antrostomy has been performed to check the interior of the sinus for tumor involvement before committing to the partial maxillectomy. The cuts extend through the alveolar ridge into the floor of the nose on the contralateral side, across the septum, and posteriorly to the posterior margin of the alveolar ridge. The inset demonstrates the lateral cuts anatomically.

through the periorbita into the fat of the orbit, an orbital exenteration is needed. Similarly, if the septum is involved, the resection must extend to the contralateral nasal cavity, but if the tumor involves the contralateral nasal cavity, the medial wall of the maxillary sinus on the opposite side must be sacrificed.

The first step in the procedure is the incision and exposure, which was described in detail in Chapter 16. The infraorbital nerve can be sacrificed immediately in this procedure, which will improve the exposure. The mucosal incision above the alveolar ridge in the labial mucosa is extended posteriorly to the back of the alveolar ridge and down across the retromolar trigone onto the soft palate (Fig. 17–15). This incision is extended into the palatal incisions. If it is not necessary to sacrifice the soft palate for oncologic reasons, it is best to preserve the soft palate by extending the incision across the palate at the soft palate hard–palate junction. This incision can be made with cautery to improve hemostasis, as there will not be a mucosal closure performed. The incision is carried full thickness through the soft palate to the nasopharyngeal lumen.

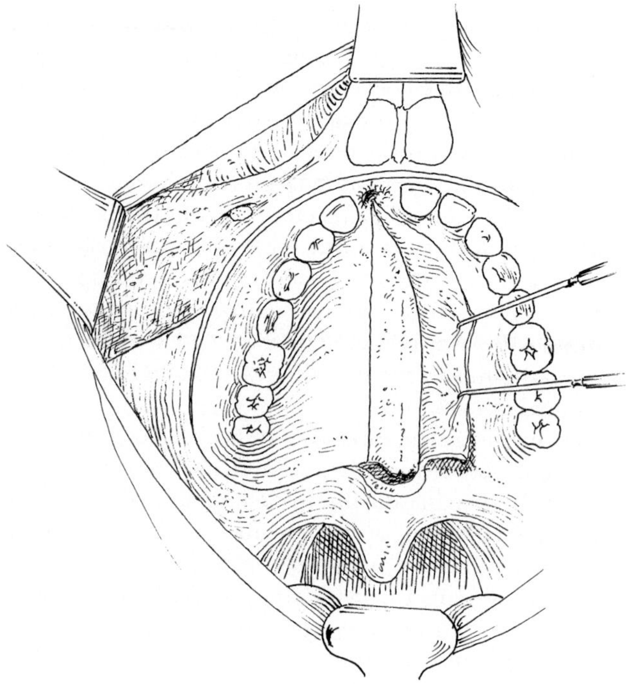

Figure 17–16. Total maxillectomy. A mucosal flap is elevated from the hard palate to widely expose the bone of the palate. This flap will be used to fold over the palatal bone edge.

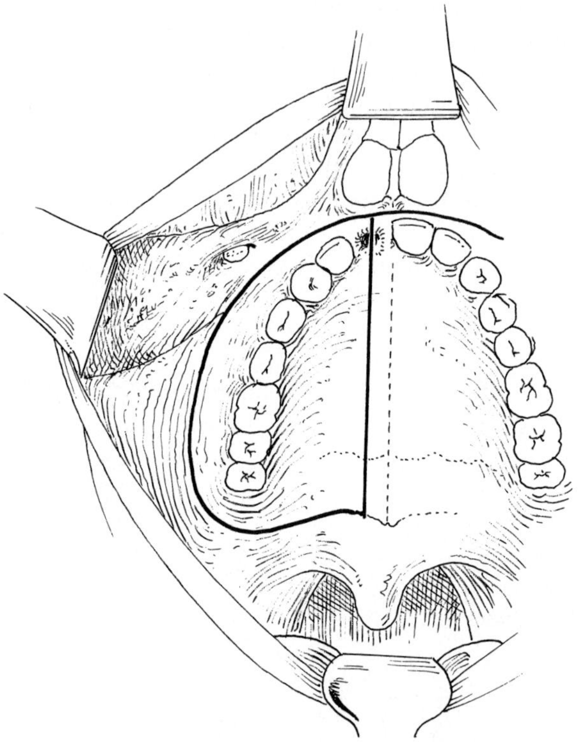

Figure 17–15. Total maxillectomy. The solid lines illustrate the mucosal incisions using the midfacial degloving approach. Anteriorly, the incision crosses through the socket of the medial incisor, which is extracted before the incision. The incision extends posteriorly on the ipsilateral side of midline to the hard palate–soft palate junction. The incision turns laterally at the hard palate–soft palate junction and crosses the retromolar trigone to join up to the gingival buccal incision of the midfacial degloving.

The mucosal incision in the hard palate is then made. In most cases of maxillary sinus cancer, the hard palate mucosa is not involved with tumor, which means that the mucosa can be largely preserved. This proves useful during reconstruction as it covers over the bone ledge of the palate to help support and cushion a prosthesis.

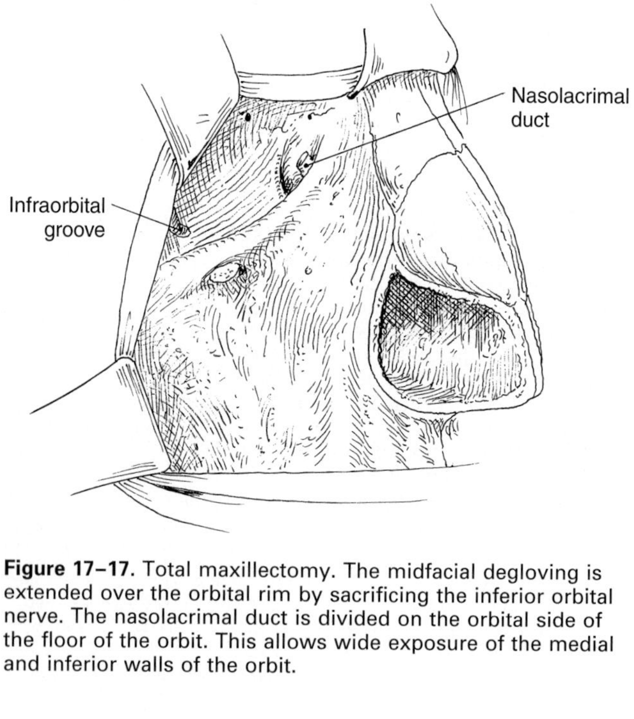

Figure 17–17. Total maxillectomy. The midfacial degloving is extended over the orbital rim by sacrificing the inferior orbital nerve. The nasolacrimal duct is divided on the orbital side of the floor of the orbit. This allows wide exposure of the medial and inferior walls of the orbit.

The incision is made about 1 to 2 cm ipsilateral to the midline using cautery directly down to the bone. The mucosa is then elevated across the midline as a flap to expose the bone of the hard palate (Fig. 17–16).

The next step is to dissect the periorbita from the floor of the orbit. Using a Freer elevator and a malleable for retraction, the plane is developed back to the inferior orbital fissure. Medially, the elevation of the orbit will cross the nasolacrimal duct. This should be divided sharply and the elevation extended onto the lamina papyracea and posteriorly back to the posterior ethmoid artery (Fig. 17–17).

At this point, the surgeon is ready to make the bone cuts. The surgeon must be prepared to move quickly from this point on, because once the first bone cut is made, the bleeding will not be controlled until the specimen is delivered. It is worthwhile to advise the anesthesiologist that the bleeding will begin to get heavier at this time and that upward of 500 mL of blood may be lost in the next 30 to 60 minutes. Adequate suction should be available, with both Frazier- and Yankauer-type tips available. Also, a large sponge or laparotomy pad should be available to place into the wound once the specimen is removed. One strategy is to soak the sponge in hydrogen peroxide. When the specimen is finally removed, the peroxide-soaked sponge can be quickly packed into the cavity. The peroxide clogs the capillaries and small vessels and helps minimize the bleeding from the resection bed.

The first cut is usually on the palate. This extends anteriorly through the alveolar ridge into the floor of the nose and posteriorly to the hard palate–soft palate junction. The best place to make this cut is through the socket of the central incisor on the tumor side (Fig. 17–18). A microsagittal oscillating saw is preferred to an osteotome. The saw is then used to cut from anterior to posterior through the hard palate into the floor of the nose (Fig. 17–19). An alternative technique is to use a Gigli saw. The cutting wire is passed through the nose and brought out the mouth. With one end through the nose and the other through the mouth, the wire is rocked back and forth under pressure. This will force the wire to cut through the bone of the floor of nose reliably in the correct line.

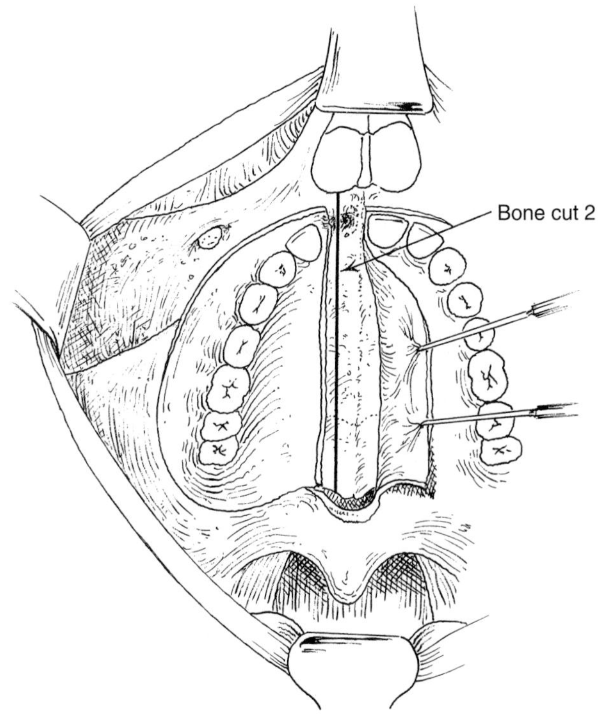

Figure 17–19. Total maxillectomy. The second bone cut is made from the alveolar ridge posteriorly to the end of the hard palate. This should extend into the floor of the nose.

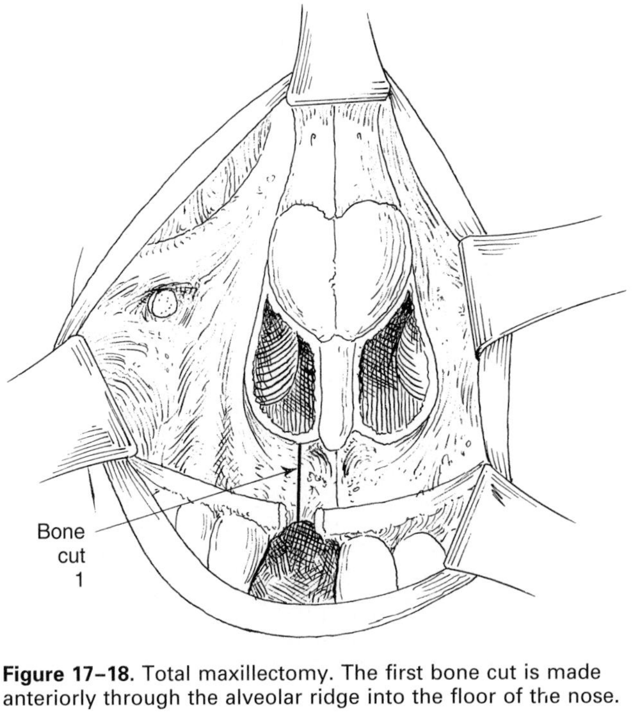

Figure 17–18. Total maxillectomy. The first bone cut is made anteriorly through the alveolar ridge into the floor of the nose.

The next cut is from the upper corner of the pyriform aperture across the medial buttress of the maxilla and across the infraorbital rim (Fig. 17–20). This cut is best made with the oscillating saw, but can also be made with an osteotome. When making this cut, the eye should be protected with a malleable retractor. With this same exposure, the cut is extended posteriorly from the orbital rim inside the orbit at the junction of the lamina papyracea and the floor of the orbit (Fig. 17–21). This cut is difficult to make with the oscillating saw and so is normally made with the osteotome. The cut should extend through the lateral wall of the nose just inferior to the ethmoid sinus and just above the medial wall of the maxillary sinus. The posterior extent of this cut is just past the posterior wall of the maxillary sinus. With

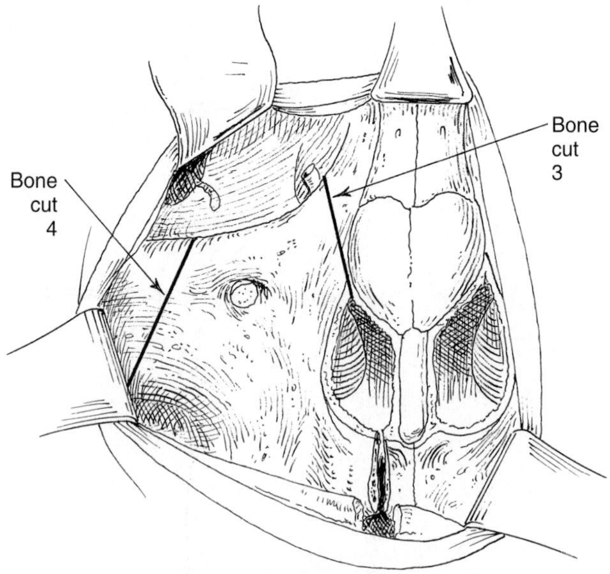

Figure 17–20. Total maxillectomy. The third bone cut extends from the pyriform aperture across the orbital rim superior to the lacrimal duct. The fourth bone cut crosses the malar eminence and orbital rim inferior to the zygomatic arch. The orbit is protected using a malleable retractor.

the osteotome directed through the orbit, the cut can be visualized through the nose to verify when the posterior extent has been achieved.

Next, attention is turned laterally to the malar eminence. At this point, the lateral buttress is cut. This cut should be made inferior to the zygomatic arch, but outside the maxillary sinus (see Fig. 17–20). The sagittal saw is the preferred instrument for this cut. The eye should again be protected with a malleable retractor. After the malar eminence is divided, the cut should be extended posteriorly along the floor of the orbit to the inferior orbital fissure (see Fig. 17–21). This is best achieved using an osteotome with the eye retracted to see the floor of the orbit. The osteotome is then angled medially to connect the two orbital floor cuts across the back of the orbit (see Fig. 17–21).

Once this last cut has been performed, the only remaining attachments are against the posterior wall of the sinus. This critical aspect of the maxillectomy is performed by feel and experience. Heavy curved Mayo scissors are used to feel around the back of the sinus and cut the attachments, which include branches of the internal maxillary artery and the pterygoid plates. It is not typically possible to view this directly. To perform this step, the maxilla, which at this point is mostly free, is grasped in one hand, while with the other hand, the scissors are reached blindly around the back of the sinus to make the cut (Fig. 17–22). With constant retraction by the noncutting hand pulling on the specimen, the attachments will be stretched, making them easier to cut. This will deliver the specimen.

With the specimen removed, a peroxide-soaked sponge is quickly packed into the wound and pressure applied. It is important to allow a few minutes at this time for the packing to control some of the bleeding and for the anesthesiologist to catch up on the blood loss. This is a worthwhile pause that helps to settle the patient, surgeon, and assistants. Although the heavy blood loss during this procedure is often disconcerting to inexperienced surgeons, the actual blood loss is rarely more than 500 to 1000 mL, which in most adult patients is not enough to require transfusion. The key to minimizing the blood loss in this surgery is to make sure that all soft tissue surgery is done with minimal blood loss, that all soft tissue bleeding is controlled before the bone cuts are started, and that the surgeon works quickly. The bleeding from the bone cuts is not avoidable or controllable until the specimen is removed. Therefore, the longer the time of resection from the first bone cut to the end, the greater the blood loss.

Hemostasis is achieved by clamping and ligation of the branches of the internal maxillary artery and vein. Smaller vessels can be controlled with bipolar or monopolar cautery. Mucosal bleeding is controlled in the end with the cavity packing. As a last resort, bleeding within the pterygoid muscles can be controlled with a prothrombotic material, such as Avitene (Davol, Boston, MA) or Surgicel (Johnson & Johnson, Arlington, TX).

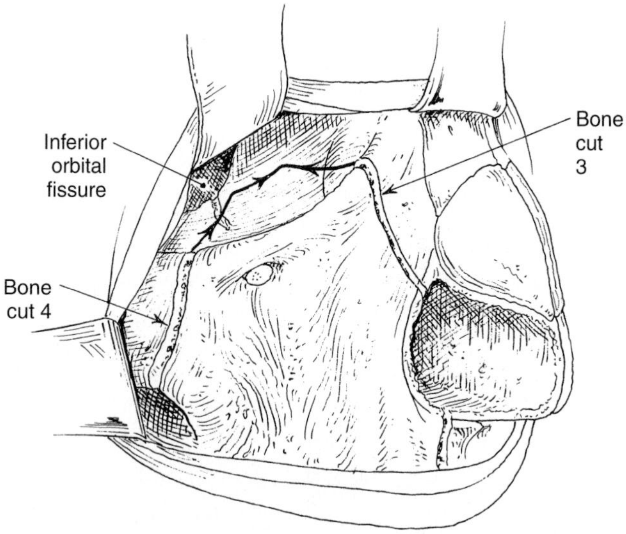

Figure 17–21. Total maxillectomy. The orbital floor cuts. The orbit is elevated with a wide malleable retractor. The medial cut extends through the lacrimal fossa posteriorly through the lamina papyracea just above the maxillary ethmoid suture. The posterior limit is the level of the posterior wall of the maxillary sinus. The lateral cut extends from the orbital rim posteriorly to the infraorbital fissure. The posterior ends of the two cuts are connected posterior to the level of the posterior wall of the maxillary sinus.

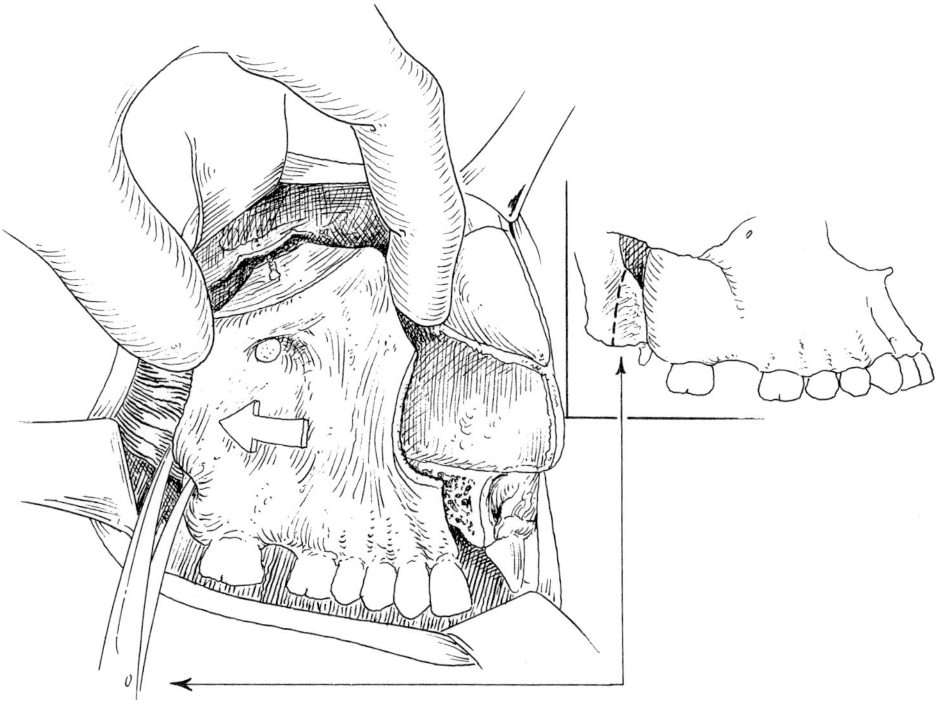

Figure 17–22. Total maxillectomy. Final delivery of the specimen. The pterygoid muscle attachments are divided and the pterygoid plates are cut with either an osteotome or heavy Mayo scissors. This step is facilitated by grasping the maxilla with one hand and rocking it forward while the scissor cuts are made with the other hand.

Total Maxillectomy with Orbital Exenteration

The primary indication for this variation of the standard total maxillectomy is an otherwise resectable maxillary sinus cancer that extends into the orbit and involves the orbital fat or extraocular muscles. The most important consideration is that the tumor must be clearly resectable in other areas. The rather significant step of exenterating an orbit should only be undertaken in the context of a potentially curable cancer. The decision to exenterate the orbital contents is made based on confirmed extension of the tumor into the orbit. If the tumor is up against the bone of the orbit without erosion, the bone will serve as the margin and the periosteum can be preserved. If the bone is eroded, it is assumed that the periosteum is involved but can be sacrificed as the margin. A biopsy of the orbital fat is then performed to confirm that there is no direct involvement of the orbital contents. However, if the tumor extends into the soft tissues of the orbit, exenteration is required.

Usually it is possible on imaging studies to determine the level of orbital involvement. Both CT scanning and MRI contribute to this differentiation. The CT scan evaluates the presence of bone erosion, whereas MRI can detect soft tissue involvement of the orbit. In rare instances in which the findings are equivocal, a careful exploratory dissection is performed. If bone erosion is equivocal, the dissection is carried out between the orbit and the periosteum. A biopsy specimen of the periosteum is taken from the suspicious area to assess the involvement, and a frozen section diagnosis is attempted. If the biopsy study yields negative results, the periosteum is preserved; if it is positive, the periosteum is resected. When the involvement of the orbital fat is equivocal, the dissection is carried out in the plane between the fat and the periosteum. A biopsy specimen of the fat is taken to assess the tumor extent. A negative biopsy result implies that the orbit is preserved with the periosteum as the margin; a positive fat biopsy confirms that the orbit must be exenterated.

In most cases of orbital exenteration, the skin of the eyelids can be preserved but the adnexal structures, including the conjunctiva and lacrimal apparatus, are resected. To accomplish this, the incision is designed to encircle the adnexal structures just outside the lash line of the eyelids (Fig. 17–23). This incision is usually performed before the maxillectomy to prepare the orbit for resection before the bone cuts are started. The incisions are made and carried down through the orbicularis muscle layer. A submuscular dissection is performed to the orbital rims superiorly and inferiorly on the surface of the orbital septum. The eyelid skin and muscle become a flap that is later used to help in the reconstruction by lining the orbital cavity (Fig. 17–24).

Once the orbital rims are reached, the periosteum is incised circumferentially around the orbit down to the bone. The orbital contents are dissected from the orbital walls medially, superiorly, and laterally, preserving the attachments of the orbital contents to the floor.

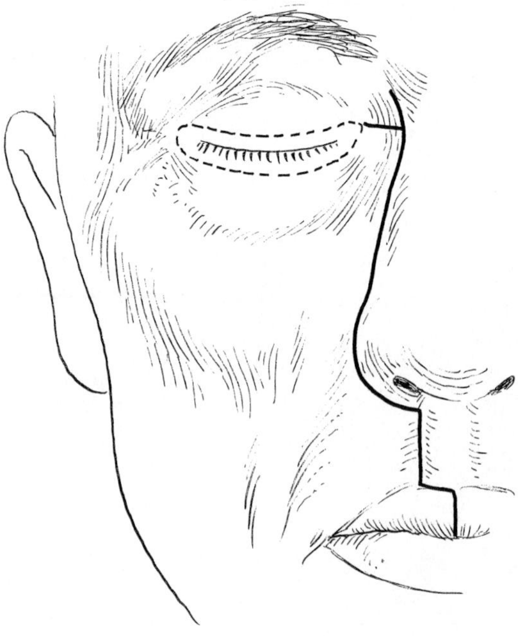

Figure 17–23. Total maxillectomy with orbital exenteration. Extended Weber-Fergusson incision. The incision encircles the margins of the eyelids.

This is done to avoid violating the tumor by attempting to dissect through the plane where the tumor penetrates the orbital floor. During the medial dissection, the anterior and posterior ethmoid arteries must be identified and ligated and the lacrimal sac elevated from the fossa. The lacrimal sac is left pedicled to the nasolacrimal duct, which can be completely included in the resection. When elevating the superior periosteum, the supraorbital nerve and vessels must be identified and ligated and the trochlea transected. Laterally, on the superior wall, the lacrimal gland must be elevated. As the dissection proceeds, the globe is mobilized but remains firmly attached by structures in the optic canal and superior and inferior orbital fissures.

The optic canal is best reached from a superior and medial approach. It can be found 5 to 10 mm posterior to the posterior ethmoid artery. With wide exposure both superiorly and medially, the eye is compressed under a malleable retractor to visualize the optic nerve (Fig. 17–25). The nerve is then clamped with a long curved hemostat, such as a tonsil clamp, and then transected with a scalpel. The stump of the nerve is tied off with a 2-0 silk suture. With this accomplished, the eye will roll forward. The dissection can then proceed in the subperiosteal plane to the superior orbital fissure. The contents of the fissure are clamped, divided, and ligated. The final step is to divide the contents of the inferior orbital fissure. This is best accomplished from the lateral side. When this is completed, the orbital dissection is finished and the eye should be pedicled only on the floor of the orbit.

The maxillectomy then proceeds as described earlier, including the soft tissue cuts on the soft and hard palate

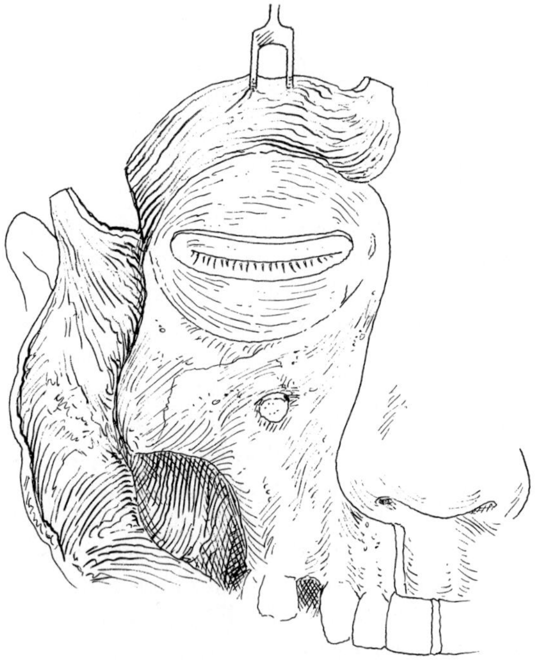

Figure 17–24. Total maxillectomy with orbital exenteration. Completed exposure. The skin flaps are dissected over the orbits on the surface of the orbital septum. At the inferior orbital rim, the periosteum is incised to connect the eyelid skin to the remainder of the flap, which is dissected in the subperiosteal plane.

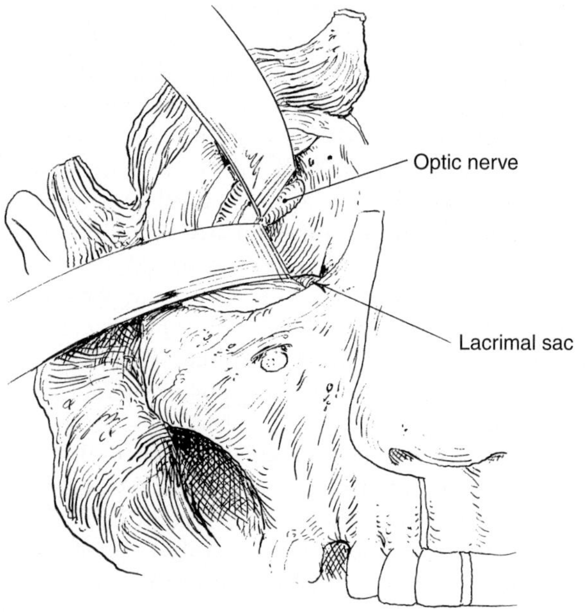

Figure 17–25. Total maxillectomy with orbital exenteration. The orbit is dissected from the superior, medial, and lateral walls of the orbit. The lacrimal duct and inferior wall are left intact to be included in the en bloc resection. The optic nerve is exposed by lateral and inferior retraction of the orbit.

and the anterior and palatal bone cuts. In making the bone cut from the nose to the orbit, the line should be superior to the nasolacrimal duct. The anterior to posterior cut on the medial floor of the orbit must be kept superior to the floor to avoid inadvertent entry into the sinus or tumor. The lateral cut through the malar eminence is the same as previously described. The anterior to posterior cut on the lateral wall of the orbit is also accomplished as before. When the time comes to cut the bone of the posterior orbit, this is done from above, pushing the orbit forward and down. Once this is accomplished, the final attachments are along the posterior wall of the sinus. This is handled identically to that described for radical maxillectomy. The tumor is then delivered with the orbital contents attached to the roof of the sinus. Hemostasis is achieved as described in the previous section.

Closure

After resection is completed and hemostasis is ensured, the maxillectomy cavity is prepared for reconstruction by proper closure. The first step is to smooth out the edges of all bony surfaces. This can be done with a bone rongeur or a drill with a diamond or cutting burr. One of the critical areas to address is the medial surface of the residual hard palate. Too sharp an edge here will create problems with the bone cutting through the overlying mucosa when the prosthesis is applied. Ideally, mucosa from the hard palate was preserved during the procedure as a flap that can be folded over the rounded bone edge and sutured to the mucosa of the floor of the nose or sinus. A raw edge that is left uncovered will eventually heal, but will leave a fragile, thin mucosa to support the prosthesis.

The area of the pterygoid muscles and posterior wall of the cavity usually presents a large raw soft tissue surface. This is customarily covered with a split-thickness skin graft from the leg. The skin graft is usually cut at 15 thousandths of an inch and left as an intact sheet and not expanded or pie-crusted. The graft is sutured to the edges of the grafted area and plicated to the underlying muscle to avoid slippage or shearing.

One of the most critical aspects of closure and reconstruction after maxillectomy is resuspension of the orbit. If the floor of the orbit is resected, the eye will tend to prolapse into the defect, resulting in enophthalmos and diplopia. To prevent this, the eye must be resuspended into the preoperative position. This can be done in one of several ways. The simplest way is to use a skin, dermal, or fascial graft sutured across the floor. This should be anchored posteriorly to the bone of the orbit by drilling small holes through the bone to hold the sutures. Medially, the graft is sutured to the medial orbital wall and laterally to the inferior edge of the lateral orbital wall. Alternatively, bone grafts can be placed. Split calvarial grafts serve best in this situation. The graft is fixed to the medial and lateral orbital walls and lies against the undersurface of the eye. The final option is to use a temporalis muscle flap. This is elevated from the temporal fossa and turned over the zygomatic arch, tunneled under the eye, and fixed to the medial orbital wall (Fig. 17–26).

After the grafts are in place and the orbit is suspended, a large pack is placed over the graft to fill the cavity from the level of the palate superiorly to the orbit and skin graft. This pack must apply enough pressure to achieve hemostasis and push the graft up against the underlying muscle. The preferred pack is a large cotton wad soaked in mineral oil and then wrapped with an iodine-impregnated sheet gauze (Xeroform, Sherwood Medical, St. Louis, MO). The pack is pushed up into place and then held in place with either retention sutures or an immediate palatal obturator. The latter is the preferred option as it allows the patient to begin oral alimentation early in the postoperative course.

If orbital exenteration has been performed, the orbital cavity must also be prepared. Ideally, the upper eyelid skin will have been preserved and can be draped back over the superior rim to help line the orbital roof. The inferior eyelid skin is folded back onto the undersurface of the face to partially cover the exposed soft tissue there. The remainder of the orbital bone and cavity should be covered with a skin graft and then filled with a conforming pack.

The final closure will depend on the technique used for the approach. The details of closing both the midface degloving incisions and the lateral rhinotomy incisions are covered in detail in Chapter 16.

Reconstruction

Reconstruction of the postmaxillectomy defect can be achieved in one of two ways: vascularized free tissue transfer or prosthetics. For patients undergoing standard unilateral maxillectomy without orbital exenteration, prosthetic reconstruction provides improved functional, cosmetic, and rehabilitative outcomes. This statement is predicated on the ability of the maxillofacial prosthodontist to fit and stabilize the appliance properly. The ideal surgical candidate will have a full set of properly maintained and restored dentition on the contralateral side. The greater the number of stabile teeth to anchor the prosthesis against, the better the retention will be. The edentulous maxilla poses special challenges for prosthetic rehabilitation. In this case, not only does the prosthesis need to replace the resected teeth, but it must also replace the contralateral teeth, all without clasps. The likelihood of a successful outcome in this situation is significantly diminished.

In addition to the dentition, the preparation of the cavity during closure of the surgical procedure will have

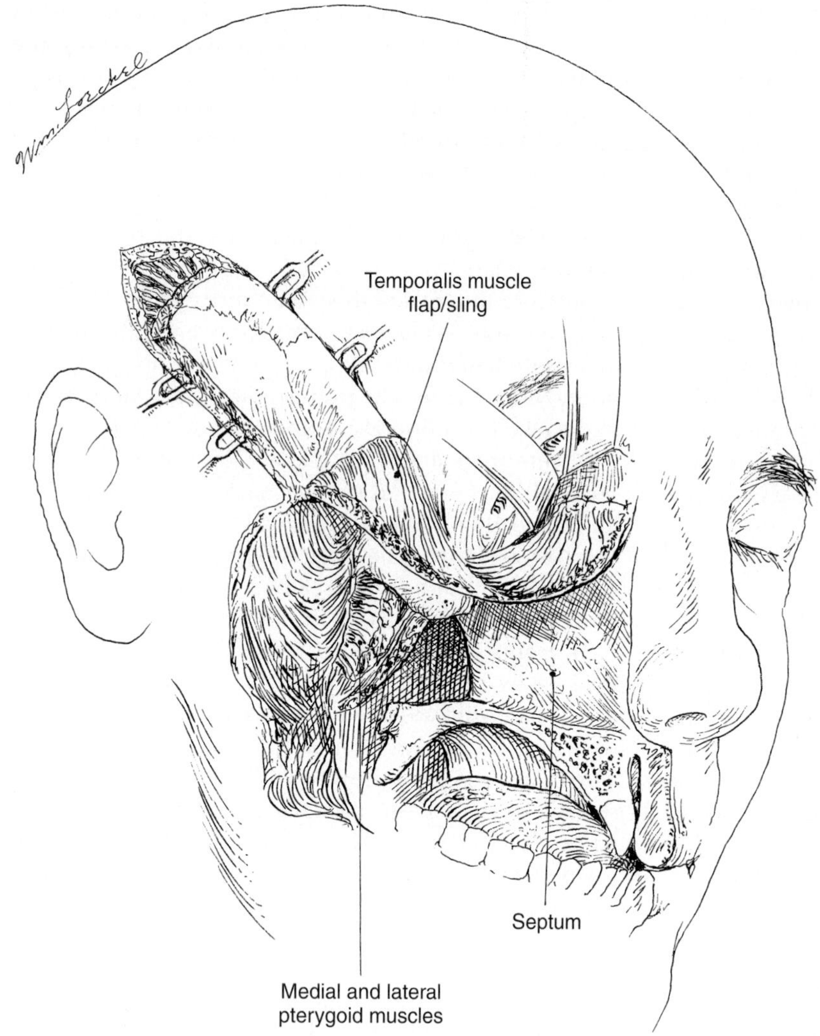

Figure 17–26. Temporalis flap. After total maxillectomy with orbital preservation, the orbit is suspended by a pedicled temporalis myofascial flap. The flap is folded over the zygomatic arch and sutured to the medial orbital wall. Drill holes through the lamina papyracea provide anchor points to suspend the flap.

a major impact on the quality of the rehabilitation. Proper rounding of the bone edges and coverage of the cavity with skin grafts will significantly aid in prosthetic fitting and retention. In the best situation, a stabile flat shelf is created medially and a circular scar band forms on the lateral surface at the edge of the buccal mucosa where it adjoins the skin graft. These points provide a foothold upon which to rest the prosthesis. Most prosthodontists consider preservation of the soft palate to be helpful also. A healthy soft palate is a third tissue shelf on which to rest the obturator.

The process of creating a quality maxillectomy appliance begins before the surgery with the creation of both upper and lower impressions. These allow the prosthodontist to have input into the selection of marginal teeth for preservation or extraction. The preoperative impression also allows for the fabrication of a temporary palatal prosthesis. This can be created with clasps to fix to remaining teeth and holes to permit placement of screws through the appliance into the residual hard palate. This temporary obturator is secured into position during the surgery and left in place for the first 5 to 7 days after the surgery. After this point, the temporary prosthesis is removed to allow removal of the packing; it can then be replaced to facilitate continued oral intake.

After the cavity has matured for several weeks, an interim obturator is fabricated. This will serve the patient for the next several months during postoperative radiation therapy until the final healing of the cavity is achieved. The interim obturator has a mound on the back that protrudes up into the cavity and helps to maintain facial contour. This mound also helps anchor the prosthesis by folding over the edges of the palatal defect. A final obturator is fashioned from a recasted mold of the upper jaw that includes an impression of the final shape of the defect.

The alternative to the palatal prosthesis is a revascularized free tissue transfer. It is possible to harvest tissue from a distant site and reconstruct the palate with vascularized bone grafts. The preferred site for palatal repair is the wing of the scapula. This can be harvested with a blood supply that can be anastomosed to vessels in the neck. The technical details of this procedure are beyond the scope of this book, but the rhinologic surgeon should be familiar with the possibilities, if not the details, of how to accomplish this technique. For most patients, this will not be the preferred option. However, in cases of edentulous patients or resection well past the midline, prosthetic reconstruction may be more difficult and less rewarding.

The other situation in which prosthetics are a less-than-optimal choice is after maxillectomy with orbital exenteration. In this situation, the orbital cavity can be covered with a painted, fabricated mold that initially simulates the appearance of the face. However, these prostheses rarely maintain their form and color, and they may slip or come loose. The result is that the quality of the repair degenerates over time. The alternative is to fill the cavity with a revascularized free tissue transfer, which is usually anastomosed to the superficial temporal vessels. Either the latissimus dorsi flap or the rectus abdominis flap are the best sources. In either case, the flap fills the orbital cavity. This approach has the advantage of eliminating the need for frequent cleaning of the cavity, and it can be covered with an eye patch or left open. The reconstruction does not resemble a normal face, but it does accomplish coverage and avoids some postoperative care problems. Ultimately, the choice of which technique to use will rest with the individual patient and physician. The best choice is what is right for that particular clinical and personal situation.

POSTOPERATIVE CARE

Good functional results with complete recovery from maxillectomy can only be achieved with high-quality postoperative care. The first issue is management of the airway and arousal from anesthesia during the immediate recovery period after surgery. Most patients will be anesthetized for only 4 to 6 hours and will be able to awaken and be extubated while still in the operating room. Most of these patients will have normal airway function and protective mechanisms, so they can be treated like non–head and neck surgery patients in terms of airway management. The one main concern is that the amount of secretion into the airway from the maxillectomy cavity may be more than the usual and may pose an aspiration risk. To guard against this risk, it is usually only necessary to make sure that the patient is fully reversed from muscle relaxants and sufficiently awake to protect the airway. If the patient fails to awaken rapidly after the surgery, they can be taken to the recovery room intubated and allowed to come around more slowly. Overnight intubation to protect the airway and support respiration is rarely necessary after maxillectomy.

As long as no complications occur, monitoring in the intensive care unit after surgery is generally not required. In some instances, when the patient has additional medical risk factors, overnight stay in the recovery room or intensive care unit may be desirable. In other cases, if extensive pharyngeal resection or neck dissection is performed, observation in the intensive care unit is advisable. However, most patients can be transferred to a regular surgical nursing unit the day of surgery after a prolonged 3- to 4-hour stay in the recovery room. In the first hours after surgery, it is advisable to obtain a hemoglobin level to determine the need for transfusion. The posterior pharynx should be examined several times in the first few hours after surgery to evaluate for ongoing hemorrhage.

Postoperative medications should include both analgesics and antibiotics. Analgesics should be prescribed to effect. Patient-controlled analgesia (PCA) is possible, but is reserved for severe pain management once the patient is fully recovered from anesthesia and able to control the administration adequately. Maxillectomy is not usually a severely painful operation. Intravenous morphine, in dosages of 2 to 5 mg per hour, is usually sufficient for the first days after surgery. Within 48 to 72 hours, pain can usually be managed by mild oral narcotics, such as hydocodone or codeine with acetaminophen. Antibiotics should be administered intravenously until the patient can maintain reliable oral intake. Although there are no studies demonstrating the efficacy of prophylactic antibiotics in maxillectomy, the possibility of infection from packing that is in place for 5 to 7 days is enough reason for most surgeons to recommend continued antibiotics. Also, it is helpful to continue antibiotic therapy during the prolonged healing phase until the cavity is completely mucosalized to avoid secondary infection from mucous stasis. The usual antibiotic choices for sinus pathogens are applicable in this case.

Activity is limited to strict bed rest the first night after surgery to help control the bleeding. However, as soon as the morning after the operation, the patient should begin to ambulate. This will help avoid atelectasis, pneumonia, and deep venous thrombosis. Patients who undergo orbital exenteration will require special attention when initiating ambulation owing to distortion in the visual field that results from eye removal. Depth perception is profoundly affected and balance and orientation may be altered as well. Specific physical and occupational therapy should begin as soon as the patient is able to understand and participate in the rehabilitation.

With a functioning palatal prosthesis, most patients are able to begin oral intake as early as the morning after surgery. With tissue reconstruction rather than a prosthesis, most surgeons would agree that the patient should remain without oral intake until after initial healing is ensured. Generally, this will be somewhere between 5 and 10 days after surgery. In the event that the cavity is not filled by either a soft tissue reconstruction or a prosthesis, the patient will be unable to tolerate oral alimentation until some form of closure of the cavity is achieved. In this case, a feeding tube will be needed.

The unique and difficult aspects of managing the postmaxillectomy patient involve caring for the cavity. The greatest advantage to free tissue transfer is that cavity care is not needed. In the absence of flap closure, care needs to begin as soon as the initial pack is removed. Patients are instructed to irrigate the cavity 2 to 3 times per day with sterile saline. In addition, manual debridement of the cavity is necessary until complete healing has been achieved. The cavities tend to accumulate thick, dried secretions that can become malodorous if left for too long. The more thorough the irrigations, the less must be removed manually by the surgeon. Cavity cleaning should be performed every 1 to 2 weeks early in the postoperative course; as time progresses, intervals between cleanings can be increased. Some patients develop a self-cleaning cavity. The prosthesis and irrigations assist in maintaining the cleanliness of the cavity, but this alone will not make the cavity self-cleaning. The key to this result is achieving a functioning mucous membrane that can clear secretions through ciliary activity. Some patients never achieve this result and subsequently require long-term maintenance programs.

COMPLICATIONS

The complications of maxillectomy, as for all surgical procedures, can be classified as either immediate or delayed. In addition, the various procedures just described have both common or general complications and those that are specific to the individual procedure. The following section covers the general complications common to all maxillectomy procedures, after which the specific complications associated with each individual variation are presented.

General Complications

As a major surgery requiring prolonged anesthesia with possibly significant blood loss, maxillectomy may be associated with a number of medical complications, including hypotension, myocardial infarction, and cerebrovascular accident. The incidence of complications is typically low in this patient population, especially with modern methods of anesthesia and intraoperative monitoring. However, these major medical complications do occur with a predictable incidence of 1% to 2%, accounting for most of the mortalities after maxillectomy operations.[35, 36] Other medical complications, such as pneumonia, urinary tract infection, catheter sepsis, deep venous thrombosis, and others, are also possible. When counseling patients about the risk of maxillectomy, it is easy to overlook these problems. The fact that these complications do occur is not a major concern for most patients as the chances of occurrence are individually low and usually treatable.

Massive hemorrhage, either during the operation or after, may be seen. Transfusion during the perioperative period is relatively common. In fact, depending on the preoperative hemoglobin of the patient, blood transfusion may be necessary for most patients undergoing maxillectomy. In today's medical practice, with the risk of transmission of both hepatitis and human immunodeficiency virus infections to the recipient, the need for transfusion should be discussed with the patient. Bleeding is almost never life-threatening and can be controlled by packing and pressure in most cases. As a treatment for uncontrolled postoperative bleeding, embolization in the neuroradiology invasive laboratory is a successful and valuable last resort.

Postoperative wound infection is a low risk for these patients because the cavities are typically left open. The patients at greatest infection risk are those undergoing free vascularized tissue transfer when the cavity is obliterated. In these cases, the contaminated wound bed is covered over with a sterile bone or soft tissue graft. The space under the graft is, therefore, at risk for infection. As with any nasal procedure requiring packing, there is a risk of toxic shock syndrome but, to date, no reports of this occurring in maxillectomy patients have been published.

Postoperative pain is a reality for all postmaxillectomy patients. In most cases, this can be controlled with moderate doses of narcotic analgesics. Once the patient is fully aroused after the operation, PCA is a beneficial approach to pain management. Most patients prefer this approach because it offers immediate relief when pain develops.

Medial Maxillectomy

Medial maxillectomy, especially when performed with en bloc ethmoidectomy, can lead to orbital injury. The possibilities range from simple orbital penetration with ecchymosis to retrobulbar hemorrhage and blindness. Injury to the inferior or medial rectus with subsequent diplopia is possible, as is damage to the lacrimal system with resultant epiphora from lacrimal stenosis. These all are uncommon complications and have not been experienced in the author's practice with the exception of one patient who developed delayed-onset epiphora.[37] This was resolved by a simple dacryocystorhinostomy.

The most likely complication of medial maxillectomy relates to nasal vestibular stenosis.[38, 39] Scar bands that encircle the nasal vestibule can form as a result of the midface degloving incision, as discussed in detail in

Chapter 16. The sinuses are a second common problem area. Scarring in the sinuses can lead to frontal obstruction, which requires reoperation. If left untreated, stenosis may eventually lead to the development of a mucocele. Significant osteitis of the maxilla is also possible. In this setting, the sinus can completely fill in with new bone formation, trapping small fragments of mucosa within the new bone. This can result in chronic infection and the failure to achieve a well-healed cavity.

Finally, medial maxillectomy may be associated with significant problems with nasal crusting. This may range from a minimal problem of needing to irrigate daily to full-blown atrophic rhinitis. In the latter case, there is little that can be done to reverse the problem. In milder cases, topical care with irrigation and antibiotic ointment in the nose can greatly relieve the problem. The incidence of this problem is actually surprisingly low. In the author's experience to date, of more than 15 patients undergoing medial maxillectomy for inverting papilloma with a range of follow-up evaluation of 1 to 7 years, no case of prolonged infection or crusting has occurred. The reason for this is not readily apparent. The critical loss of mucosa of the inferior turbinate without the development of a mucosal clearance problem is hard to understand. However, it is apparent that the cavity routinely becomes self-cleaning, at least in the short term. It is possible, too, that the time of onset for problems is longer than 7 years, and that atrophic disease will manifest in these patients in the future.

Posterior Maxillectomy

The specific complications of posterior maxillectomy are caused by the palatal defect. Nasal reflux and hypernasal speech are to be expected when the patient is neither reconstructed or obturated with a prosthesis. The reflux may be severe enough to prohibit oral intake without some method of plugging the hole. As most of the patients undergoing this surgery will be rehabilitated with a palatal prosthesis, the complications of prosthetic wear are also included with this procedure. These include erosions of the mucosa, sinus infections, and possible osteoradionecrosis of the maxilla if the patient is also irradiated.

Other problems are associated with other aspects of the surgery. Many patients will develop trismus owing to the involvement of the pterygoid muscles in the operation. With healing and scarring of the muscle, contracture is possible. If trismus does occur, it can be difficult to overcome. Physical therapy with jaw-stretching exercises is painful and results in slow progress. However, in most cases, some improvement is achieved. Finally, there are potential problems with damage to the sensory nerves supplying the maxilla and teeth. These include the infraorbital nerve and the superior alveolar nerve. Both can be damaged during this surgery, resulting in anesthesia of the upper lip and teeth. This deficit can cause significant problems with lip biting, dental hygiene, and mastication. In addition, the palate usually becomes anesthetic. This predisposes the patient to burn injuries from hot foods and makes control of the food bolus more difficult.

Inferior Maxillectomy

The inferior maxillectomy is associated with all of the complications described for the posterior maxillectomy. Additional problems relate to interference with nasal function, leading to an increased incidence of sinus problems. Also, there is an increasing risk of contracture of the upper lip owing to the loss of the underlying alveolar ridge to supply support. Depending on the location of the medial cut, some of the underlying support for the nose may also be lost. This can lead to turning of the nose to the side of the surgery and loss of vertical projection of the nasal tip.

Total Maxillectomy

In addition to the problems discussed in the previous sections, the total maxillectomy is associated with an increased incidence of crusting problems and atrophic effects in the nose. Long-term management of nasal and sinus crusting is required. For some patients, there may be subtle or overt enophthalmos. Removal of the floor of the orbit with the periosteum increases the risk of these problems. Enophthalmos is usually accompanied by diplopia and epiphora, and may lead to stretching of the optic nerve and visual loss. Secondary correction of enophthalmos is possible with the use of temporalis flaps and bone grafts. The cosmetic appearance of patients undergoing total maxillectomy is typically less than optimal. There is usually a hollowness to the cheek, a turning and drooping of the nose, and potentially, enophthalmos, all of which can alter the patient's appearance.

The postmaxillectomy patient has a significant psychological burden as well. They not only have to manage the issues related to the tumor, but must deal with a change in appearance and function. This is particularly true for patients having orbital exenteration. The long-term effects on the emotional and psychological health of survivors of this surgery have not been well studied. However, it is clear that these patients suffer from severe depression and a change in self-image that devalues their feelings of self-worth. Surgeons who perform these procedures would do well to keep this in mind.

REFERENCES

1. Fleming ID. Head and Neck Section: AJCC Cancer Staging Manual, 5th ed. Philadelphia: Lippincott-Raven, 1997, pp. 21–64.

2. Yoskovitch A, Braverman I, Nachtigal D, et al. Sinonasal schneiderian papilloma. J Otolaryngol 27(3):122, 1998.
3. Lueg EA, Irish JC, Roth Y, et al. An objective analysis of the impact of lateral rhinotomy and medial maxillectomy on nasal airway function. Laryngoscope 108(9):1320, 1998.
4. Raveh E, Feinmesser R, Shpitzer T, et al. Inverted papilloma of the nose and paranasal sinuses: A study of 56 cases and review of the literature. Isr J Med Sci 32(12):1163, 1996.
5. Weisman R. Lateral rhinotomy and medial maxillectomy. Otolaryngol Clin North Am 28(6):1145, 1995.
6. Lawson W, Ho BT, Shaari CM, et al. Inverted papilloma: A report of 112 cases. Laryngoscope 105(3 Pt 1):282, 1995.
7. Bielamowicz S, Calcaterra TC, Watson D. Inverting papilloma of the head and neck: The UCLA update. Otolaryngol Head Neck Surg 109:71, 1993.
8. Pelausa EO, Fortier MA. Schneiderian papilloma of the nose and paranasal sinuses: The University of Ottawa experience. J Otolaryngol 21:9, 1992.
9. Spiro RH, Strong EW, Shah JP. Maxillectomy and its classification. Head Neck 19(4):309, 1997.
10. Kondo M, Ogawa K, Inuyama Y, et al. Prognostic factors influencing relapse of squamous cell carcinoma of the maxillary sinus. Cancer 55:190, 1985.
11. Jiang GL, Ang KK, Peters LJ, et al. Maxillary sinus carcinomas: Natural history and results of postoperative radiotherapy. Radiother Oncol 21(3):193, 1991.
12. Sakata K, Aoki Y, Karasawa K, et al. Analysis of the results of combined therapy for maxillary carcinoma. Cancer 71(9):2715, 1993.
13. Tiwari R, van der Wal J, VanderWaal I, Snow G. Studies of the anatomy and pathology of the orbit in carcinoma of the maxillary sinus and their impact on preservation of the eye in maxillectomy. Head Neck 20(3):193, 1998.
14. Wu X, Tang P, Qi Y. Management of the orbital contents in radical surgery for squamous cell carcinoma of the maxillary sinus. Chin Med J 108(2):123, 1995.
15. Stern SJ, Goepfert H, Clayman G, et al. Orbital preservation in maxillectomy. Otolaryngol Head Neck Surg 109:111, 1993.
16. Catalano PJ, Hecht CS, Biller HF, et al. Craniofacial resection. An analysis of 73 cases. Arch Otolaryngol Head Neck Surg 120(11):1203, 1994.
17. Lund VJ, Howard DJ, Wei WI, et al. Craniofacial resection for tumors of the nasal cavity and paranasal sinuses—A 17-year experience. Head Neck 20(2):97, 1998.
18. Osguthorpe JD, Patel S. Craniofacial approaches to sinus malignancy. Otolaryngol Clin North Am 28(6):1239, 1995.
19. Kraus DH, Sterman BM, Levine HL, et al. Factors influencing survival in ethmoid sinus cancer. Arch Otolaryngol Head Neck Surg 118(4):367, 1992.
20. Jackson IT. Craniofacial approach to tumors of the head and neck. Clin Plast Surg 12(3):375, 1985.
21. Donald PJ. Recent advances in paranasal sinus surgery. Head Neck Surg 4(2):146, 1981.
22. Shah JP, Galicich JH. Esthesioneuroblastoma. Treatment by combined craniofacial resection. NY State J Med 79:84, 1979.
23. Keane WM, Atkins JP Jr, Wetmore R, Vidas M. Epidemiology of head and neck cancer. Laryngoscope 91:2037, 1981.
24. Klintenberg C, Olofsson J, Hellquist H, Sokjer H. Adenocarcinoma of the ethmoid sinuses. Cancer 54:482, 1984.
25. Itami J, Uno T, Aruga M, et al. Squamous cell carcinoma of the maxillary sinus treated with radiation therapy and conservative surgery. Cancer 82:104, 1998.
26. Kubo K, Furukawa S, Fuchilhata H, et al. Treatment results of maxillary sinus carcinoma. A retrospective study. Nippon Acta Radiol 50(7):804, 1990.
27. Sakai S, Mori N, Miyaguchi M, et al. Combined therapy for maxillary sinus carcinoma with special reference to extensive Denker's operation. Auris, Nasus, Larynx 18(4):367, 1991.
28. Ochi JW, Harris JP, Feldman JI, et al. Rhinocerebral mucormycosis: Results of aggressive surgical debridement and amphotericin B. Laryngoscope 98(12):1339, 1988.
29. Blitzer A, Lawson W, Meyers BR, Biller HF. Patient survival factors in paranasal sinus mucormycosis. Laryngoscope 90:635, 1980.
30. Stankiewicz JA, Girgis SJ. Endoscopic surgical treatment of nasal and paranasal sinus inverted papilloma. Otolaryngol Head Neck Surg 109(6):988, 1993.
31. Kamel RH. Conservative endoscopic surgery in inverted papilloma: Preliminary report. Arch Otolaryngol Head Neck Surg 118:649, 1992.
32. Waitz G, Wigand E. Results of endoscopic sinus surgery for the treatment of inverted papillomas. Laryngoscope 102:917, 1992.
33. McCary WS, Gross CW, Reibel JF, et al. Preliminary report: Endoscopic versus external surgery in the management of inverted papilloma. Laryngoscope 104:415, 1994.
34. Cooter MS, Charlton SA, LaFreniere D, et al. Endoscopic management of an inverted nasal papilloma in a child. Otolaryngol Head Neck Surg 118(6):876, 1998.
35. Cantu G, Mattavelli F, Salvatori P, et al. Combined transfacial and infratemporal approaches for T3-T4 malignant maxillary tumors. Acta Otorhinolaryngol Ital 15(5):345, 1995.
36. Bernard PJ, Biller HF, Lawson W, et al. Complications following rhinotomy. Review of 148 patients. Ann Otol Rhinol Laryngol 98(9):684, 1989.
37. Osguthorpe JD, Weisman RA. Medial maxillectomy for lateral nasal wall neoplasms. Arch Otolaryngol Head Neck Surg 117(7):751, 1991.
38. Maniglia AJ, Phillips DA. Midfacial degloving for the management of nasal, sinus, and skull-base neoplasms. Otolaryngol Clin North Am 28(6):1127, 1995.
39. Esteban F, Jurado A, Cantillo E, et al. Facial degloving as a versatile approach to paranasal sinus tumors. Acta Otorhinolaryngol Esp 48(6):457, 1997.

CHAPTER 18

Craniofacial Resection

The resection of advanced tumors of the nose and sinuses using combined neurosurgical and otolaryngologic approaches is one of the major surgical advances in the field of head and neck oncology in the last 30 years. This operation allows the complete resection of tumors involving the cribriform plate, ethmoid sinus, and even intracranial structures with a high degree of local control and reasonable risk of morbidity. Craniofacial resection is included in the contents of this book because of the importance of the procedure in the modern management of tumors of the nose and sinuses. Most typically, craniofacial resection is performed by head and neck oncologic surgeons with special training in skull base surgery. Many rhinologists will not perform this surgery. However, the well-trained rhinologist should be knowledgeable about craniofacial resection and be able to select candidates appropriately for the surgery.

HISTORICAL PERSPECTIVES

Craniofacial resection for treatment of orbital tumors was first described by Dandy in 1941.[1] However, it is Ketcham who is usually credited with introducing the technique of combined intracranial and extracranial surgery for tumors of the nose and sinuses.[2] His original publication in 1963 provoked widespread interest in this new and interesting surgery. Edgerton and Snyder suggested a two-stage technique for reconstruction.[3] However, this did not gain popularity owing to the success of the one-stage procedure. Johns et al., in 1981, described the inferiorly based pericranial flap for closure of the skull base defect.[4] This opened the way for more aggressive surgeries involving the anterior cranial base. Terz and colleagues, as cited in Arbit et al.,[5] first reported that the procedure could be extended for tumors involving the pterygomaxillary fissure. In 1981, Donald suggested that tumors of the cavernous sinus could also be approached.[6] Sasaki et al. reported the use of the pectoralis major myocutaneous flap for reconstruction of the skull base after craniofacial resection in 1985.[7] This opened the way for a wide variety of pedicled and free tissue transfers for reconstruction.[8–10]

INDICATIONS

Malignant Tumors

The most common reason for performing craniofacial resection is to completely resect a malignant lesion of the nose or sinuses. This indication comprises a wide variety of tumor sites, stages, and histologic features. Most series of craniofacial resections include a variety of histologic tumor types. The most common tumors vary from series to series, but the top four usually include adenocarcinoma, esthesioneuroblastoma (olfactory neuroblastoma), squamous cell carcinoma, and sarcoma. Adenocarcinoma tends to predominate in Europe, whereas esthesioneuroblastoma and squamous cell carcinoma are more common in the United States. Other tumors involving the nose and sinuses may occasionally be indications for craniofacial resection, including sinonasal undifferentiated carcinoma (SNUC), adenoid cystic carcinoma, melanoma, and various salivary gland histologic types.[11–14]

Esthesioneuroblastoma

The esthesioneuroblastoma is perhaps the best indication for craniofacial resection. This is a tumor that arises from the olfactory epithelium on the nasal side of the cribriform plate or on the superior aspect of the septum or superior turbinate. The cell of origin is thought to be a neural crest derivative, which gives the tumor its characteristic qualities on immunohistochemical stains. Esthesioneuroblastoma has a variety of histologic differentiations ranging from well defined and low grade to poorly defined and high grade. It tends to spread aggressively through bone and into the surrounding structures and has the potential to seed the cerebrospinal fluid (CSF), leading to meningeal metastases.[15] It does have the capability to metastasize to cervical lymph nodes and distant sites, but usually does so only late in the disease course.[16–18] These tumors tend to have a mixed response to radiation therapy, with early tumors faring much better than more advanced tumors. Newer, combined chemotherapy and radiation protocols have been successful in eradicating the more advanced tumors, offering the hope that, in the future, effective nonoperative therapy may be developed.[19] Overall, patients with esthesioneuroblastoma are good candidates for craniofacial resection because of the disease's late spread and ability to resect the tumor completely. Five-year, disease-free survival rates in most series exceed 50%.[11–18]

Squamous Cell Carcinoma

Squamous cell carcinoma may arise from any of the sinuses or the nasal structures. There is not a high degree of correlation to cigarette smoke, but this tumor may be associated with heavy metal exposure in factory workers, especially nickel workers, and there is an association with inverted papilloma. The association of squamous cell carcinoma with inverted papilloma is well established and occurs in approximately 10% of cases of inverted papilloma.[20–23] There is continued debate about whether this is attributable to malignant degeneration of the papilloma into a carcinoma or whether this is a coincidental association due to common underlying etiology. It has been observed that malignant disease is more highly associated with inverted papillomas that are either neglected for long periods or are recurrent after initial resection. Squamous cell carcinomas of the nose and sinus behave similarly to those of other head and neck sites, with a high degree of local invasion, spread along nerves and into small vessels, and early metastasis to lymph nodes and distant sites. Squamous cell carcinomas of the nose and sinuses, like other squamous cell carcinomas, tend to respond well to radiation therapy and platinum-based chemotherapy. However, most patients will eventually fail nonoperative therapy, leaving a serious local control problem. For this reason, the primary therapy for these tumors remains surgical resection if possible. However, before embarking on craniofacial resection for a squamous cell carcinoma of the nose and sinuses, a very careful evaluation of the local extent of disease and the presence of distant metastases must be conducted. Signs of distant spread or unresectable tumor should be carefully heeded as indications to avoid surgery.

Sinonasal Undifferentiated Carcinoma

SNUC is a high-grade tumor of uncertain etiology that exhibits poorly differentiated histologic characteristics not definable as one particular tumor type. Immunohistochemical stains are usually positive for keratin but otherwise negative. The key differential point is to distinguish SNUC tumors from lymphoma. The use of special stains for B-cell and T-cell markers is usually adequate to establish this diagnosis. This tumor exhibits rapid local growth through bone and into surrounding structures.[24] Perineural spread and microvascular invasion are often seen. Lymphatic and distant metastases are seen in a high percentage of patients. Results with nonoperative therapy for this tumor type have been discouraging, and cure rates with surgery have not been as good as for the more predictable esthesioneuroblastoma.[14] Patients with SNUC may be candidates for craniofacial resection using the same criteria for resection as used for squamous cell carcinoma.

Other Tumors

Among the other tumor types, most are amenable to craniofacial resection as long as anatomic criteria are met. Adenocarcinomas, sarcomas, and melanomas are, in general, poorly responsive to nonoperative therapy, so attempts at cure often depend on complete surgical resection. The exception to this is pediatric rhabdomyosarcoma of the orbit, which is always treated with chemotherapy and radiation therapy before considering ablative surgery. Adenoid cystic carcinoma is a tumor with unusual biological behavior. It has a great propensity for perineural spread and distant metastasis without a high incidence of lymphatic metastasis. Adenoid cystic carcinoma has been shown to have a unique sensitivity to neutron beam radiation with series reporting long-term local control in patients with unresectable tumors and in those with incomplete resection. The limitations of the modality are that it is highly toxic to normal tissue, and the central nervous system and optic nerves cannot tolerate a high dose of neutron radiation. Complications, such as cerebral necrosis and blindness, have been observed. For this reason, surgery remains the primary modality for resectable tumors.

Small Cell Carcinoma

Small cell neuroendocrine carcinoma is a rare tumor variation found in the nose and sinuses. This tumor may sometimes be confused with high-grade esthesioneuroblastoma, SNUC, and lymphoma. However, many pathologists consider this to be a distinct tumor type of the same derivation as small cell carcinoma of the lungs. Reliable information on the management of this tumor is lacking owing to the rarity of identifying it by histologic examination. However, it seems reasonable to consider the biology of this tumor to be analogous to similar tumors in the lungs, which are primarily treated by chemotherapy and irradiation. In the nose and sinuses, the small cell neuroendocrine carcinoma may be resected by craniofacial resection if no evidence of distant spread is found and the tumor is well localized. For larger tumors, induction chemotherapy, followed by assessment for response, can dictate whether or not radiation therapy or surgery should be employed.

Lymphoma

The one tumor type that is never an indication for craniofacial resection is lymphoma. As with all other tumor sites, lymphoma is best treated with chemotherapy and radiation therapy. High rates of remission and local control are achieved with this therapy. The primary determinants of survival will be the overall stage of the lymphoma as well as the growth pattern. Disseminated, high-grade, non-Hodgkins lymphoma is almost never cured, whereas stage I Hodgkins lymphoma is almost always cured.

Benign Tumors

In most circumstances, benign tumors can be resected with preservation of the roof of the ethmoid and cribriform plate. For this class of lesions, a wide cuff of normal tissue is not necessary to achieve local control and potential cure. However, there are circumstances when even benign tumors exhibit aggressive local spread and may require craniofacial resection for complete removal. The most common benign tumor to involve the nose and sinuses is the inverted papilloma.[20–23] This tumor is thought to be caused by infection with a subtype of the human papillomavirus, although this point remains somewhat controversial and has not been definitively established. It has a classic histologic appearance of inward-growing fronds of the mucosal lining. The mucosa may exhibit a variety of dysplastic changes extending all the way up to high-grade dysplasia or in situ carcinoma. In 10% of cases, a distinctly malignant morphology is demonstrated, with frank invasion through the lamina propria into the underlying submucosa. When this occurs, the tumor behaves similar to any squamous cell carcinoma, with the ability to spread along nerves and lymphatics and develop distant metastases.

Despite the typically benign histologic features of inverted papilloma, this tumor demonstrates very aggressive local growth through adjacent bone and sinus mucosa. Usually, the tumor originates in the area of the ethmoid infundibulum or anterior middle meatus. The tumor normally grows into the maxillary sinus and middle meatus, presenting as a unilateral nasal polyp. With prolonged neglect, the tumor can spread into the eye, ethmoid sinus, frontal sinus, and even intracranially. In most cases, however, the tumor is diagnosed at an earlier stage and treated by surgery while it is still confined to the medial wall of the maxillary sinus. Appropriate treatment at this stage is highly curative, with most series demonstrating at least an 85% cure rate. Attempts to treat the lesion by simple polypectomy are associated with a high rate of recurrence, and these are the tumors that may recur in the ethmoid sinus and extend into the skull base.

In the author's experience, two patients with inverted papilloma have required craniofacial resection; both had benign disease. The first was a patient with recurrent tumor 4 years after an original suboptimal resection. At this stage, she had disease that was accessible to resection by a radical maxillectomy. However, she refused this treatment and was lost to follow-up evaluation for 15 months. She returned when she lost vision in her eye. Scans at this time demonstrated extension of the tumor into the orbit and through the ethmoid roof. She underwent craniofacial resection with orbital exenteration and postoperative radiation therapy, but the tumor recurred 8 months later intracranially. She subsequently died 18 months after that surgery from extensive intracranial spread.

The second patient presented with a 2-year history of nasal obstruction and a tumor extending through the ethmoid into the frontal sinus and through the posterior wall of the frontal sinus. He underwent craniofacial resection with orbital preservation. He achieved long-term local control, but went back to heavy alcohol abuse and died of aspiration pneumonia after a prolonged alcohol binge.

Other benign tumors may occasionally become candidates for craniofacial resection in extreme circumstances. These include osteoma and other bone-forming tumors, meningioma, juvenile nasopharyngeal angiofibroma, and neurofibroma.[12] Osteomas are a particularly interesting indication for craniofacial resection. These tumors are very slow-growing and always benign lesions. In most cases, a simple transnasal approach or osteoplastic approach will allow complete excision without requiring craniofacial resection. However, there are cases when the tumor may extensively involve the posterior table of the frontal sinus or the roof of the ethmoid and so cannot be removed safely without an intracranial approach.[25, 26] The key to minimizing the morbidity of these procedures is limited intracranial dissection and brain retraction with careful reconstruction.

Inflammatory Diseases

In several of the large series of craniofacial resection, there is mention of a rare inflammatory disease that is addressed by craniofacial resection.[12, 27] The two principle diagnoses for craniofacial resection for inflammatory conditions are destructive granuloma and infection. Infections may be osteomyelitis of the skull base or invasive fungal infections. Mucormycosis is a fulminant infection, caused by the fungus Mucor, that extends rapidly through the sinuses by invading blood vessels and causing ischemic necrosis. Radical debridement of involved tissues is considered to be the only method of potentially curing the disease. If the skull base is involved, most surgeons would consider the case incurable and advise intravenous amphotericin and supportive care. However, in just the right circumstances, it may be possible to attempt craniofacial resection to achieve cure.

Destructive granulomas are rare and may be identified as cholesterol granuloma, reparative granuloma, or Wegener's granulomatosis. Wegener's granulomatosis is an idiopathic inflammatory condition involving multiple systems including the nose and sinuses. Its hallmark histologic findings are giant cell granulomas and perivascular inflammation. It has a tendency to cause destruction of the nasal septum, turbinates, and sinuses, leading to granulation tissue, crusting, and chronic infection. It is usually treated medically with trimethoprim/sulfamethoxasole, systemic steroids, or cyclophosphamide. Repeated debridement of granulation tissue and crust, as well as nasal irrigations with antibiotic solutions, is the mainstay of nasal care. In the worst cases, craniofacial resection has been proposed as a beneficial means of eliminating the nasal mucosa and the local source of infection, pain, and bleeding. The author has no experience with this rather aggressive approach, but it reportedly has been beneficial.

TABLE 18–1
Staging of Ethmoid Sinus Tumors

Tumor Staging

T1: Tumor confined to the ethmoid, with or without bone erosion

T2: Tumor extending into the nasal cavity

T3: Tumor extending into the anterior orbit or the maxillary sinus

T4: Tumor with intracranial extension, orbital extension including the apex, involving the sphenoid, involving the frontal sinus, or involving the skin of the external nose

Nodal Staging

N0: No regional nodal metastasis

N1: Metastasis in one ipsilateral lymph node measuring 3 cm or less in greatest dimension

N2a: Metastasis in one ipsilateral lymph node measuring greater than 3 cm but less than 6 cm in greatest dimension

N2b: Metastasis in multiple ipsilateral lymph nodes, none of which exceeds 6 cm in greatest dimension

N2c: Metastasis in bilateral or contralateral lymph nodes, none of which exceeds 6 cm in greatest dimension

N3: Metastasis in a lymph node measuring greater than 6 cm in greatest dimension

Distant Metastasis

M0: No distant metastasis

M1: Distant metastasis

Tumor Staging

Staging of tumors of the sinuses and anterior skull base does little to assist the surgeon in determining operative therapy. In contrast to other head and neck tumor sites, for which staging can help direct treatment and surgical approach, in sinus and nasal tumors, the histologic features and tumor location are more critical. To date, there has not been a universally accepted staging for nasal or ethmoid sinus tumors. Most of the reported series of patients undergoing craniofacial resection make no mention of tumor staging, although a number of staging systems have been proposed. The staging system for maxillary sinus cancer has been well established and is presented in Chapter 17. For ethmoid and nasal tumors, the author favors using the tumor, nodes, and metastases (TNM) system that has been adopted universally for other head and neck tumor sites (Table 18–1). In the future, perhaps reports of treatment for nasal and sinus tumors will use a staging system to report the results. This will help clarify treatment issues.

Tumor Extent

Staging and histologic diagnosis of the tumor aside, the principle factor for determining whether craniofacial resection is an appropriate approach to treatment rests on the tumor extent. The indications to proceed with craniofacial resection can be loosely defined as any tumor that requires removal of the cribriform plate, roof of the ethmoid, or posterior wall of the frontal sinus to achieve complete resection of the tumor. Depending on the origin of the tumor, this can occur at early or late tumor stages. For esthesioneuroblastoma arising from the cribriform plate, the earliest detectable tumor may require craniofacial resection, whereas for maxillary sinus cancers, extension into the nose and up to the cribriform or ethmoid roof may occur after prolonged growth and with a much greater tumor volume. Most cancers that extend into the ethmoid sinus or encroach on the cribriform plate fit this criterion. It is difficult to completely resect a malignant tumor involving the ethmoid sinus by cutting through the cells of the sinus below the skull base. Only with minimal extension into the lower cells would this be possible. Similarly, removal of a tumor with preservation of the cribriform plate in a patient with extension onto the olfactory epithelium of the superior turbinate, septum, or cribriform area would require peeling the mucosa from this area. This would tend to cause significant cerebrospinal fluid (CSF) leak and may be less than optimal from an oncologic standpoint.

Craniofacial resection may include any portion of the nose or ethmoid, maxillary, or frontal sinus. The location of the bone cuts is based on careful preoperative assessment of the extent of the tumor. Usually, involvement of the ethmoid sinus requires resection of the entire width of the ethmoid on that side; the anterior-to-posterior dimensions of the resection are based on the exact location of the tumor within the sinus. Either partial medial or complete maxillectomy can be performed depending on the involvement of the maxilla, and palatal and alveolar ridge resection is also possible but tailored to the individual case. The frontal sinus is usually included in the anterior bone flap, but can be included in the resection if necessary.

Orbital exenteration can be added as an extension. The management of the orbit depends on the extent of tumor into the orbit, as outlined in Chapter 17. The principles are the same. Extension up to the orbital bone requires excision of the bone. Erosion of the bone requires excision of the periorbita. Direct extension into the orbital fat or muscle requires orbital exenteration.

The contraindications to surgery are controversial. Extension of the tumor into the pterygomaxillary fissure and infratemporal fossa is a relative contraindication to surgery. The prognosis for cure is not as good when these areas are extensively involved, but the resection is still technically possible. Pterygomaxillary fissure involvement can be handled by dissecting this area from the skull base at the end of the procedure, whereas infratemporal fossa involvement requires a lateral skull base approach prior to the craniofacial resection. Involvement of the dura is not seen as a contraindication for surgery by most surgeons. However, it may be advisable to offer postoperative intrathecal chemotherapy to help prevent meningeal seeding. Frank involvement of the brain parenchyma is a possible contraindication. Clearly, extensive resection of the frontal lobe would lead to a major personality alteration in the patient. However, limited involvement with limited resection of the frontal lobes is normally well tolerated. The brain that is directly infiltrated by tumor is unlikely to function and may be an epileptogenic focus if left alone.

Most surgeons would consider involvement of the bone of the sphenoid sinus or direct invasion into the cavernous sinus to be a contraindication to surgery. These areas cannot be resected with a traditional en bloc approach. However, some surgeons have noted that piecemeal dissection of this area is possible, and that complete tumor resection can still be achieved. The advisability of this technique has yet to be definitively established.

Direct involvement of the nasopharynx, orbital apex, optic canal, carotid artery, or middle cranial fossa is widely accepted as a contraindication to surgery. Complete resection of tumor extending into these areas is not possible in a single surgery, and there is probably little or no chance of cure from this disease. In these cases, irradiation and chemotherapy offer some hope without exposing the patient to the high risks of attempting a craniofacial resection in this setting.

PREOPERATIVE CONSIDERATIONS

Extensive evaluation of patients who are being considered for craniofacial resection is imperative. The surgical and medical suitability of the patient for the surgery must be considered carefully before scheduling surgery, and extensive discussion with the patient and family about potential complications and alternative therapies is vital. No patient should be taken to the operating room for craniofacial resection without complete agreement of the patient, family, and treating physicians. The first step, though, is to evaluate the tumor. Before biopsy of any intranasal or sinus mass, computed tomography (CT) scans and, often, magnetic resonance imaging (MRI) are necessary. These are important in establishing the anatomic extent of the tumor before biopsy and in ensuring that the mass is not an encephalocele or similar lesion that may have intracranial connection. Unsuspected biopsy in this setting could lead to CSF leak or intracranial bleeding.

For any patient under serious consideration for craniofacial resection, both CT and MRI are necessary. These studies provide complementary information about the extent of the tumor. Coronal CT using bone algorithms will demonstrate the degree of bone erosion throughout the sinuses. This is critically important in evaluating the orbit, cribriform plate, and walls of the frontal and sphenoid sinuses. MRI delineates the soft tissue extent of disease and will reveal such vital information as orbital fat involvement, brain involvement, cavernous sinus involvement, and extension along nerves. These are the factors that determine the need for craniofacial resection, resectability of the tumor, and actual extent of the tumor resection. In many cases, a magnetic resonance angiogram or classical four-vessel carotid angiogram is required. These studies will delineate the vascularity of the tumor, as well as the relative encroachment on such structures as the anterior cerebral vessels and carotid arteries. If a risk to the carotid artery is present, angiography may help determine whether the artery can be safely sacrificed or would require bypass grafting.

Biopsy of the tumor is the next consideration. In most cases, it is best not to perform a biopsy before adequate scans are available. Once the tumor has been clearly defined, however, it is necessary to make a specific diagnosis before therapy can be considered. In many cases, a simple cup forceps biopsy in the office will be possible. Adequate tissue should be sampled to allow standard hematoxylin-eosin stains, as well as special immunohistochemical stains. Occasionally, a large benign polyp will present in front of a neoplastic lesion. In other cases, the tumor will not be accessible by anterior rhinoscopy or office endoscopy. In these situations, an intraoperative biopsy is required. In almost every case, this can be performed by a transnasal endoscopic technique. The advantages of this technique are that an opening into the sinus through an external incision is avoided. This avoids not only a scar, but the possibility of implantation and spread of the tumor.

In addition to the local tumor work-up, a thorough search for distant metastases and synchronous primary cancers is required. This should include a complete physical examination, including neck, breast, rectal, and pelvic examinations. If the head and neck surgeon does not feel comfortable with this evaluation, a medical or gynecologic consultation can be requested. Blood testing should include carcinoembryonic antigen (CEA) in appropriate cases, as well as complete blood count with differential, calcium, and liver function tests. The radiologic examination should include at least a chest x-ray study, but a CT scan of the chest is preferred. Abdominal and bone scans are optional but may be advisable in certain cases.

The preoperative medical evaluation should also be thorough. All patients should undergo a complete history and physical examination. Laboratory analysis, including urinalysis and blood testing for electrolytes, glucose, and coagulation factors, is advisable. In most patients older than 50 years of age, a cardiology evaluation is in order. This should include not only an electrocardiogram, but also an echocardiogram and stress test if indicated. If respiratory disease is present, pulmonary function testing may be useful to determine the severity of the problem. Many cases of perioperative mortality are related to respiratory or cardiovascular failure, not surgical complications. For this reason, patients with marginal health status or serious cardiac or respiratory illnesses are not suitable candidates for the operation.

Before discussing the case in detail with the patient, it is necessary to involve the appropriate neurosurgeon. Most institutions have one or two neurosurgeons who specialize in these operations, and a close rapport usually develops. Both otolaryngologist and neurosurgeon should view the preoperative studies together and formulate a detailed plan for the surgical approach. This plan should include the sequence of steps, individual surgeon's responsibilities during the procedure, location of the bone cuts during the resection, and method of reconstruction. If a free flap or other complex reconstruction is anticipated, a third surgical member of the team is recruited. This type of close cooperation is essential for the operation to proceed smoothly and for the operating surgeons to function together as a team.

Once all of the data have been collected, it is customary to have a conference with the treating physicians, patient, and family members. At this conference, the nature of the tumor, plan for resection, prognosis, and potential alternative therapies are discussed in detail. This should take place in a comfortable environment without time constraints or interruption. It is best to include all potential treating physicians in the discussion rather than only the surgeon. The risks of complications must be addressed in an open and honest fashion. Although it is not the intention to scare off patients with this discussion, the true nature of the surgical endeavor should be fully disclosed with some discussion of the risk of mortality, stroke, and brain damage. It is surprising how often this discussion will affirm a patient's decision to undergo surgery, rather than dissuade him or her from proceeding.

After the patient decides to undergo craniofacial resection, the final preparations can be made. These include consultation with the anesthesiologist and arranging the scheduling of the operating room, surgeons, and intensive care unit beds. At least 4 units of packed red blood cells should be available in the operating room before surgery. Invasive monitoring is appropriate, including at least a urinary catheter, arterial line, and central venous line. A pulmonary artery line is possible, if needed, and continuous neurologic monitoring can be set up if desired. Normally, though, this is not necessary for craniofacial resection.

A lumbar drain is always placed prior to surgery in case it is needed after surgery for CSF drainage and monitoring. Intravenous steroids and mannitol are considered for perioperative management. These agents are helpful in minimizing brain edema and may be administered to help prevent complications. Seizure prophylaxis can be initiated 2 to 3 days before the surgery to ensure that adequate levels of the antiseizure medication have been achieved by the time of surgery. Finally, antibiotics are prescribed to cover nasal and sinus bacteria and provide good intracranial penetration. These should be selected in consultation with the neurosurgeons and the infectious disease consultants in the local hospital.

TECHNIQUE

Approach

Craniofacial resection is always performed through a combined bicoronal and transfacial incision. Although the bicoronal incision is common to all cases, the transfacial incision may be either a midfacial degloving or a lateral rhinotomy incision. The determining factors and technique for both the lateral rhinotomy and midface degloving approaches have been presented in detail in Chapter 16.

The bicoronal incision was described in detail in Chapter 11 in connection with osteoplastic frontal sinusectomy. The technique will not differ substantially in this setting. Several issues are important to consider when performing the bicoronal incision. The first is to take into account the method of reconstruction to be used. Most of these procedures will depend on a variation of the pericranial flap or temporalis flap to reconstruct the skull base after the resection. The appropriate plane of elevation must be maintained during this elevation to avoid damaging the blood supply to the reconstructive flap. The second main issue in developing the bicoronal flap is the inferior extent of the dissection. As opposed to the osteoplastic flap procedure for chronic sinusitis, when performing craniofacial resection, the supraorbital nerves must routinely be identified and released from the bony canals. This allows complete exposure of the supraorbital rims, the superior and medial orbital walls, and the nasal dorsum. To ensure that the bicoronal flap will rotate inferiorly to the fullest extent, the incision should be brought inferiorly to the preauricular crease, below the level of the zygomatic arch.

Pericranial Flap

The standard pericranial flap is useful for reconstruction in most cases of craniofacial resection in which the frontal sinus and both orbits are preserved. As the flap is based on the supraorbital arteries, it is, therefore, a vascularized and reliable flap. In most cases, the pericranial flap need only be the thickness of the pericranial periosteum. This is achieved by elevating the bicoronal flap from the incision to the orbits and nose in the subgaleal plane. Laterally, this equates to the plane just on the surface of the temporalis fascia. The galea and frontalis muscle are incorporated into the overlying scalp in a single layer. It is not necessary to elevate the scalp flap all the way to the inferior extent of the orbital rims. Preferably, the elevation stops at the top of the orbital rims to avoid injuring the blood supply to the pericranial flap. During elevation of the scalp, it is important to make sure that the periosteum is maintained fully and as thickly as possible. To achieve this, the dissection should be kept against the frontalis muscle. Either sharp dissection or cautery dissection should be used to avoid peeling the flap up bluntly. Peeling the flap tends to split the fascial plane, tearing some of the thickness of the pericranial flap off into the scalp. Once the scalp is elevated inferiorly, as described in Chapter 11, to the level of the orbital rims, the pericranium is incised. A scalpel is used and the flap is outlined, maintaining the full width and height possible (Fig. 18–1). This extends the pericranial flap laterally to the

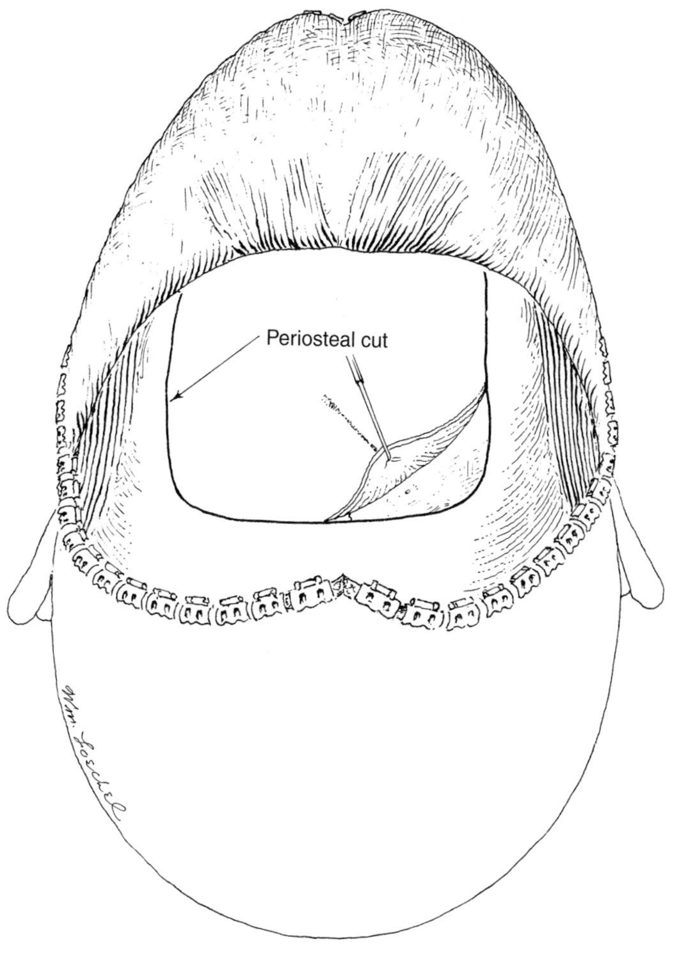

Figure 18–1. Pericranial flap design. The flap is maintained as wide and long as possible.

temporal fossa on each side and superiorly to the level of the incision. The flap is then carefully elevated from the underlying bone using any wide periosteal elevator.

One variation of the pericranial flap that can be used to increase the thickness and vascularity of the flap is to include the galea and frontalis in the flap. The risks of this technique are that the overlying scalp flap will be devascularized and that the distal edge will become ischemic and necrotic. For this reason, it is not often used. The technique involves elevating in the plane just superficial to the galea and frontalis muscle. This plane does not dissect easily, like the subgaleal plane, and so requires sharp dissection with a scalpel. A bipolar forceps is used to control bleeding points on both sides of the plane during the elevation. To make this flap useful, the elevation must continue down to the level of the orbital rims. Otherwise, the flap is tethered to the frontal skin and is overly shortened.

Temporal Galeal Flap

In addition to the standard pericranial flap, a temporal galeal flap can be employed to help reconstruct the skull base after craniofacial resection. This flap is indicated when there is an extensive defect requiring a large flap to reconstruct and to fill space. One such instance is when an orbital exenteration with resection of the roof of the orbit is performed. In this instance, a pericranial flap will be inadequate by itself to support the entire anterior cranial vault on one side. One possible reconstructive approach utilizes a temporal galeal flap. If this flap is intended to be used, it must be designed into the incision and initial bicoronal flap elevation. Instead of cutting down through the galea and elevating in the subgaleal plane, the incision must also stop superficial to the galea, and the initial elevation inferiorly must also stay superficial to the galea (Fig. 18–2). When the main portion of the frontalis muscle is reached, the muscle is incised and the subgaleal plane entered. The remainder of the bicoronal flap can be elevated in the usual way. To elevate the pericranial flap, the pericranium is incised down to bone at the junction of the pericranium with the galea just described. This shortens the pericranial flap somewhat, but will make the temporal galeal flap possible.

At the end of the operation, when the reconstruction is to be performed, the flap is developed. The galea can be followed over the vertex of the skull to the contralat-

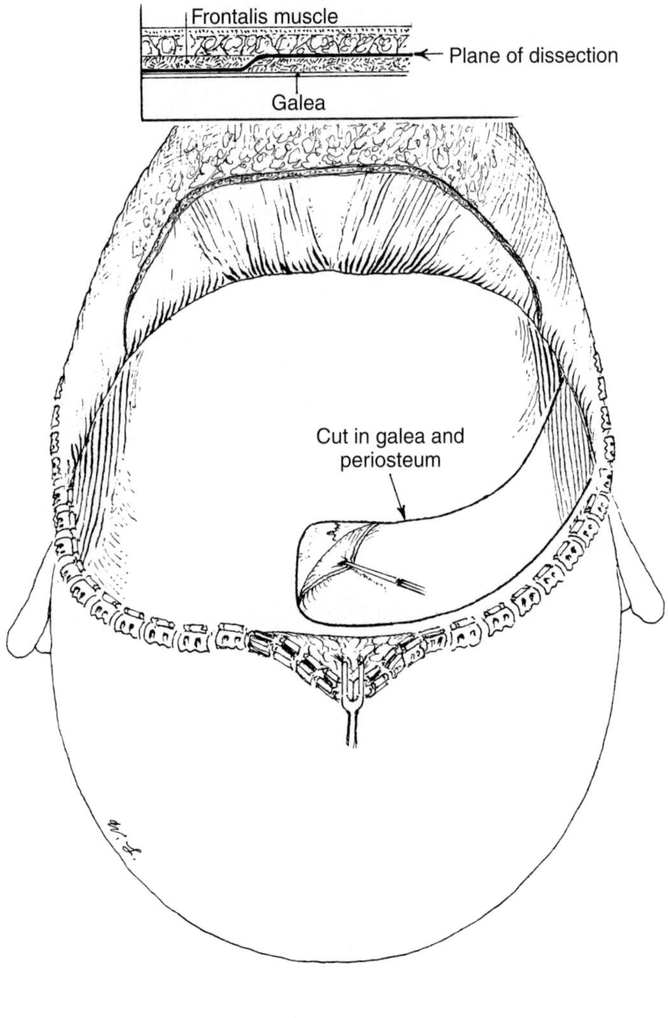

Figure 18–2. Temporal galeal flap. The figure shows the outline of the flap, which can be lengthened and widened to the extent required. The inset shows the plane of dissection superficial to the galea initially; at the inferior edge of the defined width of the flap, the plane changes to the deeper subgaleal/submuscular plane.

eral side. The flap is then outlined and the galea incised down to bone. The flap is elevated from contralateral to ipsilateral under the pericranium on the surface of the skull. At the level of the temporalis muscle, the entire muscle is elevated from the temporal fossa from superior to inferior and from posterior to anterior. The vascular supply for the flap in this case is derived from both the superficial temporal artery, if it can be preserved, and the deep temporal arteries that emanate from the internal maxillary artery and enter the undersurface of the muscle medial to the zygomatic arch. This flap, when maximized, can extend across the midline to the opposite orbital roof and from the orbital rims anteriorly to the sphenoid posteriorly.

Frontal Craniotomy

The next step in most procedures is to perform a frontal craniotomy. This is normally done by the neurosurgeon, but a brief discussion of the design and technique of this part of the procedure is warranted. The first decision is how to design the bone flap. This depends on the nature of the resection planned. In the typical case without resection of the frontal sinus or any part of the superior orbital rim, a standard bifrontal craniotomy is adequate (Fig. 18–3). This bone flap courses above the supraorbital rims as close to the rims as possible. Placing the inferior cut significantly above the rims would leave a ridge of bone blocking the view to the floor of the anterior cranial fossa. This is particularly important in the posterior aspect of the resection in the regions of the sphenoid sinus and the optic canals. The lateral edges of the flap extend to the edge of the temporal fossa. The superior limit is taken only as high as necessary to create the exposure required. The farther posterior the resection extends, the more superior the bone flap must be. In most cases, this will be well anterior to the frontoparietal suture line.

The bone flap is created by first developing burr holes at the corners of the flap. A bone saw is then used to connect the burr holes. The Midas Rex drill, with the various attachments available, is ideal for these functions. Special attention must be directed toward preventing damage to the sagittal sinus when crossing the midline. A second point of concern is the inferior cut, which must cross the base of the frontal sinus. This cut can

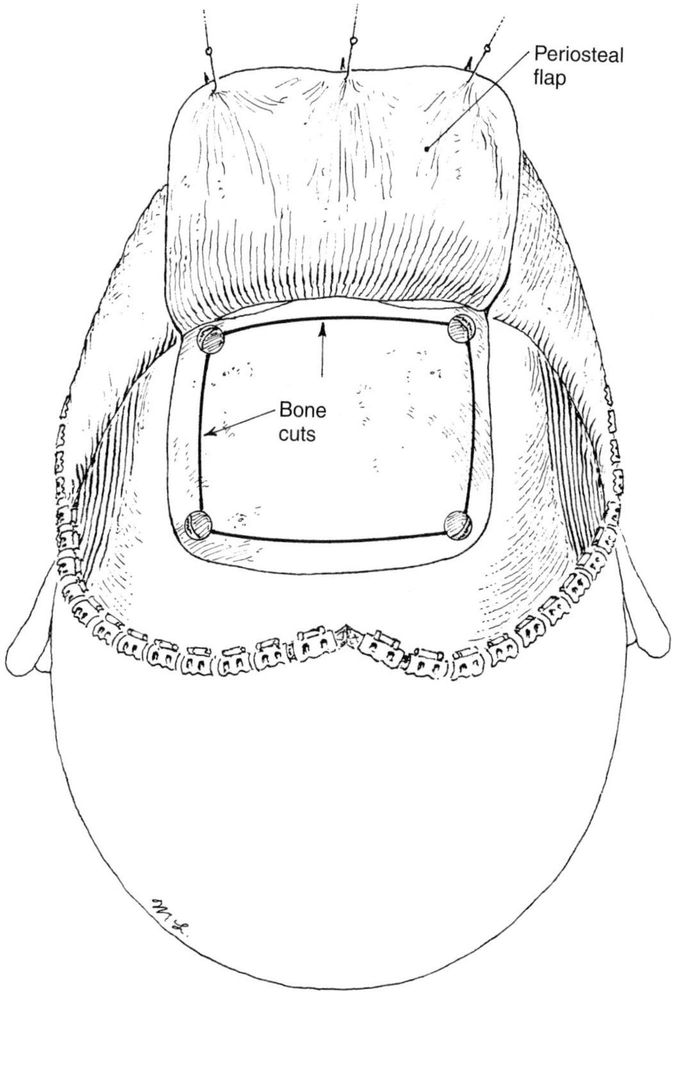

Figure 18–3. Bifrontal craniotomy. The pericranial flap is elevated, and burr holes are created at the corners of the bone flap. The drill is used to cut the bone along the indicated line from one burr hole to the next.

be extended through the anterior then posterior walls of the frontal sinus with the proper footplate attachments. During creation of these bone cuts, it is important to avoid injury to the underlying dura. Rents in the dura may occur, but lead to time-consuming dural repairs and increase the risk of postoperative CSF leak. After the bone cuts are made, the bone flap is gently elevated from the dura and removed.

In most cases, craniofacial resection will require cranialization of the frontal sinus. This is conveniently performed with the frontal bone removed by using a rongeur to take off the posterior wall of the sinus. A drill is then used to remove the mucosa on the inside of the anterior wall. The bone flap is then placed in cold saline to preserve it until it can be replaced at the end of the operation. Any residual posterior wall of the frontal sinus is removed at this point (Fig. 18–4). A small bone rongeur is usually adequate to complete this task. Residual mucosa from the inside of the sinus and frontal recess is easily removed with this exposure. At the end of the operation, the nasofrontal connection will be plugged and the pericranial flap will overlay this area to complete the separation of the sinuses from the anterior cranial fossa.

The main adaptations of this standard bone flap are for resection of part of the frontal sinus or for combined anterior and middle fossa approaches. The most common extension is for removal of all or part of the frontal sinus. This is accomplished merely by placing the inferior edge of the frontal craniotomy at a higher level on the frontal bone. If necessary, the osteoplastic technique of using a bone template to outline the sinus can be utilized. Careful interpretation of the preoperative imaging studies and cooperation between the neurosurgeon and otolaryngologist are essential to locate the bone cuts properly in these cases. The second adaptation of the standard bone flap is when combined middle and anterior fossa surgery is planned. In this case, the craniotomy must be extended down onto the greater wing of the sphenoid bone and the squamous portion of the temporal bone. This is rarely indicated for nasal and sinus tumors.

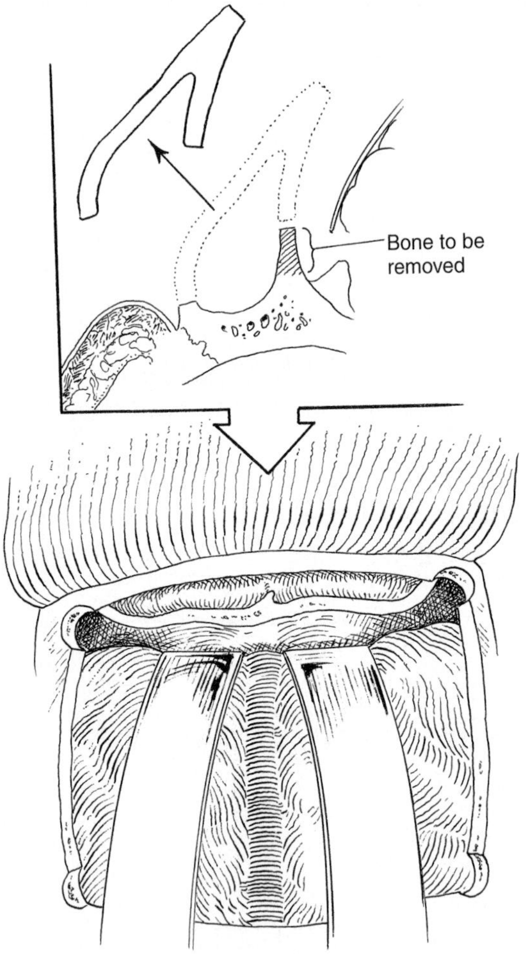

Figure 18–4. Exposure of the frontal sinus. A small residual ridge along the posterior wall of the sinus remains after the bone flap is removed. This can be removed with either a cutting drill or a bone rongeur.

Dural Elevation

Once the craniotomy is complete, the intracranial portion of the dissection must be performed. The goal here is to separate the brain from the tumor. If the tumor is isolated to the nasal side of the skull base, the dissection can be performed extradurally. However, if the tumor penetrates the skull base, a portion of the dura must be resected as a margin. If the tumor directly invades the brain, then a cuff of brain is resected around the tumor to provide the necessary margin. Extradural dissection is the simplest to perform. In this situation, the dura is separated from the underlying bone using an elevator. The dissection proceeds from anterior to posterior using malleable retractors to hold the dura and brain back out of the way. The goal is to expose the entire floor of the anterior cranial fossa as far posteriorly as the optic nerves laterally and the anterior clinoid process in the midline. The wide dissection will improve exposure in the area of the sphenoid sinus and improve positioning of the bone cuts during the resection by establishing definitive landmarks. When this dissection is performed extradurally, a small incision is normally created away from the skull base to drain the CSF. This is necessary to allow the brain to be elevated without undue force on the retractors. This small incision is easily closed when it is no longer needed.

The surgeon has to pay special attention to the elevation of the dura over the cribriform plate. In this area, the olfactory nerves penetrate the dura and enter the nose through the cribriform plate. The dura tends to invaginate into the cribriform plate around the olfactory nerves. Using good retraction, the nerves will tent up as they are reached during the dissection. The surgeon should cauterize the nerves with bipolar forceps and then cut them. After completing the dissection of this area, there is a small defect in the dura. This defect should be repaired immediately before proceeding to the next step.

When dural resection is necessary because of tumor involvement, the dissection of the brain away from the skull base proceeds inside the dura. Initially, the dura is elevated from the skull base until the area where the dura must be resected is reached. At this point, the dura is incised, and the remainder of the dissection is performed intradurally. The brain will usually elevate easily from the dura. After the area of resection is passed, the dura is incised from the inside to get back to the plane of the bone. The final appearance after completion of the dissection is shown in Figure 18–5. If brain resection is necessary, this is accomplished in a similar fashion. However, instead of separating the dura from the pia, the dissection enters the brain parenchyma. Resection of the desired portion of brain is accomplished with this tissue left attached to the skull base and dural cuff.

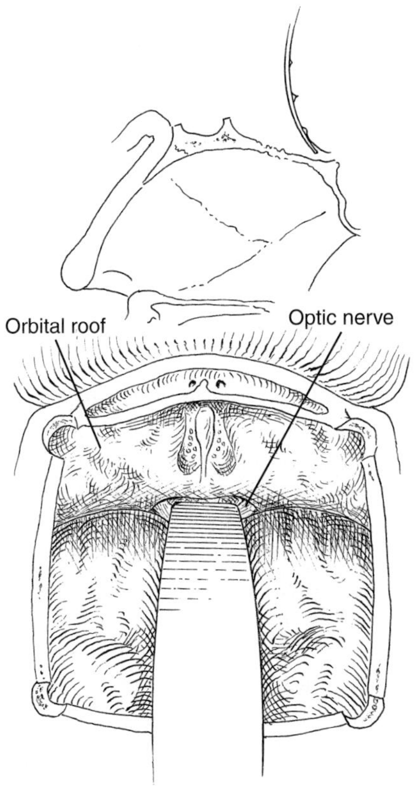

Figure 18–5. Exposure of the cribriform plate. Following extradural elevation of the frontal lobes, the floor of the anterior cranial fossa is exposed across the orbital roofs back to the optic chiasm. This extent of elevation is not always necessary but is helpful in identifying the positions of the optic nerves and sphenoid sinus.

Dural Repair

Before proceeding onto the bone cuts, it is best to repair the dura. The preferred method is to apply a fascial patch graft. The fascia can obtained from the temporalis muscle or fascia lata from the lateral thigh, or artificial dura can be used. The graft is sutured to the dural edges circumferentially around the graft. Either interrupted or continuous sutures may be used. The preferred suture is a 4-0 Neurolon (Ethicon, Inc., Somerville, NJ). Alternative techniques for dural repair include primary closure and vascularized flaps. Occasionally, primary closure can be attempted. This is limited to situations in which the dura is not involved and the only defect is from the area of the cribriform plate. The risk of primary closure is that this will constrict the brain and increase intracranial pressure. During closure, the degree of brain constriction is not apparent because the CSF has been removed. However, after the surgery, as the brain swells and the CSF reaccumulates, the intracranial pressure may increase.

The surgeon may utilize a free vascularized flap when the defect is very large. In this situation, free patch grafts may fail, with subsequent CSF fistula formation. Numerous possibilities are available for this purpose, depending on the exact nature of the defect. In the case of a large dural defect in conjunction with orbital exenteration, the entire cavity and dura can be closed using either a rectus abdominis or latissimus dorsi flap. If only the skull base and dura require repair, then a radial forearm flap may be applicable. An omental free flap is an alternative in this situation, but this requires a laparotomy, which complicates the postoperative management of the patient. Finally, in some cases, it may be desirable to perform repair of the bony defect as well as the dura. In this case, either an iliac or scapular flap could be chosen. With all of these flaps, it is best to perform them after the resection is complete to avoid misjudging the size or nature of the defect.

Intracranial Bone Cuts

The exact position of the intracranial bone cuts will be adjusted for the specific tumor under consideration. In the case of a unilateral esthesioneuroblastoma without orbital involvement, the bone cuts will fall along classical lines. The first cut will enter the orbit on the side of the tumor (Fig. 18–6). This cut can be made with a Midas Rex drill or with an osteotome and mallet. It is best to err on the side of the orbit in this instance to make sure that the tumor is not entered. Using the osteotome allows the surgeon to achieve improved control of the bone cut. This step need not be hurried, and the additional accuracy of the osteotome is worth the few extra minutes of surgical time. After making the initial cut in the orbital roof, a rongeur can be used to

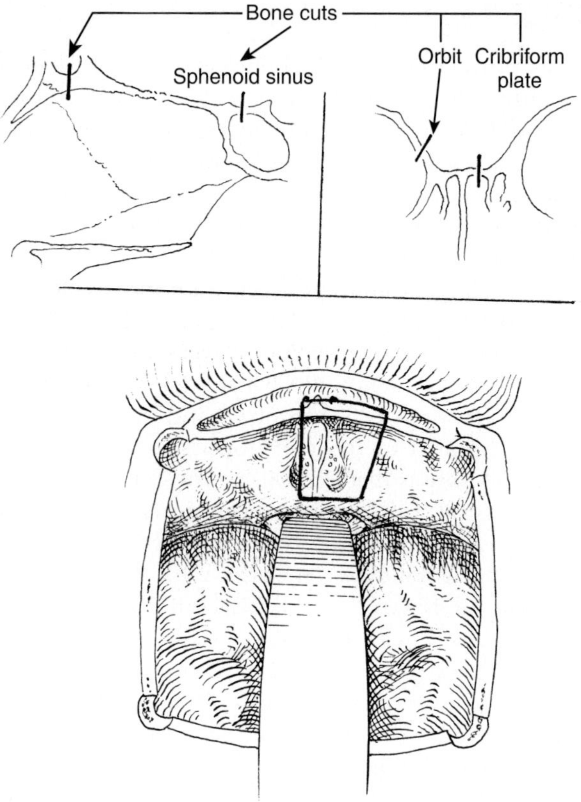

Figure 18–6. Intracranial bone cuts on the floor of the anterior cranial fossa. The surgical view and insets show the four cuts used in a standard unilateral ethmoidectomy.

remove any orbital bone on the medial side of the cut in order to identify the exact position of the medial orbital wall. By following this landmark posteriorly, the location of the anterior wall of the sphenoid sinus can be established.

The second bone cut is just posterior to the anterior wall of the sphenoid sinus (see Fig. 18–6). This cut must be connected laterally to the orbital roof cut. The risk with this step is injury to the optic nerve. In most patients, the optic nerve crosses the lateral wall of the sphenoid sinus well posterior to the anterior wall of the sinus. In these cases, the orbital cut will be able to connect to the sphenoid cut without injuring the optic nerve. In a small percentages of patients, however, the optic nerve crosses the posterior aspect of the ethmoid sinus. In these cases, it is possible to damage the optic nerve when connecting the sphenoid cut to the orbital roof cut if this cut is made too deeply. In these situations, the cut should be made very superficially; then, the orbital contents can be dissected away from the ethmoid bone before completing the cut.

The third cut is made from posterior to anterior on the contralateral side of midline (see Fig. 18–6). In the patient with a unilateral tumor, this will be through the cribriform plate just along the midline. This cut is through fairly thick bone and is best made with a saw or with a drill. By placing the cut on the side opposite the tumor, the nasal septum will be included in the specimen. This is essential for complete tumor removal. The last cut is anterior. This should be just anterior to the posterior wall of the frontal sinus to be sure to incorporate any anterior ethmoidal air cells (see Fig. 18–6). As this bone is also very thick, it, too, is best cut with a saw or drill.

Numerous modifications of this basic resection are possible. The contralateral anterior-posterior cut can be placed through the roof of the ethmoid sinus or orbit to include the entire nasal cavity and both ethmoid sinuses in the resection. The anterior cut can be placed through the nasal dorsum to include the frontal sinus floor in the resection. To include the orbital roof in the resection, as in the case of complete orbital exenteration, the lateral bone cut is placed on the lateral aspect of the orbit. Once the basic resection is mastered, these modifications place little additional burden on the surgeon.

Transfacial Approach

After the intracranial bone cuts are completed, the otolaryngologist takes over the surgery to perform the transfacial portion of the operation. The initial approach may be made through either the midfacial degloving or the lateral rhinotomy technique. These approaches are covered in detail in Chapter 16. The midfacial degloving approach is preferred for resections that preserve the eye because it is cosmetically superior and allows adequate exposure. If orbital exenteration is required, the lateral rhinotomy technique is used, as the additional facial incisions will not have an appreciable impact on facial appearance.

Total Ethmoidectomy

The basic minimal craniofacial resection is performed to remove a tumor limited to the area of the cribriform plate and ethmoid sinus on one side. The following section outlines the steps to complete this procedure. After the intracranial surgery and the midfacial degloving is complete, the orbital dissection must be accomplished. If the periorbita is to be preserved, the orbital periosteum is dissected away from the medial orbital wall. The eye is retracted with a malleable, and the periorbita is carefully elevated from the bone. This is similar to the dissection for an external ethmoidectomy, as described and illustrated in Chapter 9. The anterior and posterior ethmoidal arteries are coagulated with bipolar forceps and then divided. The lacrimal sac is elevated from the lacrimal fossa but left attached to the nasolacrimal duct as it enters its bony canal inferiorly.

The orbital bone cuts are made next. The superior cut has already been made from above through the intracranial approach. The anterior cut should extend from the anterior end of the superior cut inferiorly at the junction of the nasal bone and the frontal process of the maxilla to the level just superior to the nasolacrimal duct (Fig. 18–7). The inferior cut parallels the superior cut and extends from the inferior end of the anterior cut posteriorly along the junction of the maxilla and the lamina papyracea (see Fig. 18–7). This cut should extend posteriorly to the level of the posterior ethmoid artery. The posterior cut will connect the posterior ends of the superior and inferior cuts (see Fig. 18–7).

To complete the resection, intranasal cuts are all that remain. Usually, there will be some remaining attachments of the ethmoid block to the lateral nasal wall. These attachments can be cut with scissors. This is accomplished first at the anterior cut by dividing the mucosa just posterior to the nasolacrimal duct at the anterior attachment of the middle turbinate. The inferior cut is next completed with one tine of the scissors in the nose and the other in the orbit. The next step is to cut the nasal septum at the desired level. This may be along the floor of the nose, or it can be at any level of the septum providing an adequate margin of resection. After this last cut, the specimen will be attached only posteriorly. To deliver the specimen, it is gently rocked back and forth while pulling from below and pushing from above. The posterior attachments will become isolated and can then be divided. Care should be taken to ensure that the optic nerves are protected at this last step to avoid injury. This will deliver the specimen into the nasal cavity, where it can be removed.

Extensions to the Basic Resection

The possible extensions to the minimal craniofacial resection are numerous. The most common include medial maxillectomy, radical maxillectomy, orbital exenteration, bilateral ethmoidectomy, frontal sinus resection, and rhinectomy. These extensions can also be combined in almost any way. To illustrate the versatility of this procedure, a few specific cases from the author's experience are described as follows.

A 65-year-old woman presented with a recurrent inverted papilloma of the left ethmoid and maxillary sinus. The tumor extended through the floor of the maxillary sinus into the orbit and through the roof of the ethmoid intracranially. The resection was planned to include the unilateral ethmoid with radical maxillectomy and orbital exenteration. The procedure was performed through the midface degloving approach with a circumferential incision around the eyelids. The intracranial bone cuts were through the right cribriform plate, the left orbital roof just inside the orbit, just posterior to the anterior wall of the sphenoid sinus, and anterior to the posterior wall of the frontal sinus. The palatal bone cut was made through the right floor of the nose and right central incisor. The orbital bone cuts were made at the junction of the floor and the lateral wall, posteriorly into the pterygomaxillary fissure at the level of the inferior orbital fissure, and along the junction of the left nasal bone and frontal process of the maxilla. The defect was repaired with a standard pericranial flap and a split-thickness skin graft.

A 45-year-old man had a squamous cell carcinoma of the left frontal and ethmoid sinuses without intracra-

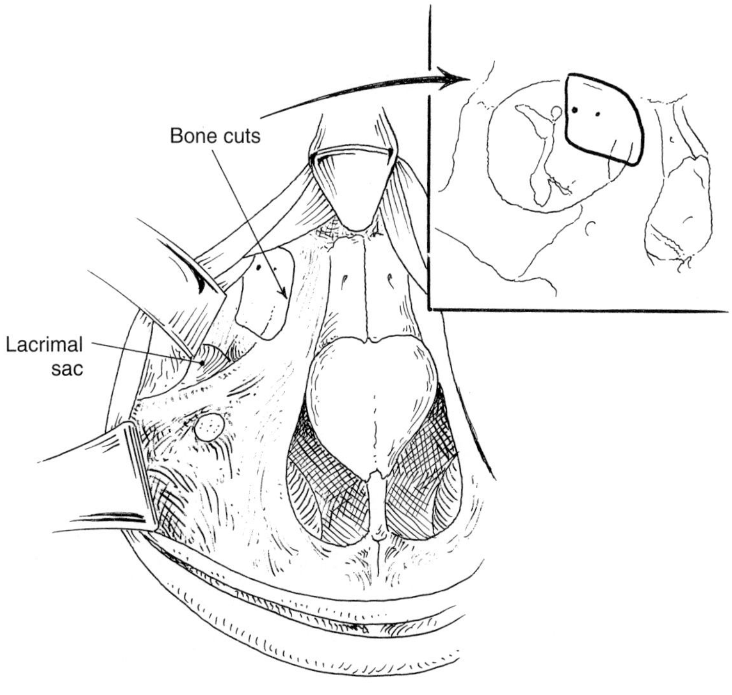

Figure 18–7. Orbital wall bone cuts for the standard unilateral ethmoidectomy. Note that this exposure is through a midfacial degloving approach, but it could be achieved through a lateral rhinotomy. The bone cuts incorporate the entire lamina papyracea.

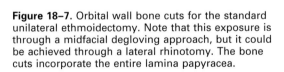

nial or orbital extension (Fig. 18–8). The surgical approach was through midfacial degloving and a bicoronal incision. The frontal bone flap extended around the left frontal sinus and down to the supraorbital rim to the right of midline. The intracranial bone cuts were made through the right cribriform plate and through the frontal sinus to connect to the frontal bone flap and were anterior to the sphenoid sinus. On the left side, bone cuts were made through the left orbital roof just inside the orbit up to the frontal sinus posterior wall, along the posterior wall of the frontal sinus, and anterior to the left orbital rim lateral to the frontal sinus. Reconstruction of the forehead was accomplished with split calvarial bone grafts. The skull base was repaired with a pericranial flap.

A 42-year-old man presented with massive recurrence of a basaloid adenocarcinoma after partial rhinectomy. The tumor filled the entire nasal cavity, extending through the nasal bones and skin, through both ethmoid sinuses up against the periorbita bilaterally, and through the cribriform plate, tenting up the dura but not through the dura. A complete resection was performed that included near-total rhinectomy, preserving the nasal tip only and bilateral ethmoid sinuses, resecting both periorbita but preserving both eyes (Fig. 18–9). The intracranial bone cuts were through the roof of both orbits, just inside the orbit anteriorly, through the orbital rims, and through the sphenoid sinus posterior to the anterior wall. The orbital dissection was inside the periorbita bilaterally, excising the entire medial wall, and through both inferior orbital rims medially into the pyriform aperture. Reconstruction was performed by a rectus abdominis free flap.

Reconstruction

Reconstruction requires several different considerations. The first consideration is management of the frontal sinus. In most cases, the sinus is cranialized. The upper part of the posterior wall is removed from the back of the frontal bone flap. The inside of the bone flap is then drilled down with a burr to remove any possible mucosal elements. Any residual posterior wall attached to the nasal frontal recess is removed with a rongeur. The ducts must then be obliterated. The mucosa within the ducts can be dissected from the walls and folded down into the nose. The recess can be blocked with bone chips, muscle, or fascia.

In all cases, intracranial reconstruction is necessary to separate the cranial cavity from the nasal cavity. In the minimal circumstance, a narrow cleft, essentially the width of the ethmoid sinus on one side, is needed. This

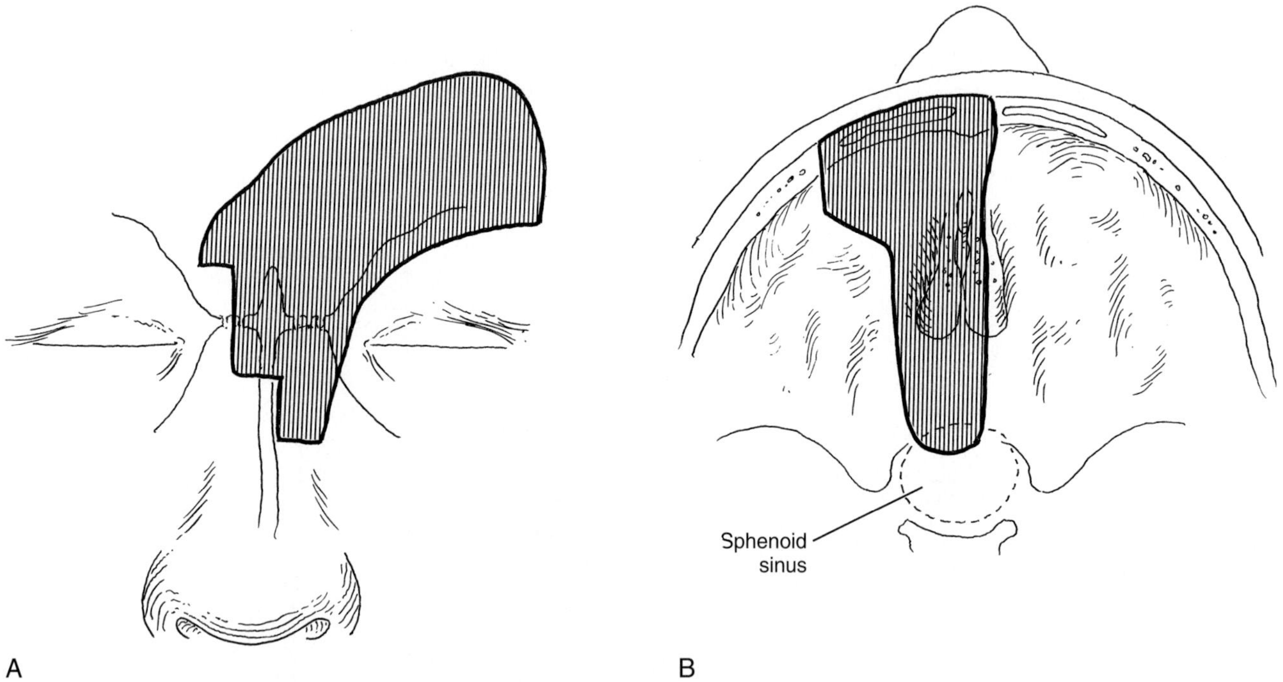

Figure 18–8. Craniofacial resection for a frontoethmoid sinus tumor. *A,* The anterior view demonstrates incorporation of the entire frontal sinus on the side of the tumor with the orbital rim and unilateral ethmoid sinus. The inferior edge of the frontal bone flap coincides with the planned superior cut of the resection. A frontal sinus template was used to delineate the line of resection. *B,* Bone cuts on the floor of the anterior cranial fossa. Note that this approach created a large skull base defect that was subsequently repaired by a split calvarial bone graft.

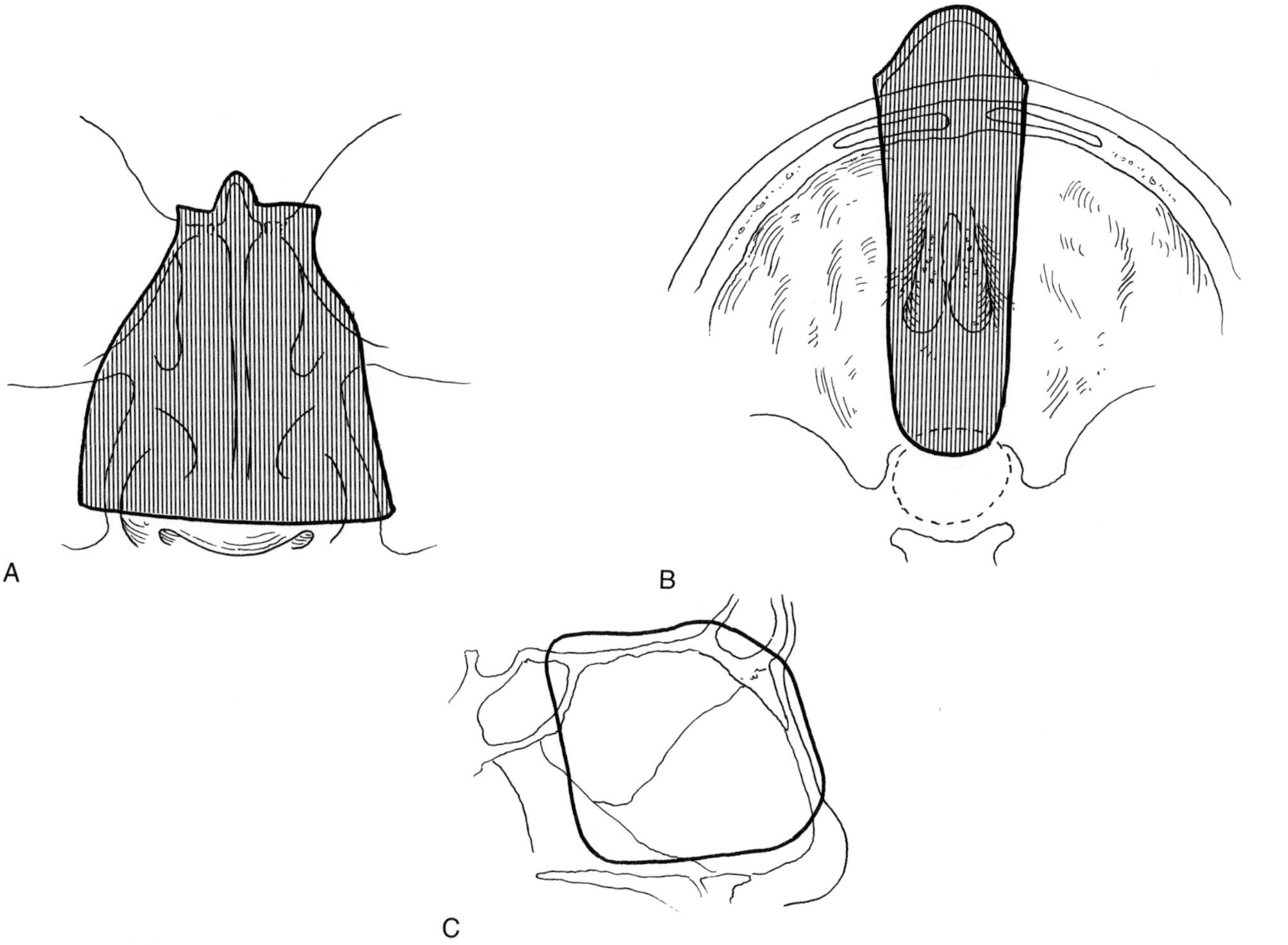

Figure 18–9. Craniofacial resection of a massive nasal tumor with near-total rhinectomy. *A,* Coronal view of the resection margins. Note the bilateral preservation of the orbits with resection of the lamina papyracea. *B,* Resection of the floor of the anterior cranial fossa. This included both ethmoids and the central skin of the glabella and nose. *C,* Midsagittal view showing inclusion of the nose up to the glabella and sparing of the nasal tip. Contrary to what is shown in the figure, the central portion of the hard palate was included in the resection.

is adequately reconstructed using a standard pericranial flap. The pericranial flap is elevated during initial bicoronal exposure. During reconstruction, the flap is laid down over the anterior skull base, covering the defect. The flap is sutured to the dura posterior to the defect or the posterior bone ledge of the skull base defect (Fig. 18–10). The undersurface of the flap can be covered with a split-thickness skin graft, and packing is placed to fill the nasal cavity. A large defect may require an additional layer to help support the frontal lobe, thereby preventing herniation. One possibility is to use both the pericranial flap and a temporal galeal flap. The temporal galeal flap is pulled down across the defect, sewing the flap to the edges as needed to stabilize the flap. The pericranial flap is placed as described earlier.

An alternative possibility for reconstructing the skull base is to use split calvarial bone grafts. This option is not normally required to provide adequate support for the skull base. However, if the defect is very large, bone grafts may lend a degree of additional security. The key to successful use is to make sure that the bone grafts are not open to the nasal cavity and are covered by vascularized tissues. The grafts do not need to be wired or plated in place, as the weight of the frontal lobe will hold the grafts in place. Defects in the supraorbital rims and frontal bone can be reconstructed with split calvarial bone grafts. In this case, the overlying bicoronal skin flap provides the vascular supply to the grafts. In this location, the grafts must be stabilized with wires or microplates.

In most cases, intranasal reconstruction is accomplished by lining the cavity with split-thickness skin grafts. The grafts are placed against the undersurface of the pericranial flap, against the orbital soft tissues, and against the pterygomaxillary fissure if exposed. The grafts are sutured into place using absorbable suture

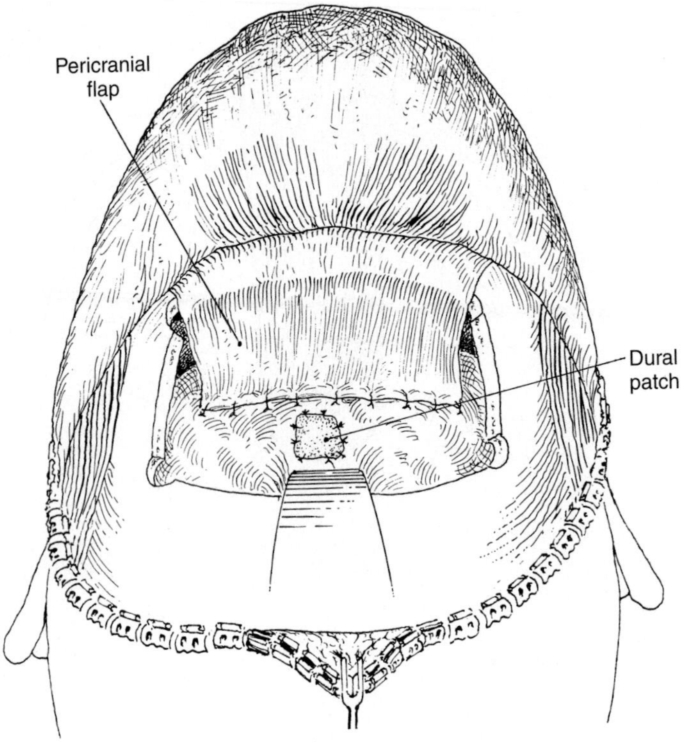

Figure 18–10. Reconstruction of the skull base with a pericranial flap. The flap is folded over the frontal sinus and sutured to the dura or bone posterior to the dural defect. The dural defect is then patched with a free fascial graft.

and are held against the surfaces by sufficient packing to fill the cavity.

Orbital reconstruction of the medial wall is sometimes required. This is especially true if the entire medial wall and adjacent periorbita is resected. In this case, without reconstruction, the orbit would sublux into the nose, resulting in enophthalmos and diplopia. The possibilities are to use a temporal galeal flap, a free fascial graft, or free bone grafts. The preferred technique is to use the temporal galeal flap. The flap is laid over the roof of the orbit, pulled over the medial orbit, and sutured to the bone of the floor of the orbit (Fig. 18–11). Free fascial grafts can be used if the temporal flap is not available. The grafts are sutured to the bone above and below the medial wall under enough tension to push the eye into the desired position. The final alternative is to use a split calvarial bone graft. This is wedged under the bone of the floor of the orbit and levered against the opposite orbit (Fig. 18–12).

Finally, there is a possibility of using revascularized free tissue transfer. These flaps are most useful in the case of large facial defects including orbital exenteration or when significant skin resection is required. In these cases, the options for reconstruction are either a free flap or a prosthetic device to fill the defect. The advantage of the free flap is that it minimizes postoperative care and cleaning. The cosmetic appearance is less than optimal, but can be masked by an eye patch. Prosthetic reconstruction simulates the normal appearance initially, but the prosthesis tends to slip, wear, and discolor over time. For this reason, many experienced skull base surgeons have come to prefer free flap reconstruction after orbital exenteration.

Prior to beginning closure, the final step in the reconstruction is to address the dead space anterior to the frontal lobe. Some surgeons maintain that it is not necessary to do anything. The theory is that this space between the frontal lobe and the frontal bone flap will fill in with serum, which will eventually be replaced by fibrous tissue and forward expansion of the frontal lobe. This process is uncertain and uncontrolled, however. For this reason, obliterating the dead space with a free fat graft has been suggested as an alternative.

Closure

The first step in closure is to replace the frontal bone flap. This will usually fit snugly back into the proper position. It is important to make sure that the inferior edge of the bone flap does not constrict the pericranial flap. The pericranial flap folds down over the supraorbital rim and under the bone flap. If the bone flap is pulled too tightly against the supraorbital rims, the pericranial flap can be compromised. It may be necessary to use a cutting burr to create a gap. The flap can be secured with any of several different techniques. The simplest method is to use wires. Small drill holes are placed in the bone flap and adjacent stationary skull. The wire is passed through both holes and twisted down to hold the bone flap in place. An alternative is to use

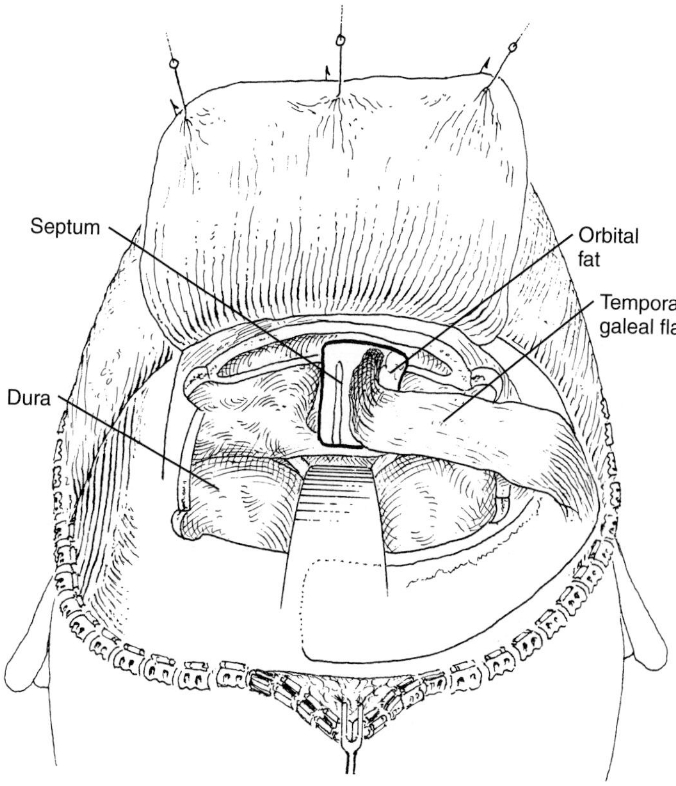

Figure 18–11. Reconstruction of the medial wall of the orbit with a temporal galeal flap. The flap is tucked through the defect and sutured to the floor of the orbit to recreate the medial orbital wall.

microreconstruction plates. These plates can be placed at various points around the bone flap. The plate is molded into position and a drill is used to place holes into the bone. Monocortical screws are then used to stabilize the plate. A third option is to use micromesh. Several small pieces of mesh can be shaped to overlap the osteotomy site. Each piece of mesh requires 6 to 10 screws to be effective. The advantages of the plates and mesh are that they are flat, have a low profile, and provide excellent stabilization.

After the bone flap is in place, the bicoronal incision can be closed. This is done in two layers: a deep layer of 3-0 absorbable interrupted sutures and staples for the skin layer. The deeper layer should approximate the galea, but does not need to include the dermis. Placing the sutures too superficially results in a high rate of extrusion of the sutures postoperatively. Normally, the bicoronal flap is drained by two suction drains. After craniofacial resection, however, this is inadvisable, as the drains may pull air or nasal contents through the skull base into the subcutaneous plane. This can lead to infection and late intracranial complications. It is better, therefore, to minimize postoperative bleeding by ensuring meticulous hemostasis.

Before the facial incisions are closed, the cavity must be packed from below. The operative cavity should be completely filled to apply pressure against the skin grafts and bone surfaces. This will improve the hemostasis, stabilize the skin grafts, and prevent air leakage into the intracranial cavity. This last aspect is very important, especially if a lumbar drain is going to be used. If an air leak is present and a lumbar drain is in place, the patient will develop a pneumocephalus. This is discussed in detail in the later section on complications. Several different packing materials can be used for the resection cavity. One possibility is to use cotton or a synthetic conforming fiber that acts like cotton. This can be soaked with mineral oil and wrapped with iodine-impregnated gauze. Traditional nasal packing is also a possibility. Six-foot lengths of Vaseline-coated strip gauze is available commercially in plastic tubes or in 12-foot lengths in bottles. In either case, most cavities are large enough to require several lengths tied together. The advantage of the strip gauze is that it conforms perfectly to the shape of the cavity, allowing the pack to be tight and occlusive.

The final closure of the facial incisions is performed last. This is described in detail in Chapter 16 in the section on skull base approaches. If the midface degloving approach has been used, the sublabial sutures are placed and then the intranasal sutures are sewn to complete the procedure. If the lateral rhinotomy has been used, the lip is closed at the vermilion border and then a two-layer closure of the incision is performed. The procedure is completed by placement of a nasal splint over the dorsum and a dressing over the head. When a head dressing is used, a classic Barton's-type head wrap is placed.

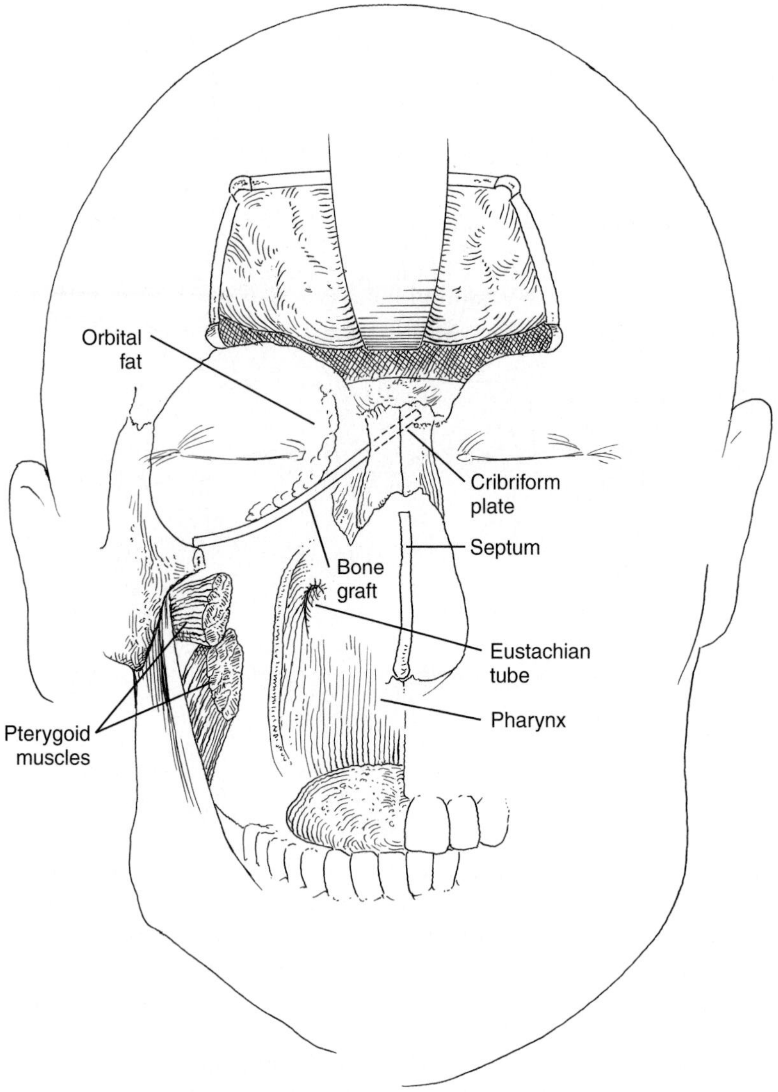

Figure 18–12. Reconstruction after a maxillectomy with craniofacial resection and orbital preservation. A split calvarial graft is levered between the lateral orbital wall and the opposite cribriform plate. If possible, the undersurface of the bone graft should be covered with a temporal muscle flap folded over the zygomatic arch and under the eye.

POSTOPERATIVE CARE

The postoperative care of the patient undergoing craniofacial surgery is among the most complicated in all of medicine. Intensive care unit (ICU) monitoring is mandatory for all patients for a minimum of 2 days. Most patients will require 3 to 5 days of such monitoring before being transferred out of the ICU. Management considerations include virtually all body systems, each of which is covered in brief.

All such patients arrive in the ICU with mechanical ventilation. The airway is maintained by either an oral endotracheal tube or a tracheostomy. Tracheostomy is not routinely performed, but may be necessary for certain patients. In the absence of a tracheostomy, the endotracheal tube can be removed as early as the morning after surgery. The night of surgery, it is best to maintain mechanical ventilation of the patient, with adequate sedation provided to ensure comfort. This approach has the advantages of allowing hyperventilation, maintaining adequate oxygenation, and protecting the airway from blood and secretions. The morning after surgery, if everything is otherwise stable, the sedation can be discontinued and the patient allowed to wake up fully. If the patient attains normal mental status, a ventilatory wean can be initiated. If the mental status is not normal, this may be attributable to cerebral edema, in which case continued mechanical ventilation is required until the mental status clears.

Intracranial pressure (ICP) must be carefully controlled after surgery. The degree of elevation of the ICP depends largely on the nature of the surgery. The elevation of ICP after these procedures is directly related to the amount of cerebral edema that occurs. If the operation remains extradural and brain retraction is minimal, cerebral edema may be absent and the ICP may not be elevated. However, when extensive dural resection is necessary and prolonged brain retraction is required, cerebral edema may be significant, and the ICP may be substantially elevated. In most cases, treatment to minimize cerebral edema is advisable. This will help the patient recover more quickly and will help to avoid brain damage. Measures to minimize the ICP include hyperventilation, CSF drainage, and administration of steroids and/or mannitol. Hyperventilation is effective because it leads to vasoconstriction of the cerebral vessels. Hyperventilation is achieved by increasing the respiratory rate on the ventilator to a level sufficient to lower the P_{CO_2} to within the range of 30 to 35. More drastic hyperventilation is generally not advocated. CSF drainage is normally achieved by a lumbar catheter, which is placed before the surgery. After the operation, 20 mL of CSF is drained every 2 hours. This decompresses the ventricles and also minimizes the risk of CSF leak. Steroids have a systemic effect of decreasing tissue edema and also carry the benefit of minimizing brain edema. Finally, mannitol draws fluid out of the interstitial spaces of the brain tissue, which has the direct effect of decreasing brain size and minimizing edema and ICP.

When the patient is slow to wake up or has a diminished level of consciousness, increased ICP is indicated. Immediate evaluation is necessary. The most important test is to obtain an emergency CT scan. The CT scan may demonstrate diffuse edema, hematoma, cerebrovascular accident, or pneumocephalus. Other tests may include CSF sampling for blood and meningitis, and electroencephalography (EEG). These tests can exclude infection and seizures as the cause of the mental status changes. Finally, an arteriogram or MRI (MRA) can be obtained if other tests indicate a possible vascular problem.

To prevent seizures, most patients receive phenytoin in the operating room or before surgery. The phenytoin is continued for the first few weeks or months after the surgery until the risk of seizures is determined to be minimal. If the patient has a known hypersensitivity to phenytoin, an alternative agent can be used.

Control of blood pressure and monitoring of the heart function are also critical. Patients with any history of cardiac disease should have a Swan-Ganz catheter placed for optimal monitoring. Other patients should at least have a central venous line in place to monitor the central venous pressure. This is necessary to maintain proper hydration status. To minimize cerebral edema, mannitol is administered. This is a diuretic and will have a tendency to lower the intravascular volume. Central monitoring is necessary to make sure the central venous pressure is maintained at adequate levels to keep cardiac performance optimal. Continuous arterial pressure monitoring through a radial arterial catheter helps to control the blood pressure. It is important to keep the blood pressure at normal levels to decrease the risk of bleeding. Even moderate hypertension can lead to development of a hematoma, requiring reoperation. If needed, medication to control the blood pressure is given. A bladder catheter to monitor urinary output is always used.

All of the available information is used to help determine the appropriate amount of intravenous fluid to deliver. This determination is critical to the effective postoperative management of the patient undergoing craniofacial surgery. Excess fluid can lead to prolonged cerebral edema, heart failure, and difficulty with oxygenation. These factors all have the potential of increasing the severity of brain damage. Inadequate fluid may lead to low urine output, uremia, hypotension, and poor cerebral perfusion. This complex situation requires an experienced ICU team to manage the patient properly.

Wound management begins in the operating room with proper packing and dressing of the bicoronal incision. The dressing should be changed the first day after surgery to allow inspection of the bicoronal flap and incision. After 48 hours, the dressings are discontinued, as they are no longer necessary to help prevent hematoma. The incisions are cleaned and covered with antibiotic ointment twice each day. Packing is usually left in place for 5 days, which is the optimal duration for protecting the skull base closure, allowing sufficient healing to prevent CSF leak, and ensuring hemostasis. Longer periods increase the risk of packing-related infection. The packing is grossly contaminated, so after about 5 days, it will begin to become a source of bacteria that can infect the skull base closure. When the packing is removed, cavity care must begin. On the first day after packing removal, only suctioning of secretions and blood clots is necessary. After this, manual cleaning of the cavity is required weekly. Irrigating the cavity can begin once the skull base is healed and CSF leak is no longer a concern. The irrigations will help the cavity heal and will decrease the amount of crust that accumulates. However, many patients with craniofacial resection will have long-term problems associated with crusting within the cavity. Cleaning the cavity, therefore, may become a regular and necessary postoperative regimen carried out by the surgeon.

Postoperative pain is a major issue for the patient. Early after the surgery, while the patient is in the ICU, intravenous morphine is favored. Under these conditions, pain can be optimally controlled by allowing the nurse to interact with the patient to determine the interval and dose that will be most effective. However, when the patient leaves the ICU, nursing care is not constant and frequent intravenous injections by the ward nurse are not possible. At this point, patient-controlled analgesia (PCA) is a favored option. This gives the conscious and oriented patient the ability to control the dosing. After the first week, the patient is usually converted to an oral agent for pain control. At this time, the intensity of the pain is often decreased enough to allow a codeine combination or equivalent-strength medication to suffice. Some patients will develop long-term chronic head pain after craniofacial resection. These patients will require a more sophisticated approach to pain management, including referral to a head pain clinic.

Nutrition is a major concern for the postoperative patient. Whenever possible, it is best to utilize the normal gastrointestinal tract for nutrition. Unfortunately, it is not possible to use a nasogastric tube in any of these patients. Early after the surgery, if the patient is unable to tolerate an oral diet, some type of nutritional support will be required. One possibility is to use an oral gastric tube. Alternatively, a gastrostomy tube can be placed. If a gastric tube feeding is not possible, the patient can receive intravenous alimentation. These options should be considered before the surgery and specific plans made to avoid long delays in instituting nutritional support.

COMPLICATIONS

Mortality

Craniofacial resection is one of the most morbid operations performed in all of surgery. For otolaryngologists, and specifically for rhinologists, this is perhaps the riskiest operation performed. Overall complication rates range from 25% to 63%,[28–31] with perioperative mortality rates ranging from 1.3% to 7.7%.[11, 12, 32] In most series, the predominant cause of death is intracranial complications. Although the risk of mortality is low in most series, the surgeon cannot escape the fact that all of the largest series in the literature report mortalities. This is important information to convey, not to dissuade the patient from undergoing the procedure, but to make sure that proper informed consent is obtained and that the decision to pursue this type of surgery is carefully thought out in advance.

Intracranial Complications

The complications of craniofacial resection can be divided into intracranial complications, extracranial complications, and systemic complications. The possible intracranial complications include cerebral edema, intracranial bleeding, cerebrovascular accident (CVA), CSF leak, pneumocephalus, meningitis, brain abscess, seizures, and altered mental status.

Cerebral edema, to some extent, is expected after craniofacial resection. The degree is usually related to the duration of brain retraction and the amount of cerebral resection. Some patients, however, develop cerebral edema unrelated to these factors. The reasons for this are probably poor fluid management, rough retraction, or injury during the craniotomy. Cerebral edema is managed by CSF drainage, steroids, mannitol, and hyperventilation. In most cases, this will result in eventual resolution of the edema. The amount of time necessary to resolve cerebral edema will vary with the severity of the problem, but may take as little as 1 day or as long as several weeks.

Intracranial bleeding can occur in the subdural space, the subarachnoid space, or within the brain parenchyma. This is a rare but potentially devastating complication and that is one of the most common causes of death or severe brain damage in patients undergoing craniofacial resection.[11–13] Bleeding may occur as a result of technical mistakes in attaining hemostasis or from coagulopathy. Fortunately, the incidence rate is low, ranging from less than 1% to 4.4%.[11, 12] When hematoma is diagnosed, this is always an indication for reoperation to drain the hematoma.

CVA is a surprisingly infrequent complication of craniofacial resection. It is seen in less than 1% of cases in most series.[12] The cause of all CVAs is cerebral ischemia. The incidence of this problem is related to the degree of retraction on the brain. The greater the retraction, the higher the risk of prolonged ischemia and, eventually, infarction. The diagnosis of CVA is suggested when the patient is slow to wake up after the operation or demonstrates focal neurologic deficits. A CT scan or MRI will reveal a focal lucency in the brain parenchyma. Management of CVA includes minimizing cerebral edema and eventual rehabilitation.

CSF leak is a well-known complication of craniofacial resection. Every patient who has this operation is at risk for this problem owing to the elevation of the dura over the cribriform plate. This results in cutting the olfactory nerves, which opens the subarachnoid space. The skull base repair is normally successful, with the multilayered reconstruction including primary closure of the dural defect, pericranial flap, and skin graft. However, owing to failure of the closure, CSF leak can be expected to occur periodically. Some series do not report any CSF leaks.[13, 14] However, most series report a significant incidence ranging from 3.8% to 13.7%.[11, 12, 30] The reason for this fairly broad range is unknown. Differences in technique and/or case selection are probably the primary reasons. Patients with relatively small defects who have not had previous irradiation and surgery are more likely to heal. Conversely, postradiation patients and those with larger defects are more likely to have problems with wound healing including CSF leak. The key to management of a CSF leak is to control the leak before the patient develops meningitis. Treatment is with lumbar drainage and direct repair of the defect if it does not stop within 5 to 7 days after surgery. Repair of CSF leak is covered in detail in a later chapter. Such leaks may require subsequent craniotomy or a free flap if transnasal repair is not possible.

Pneumocephalus is a rare but serious complication. Cantu and colleagues, in their series of 91 patients, had the highest reported incidence at 7%, whereas other series have failed to report any cases.[11–14] Pneumocephalus may occur from the patient coughing, blowing the nose, or sneezing before the skull base is healed. An alternative etiology is related to an imperfect seal of the skull base with continuous lumbar drainage that pulls air through the skull base intracranially. Pneumocephalus is indicated by a sudden change in mental status in the postoperative period. A CT scan will show the obvious intracranial air in locations not expected. Air can sometimes be seen in the frontal area for a few days or weeks after the surgery. However, air should not be located in the ventricles or along the skull base after the first few hours after the operation. Treatment involves discontinuing the lumbar drain and packing the cavity to prevent air leakage. One rare variation of this complication is tension pneumocephalus.[33] This occurs when a ball-valve mechanism traps air under pressure in the epidural space. Prompt recognition and treatment by aspiration of the air and diversion of the airway is necessary to prevent brain damage.

Perhaps the most feared complication of craniofacial resection is meningitis. Because of the intraoperative connection between the nasal cavity and the intracranial space, the risk of meningeal infection is always present. Meningitis occurs most frequently when the patient develops a CSF leak. However, it can also be caused by direct contamination during the surgery, by spread of a sinus infection after the procedure, or from contamination by the lumbar drain. Meningitis occurs in less than 5% of patients in most series, but the incidence has been reported to be as high as 14%.[30] The diagnosis is suggested by fever, nuchal rigidity, and altered mental status. Diagnosis is confirmed by obtaining CSF for cell count, glucose and protein levels, and culture. The glucose level is usually low, the protein level is usually high, and the cell counts show increased lymphocytes and neutrophils. Although gram staining may initially yield negative results, culture results should be positive. The most common organisms are those common to sinusitis. Treatment is by adequate intravenous antibiotics, guided by the results of gram stains and cultures, and subsequent repair of any ongoing CSF leak.

Brain abscess is a rare complication of craniofacial resection[12] that occurs only if infection spreads into the brain from an external source, such as the sinuses, from meningitis, or from a blood-borne organism from a distant site. The diagnosis is suggested by spiking fevers, headache, and altered mental status. CT scan will reveal a ring-enhancing mass in the brain parenchyma. Treatment consists of intravenous antibiotics and, usually, drainage of the abscess.

Seizures after these operations are always a possibility. Seizure activity in the brain can be initiated as a result of irritation, inflammation, or brain damage. Systemic alterations in electrolytes or calcium level can exacerbate or cause seizures. To prevent this problem, all patients are treated with prophylactic antiseizure medication, the most common of which is phenytoin. If phenytoin is not applicable to an individual patient, many alternatives are also available. It is important to make sure that the serum levels of the drug are optimal to prevent seizures. An optimal duration of treatment has not been well established. Often, the medication is started 2 to 3 days before the operation in order to ensure that adequate levels have been achieved at the time of surgery. After the operation, at least 2 to 3 weeks of continued treatment is advisable.

The final intracranial complication is altered mental status. This does not refer to the short-term effects of the medications and cerebral edema, but the permanent changes that can occur. This is the single most common problem associated with this surgery. The reported rate of mental status alterations varies from as low as 3%[12] to as high as 22%.[30] The differences in these rates may be related to the type of resections that are performed, as well as the threshold for determining changes. If careful memory and personality evaluations are conducted, perhaps as many as one third of these patients will have some measurable change in mental capacity. However, the number of patients that develop significant alterations in mental status is much less. The minimal effect observed is a mild alteration in personality. This can vary from emotional lability to blunting of affect. Loss of some degree of short-term memory is fairly common and may be manifested as forgetfulness, rather than loss of orientation. The causes of this problem are numerous and can include direct trauma during surgery, actual brain resection, or any one of the intracranial complications discussed earlier. There is no specific treatment for this loss of mental capacity. Sometimes, rehabilitation will help the patient regain some function. Time seems to be the best remedy available.

Extracranial Complications

The extracranial complications include those associated with the surgery itself and those related to medical complications. The surgical extracranial complications include bone flap, facial, and sinus infections; wound healing problems; orbital complications; cranial nerve injuries; bleeding problems; and cosmetic alterations. The most important local infectious complication of craniofacial resection is infection of the frontal bone flap. This usually only occurs if there is breakdown of either the bicoronal flap or the skull base closure, leading to late contamination of the bone flap. However, there are cases when the bone flap becomes infected during the surgery. The incidence of infection of the bone flap varies from 2% to 11% depending on the series.[11–14, 30] When it does occur, this is a major problem. Treatment requires removal of the bone flap, long-term antibiotic therapy, and delayed reconstructive cranioplasty. There is a high risk of meningitis when the bone flap is infected. Prevention of the spread of this infection to a life-threatening intracranial infection is dependent on early recognition and prompt, aggressive intervention.

Other infections include sinusitis, facial soft tissue infection, and neck infection. The most common of these infections is sinusitis. The short- and long-term rates of sinus infection after craniofacial resection are not precisely known. Many patients have low-grade, chronic infections that never become clinically severe enough to warrant specific treatment; severe, acute infections are probably rare. Facial soft tissue and neck infections are very rare. These problems may be related to wound infection of the lateral rhinotomy incision. Treatment is best effected by draining the wound and administering appropriate intravenous antibiotics.

Wound healing problems are among the most common complications after craniofacial resection. Cavity problems are common enough not to be considered complications. Failure of skin grafts occurs to some extent in most patients. This is managed by frequent cleaning of the cavity and daily irrigation to remove crust and debris. Seroma and hematoma under the bicoronal flap are also common. Most of the time, these fluid collections can be aspirated without risk of recurrence or infection. Localized breakdown of the skin incisions is not common, but can occur. When it does occur, routine dressing changes will normally result in healing within a few weeks.

Orbital complications may occur when the eye is preserved. Indeed, with orbital preservation, the eye is at risk for numerous problems, including epiphora and diplopia. Double vision can occur owing to displacement of the orbit secondary to the loss of medial and, in some cases, inferior support. To prevent diplopia, the eye must be resuspended to the normal anatomic position using fascial and skin grafts. This is particularly challenging when the orbital wall and orbital periosteum are both removed during surgery. The other limiting factor is the amount of orbital wall that is removed. The greater the portion of the orbital floor that is removed, the harder it is to suspend the eye in the precise position necessary to avoid diplopia. Other orbital problems include hematoma, optic neuritis, and infections. Hematoma can be caused by bleeding from the anterior and posterior ethmoid arteries or from the orbital fat. Immediate recognition and orbital decompression are necessary to save the eye. Optic nerve inflammation or injury can be caused by retraction damage, direct trauma to the nerve, or infection in the orbit. Management of optic nerve problems requires ophthalmologic consultation, and steroid and antibiotic therapy is often prescribed. Infection in the orbit may involve the conjunctiva or orbital soft tissues. Antibiotics and ocular drops are usually prescribed to treat this. The final orbital complication is lacrimal obstruction leading to epiphora. This occurs because the nasolacrimal duct is often transected during surgery. In this situation, the duct usually remains open. If lacrimal obstruction does occur, dacryocystorhinostomy is performed to correct the problem.

Cranial nerve injuries are common after craniofacial resection. In all cases, cranial nerve I, the olfactory nerve, is transected. This is part of the procedure and so is not considered a complication. However, depending on the nature of the procedure, cranial nerves II through VI could be removed in the operation. The frontal branch of the facial nerve is susceptible to injury during the elevation of the bicoronal flap. Lower cranial nerves are only at risk if the neck or the posterior fossa is involved in the surgery. Even when the lower cranial nerves are not directly involved in the operation, patients may still have problems with pharyngeal function owing to altered mental status or intracranial injury to the brain resulting in loss of nerve function.

Postoperative bleeding is a rare problem after craniofacial resection. This is because the resected cavity is always firmly packed after the operation. Despite this, there have been rare reports of significant bleeding in the postoperative period. Such bleeding must be controlled immediately either by coagulation, ligation, or packing.

Cosmetic problems are very common after these operations. Aside from the defect associated with orbital exenteration, facial asymmetry is the most likely result. In addition, there are potential problems with defects of the forehead skull owing to burr holes and osteotomies. Frontal bossing and concavity may be caused by either frontal periosteal reaction or reabsorption. Problems associated with closure of the lateral rhinotomy, covered in detail in Chapter 16, include lip notching, hypertrophy, and retraction of the cheek or medial canthus.

Medical Complications

Medical complications are particularly common after craniofacial resection. The most serious of these is myocardial infarction. The risk of myocardial infarction is related to the preoperative condition of the heart. Heart failure, unstable angina, arrhythmia, and previous myocardial infarction in the last 6 months are associated with an increased risk of cardiac morbidity with general anesthesia, regardless of the surgery. The presence of any of these risk factors is a relative contraindication to surgery.

The most common medical problem after major head and neck surgery is pneumonia. This is caused by aspiration. Patients who have secretions in the pharynx, are in a supine position, or have altered mental status are at high risk for aspiration. Fever, productive cough, and physical signs of pneumonia on chest auscultation support the presumptive diagnosis. A chest radiograph is confirmatory. Treatment includes intravenous antibiotics guided by sputum cultures, incentive spirometry, and chest physiotherapy. Respiratory support, including oxygen or mechanical respiration, is provided as needed.

Other infections may also occur, including urinary tract infection and infection of an intravenous catheter site. These relatively common problems may be diagnosed by urinalysis with urine culture and physical examination of the intravenous site, respectively. Treatment of the urinary infection requires appropriate antibiotics. Infected thrombophlebitis is treated by removal of the catheter and subsequent antibiotics.

Finally, there are a number of medical complications that occur only rarely. Deep vein thrombophlebitis, renal failure, and liver failure are among the possibilities. Prophylaxis for deep vein thrombophlebitis is widely advocated to avoid this problem. In most centers, sequential compression stockings are now preferred over subcutaneous, low-dose heparin or aspirin suppositories. This specialized compression apparatus places an inflatable plastic garment around the patient's legs up to the level of the groin. The compression stockings are attached to a pump that sequentially inflates the lower, then the upper portion of each leg to "milk" the blood out of the legs. As soon as the patient is able to ambulate, these stockings are removed and the period of risk should be over. Renal failure and liver failure have no specific relationship to this surgery but can occur with any major surgery in the presence of other complications that affect renal or liver function.

REFERENCES

1. Dandy WE. Orbital tumors: Results following the transcranial operative attack. New York: Oskar Priest, 1941, p. 1554.
2. Ketcham AS, Wilkins RH, Van Buren JM, et al. A combined intracranial facial approach to the paranasal sinuses. Am J Surg 106:698, 1963.
3. Edgerton MT, Snyder GB. Combined intracranial-extracranial approach and use of the two stage split flap technique for reconstruction with craniofacial malignancies. Am J Surg 110(4):595, 1965.
4. Johns ME, Winn HR, McLean WC, et al. Pericranial flap for the closure of defect of craniofacial resection. Laryngoscope 91(6): 952, 1981.
5. Arbit E, Sundaresan N, Galicich JH, et al. Craniofacial resection following chemotherapy. Surg Neurol 13(5):395, 1980.
6. Donald PJ. Recent advances in paranasal sinus surgery. Head Neck Surg 4(2):146, 1981.
7. Sasaki CT, Ariyan S, Spencer D, et al. Pectoralis major myocutaneous reconstruction of the anterior skull base. Laryngoscope 95(2):162, 1985.
8. Schaefer SD, Close LG, Mickey BE. Axial subcutaneous scalp flaps in the reconstruction of the anterior cranial fossa. Arch Otolaryngol Head Neck Surg 112(7):745, 1986.
9. Bridger GP, Baldwin M, Gonski A. Craniofacial resection for paranasal sinus cancer with free flap repair. Aust NZ J Surg 56(11):843, 1986.
10. Angel MF, Bridges RM, Levine PA, et al. The serratus anterior free tissue transfer for craniofacial reconstruction. J Craniofac Surg 3(4):207, 1992.
11. Canto G, Solero CL, Mariani L, et al. Anterior craniofacial resection for malignant ethmoid tumors—A series of 91 patients. Head Neck 21:185, 1999.
12. Lund VJ, Howard DJ, Wei WI, et al. Craniofacial resection for tumors of the nasal cavity and paranasal sinuses— A 17-year experience. Head Neck 20:97, 1998.
13. Shah JP, Kraus DH, Bilsky MH, et al. Craniofacial resection for malignant tumors involving the anterior skull base. Arch Otolaryngol Head Neck Surg 123:1312, 1997.
14. Levine PA, Debo RF, Meredith SD, et al. Craniofacial resection at the University of Virginia (1976–1992): Survival analysis. Head Neck 16:574, 1994.
15. Harrison DFN. Surgical pathology of olfactory neuroblastoma. Head Neck Surg 7:60, 1984.
16. Eden BV, Debo RF, Lamer JM, et al. Esthesioneuroblastoma. Long-term outcome and patterns of failure—The University of Virginia experience. Cancer 73:2556, 1994.
17. Dulguerov P, Calcaterra T. Esthesioneuroblastoma: The UCLA experience 1970–1990. Laryngoscope 102:843, 1992.
18. Morita A, Ebersold MJ, Olsen KD, et al. Esthesioneuroblastoma: Prognosis and management. Neurosurgery 32:706, 1993.
19. Bhattacharyya N, Thornton AF, Joseph MP, et al. Successful treatment of esthesioneuroblastoma and neuroendocrine carcinoma with combined chemotherapy and proton radiation. Results in 9 cases. Arch Otolaryngol Head Neck Surg 123:34, 1997.
20. Yoskovitch A, Braverman I, Nachtigal D, et al. Sinonasal schneiderian papilloma. J Otolaryngol 27(3):122, 1998.
21. Raveh E, Feinmesser R, Shpitzer T, et al. Inverted papilloma of the nose and paranasal sinuses: A study of 56 cases and review of the literature. Isr J Med Sci 32(12):1163, 1996.
22. Lawson W, Ho BT, Shaari CM, et al. Inverted papilloma: A report of 112 cases. Laryngoscope 105(3 Pt 1):282, 1995.
23. Bielamowicz S, Calcaterra TC, Watson D. Inverting papilloma of the head and neck: The UCLA update. Otolaryngol Head Neck Surg 109:71, 1993.
24. Phillips CD, Futterer SF, Lipper MH, et al. Sinonasal undifferentiated carcinoma: CT and MR imaging of an uncommon neoplasm of the nasal cavity. Radiology 202(2):477, 1997.
25. Chang SC, Chen PK, Chen YR, et al. Treatment of frontal sinus osteoma using a craniofacial approach. Ann Plast Surg 38(5): 455, 1997.
26. Chang SC, Chen PK, Chen YR, et al. Treatment of frontal sinus osteoma using a craniofacial approach. Ann Plast Surg 38(5): 455, 1997.
27. Kumon Y, Zenke K, Ohta S, et al. Operative results in fourteen cases of paranasal sinus and anterior cranial fossa lesions surgically treated by an extended transbasal approach. No Shinkei Geka 23(10):889, 1995.
28. Irish J, Dasgupta R, Freeman J, et al. Outcome and analysis of the surgical management of esthesioneuroblastoma. J Otolaryngol 26:1, 1997.
29. Bilsky MH, Kraus DH, Strong EW, et al. Extended anterior craniofacial resection for intracranial extension of malignant tumors. Am J Surg 174(5):565, 1997.
30. Catalano PJ, Hecht CS, Biller HF, et al. Craniofacial resection. An analysis of 73 cases. Arch Otolaryngol Head Neck Surg 120(11):1203, 1994.
31. Van Tuyl R, Gussack GS. Prognostic factors in craniofacial surgery. Laryngoscope 101(3):240, 1991.
32. McCutcheon IE, Blacklock JB, Weber RS, et al. Anterior transcranial (craniofacial) resection of tumors of the paranasal sinuses: Surgical technique and results. Neurosurgery 38(3):471, 1996.
33. Wanamaker JR, Mehle ME, Wood BG, et al. Tension pneumocephalus following craniofacial resection. Head Neck 17(2):152, 1995.

CHAPTER 19

Approaches for Pituitary Surgery

Pituitary surgery is traditionally within the realm of the neurosurgeon. However, since the reintroduction of the transseptal transsphenoidal approach to the sella turcica for resection of pituitary adenoma, otolaryngologists have been active partners in the surgical management of these patients. Originally performed entirely by neurosurgeons, in the past decades, otolaryngologists have lent their expertise in nasal and sinus surgery, assisting the neurosurgeon with the operation. The otolaryngologist has the advantage of familiarity with the techniques and instruments used to gain exposure of the sella turcica. In most centers today, pituitary surgery is performed jointly by a neurosurgeon and an otolaryngologist. The otolaryngologist provides the exposure, and the neurosurgeon resects the tumor. Then, the otolaryngologist returns to close the wounds and repair any damage to the nasal structures. Such collaboration has resulted in decreased rates of septal perforation, cerebrospinal fluid (CSF) leak, and functional nasal problems.[1–3]

HISTORY

The first pituitary surgeries were performed in the late 1890s through a middle cranial fossa approach.[4] This technique quickly gave way to variations of the transseptal approach as described by Hirsch and Kanavel.[5, 6] Cushing later refined the sublabial transseptal approach, decreasing the mortality rate to 5.6%.[4] However, refinements in intracranial surgery soon led to the development of the subfrontal approach. In 1939, Henderson reported improved tumor control rates with the subfrontal approach.[7] This became the dominant technique until Hardy reintroduced the sublabial approach in 1968.[8] Since Hardy's contribution, continuing developments in technology and technique have led to the transnasal approaches becoming established as the standard of care for most cases of hypophysectomy today.

DIAGNOSIS

Pituitary tumors can be classified by either function, histologic features, or tumor extent. Functional classifications are based on the hormone that is secreted by the tumor. The most common are the nonsecreting tumors and the prolactin-secreting tumors (prolactinomas). Adrenocorticotropin (ACTH)-secreting tumors cause Cushing's disease, whereas growth hormone (GH)–secreting tumors are associated with acromegaly. Thyroid-stimulating hormone (TSH)–secreting tumors are rare but have been described.[9] The histologic classification of pituitary tumors is based on the staining characteristics of the predominant cell type. This classification includes chromophobes, eosinophilic (acidophilic), and basophilic tumor types. Typically, the chromophobes are nonsecreting or prolactin-secreting tumors, the ACTH-secreting tumors are basophilic, and the GH-secreting tumors are acidophilic. These associations are tendencies, and are not absolute. Mixed populations and atypical patterns are frequently found. Finally, these tumors can be classified based on the extent of the tumor (Table 19–1). Each of these classifications is found in the literature. For clinical purposes, they describe different aspects of the tumor and are complementary, not exclusive.

Pituitary tumors may be suspected on the basis of local effects of the tumor, the presence of one of the hormone-secreting syndromes, or incidentally, as a finding on a brain scan. In the case of a hormone-secreting tumor, the diagnosis is suggested by a clinical syndrome and confirmed by an imaging study and serum hormone levels. There are three well-known hormonal syndromes associated with pituitary adenomas.

TABLE 19–1
Staging of Pituitary Tumor

I. Enclosed microadenoma—normal sella
II. Enclosed adenoma—sella enlarged, but intact
III. Localized invasive adenoma—sella enlarged with focal erosion of the floor
IV. Diffuse invasive adenoma—erosion of the entire floor of the sella
  A. Small amount of suprasellar extension filling only the suprachiasmatic cistern
  B. Large suprasellar extension deforming the third ventricle

Prolactinemia is the most common pituitary dysfunction.[10] In women, this causes amenorrhea, galactorrhea, infertility, estrogen deficiency leading to hot flashes, dyspareunia, and hirsutism. In men, this can cause impotence, infertility, gynecomastia (in 15% of cases), and rarely, galactorrhea. Serum prolactin levels are typically elevated to more than 200 ng/mL. The evaluation of prolactinemia always includes a brain scan to look for pituitary adenoma.

ACTH-secreting tumors are the most common cause of primary Cushing's syndrome.[11, 12] This syndrome can be recognized by the findings of truncal obesity, moon facies, abdominal striae, hypertension, diabetes, osteoporosis, polycythemia, hirsutism, amenorrhea, acne, weakness, and emotional lability. No single hormone test confirms the presence of the condition, but the most reliable tests are the 24-hour urine cortisol level and a dexamethasone suppression test that shows no suppression.

The excess secretion of GH causes a syndrome in adults known as acromegaly.[13, 14] In children, excess GH may cause gigantism, but this is rare compared to acromegaly. Acromegaly is recognized by postmaturity growth of bone and soft tissues, manifesting in adults as enlargement of the feet and hands, mandible, skull, and orbital ridges. Typically, the heart enlarges, which can lead to heart failure. The diagnosis is confirmed by elevation of serum GH to levels exceeding 5 ng/mL.

In all cases, the diagnosis is confirmed by an imaging study. Both computed tomography (CT) and magnetic resonance imaging (MRI) are used to evaluate pituitary tumors. The preferred technique is MRI. This study defines the anatomy of the sellar region, the morphologic characteristics of the tumor, and the extent of the tumor. By contrast, CT does not delineate the tumor as well, but provides a superior means of evaluating the nose, sinuses, and bone around the sella.

Nonsecreting tumors are diagnosed either because of symptoms from local spread of the tumor or as an incidental finding on CT or MRI studies. Owing to the proximity of the pituitary to the optic chiasm, one of the common ways to detect nonsecreting tumors is by compression of the chiasm, which results in visual loss, blurred vision, or optic field cuts. Subsequently, the patient usually consults an ophthalmologist, who then orders a scan and makes the initial diagnosis of the tumor. Other patients may initially experience headaches, and their physician eventually orders a scan that reveals the tumor. There is no classic headache that suggests a pituitary tumor. However, a sphenoid headache that is felt at the vertex or occiput is most common. Other symptoms may relate to focal neurologic deficits from suprasellar spread of the tumor and/or involvement of the cranial nerves or the brain parenchyma.

One rare but important diagnostic presentation of pituitary tumors is a sudden neurosurgical emergency known as pituitary apoplexy. This results from hemorrhage into a tumor that causes rapid expansion and sudden development of neurologic symptoms. A scan reveals a cystic tumor indicative of the hemorrhage and confirming the diagnosis.

INDICATIONS FOR SURGERY

In most circumstances, the decision to perform surgery is made by the neurosurgeon, often in consultation with an endocrinologist. Otolaryngologists may be called upon to assist in the surgery and management of the patient after the surgery. The indications for surgery for a pituitary tumor can be grouped into structural and medical indications. The structural indications relate to the local spread of the tumor and its associated effects. The medical indications are based on the presence of a particular pituitary hormone syndrome that may be best treated by surgery. One of the key determinations is the diagnosis of the tumor type. This is established on the basis of the clinical context and the chemical profile of the patient. Most pituitary tumors are either hormone-secreting or nonsecreting benign adenomas. However, other possibilities exist, including craniopharyngioma, meningioma, shwannoma, and malignant tumors. This latter group may be suggested based on the MRI and CT appearance, but usually they are confirmed only at surgery based on frozen section biopsy studies.

Structural indications for surgery are common for the nonsecreting adenomas and the prolactin-secreting tumors. These tumors tend to be detected only because of symptoms caused by tumor extension, such as visual disturbances, headache, epistaxis, and cranial nerve abnormalities. Visual disturbances may involve visual field cuts or loss of visual acuity. These occur because of superior extension of the tumor, which may press on the optic chiasm. Most often, this results in a peripheral field cut secondary to the loss of the medial retinal fibers as they cross through the chiasm. In most cases, when visual field cuts or loss of acuity is present, the best option is hypophysectomy.

Extension of the tumor intracranially or into the sphenoid sinus may result in headache. In extreme cases, there may be increased intracranial pressure from tumor bulk. In these cases, the transsphenoidal approach may be the best alternative. When the tumor erodes the floor of the sella turcica and extends into the sphenoid sinus, this may cause epistaxis. Surgery is the best choice of therapy in this situation to ensure that the floor is reconstructed. Significant tumor shrinkage through radiation or medical therapy may leave a defect, resulting in CSF leak.[15] Rarely, a tumor will extend into the cavernous sinus, causing cranial nerve deficits. In this setting, a malignant lesion should be suspected, and surgery is indicated to establish the diagnosis and, possibly, to treat the tumor.

Most prolactin-secreting tumors are initially treated with a course of medical therapy using bromocriptine. These tumors are diagnosed either by identification of prolactinemia, as described earlier, or by hormone evaluation after discovery of a pituitary tumor. If medical therapy is attempted, bromocriptine is usually prescribed and the patient is monitored for several months. Surgery is indicated if the medication fails to suppress the prolactin level or halt the growth of the tumor.

Other hormone-secreting tumors are usually treated with surgery as the primary option. The ACTH-secreting tumors associated with Cushing's disease are usually caused by microadenoma. These tumors may be undetectable on CT scan but most will usually present as a small lesion on MRI. Prior to the availability of CT scans and MRI, patients would typically undergo surgery without confirmatory radiographic studies. The diagnosis would be suggested by the clinical syndrome, but it would not be confirmed until the patient improved after surgery. Today, the presence of a microadenoma on MRI and the clinical syndrome of Cushing's disease are sufficient signs to warrant surgery. Those with acromegaly similarly respond best to removal of the tumor. Microadenomas may also be found in this situation, but again, MRI is usually confirmatory.

Once the patient and surgeon agree that an operation is indicated, an appropriate surgical technique must be selected. The preliminary choice is between a frontal craniotomy and an anterior transnasal approach. For most patients, the anterior approach is preferred. The traditional anterior approach to the sella turcica for hypophysectomy is the sublabial transseptal transsphenoidal operation. This is indicated for most pituitary tumors. This approach combines a cosmetically and functionally adequate surgery with the widest possible anterior exposure of the sella turcica. This procedure allows bimanual instrumentation under microscopic control. Specialized instruments have been designed to provide exposure, dissection, resection, and bipolar cautery.

The contraindications to this procedure include absence of the sphenoid sinus, nasal stenosis, and suprasellar extension into the surrounding structures. Absence of the sphenoid sinus, although rare, makes transnasal surgery difficult owing to the lack of orientation. However, with modern computer-assisted surgical techniques, it may still be possible to drill through the thick bone of the sphenoid. Nasal stenosis is another rare anatomic formation that, if present, can make transnasal surgery impossible. The most common anatomic contraindication to this procedure is superior extension of tumor. Most tumors that have suprasellar extension are operable by the transsphenoidal approach. As the tumor is removed from below, the superior extension tends to drop into the sella, allowing further resection. However, in cases of massive intracranial spread or involvement of critical structures, it is not possible to resect the tumor through this route. In these cases, the frontal craniotomy approach is preferred.[16, 17]

Alternative techniques for the anterior approach are becoming increasingly common. The possibilities include the external rhinoplasty approach,[18] the transnasal transseptal approach,[19] and the transnasal endoscopic approach.[20–22] The external rhinoplasty technique affords a rapid, safe approach to the septum. Normally, the small incision heals well without discernible scar, and the more superior angle of the approach has some advantages for the neurosurgeon. Many surgeons, however, believe that this approach risks cosmetic problems with the nasal tip. This concern, which is possibly unfounded, makes this approach less popular. The transnasal transseptal approach enters the septum through a Killian or hemitransfixion incision. This is both fast and safe, and duplicates the angle of the external rhinoplasty technique. However, the nose is too small in most patients to tolerate this, so alar incisions are necessary to achieve full exposure, thereby negating the advantages of this approach.

The endoscopic transnasal transsphenoidal approach is becoming increasingly popular. It is rapid and easy to close and avoids septal dissection completely. In addition, the angled endoscopes provide excellent visualization into the sella turcica, particularly any suprasellar extension of the tumor. The downside to the endoscopic approach is the unfamiliarity of the neurosurgeon with endoscopic surgery and the difficulty with hemostasis. Because the exposure is narrow, it is not easy to manipulate a bipolar instrument into the sella turcica to control bleeding. Also, the surgeon has only one hand to control instruments, making bleeding problems harder to manage. The exact role of these techniques will undoubtedly be clarified over the next several years.

PREOPERATIVE CONSIDERATIONS

Before committing to transsphenoidal hypophysectomy, the consulting otolaryngologist should fully evaluate the patient. Several issues are of concern. The first consideration is whether the surgery is technically possible to perform via the transsphenoidal route. The minimal requirement is that the patient must have an aerated sphenoid sinus. It is preferable that the patient have normal adult anatomy with symmetrical, well-aerated sinuses, a well-defined anterior wall of the sella turcica, and a straight nasal septum with a wide nasal passage. However, significant abnormalities can be overcome. Specifically, a deviated septum can be straightened during the approach or avoided completely by performing a transnasal endoscopic procedure. An asymmetrical sphenoid sinus can be overcome by using intraoperative fluoroscopy. A thick sphenoid bone can be drilled down to reach the sella turcica.

In patients with acromegaly, it is important to obtain a CT scan before committing to surgery. Some patients with this syndrome may have such a deep nose that the instrumentation may be inadequate to perform the procedure. In addition, the bones of the sphenoid sinus may be excessively thick. This may not be a contraindication, but it is important to be aware of such problems before starting the operation.

The second consideration in determining the appropriateness of the transsphenoidal approach is the presence of sinusitis. Active acute or chronic sinusitis is a contraindication to this approach. In some cases, medical treatment may clear the infection, making subsequent operation feasible. Conversely, if the infection cannot be completely resolved, an intracranial approach may be selected. Patients with chronic polyposis also should not be treated by the transsphenoidal approach.

A general medical evaluation is warranted to verify that the patient is fit for surgery. For this operation, it is important to ensure that the patient does not suffer from coagulopathy or other bleeding disorder. Patients with hormone-secreting tumors may be subject to a wide variety of medical conditions that can complicate the surgery and anesthesia. Complete evaluation and careful perioperative management are necessary for a safe surgery with a favorable outcome.

Hypophysectomy is performed exclusively under general anesthesia. However, intranasal topical and local anesthetics are always used to enhance hemostasis. The topical and local anesthetic is applied in a manner identical to that described for septoplasty (see Chapter 12). In addition to intranasal anesthesia, sublabial local anesthetic is injected to minimize bleeding from the sublabial incision. Before starting the operation, it is advisable to place a lumbar drain. This will be used to instill fluid into the subarachnoid space, pushing the tumor into the sphenoid. If a CSF leak has occurred during the procedure, the lumbar drain can be used to decompress the sella turcica to help prevent persistent CSF leak after surgery.

Prophylactic antibiotics are worthwhile for patients undergoing transsphenoidal hypophysectomy. The best choice of agent is one that covers routine sinus flora. Amoxicillin/sulbactam, cefuroxime, or a broad-spectrum combination agent are all suitable choices. Facial preparation before surgery is not performed routinely for intranasal or sublabial surgery. However, in light of the intracranial exposure achieved during this surgery, an iodine facial skin preparation is recommended.

TECHNIQUE

Sublabial Transseptal Transsphenoidal Approach

For sublabial transseptal transsphenoidal procedures, most surgeons prefer that the patient be positioned supine with the head turned toward the right (Fig. 19–1). Some surgeons prefer a semi-Fowler's position, or at least a partially upright posture to about 30 degrees. This changes the angle of view into the nose, which may help some neurosurgeons to remain oriented and may aid visualization of the sellar area. Some surgeons prefer to stabilize the patient's head with a Mayfield-type head holder using pins in the posterior skull. Prior to initiating prepping and draping procedures, a C-arm fluoroscope is often positioned and aligned to demonstrate the sphenoid anatomy. Alternatively, the C-arm fluoroscope may be used only in cases when it is actually needed. This is primarily the choice of the neurosurgeon. The patient's face should be prepped with an iodine-containing solution. This is done to sterilize the skin around the nose so that the instruments that enter the nose will not carry exogenous bacteria into the surgical field. Prophylactic antibiotics are required for these cases to help prevent infection. They should be started at least 1 hour before proceeding with surgery.

Some surgeons prefer to perform the initial dissection through the familiar hemitransfixion incision in the nasal columella. This is unnecessary, as the dissection is easily performed though the sublabial incision. After the approach becomes familiar, this incision actually provides wider exposure to the septum for the dissection.

A sublabial incision is made in the lip 5 mm above the gingival labial sulcus. It is important to maintain this cuff of mucosa to ensure strong closure at the end of the operation. The incision should extend across the width of the pyriform aperture. The initial incision is made with a scalpel. Once the mucosa is incised, cautery can be used to divide the labial muscles down through the periosteum to the bone of the premaxilla. A Freer

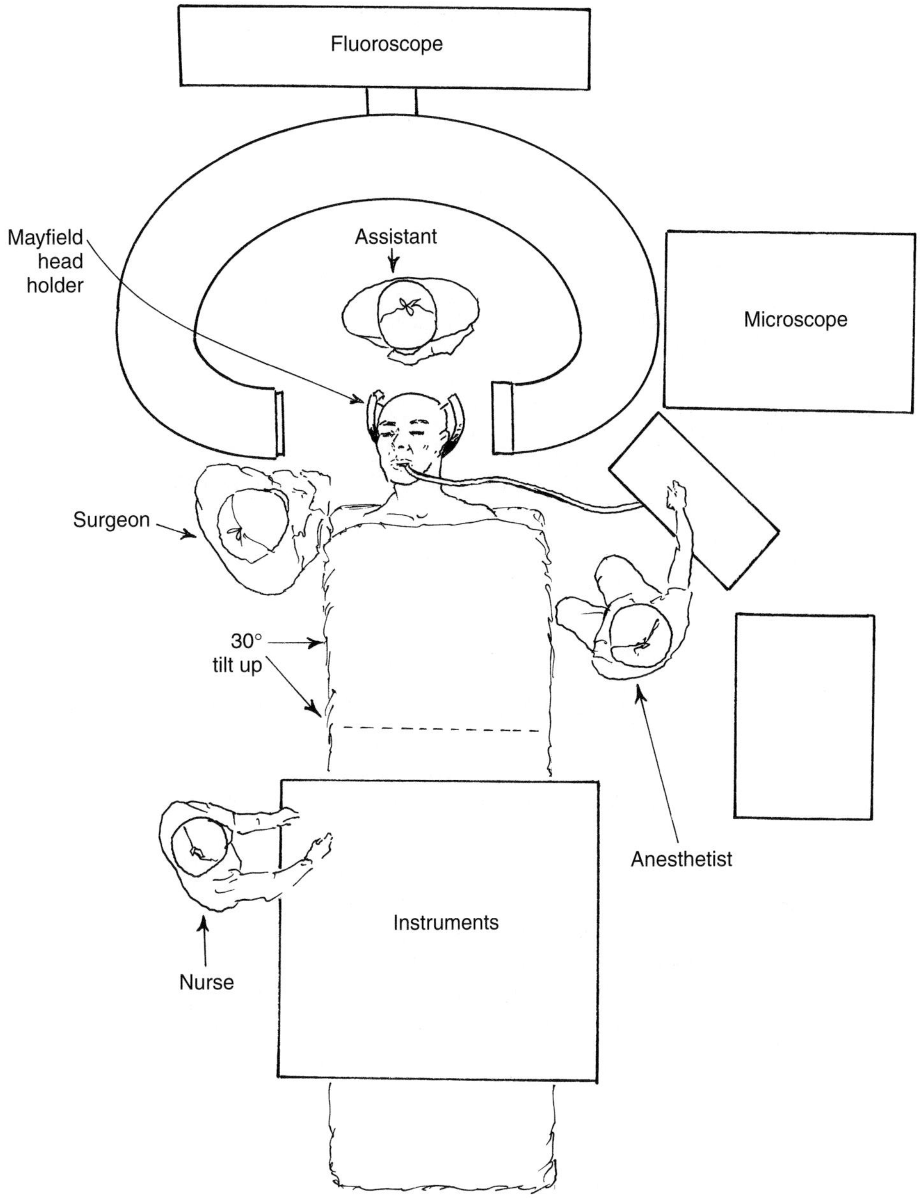

Figure 19–1. Operating room set-up for transsphenoidal resection of a pituitary adenoma. The patient is in a semi-Fowler's position and the head is turned to the right and held with a Mayfield head holder. The fluoroscope is optional but can be draped into the surgical field.

elevator is then used to elevate the periosteum to the pyriform aperture (Fig. 19–2). The pyriform aperture should be exposed laterally and superiorly about 1 cm from the floor of the nose. This allows increased retraction and facilitates exposure of the surgical field.

The next step is to expose the caudal end of the septum. This is done by dividing the soft tissues of the lip over the septum (see Fig. 19–2). Any sharp technique will work, but cautery is preferred as it helps to maintain a bloodless surgical field. The cautery is used in coagulation mode to incise the soft tissues right onto the anterior nasal spine and caudal end of the septum. At this point, the periosteum should be elevated from the nasal spine and caudal end of the septum (Fig. 19–3). The tissues are very densely adherent in this area. Careful technique is important to avoid tearing the mucosa. A curved iris scissors is useful for spreading sharply through this fibrous tissue. Once the subperichondrial plane of the quadrilateral cartilage is reached, the dissection proceeds with complete elevation of the mucosa from the left side of the septum. As with septoplasty, a Cottle elevator is used for this maneuver. Initially, the sharp end of the instrument is used to elevate the mucosa from the quadrilateral cartilage. The dissection extends posteriorly over the vomer and perpendicular plate to the sphenoid rostrum. When elevating over the bony septum, the blunt end of the Cottle elevator is preferred, as this minimizes the risk of perforating the flap.

Once the left anterior and posterior tunnels have been completed, the dissection must extend over the maxillary crest onto the floor of the nose. Direct elevation over the maxillary crest to the floor of the nose is avoided to make sure that the mucosa is not perforated.

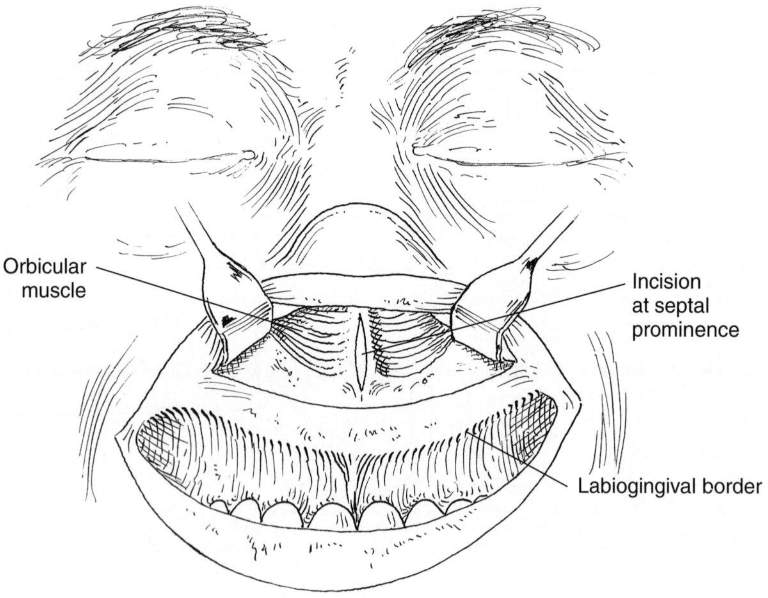

Figure 19–2. Sublabial exposure of the caudal end of the septum. The periosteum has been elevated laterally and superiorly around the pyriform aperture. An incision is made on the caudal end of the septum.

Instead, an inferior tunnel is created. By using the sublabial exposure, the pyriform aperture is in clear view (Fig. 19–4). The curved Cottle elevator is then used to lift the mucosa from the floor of the nose, dissecting along the floor from anterior to posterior to the level of the posterior choana. The inferior tunnel is then widened from the lateral wall up to the fibrous attachments at the maxillary crest. At this point, the mucosa is attached to the left side of the septum only along the edge of the maxillary crest. This is the area of greatest risk for perforating the mucosal flap. To avoid perforation, the dissection is performed from anterior to posterior with retraction of the anterior and inferior tunnels. This places the mucosa to be elevated under tension, facilitating dissection. A hockey stick is recommended for this step.

At this point, the entire left mucosal flap has been elevated from the septum and floor of the nose. The next step is to divide the bony cartilaginous junction to allow the dissection to cross over to the right side of the septum. The bony cartilaginous junction between the quadrilateral cartilage and the vomer and perpen-

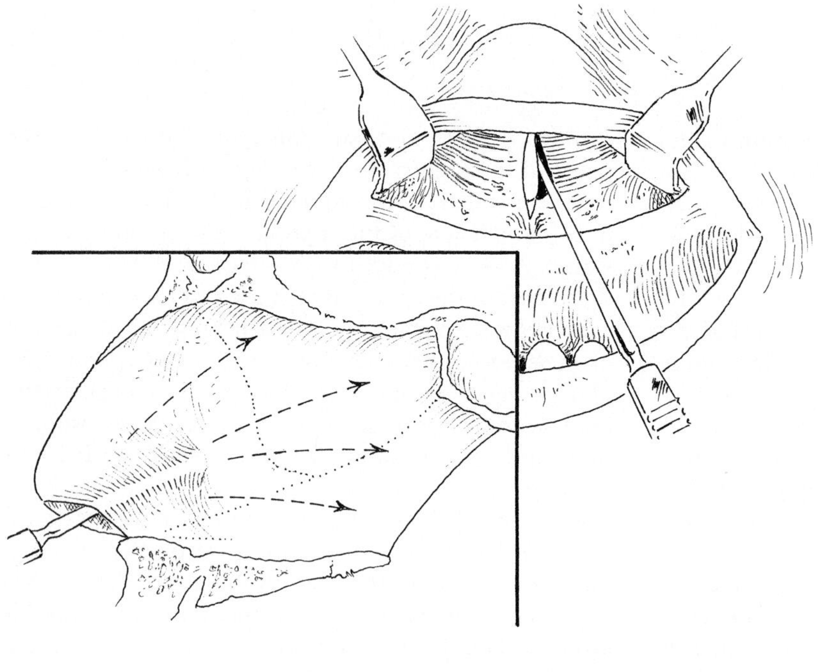

Figure 19–3. Creation of the left anterior tunnel. The subperichondrial plane is entered and the mucosa is elevated with a Cottle elevator.

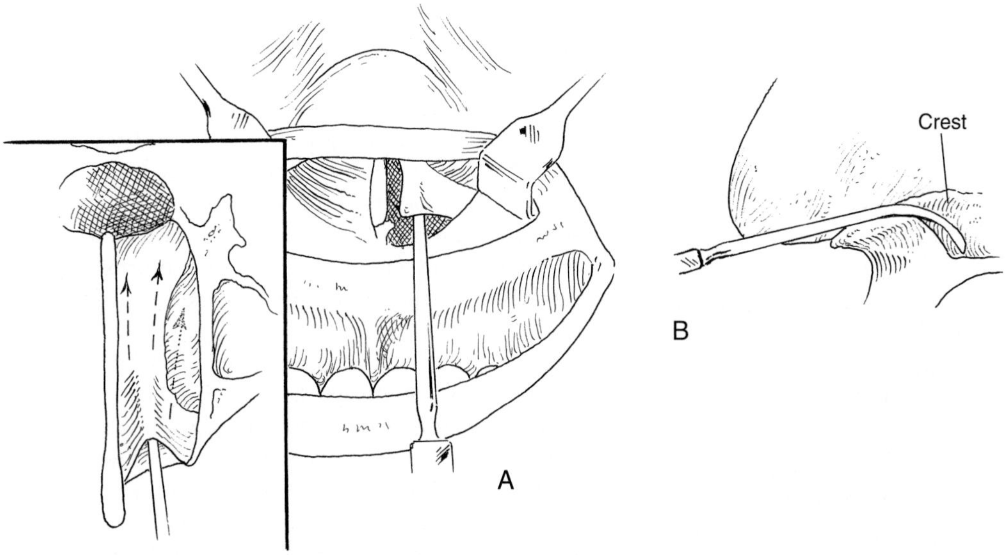

Figure 19–4. Creation of the left inferior tunnel. A curved Cottle elevator is used to elevate the mucosa in the subperichondrial plane. *A,* Anterior view. *B,* Lateral view. *Inset,* View from the superior aspect, looking down on the floor of the nose.

dicular plate is bluntly separated (Fig. 19–5). A gentle sawing motion using the sharp end of the Cottle elevator is generally effective. The cartilage should be separated from the bony septum all the way from the maxillary crest inferiorly to the nasal dorsum superiorly. At this point, the mucosa on the right side of the septum is elevated from the crossover point at the bony cartilaginous junction posteriorly to the sphenoid rostrum (right posterior tunnel). This is done using the blunt end of the Cottle elevator.

The next step is to remove a strip of cartilage from the quadrilateral cartilage at the inferior attachment to the maxillary crest (Fig. 19–6). Working through the left side of the nose through the exposure created by

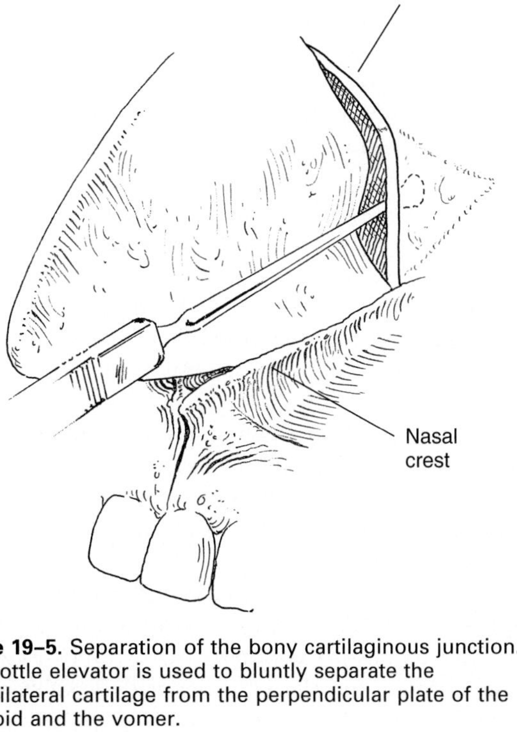

Figure 19–5. Separation of the bony cartilaginous junction. The Cottle elevator is used to bluntly separate the quadrilateral cartilage from the perpendicular plate of the ethmoid and the vomer.

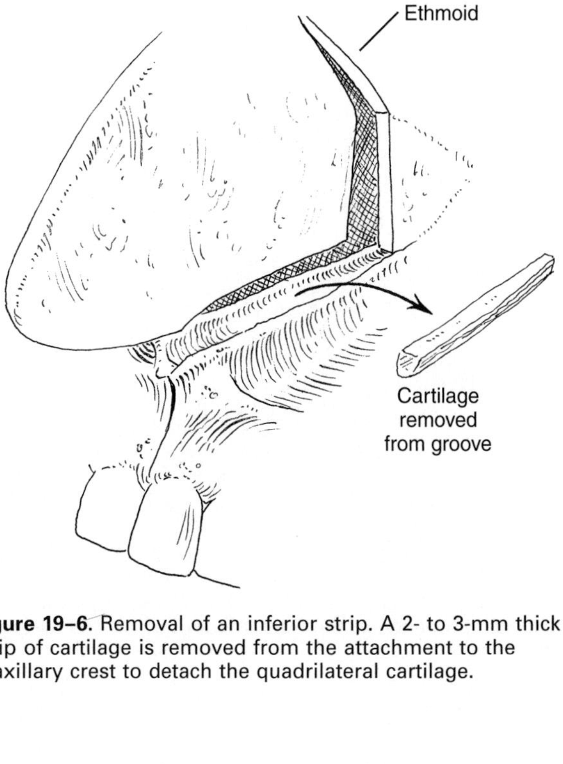

Figure 19–6. Removal of an inferior strip. A 2- to 3-mm thick strip of cartilage is removed from the attachment to the maxillary crest to detach the quadrilateral cartilage.

elevating the left-side mucosa, a cartilage knife is used to incise the cartilage. This instrument is also called the half-round knife, a D-knife, or Freer cartilage knife. A 2- to 3-mm thick strip of cartilage is incised along the maxillary crest, working from posterior to anterior. The inferior cartilage strip is then removed from the maxillary crest. It is important to take care not to perforate the mucosa on the right side of the septum during this maneuver, as the mucosa on the right side of the septum has not yet been elevated. Following this step, the cartilaginous septum is freed from all bony attachments except for those to the nasal dorsum superiorly. This allows the septum to swing over to the right lateral nasal wall.

The inferior tunnel on the right side of the nose is raised at this point using the same technique as that described for the left side and using the curved Cottle elevator. The inferior tunnel is elevated from anterior to posterior along the floor of the nose and then widened by dissecting laterally and medially to the fullest extent possible (Fig. 19–7). After this is accomplished, the last step in the septal dissection is to divide the attachments of the mucosa to the right side of the septum along the maxillary crest. This is accomplished by retracting the mucosa of the floor of the nose on the right side, pushing the septum to the right, and using the hockey stick to elevate the attachments from the maxillary crest.

The quadrilateral cartilage can then be displaced to the right lateral wall to expose the bone of the vomer and perpendicular plate. To expose the anterior wall of the sphenoid sinus, this bone must be resected. A dorsal bone scissors is used to cut the perpendicular plate high enough to ensure complete exposure of the sphenoid rostrum (Fig. 19–8*A*). The inferior cut is made through the vomer along the floor of the nose using a straight, 4-mm osteotome (Fig. 19–8*B*). The septal bone is grasped with Ferris Smith forceps and gently twisted and removed. It is important to harvest the septal bone in as large a piece as possible, as this will be used to reconstruct the sella turcica and sphenoid at the end of the procedure. After removal of the main plate of bone, any residual pieces of the bony septum still attached to the sphenoid can easily be removed using Takahashi forceps.

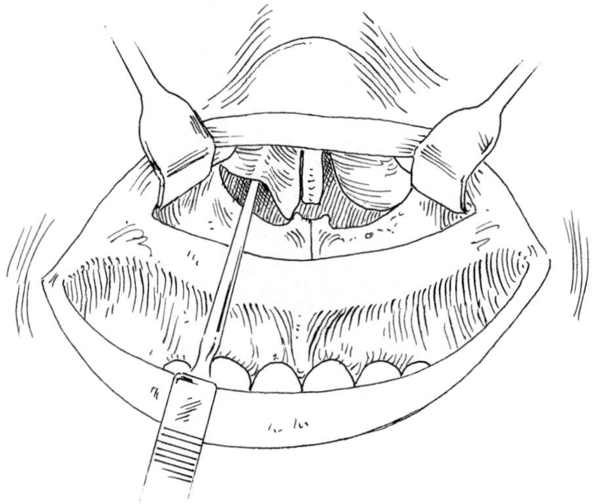

Figure 19–7. Creation of the right inferior tunnel. The curved Cottle elevator is used to elevate the mucosa from the floor of the nose.

At this point, the transsphenoidal retractor is introduced. For most techniques, the sphenoid rostrum is exposed using one of the self-retaining retractors made for transsphenoidal surgery (Fig. 19–9). There are a number of variations of retractor available. The lengths, heights, and amount of flaring of the tip differ depending on the specific retractor. It is wise to have a variety of these retractors available in the surgery set to accommodate individual anatomic variations. For most patients, a retractor with a minimally flared tip is best. This helps to increase the lateral extent of the exposure. Retractors with highly flared tips provide the greatest amount of lateral exposure, but are difficult to place without damaging the mucosal flaps. In most cases, the retractor is placed in such a way that the handle is superior. This keeps the handle out of the way of the surgery and helps to retract the lip. To place the retractor, the lip is pulled up and cushioned with a 4 × 4 gauze sponge. The left mucosal flap is retracted laterally with a Freer elevator while the transsphenoidal retractor is slid in against the cartilage and right flap. It is important to make sure that, as the retractor is opened, the mucosa is not torn. With experience, the positioning of the retractor will become easier.

The next step is to identify the natural ostia of the left and right sphenoid sinuses. The normal position of the sphenoid ostium is 30 degrees elevated from the floor of the nose, approximately 5 to 10 mm lateral to the midline (Fig. 19–9). It may not be possible to visualize the ostia directly through this approach at this stage owing to the mucosa covering the area. The best technique is to palpate the area of the sphenoid rostrum using straight Frasier suction. When the ostia are identified, the rotating sphenoid punch is used to remove the bone of the anterior wall of the sphenoid sinus. The first bites are usually made in an inferior direction, and then are spread out in all directions. When the anterior walls are removed to the limits of the sinuses, the intersinus septum is grasped with Takahashi forceps and excised (Fig. 19–10).

The final step in the transsphenoidal approach is to completely remove the mucosa from the inside of the sinus. The mucosa is elevated with a Freer or other suitable elevator and then grasped with Takahashi forceps and removed. If the mucosa is pulled gently

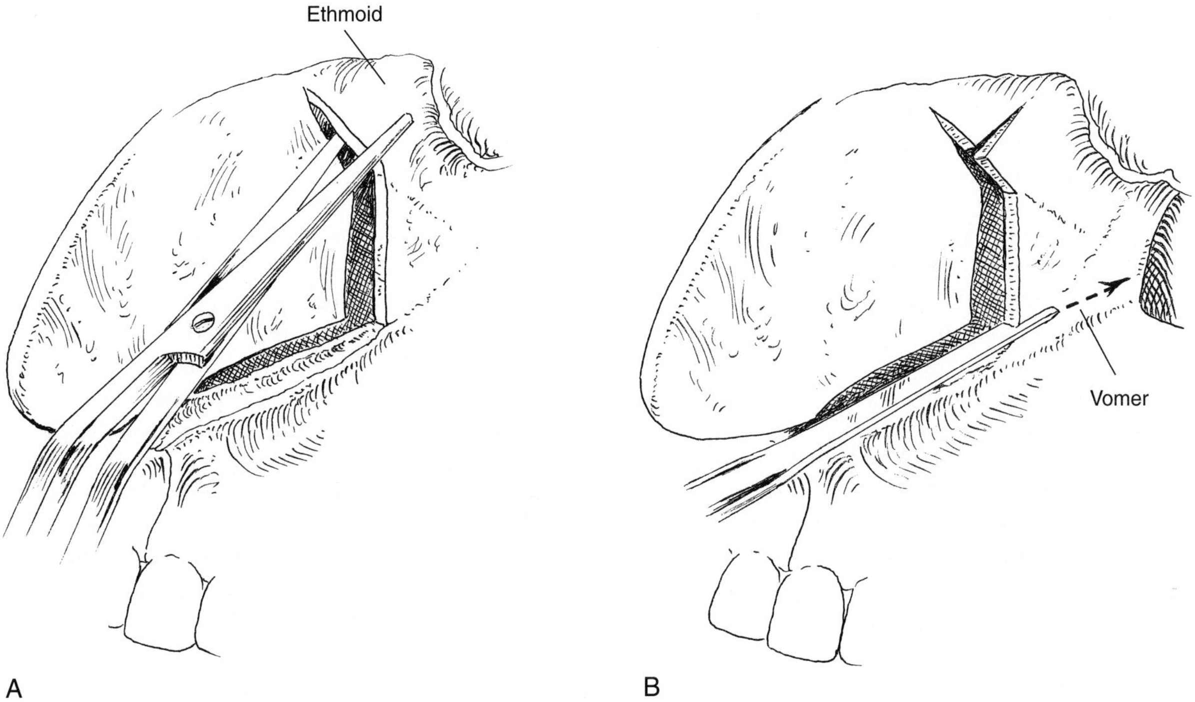

Figure 19–8. Resection of the bony septum. The bony septum is removed in one large piece. *A,* The upper cut is made with dorsal bone scissors. *B,* The inferior cut is made with an osteotome.

enough, it is possible to strip the entire sinus lining out in a single piece. This will ensure that complete removal is achieved. If this is not successful, careful dissection of the residual mucosal remnants is necessary. The risk of leaving residual mucosa is that, after obliteration, retained mucosa can lead to mucocele formation. This potentially serious late complication can be avoided by complete removal of the mucosa at this stage of the surgery.

Before turning the procedure over to the neurosurgeon, it is worthwhile to identify the landmarks within

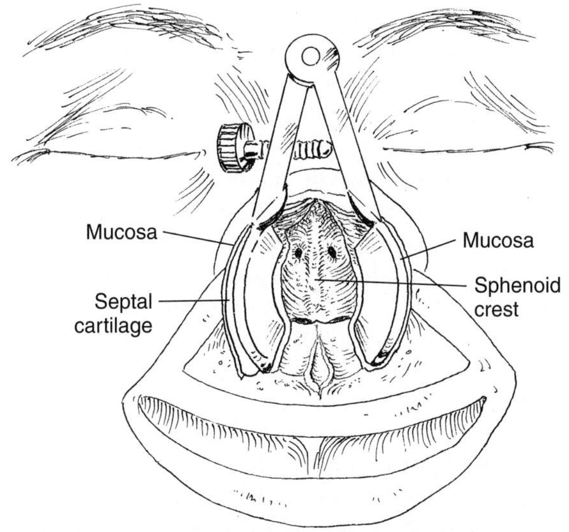

Figure 19–9. Exposure of the sphenoid rostrum. The transsphenoidal retractor has been inserted, and the midline of the sphenoid rostrum is visualized. In this example, both ostia of the sphenoid sinuses are clearly seen. Often, the ostia are hidden by mucosa and must be located by palpation.

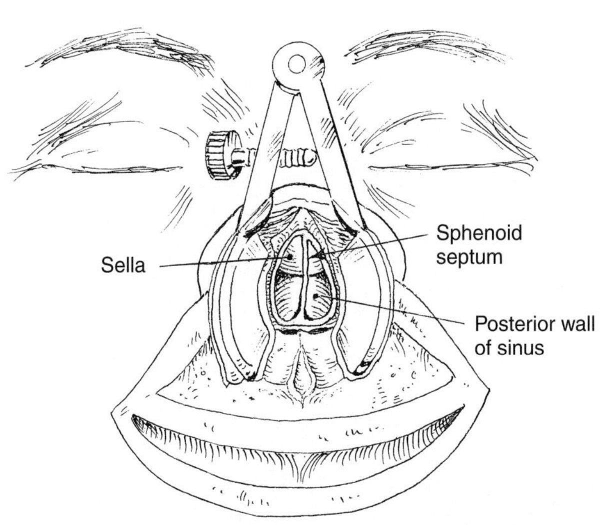

Figure 19–10. Exposure of the inside of the sphenoid sinus. The anterior walls of the sinuses have been removed, exposing the intersinus septum. This is removed with Takahashi forceps. The sella turcica is seen in the posterior superior sinus.

the sinuses. These include the optic nerves, carotid arteries, and sella turcica. By identifying these structures, the surgeon will be oriented to the entry into the sella turcica. Many operating teams utilize fluoroscopy at this point to verify the anatomy before entering the sella.

In most centers, entry into the sella turcica, incision into the dura, resection of the tumor, and reconstruction of the sella turcica are performed by the neurosurgeon. A detailed description of these procedures is available in other texts. Briefly, the bone of the sella turcica is incised with a small osteotome and flaked off with an elevator to initiate the opening. A small Kerrison rongeur is used to complete removal of the bone. The dura is coagulated using bipolar forceps, and a cruciate incision is made. The dural flaps are folded back to expose the pituitary. Usually, the tumor is easily visualized, in which case a biopsy specimen of the tumor is obtained. A combination of curetting and suctioning is then used to complete the tumor removal. Hemostasis is maintained with microbipolar cautery and packing soaked with thrombin.

Once tumor removal is completed, reconstruction is performed. The sella turcica is usually packed with a small fat or fascial graft. This is reinforced with a layer of fascia that can be sealed with fibrin glue. A bone graft from the septum is placed inside the sella turcica to hold the fat and fascia inside the sella. These bone grafts are then turned sideways and wedged into position (Fig. 19–11).

The remaining procedures are performed by the otolaryngologist. The lumen of the sinus cavity is filled with an adequate fat graft to occupy the entire inside of the sinus. Incomplete packing will lead to aeration of the sinus and failure of the obliteration. After the fat graft

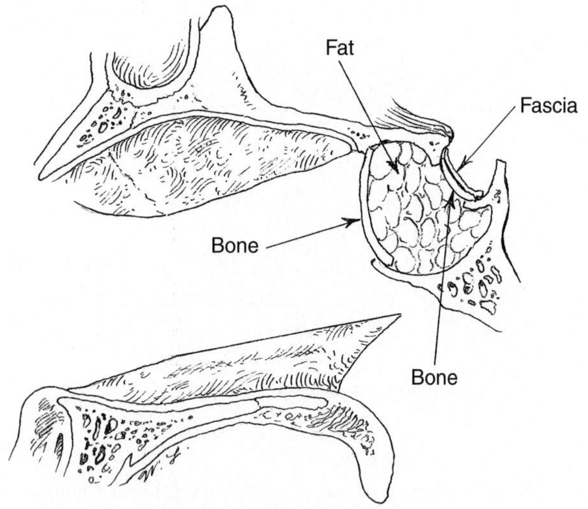

Figure 19–11. Obliteration of the sphenoid sinus. The sella turcica is sealed with fascia and bone, the sinus is packed with fat, and the sinus is closed with bone from the septum.

is placed, the anterior wall of the sphenoid is reconstructed using bone from the septum. Usually, there is a residual ledge around the outside of the sinus to hold the bone graft in place (see Fig. 19–11).

The retractor is removed and the septal space is evacuated of any blood clots. The sublabial incision is then closed. A row of simple interrupted sutures is used to approximate the incision. As with other sublabial incisions, the most popular suture is a chromic 3-0 suture on a tapered needle. The author prefers a Vicryl (Ethicon, Inc., Somerville, NJ) suture instead to help avoid the suture line pulling apart prematurely.

At this point, it is important to inspect the mucosal flaps of the septum for lacerations or tears. Significant tears should be repaired using 4-0 chromic sutures. The last step is to place a nasal pack or splints. Doyle II airway splints (Xomed, Inc., Jacksonville, FL) are preferred. These are secured by a 3-0 nylon horizontal mattress suture. If splints are used, nasal packing is generally not necessary. However, if there is any bleeding at this point, packing can be placed.

Technical Modifications

There are a number of variations of the standard transseptal transsphenoidal approach, including three different access techniques other than the straight sublabial incision. The first of these is to perform a hemitransfixion incision in the columella. This allows direct access to the septum to elevate the mucosal flaps. After the mucosal flaps are developed, the sublabial incision is created and connected to the septal tunnel. The remainder of the procedure is as described earlier.

An alternative approach is to use a strictly transnasal technique. This is accomplished either by using the external rhinoplasty approach or by performing an alar release procedure. The incision for the external rhinoplasty approach is marked out and injected as outlined in Chapter 13. The incision is performed and the columellar skin is elevated. The caudal end of the septum is exposed by separating the medial crura of the lower lateral cartilages. In some cases, to enhance exposure, it may be necessary to divide the medial crura transversely. This increases the width of the access to the caudal septum. At the end of the operation, the medial crura are repaired with horizontal mattress sutures. The remainder of the procedure is just as described for the standard approach.

A direct transnasal approach is possible to perform through a Killian incision in the anterior septum. In this procedure, the septal incision is carried inferiorly onto the floor of the nose and extended laterally to the alar attachment. To create enough space to allow the transsphenoidal retractor to be inserted, the alar rim usually must be released. This requires an incision similar to that performed during alar repositioning, as discussed in Chapter 13. This technique shortens the distance to the sphenoid sinus by about 1 cm and may be preferred in patients with acromegaly if the length of the nose is excessive.

One modification in the repair after resection is to preserve the sphenoid sinus instead of obliterating it. It is occasionally possible to leave the sinus open if there has not been a CSF leak during resection of the pituitary tumor and if the floor of the sella turcica has been well reconstructed. In this setting, postoperative CSF leak is not a concern, so it is permissible to leave the sinus open. In this situation, the floor of the sella turcica is carefully repaired and a free mucosal graft is placed against the defect in the sella and packed into position. After 1 to 3 weeks, the pack is removed, at which time the graft should be healed. In this case, the sinus must have an adequate opening into the nose to allow normal drainage of mucus.

Transnasal Microscopic Approach

The transnasal microscopic approach employs the same transsphenoidal retractors used in the transseptal approach except that the retractor is placed directly through the nasal cavity. This avoids dissection through the septum. This approach is not widely used as a primary technique. The angle of surgery is somewhat off-center, and the approach often requires a lateral alar incision. For these reasons, it is not favored. However, in the case of revision surgery, it is one of the best options, as reoperation through the septum after complete resection of the septal bone is difficult and is likely to result in significant tears in the flaps. This can be avoided by the transnasal route.

The face and nose are prepared as for the transseptal procedure just described. The first step is to incise the lateral alar rim to expand the nose, thereby allowing the retractor to be placed. A full-thickness incision is made around the soft part of the ala. This is carried across the nasal sill into the nose at the junction of the nasal rim with the face. With the rim incised, it is possible to place the transsphenoidal retractor through the nose, pointing directly to the sphenoid rostrum. In order to achieve bilateral exposure, the posterior 5 to 10 mm of the septum is resected. This is easily done by incising the septum vertically with a scalpel. The superior and inferior attachments of the posterior septum can be incised with angled scissors, and this part of the septum can then be removed without difficulty. At this point, a microscope is introduced to improve visualization of the sphenoid area.

The next step is to identify the sphenoid sinus. If this is a primary surgery, suction is used to palpate the area of the rostrum. The ostia are identified as defects in the wall of the sphenoid. In revision surgery, the entire face of the sinus may be soft owing to the previous resection, or it may be solid bone if reconstructed with a septal bone graft. In either case, the anterior wall can be removed using whichever instruments are best suited for the particular case. In primary surgery, the intrasinus and intrasellar aspects of the surgery are the same as described previously. In revision surgery, the contents of the sinus must be carefully dissected. There may be a fat graft in place, and the position of the sella turcica may be difficult to ascertain. Bipolar forceps and frequent use of fluoroscopy may facilitate the dissection.

At the conclusion of the procedure, the sinus and sella turcica are handled as before. The retractor is removed, and the alar incision is repaired. Nasal packing may be necessary to reinforce the sphenoid to help prevent CSF leak.

Transnasal Transsphenoidal Endoscopic Approach

The endoscopic approach to the sella turcica is a straightforward modification of the standard transseptal operation that has been increasingly applied to hypophysectomy. For surgeons accustomed to using endoscopy for sinus surgery, this is an easy and natural extension of those techniques. The advantages of the endoscopic approach are that it avoids an incision, can be performed quickly, and provides improved visualization of the suprasellar components of the tumor by using angled 30- and 70-degree endoscopes. Its disadvantages are limited exposure and the fact that this technique requires the surgeon to operate with only one hand. (One hand is needed to hold the endoscope and the other hand must perform all of the surgery.) Moreover, the limited exposure and one-handed surgery make it difficult to control bleeding. The other main disadvantage is that the view through the endoscope is a two-dimensional "fish eye" view. Microscopic surgery allows binocular vision with true depth perception. The endoscopic view is monocular and, therefore, lacks true depth perception. Despite these limitations, the procedure has gained rapid acceptance and popularity.

The endoscopic approach is indicated as an alternative in virtually every case that can be performed by a transsphenoidal route except in the case of patients with significant deviation of the septum. In these patients, the nasal cavity may be physically blocked, preventing an endoscopic procedure. It would be possible to perform a septoplasty and then proceed with the endoscopic operation. However, if a septoplasty is being performed already, the advantages of the endoscopic approach are lost and a transseptal microscopic procedure should be done.

To perform the procedure, the nose is initially decongested with cocaine flakes and injected with lidocaine with epinephrine, as described in Chapter 8. For most of the procedure, a 0-degree, 4-mm endoscope is used. In many patients, the anatomy is favorable for easy visualization of the sphenoid rostrum. This allows the middle and superior turbinates to be preserved. In other patients, it may be necessary to resect part of the middle and superior turbinates in order to gain adequate visualization (Fig. 19–12). In these cases, the turbinates are addressed before considering the sphenoid sinus. The posteroinferior middle turbinate is resected with endoscopic scissors. After this, the inferoposterior aspect of the superior turbinate is similarly resected (see Fig. 19–12). At this point, the exposure of the sphenoid rostrum should be excellent.

The next step is to resect the posterior aspect of the septum (Fig. 19–13). An incision is made toward the back of the septum, about 1 cm anterior to the sphenoid rostrum. The bone of the septum is then cut using either a sickle knife or, if this is not strong enough, a chisel. The septal bone over the rostrum is removed and the mucosa on both sides are resected to widely expose the area of the sphenoid rostrum (see Fig. 19–13). At this point, it should be possible to identify the two ostia of the sphenoid sinus. The ipsilateral ostium is enlarged using a rotating sphenoid punch; this is followed by enlargement of the contralateral ostium. The intervening midline septum is removed using Blakesley forceps. This should result in wide exposure of the inside of the sinus, including the floor of the sella turcica (Fig. 19–14).

The endoscopic procedure differs from the transseptal procedure in that the sphenoid is not obliterated following the endoscopic operation. For this reason, the sinus mucosa should not be completely stripped, but rather should be resected conservatively over the sella. This can be accomplished using an elevator or curette. Once the sella turcica is exposed, the bone is removed, the dura is incised, and the tumor is resected as previously described. Again, the principle difference in this technique is that the surgeon must operate with one hand.

Following tumor resection, the sella is packed with fat or fascia, and the floor of the sella is covered with a mucosal graft. An alternative reconstruction approach is to use a middle turbinate composite bone and mucosal graft (Fig. 19–15). This has the advantage of providing both bone and mucosa to heal the defect. The sinus should then be packed with a layer of Gelfoam, followed by a gauze pack to hold the graft in place. The nose is packed with a standard absorbent sponge.

POSTOPERATIVE CARE

Following hypophysectomy, patients should be observed in the intensive care unit (ICU) for at least 24 hours. Despite an extremely low incidence of serious complications, patients are at risk for intracranial bleeding and acute hormonal changes secondary to the loss of pituitary function. To control for these problems, ICU monitoring is worthwhile. Continuous monitoring of arterial oxygen saturation, blood pressure, and pulse will detect any significant hemodynamic changes before they become serious.

One of the main concerns is the possibility of CSF leakage after surgery. This is a potentially serious complication owing to the risk of meningitis with persistent

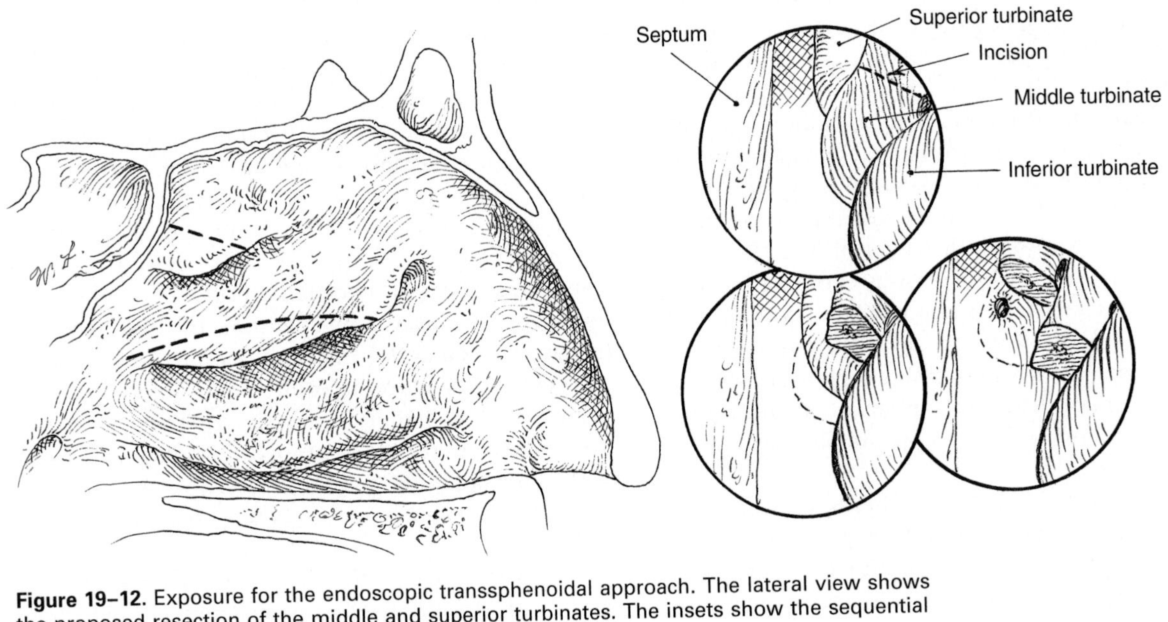

Figure 19–12. Exposure for the endoscopic transsphenoidal approach. The lateral view shows the proposed resection of the middle and superior turbinates. The insets show the sequential resection of the turbinates from the endoscopic view.

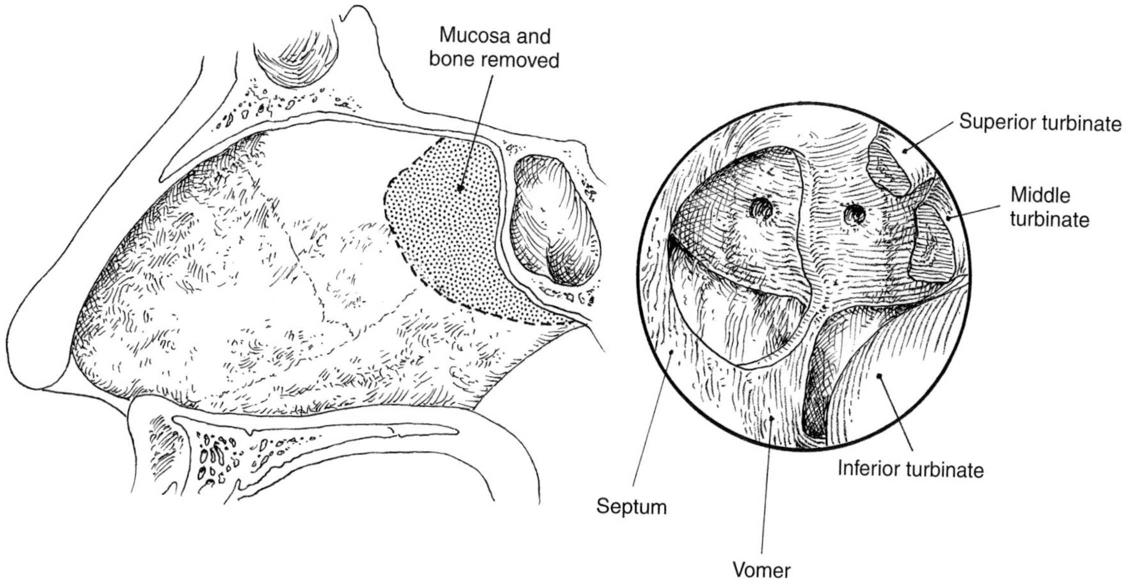

Figure 19–13. Resection of the posterior aspect of the septum. The lateral view shows the proposed resection (shaded area). The inset demonstrates the endoscopic view after resection of the posterior aspect of the septum.

CSF rhinorrhea. If the resection has not violated the diaphragm of the sella turcica, there is no risk of leak and no specific management is necessary. However, if the patient has had intraoperative CSF leakage, measures are recommended to prevent further leakage and to facilitate primary healing. The use of a lumbar drain is controversial. Drainage of CSF by a lumbar drain can decompress the repair and prevent leakage. The drain can lead to complications, though, including pneumocephalus secondary to the pulling of air into the subarachnoid space through the sella, and meningitis secondary to contamination of the lumbar site. On balance, the drain is warranted if the surgeon believes that there is a significant intraoperative leak and the repair is less than optimal. For the routine case, a lumbar drain is probably not necessary for postoperative management.

Antibiotics and pain medication are prescribed for all patients. Other medications for blood pressure control are used as indicated for the individual case. After surgery, hormonal replacement therapy should be initiated within the first few days. For patients with large tumors, panhypopituitarism should be expected. Patients with microadenomas may have no hormonal deficiencies. If the patient is expected to require replacement therapy, replacement of all hormones may be necessary. These include glucocorticoid steroids, thy-

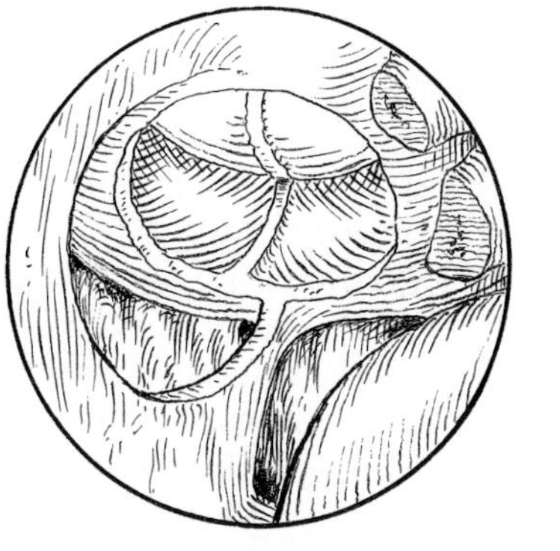

Figure 19–14. Completed exposure of the sella turcica. The anterior wall of the sphenoid has been removed to expose the inside of the sinus.

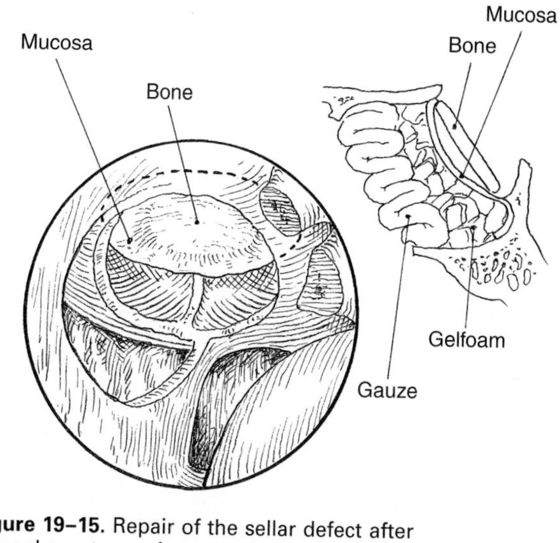

Figure 19–15. Repair of the sellar defect after hypophysectomy. A composite bone and mucosal graft is harvested from the middle turbinate and placed into the defect. The inset shows the layers of grafts and packing used to seal the sella.

roid hormone, growth hormone, antidiuretic hormone, and estrogen replacement in women. The most common hormonal problem encountered in the immediate postoperative period is diabetes insipidus. This is caused by a lack of antidiuretic hormone, which leads to severe polyuria. Patients may lose large volumes of urine in excess of 200 mL per hour. Initial management is aimed at replacing the free water and monitoring the electrolytes, replacing these as necessary. Early replacement therapy using DDAVP (1-(3-mercaptoproprionic acid)-8-D-arginine vasopressin) in either the oral or nasal spray form is the primary treatment for diabetes insipidus. DDAVP is a synthetic analogue of antidiuretic hormone. Consultation with an endocrinologist is recommended to help manage the hormonal therapy in any patient developing significant hormonal disturbances after hypophysectomy.

Nasal packing and splints are removed within the first week after surgery. If packing has been used in addition to the nasal splints, this can be removed after 48 hours. The nasal splints should be maintained for 4 or 5 days to ensure that adequate healing occurs. Once the splints are removed, normal saline mist therapy should be started and continued for several weeks. Patients undergoing the endoscopic technique are managed according to the protocol for endoscopic sinus surgery discussed in Chapter 8. However, it is important to avoid aggressive cleaning of the sphenoid sinus early on, as this may lead to inadvertent debridement of the mucosal graft. The sublabial incision requires only minimal care with occasional oral rinses. The sutures are dissolvable, but may persist for up to 2 months when Vicryl sutures are used.

COMPLICATIONS

The complications of pituitary surgery include both complications of the surgery and those of the disease process itself. Surgical mortality is rare. Series from around the world consistently report mortality rates of less than 1% for the transsphenoidal approach.[2, 12, 14, 23] This compares favorably with those of any other technique.

The surgical complications include both medical and surgical problems. CSF leakage is an important risk of surgery. The incidence of CSF leakage varies with the surgeon, techniques, and series of cases presented. For most experienced surgeons, the risk should be less than 5%.[12, 24] CSF leakage is more likely to occur in cases when the diaphragm of the sella turcica is violated or when the quality of repair of the sellar floor and the anterior wall of the sphenoid sinus is less than optimal. The cause is usually technical failure in completely sealing the sella and sphenoid sinus after surgery. This can also occur if infection causes the grafts to fail. Management of CSF leak will be covered in detail in Chapter 20.

Other intracranial complications are even less frequent than CSF leak, but include intracranial bleeding, injury to cranial nerves in the cavernous sinus, and optic nerve injury. Intracranial bleeding from transsphenoidal hypophysectomy may be a fatal complication.[25, 26] Early recognition and management is the only way to prevent catastrophic injuries. Cranial nerve injuries can occur if the dissection strays into the cavernous sinus. In attempting to control the bleeding, trauma to the cranial nerves is possible. The optic nerves are intimately associated with the pituitary. In most patients, the optic chiasm is anterior and superior to the sella turcica and is not accessible through the sphenoid. However, if there is suprasellar extension of the tumor, it is possible to injure the optic chiasm. This is one of the reasons that some neurosurgeons advocate the transfrontal approach for tumors with significant suprasellar extension.

Infectious complications of transsphenoidal hypophysectomy are surprisingly uncommon; however, the risk persists for many years.[15] The nose and sublabial mucosa are contaminated surfaces that have the potential to contaminate the sphenoid and sella turcica. Furthermore, the nose is packed after surgery, which can also lead to sinus infections, and which, in turn, can lead to infection of the sella. Despite these factors, infections are decidedly rare. The reasons for this are not totally clear. Prophylactic antibiotics are probably beneficial. Local immunity and low infectivity of the mucosal flora are also probable factors.

Some degree of epistaxis occurs after surgery in all patients. In most cases, the bleeding is self-limited and minimal. Placing intranasal splints on the septum at the end of the procedure will minimize the bleeding. If there has been more than the usual amount of bleeding during the operation, additional packing in the nose will usually control this. Excessive postoperative epistaxis can be controlled in most cases simply by adding nasal packing. If this fails to control the bleeding, it is necessary to ascertain the source of bleeding and take specific measures to control the bleeding. Examination is the first step. Angiography or magnetic resonance angiography (MRA) are possible strategies. The bleeding may be able to be controlled by endoscopic cauterization or ligation of specific vessels. Alternatively, embolization may be required if the area of bleeding cannot be accessed through transnasal approaches.

Septal perforation is a risk in all transseptal surgeries. The reported rates of perforation vary widely from 0% to 20% depending on the technique used.[1, 2, 27, 28] The risk of perforation is higher for these procedures than for routine septoplasty owing to the placement of the transsphenoidal retractor. This retractor stretches the mucosal flaps maximally and may cause tears in the flaps. Anterior perforation should be rare if the septal cartilage is preserved and is left attached to the right mucosal flap. However, it is possible for an ischemic area to develop in the middle of the anterior septum from pressure during the surgery. In most such cases, the perforation will be posterior. These perforations are typically asymptomatic owing to their location in the posterior septum, which is out of the main air stream and in which there is a high level of humidification. These factors help to keep the amount of crusting to a minimum. Repair may be possible if the perforation is symptomatic and amenable to surgery.

Long-term complications of the transsphenoidal approach include sinusitis and mucocele formation.[29] The incidence of these problems increases over time, but the exact rate is unknown. Long-term follow-up evaluation of these patients is difficult for the otolaryngologist because the neurosurgeon and endocrinologist generally manage the patient's course as primary physicians. In cases when the sphenoid sinus is not obliterated, the risk of mucocele or infection is minimal. In cases when the sinus is obliterated, any retained mucosal elements can be the source of a mucocele. Mucoceles can manifest at any time in the life of the patient. For this reason, it is necessary to monitor the patient indefinitely. If mucocele does occur, the preferred management is by endoscopic drainage.

The most common medical complications of the surgery are related to hormonal disturbances caused by resection of the pituitary. The risk of complications from these problems is minimized by involvement of an experienced endocrinologist. As with all surgery, patients undergoing transsphenoidal hypophysectomy are at risk for complications related to anesthesia, cardiovascular complications, pneumonia, and internal organ failure. Fortunately, these complications are unusual in routine cases.

REFERENCES

1. Urquhart AC, Bersalona FB, Ejercito VS, et al. Nasal septum after sublabial transseptal transsphenoidal pituitary surgery. Otolaryngol Head Neck Surg 115:64, 1996.
2. Kern EB. Transnasal pituitary surgery. Arch Otolaryngol 107: 183, 1981.
3. Lee KJ. The sublabial transseptal transsphenoidal approach to the hypophysis. Laryngoscope 88 (Suppl 7), 1978.
4. Ciric IS, Tarkington J. Trans-sphenoidal microsurgery. Surg Neurol 2:207, 1974.
5. Hirsch O. Endonasal method of removal of hypophyseal tumors. JAMA 55:772, 1910.
6. Kanavel AB. The removal of tumors of the pituitary body by an infranasal route: A proposed operation with a description of the technique. JAMA 53:1704, 1909.
7. Henderson WR. The pituitary adenomata: A follow-up study of the surgical results in 338 cases. Br J Surg 26:811, 1939.
8. Hardy J. Transsphenoidal microsurgery of normal and pathologic pituitary. Clin Neurosurg 16:185, 1968.
9. Reschke K, Rohrer T, Kopf D, et al. Hyperthyroidism in TSH-producing hypophyseal adenoma. Detsch Med Wochenschr 122(6):150, 1997.
10. Pearson OH, Brodkey JS, Kaufman B. Endocrine evaluation and indication for surgery of functional pituitary adenomas. Clin Neurosurg 21:26, 1974.
11. Salassa RM, Laws ER Jr, Carpenter PC, et al. Transsphenoidal removal of pituitary microadenoma in Cushing's disease. Mayo Clin Proc 53:24, 1978.
12. Knappe UJ, Ludecke DK. Transnasal microsurgery in children and adolescents with Cushing's disease. Neurosurgery 39(3): 484, 1996.
13. Becker DP, Atkinson R, Sakalas R, et al. Trans-sphenoidal microsurgery for acromegaly. Clin Neurol 36:101, 1974.
14. Su C, Ren Z, Wang W, et al. Transsphenoidal microsurgical removal of GH-secreting pituitary adenoma: A report of 200 cases. Chung Kuo I Hsueh Ko Hsueh Yuan Hsueh Pao 17(5):333, 1995.
15. Fiad TM, McKenna TJ. Meningitis as a late complication of surgically and medically treated pituitary adenoma. Clin Endocrinol 35(5):419, 1991.
16. Dolenc VV. Transcranial epidural approach to pituitary tumors extending beyond the sella. Neurosurgery 41(3):542, 1997.
17. Patterson RH. The role of transcranial surgery in the management of pituitary adenoma. Acta Neurochir (Suppl) (Wien) 65:16, 1996.
18. Arnott RD, Pestell RG, McKelvie PA, et al. A critical evaluation of transsphenoidal pituitary surgery in the treatment of Cushing's disease: Prediction of outcome. Acta Endocrinol 123(4):423, 1990.
19. Wei S, Zhou D, Zhang J. A direct transnasal transsphenoidal approach to pituitary tumors. Chin J Surg 34(9):572, 1996.
20. Dharambir SS, Pillay PK. Endoscopic pituitary surgery: A minimally invasive technique. Am J Rhinol 10:141, 1996.
21. Carrau RL, Jho H-D, Ko Y. Transnasal-transsphenoidal endoscopic surgery of the pituitary gland. Laryngoscope 106:914, 1996.
22. Aust MR, McCaffrey TV, Atkinson J. Transnasal endoscopic approach to the sella turcica. Am J Rhinol 12:283, 1998.
23. Yang SY, Zhu T, Zhang JN, et al. Transsphenoidal microsurgical management of pituitary adenoma. Microsurgery 15(11):754, 1994.
24. Koltai PJ, Goufman DB, Parnes SM, et al. Transsphenoidal hypophysectomy through the external rhinoplasty approach. Otolaryngol Head Neck Surg 111(3 Pt 1):197, 1994.
25. Chen G, Zuo H, Tian H. Transsphenoidal microsurgery for pituitary adenoma: Analysis of three fatal cases. Chin J Otorhinolaryngol 31(5):268, 1996.
26. Ni D, Wang Z, Yan J. Bleeding and complications related to hemorrhage during transsphenoidal removal of pituitary tumor. Chin J Otorhinolaryngol 29(4):206, 1994.
27. Gammert C. Rhinosurgical experience with the transseptal-transsphenoidal hypophysectomy: Technique and long-term results. Laryngoscope 100(3):286, 1990.
28. Soldati D, Monnier P. Endonasal sequelae after hypophysectomy. Ann Otolaryngol Chir Cervicofac 115(2):49, 1998.
29. Herman P, Lot G, Guichard JP, et al. Mucocele of the sphenoid sinus: A late complication of transsphenoidal pituitary surgery. Ann Otol Rhinol Laryngol 107(9 Pt 1):765, 1998.

SECTION

FIVE

Special Procedures

CHAPTER 20

Cerebrospinal Fluid Leak

Cerebrospinal fluid leak through the nose (CSF rhinorrhea) is an uncommon but critical problem facing the rhinologic surgeon. Historically, CSF rhinorrhea has been related to trauma, tumors, or idiopathic processes. However, in modern times, most cases are iatrogenic. With the current widespread use of sinus surgery and skull base surgery, the incidence of iatrogenic injuries to the skull base resulting in CSF leak has risen dramatically. This increase in incidence has forced the rhinologist to become involved in the management of patients with CSF rhinorrhea. In practice, not all otolaryngologists or rhinologists need to be able to repair CSF leaks, but it is essential that all rhinologic surgeons be well versed in the diagnosis of the condition and initial management principles. In this chapter, the details of diagnosis and management of CSF leak are thoroughly covered.

ETIOLOGY

CSF is the clear, watery fluid that cushions and bathes the central nervous system. It is produced by the choroid plexus within the cerebral ventricles and circulates through the ventricles into the subarachnoid space from the fourth ventricle through the paired foramina of Luschka and the midline foramen of Magendie.[1] The CSF is absorbed through the arachnoid villi spread throughout the subarachnoid space, but which are particularly abundant in the various cerebral cisterns. The total CSF volume is often quoted as being 135 to 140 mL, with about half in the spinal subarachnoid space, 20 mL in the ventricles, and the remainder in the intracranial subarachnoid space. CSF is produced and absorbed throughout the central nervous system at the rate of about 20 mL per hour.[1] This creates a natural turnover of the CSF and a flow from the ventricles to the cerebral cisterns.

CSF rhinorrhea can only occur when there is a connection between the subarachnoid space and the lumen of the nose or sinuses. Anatomically, this requires a defect in the arachnoid, dura, bone of the skull base, and the mucosa. This may occur anywhere throughout the skull base, including the middle cranial fossa. In this case, the CSF can flow through the mastoid air cells into the middle ear and down the eustachian tube into the nasopharynx, presenting as CSF rhinorrhea. The most common sites and causes of leakage vary according to the series reported. These reports differ widely based on the time period of the report, the location of the reporting physicians, and the subspecialty of the physicians. Older series report trauma and tumors as the primary causes, whereas more contemporary series most often report iatrogenic etiologies.[2–5] Urban centers have a higher incidence of penetrating injuries compared to rural locations, in which blunt trauma is a more frequent etiology. Neurosurgeons and trauma specialists focus on trauma and skull base surgeries as the primary etiologies, whereas otolaryngologists report iatrogenic injuries from ethmoidectomy.

In a series of cases reported by the author, iatrogenic injuries to the skull base and spontaneous CSF leaks were the most common.[6] In eight patients, the onset of CSF rhinorrhea had no known cause. Clinical findings in these cases varied from encephalocele to leakage around olfactory neurons through the cribriform plate. Five patients had CSF leaks as a result of endoscopic sinus surgery. In three of these, the condition was detected intraoperatively (2 of the author's patients, 1 patient from another surgeon's series in the same hospital), two patients were referred for delayed repair. In these cases, the site of injury was the cribriform plate in four of the cases and the posterior ethmoid skull base adjacent to the posterior ethmoid artery in the other case.

The areas of the skull base that are at highest risk for injury during endoscopic sinus surgery, or ethmoidectomy in general, are the cribriform plate and the anterior ethmoid skull base.[7, 8] The cribriform plate contains numerous perforations with olfactory nerves protruding through these perforations. The olfactory nerves are wrapped in dura and arachnoid, and often this covering extends into and even through the cribriform plate into the nose. CSF leakage can occur from injury to these nerves and tearing of the dura and arachnoid. In patients with extensive polyps, it is easy to lose orientation and follow the polyps directly into this mucosa, causing a CSF leak without injury to the skull base. The anterior ethmoid skull base may be extremely thin, especially in the area adjacent to the attachment of the middle turbinate. In this area, the slope of the skull base may be exaggerated, placing the skull base at increased risk.

The incidence of CSF leakage during sinus surgery has been reported in a number of series, as discussed in Chapter 8. The average rate appears to be somewhere between 0.1% and 1%, depending on the surgeon and type of cases presented.[9–11] Risk factors associated with CSF leak include revision surgery, frontal sinus surgery, and the presence of polyps. It has not been demonstrated that the experience of the surgeon greatly affects the risk of CSF leak.[12] This may be because less experienced practitioners tend to perform the more basic cases and are more conservative in their dissections, whereas the more experienced surgeons may take on the more difficult cases and perform more complete dissections.

In addition to endoscopic sinus surgery, other iatrogenic causes include neurosurgical operations and traditional (nonendoscopic) sinus surgery. In the author's experience, neurosurgical cases that have led to CSF leak include aneurysm clipping, transsphenoidal hypophysectomy, and resection of sphenoclival meningioma. However, any procedure that involves operating on the skull base from either above or below could result in CSF leak.

Other than trauma and iatrogenic causes, the most common etiology of CSF leak is idiopathic.[13, 14] Also known as spontaneous CSF leak, this is an uncommon condition that is nonetheless seen in virtually every series reported. This condition poses a significant problem for the otolaryngologist in terms of confirming and localizing the leak. Most often, the leak occurs through the cribriform plate or through one of the neural foramina (e.g., foramen rotundum to the sphenopalatine foramen). The proposed pathogenesis of this phenomena is leakage through one of the perforations in the cribriform plate around an olfactory nerve. This may occur either as a result of a sheer injury of the nerves on the superior surface of the skull base or atrophy of nerve secondary to some other cause.

Tumors and encephaloceles may cause CSF leak by eroding the skull base. With tumors, the leak normally does not occur unless something also happens to open the dura. The most common scenario is that the patient undergoes radiation therapy. As the tumor shrinks, a dural dehiscence develops where the tumor has invaded through the dura. Spontaneous encephaloceles are rare, but are often diagnosed when the patient manifests CSF rhinorrhea. In these cases, intracranial pressure causes rubbing on the skull base. Over a long period of time, this results in a bony defect. As the encephalocele enlarges through the defect, the fibers of the dura separate, allowing the leak to occur.

Prior to the popularization of endoscopic sinus surgery, trauma was the most common cause of CSF leak.[15–17] This can occur from a penetrating injury of the skull base, most commonly a gunshot wound, or it may result from blunt trauma leading to a displaced fracture of the skull base. CSF rhinorrhea has been estimated to occur in as may as 5% of patients with skull base fracture and up to 25% to 50% of patients with fractures of the anterior skull base.[15–20] Because most of these injuries do not require operative repair, they are not included in the series of patients undergoing surgery, and are less frequently reported.

DIAGNOSIS

In certain patients, CSF rhinorrhea may be clearly apparent, but in most cases, it is a challenge to diagnose and localize. The history of a patient with CSF leak is typically one of an intermittent, watery, nasal discharge that emanates from the front of the nose when the patient arises from a supine position or bends forward. As stated, the discharge is most often described as a clear, watery fluid. Often, it is reported by patients to have a sweet, rather than a salty taste. The amount of drainage varies from a few drops to a gush or stream of clear fluid.

Most cases of CSF leakage involve intermittent drainage. There are several reasons for this. One reason for intermittent drainage is because the fluid drains into the sinuses, where it is temporarily trapped. Upon a change in position, the fluid is released, draining suddenly. In certain cases, there may also be a ball valve–type mechanism that can lead to intermittent discharge. When the patient is upright, the brain sits on the anterior skull base and can plug the defect, preventing the leak. When the patient assumes a supine position, the brain pulls away from the skull base, allowing the CSF to seep out. A third mechanism that can contribute to the intermittent nature of the leak is a pressure-sensitive leak. In this case, the CSF only leaks out when the CSF pressure rises above a certain level. When the pressure is above the threshold, the fluid leaks out until the pressure drops below the threshold. At this point, the leak stops until the pressure reaccumulates.

In a patient suspected of having a CSF leak, it is important to elicit a history of a predisposing condition. This would include previous surgery, closed head trauma, nasal or sinus tumor, or any event or condition that could lead to a sudden increase in intracranial pressure. This includes such activities as lifting heavy weights, hard coughing, and frequent sneezing. A history suggestive of allergic rhinitis, viral rhinitis, and sinusitis would tend to weigh against a leak.

The difficulty in diagnosing CSF rhinorrhea stems from the fact that clear drainage from the nose is common and rarely indicates a CSF leak. Most often, the clear drainage is either mucus or tears. Mucus tends to have a greasy or slimy consistency and a salty taste, whereas tears are thin, watery, and very salty. Despite these characteristics, both tears and mucus can masquerade as CSF. Therefore, the diagnosis of CSF rhinorrhea rarely rests with a history of clear nasal discharge.

Examination of CSF leak patients is often unrevealing. Normally, there are no external indications that a leak has occurred unless the patient is a victim of recent trauma. Routine nasal examination with anterior rhinoscopy may be consistent with previous surgery or trauma or may be normal. Identifying the presence of CSF in the nose is difficult unless the leak is profuse.

In the case of a suspected leak after trauma, one can look for the so-called double-ring sign. This occurs when a combination of blood and CSF leaks out together. If some of this discharge is collected on a piece of filter paper or even a bed sheet, the CSF migrates farther out from the center of the spot than the blood. This results in an inner ring of red blood and an outer ring of clear CSF.

Attempts to stimulate clear drainage can be performed. One of the most successful is to bend the patient forward while the patient performs a Valsalva maneuver. This increases intracranial pressure and leads to leakage. Other methods that can be used to stimulate the leak include pushing against a rigid object and rolling the patient while in a head-down position.

If a leak can be stimulated, it is important to collect a sample of the fluid. There are a number of tests that can be performed to verify that the fluid is CSF as opposed to nasal mucus or tears. The easiest is to measure the glucose level using a urine or blood dipstick. Dipsticks are readily available owing to their common use in monitoring diabetes. Placing a drop of the nasal discharge on the dipstick should lead to detection of low levels of glucose. However, this test is highly subjective and has a low sensitivity.[21, 22] A quantitative glucose assay is more accurate. In this test, a small amount of the fluid is collected and assayed for glucose level, similar to a serum blood test. The test is positive for CSF if it reveals a level of 30 mg/dL or higher; results should be less than 10 mg/dL for nasal mucus and tears.[23] Unfortunately, this test is only a guideline and is not considered to be definitive because of variations in the glucose level in CSF. In some individuals, the glucose concentration of the fluid may be diluted by mucus or tears or the CSF glucose level may be low enough to be confused with nasal mucus. This is particularly true if the patient has meningitis, in which case the glucose level would be expected to be low. The glucose test can be made more accurate by performing a simultaneous lumbar puncture and collecting CSF for glucose determination. In this setting, the comparison of the nasal discharge glucose level to the CSF glucose level, obtained by lumbar puncture, should be highly diagnostic of a true CSF leak.[17]

The most reliable test for confirming CSF leak is to measure the beta$_2$-transferrin level of the discharge fluid. This test can be performed on as little as 50 μL of fluid and is highly specific and sensitive. Beta$_2$-transferrin is a protein found almost exclusively in CSF.[24, 25] None of the other fluids found in the nose can potentially contain this compound. For this reason, detection of beta$_2$-transferrin is considered to be diagnostic of CSF.[26, 27] The difficulty with this test is that it requires a specialty laboratory prepared to perform the test. Many hospitals are not able to offer this test routinely, limiting the utility of the beta$_2$-transferrin test.

For patients with a suspected leak, it is important to confirm the presence of the leak and to localize the skull base defect. There are a number of options available for detection and localization. The simplest method is to use nasal endoscopy. After thorough decongestion, the nose is examined with the 0-, 30-, and 70-degree endoscopes to attempt to identify the leak. This can be combined with Valsalva maneuver and positioning of the patient to attempt to stimulate the leak. In many cases, this will not be successful, in which case endoscopy can then be combined with intrathecal fluorescein.[28, 29] Fluorescein is a dye that has been used for contrast enhancement intrathecally, on the conjunctiva, and intravascularly. Under an ultraviolet light, the dye fluoresces, producing a bright yellow color. The concentrate is diluted to make a 5% solution and 1 to 2 mL is injected into the lumbar subarachnoid space. The patient is placed in a Trendelenburg position for about 30 minutes, and the nose is then examined endoscopically. The fluorescein dye leaks out of the defect and glows bright green or yellow. This helps to localize the site of the leak. Alternatively, the nose can be packed with pledgets that can be examined under ultraviolet light to further enhance detection. The problem with this test is that intrathecal fluorescein can cause seizures. The company that produces the product has now placed a warning label on the vial that states that the product is not intended for intrathecal injection. However, used in the low doses recommended here, it is reasonably safe. In the largest series reported on the use of intrathecal fluorescein, there was an overall incidence of 0.3% of complications using the techniques outlined here.[29] Seizures with intrathecal fluorescein are generally associated with either too high a dose or too high a concentration of the fluorescein. Ultimately, the decision to use fluorescein has to be made after weighing the risks against the diagnostic benefits. In cases when the fluorescein can resolve an otherwise undiagnosed situation, the value of the test probably outweighs the minimal risk of seizures.

In almost all cases of CSF leak, a computed tomography (CT) scan of the sinuses is obtained. This is necessary for anatomic definition of the skull base defect and may aid in confirming and diagnosing the leak. The scan should be performed using direct coronal cuts with bone windows, high-resolution technique, and thin cuts. This is the best technique available for anatomically detecting defects in the skull base. In many cases, this test alone, in the presence of an obvious leak, will complete the evaluation. However, in cases when the leak is difficult to confirm or localize, the CT scan can be combined with intrathecal contrast studies, referred to as CT cisternograms.[30–34] To perform this test, a suitable contrast material is injected into the subarachnoid space, often in the cisterna magna at the base of the skull posteriorly. The patient is then placed in the Trendelenburg position for 30 to 60 minutes before performing the CT scan. Obtained under these conditions, this test not only can detect a leak but also can localize the leak with a high degree of specificity. Some studies have reported an 85% success rate with this test. This procedure has the disadvantages of discomfort, time, and expense that must be considered in relation to other, less invasive methods. In addition, the CT cisternogram has the limitation of requiring an ongoing leak. A leak that is intermittent may not be manifested during the interval of the scan and could be missed.

Radionuclide cisternography is an alternative to endoscopy with fluorescein and CT cisternography for confirming leaks in difficult cases.[35–37] In this procedure, preweighed pledgets are placed in various locations in the nose. Usually, this includes along the cribriform plate, against the eustachian tube, and under the middle turbinate on each side of the nose (Fig. 20–1). A cisternal tap or a lumbar catheter is placed and an aliquot of radiotracer material is injected into the CSF. The patient is placed in a Trendelenburg position for 20 to 30 minutes, and over the next several hours, the patient is repeatedly scanned to determine whether any of the tracer material has leaked into the nose or down the throat into the stomach. The next day, the pledgets are removed and weighed and then scanned for the number of counts per minute. A sample of serum is collected at the time the pledgets are removed as a control. The number of counts per milliliter of fluid per minute is determined. A positive result is reported if one of the pledgets has a ratio of greater than 3:1 when compared to the serum control. This test has been reported to have a sensitivity of 85% to 90%. The problem with the radionuclide cisternogram test is that it has a relatively low specificity compared to the other methods of evaluation because of a significant incidence of false-positive results. In patients with rhinitis or sinusitis, there can be accumulation of the tracer in the pledgets, leading to the perception of a positive result. The test is more reliable if only one of the nasal pledgets is positive or if only one side has positive pledgets. The other problem with the radionuclide test is that it does not localize the leak. Because the pledgets do not identify the exact location of the leak, even in clearly positive cases when the pledgets have a high ratio of counts to the serum control, other methods are needed to localize the skull base defect. For this reason, it is not the preferred method.

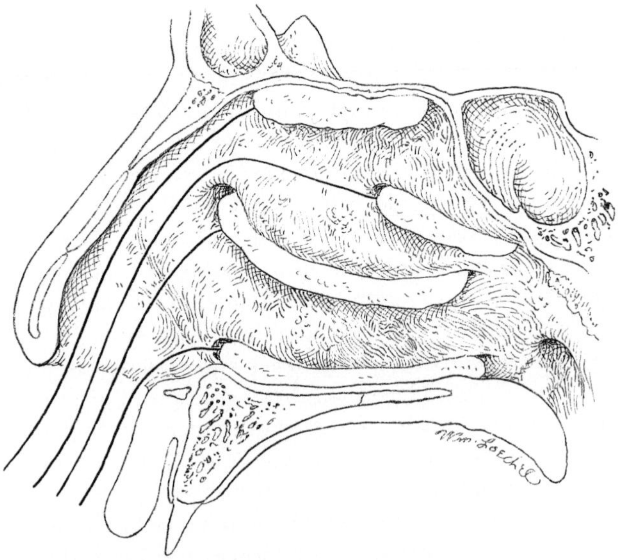

Figure 20–1. Placement of nasal pledgets. Pledgets are placed to collect extravasated CSF containing either fluorescein or a radiotracer material. The pledgets are placed along the cribriform plate, in the superior meatus and the middle meatus, and along the floor of the nose.

The newest option available for diagnosis of CSF rhinorrhea is magnetic resonance imaging (MRI) and MRI cisternography.[38–41] This test relies on the ability of T2-weighted images to enhance intensely the signal of any fluid including CSF. Early results with this technique suggest that it is highly sensitive and accurate in diagnosing the presence of leakage and in identifying the site of the leak, even in cases when the patient is not actively leaking.[41] If these results hold up over time, MRI as a noninvasive, nonionizing test will replace all other methods of detection and localization.

MEDICAL MANAGEMENT

In certain circumstances, the initial management of a confirmed CSF leak may involve medical therapy. The steps used in controlling a CSF leak nonsurgically are well described and highly successful when indicated.[19,42] The situations when conservative therapy may be successful are cases when an acute leak is detected at the time when it is caused or shortly thereafter. In these circumstances, there is a chance that, if conditions are optimized, the leak may heal. The most applicable cases are following blunt skull base trauma, such as after a motor vehicle accident. Conservative therapy is normally successful in these cases and should always be attempted before surgery is performed.[43,44] In iatrogenic cases (most commonly, after endoscopic sinus surgery), healing may occur if the leak is not detected and repaired at the time it is caused. As long as the size of the defect is not too large, healing can be anticipated in these cases. In all cases, a high-resolution CT scan should be obtained before electing medical therapy over surgery. The keys to success in nonoperative therapy are the presence of a small to moderate-sized defect and prompt application of the treatment protocol before the leak can become well established. No absolute size criteria exist, but the larger the defect, the less likely spontaneous healing will occur.

The most important aspect of the protocol for medical therapy for CSF leak is bed rest. The patient should be hospitalized and restricted to bathroom privileges. The head of the bed should be kept elevated to at least a 30-degree incline. This combination of bed rest and the upright positioning takes the pressure off of the area of the leak, promoting spontaneous healing.

Several adjunctive therapies help to promote healing. One is to administer stool softeners and, possibly, laxatives. This helps to avoid the increased intracranial pressure associated with bearing down during defecation. Along similar lines, patients should receive antitussives if a cough is present. Coughing is associated with sudden increases in intracranial pressure. Antitussives help to decrease the incidence and severity of coughing. Additionally, drug therapy designed to decrease intracranial pressure can be prescribed. One of the commonly used adjunctive agents is mannitol. This is a diuretic that works by osmotic pressure. By increasing the serum osmolality, mannitol helps to draw fluid out of the brain and CSF, which results in a lowering of the intracranial pressure. The other medication commonly used to lower intracranial pressure is acetazolamide. This agent is a carbonic anhydrase inhibitor that has been found to inhibit the production of CSF by the choroid plexus. By decreasing production of CSF, acetazolamide can decrease CSF and intracranial pressure. Finally, systemic steroids, usually dexamethasone, can be added. These agents help decrease any edema and usually lower intracranial pressure.

If this combination of therapies is not successful after 5 to 7 days, a lumbar drain may be added.[45,46] The use of a lumbar drain in this circumstance is somewhat controversial. A lumbar catheter is placed into the subarachnoid space and 10 mL of CSF per hour (20 mL every 2 hours) is drained to decrease CSF pressure. This rate of drainage corresponds to the average rate of production of CSF. The advantage to using a lumbar drain is that it can significantly lower the intracranial pressure, which promotes spontaneous healing. However, controversy exists because prolonged lumbar drainage is associated with a risk of meningitis, pneumocephalus, and severe spinal headache.[47] The spinal headache can usually be alleviated by injecting 5 to 10 mL of the patient's blood into the area of the lumbar catheter entry site into the subarachnoid space. This procedure is the so-called "blood patch." The blood presumably seals the lumbar site, preventing further leaking in this area and thus alleviating the spinal headache. The risk of meningitis from the lumbar catheter can be minimized by meticulous sterile technique in placing the drain and maintaining the drain.

The final decision of whether or not to use a lumbar drain must be individualized, with the patient participating in the decision. On balance, the lumbar drain is not recommended as part of nonoperative treatment for CSF leak in most patients. The risk of prolonged lumbar catheterization is high compared to the low probability that the use of the lumbar catheter will result in resolution of the leak after failure of medical therapy and bed rest, as described earlier. For most patients who fail the full nonsurgical protocol, the risk : benefit analysis will favor direct surgical repair.

INDICATIONS FOR SURGERY

The protocol for management of many patients with CSF leak is to attempt medical management initially. This protocol applies to patients with posttraumatic leak and delayed diagnosis of iatrogenic leak. These conditions are examples of situations when the leak may respond to nonsurgical treatment. Trauma patients who present at the time of injury with CSF rhinorrhea have a high rate of control without surgery. In these patients, the full week of hospitalization with bed rest will usually result in stoppage of the leak. If, after a full week of observation, the leak continues, addition of the lumbar catheter is considered. Depending on the findings on CT scan, the leak will be more or less likely to resolve. In linear leaks without significant displacement of the skull base fracture, a lumbar drain is recommended, as these leaks have a good prognosis for resolution. Conversely, a patient with a significantly displaced skull base fracture who has not responded to bed rest alone may not have such a good prognosis, and surgery should be considered rather than continued observation with a lumbar drain.

Patients who have iatrogenic leaks, especially after endoscopic sinus surgery, are frequently not diagnosed until the packing is removed several days after the surgery. In these cases, conservative treatment may also be successful. If the defect is large or the initial trial of bed rest is unsuccessful, a surgical procedure is warranted. However, if a CSF leak is detected during an endoscopic surgery, it is worthwhile to attempt repair immediately. In most cases, the repair will lead to primary healing and avoid the need for prolonged postoperative care or repeat surgery.[6, 9]

Patients who have idiopathic leak or CSF leak related to tumor are unlikely to respond to nonsurgical management. It is not dangerous or inappropriate to attempt conservative management in these cases, but it is unlikely to be successful. Proceeding directly to operative repair in these cases is advisable.

Regardless of the etiology of the CSF leak, if the complete nonsurgical protocol is used and the leak persists, surgery is indicated. The type of surgery selected depends on the cause of the leak, the location of the defect, and the size of the defect. Almost all defects can be successfully repaired using endoscopic surgery. However, there are specific contraindications to endoscopic repair. One of these is if the leak is located in an area inaccessible to the sinus endoscope. The best example of this is the posterior wall of the frontal sinus.[48, 49] This area is generally inaccessible to repair by sinus endoscopy. The other site that may not be accessible by endoscopy is inside a lateral recess of the sphenoid sinus.[50]

Another category of patients who are not usually candidates for endoscopic repair are patients with tumors. If the CSF leak is caused by a tumor extending through the skull base, the best approach is through a craniofacial surgical resection. Endoscopic repair is unlikely to be successful if the graft has to heal to a tumor bed. If the leak manifests only after successful radiation therapy for the tumor, it may be possible to attempt an endoscopic repair, but this is a rare circumstance.

The last situation in which an endoscopic repair may not be successful is if the defect is too large. What constitutes too large a defect is a rather subjective determination. Some surgeons have been successful in repairing defects up to 3 cm in length using an endoscopic technique. The largest defect the author has repaired using endoscopy is about 2 cm in length. Defects larger than 2 cm can be approached endoscopically if the circumstances suggest probable success.

Virtually all other patients with CSF rhinorrhea can successfully be repaired endoscopically. The choice of whether to perform an endoscopic approach or a transcranial approach is rather straightforward. Most older textbooks suggest that the transcranial approach is the safest technique with the highest chance of success. However, with the advent of endoscopic repair, this has changed. Numerous authors have published series of patients with CSF leaks repaired by endoscopy, all of which have demonstrated a high rate of success.[3, 4, 6–9, 51–67] In the series reported by the author, all of the patients operated on had initial healing of the graft with leak resolution. Only 1 of 19 patients developed recurrence of CSF leak. None of the series reported has described significant complications. The author is aware of one case not reported in the medical literature in which the patient developed intracranial bleeding after repair of a cribriform plate defect. The problem was not identified until the patient did not wake up in the recovery room. By the time the patient was returned to the operating room and a craniotomy was performed, it was too late and the patient died.

By comparison, the risks of craniotomy are significant. Craniotomy is associated with anosmia in all patients, frontal lobe injury with blunting of the patient's affect in many, and a 1% to 2% risk of mortality. Most series of cases also suggest only an 85% to 90% success rate for controlling the CSF leak with transcranial repair.[68–70] In comparison to endoscopic repair, craniotomy is clearly a secondary option. An appropriate algorithm for case selection for repair of CSF rhinorrhea is as follows. For leaks arising from the posterior table of the frontal sinus, osteoplastic flap and sinus obliteration is indicated. For all other leaks from the ethmoid or sphenoid, an endoscopic repair should be performed, with few exceptions, as the first option. One exception is that for certain leaks from the sphenoid, a transseptal transsphenoidal repair may be the best technique. Other exceptions include a defect greater than 2 cm in diameter and the rare circumstance in which an endoscopic approach is technically impossible. In these cases, it is appropriate to proceed directly to craniotomy. The final indication for craniotomy repair of CSF rhinorrhea is failure of endoscopic repair. Rarely, an external ethmoidectomy or a microscopic transnasal approach may be attempted.

PREOPERATIVE MANAGEMENT

The preoperative management depends on the type of repair planned. In all cases, it is important to consult a neurosurgeon before the operation. Regardless of the type of repair to be performed, a neurosurgeon's participation is important for monitoring, lumbar drainage, and backup should anything go wrong and a craniotomy be required. It is also important for a complete neurologic examination to be performed before the surgery in case there is need for a comparison to baseline after the operation.

A routine laboratory and medical evaluation is conducted based on the operation planned. For an endoscopic procedure that may take 1 to 2 hours to perform, a minimal work-up is required. When a craniotomy is planned, a complete evaluation is necessary to identify any potentially complicating factors.

One of the important considerations is whether or not to utilize a lumbar catheter for CSF drainage. During the surgery, this can help increase or lower the intracranial pressure depending on the circumstance. If the leak is not immediately apparent, sterile saline can be introduced to increase the intracranial pressure, thereby helping to reveal the site of the leak. Alternatively, intrathecal fluorescein can be used to help identify the site of the leak. If the brain is prolapsing through the defect, removal of CSF can decrease the intracranial pressure and help spontaneously reduce the brain prolapse. After the surgery, lumbar drainage can help decrease the intracranial pressure, minimizing the strain on the repair and the chances of failure. The negative aspects of using a lumbar catheter include the risks of meningitis and severe spinal headache. On balance, the author has advocated the use of lumbar drains for most cases of delayed repair of an established CSF fistula. In cases when a leak is detected during the primary surgery, immediate repair is performed and lumbar drainage is not necessary.

As discussed in the preceding sections, CT scan of the sinuses is mandatory for preoperative evaluation of patients undergoing repair of CSF rhinorrhea. However, there are instances in which additional radiologic studies are helpful or necessary. In isolated cases, the use of computer-guided surgery may be helpful. This should be decided on on a case-by-case basis. Computer-guided surgery has the advantage of allowing real-time localization of anatomic points on a multiplanar CT scan. This technology is particularly advantageous when the leak is in a location that is difficult to access, such as the lateral wall of the sphenoid sinus, or when a large defect is approached. In cases of encephalocele, it is worthwhile to consider an arteriogram or magnetic resonance arteriogram (MRA). These studies have the ability to delineate the relationship of the cerebral vasculature to the encephalocele. This is necessary to avoid vascular injury in these cases.

Prophylactic antibiotics are routinely prescribed to help prevent sinus infection, meningitis, and toxic shock syndrome in patients undergoing surgical repair. The use of antibiotics in patients undergoing nonoperative therapy is more controversial. However, a recent meta-analysis of the published studies on the use of prophylactic antibiotics for CSF rhinorrhea after trauma favored their use.[71] The best choice for antibiotics is unclear. A first-generation cephalosporin is probably the best agent for preventing toxic shock syndrome. Amoxicillin/clavulinic acid is probably the best overall option for prevention of sinusitis and meningitis and is adequate for prevention of toxic shock syndrome.

A final consideration is the form of anesthesia used for the procedure. Although it is possible to perform repair of a CSF leak under local anesthesia with sedation, in practice, this is not recommended. For this critically important surgery, the surgeon's comfort takes precedence over the theoretical benefits of local sedation. With the use of general anesthesia, the surgeon can perform the operation without concern for patient motion or intraoperative discomfort.

TECHNIQUES

Intranasal Repair

There are a large number of techniques described in the literature for intranasal repair of CSF leaks. All of these techniques have several factors in common. These include meticulous technique, careful site preparation, complete coverage of the defect by a graft, and graft stabilization. If all of these factors are successfully attended to, the procedure has an outstanding chance of success. In this section, the procedure described for intranasal repair is that practiced by the author. This technique utilizes endoscopic visualization, middle turbinate graft, stabilization with multiple layers of nasal packing, and a lumbar drain.

As stated, the author uses endoscopic guidance for repair of CSF leaks. Headlight illumination and microscopic visualization are alternatives that predate the endoscopic method, and most of the techniques used endoscopically can be performed with either of these two adjuncts. However, there are significant advantages to the endoscopic technique over both of the other forms of visualization. Using a headlight has the advantage of simplicity. Other than this, there are no reasons to prefer this method. Endoscopic surgery is superior for several steps, especially in exposing and preparing the defect site for grafting. This requires careful and meticulous dissection, which is best facilitated by the magnified view of the endoscope. Microscopic surgery is a traditional and viable alternative to endoscopy. The microscope provides a magnified view and bimanual dexterity. Its disadvantages are that the microscope is difficult to use in the nose, and the optical angle of the visual axis limits the field of view to defects of the cribriform plate, posterior ethmoid, and sphenoid sinus.

Endoscopic Technique

As stated earlier, the underlying principles for repair of CSF leaks using endoscopic technique are to use meticulous technique, expose the defect, place a graft over the defect, and stabilize the graft. The first step is to set up the patient properly with a lumbar drain and correct positioning. The inside of the nose should be decongested and injected with local anesthetic. The technique is as described in Chapter 8 for standard endoscopic sinus surgery. Cocaine flakes (crystalline cocaine) are used as a decongestant and to help block the sphenopalatine ganglion. Typically, only one side will be operated on, so the full 300 mg of cocaine flakes can be used on the one side. This will help to achieve maximal hemostasis. The cocaine is applied on cotton-tipped applicators to three points: above the anterior attachment of the middle turbinate, lateral to the middle turbinate, and above the posterior end of the middle turbinate. Lidocaine (1%) with epinephrine (1:100,000) is used as the local anesthetic for injection. A dose of up to 10 mL is injected in three or four spots for maximum effect without causing excessive bleeding points. These areas include the anterior attachment of the middle turbinate, the anterior attachment of the uncinate process, and the posteroinferior edge of the middle turbinate. If desired, 2 mL of local anesthetic can be injected directly into the sphenopalatine ganglion. This can be accomplished by locating the sphenopalatine foramen directly behind the posterior attachment of the middle turbinate or by injection through the greater palatine foramen medial to the first molar on the hard palate.

Approach

After the local anesthetic has had adequate time to take effect, the first step is to perform a complete ethmoidectomy. Depending on the location of the CSF leak, some variation in the degree of ethmoidectomy is possible. The guiding principle is that areas adjacent to the leak must be completely dissected to expose the surrounding skull base; however, areas distant from the leak can be preserved. A second principle is that sufficient dissection must be performed to ensure that further surgery is not necessary. Once the CSF leak is repaired, additional surgery for recurrent sinusitis would risk recurrence of the leak and so should be strictly avoided.

Adequate dissection usually means performing a complete ethmoidectomy, sphenoidectomy, frontal sinusotomy, and wide antrostomy. However, if the frontal sinus or sphenoid is completely normal, these areas can be avoided under certain circumstances. If the CSF leak is located along the cribriform plate, a complete ethmoidectomy sparing the frontal recess and the sphenoid sinus is performed. For CSF leaks arising from the anterior ethmoid roof, a complete ethmoidectomy, including dissection of the frontal recess, is required, but the sphenoid can be preserved. For CSF leaks from the posterior ethmoid or sphenoid sinus, a complete ethmoidectomy and sphenoidectomy is performed, but the frontal recess need not be dissected.

In many cases of CSF rhinorrhea, the cause of the leak will be previous sinus surgery. In these cases, a complete revision ethmoidectomy with sphenoid, frontal, and maxillary sinusotomies should be performed. A more conservative ethmoidectomy should not be performed as the risk of recurrent sinus infection with preservation of certain areas is too high to warrant conservation.

A complete description of endoscopic ethmoidectomy is outlined in Chapter 8. In cases of CSF leak, the procedure is complicated by a preexisting defect somewhere along the skull base. For this reason, it is important to approach the area of the defect with extreme caution. Slow and careful technique should be used, with each bite of tissue being carefully considered. Sharp, through-cutting instruments or a microdebrider should be used. Standard Blakesley-type instruments that tear the mucosal edges should be avoided around the area of the defect so as to prevent inadvertent injury to the dura.

In patients who have not undergone previous surgery or who have had only minimal surgery, the standard anterior-to-posterior approach can be used. Uncinectomy is performed or completed. The ethmoidectomy then proceeds through the bulla and the ground lamella. While proceeding from anterior to posterior, the first landmark to identify is the lamina papyracea. The skull base is identified in the posterior ethmoid sinus. The lamina papyracea and skull base are then skeletonized to remove any residual cells or bone fragments. It is not necessary to remove the mucosa from the skull base or lamina papyracea. On the contrary, it is preferable to preserve this mucosa if possible. When skeletonizing the skull base, special attention should be paid to the area of the suspected defect. This should be left for the end of the case, leaving any capsule or mucosa over the defect until that time.

If a sphenoidotomy is to be performed, the preferred technique is to identify the ostium and enlarge the ostium inferiorly and laterally to remove the anterior wall of the sphenoid. To identify the ostium, the posterior and inferior aspects of the superior turbinate are removed. This exposes the sphenoid rostrum, allowing the ostium to be identified by palpation with a suction catheter. A rotating sphenoid punch is used to enlarge the opening.

The remainder of the ethmoid cells can easily be exenterated once the sphenoid sinus is opened and the skull base and lamina papyracea are well delineated. At this stage, it is best to work from the sphenoid anteriorly to the frontal recess. In this way, the anterior ethmoid artery can usually be identified along the anterior ethmoid roof. This is a key landmark in the dissection of the frontal recess.

The frontal recess dissection is performed next. The agger nasi cell is opened by removing the anterior wall of the cell in the root of the middle turbinate. The opening of the frontal sinus is usually found in the space between the anterior ethmoid artery and the posterior wall of the agger nasi cell. To widely expose this area, the posterior wall of the agger nasi is removed using giraffe forceps or an angled cutting instrument on the microdebrider. If it is necessary to enlarge the ostium further, this is accomplished by removing the anterior rim of the ostium.

The last step in the preliminary dissection of the sinus is to perform a wide middle meatus antrostomy. After removing the uncinate process, it is usually possible to identify the natural ostium of the sinus. The ostium is enlarged by sharply removing the posterior fontanelle.

If the defect is located in the cribriform plate, an additional step is required. In these cases, it is necessary to remove the middle turbinate completely up to the skull base. This allows access to the cribriform plate, which otherwise would be difficult to accomplish. This also provides a wide, flat surface on which to place the graft, with increased room for overlap of the graft onto normal bone.

Defect Preparation

Once the sinuses are completely dissected, the defect site must be prepared to accept a graft. Any mucosa covering the defect must be carefully removed. In some cases, it may not be possible to ensure complete removal of all mucosal remnants. In this situation, bipolar cautery can be used to coagulate the surface of the defect to destroy any fragments still attached to the dura.

A clean surface of bone around the defect is necessary for proper graft adherence. Approximately 0.5 to 1 cm of mucosa should be removed completely around the skull base defect (Fig. 20–2). A Freer or Cottle elevator can be used to lift the mucosa from the bone, allowing easy removal. In some cases, developing the bony circumference requires extension onto the septum or lamina papyracea. In these cases, portions of the mucosa over these areas can also be removed.

Many patients will have some degree of prolapse of intracranial contents into the nose. This may range from a slight bulge to true encephalocele. The slight bulge can be managed by removal of CSF through a lumbar drain, which will cause the prolapse to pull back intracranially. Encephalocele, however, must be resected before repair can be achieved. This is accomplished by using bipolar cautery to slowly transect the base of the encephalocele. Alternating cautery and small snips with endoscopic scissors will allow slow progress across the base.

One area of controversy in repair of CSF leaks is whether or not to place the grafts intracranially. Some may argue that the intracranial graft provides superior support and has a higher success rate. However, many authors, including this one, who have experience with overlay techniques have found equivalent success rates with this technique. Regardless of one's preference, it is impossible to argue that intracranial dissection does not carry some risk. There have been reports of intracranial bleeding following repair of CSF leaks that may be attributable to this type of intracranial dissection. For this reason, the overlay technique is preferred for most cases. One exception to this is a large defect with a diameter greater than 1.5 cm, in which case significant prolapse and late recurrence are real possibilities.

If intracranial dissection is performed, the best technique is to use either a Woodson or curved Cottle eleva-

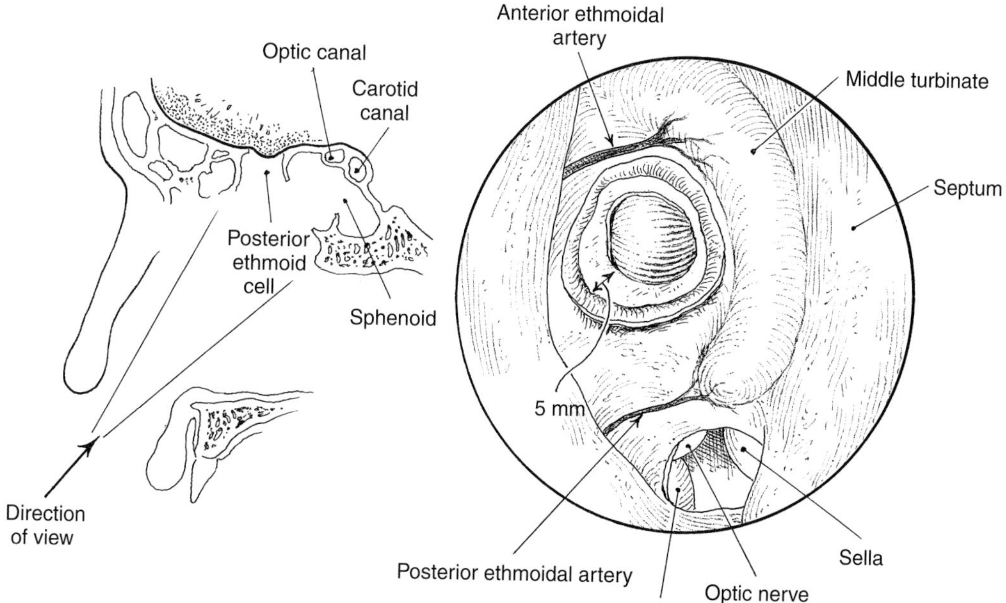

Figure 20–2. Defect preparation. Example of defect preparation from the area of the roof of the anterior ethmoid sinus. A complete sphenoethmoidectomy has been performed and the mucosa is elevated around the defect for at least 5 mm.

tor to carefully elevate the dura from the skull base on the intracranial side. This is done under close endoscopic visualization through the defect. The elevation should extend circumferentially around the defect for about 5 mm in each direction. This is not possible over the cribriform plate without cutting the olfactory nerves, so it is avoided and an overlay is always used.

Grafting

The type of graft used to repair CSF leak is also controversial. A variety of methods have been described. The surgeon can use a mucosal graft, bone graft, cartilage graft, fascial graft, or a commercially available graft material. The choices for mucosal grafts include free septal mucosal grafts, septal mucosal rotation flaps, free buccal mucosal grafts, inferior turbinate mucosal grafts, and middle turbinate mucosal grafts. Bone grafts can be obtained from the calvarium, septum, hip, or turbinate. Cartilage grafts can be obtained from the septum or auricle. Fascia is available primarily from the temporalis muscle or thigh, or is commercially available as artificial fascia. Of all of these options, the author prefers the middle turbinate as the source of the graft. The reasons for this are that the turbinate is local within the field, easy to harvest, provides both mucosa and bone, and often must be removed to facilitate the repair. All of the options have their advocates, but none of these other options combines all of the benefits of the middle turbinate as a donor site. If, for some reason, the middle turbinate is not available, the septum is an acceptable second alternative.

The exact type of graft to be used will depend on the defect to be repaired. For linear cracks or small defects measuring less than 5 mm in diameter, a mucosa-only overlay graft is used (Fig. 20–3*A*). For defects measuring between 5 and 15 mm, a composite bone and mucosal graft is used (Fig. 20–3*B*). For larger defects with a diameter greater than 15 mm, separate bone and mucosal grafts are used, with the bone placed intracranially and the mucosa used as an overlay (Fig. 20–3*C*). This protocol has been used successfully by the author with the middle turbinate used as the donor for all cases.

The graft is harvested from the middle turbinate after the ethmoidectomy using curved endoscopic scissors. The entire turbinate need not be removed if this is not necessary for exposure or repair of the defect. Only that portion required for the graft is excised, making sure that some excess is harvested to ensure that an adequate graft is developed (Fig. 20–4*A*). Once the turbinate is removed, the mucosa is dissected from the lateral surface of the turbinate from the cut edge toward the inferior edge, keeping the mucosa attached to the medial surface of the bone (Fig. 20–4*B* and *C*). If a mucosa-only graft is harvested, the bone is removed from the medial surface and the mucosa is trimmed to the size required. If separate bone and mucosal grafts are used, they are separated and each is trimmed to the appropriate size. When a composite graft is indicated, the mucosa is left attached to the medial surface of the bone

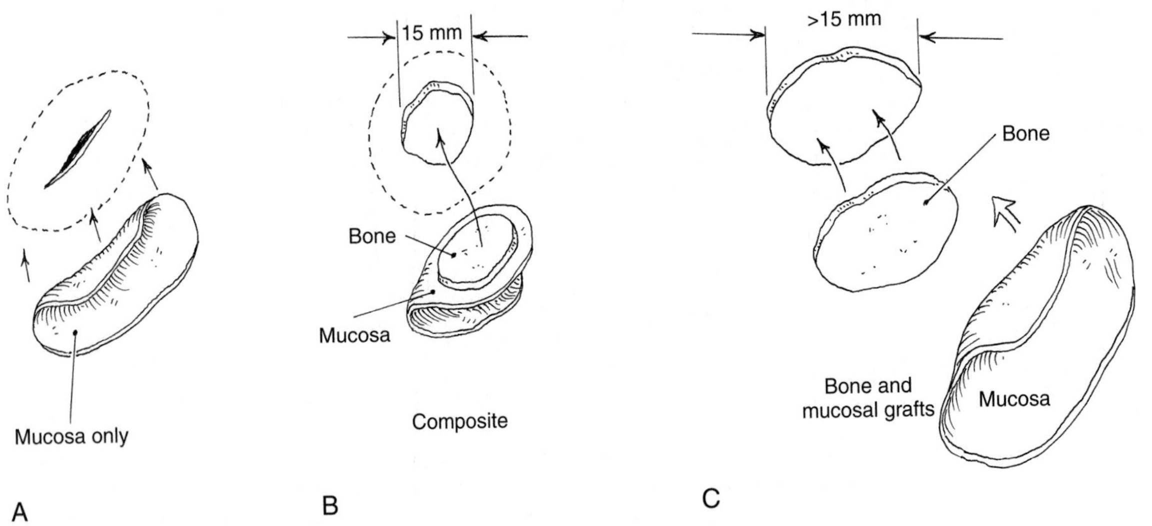

Figure 20–3. Grafting techniques. *A,* Free mucosal graft used for linear defects and defects measuring less than 5 mm in diameter. *B,* Composite bone and mucosal grafts used for defects with diameters of between 5 and 15 mm. *C,* Separate bone and mucosal grafts used for defects greater than 15 mm in diameter.

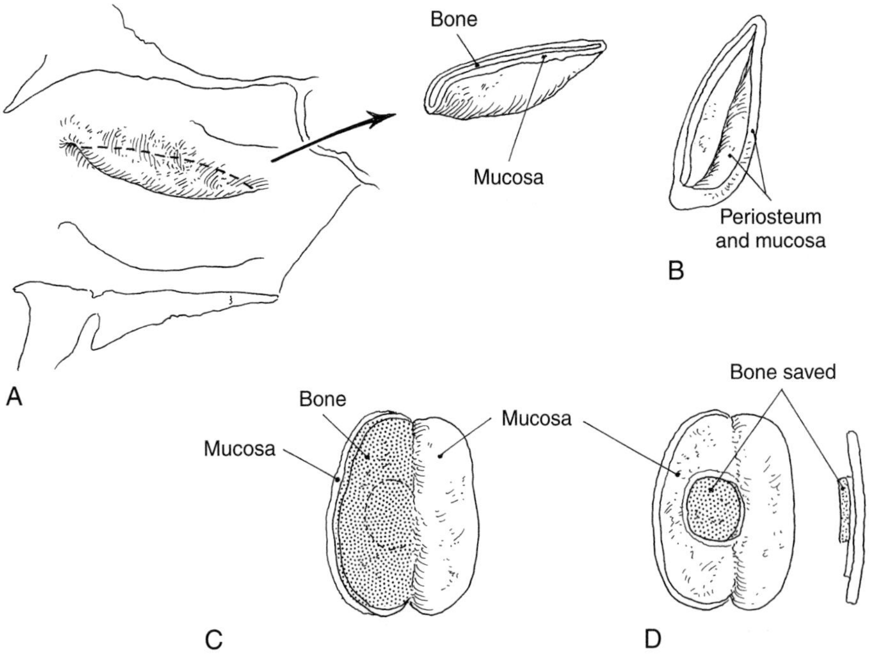

Figure 20–4. Middle turbinate graft preparation. *A,* Resecting the inferior portion of the middle turbinate. *B,* Elevating the mucosa from the lateral surface of the turbinate from the cut edge inferiorly. The mucosa remains attached to the medial surface around the inferior free edge of the turbinate. *C,* Completed mucosal elevation with the mucosal graft size twice the size of the bone. *D,* Finished graft after the bone is trimmed to the defect size seen in straight-on and lateral view.

and the bone is then trimmed to the size of the defect while still attached to the mucosa (Fig. 20–4*D*). This is accomplished by slowly elevating from the edge and trimming the bone back with scissors.

The bone graft or composite graft is manipulated into position and the bone is wedged into the defect. Bone of the middle turbinate is thin and spongiform and can easily be compressed to conform to the defect's size and shape. The mucosal grafts, if separate, are then placed over the bone and defect, making sure that the mucosal graft completely overlays the entire defect. A J-shaped curette is useful in manipulating these grafts into position. Complete hemostasis is essential during this stage of the procedure. Any bleeding points from the dura, bone, or mucosa of the skull base should be carefully controlled with bipolar cautery to facilitate graft placement and to avoid the possibility of intracranial bleeding.

Alternatives to the middle turbinate graft include free mucosal grafts from the septum or inferior turbinate and a pedicled septal mucosal flap. The septal flap can be developed based anteriorly or posteriorly, or a septal hinge flap can be used. The anterior and posterior flaps are twisted at the pedicle to lie against the skull base. The septal hinge flap is created by making full-thickness cuts through the septum to create a superiorly based flap. The mucosa and cartilage on the side of the defect are removed and the mucosa from the opposite side of the nose is folded over the cribriform plate. These flaps are primarily indicated for defects of the cribriform plate and are usually reserved for revision cases when a primary repair has failed.

If an intracranial fascial graft is to be used, this is placed before the mucosal graft. The fascia is harvested and trimmed to a size that is about 1 cm larger than the defect. This is tucked into the defect between the bone of the skull base and the dura. This should completely cover the defect and the dura. Following this placement, either a bone graft or mucosal graft can be placed over the fascia, as described earlier. Alternatively, the fascial graft placed intracranially can be used as a single-layer repair. Although the author does not advocate this technique, other surgeons have found this to be equally successful.

Graft Stabilization

One of the keys to successful repair of CSF leaks is proper stabilization of the graft. This ensures that shearing forces do not displace the graft until mucosal healing occurs, permanently sealing the leak. Over the last few years, several authors have advocated using fibrin glue to help fix the graft in position. Fibrin glue is created by the combination of blood-derived fibrin and serum and must be prepared fresh for each use. When combined, the components create a natural fibrin clot that can be applied, like a glue, to hold the graft in position. Fibrin glue has the advantages of easy application, commercial availability, and effectiveness in the short term, making this product useful in achieving stabilization. However, this substance is not a substitute for good technique and will not by itself permanently close a CSF leak.

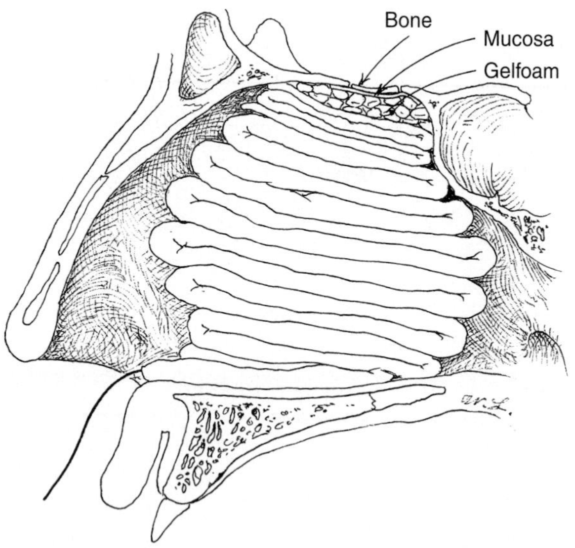

Figure 20–5. Three-layered packing for graft stabilization. The first layer is Gelfoam, the second layer is a gauze pack covering only the Gelfoam and the immediate area, and the third layer fills the nasal cavity.

The more traditional technique for stabilizing the graft is by using nasal packing. The author uses a multilayered pack that is removed over the course of 2 to 3 weeks (Fig. 20–5). The first layer, placed up against the graft, consists of multiple pieces of Gelfoam (Xomed Corp., Jacksonville, FL). The Gelfoam can be coated with antibiotic ointment. This layer helps to keep the subsequent packing from sticking to the graft. The second layer is strip gauze covered by Vaseline (Cheeseborough Ponds, Inc., Greenwich, CT) or antibiotic ointment. This pack should be just long enough to cover the graft and Gelfoam layer completely. For a sphenoid sinus leak, this will fill the sinus, whereas for an ethmoid or cribriform plate leakage site, this pack will fill the upper nasal vault. The final pack fills the remainder of the nasal and sinus cavities on the operative side and consists of the same antibiotic-coated strip gauze.

This type of occlusive packing is not uniformly advocated by other surgeons. Recommendations in the literature vary from fibrin glue, Gelfoam, and a Merocele sponge (Xomed, Jacksonville, FL) to fibrin glue alone. These variations in technique are largely related to the experience of the surgeon and the technique used to close the defect. If an intracranial fascial graft and free mucosal overlay graft are used, less occlusive packing may be required. The advantages of less packing and a potentially more stable graft are offset by the increased risk of the intracranial dissection required for this type of graft placement. The author's overlay technique has proven equally successful as an intracranial graft technique, but this safer method requires a more occlusive pack to stabilize the graft and seal the defect area. The ultimate choice is left to the individual surgeon, but in the absence of other intervening factors, the author recommends the safer overlay technique.

External Ethmoidectomy

The external ethmoidectomy approach for CSF leak repair is rarely indicated in modern rhinology. At one time, it was one of the primary options for extracranial repair of CSF leaks. However, since the advent of endoscopic sinus surgery, this procedure is not indicated for most situations. The cases when it may be appropriate include after trauma when the lamina papyracea is fractured and the orbit has prolapsed into the ethmoid sinus. In this situation, the external approach will allow retraction of the orbit to gain improved exposure of the skull base. Other possibilities may be encountered, but will be individually unique.

When this approach is used, it is performed through a standard Lynch incision, as described in Chapter 9. The initial steps are to perform an external ethmoidectomy as described in Chapter 9. Once the skull base is identified, the defect is prepared as for the endoscopic technique. Usually, a microscope will be used to enhance visualization during this step. The graft is harvested from the septum through a transnasal route; alternatively, a septal mucosal flap can be used (Fig. 20–6). The graft is then placed in an overlay position and stabilized as described earlier.

Repair by Obliteration

CSF leaks from the sphenoid and frontal sinuses can be controlled by obliterating the sinus. For sphenoid sinus leaks, this is performed through the standard transseptal approach. This procedure is described in detail in Chapter 19. The favored technique is through

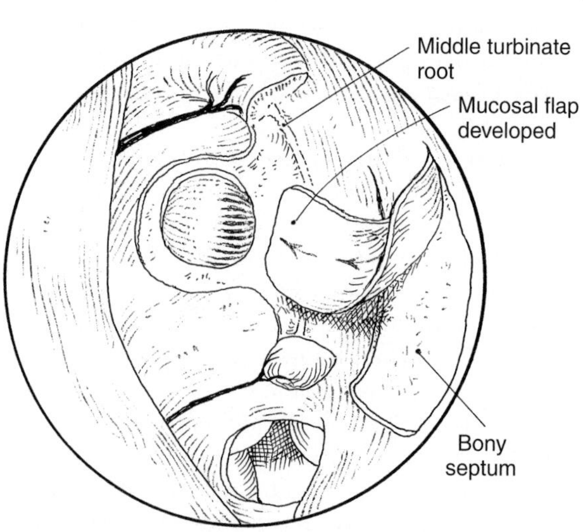

Figure 20–6. Septal mucosal graft. This graft is rotated over from the septum, attached either posteriorly or superiorly.

a sublabial incision with deflection of the quadrilateral cartilage to the right and resection of the vomer and part of the perpendicular plate to expose the sphenoid sinus through the midline. The anterior wall of the sphenoid sinus is removed to expose the inside of the sinus, leaving a shelf around the circumference of the anterior wall. The midline septum is then removed. All of the mucosa of the sphenoid sinus should be meticulously removed. If the defect is in a favorable position, it can be repaired with a fascial graft; if this is not possible, direct repair of the defect can be deleted. In this case, the sinus is filled with a fat graft that seals the defect. The graft is held in place by wedging bone from the septum across the face of the sinus.

Defects or leaks from the frontal sinus can be repaired by either obliteration or cranialization of the frontal sinus. This procedure is described in detail in Chapter 11. Usually, this is performed through a bicoronal incision and an osteoplastic flap. The defect does not need to be repaired directly. However, if the dural defect is easily repaired by direct suturing, this can be accomplished. The mucosa must be completely removed and the underlying bone drilled down to ensure complete removal. The frontal ostia are then obstructed with a multilayered plug consisting of muscle, bone, and then fascia. The sinus is filled with fat from either the abdomen or thigh. If the posterior wall of the sinus is severely damaged from trauma, cranialization should be performed. For this procedure, the posterior wall is completely removed and the frontal ostia are blocked by a muscle plug and covered by a pericranial flap. The sinus lumen should be filled with a fat graft, as with the obliteration.

Repair by Craniotomy

The indications for repair of a CSF leak by craniotomy have been discussed in the earlier section on indications for surgery. To reiterate, craniotomy is rarely a first choice for repair of CSF leak. The appropriate indications are defects measuring greater than 2 cm in diameter, endoscopically inaccessible defects, and cases in which endoscopic repair has already failed. This operation is exclusively performed by neurosurgeons. The details of the procedure are beyond the scope of this textbook. However, it is worthwhile for rhinologists to understand the basic steps.

The procedure is performed through a bicoronal approach. It is not necessary to extend the flap as low as the zygomatic arches, so there should be minimal risk to the facial nerve. A wide-based pericranial flap is developed pedicled to the orbital rims. A bifrontal craniotomy is performed to expose the frontal lobes. The dura is then elevated from the floor of the anterior cranial fossa. As elevation proceeds, the olfactory epithelium will need to be elevated. In performing this elevation, the olfactory nerves will be divided, along with the investing dura around these nerves. If possible, only the side of the defect should be elevated, as bilateral elevation will result in complete anosmia. When the area of the defect is reached, the brain is carefully retracted from the defect to avoid lacerations in the parenchyma.

Once the elevation is complete, the primary dural repair is performed. The perforation over the olfactory bulbs is closed primarily. The actual defect is then repaired directly. This may be achieved by primary closure, or a free temporal fascial graft may be required. Depending on the size of the defect, it may be desirable to place a bone or fascial graft into the actual defect. Alternatively, it can be filled with an inert substance, such as bone wax, methyl methacrylate, or ionomer cement.

Before the repair is concluded, the frontal sinus must be cranialized. This requires that the posterior wall be removed and that the mucosa of the sinus be completely removed. The frontal ostium is then obstructed with a muscle plug and bone chips, as described in Chapter 11. The pericranial flap is then folded down over the skull base and sutured to the dura posterior to the defect. The bone flap is replaced and secured by whatever technique is preferred.

POSTOPERATIVE CARE

The postoperative care of patients with frontal sinus obliteration and craniotomy is covered in other chapters in this book. Here, the aftercare of patients undergoing intranasal repair is covered.

After surgery and routine recovery, most patients will be stable enough to be managed either in a regular inpatient ward or as outpatients. The critical distinction is whether a lumbar drain is used. This decision is multifactorial. For patients with a linear crack or leakage around olfactory neurons discovered at the time of surgery, mucosal grafting without lumbar drain will almost always be successful as long as the graft is adequately stabilized. Conversely, for patients with large defects requiring the use of composite grafting or for patients with encephalocele, a lumbar drain is typically required.

Intermediate cases can be treated either with or without a lumbar drain. The decision may be based on several factors: the age of the leak, the location of the defect, and the size of the defect. For cases discovered during surgery, a lumbar drain tends to not be necessary, whereas cases with long-standing fistulas are more likely to heal with CSF decompression. Defects that are in the sphenoid sinus can be secured by a firm pack; with defects in the frontal recess or anterior ethmoid, the pack tends to slip and may expose the graft. Defects smaller than 5 mm develop little or no pressure on the graft from bulging of the dura, but high pressures may be generated by larger defects, especially those greater than 1 cm in diameter. The final decision, therefore, must be individualized. The author applies the principle of "it is better to be safe than sorry," using a lumbar drain in any case when there is a question of its necessity.

When the lumbar drain is used, the patient must be admitted to a nursing unit skilled in the care of these drains. For most patients, the drain is kept in place for a 5-day period. While the drain is in place, the patient is kept on bed rest with the head of the bed elevated to between 15 and 30 degrees. Stool softeners, cough suppressants, and other medications necessary to keep the patient comfortable are prescribed. This may include treatment for the spinal headache that often accompanies the lumbar drain. Patient-controlled analgesia using intravenous morphine is one option that has worked well for this situation. Alternatively, intermittently dosed oral or intramuscular medicines may be effective. The CSF is drained at a rate of 10 mL per hour. Rather than draining at a continuous low flow, draining 20 mL over a few minutes every 2 hours is safer and easier to manage outside an intensive care unit.

The nasal packing should be placed in three layers. The first layer is Gelfoam pieces placed over the graft. The second layer is Vaseline-coated strip gauze to fill the affected sinus to cover the graft. The last layer fills the remainder of the sinus and nasal cavity. The lowest level of packing is removed on the fifth postoperative day. This opens the nasal cavity, allowing the patient to breathe through the nose, thereby increasing comfort. The second layer of packing is left in place for 2 to 3 weeks as tolerated. In most cases, there is no significant problem with keeping this layer of packing in place for up to 3 weeks. The exception to this is if the defect is in the frontal recess or anterior ethmoid area. Packing that is left in place in this area will probably lead to frontal sinus stenosis. For this reason, the second pack should be removed in these patients within 2 days of the removal of the lower pack. Following this, the patient is treated with nasal irrigations and steroid nasal spray as per the protocol for routine endoscopic sinus surgery. Sinus debridement should be performed under endoscopic visualization when the packing is removed, and then every 2 weeks until the mucosal graft is well healed. Extreme care must be taken during these debridements to ensure that the graft is not disturbed.

During the time the packing is in place, the patient should receive oral or intravenous antibiotics. While in the hospital, intravenous antibiotics are maintained. After discharge, conversion to oral antibiotics is acceptable. The usual choices are either ampicillin/sulbactam or a second-generation cephalosporin that will cover staphylococci well. However, in cases of active sinus infection, an agent that will cover the cultured bacteria should be selected.

Long-term follow-up evaluation of these patients is essential to recognize recurrence if it occurs. Return visits are scheduled for 2 weeks, 4 weeks, 2 months, 3 months, 6 months, 1 year, and each year after that. At each return appointment, an endoscopic examination is performed. The graft should be inspected and evidence of CSF leakage assessed. Postoperative CT scans are not required but may be ordered if indicated.

COMPLICATIONS

Complications of CSF rhinorrhea can be divided into complications of the leak itself and complications of the treatment to repair the leak. The most important complication of CSF leakage is meningitis. Meningitis is caused by ascending infection from the sinuses that involves the meninges and the CSF space itself. The risk of meningitis varies with the etiology of the leak and the location of the leak. The lowest risk is in patients with spontaneous CSF leak from the sinuses without sinus infection. In these patients, the leak may be present for many years without causing ill effect.[13] These cases pose a low risk of meningitis over the short term; however, over the long term, the risk mounts and so repair is still indicated. Patients with posttraumatic CSF leak have an intermediate level of risk of meningitis. These patients develop anatomic abnormalities from the fractures that may predispose them to developing sinusitis; this, in turn, may progress into meningitis. The risk of meningitis posttrauma has been found to be in the range of 5% to 10% over the first few weeks after the injury.[44, 71, 72]

The highest risk of meningitis is in patients that develop CSF leak during surgery for sinus infection. In these patients, there is already infection in the sinuses, and there is a high risk of subsequent sinusitis. Infection in direct connection to the dura progresses rapidly to meningitis. In cases when the CSF leak is not discovered during the initial operation, meningitis may be the initial manifestation of CSF leak. For CSF rhinorrhea that develops after sinus surgery, the risk of meningitis may increase to 50% or more.

If meningitis does occur, it is usually suggested by headache, fever, and nuchal rigidity. The diagnosis is confirmed by performing a lumbar puncture to sample the CSF. This should be performed in any patient who presents with fever and headache after sinus surgery. CSF fluid that has a low glucose level, high protein level, and an elevated white blood cell count is indicative of bacterial meningitis. This is ultimately confirmed by a positive culture or the detection of bacteria on Gram stain. If left untreated, the consequences of meningitis are severe, and include brain damage, deafness, seizures, and even death. The mortality rate of meningitis varies significantly with the circumstances of the individual case. Mortality rates in series reported in the literature depend on the etiology of the infection, the time period of the study, and the stage of the infection at the time of diagnosis.

Treatment of meningitis is dominated by the selection of the appropriate antibiotics. The antibiotic should cover the suspected bacteria or those documented by culture or Gram stain. If no specific data are available, the antibiotic should cover both gram-positive and gram-negative bacteria and have good CSF penetration. The patient should be observed closely until the infection is controlled. Antiseizure medication, adequate oxygenation, and monitoring of vital signs are imperative. The antibiotic may be continued for up to 6 weeks or more if necessary.

Besides meningitis, CSF leak can cause other intracranial complications as well, including pneumocephalus, brain abscess, epidural abscess, and subdural abscess. Pneumocephalus occurs when intranasal air pressure rises acutely, forcing air intracranially. The air can dissect over the inside of the skull base or can enter the ventricular system. Air can act similarly to blood or mass lesions, resulting in brain compression. This is usually marked by a sudden change in mental status, level of consciousness, or neurologic function. The treatment is to intubate the patient immediately to prevent further air entry and to evacuate the air, if necessary, to resolve symptoms.

The risks of CSF repair are related to the procedure performed. Craniotomy complications are beyond the scope of this book. However, the risk of anosmia following bifrontal craniotomy is essentially 100%. This fact should always be kept in mind when considering surgical options.

Transnasal repair of CSF leak poses significant risks. In the author's series, there were no significant complications.[6] However, this does not equate to the absence of risk. The most feared risk is intracranial bleeding. This can occur as the result of mucosal bleeding on the outer surface of the skull base or from dural vessels. Liberal use of bipolar cautery is necessary to prevent these problems. The risk of intracranial bleeding should be low but is increased by excision of encephalocele or intracranial elevation of the dura. Intracranial bleeding during this procedure is a potentially catastrophic complication. Accumulation of blood can lead to brain compression and, eventually, herniation and death. Treatment requires immediate neurosurgical consultation and intervention. Attempts to control the bleeding from below may result in penetration into the brain and brain damage.

Other intracranial complications may include mucocele or inflammatory granuloma. These problems are caused by trapping of graft elements intracranially. Resolution of these problems will require removal, possibly through craniotomy.

Extracranial bleeding is also a possibility, but this is a risk of any sinus surgery and the risk is probably not increased in repair of CSF leak. Most series of endoscopic sinus surgery report the risk of postoperative bleeding to be 1% to 2%.[11, 12] Management is by conservative means, with packing attempted first. If this does not control the bleeding, direct cauterization is the second step. Finally, if this is not successful, ligation of the feeding vessel, either surgically or by arteriogram and embolization, can be tried.

Perhaps the most common complication of CSF leak repair is formation of scar tissue in the sinuses. This can lead to nasal obstruction or, more likely, obstruction of one of the sinus ostia. This may result in sinusitis or, eventually, mucocele. Correction of this problem may be tricky. If the scar tissue is in close approximation to the intracranial defect and the graft, revision can reopen the defect and cause recurrence of the CSF leak. If this is a risk, the sinus may need to be treated through an external approach, possibly with obliteration. The author has treated two such patients. In both cases, defects in the frontal recess area were repaired and the repair resulted in frontal sinus stenosis. Both patients were treated with frontal sinus obliteration to resolve the situation.

Postoperative sinus infection is more directly related to the underlying condition rather than the repair of a CSF leak. Because the most common cause of CSF leak is sinus surgery for polyps or severe sinusitis, these patients are at natural risk for recurrent infection. Other infections, such as meningitis, are unusual. Meningitis may be caused by infection trapped under the graft or infection of the graft itself. This has not been seen in the author's experience. Graft loss would seem to be a greater risk, but should be rare. If the graft becomes necrotic or nonviable, it is better to remove it than to leave it in place and risk exposing the patient to meningitis.

Finally, failure of the leak repair is a significant risk. Most series report successful repair in more than 90% of cases. In the author's experience, 18 of 18 patients underwent successful initial repair; 1 patient developed a recurrence of CFS leak 6 months after the initial repair.[6] All patients should be advised of this possibility, and should be closely monitored for several years to detect recurrences as early as possible.

REFERENCES

1. Hollinshead WH. Anatomy for Surgeons: The Head and Neck, 3rd ed. Philadelphia: JB Lippincott, 1982, pp. 1–30.
2. Persky MS, Rothstein SG, Breda SD, et al. Extracranial repair of cerebrospinal fluid otorhinorrhea. Laryngoscope 101(2):134, 1991.
3. Wax MK, Ramadan HH, Ortiz O, et al. Contemporary management of cerebrospinal fluid rhinorrhea. Otolaryngol Head Neck Surg 116(4):442, 1997.

4. Lanza DC, O'Brien DA, Kennedy DW. Endoscopic repair of cerebrospinal fluid fistulae and encephaloceles. Laryngoscope 106(9 Pt 1):1119, 1996.
5. Charles DA, Snell D. Cerebrospinal fluid rhinorrhea. Laryngoscope 89:822, 1979.
6. Marks S. Middle turbinate graft for repair of CSF leak repair. Am J Rhinol 12:417, 1998.
7. Dodson EE, Gross CW, Swerdloff JL, et al. Transnasal endoscopic repair of cerebrospinal fluid rhinorrhea and skull base defects: A review of twenty-nine cases. Otolaryngol Head Neck Surg 111(5):600, 1994.
8. Anand VK, Murali RK, Glasgold MJ. Surgical decisions in the management of cerebrospinal fluid rhinorrhea. Rhinology 33(4):212, 1995.
9. Stankiewicz JA. Cerebrospinal fluid fistula and endoscopic sinus surgery. Laryngoscope 101(3):250, 1991.
10. May M, Levine HL, Mester SJ, et al. Complications of endoscopic sinus surgery: Analysis of 2108 patients—Incidence and prevention. Laryngoscope 104(9):1080, 1994.
11. Vleming M, Middleweerd RJ, de Vries N. Complications of endoscopic sinus surgery. Arch Otolaryngol Head Neck Surg 118: 617, 1992.
12. Marks S. Learning curve in endoscopic sinus surgery. Otolaryngol Head Neck Surg 120(2):215, 1999.
13. Beckhardt RN, Setzen M, Carras R. Primary spontaneous cerebrospinal fluid rhinorrhea. Otolaryngol Head Neck Surg 104(4): 425, 1991.
14. Benedict M, Schultz-Coulon HJ. Spontaneous cerebrospinal rhinorrhea. HNO 39:1, 1991.
15. Lewin W. Cerebrospinal fluid rhinorrhea in closed head injuries. Br J Surg 42:1, 1954.
16. Briant TDR, Bird R. Extracranial repair of cerebrospinal fluid fistulae. J Otolaryngol 11:191, 1982.
17. Park JL, Strelzow VV, Friedman WH. Current management of cerebrospinal fluid rhinorrhea. Laryngoscope 93:1294, 1983.
18. Calcaterra TC. Extracranial surgical repair of cerebrospinal rhinorrhea. Ann Otol Rhinol Laryngol 89:108, 1980.
19. Spetzler RF, Zabramski JM. Cerebrospinal fluid fistulae: Their management and repair. In Youmans JR (ed). Neurological Surgery. Philadelphia: WB Saunders, 1990, pp. 2269–2289.
20. Mathog RH, Rosenberg Z. Complications in the treatment of facial fractures. Otolaryngol Clin North Am 9:533, 1976.
21. Steedman DJ, Gordon M. CSF rhinorrhea: Significance of the glucose oxidase strip test. Injury 18:327, 1987.
22. Hull HF, Morrow G. Glucorrhea revisited. JAMA 234:1052, 1975.
23. Kosoy J, Trieff NM, Winkleman P, et al. Glucose in nasal secretions. Arch Otolaryngol 95:225, 1972.
24. Meurman OH, Irjala K, Suonpaa J, et al. A new method for the identification of cerebrospinal fluid leakage. Acta Otolaryngol 87:366, 1979.
25. Fransen P, Sindic CJM, Thauvoy C, et al. Highly sensitive detection of beta-2 transferrin in rhinorrhea and otorrhea as a marker for cerebrospinal fluid leakage. Acta Neurochir 109:98, 1991.
26. Nandapalan V, Watson ID, Swift AC. Beta-2 transferrin and cerebrospinal fluid rhinorrhoea. Clin Otolaryngol Allergy Sci 21(3):259, 1996.
27. Blennow K, Fredman P. Detection of cerebrospinal fluid leakage by isoelectric focusing on polyacrylamide gels with silver staining using the PhastSystem. Acta Neurochir 136(3–4):135, 1995.
28. Oberascher G. A modern concept of cerebrospinal fluid diagnosis in oto- and rhinorrhea. Rhinology 26:89, 1988.
29. Wolf G, Greistorfer K, Stammberger H. Endoscopic detection of cerebrospinal fluid fistulas with a fluorescence technique. Report of experiences with over 925 cases. Laryngol-Rhinol Otol 76(10):588, 1997.
30. Ozgen IH, Tekkek A, Erzen C. CT cisternography in evaluation of cerebrospinal fluid rhinorrhea. Neuroradiology 32:481, 1990.
31. Chow JM, Goodman D, Mafee M. Evaluation of CSF rhinorrhea by computerized tomography with metrizamide. Otolaryngol Head Neck Surg 100:99, 1989.
32. Ahmadi JA, Weiss M, Segall H. Evaluation of cerebrospinal fluid rhinorrhea by metrizamide computed tomographic cisternography. Neurosurgery 16:54, 1985.
33. Nabawi P, Mafee M, Phillips J, et al. The success rate of metrizamide CT in the evaluation of cerebrospinal fluid rhinorrhea. Comput Radiol 6:343, 1982.
34. Colquhoun IR. CT cisternography in the investigation of cerebrospinal fluid rhinorrhoea. Clin Radiol 47(6):403, 1993.
35. Yamamoto Y, Mutsuga N, Aoki T. Identification of CSF fistulas by radionuclide counting. AJNR 11:823, 1990.
36. Flynn BM, Butler S, Quinn R. Radionuclide cisternography in the diagnosis and management of cerebrospinal fluid leaks. Med J Aust 146:82, 1987.
37. Mamo L, Cophignon J, Rey A, et al. A new radionuclide method for the diagnosis of posttraumatic fistulas. J Neurosurg 57:92, 1982.
38. Elijamel MS, Pidgeon CN, Toland J, et al. MRI cisternography, and the localization of CSF fistulae. Br J Neurosurg 8(4):433, 1994.
39. El Gammal T, Brooks BS. MR cisternography: Initial experience in 41 cases. AJNR 15(9): 1647, 1994.
40. Levy LM, Gulya AJ, Davis SW, et al. Flow-sensitive magnetic resonance imaging in the evaluation of cerebrospinal fluid leaks. Am J Otol 16(5):591, 1995.
41. Johnson DB, Brennan P, Toland J, et al. Magnetic resonance imaging in the evaluation of cerebrospinal fluid fistulae. Clin Radiol 51(12):837, 1996.
42. Burgio DL, Marks SC. Cerebrospinal fluid fistula. In Mathog R, Arden R, Marks C (eds). Trauma of the Nose and Paranasal Sinuses. New York: Thieme, 1995, pp. 156–170.
43. Marentette LJ, Valentino J. Traumatic anterior fossa cerebrospinal fluid fistulae and craniofacial considerations. Otolaryngol Clin North Am 24:151, 1991.
44. Clemenza JW, Kaltman SI, Diamond DL. Craniofacial trauma and cerebrospinal fluid leakage. A retrospective clinical study. J Oral Maxillofac Surgery 53(9):1004, 1995.
45. Shapiro SA, Scully T. Closed continuous drainage of cerebrospinal fluid via a lumbar subarachnoid catheter for treatment or prevention of cranial/spinal cerebrospinal fluid fistula. Neurosurgery 30:241, 1992.
46. Swanson SE, Chandler WF, Kocan MJ, et al. Flow-regulated continuous spinal drainage in the management of cerebrospinal fluid fistulas. Laryngoscope 95:104, 1985.
47. Eljamel MS, Pidgeon CN, Toland J, et al. MRI cisternography, and the localization of CSF fistulae. Br J Neurosurg 8(4):433, 1994.
48. Mayfrank L, Gilsbach JM, Hegemann S, et al. Osteoplastic frontal sinusotomy and extradural microsurgical repair of frontobasal cerebrospinal fluid fistulas. Acta Neurochir 138(3):245, 1996.
49. Mathog RH, Rosenberg Z. Complications in the treatment of facial fractures. Otolaryngol Clin North Am 9:533, 1976.
50. Landreneau FE, Mickey B, Coimbra C. Surgical treatment of cerebrospinal fluid fistulae involving lateral extension of the sphenoid sinus. Neurosurgery 42(5):1101, 1998.
51. Nallet E, Decq P, Bezzo A, et al. Endonasal endoscopic surgery in the treatment of spontaneous or post-traumatic cerebrospinal fluid (CSF) leaks. Ann Otolaryngol Chir Cervicofac 115(4):222, 1998.
52. Ng M, Maceri DR, Levy MM, et al. Extracranial repair of pediatric traumatic cerebrospinal fluid rhinorrhea. Arch Otolaryngol Head Neck Surg 124(10):1125, 1998.
53. Wormald PJ, McDonogh M. Bath-plug technique for the endoscopic management of cerebrospinal fluid leaks. J Laryngol Otol 111(11):1042, 1997.
54. Hughes RG, Jones NS, Robertson IJ. The endoscopic treatment of cerebrospinal fluid rhinorrhoea: The Nottingham experience. J Laryngol Otol 111(2):125, 1997.
55. Liu G, Zhao C, Wang S. Treatment of cerebrospinal rhinorrhea under nasal endoscope with EC ear-head adhesive. Chin J Otorhinolaryngol 31(1):16, 1996.
56. Righnini C, Reyt E, Lavieille JP, et al. Surgical treatment under endoscopic control of cerebrospinal fluid rhinorrhea of sphenoid origin. Apropos of 5 cases. Ann Otolaryngol Chir Cervicofac 113(4):188, 1996.
57. Sethi DS, Chan C, Pillay PK. Endoscopic management of cerebrospinal fluid fistulae and traumatic cephalocoele. Ann Acad Med Singapore 25(5):724, 1996.
58. Kelley TF, Stankiewicz JA, Chow JM, et al. Endoscopic closure of postsurgical anterior cranial fossa cerebrospinal fluid leaks. Neurosurgery 39(4):743, 1996.

59. Gjuric M, Goede U, Keimer H, et al. Endosnasal endoscopic closure of cerebrospinal fluid fistulas at the anterior cranial base. Ann Otol Rhinol Laryngol 105(8):620, 1996.
60. Weber R, Keerl R, Draf W, et al. Management of dural lesions occurring during endonasal sinus surgery. Arch Otolaryngol Head Neck Surg 122(7):732, 1996.
61. Budrovich R, Saetti R, Pagano G. Endoscopic treatment of iatrogenic rhino-CSF fistulas: Notes of surgical techniques. Acta Otorhinolaryngol Ital 15:51, 1995.
62. Xu G, Yang Z, Peng A. Intranasal endoscopic management of cerebrospinal rhinorrhea. Chin J Otorhinolaryngol 29(4):231, 1994.
63. Zeitouni AG, Frenkiel S, Mohr G. Endoscopic repair of anterior skull base cerebrospinal fluid fistulas: An emphasis on postoperative nasal function maximization. J Otolaryngol 23(3):225, 1994.
64. Handley GH, Goodson MA, Real TH. Transnasal endoscopic closure of anterior fossa cerebrospinal fluid fistula. South Med J 86(2):217, 1993.
65. Bouton V, Sanson J. Meningeal injury during surgery of the ethmoid sinus: Endoscopic treatment using surgical glue. Acta Otorhinolaryngol Belg 45(3):319, 1991.
66. Hoseman W, Nitsche N, Rettinger G, et al. Endonasal, endoscopically controlled repair of dura defects of the anterior skull base. Laryngol Rhinol Otol (Stuttg) 70(3):115, 1991.
67. Mattox DE, Kennedy DW. Endoscopic management of cerebrospinal fluid leaks and cephaloceles. Laryngoscope 100(8):857, 1990.
68. Aarabi B, Leibrock LG. Neurosurgical approaches to cerebrospinal fluid rhinorrhea. Ear Nose Throat J 71(7):300, 1992.
69. Surmacz L, Wicentowicz Z, Moskwa M. Immediate and late results of the treatment of cerebrospinal rhinorrhea at the Department of Neurosurgery of the District Hospital in Rzeszow. Neurol Neurochir Pol [Suppl] 1:300, 1992.
70. Zukiel R, Nowak S, Liebert W, et al. Post-traumatic cerebrospinal rhinorrhea managed surgically. Clinical analysis of of cases. Neurol Neurochir Pol 32:91, 1998.
71. Brodie HA. Prophylactic antibiotics for posttraumatic cerebrospinal fluid fistulae. A meta-analysis. Arch Otolaryngol Head Neck Surg 123(7):749, 1997.
72. Eljamel MS. Antibiotic prophylaxis in unrepaired CSF fistulae. Br J Neurosurg 7(5):501, 1993.

CHAPTER 21

Orbital Surgery

The rhinologist is occasionally called upon to perform orbital surgery. These procedures are all shared jointly with ophthalmologists trained in orbital surgery. Both specialists have training that is helpful in the management of these patients. The rhinologist is familiar with the anatomy, surgical instruments, and approaches for the surgery, whereas the ophthalmologist has the knowledge of the ocular disease processes that is necessary to make decisions about therapy. Increasingly, ophthalmologists are taking sole responsibility for these patients. In order for otolaryngologists to maintain a role in the management of patients with orbital diseases, a thorough knowledge of the anatomy and expert surgical skills in performing these procedures are critical.

The procedures covered in this chapter include orbital decompression, optic nerve decompression, and dacryocystorhinostomy. Each of these operations can be performed by an endoscopic or open surgical approach. The rhinologic surgeon should be able to perform the procedure through either approach and understand the indications and appropriate application for each.

ORBITAL DECOMPRESSION

Indications

Graves' Disease. Orbital decompression is an operation that is most often performed for Graves' ophthalmopathy. Graves' disease is the condition of thyrotoxicosis or chronic hyperthyroidism. It is thought to be caused by an autoimmune condition secondary to the production of antithyroid autoantibodies.[1] This leads to diffuse enlargement of the thyroid gland and uncontrolled secretion of thyroid hormone into the blood. The consequences of this hypersecretion are the classic signs and symptoms of Graves' disease: nervousness, restlessness, palpitations, hypertension, diarrhea, hair loss, weight loss, and in some patients, hypertrophy of the extraocular muscles within the orbit.

Hypertrophy of the extraocular muscles is thought to be secondary to deposition of immune complexes.[2] This results in the pathologic findings of inflammation, edema, and fibrosis of the orbital muscles and fat.[3] Graves' ophthalmopathy occurs in about 50% of all patients with Graves' disease,[4] but only 50% of these patients are symptomatic and only about 5% of affected patients develop severe ophthalmopathy.[5, 6]

Most patients with Graves' disease have bilateral involvement of the extraocular muscles. However, a percentage of patients can have unilateral involvement only. The reasons for these differences are unknown. Because the antibody that causes Graves' disease is systemic and the excess thyroid hormone is systemic, it stands to reason that the effects on ocular muscles would be diffuse and not localized. However, as stated, this is not the case in some patients, leading one to infer that some cofactor is necessary to incite the hypertrophic inflammatory response in the ocular muscles.

The effect of hypertrophied extraocular muscles is to cause compression of the globe from the orbital apex, which results in the eye being pushed out of the orbit. This is known as exophthalmos. As the exophthalmos increases, the classic appearance of the Graves' patient develops. This is manifested by increased scleral show to the extent that, in severe cases, the sclera is visible circumferentially around the limbus.

When this degree of exophthalmos occurs, the patient's vision can be at risk from a number of mechanisms. The first is exposure keratopathy. The eyelids do not completely close around the cornea, resulting in drying and, possibly, ulceration and clouding of the cornea. The second problem is diplopia. When the eyes bulge out significantly, they lose coordination. In addition, the eyes may suffer from differing degrees of exophthalmos. Finally, in the most severe cases, the eye can protrude to such an extent that the optic nerve becomes compressed or stretched beyond its limit of tolerance. This may result in optic nerve dysfunction and, eventually, blindness.

The first treatment of Graves' ophthalmopathy is prevention. The consequences of chronic hyperthyroidism can be prevented by early diagnosis and treatment. Exophthalmos occurs rather far along in the course of hyperthyroidism. Most patients can be diagnosed based on the symptoms of nervousness, palpitations, hair thinning or loss, and diarrhea. The diagnosis can then be confirmed by determining serum thyroid hormone levels. Hyperthyroidism is diagnosed by the combination of elevated triiodothyronine (T_3) resin uptake and thyroxine (T_4) serum level and low thyroid-stimulating hormone (TSH) level.

Once the diagnosis is confirmed, most patients will be started on medical treatment. A number of medications are available to suppress thyroid function, including propylthiouracil (PTU) and methimazole. An endocrinologist should be consulted to manage this aspect of care. In cases when medical therapy fails to control the hyperthyroidism, ablative procedures are possible. Most patients now receive radioactive iodine treatments for ablation of the thyroid. Surgical treatment with total thyroidectomy is the main alternative. For a complete discussion of these treatment modalities, an appropriate textbook of medicine or endocrinology should be consulted.

For patients that develop significant exophthalmos either prior to diagnosis or despite treatment, a number of therapeutic options are available. Some patients may respond to systemic corticosteroids. External beam irradiation has been advocated by some.[7, 8] Plasmapheresis has been recommended by others, but the improvement from this treatment is usually temporary.[9] In addition to these treatments, orbital decompression is an option. When surgery is considered, the goals of the surgery are to prevent all of the complications of this condition, including visual loss, exposure keratopathy, and diplopia. Surgery should be contemplated in patients who have progressive exophthalmos despite adequate therapy, or in any patient who develops any complications. Alternatively, some patients may undergo orbital decompression for cosmetic reasons. Exophthalmos is a cosmetically unappealing deformity for which patients are justified in seeking surgical treatment.

Prior to performing decompression for Graves' ophthalmopathy, it is important to measure the degree of exophthalmos. This is important to determine the procedure necessary to achieve the degree of retrusion desired. Each procedure has an expected range of retrusion that occurs after the surgery. Decompression can be achieved by removal of any of the walls of the orbit. Practically, though, only the medial and inferior walls can be removed. Surgery on the lateral wall of the orbit requires a lateral skull base approach. A transorbital approach to the lateral orbit is conceivable, but this limited exposure would be suboptimal for decompression. The superior wall could be removed through either a transfrontal or transorbital approach. However, removal of the superior orbital wall is accompanied by problems related to the translation of cranial pulsations to the eye, causing visual disturbance.

Historically, a number of procedures gained favor for orbital decompression, but most surgeons eventually came to favor the procedure popularized by Ogura.[10] This procedure combines medial and inferior decompression performed through an external ethmoidectomy with a Caldwell-Luc approach. This combined procedure has been reported to result in a retrusion of 5 to 7 mm of globe position. The medial decompression alone achieves 2 to 3 mm of retrusion, and the inferior decompression adds another 3 to 4 mm.

This combined external technique was the procedure of choice until endoscopic decompression was described in 1990 by Kennedy and co-workers.[11] Their procedure involves a complete medial decompression all the way to the infraorbital nerve, with incisions in the periorbita to increase retrusion. This is usually combined with lateral canthotomy with inferior cantholysis to achieve a combined retrusion of 4 to 6 mm.[12, 13] For most patients, this is a preferable option because it results in adequate decompression without external incisions or the risk of permanent injury to the infraorbital nerve. Currently, the external procedure is considered the primary option only in cases in which retrusion of greater than 6 mm is needed.

Orbital Inflammation. Orbital decompression is also performed for treatment of various forms of orbital inflammation. Chandler and colleagues, in 1970, classified orbital inflammation into five categories.[14] Table 21–1 presents this classification scheme. Preseptal cellulitis is recognized by edema and erythema of the eyelids without any signs of true orbital inflammation. Orbital cellulitis is a condition characterized by signs of orbital infection, such as chemosis, scleral injection, proptosis, or decreased extraocular motion, without the presence of abscess. Subperiosteal abscess is present when a discrete collection of purulent infection is trapped between the periorbita and the lamina papyracea. Orbital abscess is present when there is a collection of fluid inside the periorbita. The final stage is cavernous sinus thrombosis, which occurs when the infection spreads

TABLE 21–1
Classification of Orbital Infection

Stage 1: Periorbital (preseptal) cellulitis
Stage 2: Orbital (postseptal) cellulitis
Stage 3: Subperiosteal abscess
Stage 4: Orbital abscess
Stage 5: Cavernous sinus thrombosis

into the cavernous sinus. This may be recognized by total ophthalmoplegia and anesthesia of the first division of the trigeminal nerve.

These categories were initially intended to represent stages of advancing infection in the orbit secondary to sinus infection. Today, it is recognized that there is not typically a progression through these stages. Each of these orbital complications can occur without any of the other stages preceding it. However, each of these clinical syndromes can also progress and result in severe complications, including visual loss, meningitis, and death, if not treated appropriately.

Treatment begins with accurate diagnosis. All of these conditions present with lid edema. When a patient with sinusitis presents with lid edema, the first step is a complete ophthalmologic evaluation. If everything in the eye is completely normal, the diagnosis is established as preseptal cellulitis. The presence of any abnormality implies, at the very least, orbital cellulitis. Severe proptosis and visual loss usually indicate abscess, whereas complete ophthalmoplegia and anesthesia of cranial nerve V1 suggest cavernous sinus thrombosis.

In all of these cases of more advanced orbital inflammation, a computed tomography (CT) scan is indicated to confirm the diagnosis.[15,16] The CT scan should be performed in the axial and coronal planes with both soft tissue and bone windows and intravenous contrast enhancement. Thin, 2-mm cuts should be obtained throughout the orbit to maximize the chances of detecting a fluid collection or abscess. Following the CT scan and examination, it should be possible to classify the orbital inflammation accurately.

In all cases, immediate hospitalization and institution of antibiotic therapy are indicated. Antibiotics should be selected to provide broad-spectrum coverage for possible pathogens, including anaerobes and beta-lactamase–producing strains.[17] As long as the patient has a normal immune system, the likely pathogens are the usual bacteria causing sinusitis. These organisms are usually treated well by either ampicillin/sulbactam or cefuroxime with clindamycin. Usually, in cases of preseptal cellulitis, a course of 2 weeks of intravenous antibiotics followed by 2 weeks of oral antibiotics is sufficient to resolve the acute infection. Subsequently, endoscopic sinus surgery to exenterate the cells causing the infection should be considered.

Patients with early orbital cellulitis, characterized by normal vision and normal intraocular pressures, can be managed with antibiotics alone or antibiotics combined with endoscopic sinus surgery.[18–20] The conservative protocol calls for patients to be observed closely while on antibiotics, and to withhold surgery unless the inflammation progresses or fails to improve within 48 hours. The decision to operate on this subclass of patients has become controversial. A few authors have reported small series of patients and isolated cases of orbital cellulitis that have resolved without surgery. However, these patients are at high risk for progression to visual loss. The author is aware of several patients with orbital cellulitis who progressed from having normal vision to severe visual loss or blindness while being treated with antibiotics alone. For this reason, urgent surgery is recommended for any patient with true orbital cellulitis, regardless of the severity of the orbital inflammation or the presence of visual loss.

Orbital decompression is specifically indicated for orbital cellulitis in those patients with high intraocular pressure or visual loss. In these cases, in addition to complete endoscopic sinus surgery, orbital decompression is indicated to relieve the intraocular pressure caused by edema of the orbital tissues and to try and prevent further deterioration of vision. If decompression is performed promptly in this situation, progression of the process is usually halted. Recovery of visual loss is less certain and depends on how advanced the process is and how severe the visual loss is. As the visual loss progresses, ischemia of the optic nerve and retina can progress to nerve damage and permanent visual loss. For this reason, surgery should be scheduled as soon as possible.

Subperiosteal abscess should always be treated by surgical drainage of the abscess, ethmoidectomy, and decompression with removal of the lamina papyracea.[16,21–23] The results of this procedure in terms of the orbital complications are similar to those for orbital cellulitis with visual loss or high ocular pressure. On average, patients with subperiosteal abscess tend to present with more advanced infections and more severe visual loss. However, many patients with this form of orbital infection can be treated with complete resolution of the process without permanent damage.

True orbital abscess and cavernous sinus thrombosis are almost always accompanied by severe visual loss or blindness. These patients are typically very ill, may be septic, and may already have meningitis or altered mental status. In these patients, treatment is dependent on the severity of the overall condition. If the patient is unstable, intravenous antibiotics are administered and intensive care unit (ICU) support is rendered until the patient's condition stabilizes. Salvaging vision is of secondary importance to the survival of the patient. If there is residual vision and the patient is stable at the time of diagnosis, the best chance for saving vision is to perform emergent ethmoidectomy, drainage of the abscess, and orbital decompression by removal of the lamina papyracea.[24]

Preoperative Considerations

The essential preparation for orbital decompression, regardless of the indication and the technique being performed, is a complete ophthalmologic examination.

Careful documentation of visual acuity, extraocular movements, and fundoscopic examination are all necessary. For patients with Graves' ophthalmopathy, visual field evaluation and Hertel exophthalmography are also indicated. These evaluations are important in defining the need for surgery as well as the appropriate extent of surgery. In addition, this type of careful documentation is essential from a medicolegal perspective.

If the surgery is for Graves' disease, thyroid hormone status is an important issue. Patients with hyperthyroidism can develop hypertension or refractory tachycardia with administration of general anesthesia, a condition termed the thyroid storm. If the Graves' disease is not well controlled, surgery may be postponed. Alternatively, a combination of beta- and alpha-blockers can be given to prevent acute toxicity.

Patients with orbital infection should be assessed for hemodynamic stability. These patients may have overt shock, or may have bacteremia with impending shock. Proper invasive monitoring with an arterial line, urinary catheter, and central venous catheter should be arranged. For patients with overt septic shock, a Swan-Ganz catheter is preferred. After determining the hemodynamic status of the patient, adequate rehydration and stabilization of the patient should be achieved before starting surgery.

All patients undergoing orbital decompression should receive antibiotics before and after surgery. In patients with Graves' disease, prophylactic antibiotics should be given, starting 1 hour before the procedure and continued after surgery, as described for any sinus surgery. Patients with orbital infection are treated with therapeutic antibiotics beginning as soon as the diagnosis is made and continuing for up to 6 weeks, depending on the nature of the infection and the speed of infection resolution. During surgery, cultures should be obtained to guide antibiotic therapy after surgery based on specific sensitivities. The choice of antibiotics will reflect the standard options for sinus infection.

Technique

Endoscopic Orbital Decompression

Endoscopic orbital decompression is normally performed under general anesthesia. Local anesthesia can be attempted,[13] but the orbital periosteum is difficult to anesthetize. The innervation is derived from the first division of the trigeminal nerve. These branches enter the orbit through the cavernous sinus and the superior orbital fissure. Anesthetizing these nerves requires an orbital block, as performed for cataract or retinal surgery. This can be combined with a sphenopalatine block to allow local sedation to be used. For many surgeons, this approach involves more effort than the benefits are worth.

Regardless of the anesthetic technique, the nose should be prepared with topical and local anesthesia, as for routine endoscopic sinus surgery. This is illustrated and discussed in detail in Chapter 8. As described in Chapter 8, the preferred topical anesthetic is cocaine flakes, whereas the preferred local anesthetic is 1% lidocaine with 1 : 100,000 epinephrine. These agents do carry a small but controllable risk of cardiovascular reactions. To date, the author has not encountered any serious or prolonged reactions using the techniques described.

The first surgical steps are to perform a complete endoscopic sphenoethmoidectomy with intranasal frontal sinusotomy and wide middle meatus antrostomy. This is all necessary for varying reasons. The complete ethmoidectomy is needed to expose the entire lamina papyracea for removal. The sphenoidectomy is needed to help identify the position of the optic nerve and the position of the orbital apex. The frontal sinus dissection is important to allow room for the orbital contents to expand medially without obstructing the frontal sinus drainage. Finally, a wide antrostomy is important to access the floor of the orbit to allow decompression to extend onto the floor up to the inferior orbital nerve.

This part of the surgery can be performed using traditional techniques or using powered instrumentation. Most of these patients have no infection or inflammation in the sinuses, so whichever technique is used, the procedure is rapid and nearly bloodless. As the entire procedure is detailed in Chapter 8, only an abbreviated description is provided here.

The uncinate process is incised and removed. The ethmoidal bulla is encountered next and is completely resected. The laminal papyracea can be initially identified at this point. Posterior to the bulla is the ground lamella, which is removed from the inferior and medial portion extending superiorly and laterally. The cells of the posterior ethmoid are removed. The skull base is typically first identified in the posterior ethmoid. To complete this dissection, the lamina papyracea and the skull base are skeletonized. This is best performed from posterior to anterior, removing loose bone fragments and bony ridges.

The sphenoid sinus is next identified and opened widely. The optimal technique is to identify the ostium of the sphenoid sinus just lateral to the septum at about a 30-degree incline from the floor of the nose. This is best exposed by removing the posterior and inferior portion of the superior turbinate. The ostium can often be visualized at this point or, if not, palpated with the tip of the suction catheter. The ostium is enlarged inferiorly and laterally to remove the anterior wall of the sphenoid. Once the sinus has been opened sufficiently to allow good visualization, the rotating sphenoid punch is used to complete the removal of the entire anterior wall.

The next step in the procedure is to perform the frontal sinus dissection. By skeletonizing the skull base, it is usually possible to identify the position of the anterior ethmoid artery. This landmark is very helpful in the dissection of the frontal recess. The agger nasi cells are then opened anteriorly. This exposes the inside of the agger nasi cell. The posterior wall is thus identified and carefully removed. The frontal sinus ostium is normally located anterior to the anterior ethmoid artery and posterior to the posterior wall of the agger nasi cell. In these cases, the ostium should be left intact, with special care being taken to preserve the mucosa on the skull base on the posterior wall of the frontal recess.

The next step is to create a large middle meatus antrostomy. The natural ostium should be identified. Using curved endoscopy scissors, the posterior fontanelle is incised from anterior to posterior. The posterior fontanelle is then removed using the scissors along the superior edge of the inferior turbinate or using a backbiter along the same edge from posterior to anterior. The size of the antrostomy is maximized by enlarging the opening to the floor of the orbit, anteriorly to the nasolacrimal duct, inferiorly to the inferior turbinate, and posteriorly to the posterior wall of the maxillary sinus.

Once the sinus surgery is complete, the orbital wall is addressed. When the procedure is performed for Graves' ophthalmopathy, complete decompression with incision of the periosteum is required. If the operation is for infection, the amount of orbital decompression required varies. A subperiosteal abscess may only require focal decompression. However, if there is severe proptosis, complete decompression with periosteal incision may be indicated.

A J-curette is used to carefully lift the bone of the lamina papyracea from the orbital periosteum (Fig. 21–1). It is surprisingly easy to perform this maneuver without injuring the underlying orbital periosteum. Once an area of the bone is removed, an elevator can be used to separate the periosteum from the remaining bone (Fig. 21–2*A*). This dissection allows easy and safe removal of the bone. With the periosteum elevated, the bone can be removed using Blakesley forceps, backbiters, and the curette. Bone removal should extend from the skull base superiorly around the medial wall to the inferior orbital nerve inferiorly (Fig. 21–2*B*). The posterior extent of bone removal is the orbital apex at the junction of the sphenoid and ethmoid sinuses. The anterior extent of the dissection is the lacrimal sac.

One important point in bone removal is not to remove the bony wall of the frontal recess. Kennedy and colleagues have reported the occurrence of frontal sinus mucocele secondary to prolapse of the orbit after orbital decompression.[25] To avoid this, the bone removal

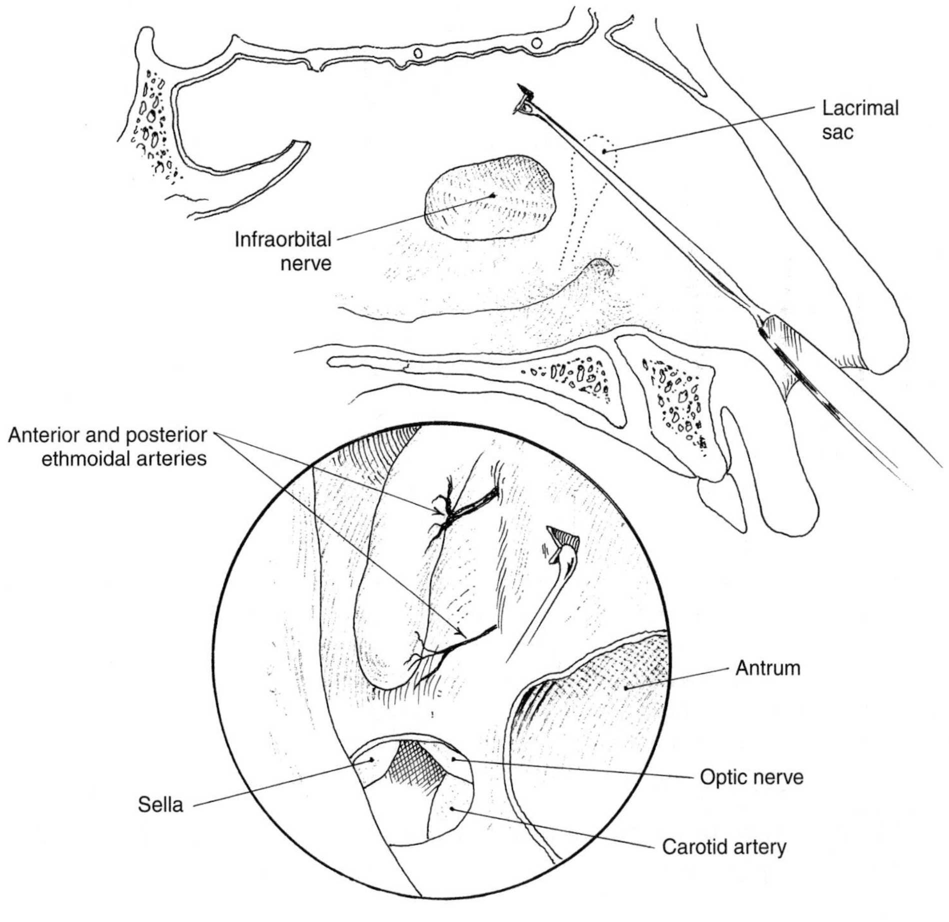

Figure 21–1. Endoscopic orbital decompression, lateral and endoscopic views. A complete sphenoethmoidectomy with frontal sinusotomy and middle meatus antrostomy has been accomplished. The bone of the lamina papyracea is removed using a curette.

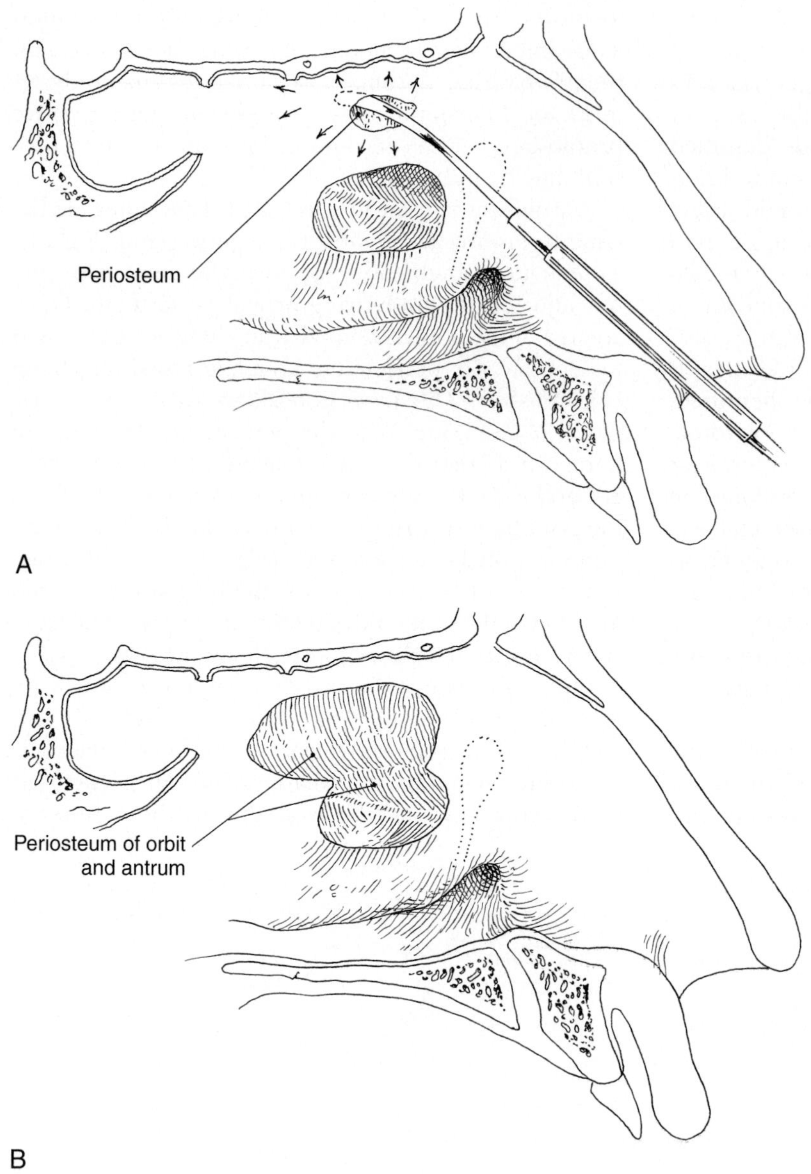

Figure 21–2. Endoscopic orbital decompression. *A,* Dissection of the periosteum from the lamina papyracea using an elevator. *B,* Completed removal of the bone from the orbital periosteum.

should not extend anteriorly to the plane of the anterior ethmoid artery along the skull base.

The final step in the procedure is to incise the orbital periosteum and tease out the orbital fat. A sickle knife is used to make multiple, parallel incisions extending from posterior to anterior (Fig. 21–3*A*). Care is taken during these incisions to make sure that the underlying orbital fat, and especially the medial rectus muscle, is not injured. The sickle knife is ideal for this since the curved blade can hook the periosteum and pull it medially away from the orbital contents. The incisions should be close enough together to facilitate removal of the intervening bands. These bands can either be cut with the knife at both ends or be snipped off with scissors (Fig. 21–3*B*).

The orbital fat is then easily teased out into the sinus cavity. A blunt pick or a curette is adequate for this technique. The final result should allow unrestricted expansion of the orbit into the sinus (Fig. 21–4). The procedure is completed by placing a sinus pack. This is usually a synthetic sponge that may be wrapped in a finger cot to help prevent the pack from sticking to the orbital fat.

Endoscopic orbital decompression is often enhanced by adding lateral canthotomy with inferior cantholysis. This technique may add an average of 2 mm of retrusion to the endoscopic decompression. The details of this procedure are described later in this chapter in the section on orbital hemorrhage.

External Orbital Decompression

External orbital decompression utilizes a medial canthal approach for medial wall decompression and the

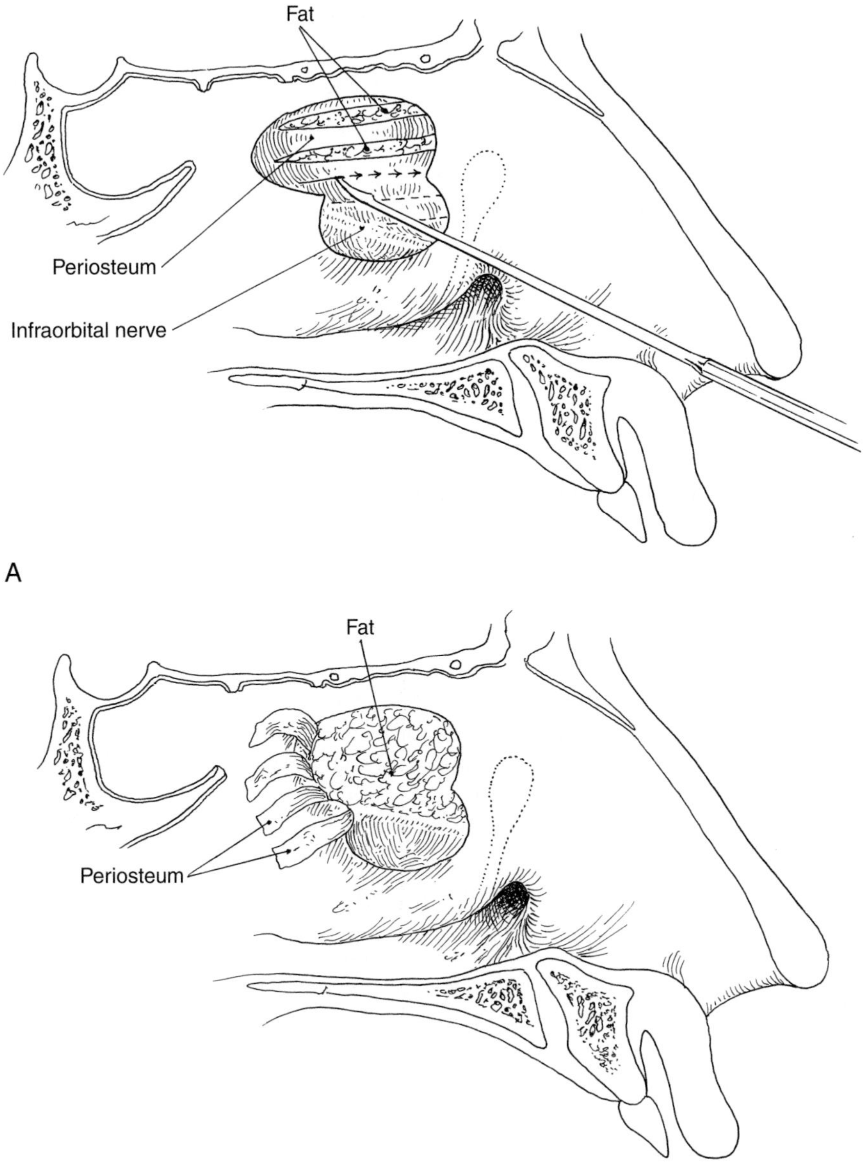

Figure 21–3. Endoscopic orbital decompression. *A,* Periosteal incisions. Using a sickle knife, incisions are made from posterior to anterior in parallel lines. *B,* Periosteal bands are removed to allow the orbital fat to medialize.

Caldwell-Luc approach for inferior wall decompression. The medial wall decompression is performed for inflammatory conditions, whereas a combined procedure is performed for Graves' ophthalmopathy. For Graves' disease, the inferior wall is decompressed first, as this accounts for most of the retrusion achieved. The medial wall decompression is added if the inferior wall procedure has not resulted in the amount of retrusion desired.

Inferior wall decompression is performed through a sublabial incision and an anterior sinus wall antrostomy. This technique is described in detail in Chapter 10. Briefly, the sublabial mucosa is infiltrated with 1% lidocaine with 1 : 100,000 epinephrine. The incision extends from the midline to about over the first molar. The incision is placed about 5 mm above the gingival labial sulcus. The incision is carried down to the bone of the maxilla, and a subperiosteal elevation of the facial soft tissues is performed. The pyriform aperture is identified, and the dissection should expose the infraorbital nerve. A 4-mm chisel is used to create an opening in the anterior wall. This opening is extended widely to expose the inside of the sinus using Kerrison forceps.

With the inside of the maxillary sinus widely exposed, the natural ostium of the sinus should be identified and enlarged by removal of the posterior fontanelle. The mucosa over the roof of the sinus should be removed carefully. The inferior orbital nerve is identified before proceeding further to make sure that it is not injured

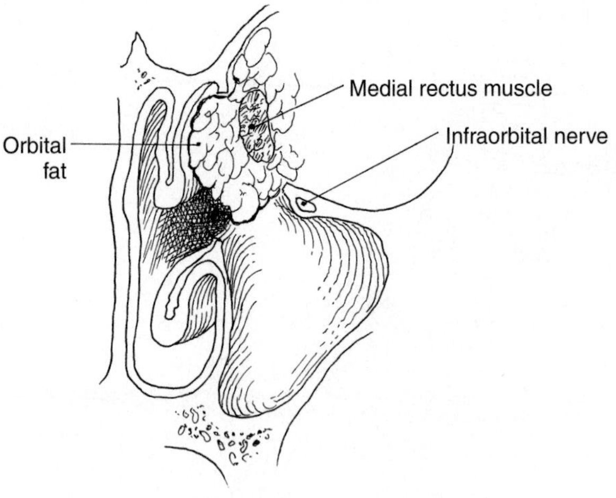

Figure 21–4. Endoscopic orbital decompression. Midcoronal view demonstrating the completed procedure.

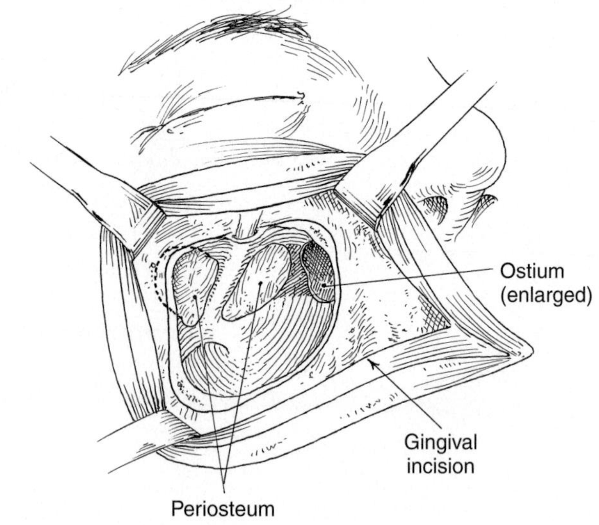

Figure 21–6. External approach for orbital decompression. The bone of the orbital floor has been removed, exposing the periosteum. The natural ostium of the sinus has been enlarged.

during the remainder of the operation (Fig. 21–5). At this point, the bone of the sinus roof is removed (Fig. 21–6). A curette is useful for beginning this elevation, which should be done carefully to avoid tearing the underlying periosteum. The curette is used to scratch through the thin bone medial to the infraorbital nerve. When a small area of the periosteum is exposed, a Freer elevator can be inserted though the gap and used to separate the bone from the periosteum. This facilitates use of a Kerrison rongeur to remove the bone rapidly and safely.

At the completion of bone removal, a large central area of the roof of the sinus is removed with the infraorbital nerve in the center. To achieve adequate subluxation of the orbit into the sinus, the periosteum is incised in parallel lines from posterior to anterior. The intervening strands of periosteum can be excised to allow unrestricted expansion (Figs. 21–7 and 21–8).

The inferior decompression is completed by packing the sinus, with the packing material coming out of the sinus into the nose through the medial wall antrostomy. The sublabial incision is finally closed in routine fashion. To ensure that the sutures hold until the wounds have a chance to heal, interrupted 3-0 Vicryl sutures are preferred over chromic sutures or continuous running sutures.

Medial wall decompression is performed by completing an external ethmoidectomy, as described in detail in Chapter 9. Briefly, this procedure is begun with a medial canthal incision. The skin is prepared with iodine solution, the incision is marked on the skin, and local anesthetic is injected. The incision is made and carried down to the bone of the lateral wall of the

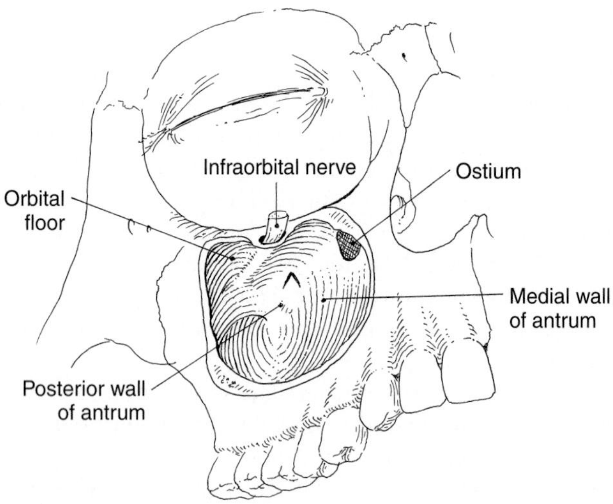

Figure 21–5. Anatomy of the maxillary sinus (right side) before proceeding with the external approach for orbital decompression.

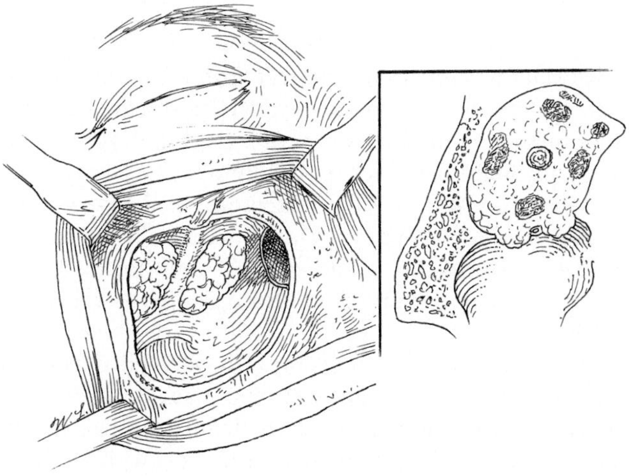

Figure 21–7. External approach for orbital decompression. The periosteum has been incised and removed. The inset shows a coronal view of the degree of prolapse.

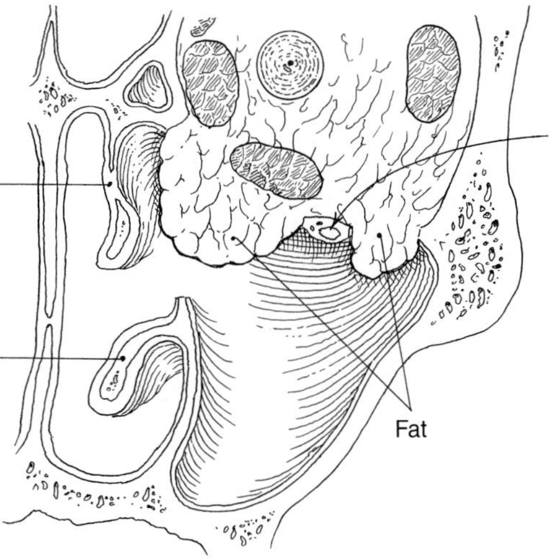

Figure 21–8. External approach for orbital decompression. A coronal view demonstrates the degree of prolapse after medial and inferior decompression. The infraorbital nerve remains in the bony canal as an island.

nose. Using a Freer elevator, the medial orbital wall is exposed. The anterior and posterior ethmoid arteries are identified, coagulated with bipolar cautery, and divided. The bone of the lamina papyracea is fractured and then removed. The complete ethmoid is removed.

Once this step has been completed, the periosteum of the orbit is incised along parallel lines and the intervening strands are removed. The ethmoid sinus is usually not packed, but if necessary, it can be packed by bringing one end of the pack out through the nose. The incision is normally drained with a Penrose drain. A cosmetic repair of the incision is performed using 6-0 nylon suture.

Postoperative Care

The postoperative care of the patient undergoing endoscopic sinus surgery is the same regardless of the exact procedure performed. This care is covered in detail in Chapter 8. For patients with Graves' disease, the only special consideration is to make sure that healing proceeds normally. Exposed orbital fat has a tendency for crusting as granulation tissue is formed on the surface. Crusts can be carefully debrided. Adherent crust should be allowed to separate as the mucosa grows along the surface of the orbit. Intensive irrigations are necessary to minimize the amount of debridement required. One area of concern is the continued patency of the frontal sinus. When the orbital fat medializes, there can be adhesions across the frontal recess, leading to blockage of the frontal sinus. The keys to avoiding this are to limit the removal of the lamina papyracea to levels posterior to the anterior ethmoid artery, and to preserve the mucosa along the skull base and lateral wall of the middle turbinate. Vigorous postoperative care is important to help ensure that any synechiae that begin to form are divided, thereby preventing dense adhesions from forming.

For patients in whom orbital infection is the indication for orbital decompression, significant medical management is required in addition to the routine postoperative care. Some patients may be unstable, requiring ICU monitoring and treatment. Others may be managed with inpatient hospitalization and prolonged intravenous antibiotic therapy. Discharge from the hospital is appropriate as soon as the patient is stable and the eye infection is controlled. This degree of progress will be apparent by a pattern of decreasing edema and erythema and improving ocular mobility. Vision should be stabilized or improved. The course of antibiotics should continue for a minimum of 6 weeks, with a least a 2-week course of intravenous antibiotics.

Postoperative care of the patient undergoing external orbital decompression resembles that for routine Caldwell-Luc and external ethmoidectomy. In orbital decompression cases, there are no substantial differences from these more classic procedures. Hospitalization is usually required only overnight, and the medical and surgical care is minimal.

Long-term follow-up evaluation of patients with orbital decompression is important. This is necessary for detection of late mucocele formation or late changes in the orbit. Mucocele is rare, but may occur long after the surgery, up to many years later. There is also a risk of late orbital problems. In Graves' disease, progression of the exophthalmos is possible. In patients with infection, there is a risk of enophthalmos occurring after all the inflammation completely resolves. In such cases, an orbital reconstruction to overcome the enophthalmos may be required.

Complications

The complications of orbital decompression can be classified as being related to the approach or being related to the decompression. The complications of the various approaches are covered elsewhere (Chapters 8, 9, and 10). The complications related to the decompression are covered here.

The most common and important side effect of the surgery is diplopia. Many of the candidates for these operations will have diplopia prior to surgery. In Graves' disease, this may be caused by asymmetrical involvement of the ocular muscles or severe involvement leading to decreased mobility. In patients with diplopia before the operation, the condition is unlikely to resolve following surgery, and in about 20% of patients, the diplopia may worsen.[12, 13]

The main concern with orbital decompression is that a patient with normal extraocular muscle function can develop diplopia after decompression. This may occur as a result of direct injury to the medial or inferior rectus muscles, but most likely, the cause is asymmetrical expansion of the orbit. This may occur in up to 40% of cases when operating for Graves' disease.[12, 13] This diplopia can be treated with corrective lenses or strabismus surgery in some cases. However, all patients undergoing this surgery should be carefully counseled about this possibility. On balance, the possibility of visual loss and the cosmetic deformity associated with Graves' disease must be weighed against the risk of diplopia. For most patients, the risk : benefit ratio favors surgery.

Aside from diplopia, there are significant risks to the eye during decompression. These risks arise from the possibility of bleeding into the orbit. Bleeding into the orbit can occur during incision of the periosteum or during removal of the bone of one of the orbital walls secondary to a tear of an orbital vessel or the anterior or posterior ethmoid artery. Bleeding into the orbit is a dire emergency that can lead to diplopia, abscess, and visual loss up to and including blindness. The risk of this is generally very low. In endoscopic sinus surgery performed for chronic sinusitis, the risk is reported to be as low as less than 1/1000. When performing orbital decompression, the risk of intraorbital bleeding is higher than for routine cases, but is still low (<1%). The management of orbital hemorrhage is covered in detail later in this chapter.

OPTIC NERVE DECOMPRESSION

Indications

Traumatic Optic Neuritis. The strongest indication for performing optic nerve decompression is for certain cases of posttraumatic optic neuritis.[26–28] Patients with severe frontal, nasal, and orbital trauma may sustain a fracture that extends into the orbital apex and, possibly, the optic canal. The incidence of significant visual loss after facial trauma is usually estimated to be 2% to 3%.[29, 30] When this occurs, the optic nerve may sustain direct injury or be injured by compression within a closed compartment.[31] The result is visual loss that corresponds to the severity of the optic nerve injury. This can vary from a minimal contusion or neuropraxia that results in only one or two lines of visual loss measured by a Snellen near-vision card, to transection and permanent, complete blindness.

Management of these injuries depends on precise diagnosis of the extent of the injury, which includes a complete ophthalmologic examination. An assessment of the visual acuity of both eyes, extraocular movements, and the anterior segment, as well as fundoscopic examination, is necessary. An optic nerve injury is suggested when the visual acuity is decreased and an afferent pupillary defect is present in the absence of injury to the anterior segment. An afferent pupillary defect is present when a light swung from the uninjured eye to the injured eye results in dilation of the pupil. The pupil dilates because the injured optic nerve perceives less light than the normal eye. This is interpreted by the brain stem as a sudden decrease in light, which causes the pupil to dilate to adjust to the change in conditions.

The fundoscopic examination is essential to confirm the diagnosis of optic nerve injury. The most common finding will be a normal retina with either a swollen optic nerve head secondary to acute trauma to the anterior optic nerve segment or a pale, atrophic, nerve head from injury to the posterior optic nerve segment. Other findings, such as retinal detachment, hemorrhage, and anterior segment injury, do not rule out optic nerve trauma, as these injuries can occur simultaneously. In the setting of combined optic nerve and other injuries to the eye, the optic nerve injury may be hard to diagnose. Fortunately, most of these injuries are isolated.

In addition to these examinations, a high-resolution CT scan of the orbits with direct coronal cuts and bone windows is necessary to define the nature of the fracture and injury. The scan may demonstrate disruption, bone fragments in the optic canal, or a nondisplaced fracture through the optic canal. In order to detect the most subtle findings, thin cuts of 1 to 2 mm through the optic canal are necessary.

Once the diagnosis of optic nerve injury is established, a management strategy must be developed and followed. Most ophthalmologists recommend immediate, high-dose, steroid therapy. One dosing regimen suggested in the literature includes a loading dose of 30 mg/kg of intravenous methylprednisolone, followed by a dosage of 15 mg/kg every 6 hours for up to 3 days.[28] These doses are suprapharmacologic and have the effect of minimizing the edema and free radical damage within the nerve. There may also be other protective effects of this type of treatment. Although there may be some temporary adrenal suppression from this course of treatment, as long as the treatment ends within 2 to 3 days, the adrenal function recovers rapidly and a prolonged taper interval is not necessary.

For patients who improve within 24 hours of initiation of steroid therapy, the course of treatment is usually extended for up to 3 days while the eye is carefully monitored. Most of these patients achieve adequate recovery, in which case surgery has no role. Patients who show little or no improvement on steroids within the first 24 hours, or who, after 3 days, have persistent, severe loss despite some improvement are candidates for decompression. For these surgical candidates, the CT scan must be examined carefully, and patients should be advised of the possibility of surgical decompression. The CT scan should indicate that the patient has either a nondisplaced or minimally displaced fracture. With total disruption of the optic canal, surgery is unlikely to be of benefit. However, if the CT scan is favorable and the patient or designated family member desires surgery, this should then be planned as soon as possible.

If optic nerve decompression is performed for traumatic optic neuropathy, the results depend on the severity of the injury and the findings at surgery. In patients with no light perception before surgery, useful vision is gained in only 10% to 50% of cases.[26–28] In patients who have light perception before surgery, some degree of improvement is seen in most patients, and useful vision is almost always regained.[26–28]

Infectious Optic Neuritis. A more controversial indication for optic nerve decompression is inflammation secondary to sinus infection. Rarely, patients with posterior ethmoid or sphenoid sinusitis may develop visual loss secondary to extension of the inflammatory infectious process through the bone of the optic canal to involve the optic nerve. Some patients with either thin-walled canals or frankly dehiscent canals may be predisposed to such an occurrence if sinusitis develops in the adjacent sinuses.

The reasons why an individual patient would develop optic neuritis as a complication of sinusitis are unclear. The possibilities include immunocompromise, virulent infection, dehiscent bone, or high intrasinus pressures. The author has managed a series of seven patients who developed optic neuritis secondary to sinusitis. Of these patients, all had one or more risk factors identified. The most common infectious agent, affecting four patients, was an Aspergillus species. The other patients had no growth. One of those with no growth had acquired immunodeficiency syndrome (AIDS), the second was a diabetic with chronic sinusitis, and the third had a large cholesterol granuloma. Of the patients with fungal infection, one had AIDS, one had allergic fungal sinusitis that became invasive, and the remaining two were both diabetic.

Among these patients, only two have undergone optic nerve decompression. One patient who had invasive fungal sinusitis was a 70-year-old diabetic woman with a fungoma of the posterior ethmoid and sphenoid sinuses. The patient had no vision in the right eye and 20/400 vision in the left eye. The patient underwent surgery for debridement of the fungoma and optic nerve decompression. At surgery, the optic canal was intact and successfully decompressed. Eventually, the patient could detect hand waving in the right eye and had 20/100 visual acuity in the left eye and was able to read with magnifying glasses. The second patient had acute visual loss associated with isolated sphenoid sinusitis and AIDS. At the time of surgery, he had no vision in the affected eye. He failed to recover any vision postoperatively. Among the other patients with visual loss, only ethmoidectomy with sphenoidectomy was performed. One patient with invasive aspergillosis and AIDS died within 48 hours from intracranial spread of the fungal infection. One patient with a large cholesterol granuloma of the posterior ethmoid and sphenoid had no vision in his left eye for 2 months. Following decompression of the cyst, he regained vision in the eye up to an acuity of 20/500. Two other patients with allergic fungal sinusitis who developed invasive fungal infection had no vision in the affected eye and did not regain vision following surgery.

In summary, once vision is lost from inflammatory optic neuritis, the chances of recovering vision are poor. Whether or not decompression of the optic nerve, performed in addition to sphenoethmoidectomy, contributes to recovery is unclear. Certainly, the optic nerve decompression adds time and considerable technical difficulty to the operation. A reasonable approach to the decision as to whether to perform optic nerve decompression is to assess the stability of the patient's condition and the duration of the visual loss. If the patient's condition is stable, the procedure can be considered. Moreover, the optimal surgical patient has a history of acute onset of visual loss of less than 1 week's duration. Finally, best results are achieved in those who, despite severe visual loss, have some residual light perception. These last criteria are designed to increase the likelihood of success of the procedure. Long-standing visual loss is unlikely to respond to decompression. In a patient with serviceable vision, the risk of damage to the optic nerve from the decompression outweighs the potential benefit of the surgery.

Optic Nerve Compression. A number of conditions that can lead to compression of the optic nerve may be indications for optic nerve decompression. These can be divided into expansile lesions of the sinuses, intracranial expansile lesions, and expansile lesions of the sphenoid bone. The sinus lesions include mucocele, cholesterol granuloma, and fungal processes. Mucocele most commonly affects the frontal and ethmoid sinuses. When the mucocele occurs in the posterior ethmoid or sphenoid, optic nerve compression can result. If this is diagnosed relatively early in the course of the condition, simple drainage of the mucocele is all that is typically necessary.

Actual optic canal decompression is not normally required. This is also true for cholesterol granuloma and fungal processes. These lesions all develop high internal pressures that lead to bone erosion and compression of the optic nerves. Simple drainage and evacuation of the lesion will remove the pressure on the nerve. No additional bone removal should be required to relieve the pressure.

A variety of intracranial lesions can erode the bone of the optic canal, leading to compression of the optic nerves. These include pituitary tumors, meningiomas, encephaloceles, and meningoceles. These lesions cause compression of the optic nerve after eroding the bone of the canal. Treatment is to remove the lesion while preserving the optic nerve. As opposed to the sinus lesions, which can be treated by drainage, the intracranial lesions must be removed.

The last category includes lesions of the sphenoid bone, the most common of which is fibrous dysplasia. This disease is an idiopathic process that can affect multiple sites (polyostotic) or a single site (monostotic). The pathologic lesion is a fibrotic expansion of the diploic space of the bone. Fibrous dysplasia is recognized on CT scan by the classic ground-glass appearance of the bone. As the pathologic process progresses, the bone expands and can involve the bone of the optic canal. This may result in compression of the nerve. In cases when visual loss becomes progressive, treatment is indicated.[32, 33] Decompression in patients with extensive orbital lesions without visual loss, when performed prophylactically to prevent visual loss, is more controversial.[34] When optic nerve compression from fibrous dysplasia is treated, bony decompression of the optic nerve or nerves is required. This is a technically challenging procedure owing to the relatively bloody dissection and the extreme thickness of the bone in this condition.

Selection of Approach

When a decision is made to proceed with optic nerve decompression, a surgical approach must be chosen. There are three basic techniques for this surgery: intracranial, transorbital, and transnasal. The intracranial approach uses a bifrontal craniotomy with elevation of both frontal lobes to expose the optic chiasm and orbital apex. The transorbital procedure uses a medial canthal incision and follows the medial orbital wall back to the optic nerve. This technique may utilize an operating microscope or surgical loupes for magnification. The transnasal approach is performed endoscopically and goes through the ethmoid and sphenoid sinuses to identify the optic nerve at the orbital apex and in the sphenoid sinus.

The intracranial approach is the original technique for performing optic nerve decompression. In modern practice, it is indicated only in cases when the optic nerve compression is caused by an intracranial lesion or if another approach is not technically feasible. This may occur in certain cases of trauma when disruption of the ethmoid sinus leads to medial prolapse of the orbit in combination with an injury to the eye itself, preventing retraction of the eye during surgery. In this case, an endoscopic approach may not be possible because of the soft tissues of the eye blocking the path to the orbital apex. An external approach is not possible owing to an anterior segment or retinal injury that makes extensive retraction too risky. Also, the intracranial approach is indicated for most cases of fibrous dysplasia. This situation requires wide exposure and identification of as many landmarks as possible to help locate the optic canal. The advantage of the intracranial approach is that the nerves can be identified at the chiasm and followed into the optic canal.

The transorbital approach is indicated for cases of trauma or infection and represents an alternative technique for surgeons who prefer this method. It is easy to pinpoint the position of the optic nerve through this approach, which is familiar to most experienced orbital and sinus surgeons. However, since the introduction of endoscopic decompression, the transorbital approach has become a secondary option. Currently, the transorbital approach is primarily indicated for patients with significant prolapse of the orbital contents into the ethmoid sinus, blocking the intranasal approach to the optic nerve.

The endoscopic approach is favored for most intrasinus pathologic conditions and for most cases of inflammation and trauma. The advantage of the intranasal approach is that it avoids an external incision and retraction on the eye. For these reasons, it will always be the first choice unless contraindicated. The primary criterion for the endoscopic approach is that the surgeon have complete mastery of the endoscopic sinus technique and the anatomy of the optic canal. If this criterion is met, then most cases will be amenable to the endoscopic approach. The few exceptions, covered earlier, include fibrous dysplasia, intracranial masses, and select cases of complex orbital and sinus trauma.

Preoperative Considerations

The most important aspect of surgical planning is to gather the proper surgical team for the particular approach selected. Otolaryngologists are involved primarily in the orbital and transnasal approaches. Whenever an optic nerve decompression is performed, an ophthalmologist should be involved. A complete preoperative examination and postoperative follow-up examination are essential. Availability of an ophthalmologist during surgery is also desirable. Clearly, a neurosurgeon is the primary surgeon in any procedure involving intracranial decompression.

Other considerations depend on the particular approach planned. For craniotomy, a complete medical evaluation is required. This information is essential for intraoperative management during the prolonged surgery. Complete intraoperative monitoring must also be arranged. Prophylactic antibiotics are required for the external orbital and cranial approaches, but are not usually needed for the transnasal approach.

Technique

Endoscopic Optic Nerve Decompression

Endoscopic optic nerve decompression requires that the bone of the optic canal be carefully drilled away to expose the nerve sheath. The key to being able to perform the procedure is to have a drill capable of removing the bone in a controlled manner. One option is to use an otologic drill with long drill bits. This drill provides optimal power for the procedure, and certain of these drills provide irrigation delivered to the tip. However, the otologic drills lack suction. This leads to rapid accumulation of irrigant in the operative field, resulting in short periods of drill application with frequent suctioning. In addition, the use of otologic drills for intranasal procedures risks causing a friction burn to the front of the nose or alar rim. The primary alternative is to use one of the commercially available sinus microresectors fitted with a cutting burr. These instruments all provide suction and irrigation at the tip, which can greatly facilitate the operation. The drill in these cases is hooded, which protects the patient from friction burns. However, these drills lack power, making bone removal a slow process. Nonetheless, the microresector is generally preferred to the otologic drill, as it is safer for the patient and, with patience, can achieve full decompression.

The procedure is performed under general anesthesia with the aid of both topical and injected anesthetics (cocaine flakes and lidocaine with epinephrine). The initial steps of the operation are to complete an anterior-to-posterior ethmoidectomy with middle meatus antrostomy and wide sphenoidotomy with removal of the entire anterior wall of the sphenoid sinus. This is accomplished in the standard fashion, as described in Chapter 8. A brief recounting of the steps is presented here.

The uncinate process is removed in its entirety to expose the ethmoidal bulla. The bulla is then entered and removed to expose the ground lamella. The ground lamella is entered medially and inferiorly and the vertical portion is removed. The posterior ethmoid cells are removed to expose the sphenoid rostrum. The ostium of the sphenoid is identified by removing the posteroinferior portion of the superior turbinate. From the ostium, the anterior wall of the sphenoid sinus is taken down inferiorly and laterally. Once this is done, the skull base and lamina papyracea are skeletonized from posterior to anterior. The last preliminary step is to enlarge the natural ostium of the maxillary sinus by complete removal of the posterior fontanelle.

The next step is to identify the optic canal within the sphenoid sinus and the posterior aspect of the orbital wall. The position of the optic canal within the sphenoid sinus is normally suggested by the location of a depression or dimple in the lateral wall caused by the crossing of the optic nerve and the carotid artery, referred to as the optic recess or cup (Fig. 21–9). The best technique for decompression of the optic nerve is to thin the bone over the nerve down to an eggshell thickness and then to flick the bone off with a curette. The nerve is identified at the apex of the orbit by first removing the bone of the posterior lamina papyracea (see Fig. 21–9). The thickest bone is located at the junction of the lamina papyracea, anterior wall of the sphenoid, and lateral wall of the sphenoid sinus.

The bony decompression should be extended posteriorly to the posterior wall of the sphenoid sinus just anterior to the optic chiasm (Figs. 21–10 and 21–11). Once the bony decompression is completed, a decision must be made as to whether to open the optic nerve sheath. If it is necessary to open the sheath to allow the edematous nerve room to expand to relieve pressure, this is accomplished by incising the sheath with a sickle knife from posterior to anterior. The fibrous sheath at the apex of the orbit is particularly thick owing to the presence of the tendinous insertions of the extraocular muscles into the orbital periosteum. This is called the annulus of Zinn (Fig. 21–11). Care must be taken in incising the sheath to avoid injuring the underlying nerve. It is this possibility that prevents incising the nerve in every case. If the reason for the surgery is to decompress an edematous nerve, then it makes sense to open the sheath. Conversely, if the reason for the decompression is to remove infected bone from the optic canal, incising the sheath may not be necessary.

The procedure is completed by placement of a hemostatic pack. Normally, a synthetic sponge is used. This should be placed to stent the middle turbinate medially, but should not be positioned against the exposed optic nerve. Otherwise, the pack could stick to the nerve, causing injury on removal.

Transorbital Optic Nerve Decompression

The transorbital or external ethmoid approach for optic nerve decompression is performed through a standard medial canthal incision with retraction of the orbit to expose the optic nerve at the apex of the orbit. A binocular microscope is used for visualization, and the bone of the optic canal is drilled away.

The procedure is performed under general anesthesia. Sterile preparation and draping is performed prior to the surgery. Either a standard curvilinear incision or

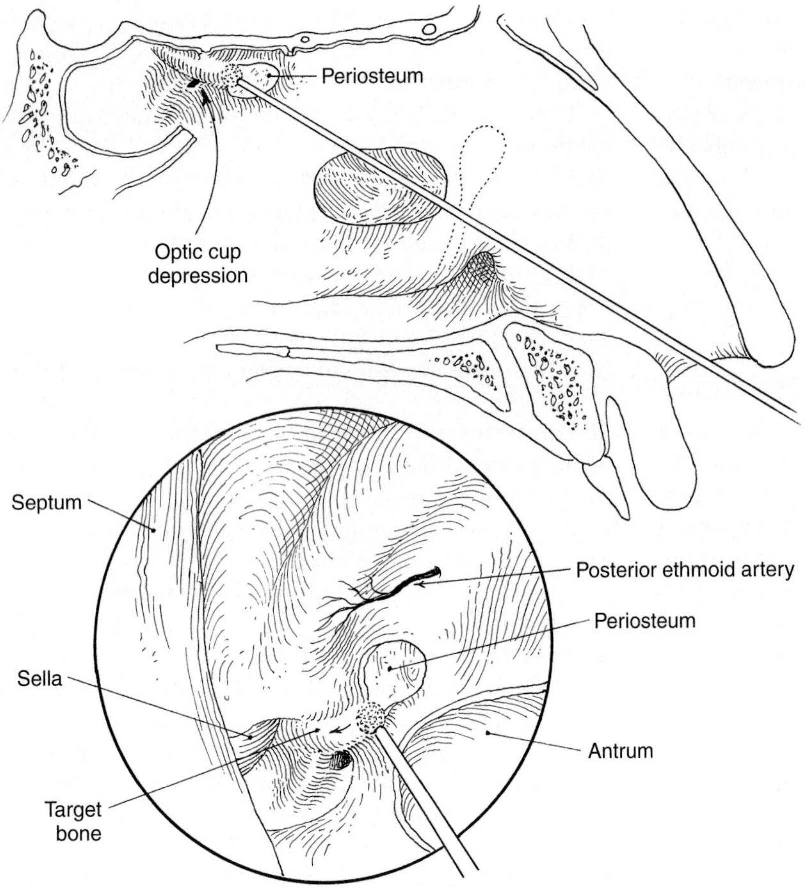

Figure 21–9. Endoscopic optic nerve decompression, lateral and endoscopic views. A complete sphenoethmoidectomy with wide antrostomy has been performed. The diamond drill is used to remove bone from the orbital apex and over the optic nerve.

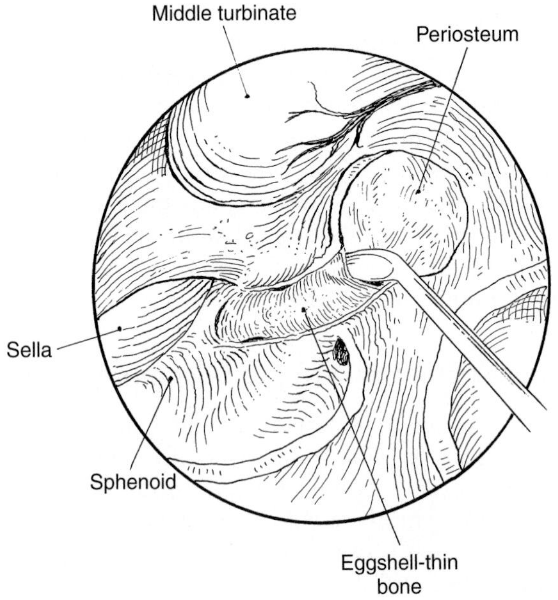

Figure 21–10. Endoscopic optic nerve decompression. The bone over the optic nerve has been thinned to eggshell thickness. The bone is then flicked off with a J-curette.

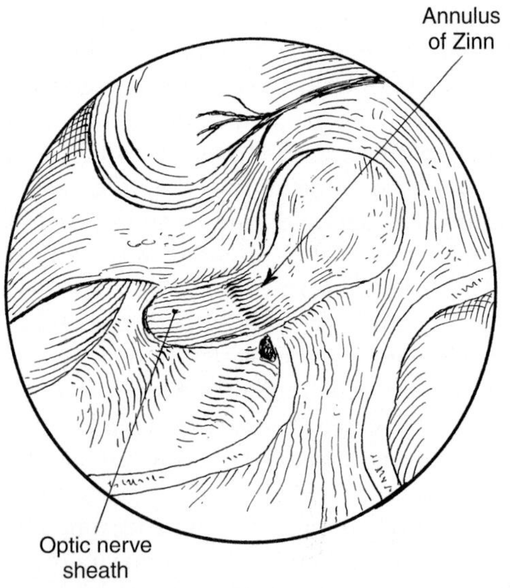

Figure 21–11. Endoscopic optic nerve decompression. The bone removal is complete and the nerve sheath is exposed. A thickening of the sheath is present at the annulus of Zinn, where the extraocular muscles insert.

a modified incision incorporating a W-plasty is marked onto the skin and injected with local anesthetic containing epinephrine (see Fig. 9–1). The incision is made through skin and subcutaneous tissue. The angular artery should be controlled either with cautery or ligation (Fig. 9–2). The soft tissues are divided through the periosteum down to bone.

A subperiosteal elevation of the orbital contents is then performed. The anterior lacrimal crest and posterior lacrimal crest are identified and the lacrimal sac is elevated from the fossa but left attached to the nasolacrimal duct inferiorly. This portion of the surgery is performed using a headlight for visualization. Retraction is best achieved using a malleable retractor. The next landmarks are the anterior and posterior ethmoid arteries. These arteries are found in the frontoethmoidal suture line. Both arteries should be coagulated with bipolar forceps. The elevation should extend past the posterior ethmoid artery to the optic foramen at the apex of the orbit. The optic foramen is approximately 5 mm posterior to the posterior ethmoid artery, but may be as close as 3 mm or as far as 10 mm.

In comparison to external ethmoidectomy, optic nerve decompression begins with bone removal posteriorly. The posterior ethmoid artery normally marks the anterior aspect of the most posterior ethmoid cell. This cell is entered and the lamina papyracea is removed outward from this point to expose the lateral aspect of the face of the sphenoid sinus (Fig. 21–12). The sphenoid sinus should be entered inferiorly and just lateral to the junction of the lamina papyracea and the anterior wall of the sphenoid sinus. After the entire anterior wall of the sphenoid sinus is removed, the view will expose the bone of the optic canal (Fig. 21–13).

At this point, the microscope is introduced and the drilling begins. A malleable retractor is held by an assistant to protect the orbit and optic nerve and to create space for the drill. The skin can be retracted by a self-retaining retractor, such as a Wheatlander. This is helpful in protecting the skin from injury during drilling. The bone is slowly removed from anterior to posterior on the medial surface of the optic nerve. As with the endoscopic procedure, the bone is thinned down to eggshell thickness, which can be fractured by gentle pressure with the back side of a J-curette. The small fragments of bone are then flicked away with the sharp edge of the curette (see Fig. 21–13).

The last step in the decompression is to incise the nerve sheath. The thickest part of the sheath is the

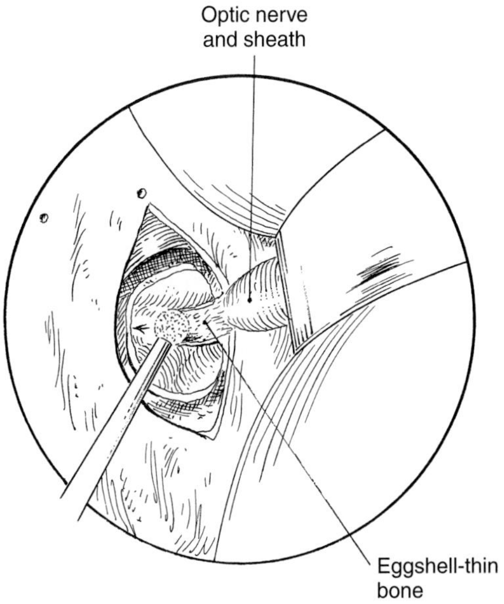

Figure 21–13. External ethmoidectomy approach for optic nerve decompression. After the sphenoid sinus is widely opened, the bone of the optic canal is drilled away.

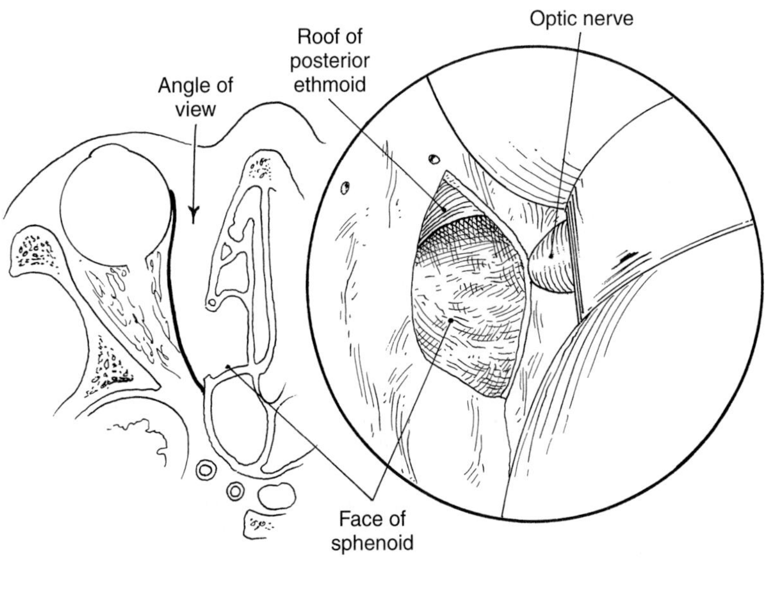

Figure 21–12. External ethmoidectomy approach for optic nerve decompression. Through a medial canthal incision, the lamina papyracea is exposed and the posterior ethmoid is entered. This exposes the face of the sphenoid sinus.

annulus of Zinn, located inside the optic foramen at the orbital apex. Care is taken to avoid injury to the nerve as the sheath is cut with a sickle knife (Fig. 21–14).

The wound is not typically packed, but can be drained if there is residual oozing at the end of the procedure. Either a 1/4-inch Penrose drain or a rubberband drain can be used to decompress the wound. The incision is closed in two layers. The deep layer must reapproximate the periosteum of the medial canthal area with at least one deep suture in the medial canthal tendon. The skin is closed with interrupted 6-0 nylon sutures. Alternatively, if a linear incision is used, a running closure is possible.

Postoperative Care

After surgery, most patients undergoing optic nerve decompression will be hospitalized for a period of days. Whether the patient is a trauma victim or has acute visual loss from infection, the patient is unlikely to be ready for discharge until significant postoperative care is rendered. The two groups of patients should be considered separately. Trauma patients undergoing decompression of the optic nerve may have associated fractures that may require surgery. These patients may also have concurrent intracranial injury, cervical spine injury, or thoracic or abdominal injury that may require substantial care.

Most patients sustaining traumatic injury to the optic nerve will receive high-dose steroids for a period of at least 24 to 48 hours after surgery. Otherwise, the care is typical for any endoscopic sinus surgery. The packing should be removed 3 to 7 days after the operation. At that time, the nose should be thoroughly suctioned of all blood clots and mucus. This is done endoscopically and can usually be performed easily in an office setting. Occasionally, however a patient will not tolerate this office procedure, in which case this first debridement can be performed in the operating room under general anesthesia.

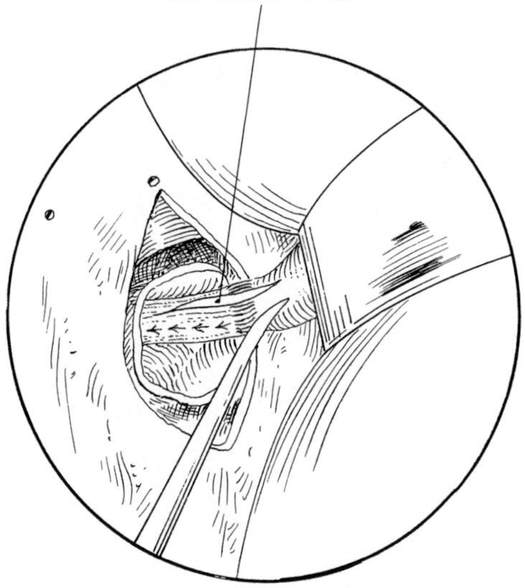

Figure 21–14. External ethmoidectomy approach for optic nerve decompression. The nerve sheath is incised to release any pressure from edema of the nerve.

Following this cleaning, irrigations with normal saline should be initiated twice each day. The irrigations are important in preventing crust from building up, which can lead to delayed healing and adhesions. Subsequent sinus debridements are performed 3 and 6 weeks after surgery as necessary. At each of these evaluations, any residual adhesions or crusts are debrided, and medical therapy is adjusted as needed.

Postoperative pharmacologic therapy includes steroids, antibiotics, nasal steroid spray, and adequate analgesics. After the first few days of high-dose steroid therapy, either the steroids are discontinued or a gradual taper is instituted. This will be determined based on the clinical course of the patient and the response, in terms of visual acuity, to the surgery and medical treatment. Antibiotics are selected to cover the usual bacteria and are continued for a minimum of 2 weeks. Additional treatment is based on the patient's clinical course and the presence or absence of mucosal inflammation. Nasal steroid spray is started after the packing is removed and is continued for 3 to 6 months to help prevent inflammation until mucosal healing is complete. Pain medication should be adjusted to the needs of the patient. For trauma patients, pain management will often be determined on the basis of the extent of the associated injuries.

The principle difference in the postoperative care of the patient with infectious optic neuropathy is the need for prolonged intravenous antibiotics. For patients with invasive fungal infection, amphotericin is usually administered up to a total dose of 2 to 3 grams. This is followed by a prolonged course of an oral antifungal agent, typically, itraconazole. Discharge from the hospital is generally delayed until the patient is clinically stable with administration of amphotericin or intravenous antibiotics and is able to continue the treatment at home.

Patients undergoing the external approach to the optic nerve typically require the same medical therapy as those in whom the endoscopic procedure is performed. However, repeated sinus debridement and sinus irrigation are not typically performed, as the sinuses are not open anteriorly. Clean healing for these patients depends on mucociliary clearance to remove blood clots and mucus from the sinus.

Complications

For the endoscopic surgical approach, the complications are basically the same as for endoscopic sinus surgery for chronic sinusitis (see Chapter 8). For patients undergoing optic nerve decompression, the additional risks of note include injury to the optic nerve and injuries related to the drill. The risk of direct injury to the optic nerve should theoretically be higher than for standard sinus surgery. Curiously, this does not appear to be the case. Probably this is due to the high skill level of most surgeons performing this operation and the extreme care taken around the optic nerve. In addition, these patients already have severe visual loss, so the effects of injury may be very difficult to detect and assess.

Drill-related problems may occur from inadvertent mucosal injuries. The shaft of the drill may erode the mucosa at the front of the nose on the medial edge of the inferior turbinate. In addition, there is a risk of thermal injury to the nasal sill if an otologic drill is used. This can be prevented by protecting the front of the nose with a moist sponge positioned under the drill.

Complications of the external or transorbital approach include cosmetic problems related to the healing of the incision. The incision may heal poorly owing to trapdoor deformities, contracture, or hypertrophic scarring. More importantly, there is a significant risk of injury to the eye, including injury to the medial rectus muscle, direct injury to the optic nerve, or bleeding into the eye causing orbital hematoma. These risks should be minimal, but are probably greatest with the transorbital approach owing to a less favorable angle of dissection and the need for significant retraction of the eye during surgery.

DACRYOCYSTORHINOSTOMY

Dacryocystorhinostomy (DCR) is an operation that is performed to re-create normal lacrimal drainage into the nose. It can be performed either endoscopically or through an external approach. The literature is replete with a variety of techniques proposed for this operation. The techniques described in this chapter are the author's adaptations of those described in the literature. As for most procedures, the results of the surgery depend more on skillful performance of the procedure than on the specific technique selected.

Indications

DCR is performed for obstruction of the lacrimal drainage system. It is most successful when the obstruction is caused by stenosis of the nasolacrimal duct. In certain cases, however, obstruction of the lacrimal sac may also be amenable to correction by DCR. In these cases, the success of DCR depends on the ability to restore lacrimal flow into the sac. Obstruction proximal to the lacrimal sac requires a conjunctivorhinostomy.

There are a wide variety of causes of nasolacrimal duct obstruction. The most common cause is dacryocystitis, or infection of the lacrimal sac and duct.[35, 36] This can lead to ulceration, scar tissue, and stenosis of the nasolacrimal duct. In current practice, an increasingly common cause is iatrogenic injury. Surgical procedures that affect the lateral wall of the nose may lead to injury to the nasolacrimal duct and subsequent scar tissue formation and obstruction. Examples of procedures that may lead to injury to the duct include inferior nasal antral window surgery, partial or total inferior turbinectomy, middle meatus antrostomy, and medial maxillectomy.[37] The incidence of lacrimal obstruction from any one of these procedures is very low, but many of these procedures are quite common, and so the total number of patients affected is significant.

Finally, there are uncommon causes of lacrimal obstruction, including trauma and tumors. Naso-orbital-ethmoid fractures, Le Fort fractures, and medial maxillary fractures can lead to traumatic injury to the duct, which may result in stenosis because of bony compression or scar tissue. Tumors of the lacrimal sac or duct are rare, but can occur. Squamous cell carcinoma, adenocarcinoma, melanoma, and lymphoma have been described. DCR is typically not one of the treatments of choice for these cancers. In most cases, wide excision with reconstruction of the lacrimal apparatus through staged procedures is often recommended. In some cases, radiation therapy and chemotherapy may be used as alternatives. If this is the case, then DCR may be necessary after treatment to manage scarring. Benign tumors and cysts of the lacrimal sac and duct have also been described. Local excision with DCR may be the therapeutic option of choice.

The decision of whether to perform an endoscopic or external approach depends on the pathologic presentation. In cases when the duct obstruction is attributable to iatrogenic injury, trauma, or infection, an endoscopic approach seems to be the best technique. The endoscopic technique has the advantages of avoiding external scars, affording easy removal of the lacrimal bone, and allowing verification of the lacrimal stent position at the end of the operation. In addition, a randomized prospective study has revealed that the success rate of the endoscopic and external procedures is statistically equivalent.[38] The only disadvantage of the endoscopic approach is that it does not allow adequate visualization of the inside of the lacrimal sac. Therefore, if a pathologic process involving the sac contributes to the lacrimal obstruction, this procedure is not applicable.

The external approach can be performed in any situation. However, it is best reserved for patients with pathologic disease of the lacrimal sac when sac exploration is required. The other main indication for the external approach is in cases in which the endoscopic approach has failed. The final indication for the external approach is in the case of a surgeon who does not have the endoscopic skills to perform the procedure intranasally.

Diagnosis and Evaluation

The predominant symptom of most patients with lacrimal obstruction is excessive tearing, known as epiphora. It is important to distinguish, by examination, between the various causes of epiphora. The least common cause is excessive production of tears or excessive lacrimation. This diagnosis is established only after exclusion of all other possibilities by documenting an increased rate of tear production. Certain medical conditions can lead to abnormally high tear production, the principal one being chronic irritation of the cornea. This can lead to hypersecretion of tears and epiphora.

The evaluation of epiphora begins with a routine, complete, ophthalmologic examination. This should include anterior segment examination using a slit lamp to assess the possibility of corneal pathology. This examination is enhanced by using topical fluoroscein to stain the tears. Defects in the cornea are then revealed as areas of pooling of the fluorescent dye, which can be seen under the slit lamp. In addition, it may be helpful to attempt to irrigate the lacrimal apparatus by cannulating the lacrimal sac through the puncta. Usually, this results in free flow of irrigant into the nose.

Jones type I and II tests are used to definitively document the obstruction of the lacrimal apparatus and the site of obstruction. The Jones type I test is performed by placing fluoroscein on the cornea. Usually, the lower eyelid is pulled down, and one or two drops of the dye are placed in the sulcus. The nose is then observed to determine whether the dye passes through the lacrimal apparatus into the nose. This test can be enhanced by the placement of a cotton pledget under the inferior meatus or in both the inferior and middle meatus if endoscopic damage to the duct is suspected. The cotton is removed after several minutes and observed under a Woods ultraviolet lamp. Under ultraviolet light, the fluoroscein glows brightly and is easy to detect. Normally, abundant fluoroscein should be seen on the cotton pledget within seconds of the dye being placed into the eye. The Jones II test is performed by cannulating the lacrimal sac and irrigating the dye directly into the sac. As with the Jones I test, the presence of dye in the nose is apparent from examination of the cotton pledgets.

A patient with an obstruction of the nasolacrimal duct will test negative on Jones type I and II tests, as the dye will not flow into the nose in either situation. However, if the Jones I test yields negative results and the Jones II test is positive for flow into the nose, this indicates that the obstruction is in the sac or lacrimal collecting apparatus. In actual clinical practice, most ophthalmologists will not use the Jones tests, but will rely on direct irrigation with saline as the diagnostic test. If the sac can easily be cannulated but irrigation does not flow into the nose, this implies that nasolacrimal obstruction is present. Surgery is generally offered to patients with obstruction that is confirmed either by failure of the Jones tests or failure to achieve irrigation.

Preoperative Considerations

For both the external and endoscopic procedures, there is very little in the way of preoperative care required. Once the diagnosis of obstruction is made and surgery is scheduled, most patients can proceed directly to surgery. Because the operation is fairly minor and can be performed rapidly in an outpatient setting, most patients who are candidates for general anesthesia will not require any special preoperative care.

General anesthesia is preferred for most patients. This provides maximal comfort for the patient and allows the surgery to be performed without delay attributable to patient discomfort. Local anesthesia with sedation is possible, however, for those patients who prefer this option or for those who cannot tolerate general anesthesia. Although it is difficult to completely anesthetize the surgical field with local anesthesia, with careful nerve blocks it is possible.

For intranasal cases, no skin preparation or prophylactic antibiotics are required. However, for external approaches it may be desirable to administer prophylactic antibiotics. It is customary to perform thorough skin preparation with either iodine solution or a suitable substitute. Iodine solution is not damaging to the eye, but iodine soap can be caustic and should be kept away from the eye.

Technique

Endoscopic DCR

For the endoscopic procedure, the nose is decongested and injected with local anesthetic, as for all endoscopic sinus surgeries. This technique, which provides maximum decongestion for visualization and hemostasis, is described in detail in Chapter 8, as well as earlier in this chapter in the section on endoscopic orbital decompression.

The first step in endoscopic DCR is to medialize the middle turbinate and examine the middle meatus. In patients who have had previous sinus surgery, the uncinate process may be partially or completely removed and the maxillary sinus ostium may have been enlarged. In others, there may be significant distortion of the anatomy, including absence (removal) of the middle turbinate. In cases when the anatomy is severely disturbed or unclear, locating the lacrimal sac may be difficult.

In these situations, a laser light probe may be helpful in identifying the lacrimal sac. These probes have either a red or white light, which can be passed through a lacrimal puncta into the lacrimal sac. The transilluminated sac can then be viewed intranasally with the endoscope to pinpoint its location. In the author's experience, this has only been necessary in one case. It is important to make this determination before surgery, however, as the probe is not part of the standard setup for sinus endoscopy.

In the case of a nose that has not previously been subjected to surgery, the anatomy is usually very clear. The uncinate process is identified and removed in its entirety, as demonstrated in Chapter 8. Essentially, an incision is made through the attachment of the uncinate to the lateral wall and the uncinate is removed. To avoid stenosis of the maxillary sinus ostium, it is advisable to enlarge the ostium by removal of the posterior fontanelle, although this procedure is not recounted here.

At this point, it is usually possible to identify the position of the lacrimal sac and the nasolacrimal duct on the lateral wall of the nose, just anterior to the attachment of the middle turbinate and ostium of the maxillary sinus (Fig. 21–15). An incision in the mucosa of the lateral wall, about 1 to 2 cm anterior to the attachment of the middle turbinate, is then made with a sickle knife (Fig. 21–16*A*). The mucosa is then undermined and excised in this area (Fig. 21–16*B*), exposing the bone over the lacrimal sac. This incision and mucosal removal can be performed with traditional instruments, electrocautery, or a laser. The advantage of the cautery and laser is that they prevent bleeding that can distort the surgical field. When the traditional instruments are used, a suction cautery unit can be applied to the mucosal edges to achieve hemostasis before proceeding.

The next step is to remove the bone of the medial wall of the lacrimal fossa. This can be performed with a rongeur or, preferably, with a drill. The drill options include an otologic drill and one of the microdebriders

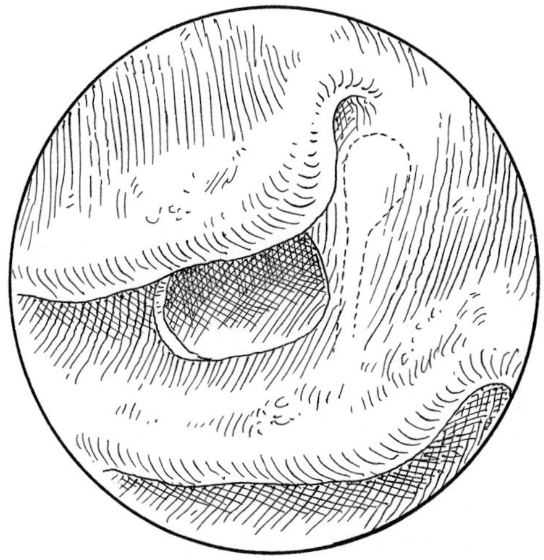

Figure 21–15. Endoscopic DCR. Anatomy as viewed from a medial perspective after preliminary antrostomy. The lacrimal sac and duct are outlined by the dashed line.

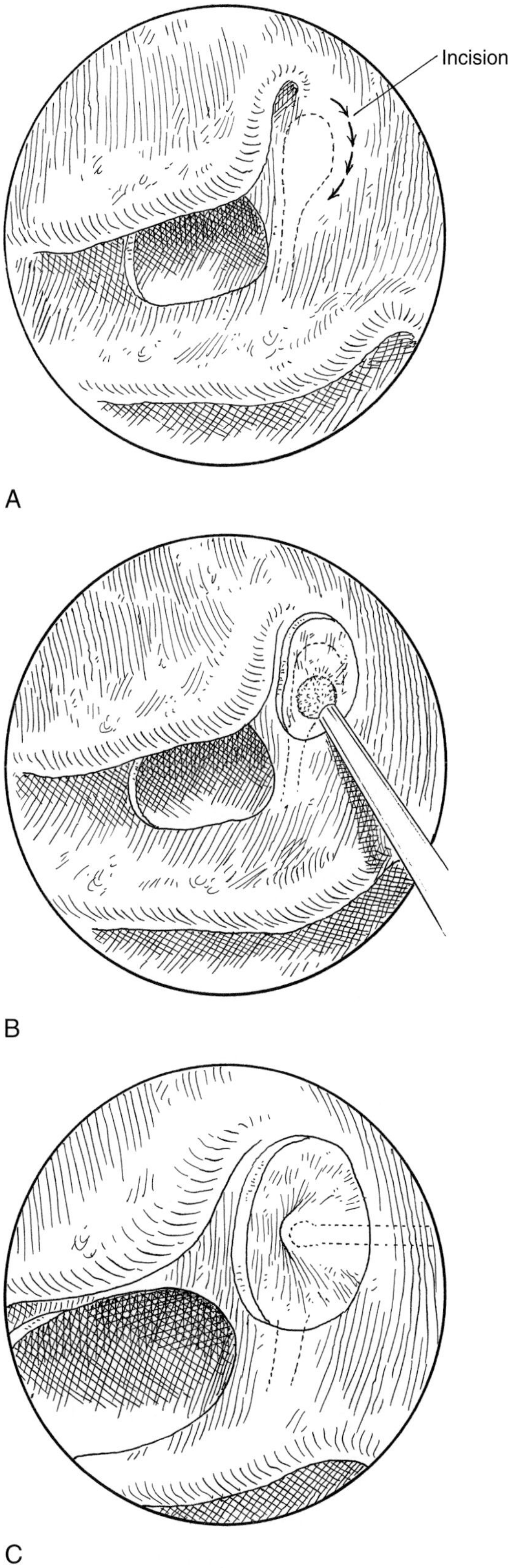

Figure 21–16. Endoscopic DCR. *A,* The arrows indicate the incision in the mucosa anterior to the position of the lacrimal sac. *B,* The bone over the sac is removed with a diamond drill. *C,* The position of the sac is confirmed by palpating the sac with a lacrimal probe placed into the sac through one of the lacrimal puncta.

used for sinus surgery that has been adapted with a cutting burr. As described earlier in this chapter, there are pros and cons for each instrument. To date, the author has always used the otologic drill because of the added power. In either case, the bone is thinned in concentric circles with the deepest point in the center (Fig. 21–16*B*). Once the bone has been removed down to the periosteum of the sac, the bone window can be enlarged with a rongeur or the drill. Alternatively, the bone over the lacrimal sac can be removed with standard instruments. This less elegant technique is nonetheless effective in exposing the sac.

Before incising into the sac, it is important to verify the exact location of the sac to make sure that the bone window is placed appropriately. Otherwise, the eye itself may be inadvertently entered. Several techniques are useful. The simplest is to palpate the lacrimal sac. By pressing on the sac directly, it can be seen on endoscopic examination to bulge into the nose. This can be potentially misleading, however, as the pressure can also be transmitted to the eye, causing the eye to bulge into the nose, mimicking the sac. A second technique is to pass a lacrimal dilator into the sac. Gentle pressure on the medial wall of the sac will be evident in the nose as the sharp point of the probe pushes into the nose (Fig. 21–16*C*). Finally, if the light probe is available, this can again be used to verify the position of the sac.

Once the position of the sac has been definitively identified, the medial wall should be incised with a sickle knife. The preferred technique is to make a cruciate incision (Fig. 21–17) or to excise the medial wall. This can be done by cutting the sac anteriorly and then making a flap from the medial wall. The flap is then easily excised. Alternatively, the medial wall of the sac can be removed with a microdebrider. Upon opening the sac, it may be possible to detect the release of a small amount of fluid or pus. Once the sac is open, the mucosal lining of the inside of the sac should be able to be appreciated.

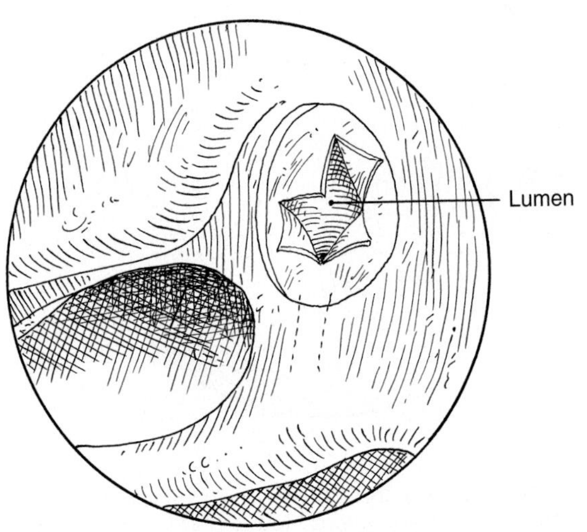

Figure 21–17. Endoscopic DCR. The lacrimal sac is opened with a cruciate incision. Alternatively, the medial wall can be excised or vaporized with a laser.

The final step in the procedure is placement of the lacrimal stents. These stents go through the lacrimal puncta, canaliculi, and lacrimal sac, and into the nose through the medial wall of the sac. These stents are essential to achieving a high rate of success with this operation. Many cases would be successful without the stents, but to achieve a greater than 90% success rate with the operation, long-term stenting is required.

The most common stents used are Crawford lacrimal tubes. These tubes have a beaded probe attached to each end of the tube to allow one end to be passed through each of the upper and lower eyelid puncta (see Fig. 21–18*B*). The Crawford tubes are made of a very soft, stretchable, Silastic material that resists breakdown. The surface of the tube acts as a conductive surface, allowing capillary action of the tears along the outside of the tubes, through the lacrimal puncta, into the sac, and then into the nose. Other options are available, including glass tubes or synthetic glass tubes, known as Jones tubes. These stents go through one punctum only. The tears pass through the lumen of these tubes or around them by capillary action.

To place the tubes, the puncta must be dilated first. A set of standard lacrimal dilators is used for this. The dilation begins with either a 000- or 00-sized dilator and proceeds through the 0, 1, and 2 sizes before an attempt is made to place the stent. This should be done very gently and carefully so as not to damage the puncta. Optimal lighting and magnification are helpful in performing this procedure. It is useful to grasp the eyelid margin lateral to the punctum to stabilize the lid before placing the end of the dilator into the punctum. Finally, when placing the stent, it is important to adjust the angle of the probe once it has entered the punctum to maneuver the probe into the lacrimal sac (Fig. 21–18*A*). The inferior canaliculus bends superiorly to enter the sac, whereas the upper lid canaliculus bends inferiorly to enter the sac. The probe is then passed through the sac, through the opening in the medial wall, and into the nose.

After both puncta are cannulated, the metal probes are cut off the tubes and the ends of the tubes are tied together with at least a half dozen throws of a square knot to secure the tubes. The tubes should be pulled down into the nose when tying them. Excess tube is then cut off after the knots are tied. When they are released, the tubes will spring back into the nose to the appropriate level (Fig. 21–18*C*). It is important to check the eyelids at this point to make sure that the tubes are not so tight that they hold the eyelids together medially. This could lead to adhesion between the lacrimal puncta. The last step of the procedure involves place-

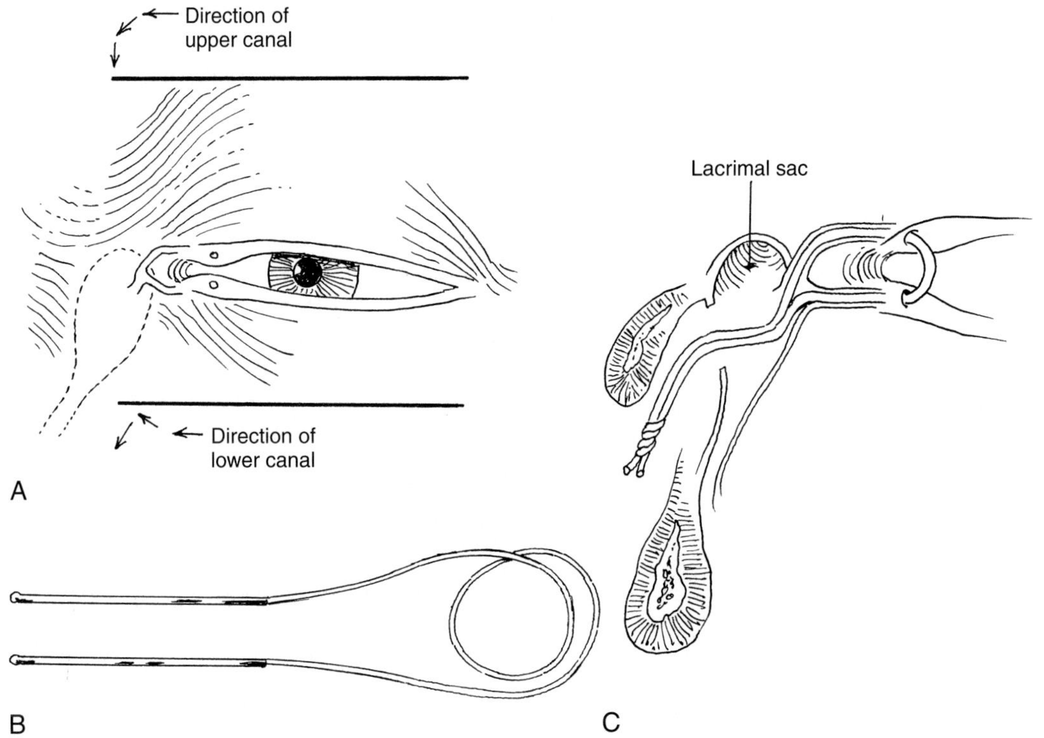

Figure 21–18. Endoscopic DCR. Stenting the lacrimal sac with Crawford tubes. *A,* Anatomy of the lacrimal canaliculi demonstrating the change in direction necessary to thread the stent into the sac. *B,* Appearance of the Crawford lacrimal tubes. *C,* Final appearance of the tubes following placement, tying of the tubes, and trimming of the excess.

ment of a nasal pack. An absorbent sponge is preferred over a traditional gauze pack.

External DCR

The incision for the external approach for DCR is typically modified from the normal medial canthal incision to a more inferior and oblique location (Fig. 21–19*A*). The incision is infiltrated with local anesthetic containing 1% lidocaine with 1 : 100,000 epinephrine. After 5 minutes, the incision is made. The soft tissues are divided through the muscle and periosteum to the bone of the medial orbital rim. The angular artery may need to be ligated if it crosses the incision. A subperiosteal dissection is performed anteriorly onto the nasal dorsum for several millimeters and posteriorly into the lacrimal fossa. The anterior lacrimal crest will be identified first, followed by the lacrimal sac within the lacrimal fossa. The sac is elevated from superior to inferior to expose the lacrimal fossa and the posterior lacrimal crest (Fig. 21–19*B*).

The next step is to create a bony window through the lacrimal fossa into the nose. A small chisel is used to open a small window, which is then enlarged using a Kerrison rongeur (Fig. 21–19*C*). The window should be as large as the main portion of the lacrimal fossa. The mucosa of the lateral wall of the nose over the lacrimal sac should be incised in a cruciate fashion or in a U-shape; alternatively, a flap may be created. In some techniques, the mucosa is formed into one to four small flaps that are sutured to the edges of the lacrimal sac incisions. In other techniques, the mucosa is merely excised. There does not seem to be a significant difference in the success rate of the operation using either technique.

The lacrimal sac is then opened. The sac should be incised from its connection to the lacrimal duct on the medial surface continuing superiorly (see Fig. 21–19*C*). Once the sac is opened, the full incision can be completed by visualizing the inside of the sac and cutting the wall under direct vision. With the sac open, the inside can be examined to rule out luminal pathology. If a flap technique is performed, the edges of the sac are sutured to the mucosal flaps of the lateral wall of the nose. These sutures are difficult to place but can be accomplished with careful technique. A 5-0 Vicryl (Ethicon) or chromic suture is recommended. If an excisional technique is used, the medial posterior wall of the sac should be removed.

The opening from the sac into the nose should be stented with Crawford tubes, as described earlier for the endoscopic technique. If a flap technique is used and good closure is achieved, the stent may be omitted, but the author's preference is to stent all cases. An intranasal

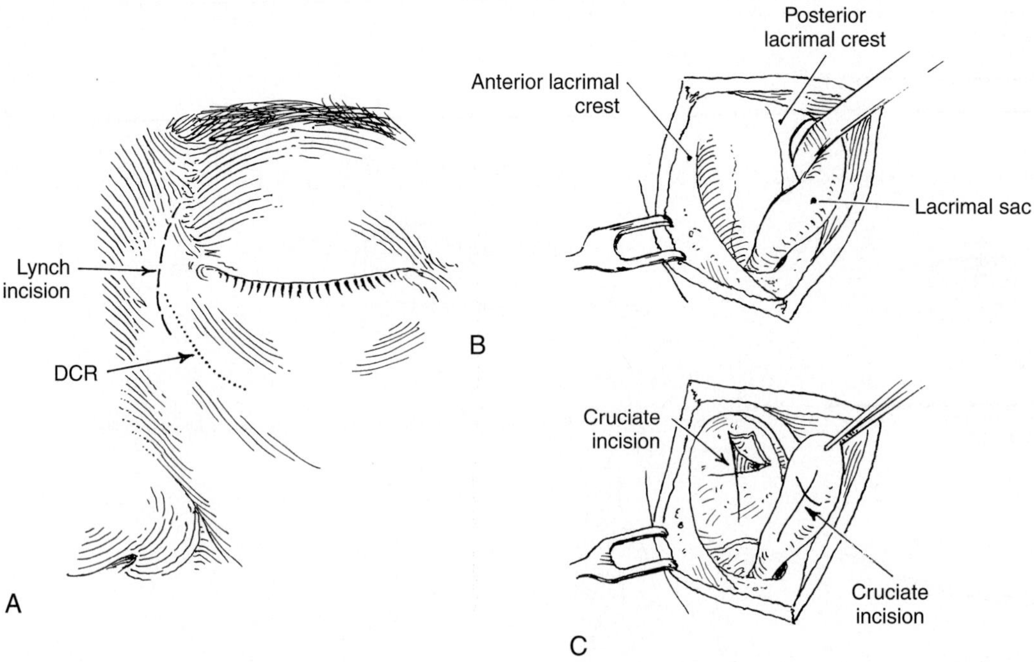

Figure 21–19. External approach for DCR. *A,* The standard medial canthal incision is indicated by the dashed line; the modified incision is indicated by the dotted line. *B,* Exposure of the lacrimal fossa. The sac is elevated from the fossa with a malleable retractor. *C,* After bone removal, the nasal mucosa and the lacrimal sac are incised. A cruciate incision is demonstrated, but a flap technique can also be used.

pack should be placed at the completion of the procedure. Either an absorbent sponge or a rolled Telfa pack can be used. The incision is closed in three layers. The first layer should reapproximate the periosteal layer with an attempt to incorporate the medial canthal tendon. The skin is then closed with a deep layer of absorbable suture and a cosmetic skin closure using 6-0 nylon sutures.

Conjunctivorhinostomy

Conjunctivorhinostomy is a technique that is performed when either the lacrimal sac is obliterated by scar or resected during tumor surgery. In such cases, the Crawford tubes can be inserted through the common lacrimal canaliculus directly into the nose, or a conjunctivorhinostomy can be performed. In the latter technique, the connection is made directly between the conjunctiva and the nose.

The first step is to resect the caruncle of the medial canthus. Through this defect, a tunnel is created into the nose. If necessary, the bone in this area can be drilled away, or it may already have been resected. A Jones tube is then inserted through the opening into the nose. The tube should be positioned so that it lays flush with the surface of the conjunctiva and extends into the nose, but not up against the septum.

This tube will allow tears to pass into the nose through the lumen of the tube, as well as by capillary action around the tube. The negative pressure of nasal airflow during inspiration is critical to the success of this procedure.

Postoperative Care

DCR, whether external or endoscopic, is performed as an outpatient procedure. After an appropriate recovery period, the patient is discharged to home on antibiotics and analgesics. The antibiotic that covers the routine sinus pathogens should be prescribed for 1 to 2 weeks. The pain relievers selected should cover the extent of the patient's pain. Typically, a combination codeine derivative is adequate. On the night of surgery, activity is limited to bathroom privileges only. Activity is then advanced to routine ambulation the next morning. Full activity, including exercise, is postponed for 2 weeks after surgery. The night of surgery, the patient's diet is restricted to liquids. The diet is advanced to regular the next morning.

The external incision is cleaned twice each day and covered with antibiotic ointment. The patient should return for packing removal 4 to 7 days after the procedure. External sutures can be removed at this time. At this time, the nose should be carefully suctioned under endoscopic control. The internal stents are examined and cleaned of debris. Irrigations with normal saline are initiated at this point and continued twice each day until healing is complete. Subsequent examinations and debridements are performed 3 and 6 weeks after surgery. In the optimal circumstance, the lacrimal stents can be removed at the 6-week postoperative visit. If there is continued inflammation, crusting, or granulation, the stents should be left in place. The stents are removed only when complete healing is demonstrated by endoscopic examination.

Complications

The most serious complications of DCR result from orbital hemorrhage. This is rare following either endoscopic or external DCR. The primary cause is inadvertent trauma to the eye from inaccurate placement of the bony window in the lateral wall of the nose. If the window is too far posterior or too far superior, the incision into the presumed lacrimal sac may instead be made into the orbital fat or medial rectus muscle. This can result in uncontrolled bleeding into the retro-orbital space. During the external procedure, there is no risk of this type of injury. However, bleeding from the sac into a closed wound can result in orbital hemorrhage. There is also a risk of injury to the eye during subperiosteal dissection of the lacrimal sac. Diagnosis and management of orbital hemorrhage is covered in detail in the next section.

Other complications of DCR include failure of the procedure, secondary ophthalmologic problems, bleeding, infection, and poor cosmetic appearance of the external scar, if present. The success rate of DCR with either approach is very high. Most series report a success rate of greater than 90%.[35,36] Failure may be attributable to inaccurate diagnosis, leading to the operation done for epiphora not amenable to DCR. In other cases, failure may be due to technical problems during the surgery. Finally, infection in the sac or intranasally after the surgery can lead to scarring in the sac or in the rhinostomy, which can result in partial or complete obstruction.

Secondary eye problems can occur when the DCR is not working properly or the wound becomes infected. In these situations, the patient may develop conjunctivitis, which can lead to corneal ulceration. There can also be direct injury to the cornea, especially during the external procedure. Diplopia can result from direct injury to any of the eye muscles. This can occur during elevation of the lacrimal sac or during the endoscopic procedure when incising the lacrimal sac.

Bleeding from DCR should be minimal, so the risk of transfusion should be close to zero. After surgery, intranasal bleeding is possible, but should be self-limiting or easily controlled by minimal packing. Infection of the lacrimal sac or lateral nasal wall from the surgery is relatively common. Crusting over the raw mucosa can lead to trapping of secretions and secondary infection. When this occurs, it can usually be treated by endoscopic debridement and antibiotics. Wound infection of the external incision is also possible, but should occur in less than 5% of cases. If infection is not controlled early in the postoperative course, it is possible for the infection to spread to the eye itself, resulting in orbital cellulitis or abscess. Treatment of severe orbital infection is as outlined earlier in the section on orbital decompression.

Finally, poor cosmetic outcome from the external incision may occur, although this should be avoidable. Inaccurate suturing or use of too heavy a suture material may be the cause. The main determinate of the cosmetic outcome is careful placement of the incision. The classical incision is the medial canthal incision or Lynch incision. This typically results in a noticeable but cosmetically acceptable scar. The modified incision illustrated in this chapter was designed to improve exposure for this procedure and to hide the incision in the shadow of the orbital rim and nasal dorsum. With careful closure, this scar should be almost invisible.

ORBITAL HEMORRHAGE

One of the most important complications of any nasal or sinus surgery is orbital hemorrhage. This may be anterior to the orbital septum, resulting in external hematoma, ecchymosis, and swelling of the eyelids. Anterior hemorrhage is usually self-limiting and generally resolves without treatment. Bleeding posterior to the orbital septum may result in retro-orbital hematoma leading to proptosis, ophthalmoplegia, and visual loss. Proper diagnosis and management of orbital bleeding can avert the consequences and save the patient's eye from permanent damage. As it is essential that the rhinologist be prepared for this possibility in every case, the details of diagnosis and management of orbital bleeding are covered here.

Etiology

A number of mechanisms can lead to orbital bleeding. External bleeding can occur secondary to retrograde bleeding from the nose through the nasolacrimal duct. Anterior or superficial bleeding may be caused by bleeding from the skin or subcutaneous tissues during any procedure that involves a medial canthal or subciliary incision. Finally, superficial hemorrhage routinely occurs, at least to some extent, in all rhinoplasty cases involving lateral osteotomies. In these last instances, the etiology is uncontrolled bleeding from areas that are anterior to the orbital septum.

Posterior or retro-orbital bleeding may occur from direct trauma. Direct trauma to the orbital tissues inside the orbital septum can occur during operations that border on or violate any of the orbital walls. Examples of this type of injury include inadvertent penetration through the lamina papyracea during endoscopic sinus surgery, laceration of the orbital periosteum while elevating during any procedure performed through an external ethmoidectomy approach, and uncontrolled extension of an osteotomy during rhinoplasty or tumor resection. The result of all of these is a tear in a blood vessel inside the orbital periosteum that bleeds into the orbital tissues.

The other mechanism of retro-orbital hemorrhage is by retraction bleeding from either the anterior or posterior ethmoidal arteries. If, during the performance of an intrasinus operation, the anterior ethmoid artery is avulsed at the lamina papyracea, the stump of the artery can retract into the orbit and continue to bleed.

Diagnosis

Orbital hemorrhage should be suspected after any nasal or sinus procedure whenever there are any signs or symptoms of a problem with the eye. The hallmark of anterior or superficial bleeding is ecchymosis. An alarming degree of discoloration may be noted. In addition, there may be significant edema of the eyelids. Anterior hematoma or hemorrhage is distinguished from more serious posterior bleeding by the absence of any signs or symptoms of true orbital involvement. In the case of anterior bleeding, the eye itself should be quiet, without chemosis, decrease in extraocular mobility, or visual loss as manifested by afferent pupillary defect. On examination, the intraocular pressures should be normal, as should the fundoscopic examination.

This is in marked contrast to retro-orbital hemorrhage and hematoma. This condition develops through a series of stages. The first signs are usually medial canthal ecchymosis and slight proptosis. At this point, there may be a slight decrease in the extraocular motions, but the intraocular pressure, visual acuity, and retinal examination should be normal. The next phase of the developing hematoma is increasing proptosis, decreasing extraocular motions, and the onset of elevation of intraocular pressure. As the process continues, visual acuity begins to decrease, chemosis and retinal changes become evident, and the intraocular pressures rise significantly. At this stage, an afferent pupillary defect should be easily detected. The final stages of progressive hematoma are marked by complete ophthalmoplegia, critical elevations of intraocular pressure, and rapidly declining visual acuity.[39, 40]

Management

The management of orbital hemorrhage is based on the severity of the rise in ocular pressure and the overall stage of the process. In all cases, the patient's head should be elevated and ice should be placed over the affected eye. In patients who have not undergone previous eye surgery, orbital massage may help as well.[41] For patients with anterior hematoma, the eye is not generally at risk and further steps are not usually needed. If the hematoma continues to expand, then it may be necessary to return the patient to the operating room for evacuation of the hematoma and isolation of the source of bleeding with direct ligation or cautery of the vessel.

The management of retro-orbital hematoma is much more complicated. In addition to ice, head elevation, and massage, nasal packing should be removed as soon as the diagnosis is made to allow additional bleeding to egress into the nose. Subsequent steps are based on the degree of involvement. If the intraocular pressures are normal and visual acuity is intact without evidence of afferent pupillary defect, then observation alone is usually adequate. As long as the intraocular pressure remains within the normal range, there is little risk that any permanent injury will result. For patients with minimal proptosis and the earliest rises in pressure, medical management is normally sufficient, including high-dose intravenous steroids, mannitol, and acetazolamide.[41]

If the patient develops an afferent pupillary defect, this indicates visual loss and immediate surgical intervention is indicated. In this situation, the first step is to perform a lateral canthotomy with inferior cantholysis.[39] This will usually suffice in controlling the intraocular pressure. As soon as the procedure is finished, the intraocular pressure should be rechecked and then monitored every 5 to 10 minutes until the bleeding stops spontaneously. If the bleeding does not stop after 15 to 20 minutes, then the surgical wound should be reexplored and the source of bleeding identified and cauterized or ligated.

In extreme circumstances, lateral canthotomy with inferior cantholysis may not normalize the intraocular pressure. In this situation, a more aggressive orbital decompression should be performed in conjunction with control of the bleeding.[42] The best approach for decompression in this setting depends on the probable site of bleeding. In the case of bleeding from the anterior ethmoid artery or medial wall of the orbit, an external ethmoidectomy approach is used. If the bleeding is from the orbital floor, the approach should be through a Caldwell-Luc or inferior subciliary incision.

Technique for Lateral Canthotomy

The lateral canthotomy is a very simple procedure that involves incising the lateral canthal tendon. This procedure is typically performed in an emergency situation and may be done in the recovery room, the emergency room, or the operating room depending on when the decision is made to proceed. The equipment required

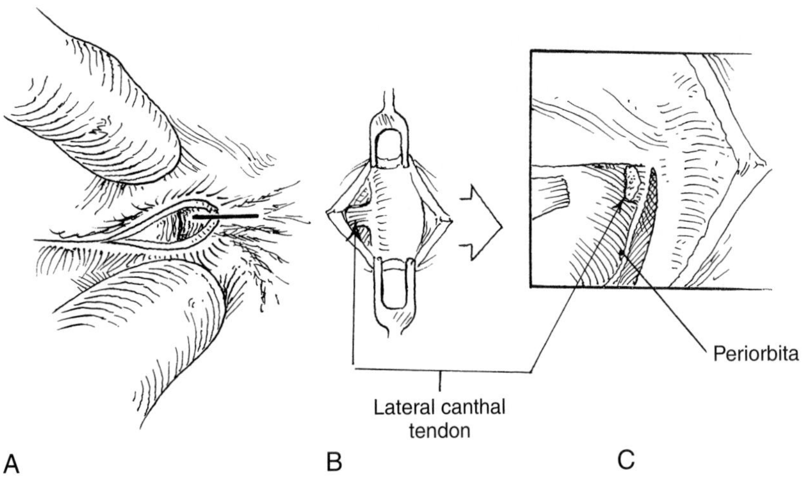

Figure 21–20. Lateral canthotomy with inferior cantholysis. *A,* The lateral canthus is stretched open with two fingers of one hand and the knife is held with the other hand. The line demonstrates the position of the incision. *B,* Identification of the inferior slip of the lateral canthal tendon. *C,* Completed inferior cantholysis.

is minimal: local anesthestic, scalpel, clamp, and curved iris scissors.

The area of the lateral canthus is injected with a minimal amount of local anesthetic. Excessive infiltration is avoided to keep from distorting the anatomy and landmarks. An incision is made in the skin that extends from the conjunctival margin in a straight line laterally (Fig. 21–20*A*). The scissors are used to incise the orbital periosteum over the lateral orbital rim. Through the incision, an inferior cantholysis is also performed. This is completed by identifying the inferior slip of the lateral canthal tendon and dividing it using the scissors (Fig. 21–20*B*).

Upon completing the procedure, the intraocular pressure should be checked. If the procedure has been successful, the pressure should normalize, vision should rapidly return to normal, and the afferent pupillary defect should resolve. This technique works by allowing the orbit to expand. There may be a small amount of blood clot released, but the primary mechanism of control is providing an outflow for the orbital pressure. The wound is not closed until the hematoma has dissipated and the eye has begun to regress into the orbit. This may occur within 24 to 48 hours. The repair is performed in the operating room. The lateral canthal tendon is reapproximated and the tendon is attached to the lateral orbital rim inside the orbital rim. The skin is closed with 6-0 nylon suture.

REFERENCES

1. Wartofsky L. Diseases of the thyroid. In Isselbacher KJ, Braunwald E, Wilson JD, et al. (eds). Harrison's Principles of Internal Medicine, 13th ed. New York: McGraw Hill, 1994, pp. 1930–1952.
2. Konishi J, Herman MM, Kriss JP. Binding of thyroglobulin and thyroglobulin-antithyroglobulin immune complex to extraocular muscle membrane. Endocrinology 95:434, 1974.
3. Riley FC. Orbital pathology in Graves' disease. Mayo Clin Proc 47:957, 1972.
4. Weisman RA, Savino PJ. Management of endocrine orbitopathy. Otolaryngol Clin North Am 21:93, 1988.
5. Garrity JA, Fatourechi V, Bergstralh EJ, et al. Results of transantral orbital decompression in 428 patients with severe Graves' ophthalmopathy. Am J Ophthalmol 116:533, 1993.
6. Rootman J. Graves' orbitopathy. In Rootman J (ed). Diseases of the Orbit. Philadelphia: JB Lippincott, 1988, pp. 241–280.
7. Petersen IA, Kriss JP, Donaldson SS. Prognostic factors in the radiotherapy of Graves' ophthalmopathy. Int J Radiat Oncol Biol Phys 19(2):259, 1990.
8. Petersen IA, Donaldson SS, Kriss JP. Orbital radiotherapy: The Stanford experience. In Wall JR (ed). Graves' Ophthalmopathy. Oxford: Blackwell, 1990, pp. 135–144.
9. Kelly W, Longson D, Smithard D, et al. An evaluation of plasma exchange for Graves' ophthalmopathy. Clin Endocrinol 18:484, 1983.
10. Walsh TE, Ogura JH. Transantral orbital decompression for malignant exophthalmos. Laryngoscope 67:544, 1957.
11. Kennedy DW, Goodstein ML, Miller RM, et al. Endoscopic transnasal orbital decompression. Arch Otolaryngol Head Neck Surg 116:275, 1990.
12. Shepard KG, Levin PS, Terris DJ. Balanced orbital decompression for Graves' ophthalmopathy. Laryngoscope 108:1648, 1998.
13. Metson R, Shore JW, Gliklich RE, et al. Endoscopic orbital decompression under local anesthesia. Otolaryngol Head Neck Surg 113(6):661, 1995.
14. Chandler JR, Langenbrunner DJ, Stevens ER. Pathogenesis of orbital complications in acute sinusitis. Laryngoscope 80:1414, 1970.
15. Handler LC, Davey IC, Hill JC, et al. The acute orbit: Differentiation of orbital cellulitis from subperiosteal abscess by computerized tomography. Neuroradiology 33:15, 1991.
16. Froehlich P, Pransky SM, Fontaine P, et al. Minimal endoscopic approach to subperiosteal orbital abscess. Arch Otolaryngol Head Neck Surg 123:280, 1997.
17. Brook I, Frazier EH. Microbiology of subperiosteal orbital abscess and associated maxillary sinusitis. Laryngoscope 106:1010, 1996.
18. Schramm VL, Myers EN, Kennerdell JS. Orbital complications of acute sinusitis: Evaluation, management, and outcome. ORL J Otorhinolaryngol Relat Spec 221, 1977.
19. Rubinstein JB, Handler SD. Orbital and periorbital cellulitis in children. Head Neck Surg 5:15, 1982.
20. El-Silimy O. The place of endonasal endoscopy in treatment of orbital cellulitis. Rhinology 33:93, 1995.
21. Younis RT, Lazar RH. Endoscopic drainage of subperiosteal abscess in children: A pilot study. Am J Rhinol 10:11, 1996.
22. Arjmand EM, Lusk RP, Muntz HR. Pediatric sinusitis and subperiosteal orbital abscess formation: Diagnosis and treatment. Otolaryngol Head Neck Surg 109:886, 1993.
23. Pereira KD, Mitchell RB, Younis RT, et al. Management of medial subperiosteal abscess of the orbit in children—A 5-year experience. Int J Pediatr Otorhinolaryngol 38:247, 1997.

24. Wolf SR, Gode U, Hosemann W. Endonasal endoscopic surgery for rhinogen intraorbital abscess: A report of six cases. Laryngoscope 106:105, 1996.
25. Hoffer ME, Kennedy DW. The endoscopic management of sinus mucoceles following orbital decompression. Am J Rhinol 8:61, 1994.
26. Kountakis SE, Maillard AAJ, Urso R, et al. Endoscopic approach to traumatic visual loss. Otolaryngol Head Neck Surg 116:652, 1997.
27. Luxenberger W, Stammberger H, Jebeles JA. Endoscopic optic nerve decompression: The Graz experience. Laryngoscope 108: 873, 1998.
28. Li KK, Teknos TN, Lai A, et al. Traumatic optic neuropathy: Result in 45 consecutive surgically treated patients. Otolaryngol Head Neck Surg 120:5, 1999.
29. Holt GR, Holt JE. Incidence of eye injuries in facial fractures: An analysis of 727 cases. Otolaryngol Head Neck Surg 91:276, 1983.
30. Turner JWA. Indirect injuries of optic nerve. Brain 66:140, 1943.
31. Steinsapir KD, Goldberg RA. Traumatic optic neuropathy. Surv Ophthalmol 38:487, 1994.
32. Chen YR, Breidahl A, Chang CN. Optic nerve decompression in fibrous dysplasia: Indications, efficacy, and safety. Plast Reconstr Surg 99:22, 1997.
33. Edelstein C, Goldberg RA, Rubino G. Unilateral blindness after ipsilateral prophylactic transcranial optic canal decompression for fibrous dysplasia. Am J Ophthalmol 126(3):469, 1998.
34. Papay FA, Morales L Jr, Flaharty P, et al. Optic nerve compression in cranial base fibrous dysplasia. J Craniofac Surg 6:5, 1995.
35. Sprekelsen MB, Barberan MT. Endoscopic dacryocystorhinostomy: Surgical technique and results. Laryngoscope 106:187, 1996.
36. Eloy PH, Bertrand B, Martinez M, et al. Endonasal dacryocystorhinostomy: Indications, technique and results. Rhinology 33:229, 1995.
37. Bolger WE, Parsons DS, Mair EA, et al. Lacrimal drainage system injury in functional endoscopic sinus surgery. Arch Otolaryngol Head Neck Surg 118:1179, 1992.
38. Hartikainen J, Antila J, Varpula M, et al. Prospective randomized comparison of endonasal endoscopic dacryocystorhinostomy and external dacryocystorhinostomy. Laryngoscope 108:1861, 1998.
39. Stankiewicz JA. Blindness and intranasal endoscopic ethmoidectomy: Prevention and management. Otolaryngol Head Neck Surg 101:320, 1989.
40. Corey JP, Bumsted R, Panje W, et al. Orbital complications in functional endoscopic sinus surgery. Otolaryngol Head Neck Surg 109:814, 1993.
41. Saussez S, Choufani G, Brutus J-P, et al. Lateral canthotomy: A simple and safe procedure for orbital haemorrhage secondary to endoscopic sinus surgery. Rhinology 36:37, 1998.
42. Rice DH, Schaefer SD. Anatomy of the paranasal sinuses. In Rice DH, Schaefer SD (eds). Endoscopic Paranasal Sinus Surgery, 2nd ed. New York: Raven Press, 1993, pp. 3–50.

CHAPTER 22

Epistaxis

Nasal bleeding is one of the most common maladies treated by otorhinolaryngologists. At one time or another, most people experience some degree of bleeding from the nose. Despite the common nature of this condition, no other medical or surgical specialty professes special knowledge or interest in the study or management of epistaxis, so epistaxis is left to the otolaryngologist and rhinologist to manage. This common problem is taken for granted by many otolaryngologists and trivialized by others. However, for many people, epistaxis is a serious and potentially life-threatening medical condition that can have a profound impact on quality of life. In this chapter, the topic of epistaxis is covered in detail, including underlying causes, co-factors, evaluation, and medical and surgical management.

ANATOMY

Nasal bleeding can conveniently be divided into anterior and posterior epistaxis. Although this classification system is somewhat arbitrary, it is based on the concept that anterior bleeding comes from the anterior blood supply, and posterior bleeding comes from the posterior blood supply. Another way of differentiating between anterior and posterior epistaxis is by where the blood goes. Anterior bleeds come out the front of the nose, whereas posterior bleeds run down the back of the nose into the pharynx.

Roughly 90% of cases of epistaxis can be classified as anterior, with most of these patients being treated as outpatients.[1] In hospitalized patients, the breakdown by bleeding site is equally divided between anterior and posterior.[2] The single most common site is the anterior aspect of the nasal septum. This area, sometimes referred to as Little's area, contains a rich capillary blood supply that is at the confluence of three different arterial blood supplies. This anastomotic area is also called Kisselbach's plexus. Other common sites of anterior bleeding include the anterior edge of the inferior turbinate and the anterior ethmoid sinus. Posterior epistaxis typically arises from vessels on the posterior septum, on the floor of the nose in the posterior choanae, or from the back of the middle or inferior turbinate.

These clinical patterns are based on the underlying vascular anatomy, which has been presented in detail in Chapter 1 and so will not be fully recounted here. Briefly, the nose is supplied by three separate arterial sources. The facial artery contributes through the septal branch of the superior labial artery, primarily supplying blood to the anterior nasal septum, anterior floor of the nose, and nasal tip structures. The internal carotid artery contributes through the ophthalmic artery, which gives off the anterior and posterior ethmoid arteries and the supraorbital artery. These vessels supply the lateral wall of the nose, ethmoid sinus, septum, and frontal sinus. The internal maxillary artery gives off numerous branches in the pterygomaxillary fissure, including the sphenopalatine artery, descending palatine, and inferior orbital arteries. These vessels supply the maxillary and sphenoid sinuses; the posterior septum, floor, and lateral wall of the nose; and the external nasal structures above the nasal tip.

CAUSES OF EPISTAXIS

Trauma

A number of factors and conditions contribute to the development, severity, and recurrence of epistaxis (Table 22–1). The most common factors involved in epistaxis are trauma and mucosal dehydration. Trauma, ranging from digital trauma to gunshot wounds, is the most common inciting factor in initiating nasal bleeding. Digital trauma is exceedingly common. Especially in children, finger manipulation of the nose is an almost ubiquitous behavior. In an attempt to remove crust, scratch an itch, or simply out of habit, humans have a propensity for digital manipulation of the nose. This can lead to mucosal abrasion and, eventually, ulceration. The most common site for this type of trauma is

TABLE 22-1
Causes of Epistaxis

Trauma
- Digital
- Nose blowing
- Blunt
- Penetrating
- Iatrogenic

Mucosal Dehydration
- Deviated septum
- Arid environment

Inflammation
- Rhinitis (allergic, viral)
- Sinusitis
- Autoimmune disorders (Wegener's granulomatosis, sarcoidosis)
- Environmental irritants (air pollutants, smoke)

Tumors
- Benign (inverted papilloma, juvenile nasopharyngeal angiofibroma)
- Malignant (nasopharyngeal carcinoma, esthesioneuroblastoma, etc.)

Hypertension

Coagulopathy
- Hemophilia
- Thrombocytopenia
- Medication-related (aspirin, coumadin, heparin)
- Renal failure
- Cancer chemotherapy

Hereditary Hemorrhagic Telangiectasia

the anterior septum. This initially leads to a small amount of blood that merely coats the ulceration, leading to a fibrous clot that dries into scab formation. Removal of the scab causes further injury to the mucosa, which can result in more significant bleeding.

A second common form of trauma is nose blowing. It is possible to cause rupture of superficial vessels of the mucosa by violent nose blowing. This can lead to bleeding from the anterior septum or other areas where there are superficial vessels. Nose blowing is an especially prominent source of trauma in patients who have undergone recent surgery on the nose or sinuses or who have preexisting bleeding sites. In these cases, it is possible to blow the clots off of a raw mucosal surface, which leads to severe and sudden epistaxis.

More severe forms of trauma are also commonly associated with epistaxis. These causes are less likely to be the cause of bleeding from the nose on a population basis. However, the frequency of epistaxis is very high in these settings. The trauma may be in the form of blunt trauma to the nose or sinuses, resulting in fracture of the septum, lateral wall, or one of the sinuses. The fracture leads to disruption of the mucosal lining, tearing of blood vessels, and bleeding. The bleeding usually occurs acutely following the injury. There may also be delayed secondary epistaxis. This results from injury to one of the major vessels, most commonly, the anterior ethmoid artery. The artery initially clots at the site of disruption. However, either the clot fails to hold, or it falls off before complete healing occurs. Penetrating trauma to the nose can result in the most severe form of nasal bleeding due to direct transection of one of the major vessels. The vessel involved may be the internal maxillary artery or vein, or the internal carotid artery. This type of bleeding is life-threatening and must be controlled within minutes or it can be fatal.

Finally, surgical trauma can result in bleeding. In every chapter in this book, intraoperative and postoperative bleeding is discussed as a complication. No matter who the surgeon is or what technique is used to prevent postoperative bleeding, a percentage of patients will still experience bleeding. In most cases, this can easily be controlled, but rarely, surgical epistaxis can be severe. One recent article estimated the incidence of the need for transfusion associated with nasal and sinus surgery to be 0.46%, or about 1 of 200 patients.[3]

Dehydration

Drying of the nasal mucosa is the second most common factor contributing to epistaxis. Whether trauma or mucosal drying is a more important factor varies from one patient to the next. Most patients will have one factor or the other as a major part of their history of epistaxis. One of the important functions of the nose is to humidify the air as it passes through the nose. The nasal mucus is essential to this function to transfer moisture and protect the mucosa by preventing drying. The function of the mucosa, especially of the inferior turbinate mucosa, is neurologically controlled. Sympathetic vasoconstriction and parasympathetic vasodilatation are balanced to adjust mucous secretion and mucosal blood flow. This is mediated by complex reflexes that attempt to optimize nasal resistance for the amount of humidity in the environment and the nasal airflow needs. In addition to the neuroregulation of the internal nasal environment, the external environmental humidity also has a profound effect on nasal dryness. Epistaxis is much less common in regions that have high ambient humidity than it is in arid regions. Epistaxis is also much more common in the northern United States in the winter owing to the combined effects of cold, dry air outside and poorly humidified, forced hot air heat inside.

In addition, there are other factors that can lead to increased dryness, the most important of which is a deviated septum. When the septum is significantly deviated, there can be an abnormally high airflow through the side of the nose opposite the deviation. In other cases, the deviation protrudes into the airflow stream, leading to abnormal drying on the point of the spur. A related factor is the surgically altered nasal airway that can no longer humidify the air adequately. This may be accompanied by an abnormally high airflow across the nasal mucosa.

Thus, environmental humidity, quality of nasal mucus, and nasal airflow combine to produce a net drying effect on the nasal mucosa. The outcome in some patients is that the mucosa dries out, leading to crusting and cracking and an increased tendency for digital manipulation.

Inflammation

In some patients, inflammatory conditions can lead to nasal bleeding. Common conditions, such as viral rhinitis, allergic rhinitis, and sinusitis, cause increased inflammation of the mucosa. This can make the mucosa more fragile and more susceptible to trauma from nose blowing and the effects of nasal drying. In addition to these common conditions, there are patients who suffer from unusual inflammatory conditions of the nose and sinuses in which epistaxis is a common complicating factor. These include Wegener's granulomatosis and sarcoidosis. These conditions lead to mucosal ulceration or extreme inflammation that may predispose the patient to crusting, abrasion, and eventually, bleeding. Also, there are environmental pollutants that can lead to inflammation and predispose an individual to bleeding. However, only heavy or frequent exposure to an irritative pollutant is likely to become significant. This most often affects factory workers employed in plants with poor air maintenance systems and high levels of airborne pollutants.

Tumors

A less common but important cause of nasal bleeding is sinonasal tumor. Epistaxis may be the presenting complaint of a patient with a tumor. Most benign tumors tend to not bleed, whereas malignant tumors have a tendency to necrose and bleed. The exception to this is juvenile nasopharyngeal angiofibroma, which classically presents as recurrent epistaxis in adolescents or young adult men. As will be discussed later in this chapter, persistent bleeding is an indication to proceed with imaging studies to evaluate the patient for possible tumor.

Hypertension

Among the most important factors to consider in the patient with epistaxis is elevated blood pressure. This condition is extremely common among adults presenting to physicians or to the emergency department. It is uncertain whether the hypertension is an etiologic factor in all of these patients. This is because the natural response to seeing blood from one's nose is to get agitated, which can directly lead to elevation of the blood pressure. Patients without a history of hypertension commonly will have a markedly increased blood pressure in the face of significant epistaxis. Studies designed to answer the question of whether hypertension is important in epistaxis have been conflicting. One recent study found the incidence of epistaxis to be unrelated to the severity of hypertension, but to be possibly related to the duration of hypertension.[4]

In some patients, hypertension appears to be an important factor. Elevated blood pressure can contribute to epistaxis in three different ways. The first is as a direct cause of the start of the bleeding. In this situation, the high pressure causes rupture of a blood vessel in the nasal or sinus mucosa, leading to epistaxis. Second, although high blood pressure may not cause the initial vascular rupture, once the bleeding starts, it can lead to significant worsening of the bleeding. Finally, hypertension can contribute by preventing an active nosebleed from slowing down or stopping owing to the high pressure in the vessels.

Coagulopathy

As with patients who are hypertensive, patients with abnormal blood clotting are predisposed to nasal bleeding. These patients are predisposed to bleeding of any kind, but more than anything, these patients tend to have much worse problems with nosebleeds than patients without coagulopathy. In this situation, it is unlikely that the blood clotting disorder causes the nasal bleeding. However, once the bleeding starts even a little bit, the result may be a severe nosebleed.

A number of conditions interfere with blood clotting and are associated with epistaxis. These include all of the various forms of hemophilia. This condition leads to unwanted bleeding due to the absence or inactivity of one of the clotting factors. These conditions are rare, but affected patients tend to have severe nosebleeds from an early age. There are also patients with inherent disorders of platelet function. These patients, too, may have severe problems with nosebleeds for many years.

In addition to the classic hemophilias and coagulopathies, there are several acquired conditions that lead to poor blood clotting and, frequently, a history of nosebleeds. The most common of these is regular aspirin use. Aspirin, by inhibiting the enzyme cyclooxygenase, interferes with platelet function. This results in significant increases in bleeding time, but should not increase the incidence of nosebleeds. Millions of Americans are currently taking a regular dose of aspirin, as prescribed by their doctors, for prevention of stroke, heart attack, and clotting in prosthetic arteries. For this reason, aspirin use is becoming an increasingly important risk factor for epistaxis in adults. Other medications that lead to prolonged clotting times are the anticlotting factors coumadin and heparin. These two agents, which work on different parts of the clotting cascade, both lead to prolonged bleeding times and increased risk of severe nosebleeds.

Patients with chronic renal failure commonly have problems with epistaxis. This is due to the two-pronged problem of regularly receiving heparin during dialysis and having poor clotting secondary to the renal failure. In these patients, epistaxis tends to occur either while the patient is undergoing dialysis or shortly after the dialysis. Patients with septic shock develop a condition of poor clotting that may progress to disseminated intravascular coagulation (DIC). This starts out as uncontrolled clotting of the blood within the vascular system and progresses to a coagulopathy secondary to consumption of all available clotting factors.

Finally, there are patients who acquire clotting deficiencies as a result of cancer therapy. This may occur secondary to high-dose chemotherapy, leading to transient decreases in the platelet count. Alternatively, the coagulopathy may be caused by depletion of bone marrow reserves of platelets due to bone marrow transplant. In both of these cases, thrombocytopenia becomes a clinical reality and epistaxis may result.

Hereditary Hemorrhagic Telangiectasia

Often known as Osler-Weber-Rendu syndrome, hereditary hemorrhagic telangiectasia (HHT) is an inherited autosomal dominant disorder of the capillaries and microvasculature of epithelial surfaces.[5–7] Affected individuals have an abnormality of the microvasculature that results in development of small vascular malformations referred to as telangiectasia. These lesions develop repeatedly over the course of time, increasing in number and size as the patient ages. Minimal trauma, such as sneezing, hard nose blowing, or even hypertension, is enough to cause the lesions to bleed.

Patients with HHT not only have refractory and recurrent epistaxis, they are prone to development of lesions in the brain, lungs, or anywhere in the gastrointestinal tract.[8, 9] For this reason, if this condition is suspected, it is important to evaluate the patient thoroughly for other sites of lesions.

HHT is an uncommon cause of epistaxis, but an important cause owing to the severity of the condition and the special measures required for treatment. In any patient with recurrent epistaxis, a careful examination of the mucosal surfaces in the nose should be performed to rule out HHT lesions. The presence of three or more suggestive vascular lesions should alert the physician to the possibility that the patient may have HHT.

EVALUATION

When the patient with epistaxis initially presents for treatment, it is important to perform a systematic evaluation. One may be tempted to proceed directly to managing the patient's symptoms without performing a careful history and physical examination. Indeed, in cases of heavy bleeding, this may be necessary. For most patients, though, a temporizing measure, such as packing the nose with Neo-Synephrine–soaked cotton pledgets, should control the bleeding sufficiently to allow the physician to perform a proper evaluation before initiating definitive treatment. This is important because the method of controlling epistaxis depends largely on the specifics of an individual case, with an entire menu of options available (Table 22–2).

History

A complete history for epistaxis should elicit all of the factors that may have a bearing on the cause of the condition and its treatment. During the initial inquiry, it is important to investigate the duration of bleeding, frequency of bleeding, and amount of bleeding. This will help the physician to gauge the severity of the problem. It also is important to determine the side of the bleeding and its primary site of origin and flow: out the front of the nose, down the back of the nose, or a combination of the two. This will suggest where the site of bleeding might be and, therefore, the primary vascular supply. Information on any previous treatment the patient has received for epistaxis, including packing, cautery, and surgery, is also important.

It may be possible during history taking to elicit information that will provide clues to the underlying cause of the bleeding. Questions pertaining to the possibility of trauma, inflammatory processes, or tumors may be

TABLE 22–2
Management of Epistaxis

Medical Management
Nasal Packing
Traditional anterior pack
Nasal sponges
Gelfoam
Traditional posterior pack
Nasal balloon
Cautery
Silver nitrate
Endoscopic electrocautery
Laser cautery
Embolization
Ligation
Transantral ligation of the internal maxillary artery
External ligation of the ethmoid arteries
Endoscopic ligation of the sphenopalatine artery
Surgery
Septoplasty
Septal dermoplasty

informative. The past medical history may include many conditions that can contribute to epistaxis, including hypertension, renal failure, cancer, or coagulopathy. A complete list of medications that the patient takes, including any over-the-counter medicines that may contain aspirin or related products, should be recorded.

Physical Examination

Of primary concern in the examination of patients with epistaxis is the intranasal examination. Aside from this aspect, a complete head and neck examination should be performed. Otoscopy may reveal hemotympanum from backflow through the eustachian tube or effusion related to a mass in the nasopharynx. An eye examination may demonstrate findings that suggest a mass involving the sinuses and eye. The oropharynx should be checked for the amount of blood draining posteriorly. The neck examination may reveal inflammatory or metastatic lymph nodes.

The initial examination of the nose should be by anterior rhinoscopy, using a head mirror and indirect lighting or a headlight. The nose is dilated with a nasal speculum. Any blood or debris within the nose should be removed to expose the underlying mucosa. The findings on examination may vary widely from normal to a large tumor, and will depend on whether the patient has acute or chronic and recurrent bleeding.

In the case of a patient with acute epistaxis, there will typically be active bleeding or blood clot in the nose. The initial task is to remove the blood clots to try and determine first the side of the bleeding, and then whether it is anterior or posterior epistaxis. The physician should inspect the patient's nose systematically, with a speculum in one hand and suction in the other. This way, it should be possible to isolate the bleeding site. If there is too much bleeding to identify the source, the nose should be decongested with a temporary pack soaked with decongestant. Usually, cotton pledgets work well in this situation. Regardless of the initial appearance, both sides of the patient's nose should be carefully examined to make sure that there is not bilateral epistaxis. The most likely finding is a superficial vessel that has eroded, leading to the bleeding. A venous bleed will usually be darker and will flow in a nonpulsatile manner. The arterial bleed typically is bright red and, with proper suction and nasal cleaning, will show evidence of pulsatile flow with a discrete stream.

For patients with chronic or recurrent epistaxis, a more thorough examination must be conducted to identify a potential bleeding source. In many cases, there will be an obvious source, either a scab or ulcer on the anterior septum. In other cases, the findings may be subtle. The examiner must carefully search the mucosa for superficial vessels, subtle ulcerations, friable patches, or vascular malformations.

Endoscopy

In cases of either acute or recurrent epistaxis without an obvious bleeding source, an endoscopic examination is indicated to attempt to identify the site. This is usually performed bilaterally and with thorough decongestion and topical anesthesia. Either a flexible or rigid endoscope can be used with approximately equal effect. The flexible scope is perhaps easier to use and less uncomfortable. However, the rigid scopes have superior optics, with better image resolution.

During endoscopic examination, most of the inside of the nose can be visualized with magnification. This should help the physician to establish a diagnosis and identify the source of bleeding. It is important to orient the endoscopy, as well as the examination in general, to the area of suspicion based on the history. This will also improve diagnostic accuracy.

Radiologic Evaluation

Routine radiologic studies have little role in the initial diagnosis of epistaxis. That is not to say that patients with epistaxis may not require computed tonography (CT) scans or later be found to have lesions that require radiologic evaluation. The imaging study of choice for initial evaluation of most nasal or sinus pathologic conditions, including epistaxis, is the CT scan. The one significant role for CT scan is in the evaluation of patients with recurrent epistaxis without a known source or cause. In these cases, sinonasal tumors are sometimes the cause of the bleeding. In this setting, a CT scan is done to try to differentiate between a tumor as a cause of bleeding and the more routine etiologies.

MANAGEMENT

Management of epistaxis depends on a number of factors, including duration of bleeding, amount of bleeding, location of the source of bleeding, the presence of co-factors, such as coagulopathy and hypertension, and previous treatment. The options include medical management, nasal packing, cautery, surgical ligation, and embolization. In Figures 22–1 and 22–2, proposed guidelines for the management of epistaxis are presented. Each of these protocols must be modified significantly if the patient has medical co-factors, such as thrombocytopenia or coagulopathy. Although it is not possible to provide exact guidelines for determining when to use each of these treatments, the well-trained otolaryngologist has all of these options available and can apply them according to the specific circumstances of the individual patient. The specific indications for each of these strategies are detailed in the following sections.

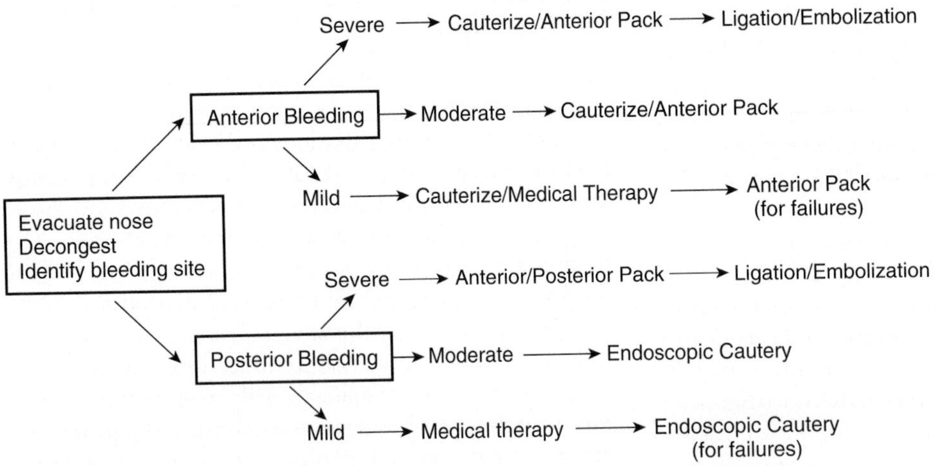

Figure 22–1. Management protocols for acute epistaxis. The upper division is for anterior bleeding, which can be divided further into mild, moderate, and severe bleeding. Initial therapy for severe and moderate bleeding is to cauterize and then place a pack. For mild bleeding, packing is not usually necessary. For severe, life-threatening epistaxis or epistaxis in which multiple transfusions are required, vessel ligation or embolization should be considered at the initial presentation. The lower division is for posterior bleeding, which can be divided into severe, moderate, and mild. Initial therapy for the severe posterior bleed is to place a pack to control the bleeding and then perform either ligation or embolization. For moderate bleeding, endoscopic cautery is appropriate. For mild bleeding, medical therapy alone can be tried, with cautery performed for those in whom medical treatment is unsuccessful.

Medical Management

For patients with recurrent or chronic epistaxis, medical management is usually the first line of therapy. Most of the time, these patients exhibit anterior epistaxis from Kisselbach's plexus of the anterior septum. The examination usually reveals signs of recent bleeding from this area, including erosions, superficial vessels, or blood clots. Often, there may be a septal deviation or a sharp spur on the anterior crest of the septum. In some cases, though, there will be no identifiable source of the bleeding. In either case, the initial management is the same.

On the first visit of a patient with minimal or moderate history of nasal bleeding, an empiric trial of medical therapy is advised. This includes several measures designed to increase humidification of the mucosa to allow the bleeding site to heal. This approach is based on the assumption that dryness is one of the most important factors causing epistaxis. The recommendations include applying an ointment to the anterior nose each morning

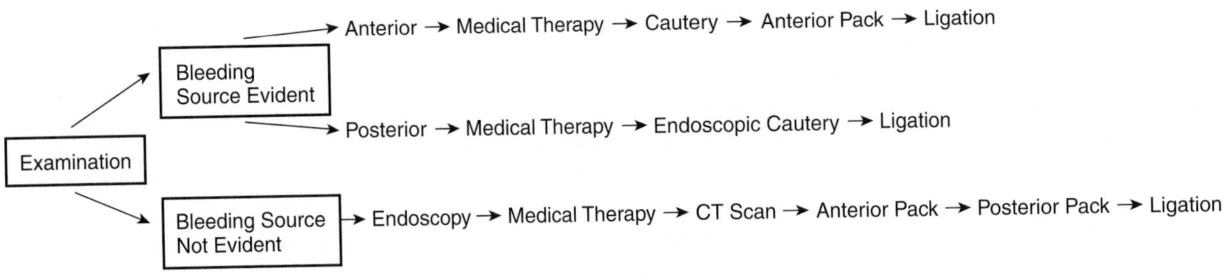

Figure 22–2. Management protocol for chronic or recurrent epistaxis. The upper division is for patients in whom the bleeding source is identified on initial evaluation; these can be further classified according to anterior and posterior bleeding sites. In both situations, medical therapy is initially tried. For patients with anterior bleeding that fails medical therapy, cautery, followed by placement of an anterior pack, followed by ligation should be considered. For posterior bleeding that fails medical therapy, cautery, followed by ligation, is recommended. The lower division is for patients in whom a site of bleeding has not been definitively identified. Endoscopy is indicated. If this fails to identify the bleeding site, a trial of medical therapy is indicated. If this approach fails to stop the bleeding, a CT scan is indicated to document the presence or absence of tumors. In the absence of a diagnosis and continued bleeding despite medical therapy, placement of an anterior pack, followed by a posterior pack, followed by bilateral vessel ligation, is indicated.

and night. In between ointment applications, nasal saline is sprayed into the nose every 2 to 3 hours. In addition, every effort should be made to humidify the air of the home environment. This usually requires using a room air humidifier in the bedroom every night. Maximum effect is achieved by running the humidifier on full with the doors and windows to the room closed.

In addition to these topical treatments, medical conditions that contribute to the bleeding should be controlled. For example, in patients with hypertension, medication should be administered to lower the blood pressure to within normal range. For patients with coagulopathy, every attempt should be made to normalize clotting function. This may require discontinuing coumadin or aspirin therapy. For patients with acute and life-threatening bleeding, platelet or plasma transfusions may be administered to reverse the bleeding disorder.

Patients with epistaxis should also minimize their activity while the nose is healing. Exercise should be deferred until the bleeding has stopped for at least 1 week. Bed rest is generally not necessary, nor is staying home from work or school. However, patients should be aware of their level of activity and take steps to avoid any activities that would elevate the blood pressure. Nose blowing should be minimized, and patients should be instructed to blow gently. Patients should also be instructed to avoid rubbing and picking at the nose. Finally, adjunctive therapy, including stool softeners and antitussives, should be considered in selected patients.

If initial attempts to control epistaxis with these conservative medical therapies fail, a more comprehensive approach to the problem should be initiated. This may include specific investigations to evaluate the hemoglobin, platelet levels, and coagulation function. An endoscopic examination, if not already performed, should also be considered. This subset of patients might also benefit from a CT scan to rule out the possibility of an occult tumor. Second-line therapy is then indicated, including nasal packing, cauterization, and vessel ligation.

Nasal Packing

Nasal packing is indicated for patients with acute epistaxis to control the bleeding and in patients with recurrent epistaxis who do not respond to medical management. Patients with acute epistaxis include those who come to the emergency room with uncontrolled bleeding, inpatients with bleeding, surgical patients, and the rare patient who comes into the office with active bleeding. In these patients, nasal packing is indicated to arrest the active bleeding. It may also be possible to stop the bleeding in these patients with a decongestant, careful cleaning of blood clots from the nose, and cautery. In many cases, though, it is best to place some type of nasal packing to prevent recurrent bleeding until complete healing can occur. Packing may also be used in patients with recurrent bleeding. This is usually reserved for patients with recurrent bleeding who fail medical management.

Standard Nasal Packing

Indications. There are numerous choices for packing material. Each of these options is appropriate in certain circumstances. Traditional nasal packing involves a layered pack of strip gauze coated with an antibiotic ointment or petroleum-based lubricant. This type of packing can be used for almost any circumstance. It is preferred for packing the maxillary sinus after a Caldwell-Luc procedure and for filling the defect after maxillectomy. For routine cases of anterior epistaxis, the full traditional anterior pack is reserved for patients in whom initial attempts to control the bleeding with simpler forms of packing fail.

Technique. Prior to placing the packing, the nose should be well decongested and anesthetized with a topical anesthetic. The preferred medication is either 4% or 10% cocaine solution. If this is unavailable, 0.25% neosynephrine with 2% lidocaine can be used as an alternative. Packing is performed with either indirect lighting using a head mirror or direct lighting afforded by a headlight. The nose is exposed with a nasal speculum and suctioning is performed with an appropriate-sized Frasier suction. A bayonet forceps is used to place the packing one layer at a time. Packing of the nose should proceed from inferior to superior and from posterior to anterior. Throughout the procedure, careful and gentle technique should be used. It is especially important to avoid injury to the mucosa as the pack is placed.

The first step is to grasp the packing about 10 cm from one end. This point is placed into the back of the nose (Fig. 22–3*A*). Loops of the packing are then placed one on top of another, gently but firmly pressing the loop onto the floor of the nose as each is placed. In this way, the pack is built up sequentially. The final pack should tightly fill the nasal cavity (Fig. 22–3*B*). The pack is placed in the same way when packing is done after maxillectomy or a Caldwell-Luc procedure. The pack is layered in from lateral to medial, from posterior to anterior, and from inferior to superior.

Follow-up Care. Assuming that the pack is able to control the bleeding, the patient can be sent home with an anterior pack in the nose. It is advisable to prescribe antistaphylococcal antibiotics for the duration of time the pack is in place as prophylaxis against toxic shock syndrome. The patient should be advised to restrict activity. Absolute bed rest is not necessary, but the pa-

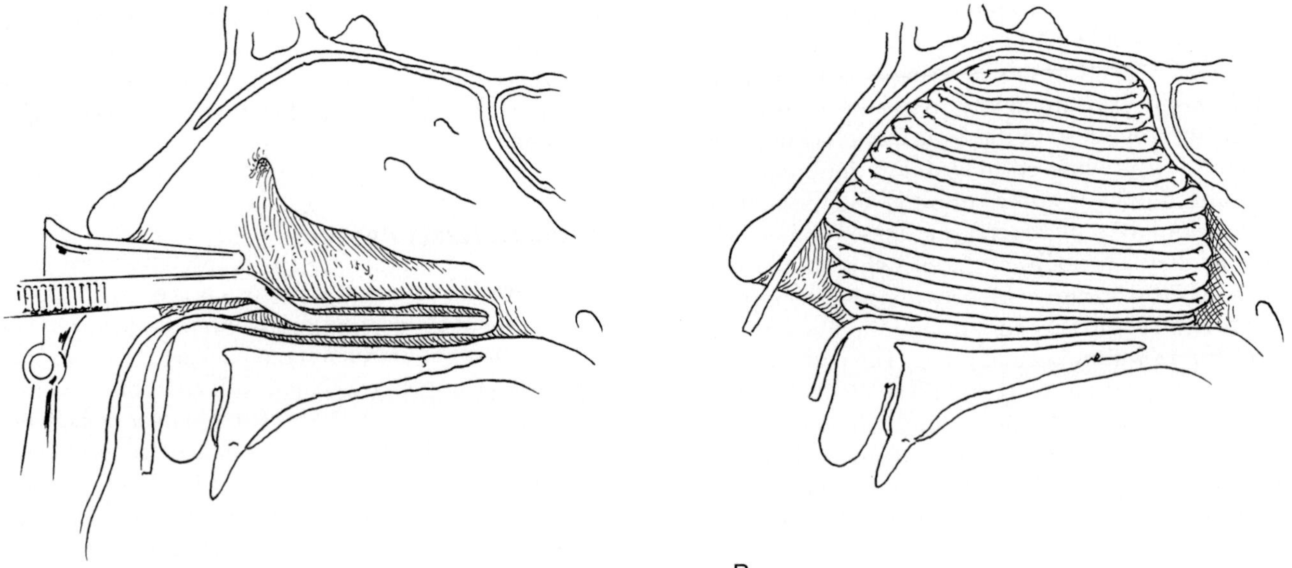

Figure 22–3. Placement of traditional or standard anterior nasal packing. *A*, The gauze is grasped 10 cm from one end and placed into the posterior choanae. *B*, The gauze is layered one length at a time to build up the pack.

tient should avoid strenuous activity and should not attempt to maintain normal activity levels.

The packing should be left in place for a period of 2 to 5 days depending on the severity of the bleed and the location. Upon removal of the packing, the nose should be decongested and cleared of any blood and secretions. If there are significant erosions on the mucosa, Gelfoam (Upjohn Co., Kalamazoo, MI) can be placed to help prevent recurrent bleeding. After removal of the packing, the patient should be started on medical therapy, including ointment, saline, and humidification.

Merocel Packing

Indications. Merocel (Merocel Corporation, Jacksonville, FL) is a synthetic sponge material that is nonreactive and well tolerated as a nasal and sinus packing material. The pack is introduced in a dehydrated state and is expanded by either instilling saline or by absorbing blood from the patient. As the material expands, it fills the nasal or sinus cavity, helping to stop the bleeding in two ways: by applying pressure against the mucosa and by providing a surface against which the blood can clot.

Merocel sponges come in a variety of shapes and sizes. Two particular styles are favored by the author for specific circumstances. The product marketed as the Kennedy sinus pack is the preferred packing after endoscopic sinus surgery. It is the ideal size to fill the ethmoid cavity. In cases when this is inadequate, two or even three packs can be placed on one side of the nose.

The Pope nasal pack is designed as a full nasal pack. The height and length are proportioned to fill the nasal cavity. This pack is ideal for controlling anterior epistaxis. Because of the ease of placement and the minimal damage caused to the mucosa when placing this sponge, it is the author's preference for first-line management of anterior epistaxis. When fully expanded, the sponge fills the nasal cavity and should control most cases of anterior bleeding. If this pack fails, it can be converted to either a full anterior pack or a combined anterior and posterior pack.

Technique. Placement of these packs is very simple. The Kennedy pack is placed through the nose lateral to the middle turbinate so that the posterior edge is up against the back of the middle turbinate. The anterior edge is directed into the notch between the anterior edge of the middle turbinate and the lateral nasal wall (Fig. 22–4*A*). The sponge is expanded by instilling 10 mL of saline into the nose with a syringe. Some surgeons prefer to place the sponge into a finger cot to help prevent it from sticking to the surrounding tissues. However, this also compromises its effectiveness as a hemostatic sponge and so is not favored by the author.

The Pope pack is placed after the nose is decongested and anesthetized with topical medications. The sponge is placed into the nasal cavity proper, medial to the turbinates and against the septum (Fig. 22–4*B*). This pack can also be expanded by instilling saline into the nose. Any desired adjustments in position should be made before the sponge is expanded.

Follow-up Care. While the packs are in place, the patient should be managed as if a full nasal pack were in place,

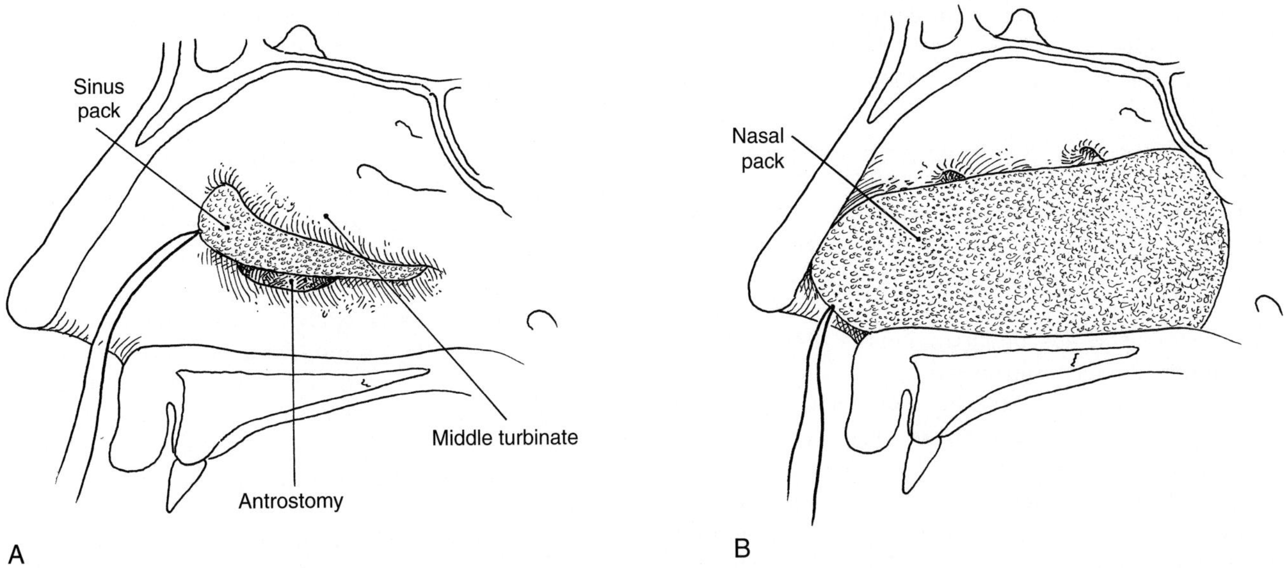

Figure 22–4. Placement of nasal sponges. *A,* A Kennedy sinus pack is placed lateral to the middle turbinate in patients who have undergone sinus endoscopy. *B,* A Pope nasal pack is placed between the septum and turbinates.

that is, with activity restriction and antibiotics. The packs are maintained for a period of 2 to 5 days depending on the circumstances. After removal of the packs, a regimen of ongoing care is recommended, including full medical treatment and irrigations for patients who have undergone sinus surgery.

Gelfoam

Indications. Gelfoam (Upjohn Co., Kalamazoo, MI) is a dissolvable synthetic matrix that has a procoagulant effect. This product is available in a variety of shapes and sizes. It is primarily used in the nose as sheets, which can be cut and folded to the desired size. As opposed to the Merocel sponges, which expand when they get wet, the Gelfoam pack tends to shrink when it gets wet. When wet, this material becomes nonadherent and begins to dissolve. It will completely dissolve in a matter of weeks, but usually will shrink and fall out before this happens.

Gelfoam is useful in a number of different situations. In patients with chronic or recurrent epistaxis with small areas of mucosal ulceration or exposed vessels, it can be used as a limited anterior pack to help promote healing. In patients with coagulopathy from any number of causes, Gelfoam is an attractive alternative to packs that must be removed, as removal of packing usually exposes areas of mucosal damage that can rebleed. The Gelfoam pack will dissolve slowly and allow complete healing without requiring removal that would expose raw areas. Gelfoam is also often placed against the bleeding site in the nose after cauterization or after a nasal pack is removed. This helps to protect the bleeding site from desiccating after the original treatment controls the bleeding. Finally, Gelfoam may be used after repair of a CSF leak as an initial layer to support the graft. This prevents the graft from sticking to the gauze or Merocel pack placed.

Technique. Gelfoam packs can be tailored to the specific needs of the individual patient. The standard size of the product that is most useful for the nose is a 6 × 2 cm piece. Before insertion, the nose is decongested and anesthetized as for other packs. The standard piece is folded in half to make a 3 × 2 cm piece and then folded along the long axis to make a 3 × 1 cm plug. This should be pressed flat. The pack is then placed into the nose against the site of bleeding. These packs can be layered one on top of the other to create progressively increasing pressure on the mucosa.

Follow-up Care. The Gelfoam pack requires somewhat different care from other packs. Like other packs, antibiotics and decreased activity levels are advised. However, these packs are usually not removed. Patients are started on nasal saline spray 24 to 48 hours after the pack is placed. Normally, within the first few days, the pack falls out. If this does not occur, the saline treatments are continued until the pack falls out. By 1 week after placement of the packing, the residual Gelfoam can be easily suctioned from the nose without causing any trauma. At this point, the bleeding site is usually healed.

Posterior Nasal Pack

Indications. Posterior nasal packing is indicated for the management of posterior epistaxis. Most patient who develop posterior epistaxis require intervention of some type. This is because the source of bleeding is usually from a major branch of the sphenopalatine artery. Bleeding is typically heavy and cannot be controlled with an anterior pack or by anterior compression of the nose. The decision to utilize a posterior pack rather than a nasal balloon, embolization, or surgical ligation is dependent on the physician and his or her training and experience. This is the traditional first-line therapy for posterior epistaxis. However, with the many options available today, many otolaryngologists prefer not to use the traditional posterior pack.

The benefits of the posterior pack are that, if properly placed, this method almost always results in control of the bleeding. If the posterior pack fails to work, then surgery to ligate the vessels would be indicated. A second advantage of the posterior pack is that it can be created with minimal supplies available in all emergency rooms and on all nursing units. A final advantage is that it can be placed in any patient. There are no absolute contraindications to placing a traditional posterior nasal pack.

There are, however, significant disadvantages to this method of controlling posterior nasal bleeding. The most important is that it is very uncomfortable to place as well as to maintain for any length of time. Even with thorough topical anesthesia and decongestion, the posterior pack is painful to place. Once in place, the pack causes intense pressure and complete nasal blockage. In addition, these packs usually must be maintained for a period of at least 3 days to improve the chances of success. Another problem is that these packs tend to cause significant injury to the nasal mucosa. Ulcerations are common and abrasions are universal.

Finally, there is a significant risk for development of hypoxia with this pack. The presence of a nasal pulmonary reflex has long been debated in otolaryngology.[10–12] Regardless of the cause, it is a common observation that patients with traditional posterior nasal packs can have significant hypoxia. The author has witnessed a full respiratory arrest in a young patient without cardiovascular disease about 30 minutes after placement of a posterior nasal pack. Because of this possibility, all patients with posterior packs should be admitted to the hospital and observed in a monitored bed for at least the first day after placement. After this, the patient should remain hospitalized until the packing is removed.

Owing to these disadvantages, the author does not use a traditional posterior pack as the first line of therapy. Rather, this type of pack is reserved for patients in whom milder forms of treatment have failed, as well as those who are not suitable candidates for surgery because of medical contraindications. The latter are most often elderly patients with a cardiac condition. Others in this category include patients in the intensive care unit or those hospitalized for chemotherapy with a medically induced coagulopathy or low platelet count.

Technique. Before placing a traditional posterior nasal pack, the patient should be well decongested and anesthetized. Transpalatal injection through the greater palatine foramen should be considered. The nose can be packed with a temporary pack of Neo-Synephrine–soaked cotton pledgets. While the nose is decongesting, the posterior pack should be prepared. The basic goal of the procedure is to wedge a nonabrading, tightly rolled pack into the nasopharynx against the posterior choanae. The pack can be made from any number of materials. A gauze sponge can be rolled up, or a cotton ball can be used. Also, the size of the pack will vary depending on whether a unilateral or bilateral pack is needed.

With the cotton ball technique, a cotton ball of the desired size is moistened with mineral oil. This makes the cotton ball malleable and compressible. The cotton is then wrapped with a nonadherent petroleum gauze and tied with 0 silk sutures. Three pieces of umbilical tape are then tied or sutured to the pack. The alternative is to use a gauze sponge rolled up and tied with the sutures or dental gauze packing prepared in the same way.

To place the pack, a red rubber catheter is placed through each side of the nose, grasped in the pharynx, and brought out through the mouth. One umbilical tape tied to the pack is tied to each of the red rubber catheters. The catheters are then withdrawn through the nose pulling the pack into the nasopharynx (Fig. 22–5*A*). The third umbilical tape is brought out through the mouth and taped to the cheek. A full anterior pack is placed in front of the posterior pack. The umbilical tape through the nose is pulled tight to add the desired pressure and is then tied around a gauze bolster over the anterior nasal spine (Fig. 22–5*B*).

Follow-up Care. After placing the posterior pack, the patient should be observed in the intensive care unit or an alternative monitored bed. If there are no problems, the patient can be transferred to a regular hospital bed after 24 hours. For the entire time that the posterior pack is in place, humidified oxygen should be administered. The percent of inspired oxygen is not as important as the humidification. As the patient will not be able to breathe through the nose, the humidification will prevent drying of the pharynx, in addition to maintaining blood oxygen saturation. Intravenous antibiotics are prescribed to prevent sinus infection and to prevent toxic shock syndrome.

The pack is normally kept in place for 3 to 5 days. The exact amount of time will depend on the severity and duration of bleeding before the pack was placed. The more serious the epistaxis, the longer the pack should remain in place. When the pack is removed, the

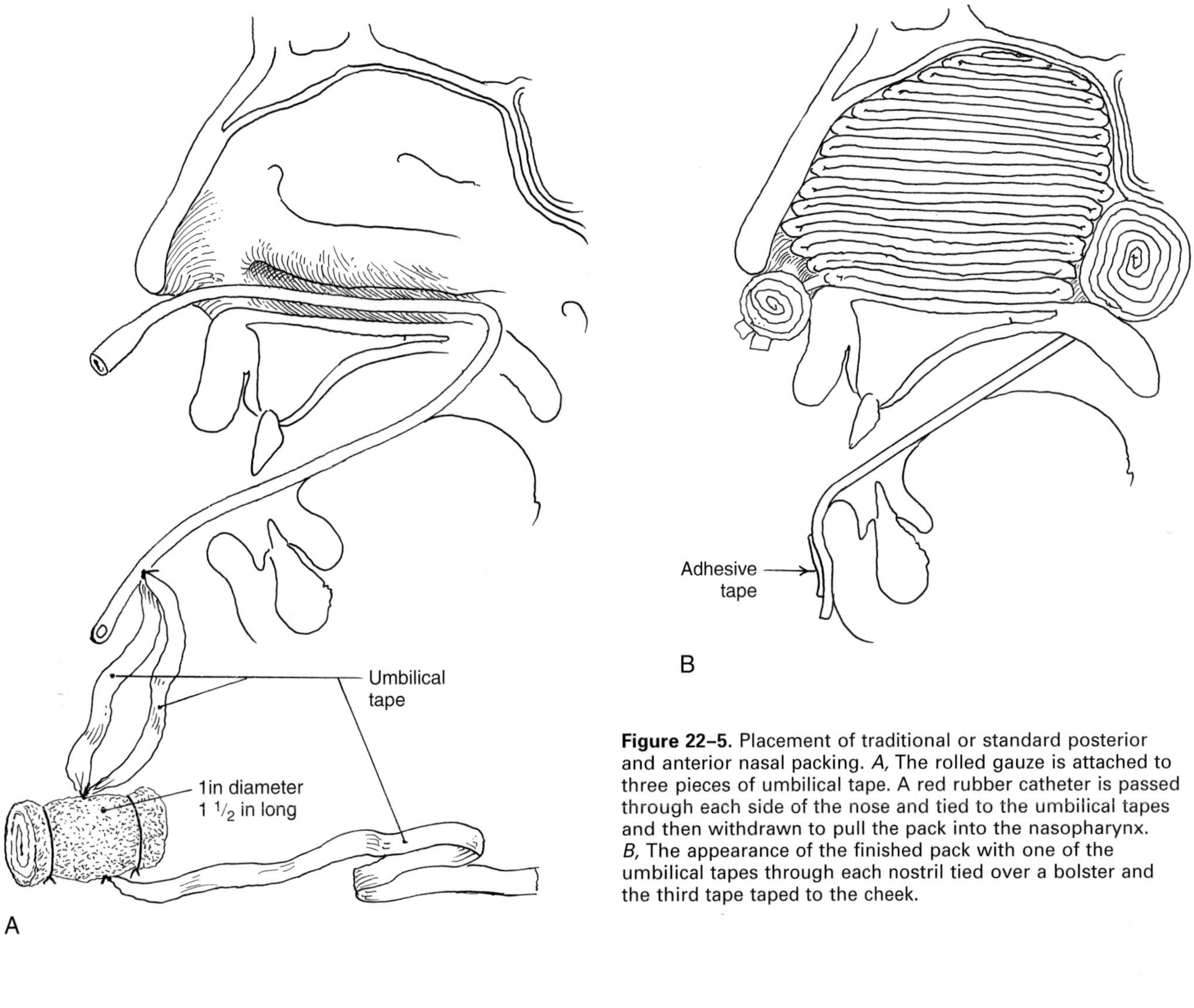

Figure 22–5. Placement of traditional or standard posterior and anterior nasal packing. *A,* The rolled gauze is attached to three pieces of umbilical tape. A red rubber catheter is passed through each side of the nose and tied to the umbilical tapes and then withdrawn to pull the pack into the nasopharynx. *B,* The appearance of the finished pack with one of the umbilical tapes through each nostril tied over a bolster and the third tape taped to the cheek.

nose should be suctioned clear of blood and mucus and thoroughly decongested. A temporary Gelfoam pack may be applied to any areas of abrasion. The patient should be started on medical therapy, including humidification, nasal saline, and ointment, to prevent recurrent epistaxis.

Nasal Balloon

Indications. Created solely for the purpose of managing posterior epistaxis, the nasal balloon is an excellent treatment option. This device is a catheter with two balloons. The posterior balloon is placed into the nasopharynx and inflated; the anterior balloon fills the nasal cavity. With both balloons inflated, pressure can be applied to the bleeding vessel, regardless of site. By adjusting the amount of inflation of the balloons, the amount of pressure on the mucosa is optimized to control the epistaxis.

There are several advantages of the nasal balloon. First, it is very simple to apply. This feature makes it possible for emergency room physicians and other nonotolaryngologists to utilize this technique. Second, placing the nasal balloon causes almost no trauma to the mucosa, so its use causes less nasal scarring and less secondary bleeding than traditional packing. A third advantage is that the balloons can be inflated to varying degrees. This allows the physician to use only the amount of pressure necessary to achieve control, even in cases of severe epistaxis. Finally, the balloons can be deflated gradually over a period of 24 hours. This gradual decrease helps to prevent the rebleeding that can occur with sudden removal of packing.

There are several disadvantages of the nasal balloon as well. Despite the fact that it is not difficult or uncomfortable to place the balloon, the patient is likely to be very uncomfortable during balloon inflation and until the device is removed. High pressures in the nose always cause pain and pressure. In addition, the patient will not be able to breathe through the nose while the balloon is in place. One of the unique problems associated with the balloon is that it causes a high rate of injury to the nasal sill or ala and the balloons cannot be used bilaterally. Finally, this form of posterior pack carries the risk of hypoxia, just as the traditional pack does.

On balance, the advantages of the balloon over the traditional posterior pack are significant. The author prefers the nasal balloon as the first option for management of posterior epistaxis. The contraindications are few and include an inability to place the balloon owing to severe deviated septum or nasal mass.

The suggested management course is to place a nasal balloon as the first line of treatment for most patients with confirmed posterior epistaxis. If, after the balloon is used, bleeding continues or recurs, a surgical option is considered.

Technique. The placement of the balloon is very simple. The nose is decongested and anesthetized. The catheter is placed through the nose into the nasopharynx. The posterior balloon is inflated with 10 mL of saline. This is the amount necessary to fill the entire nasopharynx. The catheter is then pulled outward and the anterior balloon is slowly inflated until the balloon starts to bulge out of the nose. Additional saline can be used in either balloon as needed to control the epistaxis. The hub of the catheter is wrapped with gauze to cushion the ala and to maintain tension on the nasopharynx (Fig. 22–6).

Follow-up Care. The balloon is left in place for 3 to 5 days and then gradually deflated. The protocol for withdrawal of the saline is variable. One possible method is to withdraw 2 mL from each balloon every 2 hours until the balloons are completely deflated. The catheter is then removed and the nose is decongested and suctioned thoroughly. Rebleeding is almost always an indication to proceed to surgical intervention.

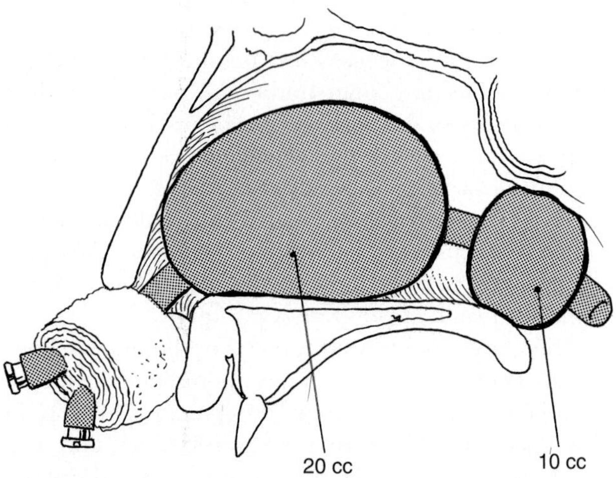

Figure 22–6. Placement of a nasal balloon. The smaller balloon is filled in the nasopharynx and pulled forward. The second balloon is filled to the extent necessary. A gauze is wrapped around the stem of the balloon to protect the front of the nose.

Cautery

Cauterization is an effective and simple way of controlling epistaxis. There are currently two methods of applying cautery in the nose. The first involves the use of silver nitrate ($AgNO_3$) and is primarily applicable to anterior epistaxis. The second is electrocautery, which can be used throughout the nose, but is primarily used for posterior epistaxis.

Silver Nitrate

Indications. As stated earlier, $AgNO_3$ is used primarily for anterior epistaxis. The most convenient and usual method of delivery is via a silver nitrate applicator stick. When touched to the mucosa, this causes a chemical burn that coagulates the tissue. The depth of the effect depends on the amount used and the duration of contact between the applicator and the tissue. Generally, the depth of the effect is minimal, with little tissue damage below the submucosa. The depth of coagulation is both an advantage and a limitation of this technique. The advantage is that there is minimal tissue damage and, therefore, minimal discomfort and rapid healing. The limitation of this method is that only superficial, small vessels can be coagulated.

The best indication for use of $AgNO_3$ is for active bleeding from an anterior nasoseptal vessel. In this situation, the chemical cautery can stop the bleeding. The procedure may also be appropriate for patients with recurrent epistaxis with an exposed vessel on the septum or a small vascular malformation in the anterior nose. This method of cautery is specifically *not* recommended for patients with recurrent bleeding without an identifiable point source, as the cautery is likely to cause more damage.

Technique. The nose is first decongested and anesthetized with topical anesthesia. Injection of local anesthetic is usually not necessary for application of silver nitrate. For actively bleeding vessels, one or two sticks are pressed against the vessel and slowly rolled to release the chemical. A piece of moistened cotton is then pressed over the area, pushing the sticks onto the vessel. After 15 to 30 seconds, the cotton and sticks are removed and any excess $AgNO_3$ is suctioned. The area of the cautery should be reinforced with Gelfoam or other suitable packing.

Follow-up Care. Patients should be started on a regimen of maximal medical therapy as outlined earlier. The Gelfoam packing is maintained until it is expelled spontaneously or dissolved. These patients should be followed closely as there is a high possibility of rebleeding.

This is especially true if the patient is not compliant with recommended medical care.

Endoscopic Cautery

Indications. Endoscopic cautery is indicated for controlling posterior epistaxis and epistaxis that stems from the septum and lateral wall, both of which lie beyond the reach of a silver nitrate stick.[13, 14] This procedure is very effective if the exact location of the bleeding vessel is known or the bleeding is active at the time of the procedure. This procedure is controversial because the success rate has not been well established. For individual surgeons adept at the technique, the success rate may be very high, in excess of 90%. However, there have yet to be any large series of unselected cases published in the literature to accurately document the success rate of the procedure. The role of this technique is, therefore, uncertain.

For those with experience and confidence in the procedure, endoscopic cautery may supplant posterior packing in most patients. Instead of placing a formal posterior pack, a temporary pack or a nasal balloon is placed and the patient is taken to the operating room as soon as this can be arranged. If successful, this management protocol can decrease the patient's discomfort and the overall cost of treatment for posterior epistaxis. Other surgeons may find no role at all for this procedure.

The author suggests that endoscopic cautery does have a role for those surgeons who are experienced in sinus endoscopy. However, because of the great utility of other options, this technique is infrequently used. The best circumstance for its use is a patient with active bleeding in whom a preliminary endoscopic examination is able to identify a specific site of bleeding. In these patients, endoscopic cauterization can prevent the need for a prolonged period of posterior packing. For those who bleed through a posterior pack or have recurrent bleeding after placement of a pack, a ligation procedure is preferred. However, for patients with coagulopathy and posterior epistaxis, cautery is the main alternative to embolization. The primary criterion is whether or not the bleeding site can be determined.

Technique. In most cases, the patient will have a temporary pack in place at the time of the procedure. Before taking out the pack, all necessary equipment should be set up and a suitable level of anesthesia should be achieved either through general anesthesia or conscious sedation. To help anesthetize the area in the instance of conscious sedation, a transpalatal block of the sphenopalatine ganglion should be performed. This will ensure that the procedure can be performed without causing discomfort.

When everything is ready, the pack is removed. The nose should be well decongested. The best way to do this is with cotton pledgets soaked with oxymetazoline. Owing to the presence of blood and mucus in the nose, it may take several changes of the decongestant packs before the nose is well decongested. Using cocaine in this circumstance may require several vials and leads to an unpredictable amount of absorption.

The nose is now examined using a 0-degree or 30-degree, 4-mm endoscope. In most cases, the site of bleeding will be identified easily. If there is no active bleeding, the exact bleeding site should have been identified preoperatively. If no bleeding site can be determined, it is possible to cauterize the main branches of the sphenopalatine artery at their takeoff near the sphenopalatine foramen.

Cautery is performed using a suction cautery unit. These catheters can be bent to give the tip a slight curve, allowing the physician to reach around the back of the inferior and middle turbinates and work against the floor of the nose. The cautery setting should be at a moderate level. The cautery is placed above the scope and advanced to the back of the nose to the area of the bleeding. The cautery current is delivered directly to the offending vessel. A light touch should be used to prevent the cautery from sticking to the mucosa. A piece of Gelfoam soaked in oxymetazoline is then placed over the treated vessel to complete the procedure.

Follow-up Care. The risk of recurrent bleeding after endoscopic cautery can be minimized by vigorous follow-up care. This should include maximal humidification, a twice-daily coating of the inside of the nose with ointment, frequent applications of nasal saline spray, and control of hypertension and coagulopathy. The patient should be observed closely the night of the procedure. If there has not been further bleeding, the patient can be discharged the next morning. For the first few days, the patient should restrict activity to minimal ambulation only. Stool softeners and cough suppressants may be indicated in selected patients.

Follow-up examinations should be performed after 5 to 7 days. At that time, the nose should be well decongested and examined endoscopically. The area of the cautery treatment should be examined, but must be handled gently to avoid causing recurrence of bleeding. Further follow-up evaluation should be scheduled in 2 to 3 weeks and thereafter as determined by the patient's clinical course.

Embolization

One of the options for severe posterior epistaxis in intra-arterial embolization.[15, 16] This procedure is usually performed in the arteriography suite of the hospital. Normally, a catheter is placed into the groin and threaded through the femoral artery, into the aorta, and then into the carotid artery. The catheter is then guided into the external carotid artery and finally, into the internal maxillary artery. A test injection is performed to identify the bleeding site. Finally, the internal maxillary artery is embolized. Various materials have been used for embolization, including Gelfoam, coils, balloons, and polyvinyl alcohol (PVA) particles. The result is that the arterial flow to the bleeding site is interrupted and the bleeding should then stop.

Embolization is a useful and highly successful technique for controlling posterior epistaxis.[15, 16] However, in all large series of carotid artery catheterization, there is an incidence of serious cerebrovascular accident (CVA) resulting in permanent neurologic deficit.[15–19] The incidence of this varies with the skill of the radiologist in performing the procedure, with an overall average of about 4%.[20] No other procedure for control of epistaxis has such a high incidence of this type of major complication. For this reason, the use of embolization for control of epistaxis is controversial. Some otolaryngologists recommend embolization as the first option for posterior epistaxis. Others limit its use to those in whom initial posterior packing fails.

The author limits the use of embolization to those patients who are not candidates for surgical intervention or who fail surgery. This would include patients with severe medical comorbidity, severe coagulopathy, or bleeding from tumors. In these settings, and especially when multiple factors are present in the same patient, embolization may be a useful means of controlling the bleeding without subjecting the patient to a surgical procedure that may be poorly tolerated.

Ligation

Transantral Ligation of the Internal Maxillary Artery

Indications. Transantral ligation of the internal maxillary artery is the traditional procedure of choice for controlling posterior epistaxis.[20–25] This procedure has been analyzed in terms of cost-effectiveness and length of hospitalization compared to traditional posterior packing for posterior epistaxis.[21] In this comparison, the surgical procedure, if performed at the time of admission for posterior epistaxis, was found to result in shorter hospital stays and lower overall cost. However, given the choice, most patients would prefer not to have a surgical procedure, and the morbidity of the transantral procedure is significant. For these reasons, early surgical intervention using this technique has not gained wide acceptance.

The author has used this procedure as the primary surgical intervention for epistaxis in patients with bleeding through a well-placed posterior pack, or with recurrent bleeding after the removal of the pack. Other indications include patients with massive bleeding, regardless of the success of the initial nasal pack, and some patients with HHT. Recently, however, the advent of endoscopic ligation of the terminal branches of the sphenopalatine artery has challenged the role of the transantral ligation procedure. For most patients, this new alternative is an attractive option that has the advantage of avoiding the sublabial incision and injury to the infraorbital nerve. A complete discussion of this procedure is presented in the following section.

Technique. Transantral ligation of the internal maxillary artery is performed under general anesthesia. The endotracheal tube should be positioned away from the corner of the mouth and taped to the mandible to avoid restricting the mobility of the upper lip. The patient is positioned supine with the head tilted slightly to the right. For surgery on either the right or left side, the right-handed surgeon should sit or stand on the patient's right. Normally, the patient comes into the operating room with a posterior pack in the nose. The first step is to remove the pack. The nose is decongested and a temporary cotton pack soaked in oxymetazoline will usually suffice to prevent the nose from bleeding during the procedure. Formal skin preparation is not necessary. The sublabial area should be anesthetized with local anesthetic containing 1% lidocaine with 1 : 100,000 epinephrine.

The sublabial incision is made with a No. 15 scalpel through the mucosa. The incision is located 5 mm above the gingival labial sulcus and extends from the midline to the first molar. The incision should extend down to the bone of the maxillary wall, angling inferiorly to avoid injuring the infraorbital nerve. The periosteum is incised and a subperiosteal elevation is performed over the anterior wall of the maxillary sinus. The maxillary sinus is entered over the canine fossa using a 4-mm osteotome and mallet. The opening is enlarged with a Kerrison rongeur. The opening should be maximized by removing the anterior wall medially to the medial buttress, laterally to the lateral wall, inferiorly to the floor of the sinus, and superiorly to the infraorbital nerve (Fig. 22–7*A*).

The mucosa of the posterior wall is removed carefully to avoid stripping the mucosa from the superior, lateral, medial, or inferior walls. Medially, the posterior wall of the maxillary sinus thickens and attaches to the pterygoid plates. The initial bone removal of the posterior wall should start in the center of the posterior wall, 1 to 2 cm below the floor of the orbit. A 4-mm osteotome is used in a controlled fashion with very light taps to fracture the thin bone of this area. A Kerrison rongeur is used to remove this bony wall, exposing the pterygomaxillary fissure (Fig. 22–7*B*). The contents of the fissure are behind the periosteum of the posterior wall. The periosteum should be cauterized with a bayonet-type bipolar forceps in a cruciate fashion. A bipolar

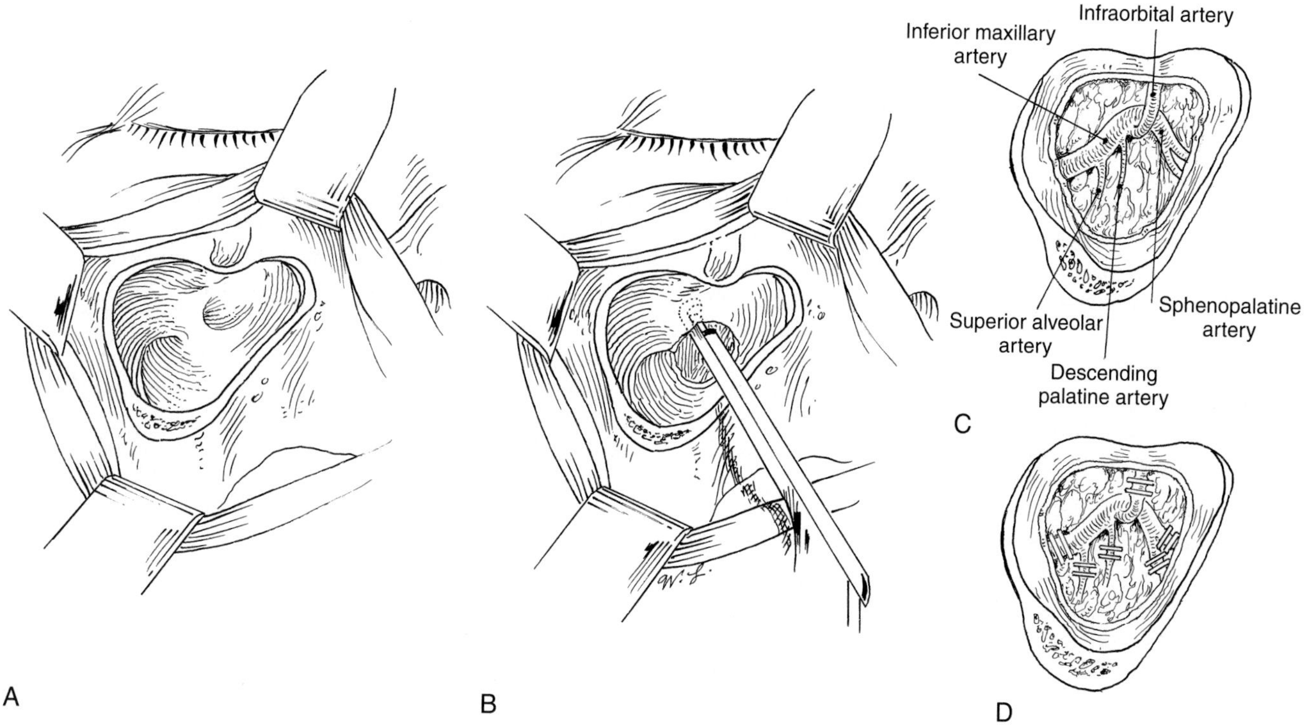

Figure 22–7. Transantral ligation of the internal maxillary artery. *A,* Completed sublabial exposure. The infraorbital nerve is preserved and the antrostomy is maximized. *B,* A small opening in the posterior wall of the sinus is made and the incision is enlarged using a Kerrison rongeur. *C,* Identification of the branches of the internal maxillary artery. Significant variation in the anatomy is possible. *D,* Completed ligation of the branches, with two microclips placed on each vessel.

forceps is used to avoid having monopolar cautery deliver current into the contents of the fissure.

The periosteum is then incised with a No. 15 scalpel mounted on a long knife handle. The periosteal flaps are folded back to expose the fat of the fissure. There are a number of techniques available to dissect the vessels from the fat. The technique preferred by the author is to use the bipolar bayonet forceps to tease the fat out. A small amount of fat is grasped and pulled out and then cauterized. This technique, performed sequentially, will begin to expose the vessels. The internal maxillary artery enters the anterior aspect of the fissure laterally and inferiorly. The vessel usually loops and then exits through the sphenopalatine foramen.

The anatomy of the vessel is somewhat variable. However, there are several branches that can usually be identified, including the descending palatine, the superior alveolar, the infraorbital, and the terminal vessel, the sphenopalatine artery (Fig. 22–7*C*). Each of these branches should be carefully dissected so that the anatomy is clear. Each of the branches is ligated with a small to medium-sized vascular clip. One or two clips can be placed on each vessel; two clips are preferred if there is room (Fig. 22–7*D*).

After the arterial branches are successfully ligated, the temporary nasal packing is removed and the nose is suctioned. A moderately sized antrostomy is performed, strip gauze packing is placed through the antrostomy into the nose, and the sinus is packed. The sublabial incision is then closed using interrupted 3-0 Vicryl (Ethicon Corp., Somerville, NJ) suture.

Postoperative Care. The postoperative care after a transantral ligation of the internal maxillary artery is similar to that for the Caldwell-Luc procedure for chronic sinusitis. After the surgery, the patient is hospitalized for continued observation. Routine care is provided, including antibiotics, analgesics, and intravenous fluid hydration. Humidified air or low-flow oxygen is delivered through a face mask or face tent. The period of hospitalization need only be an overnight stay provided there is no postoperative epistaxis.

The nasal packing can be removed 2 to 7 days after surgery depending on available follow-up appointments, the severity of the bleeding, and the patient's tolerance of the pack. In most cases, the intranasal part of the pack can be removed the morning after surgery. This will significantly improve the patient's comfort level. After the intranasal portion of the pack is removed, nasal saline spray and room air humidification should be prescribed. This regimen is continued until healing is complete and crusting subsides. The sublabial sutures do not need to be removed, but can be removed 10 days after surgery if they bother the patient.

Recurrent bleeding is possible but unusual after this operation. The primary cause of rebleeding is misdiagnosis of the source of the bleeding. The other primary cause of recurrent epistaxis is failure to ligate the appropriate vessels. The problem in the case of rebleeding is that it is difficult to distinguish between these two possibilities based on examination or history. Therefore, the recommended management of recurrent bleeding after transantral ligation of the internal maxillary artery is to perform an arteriogram. This will reliably distinguish between these situations, and it also affords the option of embolization if the source of bleeding is discovered and is amenable to embolization.

Complications. Other than recurrent bleeding, the complications of transantral ligation of the internal maxillary artery are identical to those of Caldwell-Luc surgery. Chapter 10 covers these problems in detail. The most common complications include chronic facial or dental pain or facial numbness from injury to the infraorbital nerve. Other complications may be acute or chronic infection of the sinus, fibrosis or osteitis of the sinus, and formation of a mucocele. Finally, the routine medical and surgical complications of hematoma, wound infection, and anesthetic complications can occur, but are rare.

External Ligation of the Ethmoid Arteries

Indications. The external approach for ligation of the anterior and posterior ethmoid arteries is rarely used for control of epistaxis. Most cases of recurrent or massive bleeding of the nose involve the posterior circulation. The rare case of bleeding from the anterior half of the lateral wall of the nose can usually be controlled by nasal packing. Perhaps the most common indication is in conjunction with the transantral ligation of the internal maxillary artery for bleeding from the posterior nose when the site is not well identified.[26] Some of the patients in whom conservative methods may fail, requiring ligation of the ethmoid arteries, include trauma patients with fractures through the skull base that avulse or lacerate the anterior ethmoid artery. Following endoscopic sinus surgery, some patients may develop heavy bleeding from the anterior or posterior ethmoid arteries that may not respond to packing. Most of the time, these patients can be treated with endoscopic cautery of the bleeding vessel. However, in certain cases, it may be preferable to ligate the vessel. Finally, patients with HHT may require vessel ligation to minimize the frequency or severity of epistaxis.

Technique. The external ligation of the anterior and posterior ethmoid arteries is performed through the same approach as outlined in Chapter 9 for external ethmoidectomy. Typically, this procedure is performed under general anesthesia. Local anesthesia with sedation is possible, but it is difficult to completely anesthetize the surgical field unless an orbital block is used. In most cases, the nose is packed and there may be a posterior pack or nasal balloon. If possible, it is best to leave this in place until after the procedure is finished. If the packing blocks the surgical field, the pack is removed after the anesthetic takes effect, and the airway is secured. The nose is suctioned clear, decongested, and a temporary pack to control bleeding is placed in such a way that it does not block the surgical field.

The face is prepared with either iodine or a facial disinfectant that is safe for use around the eye. The incision is marked out and injected with 1% lidocaine with 1:100,000 epinephrine to help with hemostasis. The classic incision is the curved medial canthal incision known as the Lynch incision. However, the preferred incision incorporates an M or W into the incision to help hide the scar and prevent contracture.

The incision is made and the subcutaneous tissue is divided down through the periosteum to the bone. The angular artery will be encountered in the inferior aspect of the wound and should be controlled with either ligation or bipolar cautery. The soft tissues are retracted and the eye is elevated from the orbital bone with a Freer elevator. Inferiorly, the anterior lacrimal crest will be crossed and the lacrimal sac elevated from the lacrimal fossa (Fig. 22–8). The posterior lacrimal crest is crossed to reach the lamina papyracea. As the eye is elevated, the frontoethmoidal suture line is carefully sought. This is a critical landmark, as the ethmoidal arteries are found in the suture line or just inferior to it. The anterior ethmoid artery is found about 15 to 20 mm posterior to the anterior lacrimal crest (Fig. 22–8).

The artery can be ligated using small vascular clips or cauterized with bipolar cautery. The preferred technique is to use bipolar cautery, as the clips tend to fall off and can lead to orbital hematoma. With either technique, the artery is first identified; elevation above and below the artery is then achieved so the vessel can be isolated from the surrounding structures. To use the clips, the eye is retracted laterally and one clip is placed as close to the lamina papyracea as possible; a second clip is then placed as close to the eye as possible. If enough room is available, a second clip can be placed on each side. The artery is then divided between the clips. The alternative technique is to use the bayonet bipolar cautery. The artery is thoroughly cauterized from the orbital wall to the eye. It is important to make sure that the full diameter of the artery is cauterized. Partial-thickness cauterization will lead to bleeding. Once the artery is ready, Jameson scissors are used to transect the artery in the middle, making sure that there is room to cauterize each stump if necessary (Fig. 22–8). The dissection is then carried posteriorly for another

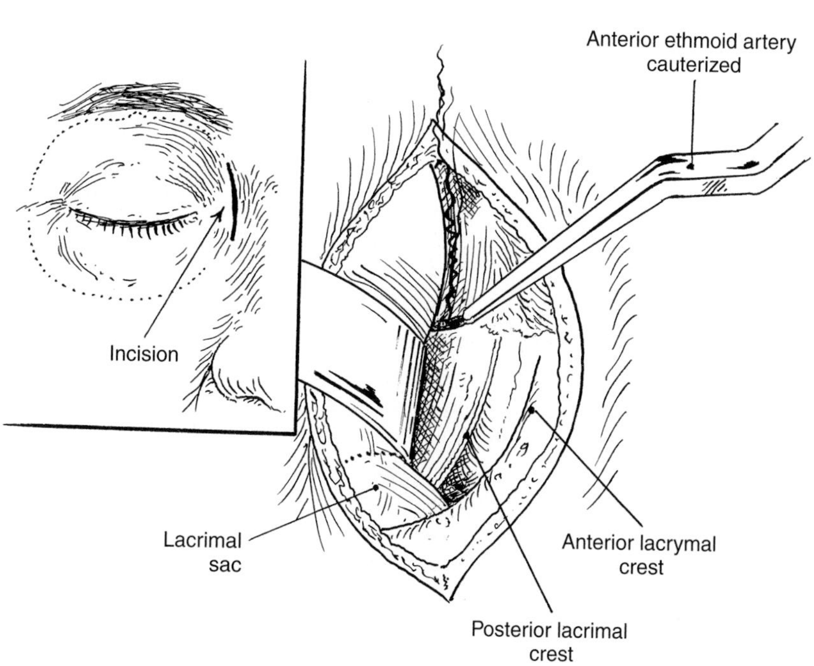

Figure 22–8. External ligation of the ethmoid arteries. The inset demonstrates the standard Lynch incision. The anterior ethmoid artery is identified at the level of the frontal ethmoidal suture, 15 to 20 mm posterior to the anterior lacrimal crest.

10 to 12 mm until reaching the posterior ethmoid artery. The same technique used for ligating or coagulating the anterior artery is also used for the posterior artery (Fig. 22–9).

After the arteries are divided, the wound is closed. Hemostasis should be achieved using bipolar cautery on the orbital tissues and monopolar cautery on the subcutaneous tissues. The incision should be closed using fine suture with careful technique. The medial canthal tendon is reapproximated with 3-0 Vicryl suture, whereas 4-0 Vicryl sutures are used on the subcutaneous

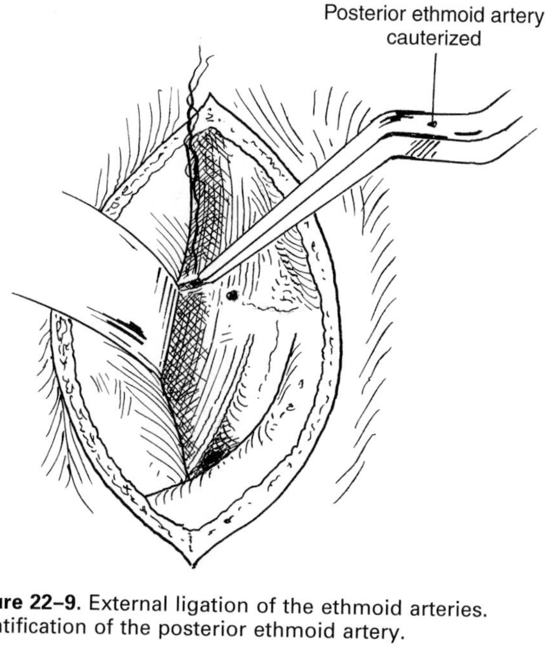

Figure 22–9. External ligation of the ethmoid arteries. Identification of the posterior ethmoid artery.

tissues at the points of the W-plasty. The skin is closed using 6-0 nylon sutures. If hemostasis is assured, no drain is needed. However, if there is any doubt, a small Penrose or rubberband drain can be used.

After the incision is closed, the nasal packing in the nose is removed. The nose is suctioned clear and decongested. There should be no further bleeding at this point. If a specific area of abrasion is of concern, this can be lined by a piece of Gelfoam.

Postoperative Care. All patients should be observed at least overnight after this surgery. There are two significant concerns: orbital hematoma and rebleeding. Orbital edema and ecchymosis are expected. However, there should not be any chemosis, true proptosis, or limitation of extraocular movements. Any of these signs suggests orbital hematoma and should be managed immediately according to the protocols outlined in Chapter 21. Rebleeding is carefully watched. If the presurgical diagnosis was correct, this should not occur.

Routine postoperative care is also provided, including antibiotics, analgesia, and intravenous fluids. Diet is resumed the morning after surgery and advanced as tolerated. As with all patients treated for epistaxis, activity should be minimized. The first night, strict bed rest is advised, with ambulation introduced the next day. Exercise is restricted until 2 weeks after the surgery; resumption of activities depends on the absence of rebleeding.

Complete medical care measures to prevent recurrent bleeding are instituted beginning immediately after the surgery. These have already been presented earlier in the chapter, but include control of hypertension, reversal of coagulopathy, and humidification of the nose with ointment, nasal saline spray, and room air humidification.

Complications. The most serious complications of external ligation result from orbital hematoma and can include ecchymosis, diplopia, and visual loss. In the event of a severe orbital hematoma, there may also be a need for further surgery to decompress the orbit or evacuate the hematoma. Other, surgery-related complications include poor scarring, wound infection, wound breakdown, and recurrent epistaxis. The standard curved Lynch incision is prone to developing noticeable scarring due to contracture. This may occur with any curved incision because of the tendency to shorten the distance along the radius from one end of the incision to the other. This results in webbing of the medial canthal area. This can be secondarily treated by performing a W-plasty. Alternatively, this modification can be incorporated into the initial incision to prevent the problem.

Wound breakdown and wound infection should be rare unless there has been bleeding into the incision, creating a hematoma. If wound infection does occur, treatment involves draining the wound of purulence and administering intravenous antibiotics. Secondary revision of the scar will be necessary but should be delayed until the scar has matured. Recurrent epistaxis is most likely attributable to misdiagnosis of the cause of bleeding. For most patients, this procedure is performed at the same time as the transantral ligation of the internal maxillary artery. With this combination, rebleeding is unlikely unless the bleeding comes from the other side of the nose. If rebleeding occurs, arteriography is recommended to identify the source of bleeding, at which time embolization may be performed if applicable.

Endoscopic Ligation of the Internal Maxillary Artery

Indications. Endoscopic ligation of the internal maxillary artery is the newest addition to the surgical arsenal of the rhinologist for posterior epistaxis. First described in the literature in 1992,[27] this operation has rapidly gained acceptance. Several articles now document the validity of this approach.[28–31] Increasing experience has found that this procedure is rapid, easy, and highly successful. Its advantages over transantral ligation of the internal maxillary artery include avoidance of a sublabial incision, avoidance of injury to the infraorbital nerve, and distal ligation of the arterial branches. Its advantage over endoscopic cautery is that the artery is ligated and so is less likely to rebleed or cause ulceration of the mucosa.

Because of these advantages, endoscopic ligation has become the procedure of choice for surgical control of posterior epistaxis. The precise indications depend on the experience and skill of the surgeon and the role for surgical control of epistaxis. For those who are comfortable with endoscopic sinus surgery and who have experience with this procedure, the indications are increased. One school of thought is that any patient who requires a posterior pack to control nasal bleeding should have the ligation procedure performed as soon as it can be arranged. Without ligation, if a posterior pack is placed, the patient would have to be admitted to an intensive care unit bed and observed for 3 to 5 days before considering removal of the pack. After removal of the pack, the patient is observed for an additional 24 to 48 hours. As an alternative, the patient who undergoes ligation within 24 hours of admission can be discharged within 24 hours of the procedure. This saves 2 to 4 days of hospitalization, as well as the obvious discomfort of the posterior pack. The disadvantages of the endoscopic ligation are the technical demands of the operation and the need for surgical intervention compared to a pack placed in the emergency department.

On balance, the author favors this alternative for most patients with posterior epistaxis. The exceptions are patients who are poor candidates for surgery owing to comorbid medical conditions or severe coagulopathies, and those without a known site of bleeding. An alternative, more conservative philosophy is to reserve all surgical interventions for patients in whom initial attempts at control using a posterior pack are unsuccessful. The author considered this approach to have merit before endoscopic ligation was available. Now that the morbidity of ligation has been reduced to that of an endoscopic procedure, however, ligation has become the best option available.

Preoperative Care. Patients undergoing endoscopic ligation will usually have a posterior pack in place at the time of surgery and will have had significant bleeding before surgery. For these reasons, it is important to determine the patient's hemoglobin level and to transfuse the patient as necessary to elevate the hemoglobin above 10 g/dL. Cross-matched blood should be standing by at the time of surgery in case it is needed. Attempts to control the blood pressure and reverse any coagulopathy should be made. Prophylactic antibiotics are administered and an assessment of anesthetic risk is made.

Technique. The patient is brought to the operating room with the posterior pack in place. General anesthesia is achieved with orotracheal intubation. Hypotensive anesthesia should be used, if possible, to minimize bleeding. Before the nasal pack is removed, a transpalatal injection of the greater palatine foramen is performed using local anesthetic containing 1 : 100,000 epinephrine. This will help minimize bleeding after the pack is removed. For this injection, a 25-gauge needle is bent about 1 cm from the end to an angle of about 45 degrees. The foramen is then palpated medial to the first molar, at the junction of the hard palate and the alveolar ridge. The needle is probed into the palate until the foramen is entered. The needle is then inserted 1 cm into the foramen and about 3 mL of local anesthetic is injected.

Once this injection has been completed, the surgeon should wait at least 5 minutes to allow vasoconstriction to occur. The patient is draped during this time period and the pack is removed. The nose should be thoroughly suctioned to remove blood clots and mucus. The nose is then packed with cotton pledgets soaked with oxymetazoline. This agent is preferred over cocaine for two reasons: the hypertensive effects of cocaine and the likelihood that, because the nose is usually moist and there may be bleeding, the cocaine would be diffused and its effect diminished. The nose is further prepared with injection of local anesthetic as for endoscopic sinus surgery (see Chapter 8).

There are two basic techniques for performing this operation. The first involves a direct approach to the sphenopalatine foramen. With this technique, the posterior attachment of the middle turbinate is identified and an incision is made in the mucosa about 1 cm anterior to this point, extending from the inferior turbinate to the ethmoid sinus. The mucosa is then dissected from the underlying bone from anterior to posterior to approach the foramen. This direct approach is faster and entails less bleeding than its alternative. However, it is a more restricted approach in that identification of the foramen is difficult and ligation will be lateral to the foramen.

As an alternative, a more transethmoidal technique can be used. With this method, the ethmoid is removed and the medial wall of the maxillary sinus is taken down to provide wide exposure to the area of the foramen. This approach allows easy identification of the sphenopalatine foramen and dissection back into the pterygomaxillary fissure for more proximal ligation of the vessels.

The initial step in this procedure is to perform an endoscopic ethmoidectomy and wide middle meatus antrostomy. This can be performed by traditional techniques or by using one of the powered instruments available. In either case, the procedure follows the same steps outlined in Chapter 8 for ethmoidectomy and antrostomy and highlighted here. The uncinate process is removed as the first step. This exposes the ethmoidal bulla. The bulla is then removed from anterior to posterior and inferior to superior. The next landmark is the ground lamella. This is perforated inferiorly and medially to enter the posterior ethmoid sinus. The skull base is identified in the posterior ethmoid and the lamina papyracea is also identified in the posterior ethmoid. These structures are skeletonized up to the anterior ethmoid artery and posteriorly to the sphenoid face.

At this point, the natural ostium of the maxillary sinus is identified by removal of any residual uncinate process. The antrostomy is enlarged by removal of the posterior fontanelle. The antrostomy is enlarged posteriorly from the natural ostium to the level of the posterior wall of the maxillary sinus. At this point, the anatomy should be quite clear. The ethmoid cavity is well formed, with easy visualization of the antrostomy and the posterior attachment of the middle turbinate (Fig. 22–10*A*).

At this point, the surgeon can proceed with the identification and dissection of the branches of the internal maxillary artery. Beginning at the posterior edge of the antrostomy, the mucosa of the lateral wall is elevated using a Freer elevator (Fig. 22–10*B*). The vessels are found almost immediately posterior to the antrostomy at the attachment of the middle turbinate. The vessels are followed laterally to the sphenopalatine foramen. The bone of the foramen is removed using a Kerrison rongeur. The vessels are followed further laterally, with additional bone removal in this fashion until the main internal maxillary artery is identified (Fig. 22–10*C*). The vessels are then carefully dissected using the Freer elevator to tease apart the vessels from the surrounding soft tissues. Once the vessels are isolated, vascular clips are applied to the main artery and the three terminal branches in the nose. Specifically, these are the sphenoid/septal branch, the inferior turbinate branch, and the middle turbinate branch (Fig. 22–10*D*).

The procedure is concluded simply by placing a Merocel sponge lateral to the middle turbinate. The nose is then reexamined endoscopically to assess for control of bleeding. If necessary, suction cautery can be used at the original bleeding site that was the cause of the epistaxis.

Postoperative Care. Patients undergoing endoscopic ligation should be hospitalized overnight for observation. Discharge can occur as early as the morning after surgery if there has been no postoperative bleeding. During the hospitalization, intravenous fluids are administered, along with humidified air or oxygen by face mask. Activity is limited to bathroom privileges only; the diet is started at clear liquids and advanced to a regular diet the next morning. Hypertension should be carefully controlled.

After discharge from the hospital, the patient's activity and diet are gradually returned to normal. Full activity, including exercise, should be avoided for 2 weeks after the procedure. Medications include adequate analgesics and oral antibiotics for at least 2 weeks.

The pack is removed in the office after a minimum of 3 days. When the pack is removed, the nose is decongested and anesthetized with topical lidocaine or a suit-

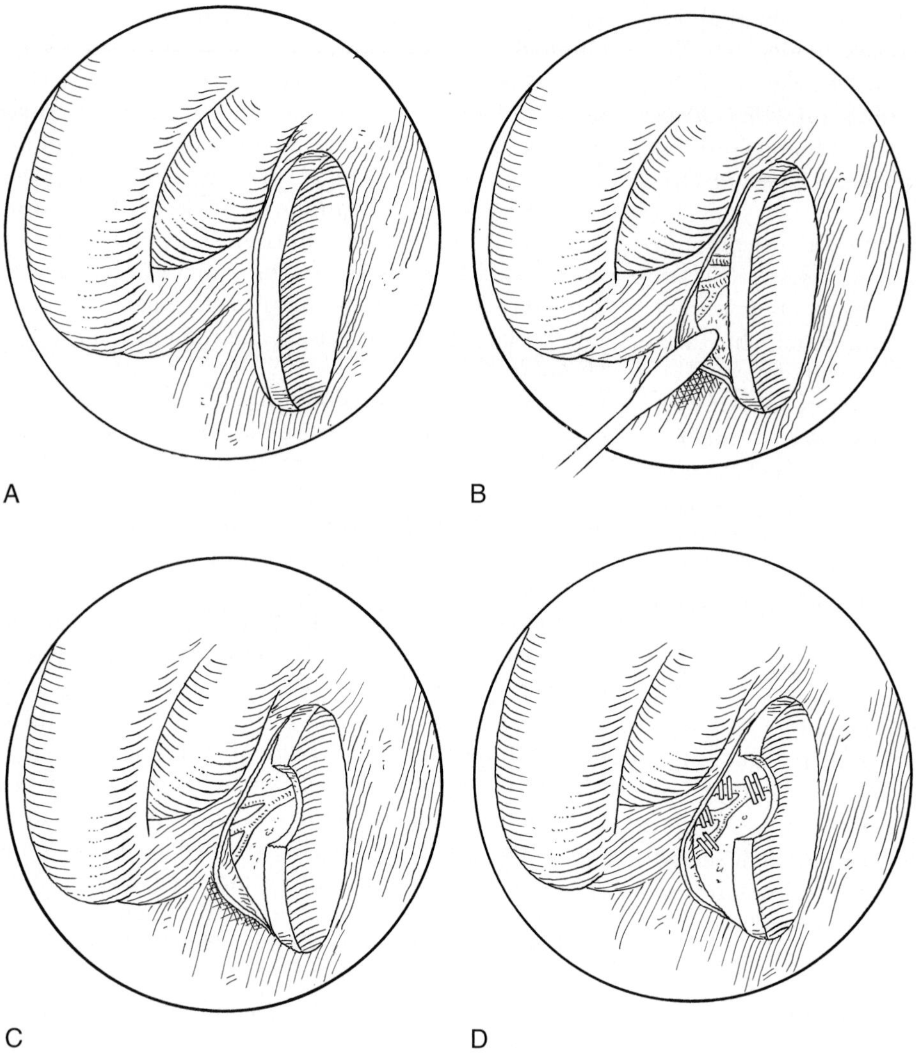

Figure 22–10. Endoscopic ligation of the sphenopalatine artery. *A,* Initial exposure after antrostomy. The ethmoid may be dissected if this is helpful to the surgeon. *B,* The mucosa immediately posterior to the antrostomy is elevated to expose the branches of the sphenopalatine artery. *C,* The bone of the sphenopalatine foramen is removed to expose the main artery. *D,* The final appearance after the artery and its main branches are ligated with microclips.

able substitute. The sinus cavity is then examined endoscopically. The sinus cavity is suctioned clear of all blood clot and any mucous debris. Extreme care must be exercised when suctioning over the area of the ligation to avoid accidentally suctioning off one of the clips. The patient is then started on saline irrigations. Detailed instructions are given to the patient as to how to mix a sterile solution of normal saline and to perform the irrigations. The care protocol calls for irrigation every morning and evening. This is accomplished using a rubber ball syringe. The syringe is placed 1 to 2 cm into the nose and angled outward and upward. Vigorous irrigation is performed with two or three syringes full of saline. The patient then carefully blows the nose and applies nasal steroid spray to the affected side. In between the morning and evening irrigations, the patient is instructed to spray normal saline spray into the nose every 2 to 3 hours.

Further examination and debridement of the sinus cavity is performed 3 weeks and 6 weeks after surgery. At each visit, the nose is decongested and anesthetized and examined endoscopically. Clots and crusts are removed and regenerative cysts and polyps are debrided. After 6 weeks, complete healing is usually noted. Further follow-up evaluation is tailored to the individual patient and the clinical course.

Complications. The most important complication of this operation is rebleeding, although the incidence of this is as yet unknown. There are not enough series reported in the literature to adequately assess the success rate. However, if the diagnosis of the site and cause of the epistaxis was correct and the procedure was technically successful, rebleeding should be rare. If the diagnosis was incorrect or if the ligation were to fail, rebleeding would be very common.

All of the complications associated with endoscopic sinus surgery are possible with this procedure. These include scarring, bleeding, infection, epiphora, recurrent sinus infection, mucocele, orbital injury, CSF leak, and intracranial bleeding. However, the risk of these complications should be lower in this setting than for routine endoscopic sinus surgery. The factors associated with an increased risk of complications during endoscopic sinus surgery include revision surgery, sinonasal polyposis, and operation in the sphenoid sinus and frontal recess. During endoscopic ligation of the internal maxillary artery, there is rarely significant inflammation or polyp tissue in the sinuses, making the dissection easy and relatively bloodless. Most of these patients have not had previous nasal or sinus surgery, and it is not necessary to open the sphenoid sinus or to dissect the frontal recess. These factors minimize the risk of serious complications.

Coagulopathy

Patients with coagulopathy form a special subset of patients with epistaxis. This group includes all patients with disorders of clotting factors or platelets that increase the bleeding time. These patients are more prone to develop epistaxis and are more likely to fail medical management than patients with normal clotting function. The options for treatment are the same as those indicated earlier for patients with normal clotting mechanisms, but the application of the techniques varies depending on the situation.

Management strategy can be divided according to whether a patient has reversible or nonreversible clotting dysfunction. In patients with reversible clotting dysfunction, the usual protocols outlined in Figures 22–1 and 22–2 will apply, with the additional step of reversing the clotting dysfunction. In patients with nonreversible clotting dysfunction, more conservative methods are indicated. In these patients, surgery and traditional packing are virtually ruled out as options. Surgery is difficult because, in the absence of natural hemostasis, the intervention can become a life-threatening misadventure. All surgeries of the nose and sinuses rely on natural clotting mechanisms to control the minor bleeding that is expected from the mucosal edges of incisions and dissections. It is not routine or even possible to maintain complete hemostasis during nasal and sinus surgery. This may then result in excessive intraoperative and postoperative bleeding, leading to severe complications. Traditional gauze packing is not advisable because it usually results in significant intranasal abrasions and ulcerations that will cause severe secondary bleeding upon removal of the packing.

For these reasons, most cases of bleeding in patients with clotting dysfunction will need to be treated by either dissolvable packing, nonabrasive packing, cautery, or embolization. In cases of mild to moderate bleeding, Gelfoam packing is tried initially. If this fails, then either a nasal sponge or a nasal balloon is used. When the nasal sponge or balloon is removed, this is usually replaced by a Gelfoam pack. If these measures fail, endoscopic cautery can be tried. This technique depends on identification of a discrete source of bleeding. When this is possible, the area of bleeding can be cauterized without significant harm to the surrounding mucosa. If all else fails, or in cases of severe or life-threatening epistaxis in this patient population, embolization is advised. Endovascular techniques are frequently performed in patients with clotting dysfunction, so this condition does not pose a significant deterrent to this modality.

Management of Hereditary Hemorrhagic Telangiectasia

The management of HHT depends on several independent factors. These include the number and location of the intranasal lesions, the severity and frequency of epistaxis, the number and location of gastrointestinal, brain, and pulmonary lesions, the number of blood transfusions attributable to the epistaxis, the effect of the epistaxis on the patient's quality of life, and the previous treatment(s) attempted.

Medical therapy for HHT, in addition to that outlined earlier for epistaxis in general, has focused on the use of estrogen and progesterone.[32, 33] This treatment was based on the observation that epistaxis tended to decrease during pregnancy among affected individuals. Antifibrinolytic therapy using aminocaproic acid has also been discussed.[34] None of these medical treatments has proven effective in completely relieving epistaxis in the long term, but some benefits have been claimed.

Because of the failure of these methods, numerous other modalities have been attempted, including sclerotherapy, brachytherapy, electrocautery, arterial ligation, embolization, septal dermoplasty, closure of the nasal cavities, and laser coagulation.[35–40] The clear implication of all of these reports is that there remains no cure for HHT and, despite all treatment attempts, recurrent epistaxis is possible.

In light of these facts, the author suggests that treatment should be designed to minimize the bleeding while avoiding complications. For this reason, extreme measures, such as brachytherapy, embolization, and invasive surgery, should be avoided. The preferred measures are to use medical therapy, if possible, and laser treatments in those patients who need transfusion or for whom epistaxis has a significant, negative effect on quality of life. The reports by Bergler et al.[35] and Lennox et al.[36] have suggested that the argon plasma laser is the preferred laser over the yttrium aluminum garnet (YAG) or KTP. Both groups report benefits to the patients with minimal or no side effects, although the report by Lennox and co-workers suggests that patients with severe epistaxis may not benefit.

For patients in whom laser therapy fails, necessitating some other approach to control the bleeding, several possibilities are available. Septal dermoplasty has been advocated in the past.[41] This procedure was described in Chapter 12. The exact indications for this operation are currently unclear, but the approach may be considered for this category of laser failures. The main alternative to septal dermoplasty is bilateral ligation of the internal maxillary arteries and ethmoid arteries. However, the success of this approach remains questionable as patients continue to form telangiectasia despite this procedure, and the potential side effects of the surgery are significant.

Closure of the nasal cavity, the so-called Young's procedure, has been tried as well.[39,42] In this operation the anterior nares are closed by developing skin flaps from the nasal vestibule. The authors claim that, if the nasal closure is complete, the result will be complete cessation of bleeding in every case. Theoretically, this is due to the absence of airflow through the nose, which means that there is no source of desiccation or trauma to the telangiectasia and thus no bleeding. This author has no experience with this technique and, therefore, can neither dispute nor confirm the published results. However, in a patient who is willing to accept complete nasal obstruction, this procedure would certainly be a consideration.

REFERENCES

1. Maceri D. Nasal trauma. In Cummings CW, Fredrickson JM, Harker LA, Krause CJ, Schuller DE, (eds). Otolaryngology—Head and Neck Surgery, 1st ed. St Louis: CV Mosby, 1986, pp. 614–623.
2. Pollice PA, Yoder G. Epistaxis: A retrospective review of hospitalized patients. Otolaryngol Head Neck Surg 117(1):49, 1997.
3. Maune S, Jeckstrom W, Thomsen H, Rudert H. Indication, incidence and management of blood transfusion during sinus surgery: A review over 12 years. Rhinology 35:2, 1997.
4. Lubianca-Neto J, Bredemeier M, Carvalhal E, et al. A study of the association between epistaxis and the severity of hypertension. Am J Rhinol 12(4):269, 1998.
5. Osler W. On a family form of recurring epistaxis associated with multiple telangiectasia of the skin and mucous membranes. Bull Johns Hopkins Hosp 2:233, 1901.
6. Weber FP. Multiple hereditary developmental angiomata (telangiectasia) of the skin and mucous membranes associated with recurring hemorrhages. Lancet 2:160, 1907.
7. Rendu H. Epistaxis repetees chez un sujet porteur de petits angiomes cutanes et muquex. Bull Mem Soc Med Hop (Paris) 13: 731, 1896.
8. Reilly PJ, Nostrant TT. Clinical manifestations of hereditary hemorrhagic telangiectasia. Am J Gastroenterol 79:363, 1984.
9. Vase P, Grove O. Gastrointestinal lesions in hereditary hemorrhagic telangiectasia. Gastroenterology 91:1079, 1986.
10. Larsen K, Juul A. Arterial blood gases and pneumatic nasal packing in epistaxis. Laryngoscope 92(5):586, 1982.
11. Jacobs JR, Levine LA, Davis H, et al. Posterior packs and the nasopulmonary reflex. Laryngoscope 91(2):279, 1981.
12. Jacobs JR, Dickson CB. Effects of nasal and laryngeal stimulation upon peripheral lung function. Otolaryngol Head Neck Surg 95 (3 Pt 1):298, 1986.
13. McGarry GW. Nasal endoscope in posterior epistaxis: A preliminary evaluation. J Laryngol Otol 105:428, 1991.
14. Wurman LH, Garry Sack J, Flannery JV, Paulson O. Selective endoscopic electrocautery for posterior epistaxis. Laryngoscope 98:1348, 1988.
15. Tseng EY, Narducci CA, Willing SJ, Silles MJ. Angiographic embolization for epistaxis: A review of 114 cases. Laryngoscope 108:615, 1998.
16. Moreau S, Goullet De Rugy M, Babin E, et al. Supraselective embolization in intractable epistaxis: Review of 45 cases. Laryngoscope 108:887, 1998.
17. Elden L, Montanera W, Terbrugge K, et al. Angiographic embolization for the treatment of epistaxis: A review of 108 cases. Otolaryngol Head Neck Surg 111:44, 1994.
18. Sinuloto MJ, Leinonen AS, Karttunen AI, et al. Embolization for the treatment of posterior epistaxis. Arch Otolaryngol Head Neck Surg 119:837, 1993.
19. Merland JJ, Melki JP, Chiras J, et al. Place of embolization in the treatment of severe epistaxis. Laryngoscope 90:169, 1980.
20. Cullen, MM, Tami TA. Comparison of internal maxillary artery ligation versus embolization for refractory posterior epistaxis. Otolaryngol Head Neck Surg 118(5):635, 1998.
21. Schaitken B, Strauss M, Houck J. Epistaxis: Medical versus surgical therapy—A comparison of efficacy, complications and economic considerations. Laryngoscope 97:1392, 1987.
22. Strong EB, Bell A, Johnson LP, Jacobs JM. Intractable epistaxis: Transantral ligation vs. embolization—Efficacy review and cost analysis. Otolaryngol Head and Neck Surg 113:674, 1995.
23. Nair KK. Transantral ligation of the internal mammary artery. Laryngoscope 92:1060, 1982.
24. Spafford P, Durham JS. Epistaxis: Efficacy of arterial ligation and long-term outcome. J Otolaryngol 21:252, 1992.
25. Welsch LW, Welsh JJ, Scogna JE, et al. Role of angiography in the management of refractory epistaxis. Ann Otol Rhinol Laryngol 99:69, 1990.
26. Singh B. Combined internal maxillary and anterior ethmoidal artery occlusion: The treatment of choice in intractable epistaxis. J Laryngol Otol 106:507, 1992.
27. Budrovich R, Saetti R. Microscopic and endoscopic ligature of the sphenopalatine artery. Laryngoscope 102:1390, 1996.
28. Snyderman CH, Carrau RL. Endoscopic ligation of the sphenopalatine artery for epistaxis. Otolaryngol Head Neck Surg 8(2):85, 1997.
29. Snyderman CH, Goldman SA, Carrau, RL, et al. Endoscopic sphenopalatine artery ligation is an effective method of treatment for posterior epistaxis. Am J Rhinol 13(2):137, 1999.
30. Bolger WE, Borgie RC, Melder P. The role of the crista ethmoidalis in endoscopic sphenopalatine artery ligation. Am J Rhinol 13(2):81, 1999.
31. White PS. Endoscopic ligation of the sphenopalatine artery (ELSA): A preliminary description. J Laryngol Otol 110:27, 1996.
32. Harrison DFN. Use of estrogen in treatment of familial hemorrhagic telangiectasia. Laryngoscope 92:314, 1982.
33. Flessa HC, Glucek HI. Hereditary hemorrhagic telangiectasia (Osler-Weber-Rendu). Management of epistaxis in nine patients using systemic hormone therapy. Arch Otolaryngol 103:148, 1977.
34. Korzenik JR, Topazian MD, White RI. Treatment of bleeding in hereditary haemorrhagic telangiectasia with aminocaproic acid. N Engl J Med 331:1326, 1994.
35. Bergler W, Riedel F, Baker-Schreyer, A. Argon plasma coagulation for the treatment of hereditary hemorrhagic telangiectasia. Laryngoscope 109:15, 1999.
36. Lennox PA, Harries M, Lung VJ, Howard DJ. A retrospective study of the role of the argon laser in the management of epistaxis secondary to hereditary haemorrhagic telangiectasia. J Laryngol Otol 111:34, 1997.
37. McCaffrey TV, Kern EB, Lake CF. Management of epistaxis in hereditary hemorrhagic telangiectasia. Review of 80 cases. Arch Otolaryngol 103:627, 1977.
38. Parnes LS, Heeneman H, Vinuela F. Percutaneous embolization for control of nasal blood circulation. Laryngoscope 97:1312, 1987.
39. Lund VJ, Howard DJ. Closure of the nasal cavities in the treatment of refractory hereditary haemorrhagic telangiectasia. J Laryngol Otol 111:30, 1997.
40. Pohar S, Maseron JJ, Ghilezan M, Le Bourgeois JP, Pierquin H. Management of epistaxis in Rendu-Osler disease: Is brachytherapy effective? Int J Radiat Oncol Biol Phys 27:1073, 1993.
41. Saunders WH. Septal dermoplasty for control of nose bleeds in hereditary hemorrhagic telangiectasia. Trans Am Acad Ophthalmol Otolaryngol 64:500, 1960.
42. Lund VJ, Howard DJ. Closure of the nasal cavities in the treatment of refractory hereditary haemorrhagic telangiectasia. J Laryngol Otol 111:30, 1997.

INDEX

Note: Page numbers in *italics* indicate figures; those followed by t indicate tables.

ISBN 0-7216-7804-1

90038

9 780721 678047